# The Handbook of Medicinal Chemistry

## Principles and Practice

## 2nd Edition

# The Handbook of Medicinal Chemistry

## Principles and Practice

## 2nd Edition

Edited by

**Simon E. Ward**

*Cardiff University, UK*
*Email: WardS10@cardiff.ac.uk*

and

**Andrew M. Davis**

*AstraZeneca, Sweden*
*Email: andy.davis@astrazeneca.com*

ROYAL SOCIETY
OF **CHEMISTRY**

Print ISBN: 978-1-78801-898-2
PDF ISBN: 978-1-83767-107-6
EPUB ISBN: 78-1-83916-588-7

A catalogue record for this book is available from the British Library



The Royal Society of Chemistry is a charity, registered in England and Wales, Number 207890, and a company incorporated in England by Royal Charter (Registered No. RC000524), registered office: Burlington House, Piccadilly, London W1J 0BA, UK, Telephone: +44 (0) 20 7437 8656.

Visit our website at books.rsc.org

# Foreword to the 2nd Edition

I am very happy to have been given the opportunity to write this Foreword to the latest edition of *The Handbook of Medicinal Chemistry*. This science whose practice we all share has a long history and looks to have a lengthy future as well – but just as it does not resemble its beginning very much by this point, its later form will surely be quite different from what we see now. Large changes are coming. "Well of course they are," you may well think, "there are always large changes coming". What's so different now? What makes this Foreword different? Perhaps a bit of history will help make the case for that statement.

## Targets and Drugs

My career as a medicinal chemist began in 1989, in a central nervous system research group. Naturally, I did not know enough to be terrified of the problems that were set before us, which were diseases such as schizophrenia and Alzheimer's. (It will immediately be noted, for example, that both of those are very much still with us and still in need of pharmacological aid). I soon learned, though, that my colleagues in the biology labs were quite excited about the G-protein coupled receptors that we had targeted in both areas, as new technology was displacing the tissue assays that had been in use for many years. It was, for example, farewell to the rabbit trachea and the rat *vas deferens* in muscarinic receptor characterization, and a look at the older literature[1,2] will clear up any suspicions that I might be inventing those. Instead, we welcomed the cloned receptor subtype membrane-binding assays, which we felt would surely clear up many of our difficulties once we all got our bearings.

This switch to such individual targets with assays enabled by molecular biology had been taking place throughout the 1980s, with the late-1970s success of captopril[3,4] as an angiotensin-converting enzyme inhibitor helping to light the way. But the idea of such targets themselves had been working its way into the practice of medicinal chemistry ever since Raymond Ahlquist proposed in 1948 that adrenergic signaling could

The Handbook of Medicinal Chemistry: Principles and Practice, 2nd Edition
Edited by Simon E. Ward and Andrew M. Davis

Published by the Royal Society of Chemistry, www.rsc.org

be explained by what he termed “alpha” and “beta” receptors.[5,6] The receptor concept caught on,[7] but even up through the 1960s you could find warnings in the literature not to take such ideas too literally.[8] That is, one was not to assume that these were necessarily defined molecular entities with real structures, but rather just useful mental models or a sort of shorthand to categorize the various mysterious classes of drug action. Even among those researchers who took receptors to have physical reality, it was unclear if they were proteins, complex carbohydrates, or who knew what. And as for how they might work? That was even more mysterious.

Receptors turned out to be real molecular species, of course – in fact, they were proteins that could be cloned and expressed once we knew how to do such things. The same went for enzymes, whose proteinaceous nature had become clear much earlier, but whose production and purification were likewise changed forever by molecular biology techniques. And thus medicinal chemistry went through one of its revolutions, with target-based drug discovery becoming the unquestioned default mode of the field. It still is. Target-agnostic phenotypic screening went into eclipse for a while, but even with its revivals over the years, the first thing that people will try to do with an interesting phenotypic hit is to ... try to identify its specific target.[9] And that's done partly so that the protein can then be expressed and turned into the subject of the non-phenotypic screening assay it would have been from the beginning, had anyone but known to look at it.

This is the world that readers of this new volume have been living in (as have I!) There's no doubt that it's been good to us. Whole classes of actionable targets have opened up over the years: enzymes such as the proteases, hydrolases, kinases, and phosphodiesterases, all ready to be inhibited, and also the receptors and ion channels to be addressed in all their profusion: agonists and antagonists, full and partial and inverse, all waiting to be discovered and exploited. A solid history of modern medicinal chemistry could be written from the perspective of watching these territories being mapped out and settled.

All of them attracted some doubters at first. With the profusion of kinase-targeting drugs that we have now, it can be difficult to remember that some very intelligent people wondered at one time whether a selective kinase inhibitor was even possible.[10] After all, wouldn't you just hit every other ATP-binding site in the whole cell? Sometimes the doubters had a point, though: the nuclear receptors have had some striking successes as drug targets, but many of those came before we even understood them very well, and not so many have arrived since. Epigenetic enzymes went through a great period of enthusiasm too, but it's been a difficult field to make progress in. No doubt many readers can provide other examples from their own experience.

For a while, it was difficult to imagine that target-based drug discovery had any real limits, but anyone who took the time to think about it knew that it must. The number of pathways in living cells is large, but most certainly finite – as is the number of proteins, and of course the number of genes coding for them. Indeed, one of the most direct reminders that there would eventually be an end to it all was provided by the Human Genome Project. The speculative frenzy around human sequencing in that era was driven by the fear that unless you reached into your pocket immediately, other people (and not you, you cheapskate) would end up owning the rights to all of those targets and all of those proteins. Patents were being filed at a ridiculous pace, many of them doubtless overlapping in what promised to become an epic tangle during prosecution. The signs were clear: the great prairie of target space had at one time stretched almost unbroken to the horizon, but now there was dust flying everywhere as fence posts were pounded in and barbed wire was hurriedly strung up.

And then that horizon suddenly got closer. The initial 2001 figure of only about 30 000 human genes in total was alarmingly short of almost all the estimates at the time, and it caused widespread consternation.[11] At that point, it seemed possible that more "genes" had been filed on than there were actual genes to be had, which is worth thinking about. At any rate, the whole patent-every-gene business model collapsed as it became clear that genes alone clearly weren't everything. Splicing variations and post-translational modification were responsible for much of the variety of the proteome, as we all should have remembered. It also became clear that the patent offices, in what has to be regarded as farsightedness, weren't going to even consider allowing the sort of patentability (and the sort of reach) for all those claims that people had been writing up.[12]

But bioinformatics was still showing everyone the end of the line. At one point, when gene sequencing was still so difficult and expensive, the question of how many human protein kinase enzymes there really were was basically unanswerable, at least if you wanted something more specific than "a lot." But as the annotations and sequences got better and better, the answer took on an extremely discrete character: there are five hundred and eighteen of them. Similarly, the other target classes began lining up and counting off. It gave a person a strange sensation at the time.

There was still plenty of frontier, though, and for that matter there still is. It was obvious that we didn't know the actual functions of many of these proteins that had been enumerated. We still don't, not to the level of detail we would like. And there were big swaths of protein space whose annotations were as thin as tissue paper (and still are), with roles that have just barely begun to be understood. Eventually another shock will have to be faced when this unexplored intellectual space starts undeniably shrinking, but that time is not yet. It will come eventually, and though it's hard to say what the effect on medicinal chemistry will be, the field of particle physics over the last fifty years might offer a preview. At one of my former companies, we amused ourselves (in somewhat cynical fashion) by coming up with possible advertising slogans for our employer. One of my favorites was "(Name Redacted) Pharmaceuticals: Where Progress is Our Only Problem." That joke, similar to a candy bar, had a chewy bit of truth in the center of it.

## Drug Mechanisms

What have we done with all these target proteins? Generally, we have tried to stop them in their tracks. Let's be honest with ourselves: it's far, far easier to throw a wrench into the cellular machinery with inhibitors and antagonists than it is to make the gears turn faster by discovering enzyme activators or selective agonists. Most of the time, most drug discoverers have looked through the biochemical pathways of disease with an eye to which parts of them could be usefully disabled. Even current hot topics such as selective protein degradation (more on which shortly) are often just new variations on the "what can we interrupt" strategy. But all that wrench-throwing has been fantastically useful and informative, not to mention (on occasion) fantastically lucrative. A large part of the mapping and exploration mentioned above has been accomplished through the use of small molecule tool compounds, a favored few of which have become actual drugs. That process will certainly continue. A good small-molecule tool can shed an extraordinary amount of light on the biochemistry of health and disease, and can be made the subject of more and various sorts of useful experiments than almost anything else in medical research.[13]

It seems clear that there are currently more new modes of therapy dawning in the clinic simultaneously than there have been at any time in at least the past thirty or forty years. It's an amazing thing to watch. Not all of these are small-molecule driven (more on that shortly as well!) but some are, and others have a place for small-molecule targeting to assist them. We have CRISPR gene editing, chimeric receptor T cells (and other cellular modifications *ex vivo*), the above-mentioned targeted protein degradation, a revival of interest in antibody-drug conjugates, and likewise a growing interest in applying the techniques of organic chemistry to large biomolecules of many types.

That last field overlaps with the area now called "chemical biology," and that brings up another point worth emphasizing. Medicinal chemistry (perhaps it would be more accurate to say medicinal chemists?) has sometimes had its scope limited by what can only be called a lack of imagination. We're not the only scientific field whose practitioners enjoy drawing boundary lines and declaring that the "real" subject only exists on this side of them, of course. But given med-chem's position at the intersection of several different sorts of biology and medicine, purity tests can be dangerous. Medicinal chemistry is where chemistry gets added to all of those other fields, and I've long maintained that if you have begun thinking of the subjects of your research as actual molecules, with shapes, sizes, charge distributions, distinct molecular weights, and all the rest of it, then you are turning into a chemist whether you realize it or not. That means that many molecular biologists are slowly becoming chemists, and I think we should let this process continue rather than scaring them all off for fear that they will dilute our own field. The era of ill-defined boxes, circles, and triangles with arrows pointing vaguely between them cannot end soon enough, and it will be finished off by understanding all these species at a molecular level. As chemists do. So my advice is for medicinal chemists to move into these new territories and bring their skills with them. We have things to offer that aren't available anywhere else, ways of thinking about molecular species that haven't yet taken hold in some of the other closely related fields and are very much needed.

Consider as an example targeted protein degradation, which as I write is attracting huge amounts of investment, interest, and labor. At the moment, the various chimeric species that are used to make TPD happen in living cells (or living patients) are somewhat mysterious. A great deal of experimentation is needed to come up with appropriately linked "business ends" to obtain the desired effects. We generally can't predict why some of these work so well (nor why others work so poorly), but it's clear that answers are out there for us if we can make our way to them. These will be found in the interaction of protein–protein surfaces, in the orientations of the target and ligase ligands, in the subtleties of entropy and enthalpy that go into the formation of a ternary complex and what we call cooperativity.

We also have a good deal to learn about the properties of the (often large and unwieldy) bifunctional molecules themselves. How do such species cross cell membranes, and what are their pharmacokinetic fates in general? We're not used to working with such things, and for now we are feeling our way. But such species, and some of the equally large and complex molecules that have made their way into the clinic as protein–protein interaction inhibitors and other classes, have (I believe it's fair to say) put a bookend on what has to be called the "Rule of Five" era.[14] A renewed attention to molecular properties was probably a good idea, considering some of the excesses of the early combinatorial libraries, but most people who lived through the entire cycle would probably agree that the whole process went a bit too far.[15] I believe that a department manager I worked with was joking when he wondered if there should perhaps be some sort of electric shock administered through the keyboard when a chemist tried to register some molecule with too many egregious rule violations. But another one was at least a little bit serious when he suggested a cap-and-trade system for the department, with every bench chemist getting a set quota of metal-catalyzed aryl–aryl coupling reactions per year.

Antibiotics, especially macrocyclic ones, were always known to be exceptions to most attempts to confine them to rules in property space. A great deal of effort has now gone into figuring out just why that might be so, with mixed results.[16] But one undeniable result has been a broadening of medicinal chemists' thoughts, with large macrocyclic closures of all sorts making appearances in clinical candidates in recent years. Perhaps we all had to put on those tight buckles and straps for a while to see the best ways out of them. But the shackles do seem to have fallen off: molecules are moving into the clinic now whose structures might have gotten you fired twenty years ago – well, from a few of the more doctrinaire organizations, anyway.

This process looks to continue for a good long time to come. There are many other ways to apply the bifunctional-molecule idea, just to pick one large-molecule area. Instead of dragging over a ubiquitinating enzyme complex to a protein of interest, why not bring in any of the other post-translational enzyme systems? Why not use a bifunctional to nail down a particular molecule's location inside a cell, or to make some protein occupy one of those locations that otherwise it would never see? Why not move beyond proteins to glycosylated surfaces? Ten or fifteen minutes of staring out a convenient window will allow a person to sketch out enough research to keep everyone busy for years.

And this is just one area! A related possibility is in the intriguing area of "molecular glues," small molecules that actually cause two otherwise unacquainted proteins to come together in unexpected ways. I will freely admit that such a mechanism would have seemed very weird and unlikely to me at one time, but here we are. For that matter, I would have furrowed my brow a bit at the bifunctional degraders, too, finding the whole concept a bit too unwieldy and brute-force. The poet Philip Larkin said that reading Thomas Hardy taught him "never to be afraid of the obvious," and that's a lesson that we all get to learn, and relearn.[17] Surprises wait for us at both ends of the scale, and the only way that we are going to run out of things to do would be through a failure of imagination.

## The Shape of Things to Come

How we do those things, though, will surely be changing. Medicinal chemistry has seen any number of fads and periods of excitement over the years, as new techniques appear. From computational drug design (in all its forms), through combinatorial chemistry, fragment-based drug discovery, DNA-encoded libraries, and more, each of these has begun with a wave of enthusiasm (and skepticism) and has eventually found its place as part of the toolbox, another one of the many things that medicinal chemists do.

But we will certainly be making new molecules; that much is sure. The reactions we use to make them now are a mixed assortment,[18] featuring some classic transformations from the earliest days of organic synthesis (such as amide formation) all the way up to the latest bond-forming catalysts from the literature. It has been demonstrated that a huge variety of diverse compounds can be prepared with simple chemistry using the great profusion of synthetic building blocks and intermediates.[19] But at the same time, there is still a need for new reactions, especially those that might move into that same category of reliable bond-forming workhorses.[20] Experienced medicinal chemists never lose sight of the fact that the chemistry itself is just a means to the end: producing a wide variety of new molecules for testing. If a new technique provides a reliable way to do that, and especially if it gives access to structures that were previously hard to synthesize, it will rapidly find a home in the labs. The relatively rapid uptake of photoredox techniques is an example, and there will surely be others.

I think, though, that we might be on the edge of some larger changes. And that takes us back to the assertions that I made in the opening paragraph of this Foreword. Let's consider what many of us have always thought of as the prerogative of a synthetic organic chemist: working out a synthetic plan to make a new molecule. Sometimes this is fairly trivial, sometimes very much not. But until now, coming up with a synthetic plan has involved one or more chemists sketching out structures and thinking about what can be made from what, and how. People bring their own experience to the process, of course, and they bring a good deal of literature searching for reactions and conditions. But in the end, it's always been a human process, full of human choices and human insights.

That's going to change. This is not a popular viewpoint, as I am reminded every time I express it in public. It's true that the various software packages that are now available to do retrosynthetic planning are often not very impressive. But what I find impressive is that they exist in the first place. And I feel certain that they will continue to improve, and to improve at a faster pace than humans do. Look, for example, at what has happened to games such as chess and Go, which were once only the province of human thought as well. There are no humans left that can beat the best programs for these games, and there never will be again. The same fate awaits every other game with set rules and strategy, and I maintain that organic synthesis is one of those games. Of course it's a game: that's why we love it so much. It has more pieces and more moves than chess, and it is played on a larger board than Go, but since when did such factors do more than slow down (for a while) a computational approach? No, for the great majority of synthetic planning, I foresee an era of what chess champion Garry Kasparov calls "chimeric" play, with humans and software cooperating to address the other's weak points.[21]

Eventually, I see the software doing more and more of the work and being able to fill in more and more chemical space with useful suggestions. It's admittedly hard to imagine a retrosynthesis program proposing a good route to palytoxin or vancomycin, but think about it: how often are any of us ever called to do such a thing ourselves?

As with the software, so with the hardware. People have been trying to automate organic synthesis for a long time now, but what some chemists might not realize is the extent to which that process has already succeeded. I refer to such familiar objects as rotary evaporators, fraction collectors, autosamplers, and the like. All of these labor-saving devices and more took over what used to be hand labor. Some of this has happened over the course of my own career: if you had shown me a modern chromatography setup, with prepacked columns running any sort of solvent mixtures from normal to reverse phase with any sort of automatically mixed gradient one might choose, with an option to only collect fractions when something actually seemed to be coming out the other end ... well, I might have had to sit down for a while. It would have seemed an unimaginable futuristic luxury, but chemists in well-appointed labs now take this sort of thing for granted.

We may well be getting closer to more direct automation of the chemistry itself. We have increased use of high-throughput experimentation already, both in the analog-making and the reaction-finding senses of the term. And for years now, various groups and companies have been trying to automate the entire thing, with robotic weighing, mixing, reacting, monitoring, and purification steps. The dream has been to realize a fully closed loop, with some sort of automated primary assay joined to the synthetic process, and the results being then fed back, perhaps, to another piece of software which will recommend the next round of analogs for the synthetic hardware to produce.[22] This may not to everyone's taste, but remember, dreams come in various types and with various degrees of enjoyment.

I'm not sure what I think about that one, either, at least in its strongest forms. But the advances in flow chemistry and in automating many regular laboratory tasks make this idea closer to realization than it has ever been. It remains to be seen how much sense (both scientific and economic) it will make for medicinal chemistry in general, but can anyone doubt that it might well be just the thing for the "go make me a hundred different amides" part of the work? That's not the most glorious feature of med-chem, true, but it's not to be sneered at, either.

And that brings up a more general point. Just as in other fields of work, all of this mechanical and electronic assistance is taking away what we would have called "grunt work", while at the same time gradually expanding our beliefs about just what constitutes grunt work in the first place. Synthetic chemists used to have to blow all their own glassware and synthesize all their reagents, little of either being commercially available. I thought nothing about packing my own chromatography columns and collecting all my fractions by hand when I was in graduate school, but many chemists now would feel differently and I'm with them. There are better uses of one's time. As the machinery advances, we will all in fact have to find those better uses. We will be gradually moved, perforce, into the areas where the robots and the software packages cannot yet help us, into higher-order problems that are less open (for now?) to computation and automation. Synthetic organic and medicinal chemists will need to get used to working at a higher level, since the lower levels will, as the years go on, be less and less our concern.

If that really is the way the future goes, then the field will end up eventually in a very different shape than it is now. When I started in industry, there were older chemists around who'd been knocking around the labs for decades, stretching back to an era I had trouble picturing at all. Some of them were content just to keep their heads down and crank out molecules at the bench – I well recall one of them telling me that he didn't want the spotlight and didn't want to be working on anything flashy or high risk. He just wanted to come in and do his work quietly and reliably on whatever ordinary chemistry needed doing. For better or worse, this type of chemist has been harder to find in medicinal chemistry departments over the years, and they look to get even rarer still. I don't foresee everyone getting more specialized, though. The jack-of-all-trades, the *débrouillard*, that sort of chemist will always have a place and may well be needed more than ever. But the trades such a person will divide his or her time among and the problems where ingenuity and insight will need to be applied – those will be different. They already are.

To borrow a line, it's not going to be chemists *versus* machines. It's going to be the chemists that use the machines productively *versus* the ones who don't. We're going to need all the help we can get. As we move into the sorts of complex mechanisms discussed earlier, it looks very much like we may be making larger, more complicated molecules, and plenty of them. We may well find ourselves spending most of our time on more complex chemistry than we tend to now, and the idea of setting up a set of amide formations yourself in a fume hood might start to sound as antiquated as going out to collect firewood.

Readers will have noticed that I have not until now been talking about molecular modeling and computational drug design *per se*. The number of failed predictions and retrospectively ironic headlines in this area gives me pause, and I don't want to add any more to the list. No other part of drug discovery seems to have had as many repeated bursts of enthusiasm, and while that has made for a bumpy ride, it remains true that there has always been a lot to be enthusiastic about. I'm fond of saying that I'm a short-term pessimist and a long-term optimist about computational drug discovery – by that, I mean that I see no reason why it eventually won't be extremely useful, but if someone walks up to me next week and says that they have solved its problems and everything is ready to go, I will still hold on to my wallet.

The timetable for when the switchover to "extremely useful" comes has slipped several times over the years, but there's still no doubt that modeling, docking, virtual screening, and all the other techniques have made a lot of progress. And it's certainly not the modelers' fault that progress has been harder to realize than people thought it would be back in the 1980s. But while (say) calculating small-molecule ligand binding to anything close to experimental error is a hard problem, it certainly doesn't seem to be an insoluble one. Betting against a field that has the increase of computational power on its side and can be advanced at any time by sudden algorithmic insights is not a wise move.

There's also the advent of machine learning and AI to consider. Even as I write this Foreword, word has come of the best results yet on calculating protein folding, and it came *via* an AI approach.[23] That result illustrates the strong and the weak points of such systems. Thus far, they are very good (sometimes terrifyingly so) at sorting through existing knowledge. The protein-folding result, for example, was not realized so much by fundamental insights into hydrogen bonding or torsional strain, but through advances in recognizing protein structural motifs in the huge archives of existing data. The application of such techniques to the retrosynthesis programs mentioned earlier should be obvious (and this is one of the reasons I think that they will be increasingly useful). What an AI will not do much of, not yet, is to help you out with things that are not already buried in what's known. But that still leaves a great deal of scope for interesting things, particularly as AI algorithms go to work on the problem of optimizing themselves.

## The End Results

But never forget, all this is in the service of great things. We medicinal chemists work on so many failed projects of various kinds that it can be difficult to stand back and look at some of the successes. Oncology is a dramatic example. Thanks to new approaches in that field, there are people out there today deciding what to order for lunch who would not even be among the living under earlier treatment regimens. The startling inside-of-a-year advent of vaccines against the SARS-Cov2 virus is another case in point. Vaccine development will clearly never be the same again, and the world will be the better for it.

The central fact of drug discovery, and of the drug industry itself, has been the horrendous failure rate in clinical trials. For many years now, it's stayed around 90% over the whole field, with some therapeutic areas doing better (cardiovascular, infectious disease) and some doing worse (oncology, CNS).[24] But think about it: if we could only manage to fall on our faces eight times out of ten, we would roughly double the number of new drugs making it to patients. That would be a tremendous outcome, and it isn't going to take anything miraculous to achieve it. A steady pace of improvements up and down the process, even though many of them might be small, will be enough. We can heal the sick, we can improve people's lives, and once in a while (as with some of the recent advances in immuno-oncology) we can nearly pull people out of the grave. Every year we get better at it; every year we know more. It is, when you think about it, a great job to be doing.

Derek Lowe

## References


1. R. M. Eglen and R. L. Whiting, *J. Auton. Pharmacol.*, 1990, **10**, 233–246.
2. H. N. Doods, M. J. Mathy, D. Davidesko, K. J. van Charldorp, A. de Jonge and P. A. van Zwieten, *J. Pharmacol. Exp. Ther.*, 1987, **242**, 257–262.
3. C. G. Smith and J. R. Vane, *FASEB J.*, 2003, **17**, 788–789.
4. D. W. Cushman and M. W. Ondetti, *Hypertension*, 1991, **17**, 589–592.
5. R. P. Ahlquist, *Am. J. Physiol.*, 1948, **153**, 586–600.
6. D. B. Bylund, *Am. J. Physiol.: Endocrinol. Metab.*, 2007, **293**, E1479–E1481.
7. H. P. Rang, *Br. J. Pharmacol.*, 2006, **147**(S1), S9–S16.
8. A.-H. Maehle, *Endeavour*, 2009, **33**, 135–140.
9. J. G. Moffat, F. Vincent, J. A. Lee, J. Eder and M. Prunotto, *Nat. Rev. Drug Discovery*, 2017, **16**, 531–543.
10. P. Cohen, *Nat. Rev. Drug Discovery*, 2002, **1**, 309–315.

11. D. R. Zerbino, A. Frankish and P. Flicek, *Annu. Rev. Genomics Hum. Genet.*, 2020, **21**, 55–79.
12. J. S. Sherkow and H. T. Greely, *Annu. Rev. Genet.*, 2015, **49**, 161–182.
13. P. Brennan and S. V. Rodriguez, *The Discovery and Utility of Chemical Probes in Target Discovery*, Royal Society of Chemistry, Cambridge, 2020.
14. M. D. Shultz, *J. Med. Chem.*, 2019, **62**, 1701–1714.
15. W. P. Walters, J. Green, J. R. Weiss and M. A. Murcko, *J. Med. Chem.*, 2011, **54**, 6405–6416.
16. B. C. Doak, B. Over, F. Giordanetto, and J. Kihlberg, Chem. Biol., 2014, 21, 1115–1142–.
17. R. Phillips, Paris Rev., 1982, 84.
18. D. G. Brown and J. Boström, *J. Med. Chem.*, 2016, **59**, 4443–4458.
19. A. Tomberg and J. Boström, *Drug Discovery Today*, 2020, **25**, 2174–2181.
20. J. Boström, D. G. Brown, R. J. Young and G. M Keserü, *Nat. Rev. Drug Discovery*, 2018, **17**, 709–727.
21. G. Kasparov, *Deep Thinking: Where Machine Intelligence Ends and Human Creativity Begins*, PublicAffairs, New York, 2017.
22. R. Mullin, *Chemical and Engineering News*, https://cen.acs.org/business/informatics/lab-future-ai-automated-synthesis/99/i11, accessed November 2021.
23. AlphaFold, https://alphafold.ebi.ac.uk/, accessed November 2021.
24. C. H. Wong, K. W. Siah and A. W. Lo, *Biostatistics*, 2019, **20**, 273–286.

# Preface to the 2nd Edition

We published the first edition of 'The Handbook of Medicinal Chemistry: Principles and Practice' in 2015, following in the footsteps of the perennially popular 'Medicinal Chemistry Principles and Practice'. Both titles were designed to complement and support the biannual Royal Society of Chemistry Medicinal Chemistry summer school which has provided inspirational training to early career medicinal chemists and others entering the world of drug discovery for over 40 years.

For the 2015 edition, we considerably expanded the scope and content of its predecessor volumes, recognising the significant shifts in both the scientific practices and the nature of institutions engaged in drug discovery and development. We divided the book into three main sections: firstly, the fundamental principles used by the medicinal chemist; secondly, the application of those tools to progress molecules through discovery into development; and thirdly, case studies to demonstrate the reduction of these principles into practice. This volume was very well received and brought together for the first time in a single volume the key enabling information for the contemporary, practising medicinal chemist.

Given this impact, why then, only seven years later, is this second edition being published? What has changed in that time to make a new volume necessary?

Of course, the most striking illustration of the speed of scientific and industrial advance and change has been the phenomenal response to develop prophylactic and therapeutic strategies to coronavirus disease. Interestingly, this second edition was conceived before we knew about severe acute respiratory syndrome coronavirus 2 (SARS-CoV-2) and the chapter writing and editing then has taken place in its shadow. The ability to respond rapidly to SARS-CoV-2 stemmed from the enormous technological and biological advances in recent years. These advances also underpin a plethora of new approaches making an impact in the discovery of new medicines.

The last seven years have seen new chemistry and synthetic methodology continuing to provide new opportunities for medicinal chemistry, alongside molecular biology developments which are providing new screening paradigms. In 2015 DNA encoded libraries were an emerging technology, they are now an established part of the lead generation

The Handbook of Medicinal Chemistry: Principles and Practice, 2nd Edition
Edited by Simon E. Ward and Andrew M. Davis

Published by the Royal Society of Chemistry, www.rsc.org

canon – available from several CRO providers and even academic institutions. PROTACS, first proposed in 2001, were still an emerging modality in 2015, but have now exploded across the drug discovery landscape, with the first examples already in clinical testing. While QSAR was already a mature discipline, who would have guessed in 2015 that the combination of machine learning algorithms with artificial intelligence would bring *de novo* design, heralded by computational chemistry in the 1980s, back as a realistic prospect. Virtual screening, also not a new technique, has vastly expanded its scope through modern algorithms and cloud computing to explore virtual spaces of up to $10^{12}$ molecules and beyond. By 2015 we had already had the human genome in our hands for more than 13 years, but the acceleration and plummeting costs of whole genome sequencing are now providing vast data-sources of millions of human genome sequences aligned to patients' clinical data to mine for genes linked to diseases, providing medicinal chemists with new, better validated (although often more challenging) protein targets. Phenotypic screening has always been a rich source of chemical tools and while not as intellectually appealing as rational design, it has continued to find fascinating and important molecules like CFTR correctors which are changing the face of CF treatment. Molecular biology has been revolutionised by CRISPR/CAS9, providing more complex tools, providing genome-wide protein knockout, or activating screens to find new targets and even offering the concept of targeted genome editing as a new drug modality. Chemical biology continues to uncover subtle and revealing modes of action, which has opened up new fields, including exome skipping and RNA targeting, alongside uncovering small molecules acting as molecular glues and molecular glue degraders. Large-scale proteomics, and techniques such as CETSA, are enabling true in-cell target engagement and target deconvolution. In the field of structural biology, breakthroughs in equipment, instrumentation and computational power have meant cryogenic electron microscopy can now achieve resolutions suitable to impact drug discovery and open out structure-based drug design to previously unattainable target classes such as ion channels and macromolecular protein complexes. Then there is single-cell transcriptomics, hydrogen–deuterium exchange, acoustic mist mass spectrometry screening, high throughput imaging, the list goes on. So much has happened in seven years!

So apart from those subjects, which we have tried to incorporate, what else has changed in the second edition? Firstly, we have kept broadly to the overall structure of the first edition given the positive reception of its structure and logical flow from target and hit discovery through to clinical development. All the chapters have been revised and updated with new information, regulatory or legislative additions and exemplified with contemporary examples and case studies. We have three new chapters:

Synthetic chemistry – which reinforces the importance of the parent discipline of synthetic organic chemistry in the day-to-day job of the medicinal chemist and importantly uses synthesis as a tool to facilitate the preparation of key design molecules, as well as recognising the role of the chemist outside traditional 'small molecule' space.

AI and machine learning – to both establish its fundamental principles from QSAR analyses and helpfully delineate the hope from the hype and outline practical applications.

New modalities – which expands horizons beyond the 'already drugged' into the chemical space between traditional chemistry and biology – oligonucleotides, complex peptides, homo- and hetero-fused molecules (such as bi-specific antibodies, PROTACS *etc.*) as well as approaches to modify processing of RNA, DNA or protein synthesis.

Some of the approaches such as targeted protein degradation (*via* PROTAC or other modality), modification of RNA splicing, ability to visualise ligand-bound protein structures of membrane-bound proteins *via* cryo-EM, routine assessment of protein activity within the cell, are now so routine, it is hard to imagine them being outside the mainstream of drug discovery at the time of writing. Indeed, the inspiring case study we're delighted to be able to include describing risdiplam for the treatment of spinal muscular atrophy – and celebrated on the cover of this book – is testament to the fusion of new biological understanding opening up previously inconceivable approaches with excellence in medicinal chemistry and iterative lead optimisation.

For the Foreword, we were delighted that one of our industry's most influential commentators, Derek Lowe, author of the 'In the pipeline' blog, provides us with a perspective on medicinal chemistry.

Alongside the last edition we also published the medicinal chemistry toolkit iPad app. It was a joint initiative between the editors, Molmatinf and the RSC. This was a successful initiative making useful everyday tools freely available on a tablet as a secure environment. We received many requests for the app to be available on other platforms. So to accompany this edition, the editors and Molmatinf, sponsored by AstraZeneca Open Innovation, have ported the dose to man component of the iPad app to a freely available secure web app on the following link:

https://molmatinf.com/medchemtoolkit

As stated in the preface to the first volume, the career of the medicinal chemist remains one of the most challenging and stimulating careers imaginable. The medicinal chemist, at the heart of a network of multidisciplinary scientists, can craft the beginnings of the journey towards a new medicine. And surely there could be no greater motivation.

We hope that this new edition will continue to train and inspire the next generation of drug discovers in the wide diversity of institutions and organisations that are striving to improve the quality of life for millions of people across the world.

Simon E. Ward and Andrew Davis

# Foreword to the First Edition

I am delighted to have been invited to write an introduction for The Handbook of Medicinal Chemistry: Principles and Practice. The editors and authors have played an outstanding role in covering all of the major components of modern medicinal chemistry in an expert and timely manner, within a comprehensive handbook relevant to newcomers and experienced scientists alike. This volume will be a pleasure to read through, and then to pick out relevant sections for in depth consultation. I am sure Principles and Practice will be in constant use, as different problems arise in drug discovery projects almost on a daily basis, and will become essential reading for medicinal chemists of whatever background and experience.

An overview of the dramatic progress we have made with healthcare quality shows that life expectancy has consistently risen over the past century with an increase from 60 to over 85 years for women in most industrialised nations. Similar trends are evident for men and equally importantly, the developing world is now moving in the same direction. While improved standards of hygiene, nutrition, housing and other factors are obviously important, it is estimated that 40% of the recent increase in life expectancy in the US is due to modern medicines largely discovered by the pharmaceutical industry:[1] powerful antibiotics are available to treat life-threatening bacterial infections; hypertension (the silent killer) can be controlled by any number of once-daily therapies; elevated cholesterol which is a major cardiovascular risk factor, is well managed with statins, while H2 antagonists and even proton pump blockers are available over the counter to treat gastric ulcers. When HIV/AIDS appeared on the scene in the early 1980s, it was considered a death sentence and control was thought to be beyond our reach due to facile transmission and potential for resistance. Today, over thirty drugs from six mechanistic classes are available, and those in the West who contract the virus have enjoyed much improved quality of life and longevity. Importantly, similar benefits are now emerging in the developing world where for example, life expectancy in Kwa Zulu-Natal has risen from 49 in 2003 to 60 years in 2011 as affordable anti-retroviral combinations became available in the public healthcare system. Hopefully, recent headlines from The Economist such as: "The end of AIDS? How 5 million lives have

The Handbook of Medicinal Chemistry: Principles and Practice, 2nd Edition
Edited by Simon E. Ward and Andrew M. Davis

Published by the Royal Society of Chemistry, www.rsc.org

been saved and a plague could be defeated" are now within sight, and a fair balance between drug pricing and health benefits will become commonplace.

Despite such outstanding success, there are still tremendous healthcare challenges facing medicinal chemists and the whole drug discovery community. We all know that cardiovascular disease (CVD) is a major risk factor responsible for over four million deaths in Europe each year, but few realise that 80% of global CVD mortality actually occurs in low- to middle-income countries which are disproportionately affected. The prevalence of obesity in US adults will grow to 50% by 2030, and it is also estimated that 92 million Chinese already suffer from Type 2 diabetes. While malaria, TB and HIV are still scourges in many parts of Africa, non-communicable diseases killed 36 million people in 2008 which represents 63% of total deaths, with the majority occurring in emerging nations. In any one year, 40% of Europeans will be affected by some type of brain disorder with total annual costs of care around Euro 800 billion, more than CVD, cancer and diabetes combined. Mental depression is responsible for 38% of all morbidity and 23% of Quality-Adjusted Life Years (QALYs) lost, whereas the corresponding figures for cancer are 3 and 16%, respectively. The WHO has forecast an impending disaster due to unchallenged increases in antimicrobial resistance, but only four new classes of antibiotics have been introduced over the past 40 years. In response to these major threats to health and well being, the demand for new medicines will continue unabated, albeit with different emphasis on quality of life or longevity depending on regional differences in economic and social development. However, new paradigms for research focus, organisation, cooperation and funding will be required, as we adjust to an ever changing scenario of contracting Pharma and withdrawal from major therapeutic areas. This introduction offers a personal perspective on some factors that may influence success and failure in drug discovery, and suggests how the sector might learn from the past and evolve in the future.

Size and organisation are key factors for innovative drug discovery which have been overlooked in endless rounds of mergers and acquisitions over the past decade, and the relentless drive to international research conglomerates. During the period when we were most productive at the Pfizer research laboratories in Sandwich, our total staffing was probably around two to three hundred, but that period witnessed outstanding discoveries such as amlodipine, diflucan, doxazosin and sildenafil. Our research was driven by dedicated scientists working together in multidisciplinary teams towards common objectives within a supportive, but focussed environment. Unusually, drug metabolism experts were also integral members of discovery projects which provided a significant competitive edge, as we did not have to beg, borrow or steal from development which was the norm throughout Pharma at that time. While we fully understood the need to compete internationally, we operated largely on a local and personal scale where a trip to the US was an annual treat, not a weekly routine. We all knew each other, managers and directors walked the job, and we were not distracted by administration. Scientists were constantly in and out of each other's laboratories as we had a hunger to generate, share and exploit new data that would drive our projects forward. Face to face discussions were the norm, and stimulated a level of intellectual challenge far beyond impersonal e-mails and text messages. The current journals section of the library was a focal point for discussions where we swapped ideas as we jostled for the latest articles, but paper copy has largely disappeared and individual online access may not generate the same thought- provoking synergies unless alternative communication networks are established. In addition, we valued our "Tribal Elders" who had "been there, done that" and freely shared their experience, but successful role models have largely disappeared in today's cost cutting climate. However, the added value generated through a mentoring and supportive culture coupled with institutionalised learning cannot be over estimated.

As we grew we had to adapt, and I became drawn to the concept of the Roman Centurion who traditionally leads and cares for 100 soldiers which seemed a sensibly sized unit, particularly in a research environment. When there were 100 chemists in my discovery group, I knew them all and what they were doing, and I was also able to engage at a personal level. However, as the group expanded it became more difficult to maintain that level of interaction, and informal discussions were diluted. Dunbar's number of 150 is an estimate of the social contacts humans can cope with, obviously at differing levels of engagement, which is roughly in line with the Centurion concept. The average size of a village in the Domesday Book of 1086 was also around 150, and any further increase stimulated migration to form new settlements. These numbers intuitively feel right as they reflect the importance of personal contact, and also address the critical mass necessary for survival. Similar considerations should underpin drug discovery organisations where large groups should be broken down into nimble, multidisciplinary units that can be managed and led on a personal scale. Teams should be largely autonomous but accountable, with innovation and a data-driven culture recognised and rewarded, rather than the consensus management and upward decision making that has ossified Pharma in recent years.

Critical mass is probably more important than size *per se* as the ability to respond rapidly to breaking science can make the difference between success and failure. For example, we quickly realised that half a dozen chemists on a lead optimisation project would not be competitive, whereas 12 to 15 could hold their own. However, we could never manage the teams of 20 to 40 that others mobilised as duplication, poor communication and a loss of personal responsibility inherent in such large groups compromised productivity and motivation. Innovative scientists often want to be different, but some can drift into peripheral activities with a lack of focus and commitment to team objectives. Crucially, the concept of critical mass and nimble research units became confused with absolute size in the fruitless drive to build the largest R&D organisations. Even before the merger with Wyeth, Pfizer had an annual R&D budget of nearly $8 billion with thousands of staff spread over eight centres on three continents, which may not be conducive to a personal or nimble approach. The negative impact of mergers and acquisitions on productivity is well documented[2] as research simply cannot be effectively managed in such massive units, nor can innovation survive, particularly with multiple locations, cultures and ever changing leadership. Technology can be expanded in a modular manner and centralised facilities for HTS, gene sequencing and other service operations are efficient and cost effective, but innovation simply does not scale. If readers were to take one key message from this introduction, it would be my strong conviction that drug discovery is a personal and shared experience, not a metrics-focused, mechanical event. So many times, successful projects are driven by a small core of dedicated champions with a burning desire to address particular medical needs, working together in a research-friendly environment not dominated by numbers.

Hype and premature over-investment in new technologies are other examples of how Pharma lost its way with the drive towards "faster, cheaper, better," but quality was lost in the pursuit of numerical goals. Most companies thought that industrialisation of drug discovery was the way of the future and that attrition need not be improved if the number of candidates entering development was significantly increased. Numbers and metrics became key drivers and innovation and personal accountability were lost in the process. Gone were the days of research proposals that laid out a biological rationale and thoughtful chemistry plans that were subject to rigorous challenge, and HTS assumed the default mode for new projects. HTS became a macho competition across Pharma with migration from 96 to 384 to 1536 well plates, and the drive to generate millions of data points over the shortest time frame. However, assays were often not robust, and quality control was poor. Compound collections contained everything chemists had registered, and it took some time to weed out frequent hitters, reactive intermediates and undesirable structural flags that were never intended to included in screening files in the first place. Unfortunately, re-building these collections also became numbers driven as it was easy to impress senior managers with the claim to synthesise millions of peptides overnight, but without adding that these compounds had little utility for drug discovery. Combinatorial libraries constructed from simple, non-peptide building blocks suffered a similar fate as focus on "what we can make" rather than "what we should make" led to large collections of closely related compounds with low value for screening, particularly as mixtures. Some Pharma companies responded by investing up to $100 million in building diverse, multi-million compound collections, but such large files are rarely screened routinely as representative sub-sets usually provide an idea of the relevance of the overall library to a particular target. However, it is encouraging that HTS has matured considerably over the past decade, where greater attention to assay reproducibility and compound quality has been rewarded with viable hit matter identified much of the time. More recently, advances in computational chemistry and structural biology have led to the integration of virtual screening with smart HTS which has further increased success rates. Such improvements are a tremendous advance, but the time-scales and resources required for new technologies to reach maturity are quite sobering.

Of course, the allure of HT-everything drove massive investments in numerous other technologies including every "omics" under the sun, often through fear of losing out to competitors rather than an appreciation of real value or time scales involved. The Gartner Hype Cycle neatly summarises new initiatives passing through a technology trigger, peak of inflated expectation, trough of disillusion, slope of enlightenment and plateau of productivity that we have all experienced. Multiple external collaborations often proved a distraction from drug discovery, and some major investments from the 1990s are still way off delivery. For example, billions have been invested in DNA- and RNA-based therapies as interest shifted from antisense to ribozymes to RNA interference, although it was obvious that delivery would be a common problem that still has not been solved generically. However, the first systemic antisense drug was approved in 2013, some 23 years from "a blank sheet of paper to market" which again brings home the timescales required for new technologies to bed-in and mature. Gene therapy involves the simple concept of introducing a gene into a cell to express a particular protein involved in disease, but the few regulatory approvals to date are limited to niche indications with return on investment still a long way off. Perhaps the highest hopes were raised over the sequencing of the human genome which was announced in draft form in 2001, with ambitious claims that this would revolutionise healthcare diagnosis and treatment. This may turn out to be the case, but more than a decade later, millions of gene sequences are in hand with "the dream" still far from reality. Maybe the fundamental thought processes outlined by James Watson in The Double Helix put such numbers-driven approaches into context. However, some genes and SNPs have shown a weak association with disease but there has been little impact on target validation or patient selection, except for particular cancers. In the latter case, identification of genetic markers of drug sensitivity has proved to be extremely powerful in patient stratification for clinical trials and targeted therapies, but there has been little progress with other diseases.

Improved candidate survival is another key issue, as the enormous cost of bringing a new medicine to market is unacceptable since it also includes wasted investment in the numerous failures that occur throughout the drug discovery and development process. Alarmingly, recent surveys suggest that less than 10% of preclinical candidates that enter development reach the market, and it is difficult to imagine that any other business sector would accept such an appalling failure rate. Reducing attrition must be a major priority for Pharma in general and medicinal chemists in particular, since even modest improvements would have a significant impact on the cost-effective output of new medicines.

The individual reasons for candidate failure have been well documented, but the dual themes of mechanism- and compound-related attrition are particularly relevant during the discovery phase. Validating a new target in the laboratory is a daunting task even with today's sophisticated technologies and realistically, only a certain level of confidence can be established that a particular pathway or mechanism will be relevant in man. To mitigate risk, mining gene families has received particular attention on the assumption that experience with one clinically-relevant member could be extended to close relatives. While this may apply to druggability, there seems to be a high level of biological redundancy such that seemingly attractive targets may not be involved in physiological or pathophysiological processes. For example, despite convincing rationale for disease relevance and the discovery of potent ligands for numerous members of the adenosine and PDE families, only a handful of drugs have actually resulted. Clearly, animal experiments are still poorly predictive of the clinical situation, particularly for CNS and cancer where above average attrition is par for the course. Mechanism-related failures may also be a consequence of evaluating new drugs in heterogeneous patient groups such that efficacy signals from responsive subsets are lost in the noise.

Reducing mechanism-related failures calls for greater innovation and investment in target validation, but animal models always have limitations and rapid progression of quality candidates to the clinic may be more informative. This will require developing robust biomarkers that confirm drug activity in relevant tissues, identifying patient subgroups that respond to a particular mechanism of action and establishing definitive clinical end points. Overall, a much better understanding and interpretation of PK/PD relationships will be required, and early enough to influence discovery projects. Some consider that these initiatives will fragment markets, but the cost of clinical trials and attrition will be significantly reduced, and surely targeting patients with a high chance of response must be a key objective? Pre-competitive collaborations for both target validation and patient selection will become more common, and there are encouraging signs that Pharma is moving in this direction.

Given such significant investment in biological and clinical sciences, medicinal chemists have a key role to play in designing high quality candidates capable of completing definitive Phase 2 proof of concept studies where full dose–response relationships can be explored. Their challenge is to optimise the physicochemical and molecular properties they so well understand to eliminate compound-related failures such that decisions on candidate progression can be made on efficacy and safety data alone. 30% of all candidate failures are due to inadequate clinical efficacy, but probing new mechanisms with sub-optimal compounds provides minimal learning at significant cost. Indeed, analysis of 44 Phase 2 programmes at Pfizer[3] confirmed that the majority of failures was due to lack of efficacy, but in 43% of those cases it was not possible to conclude that the mechanism had been properly tested due to limited exposure and target engagement.

The Lipinski Rule of Five is now part of the fabric of drug design since these data-driven guidelines summarise the physicochemical parameters that influence permeability and oral absorption. While there are exceptions, medicinal chemists who push the guidelines to the limit usually bequeath compound-related deficiencies to their colleagues at some stage in the discovery and development process, and which often come home to roost in the clinic. Various analyses have shown that molecular weights of drug candidates decrease along the development pathway which must raise at least an amber flag to those pursuing lead series with molecular weights above 400. Increasing molecular weight and lipophilicity is seductive as this allows introduction of structural diversity and novel substituents that improve potency and allow differentiation from prior art. However, while low oral doses are obviously preferred for clinical candidates, the median target affinity for current small molecule drugs is around 20 nM, so the goal of continually driving down absolute potency may be less important than focussing on ligand efficiency which reflects the average binding energy per heavy atom. Ligand lipophilicity efficiency may be even more relevant for lead optimisation as this provides a constant reminder that SARs should be developed without compromising physicochemical properties.

For compounds with high molecular weight and lipophilicity, solubility is almost invariably compromised and is often not improved during lead optimisation such that bioavailablity may be low and variable. Such compound-related limitations are significant barriers to exploring dose–response relationships in the clinic and may also have a negative impact on eventual commercialisation. Compounds at the fringes of the guidelines tend to be more susceptible to CYP oxidation/induction, which can reduce bioavailability through first pass metabolism, generate biologically active and/or toxic metabolites and lead to significant drug–drug interaction liabilities. Encouragingly, medicinal chemists now have a greater understanding of the scientific principles that control absorption, distribution and metabolism, and failure during development for pharmacokinetic factors has been reduced from 40 to below 10%.[4]

Entropy driven, non-specific interactions are important for binding between small molecules and proteins so compounds with high molecular weight and lipophilicity tend to be promiscuous with significant off–target activities. Given that safety issues in animals and man are responsible for some 30% of candidate losses, medicinal chemists should work within physi–cochemical parameters associated with success, not failure. Of course, there are exceptions such as natural products and some anti-virals for example, and larger, more complex molecules may be required to block protein–protein interactions, but passive drift outside the guidelines should be avoided.

The challenges to medicinal chemists are clear: physicochemical property inflation should be reduced; compound-related failures eliminated; and attrition significantly improved. We have a unique responsibility for discovering new drugs that will meet future medical needs and to ensure the viability of industry-based research in years to come, but personal accountability can be eroded as the drug discovery processes is broken down into compartments with "experts" assigned to artificial stages from design to candidate selection. Such fragmentation may simplify metrics, but may be personally unrewarding and less productive than a holistic approach where chemists have target laboratory and clinical profiles in mind even as they consider early hit structures.

Phenotypic screens were common in the 1970s when I joined Pfizer, and the rigorous mechanistic approach pioneered by Sir James Black was only just starting to make an impact. I became a member of the antihypertensive project where we were trying to improve on pra- zosin, a diaminoquinazoline derivative discovered by our colleagues in Groton. It had been suggested that prazosin acted as a PDE inhibitor, but the biological target was unknown so our screening sequence was alarmingly simple: synthesis then oral administration to spontaneously hypertensive rats, which actually was common practice at that time. Of course, a fall in blood pressure confirmed oral availability and perhaps our compounds were hitting a single target, but negative results were difficult to interpret and we abandoned the project. Some time later, Sandwich pharmacologists showed that prazosin was the prototype for a new mechanistic class of post-synaptic $\alpha_1$-adrenoceptor antagonists and we immediately understood why these compounds lowered blood pressure. Screening switched to functional blockade of noradrenaline-induced vascular contraction through $\alpha_1$-receptors which enabled us to rapidly identify the basic pharmacophore responsible for affinity and selectivity, while interrogation of the prior art suggested how SARs could be developed in an innovative fashion. Almost immediately, we synthesised UK33,274 (doxazosin), a potent and highly selective $\alpha_1$-adrenoceptor antagonist that was later marketed as Cardura®, a once-daily antihypertensive agent that attained annual sales of over $1 billion.

When we started our calcium antagonist project to seek a once-daily follow on to nifedipine for the treatment of angina and hypertension, we screened compounds in guinea pig hearts as we thought we should target the cardiac rigour that occurs during an ischeamic attack. We did indeed discover a novel series of anti-rigour agents, but without a trace of calcium antagonist activity. Again, when we moved to specific binding and functional screens, we made rapid progress with the discovery of UK48,340 (amlodipine), a potent and selective calcium antagonist with complete bioavailability and a 30 hour half-life in dogs. This compound is marketed as Norvasc® (Istin® in the UK) for the once-daily treatment of angina and hypertension and became the World's fourth most popular drug with annual peak sales of $5.5 billion. I am convinced that neither amlodipine nor doxazosin would be bringing benefit to patients today if we had not moved from such crude and inappropriate phenotypic screens to defined mechanistic targets, but of course one size does not fit all.

Our attempts at phenotypic screening at the animal or organ level were poorly considered and were not productive, and like most of the industry we became attracted to mechanism-based approaches. This was driven not only by difficulties in rational prosecution of lead matter, but also from our experience that "no mechanism" candidates had higher failure rates in development. In addition, there was always a lingering fear that unexpected side effects might appear in the clinic when biological targets were not defined. Accordingly, one might assume that rational, target-based approaches would dominate today's landscape but surprisingly, in my view at least, 37% of first in class NMEs approved by the FDA over the decade up to 2008 originated from phenotypic screening. A defined mechanism of action may be preferable, but it is not essential for regulatory approval where agencies focus more on efficacy and safety. Some consider that phenotypic assays are more relevant for a complex disease condition than screening against a single molecular target, but follow-up can be challenging as activity reflects multiple parameters such as access, distribution and promiscuity. In addition, Structure-Based Drug Design is not relevant and "ligand efficiency" has limited value, and the richness of prior art is often lost when targets are unknown. Despite these caveats, innovative medicinal chemists have a fine record in overcoming such challenges and translating phenotypic hits into successful clinical drugs. Traditionally, there has been a poor and well-documented return from HTS against single antimicrobial targets, and phenotypic screening has proved more appropriate. For example, the Medicines for Malaria Venture has recently coordinated screening of Pharma libraries in a phenotypic, blood-stage malaria assay where numerous, attractive leads were identified, some of which have been transformed into high-quality clinical candidates. Wider use of carefully defined phenotypic screening should be expected in future as newer technologies such as chemical proteomics have significantly facilitated target identification, and some claim up to a 70% success rate within months or even weeks.

The relative merits of small molecules and biologicals are regularly debated as if it were one class or the other, whereas both will play important roles in meeting future medical needs. It is expected that up to eight of the top ten drugs in 2014 will be biologicals which is taken by some to mark the end of small molecules, but this may be an artefact of timing in that Biotech was initially some way behind Pharma, and these products have taken time to mature. Indeed, several leading biologicals have passed or are near the end of their patent life and "The Cliff" does not respect particular molecules. Generic biosimilars will make an increasing impact, although there are still hurdles particularly in the US, but revenues may not be eroded as rapidly as for small molecules. While biologicals have been outstandingly successful for the treatment of arthritis, cancer and diabetes, for example, these molecules are expensive to make and can cost thousands of dollars each month, without offering the convenience of oral administration for chronic diseases. Dose simplification has been an important driver for the widespread acceptance of statins and for the success of anti-retroviral therapies in the developing world for example, which would be impractical with biologicals.

Regenerative medicine and stem cell therapies will also find a place for some diseases, but such approaches are likely to focus on specific patient populations, given potential high cost and specialist administration. Pressures on healthcare budgets will increase as the population ages, but there should be a continuing role for novel, small molecules that provide cost effective therapies that can be conveniently taken by mouth. Indeed, 26 of the 39 NCEs approved by the FDA in 2012 are small molecules with only two monoclonal antibodies which may be a pointer to the future, or simply a reflection of a "one off" mix of research projects initiated some ten or more years ago. Whatever the future holds, medicinal chemists will be key players addressing clinical needs not only through small molecules but also with the design and production of hybrid biological therapies, and full participation in new chemical and synthetic biology initiatives.

Pre-competitive collaborations will become more important in the future in order to reduce cost, risk and duplication. Most pharma portfolios probably share 70–80% similarity with multiple and parallel investments in the same targets, and often molecular scaffolds. For example, several companies took neurokinin and endothelin antagonists to the clinic over similar periods but with little reward, while the cumulative time and effort committed to renin inhibitors was absolutely staggering. Such duplicative failures might be avoided through pre-competitive collaborations between industry and academia for target validation, particularly given the alarming claim that far less than 50% of biological publications can be repeated by third parties. Surely, we are past the point where individual Pharma/Biotech companies can continue to make parallel investments to reach the same negative conclusions given the tremendous pressures the industry is facing? Identifying patient populations that respond to new mechanisms of action is also essential, but this will require cooperative investment from industry, academia, health services and regulators. If validated targets and patient subsets do enter the public domain earlier than at present, then responsibility for establishing a competitive edge and robust IP will depend largely on innovative medicinal chemistry which will simply become too valuable to contract out. There are signs that the community may be moving towards precompetitive collaborations with the Structural Genomics Consortium championing more open interactions and providing wide access to chemical tools to probe new targets. Medicinal chemists play a central role in such initiatives by designing prototype molecules and developing analytical capability to build our understanding of biological pathways and mechanisms, and for target validation. Strict criteria for compound potency and selectivity should be demanded for proof of concept studies, and a further frame shift in chemical innovation will be required to exploit receptors and enzymes currently considered undruggable, and for those yet to be discovered.

On a broader precompetitive front, the EU Innovative Medicines Initiative has launched a new Euro 224 million programme jointly funded with industry to channel academic and industry partners towards new classes of antibiotics that address antimicrobial resistance. A further EU Public Private Partnership will invest nearly Euro 200 million to bring together multiple partners to create a Lead Factory comprising a European Screening Centre and compound collection. Access to HTS and 0.5 million diverse structures could enhance the rate of lead generation across the community, particularly for academic researchers who have previously had difficulty in identifying tractable chemical matter. In the US, a National Centre for Advancing Translational Sciences has been established with focus on facilitating translation from the laboratory to clinic which could have significant pre-competitive impact, although there are vociferous critics of both mission and budget. Ten pharmaceutical companies have formed a non-profit organisation called TransCelerate BioPharma to accelerate the development of new medicines, while DataShare aims to create a repository of information from cancer trials carried out by Pharma, academia and public institutions that can be shared across the community. More broadly, an international AllTrials initiative is campaigning for industry and regulators to make full Clinical Study Reports available, and GSK has taken the lead amongst large Pharma by agreeing to participate. Such precompetitive collaborations in drug discovery and development not only have the potential to reduce costs and risks, but also to bring significant patient benefit.

Economic conditions will become harsher than in the past with unflinching pressures on budgets at national, regional and local levels. Healthcare costs overall and drug prices in particular will be under the closest scrutiny as we move more towards an ageing society. Continued rises in health investment as a percentage of GDP will simply not be sustainable worldwide. New medicines will have to demonstrate positive outcomes over existing treatments, with hard evidence of reduced mortality and morbidity, improved quality of life and savings in overall healthcare budgets. There will be high expectations, or more likely demands, for innovative and cost- effective medicines that will transform treatment paradigms and justify reimbursement. Although NICE in the UK has led the way in relating treatment benefits and costs to QALYs and Disability-Adjusted Life Years, such agencies are now commonplace throughout the world and criteria for reimbursement are becoming more stringent. Indeed, 2012 may prove to be a watershed with respect to pricing and reimbursement as five orphan drugs approved by the FDA have annual prices between \$100 000–300 000 while several new anti-cancers will cost from \$7000–10 000 per month, and there is already significant pushback from oncology experts. Healthcare systems may not be able to offer such expensive new therapies unless significant clinical benefit can be demonstrated, but earlier industry-agency agreement on target efficacy/safety criteria could minimise negative reimbursement decisions currently taken after years of costly investment. Encouragingly, the FDA has introduced a "breakthrough" status for fast tracking innovative new medicines based on Phase 2 data which resulted in the approval of ivacaftor for cystic fibrosis in 2012.

There have been high expectations that the developing world would provide a more welcoming environment as living standards rise, but leading countries such as China and India are driving down drug costs even more aggressively than in the West, and are tending to favour local manufacturers. Bringing cost-effective healthcare to the general population is their first priority, although expanding middle classes may be willing to pay higher prices for some new medicines. However, these markets are currently not robust enough to support investment in R&D at historical levels and few new drugs have emerged from generic companies. Given the mantra that "innovative R&D follows premium priced markets" it is unlikely that high-investment pharmaceutical research will make a major shift eastwards in the near future, particularly given worrying threats to IP that had previously been secured elsewhere. However, China has announced a five-year plan to invest $7 billion in academic projects that might lead to new drugs and eventually spawn an innovative pharmaceutical industry, although the need to build expertise and depth is openly accepted.

So what of the future? Some ten years ago, I suggested to a sceptical audience that the future pharmaceutical industry would be largely located in the US with outposts in Europe and Japan, which may well come to pass. However, even the US is in flux as budget deficits and pressure to reduce healthcare expenditure continue to force down drug costs and R&D investment. Consequently, traditional organisations are consigned to the past as the number of leading pharmaceutical companies in the US has declined from 42 in 1988 to 11 today, and all have undergone significant downsizing with major site closures. In the UK, international players such as AstraZeneca, GSK, Pfizer, Merck, Novartis, Organon (Merck/Schering) and Roche have abandoned modern research facilities, there have been thousands of job losses and the overall situation is probably still meta-stable. Indeed, decentralisation of R&D organisations is in full flow, as Pharma continues to minimise fixed costs by externalising routine research activities to CROs, and by working more closely with the academic community. For example, AstraZeneca has significantly reduced resource on neuroscience research and has moved to a virtual model where a small internal team collaborates with leading academic centres to share reward and risk. Pfizer has established Centres for Therapeutic Innovation in Boston, New York, San Diego and San Francisco to facilitate interactions with academic institutions, and has placed their own staff in collaborator laboratories. While these initiatives should provide early access to new biology, translation to successful drug discovery projects still has to be realised, and there will be the inevitable trade off between publications and IP. In addition, core expertise within Pharma, particularly medicinal chemistry, cannot be eroded too far, as successful collaborations require complementary intellectual contributions from both partners, and coherence on objectives.

Simple arithmetic suggests that given the significant scale of Pharma contraction and reduction in R&D investment, the number of new drugs reaching deserving patients will decrease, and there are also concerns that whole therapeutic areas are being abandoned. Historically, around five First in Class new medicines have been approved each year and any decline would leave major clinical needs unsatisfied. This shortfall will probably not be compensated for by Biotech where investment in early stage companies has been severely scaled back, nor is it clear that continued Pharma investment will be sustainable even at today's levels. Alternative models for R&D funding will be required involving academia, charities, governments, industry and private investors. However, given the time-scales and uncertainties traditionally inherent in drug discovery programmes, there may be pressure from funding bodies to reduce costs and risks through increased emphasis on target validation, attrition, predictive toxicology, and patient selection, and to develop more open collaborations. Funders may also need to be convinced that lessons from the past have been learned, and that cost effective and sustainable models for drug discovery can evolve to provide acceptable returns on investment.

Now would be an opportune time to strengthen drug discovery capabilities in the public sector by co-localising industry-experienced medicinal chemists alongside world class biologists and clinicians with a real commitment to the discovery of new medicines. In many cases, a fundamental change in mind set will be required for medicinal chemists to be accepted as equal partners, rather than as a service function. It will be important to build up chemistry to a critical mass as simply adding a few experienced scientists to established academic groups would not be effective. Of course, there are already research institutes and academic centres focused on drug discovery but not on the scale now required, and integration of Pharma veterans within the wider community will take time as there is little appreciation of the skills base required for medicinal chemistry. However at steady state, barriers between "academic" and "industry" researchers may soften and there would be increased permeability across previously defined disciplines and sectors. Of course, broadening individual skill sets should not be allowed to compromise quality control. Drug discovery centres would be more output-focussed than traditional academia with set objectives and goals, but rigid metrics would not be appropriate; the traditional industry dichotomy of "scientists" and "managers" would disappear, and a culture of innovation and scientific excellence would flourish. Long-term investment in the most challenging disease areas such as antibacterials and neurosciences would be encouraged and supported. There will also be important roles for Public Private Partnerships some of which have attracted significant funding for drug discovery, and have appointed scientists with industry experience who are building real and virtual R&D portfolios with multiple projects ranging from early hits to regulatory approval. These organisations and charities have traditionally focused on diseases of the developing world and cancer, but similar commitments to a wider range of therapeutic areas will be required in the future. Overall, there is a strategic and pressing need to strengthen competitive drug discovery initiatives outside Pharma and Biotech, and concerted efforts from interested parties will be required to ensure research capabilities are commensurate with future medical needs.

Drug discovery organisations will be more heterogeneous in the future, but research units could be roughly scaled in multiples of 50–100, with say a total of 200–300 multidisciplinary scientists providing an optimal balance of critical mass, personal interactions, individual accountability and potential for commercial success. Multidisciplinary teams would have disease and project focus, and would be closely integrated with clinical and academic colleagues. Medical need and scientific excellence would be fundamental drivers for project selection, which would be owned by teams through target validation, hit discovery, lead optimisation, candidate selection, biomarker PK/PD to clinical proof of concept. All team members would be actively involved in science right up to the limit of their abilities, including project leaders and directors. Skilled laboratory scientists would be recognised and rewarded with proper career progression. There would be ready access to the most relevant technologies such as HTS, protein crystallography, computational chemistry, fragment screening *etc.*, which would be expertly exploited as enablers rather than constraints or solutions *per se*. Of course, goals would be defined at group and personal levels and decisions taken with respect to portfolio priorities rather than individual preference, but the driving force would be quality not quantity. This would engender a culture of innovation and realism in which knowledge transfer and training of future generations were also highly valued. "Think global, act local" would recognise a fiercely competitive external environment, but focus on personal interactions and knowledge-based decisions would be much more effective than continual multi-site meetings, transatlantic travel and late night video conferences.

Medicinal chemists have never been in such a strong position to meet the challenges that now face drug discovery given the major scientific advances we have experienced over the past decades. We have unprecedented knowledge to design and synthesise new molecules, understand protein structure and function, and to appreciate the physico-chemical factors that control delivery, efficacy and safety. We have the tools we need to exploit the massive worldwide investment in biomedical sciences, and to be more innovative and effective in execution and decision making from idea to proof of concept. Our challenge is to work with biology and clinical colleagues within a research-driven, but sustainable environment to integrate and apply our skills to discover innovative molecules that will meet the medical needs of the twenty-first century.

S. F. Campbell, Kent, UK

## Acknowledgements

I am most grateful for the interest, encouragement and insightful comments from Julian Blagg, Duncan Campbell, Manoj Desai, David Fox and Graeme Stevenson.

## References

1. F. Lichtenberg, *NBER Working Paper*, 2003, 9754.
2. J. L. LaMattina, *Nat. Rev. Drug Discovery*, 2011, **10**, 559.
3. P. Morgan, P. H. Van Der Graaf, J. Arrowsmith, D. E. Feltner, K. S. Drummond, C. D. Wegner and S. D. A. Street, *Drug Discovery Today*, 2012, **17**, 419.
4. I. Kola and J. Landis, *Nat. Rev. Drug Discovery*, 2004, **3**, 711.

# Preface to the First Edition

Medicinal Chemistry sits at the heart of the pharmaceutical industry and the medicinal chemist has one of the most challenging and rewarding jobs imaginable. The medicinal chemist designs the drug which must balance often conflicting demands of a suitable dose, by the chosen delivery route, at a desired dose frequency to provide a therapeutic effect while maintaining margins to adverse effects throughout the dosing period. The drug molecule may be given to millions of patients all of whom may respond to the drug differently, and all of whom must be treated safely and effectively. Whilst drug discovery is undoubtedly an endeavour involving a wide range of scientific disciplines, the medicinal chemists are critical to the design and progression of a drug molecule. It is the medicinal chemist who integrates and balances the diverse inputs into a single chemical structure which has the potential to become a new medicine.

This is an enormously difficult task. Our advances in synthetic organic chemistry mean that we can respond well to the challenges of preparing and purifying new molecules and chemists can be trained in these skills during undergraduate and graduate studies. In contrast, compound design is far harder to control and requires extensive experience and knowledge to take the sometimes subjective decisions to arrive at a potential drug candidate. There are few universal rules in drug design, and barely any universally accepted guidelines, and it sometimes seems success is more a matter of chance. But, as Louis Pasteur said, "chance favours the prepared mind". However, given the current challenges and high attrition during the development phase, and the acceptance that many reasons for failure are directly attributable to the chemical structure of the drug candidate, medicinal chemists have a duty to design the best molecule possible to advance from research into development and beyond.

The aim of this book, through a series of monographs by leading scientists from across the world, from major pharmaceutical companies, biotechnology companies, contract research organisations and academia is to prepare the medicinal chemist to spot the good chances.

The Handbook of Medicinal Chemistry: Principles and Practice, 2nd Edition
Edited by Simon E. Ward and Andrew M. Davis

Published by the Royal Society of Chemistry, www.rsc.org

The book covers the whole R&D process from target validation through to late stage clinical trials, through descriptions of the background science, the process, learnings, case studies, leading references and even hints and tips.

The foreword has been written by one of our industry's most respected scientists, Simon Campbell CBE FRS, FMedSci. Simon Campbell joined Pfizer as a Medicinal Chemist in 1972, and was a key member of the teams that led to such blockbuster drugs as Cardura, Norvasc and Viagra. He went on to become Pfizer's Senior Vice President for World-wide Drug Discovery and Medicinal R&D in Europe. He was President of the Royal Society of Chemistry from 2004 to 2006 and maintains a very active and influential role in our industry. With his considerable experience Simon provides us with his personal learnings, and the undoubted opportunities for medicinal chemistry looking forward.

The early chapters describe the tools of the medicinal chemist's trade such as physical organic chemistry, computational chemistry and QSAR, library design, fragment based lead generation and structure based design.

The middle section of the book covers the supporting scientific disciplines, including assay development, receptor pharmacology and *in vivo* model development, drug metabolism and pharmacokinetics, molecular biology, toxicology and translational science, computational biology and of critical importance, intellectual property.

The later sections of the book describe the overall research and development process from target generation, lead identification and optimisation through to pharmaceutical development, clinical development and chemical development, including the importance of efficient project management.

Due to the high levels of failure faced during drug development, case studies of successful R&D are hard to find, but are invaluable as a touchstone for pathways to success. So the last three chapters provide case studies of drugs that made it into the later stages of clinical development and/or onto the market, Brilinta, Aleglitazar and Lapatinib. Even during the preparation of this book, one of our case studies was unfortunately halted during Phase III trials. As sad as Phase III failure is, few drugs reach this stage of clinical development and there are many lessons to be learnt in this story that justify its esteemed place in this section.

The book began as life as a proposal to update to a 3rd edition the Royal Society of Chemistry's long running publication "Principles and Practice of Medicinal Chemistry". The first edition was published over 20 years ago, and was a spin-out from the biannual Royal Society of Chemistry Medicinal Chemistry Summer Workshop, which itself has been running for over 40 years and has been the training ground for many of our industry's leading medicinal chemists. The 3rd edition proposal retained some distinctive features of its predecessors, being highly practitioner focused, but grew to incorporate a broader context and to reflect the changing reader demographic reflected in the changing industry and drug discovery environments. It also grew to incorporate new opportunities that did not exist 20 years ago.

Paper publishing is as valid today as it has ever been, but mobile computing and e-publishing are changing the way information can be used and presented. E-publications allow interaction with the content which cannot occur with paper. App-stores allow easy access to sophisticated software that can be delivered and updated with ease. Many tools potentially useful to medicinal chemists do not exist in an easily accessible and secure manner. So for the 3rd edition we wanted to develop, as a companion to the print book, a set of useful medicinal chemistry apps to run locally on tablet computers, and also a fully interactive e-book version to complement the paper copy. The apps would bring to life concepts described within the book chapters and allow chemists to quickly and easily find help in their design challenges.

While even 10 years ago protein structure visualisation and small molecule modelling required high-end workstations and costly software, nowadays this can be accomplished on a tablet computer. Indeed, the frontispiece image of this book was designed inside the freeware app iMolview from Molsoft on an Apple iPad3. Similarly static pictures of X-ray crystal structures within the chapters can be brought into high resolution reality, and the reader can interact with the exact data that the original medicinal chemist used in the documented design. Structures can link to ChemSpider or even Wikipedia and other online resources providing deeper context, and hyperlinks to regulatory guidance mean the medicinal chemist has access to primary information sources relevant to each chapter.

So while this 3rd edition was inspired by its predecessors, with the companion apps and the e-book format, it was time to change the book's name. We hoped the book would become an everyday companion for the practicing medicinal chemist, and so the title "Handbook of Medicinal Chemistry" seemed appropriate. With both print and electronic format and companion apps we hope that, with this handbook, we can more fully prepare the mind of the medicinal chemist to pick the right chances.

Andrew Davis and Simon E Ward

# Contents




The Handbook of Medicinal Chemistry: Principles and Practice, 2nd Edition
Edited by Simon E. Ward and Andrew M. Davis



Published by the Royal Society of Chemistry, www.rsc.org

## 17 Patents for Medicines 611

*Paul A. Brady and Andrew Cook*

## 18 Target Validation for Medicinal Chemists 653

*Matthew Thomas and Lorna Ewart*



## 19 Lead Generation 682

*Frank Narjes, Garry Pairaudeau and Dušan Petrović*

## 20 Lead Optimisation: What You Should Know! 720

*Simon E. Ward and Andrew M. Davis*

# 1 Physicochemical Properties

Andrew M. Davis*[a] and Paul D. Leeson[b]

[a]Hit Discovery, Discovery Sciences, R&D, AstraZeneca, Cambridge, UK; [b]Paul Leeson Consulting Ltd, The Malt House, Main Street, Congerstone, Nuneaton, Warwickshire CV13 6LZ, UK
*E-mail: andy.davis@astrazeneca.com

## 1.1 Introduction

Chemistry is implicitly concerned with chemical structure, but just as much of medicinal chemistry thinking is occupied with the impact of the structure on the physicochemical properties of the molecule. Optimising the shape, hydrophobicity, hydrogen bonding and charge distribution of a lead molecule to be complementary to the target binding site is central to increasing potency and selectivity. Improving solubility and permeability and other absorption, distribution, metabolism, elimination, and toxicological (ADMET) properties requires the control of bulk physicochemical properties. The control of physicochemical properties is directly related to the much used, but ill-defined, notion of "compound quality". In this chapter we shall describe some of the more common physicochemical properties, how they are calculated and measured, and their impact on medicinal chemistry optimisation.

## 1.2 Physicochemical Properties

The fundamental physicochemical properties most often used in defining compound quality are shown in Table 1.1.

The Handbook of Medicinal Chemistry: Principles and Practice, 2nd Edition
Edited by Simon E. Ward and Andrew M. Davis

Published by the Royal Society of Chemistry, www.rsc.org

**Table 1.1** Commonly used metrics for compound quality.

| Property | Description |
|---|---|
| Molecular weight (MW) | Surrogate for molecular size |
| Heavy atom count | Surrogate for molecular size |
| $\log P$ | *n*-Octanol/water partition coefficient |
| $\log D_{7.4}$ | *n*-Octanol/water distribution coefficient at pH 7.4 |
| $pK_a$ | Ionisation constant |
| Aqueous solubility | Equilibrium solubility at pH 7.4 |
| HBA or sum of O + N atoms | Count of hydrogen bond acceptors |
| HBD or sum of OH + NH atoms | Count of hydrogen bond donors |
| Ro5 | Poor solubility and permeability is more likely when MW > 500, $c\log P > 5$, O + N > 10, OH + NH > 5 |
| PSA or TPSA | Dynamic or static total polar surface area |
| $Fsp^3$ | Fraction sp$^3$ carbons = Csp$^3$/C |
| *n*Ar | Count of aromatic rings |
| Property forecast index (PFI) | Chrom $\log D_{7.4} + n$Ar |
| Intrinsic PFI (iPFI) | Chrom $\log P + n$Ar |
| LLE or LipE | Lipophilic Ligand Efficiency = *p*[Activity] − $\log P$ or $\log D$ |
| LE | Ligand efficiency = *p*[Activity] × 1.37/heavy atom count (kcal mol$^{-1}$ HA$^{-1}$) |

## 1.3 Lipophilicity

The lipophilicity of a molecule is the most important contributor to ADMET properties, and "reduce lipophilicity" has become something of a mantra to medicinal chemists. As we shall see in this chapter, and what will be apparent throughout the book, high lipophilicity is in general detrimental to achieving good drug-like properties.

The terms lipophilicity and hydrophobicity are used interchangeably in medicinal chemistry, probably erroneously, as the driving force for membrane partition, or partition of compounds into protein pockets, is hydrophobic rather than lipophilic. IUPAC provides distinct definitions:[1]

**Lipophilicity** represents the affinity of a molecule for a lipophilic environment.

**Hydrophobicity** is the association of non-polar groups or molecules in an aqueous environment, which arises from the tendency of water to exclude non-polar molecules.

While dispersion forces between non-polar surfaces do contribute to the overall partition of a compound out of water into a protein active site or non-polar environment such as the centre of a lipid bilayer, much of the driving force is hydrophobic, as we will describe further.

Thermodynamic measurements show that the free energy change governing partitioning is largely entropically driven.[2] Table 1.2 shows the thermodynamic parameters for the transfer of some simple hydrophobic groups from their liquid state to water at 25 °C. As can be seen, the free energy of transfer is dominated by the entropy term, and at 25 °C the enthalpy change is almost zero.

The origin of the hydrophobic effect is still debated, not least due to the importance of the hydrophobic effect to protein folding, but the authors favour the so-called "iceberg model".[3] In bulk water, each water molecule can donate two hydrogen bonds and

**Table 1.2** Thermodynamic parameters for transfer of hydrocarbons from pure liquid to water at 25 °C.[2]

| Compound | $\Delta G^{\circ}$ hydrocarbon to water (kJ $mol^{-1}$) | $\Delta H^{\circ}$ hc to w (kJ $mol^{-1}$) | $T\Delta S^{\circ}$ hc to w (kJ $mol^{-1}$) |
|---|---|---|---|
| 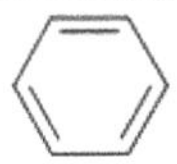 | +19.3 | +2.1 | −17.2 |
| 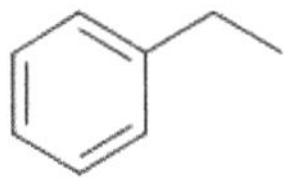 | +26.2 | +2.0 | −24.2 |
| 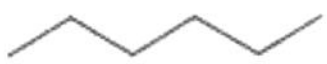 | +32.4 | +0.0 | −32.4 |

accept two hydrogen bonds through its lone pairs on oxygen, and in bulk water all four interactions are satisfied in a dynamic 3-D network. A hydrophobic group placed in water requires a cavity to be made to accommodate it, which disrupts the hydrogen bond network each water molecule makes with surrounding water molecules. In order to make a cavity in water for a hydrophobic group, some of the water molecules' hydrogen bonds are necessarily broken and the dynamic process of hydrogen bonds being made and broken in liquid water is disrupted. Those water molecules around the hydrophobic group become structured, almost ice-like, in trying to maximise their hydrogen bonding potential. When the hydrophobic group is removed from water and partitions into a hydrophobic receiver phase, the dynamic hydrogen bond network is re-established, the cavity filled, the ordered waters becoming disordered again, which is entropically favourable.[4]

For a flexible molecule, when placed in water it will try to minimise its exposed hydrophobic surface area and to maximise its hydrogen bonding potential to surrounding water molecules. When placed in a hydrophobic acceptor phase the opposite occurs, and the molecule will try minimise its potential for unpaired hydrogen bonds. For these reasons, partitioning of flexible molecules has a conformational component, and the molecule's conformation in water can be different from its conformation in the hydrophobic phase. For example, the macrocyclic immunosuppressant FK506 has different conformations in chloroform and water.[5] The phenomenon of minimising the exposure of hydrophobic surface area in water is called "hydrophobic collapse", and likewise the phenomenon of the potential to minimise unpaired hydrogen bonds in non-polar media can be termed "hydrophilic collapse". The whole process has been recently referred to as "chameleonic" efficiency.[6] The existence of hydrophobic and hydrophilic collapse may be seen by correlations of clog$P/D$ *vs.* measured log$D_{7.4}$ where the slope is often <1.0.

For partition into a protein active site, one might expect a positive contribution of dispersion forces between the hydrophobic groups on the ligand and hydrophobic side-chains in the cavity. The cavity is already preformed (unless the cavity is induced by the ligand). But where hydrophobicity drives drug binding, plots of p$K_i$ *vs.* log$P/D$ often have slopes <1.0, and not >1.0 routinely, as might be expected, suggesting little benefit in the partition into the protein active site over partitioning into *n*-octanol. A few rare examples exist.[7,8] As highlighted by Fersht,[7] the $\log(k_{cat}/K_m)$ for the chymotrypsin-catalysed hydrolysis of a series of esters of the form R–CH(NHAc)$CO_2$Me, increases with increasing hydrophobicity (as measured by *n*-octanol–water partition coefficients) with slope = 2.2. Fersht also cites the inhibition of chymotrypsin by a series of substituted formanilides, which increases with increasing hydrophobicity with a slope of 1.5.

For many years, the standard system in which to measure lipophilicity has been the partitioning of a molecule between *n*-octanol and water. The equilibrium of a neutral compound between *n*-octanol and water is measured, normally at 20 °C and the partition coefficient is reported on a $\log_{10}$ scale.

$$\log P = \log_{10}\left(\frac{[\text{drug}]_{n-octanol}}{[\text{drug}]_{water}}\right) \tag{1.1}$$

A log*P* of zero represents an equal partition between water and the *n*-octanol phase.

The solvent *n*-octanol became the standard hydrophobic phase for the partition experiment, as it is non-water miscible, UV-transparent, but has enough polarity due to its hydroxyl group to dissolve many drug molecules, unlike more hydrophobic alkane phases. While the properties of *n*-octanol have proven useful, it should be remembered that *n*-octanol–water is a model partitioning system, and its choice as a model system has some benefits, but also brings some compromises in quantifying hydrophobicity (for example, the *n*-octanol layer contains ~33% water on a molar basis[9]). Some of these benefits and compromises will be highlighted later.

*n*-Octanol–water was the solvent system chosen to quantify hydrophobicity by Corwin Hansch in the 1960s in his seminal papers at the birth of modern QSAR.[10,11] Since then, many compounds have had their log*P* values measured, and large compilations exist, which provide the basis for prediction algorithms to calculate log*P*, such as the classic clog*P* algorithm.[12] The availability of good prediction algorithms and their supplementation with new measurements to improve predictive power, have sustained *n*-octanol–water as the industry standard partitioning system in which to measure log*P*.

### 1.3.1 Measuring Log*P* and Log*D*

The standard experimental procedure for measuring partition coefficients is known as the "shake-flask" method. Traditionally this would measure the equilibration of one compound, pre-dissolved in either water or *n*-octanol, shaken in a glass laboratory bottle at constant temperature until equilibrium is attained. The mixture is then centrifuged to separate the phases, each phase sampled and the concentration of the analyte in each phase measured by UV spectroscopy. It was a highly labour-intensive measurement. The method has now been automated to run on modern laboratory automation in 96-well plates, in mixtures of up to 10 compounds using LCMS with single ion monitoring, removing the throughput bottleneck of the traditional method.[13] Due to the sensitivity of measuring concentrations in both phases to estimate the log*P*, shake flask has a dynamic range of $-2 < \log P < 4$.

*n*-Octanol–water largely only supports the partition of neutral species. When the drug molecule contains an ionisable centre (*i.e.* is an acid, base or zwitterion), the distribution of the compound between *n*-octanol and water becomes dependent upon the aqueous-phase pH, and so the equilibrium must be measured at a particular pH. The distribution coefficient, *D*, is the partition of a compound at a particular pH and is also recorded on a $\log_{10}$ scale.

For an acid:

$$\log D = \log P - \log(1 + 10^{\mathrm{pH}-\mathrm{p}K\mathrm{a}}) \tag{1.2}$$

For a base:

$$\log D = \log P - \log(1 + 10^{\mathrm{p}K\mathrm{a}-\mathrm{pH}}) \tag{1.3}$$

A theoretical plot of $\log D$ *vs.* pH for an acid with $\mathrm{p}K_\mathrm{a} = 4$ and a base with $\mathrm{p}K_\mathrm{a} = 9$, both having $\log P = 2$, is shown in Figure 1.1.

For every 1 log unit change in aqueous phase pH, either above the $\mathrm{p}K_\mathrm{a}$ of an acid or below the $\mathrm{p}K_\mathrm{a}$ of a base, the $\log D$ decreases by 1 log unit. As a standard point of comparison, the distribution coefficient is usually measured at pH 7.4, representing physiological pH. Log*D* measured at pH 6.5 is also used, as this is relevant to absorption from the lower intestine. The log*P* can still be measured if the aqueous phase pH is chosen such that the compound is largely in its neutral form, but that necessitates a bespoke experiment.

The log*D*–pH curves in Figure 1.1 are ideal curves assuming only the neutral form can partition into the hydrophobic phase in accord with the pH partition hypothesis. Experimentally, *n*-octanol–water distribution coefficients do not behave as the theoretical curves in Figure 1.1 suggest. At higher pH values for an acid or lower pH values for a base, both a few pH units away from the $\mathrm{p}K_\mathrm{a}$, distribution in *n*-octanol–water can become pH independent, suggesting distribution of the ionised form into *n*-octanol can become the dominant species over the partition of the diminishing neutral form, see Figure 1.2.

However, the plateau log*D* value is dependent upon the aqueous phase ionic strength, suggesting the partitioning species is an intermolecular ion pair, the drug molecule

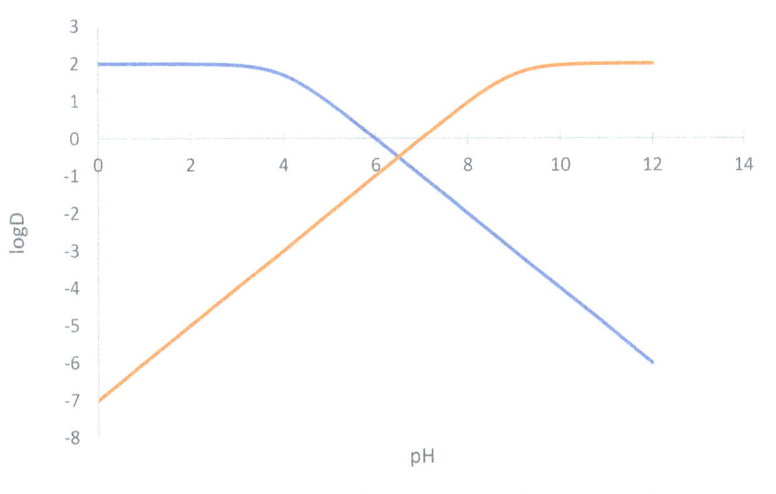


**Figure 1.1** Theoretical log*D* *vs.* pH curves for an acid, log*P* = 2, $\mathrm{p}K_\mathrm{a} = 4$ (blue curve), and a base, log*P* = 2, $\mathrm{p}K_\mathrm{a} = 9$ (orange curve).

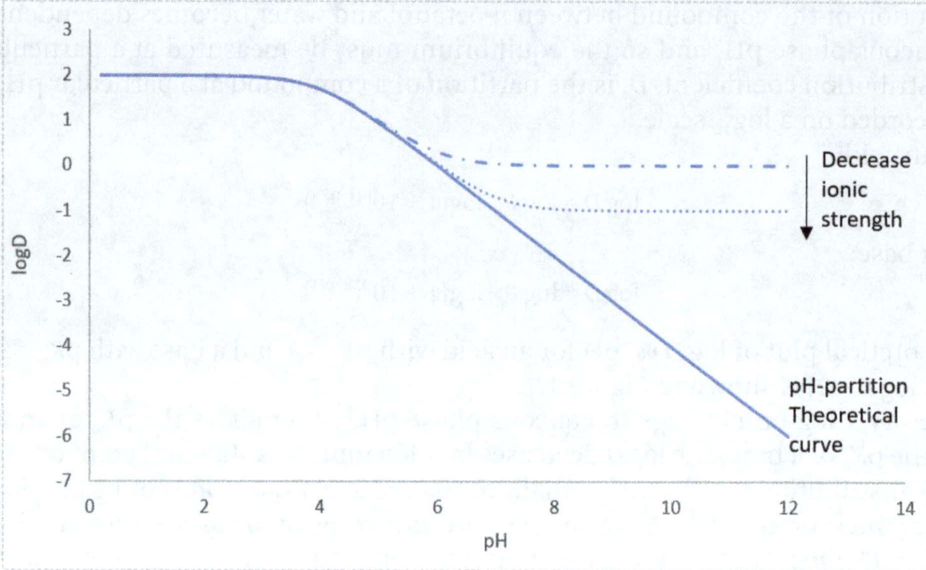


**Figure 1.2** Plot of $\log D$ *vs.* pH for an acid with $\log P = 2$ and $pK_a = 4$, theoretical curve, and a typical curve seen in *n*-octanol showing ion-pair partitioning. Decreasing ionic strength can suppress the impact when measuring $\log D_{7.4}$.

taking with it a counterion from the buffer. In a study with the acidic drug proxicromil, at pH 7.4 in *n*-octanol–water, where the water phase contained 0.15 M NaCl, more than 95% of the observed partition of proxicromil was due to the ion pair, while only 5% was due to the neutral form of proxicromil.[14]

There is little literature evidence supporting the physiological importance of intermolecular ion-pair partitioning to membrane permeability, as observed in *n*-octanol–water partitioning. In fact, introducing an intramolecular ion pair is a successful strategy to minimise passive partitioning across the blood–brain barrier, as exemplified by the development of non-sedating antihistamines.

It could be argued that the problem of ion-pair partitioning in solvents such as *n*-octanol should be embraced, and that all distribution coefficients should be determined using a physiological concentration of salt in the buffer. However, this approach should be refuted since the contribution of the ion-pairing component to the observed distribution coefficient will depend strongly on the nature of the organic solvent, being much larger for aliphatic alcohols such as *n*-octanol than for chloroform or alkanes.[15,16]

For practical purposes the existence of ion-pair partitioning seen in *n*-octanol should be treated as an artifact of the chosen partitioning system and dependent on experimental conditions. Experimentally one would try to avoid measuring a $\log Do/w$ on these ion-pair plateau. This can be done by minimising the ionic strength of the aqueous phase or extrapolation of the distribution coefficient to zero ion strength.

Ion pairing also influences the partitioning of molecules into phospholipid membranes, although the mechanism is different, and in this case, can have biological significance. Studying partitioning of proxicromil into DOPC membrane vesicles, while an increase in ionic strength leads to an increase in partitioning of proxicromil, this is almost exclusively due to the fact that increased ionic strength leads to a reduction in surface potential at the phospholipid membrane–water interface and modulation of the self-induced surface charge driven by the interfacial partitioning of proxicromil ion. This is because proxicromil can partition to organise its hydrophobic structure to dip into the membrane while leaving its carboxylic acid headgroup exposed to the membrane water interface. The ionic strength effect can be well accounted for by the Gouy–Chapman model of the electrical double layer.[14] This indicates that the increased values of $D_{mem}$ observed at higher ionic strengths are not due to the intervention of ion-pair partitioning. This is even more significant for bases, as we shall detail later.

### 1.3.2 Zwitterions

For a zwitterionic compound, which contains an acidic and a basic ionisable group, at aqueous phase pH values lying between the p$K_a$ values, partitioning is a maximum where the molecule can exist as a neutral and a zwitterionic species.

For a zwitterion the $\log D$ at a particular pH is given by:

$$\log D = \log P - \log(1 + 10^{\mathrm{p}K\mathrm{a1-pH}} + 10^{\mathrm{p}K\mathrm{a2-pH}}) \tag{1.4}$$

Log$D$ is at a maximum between the p$K_a$ values, but between the p$K_a$ values, the compound exists both as a zwitterionic form and a neutral form, the exact ratio being dependent on the microscopic p$K_a$ values of the different ionising species. As *n*-octanol–water can support the partitioning of the intramolecular ion pair and the neutral form, this may not be relevant for phospholipid bilayer partitioning, as mentioned above. If a high proportion of the neutral form is required, the separation of the p$K_a$s may also be important – as when the acid and base p$K_a$ are closer together, the proportion of the neutral form increases. Zwitterions are an important class of drugs,[17] and can achieve permeability by both passive permeability (driven by the neutral form) and active transport, Figure 1.3. The fact that non-sedating histamine receptor H1 antagonists such as fexofenadine use zwitterionic nature to minimise CNS exposure while achieving good gastrointestinal permeability due to active uptake, indicates some of the benefits of designing zwitterions.[18,19] Levodopa is a zwitterionic prodrug of dopamine, used in the symptomatic treatment of Parkinson's disease. In this case forming the zwitterion increases oral absorption and delivery to the brain, presumably by competition with natural amino acids for active transport.[20] In the brain it is decarboxylated to release dopamine, supplementing the dopamine deficit in Parkinson's patients. A number of groups have attempted to increase the delivery of levodopa to the brain by forming ester and amide prodrugs of the prodrug to increase their passive permeability.[21]

As we shall see in this chapter, and what will be apparent throughout the book, is that both high $\log D_{7.4}$ *and* high $\log P$ are detrimental. So what are good ranges to aim for? For oral drugs, $\log D_{7.4}$ values of 0–2 and $\log P$ values of 0–3 would seem good target ranges, leading to compounds with both good water and good lipid solubility. Similar targets have been cited by other authors.[22] These ranges for $\log P$ and $\log D_{7.4}$ are also

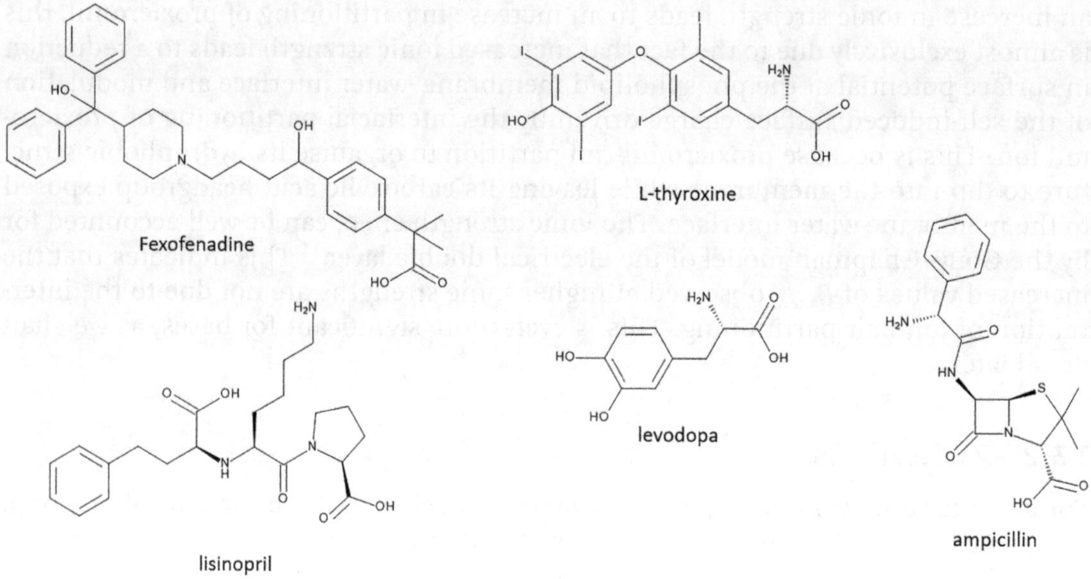


**Figure 1.3** Examples of Zwitterionic drugs.

suitable for CNS penetration, although oral, and especially CNS penetration, adds further limits on other physicochemical properties, as we shall go on to describe in the following sections.

Log$D_{7.4}$ can be lowered by either decreasing the log$P$ of the molecule, or moving the p$K_a$ of ionisable centres further away from pH 7.4 (lower for an acid or higher for a base). But lowering log$D_{7.4}$ by changing the p$K_a$ of a high log$P$ compound, by increasing the p$K_a$ of bases or decreasing the p$K_a$ of acids, at extremes could lead to highly amphoteric compounds with cell lytic properties.

## 1.3.3 Other Solvent Systems

Water–hydrophobic solvent phase partitioning as a quantitative scale of hydrophobicity goes all the way back to the birth of QSAR. Early work used olive oil–water partitioning. Hans Horst Meyer[23] first proposed and demonstrated that anaesthetic potency was related to lipid solubility. Two years later a similar proposal was made by Charles Overton.[24] They showed the narcotic effect on tadpoles was proportional to the partition coefficient of the compounds from water into olive oil, as a model for the partition of the narcotics into the biological membrane. Beginning in the 1960s, after the pioneering work of Hansch and co-workers, *n*-octanol became the dominant system, as discussed above. But other hydrophobic solvents have been chosen in which to measure partitioning with water, including alkanes, toluene, chloroform as a hydrophobic phase possessing a weak hydrogen bond donor, propylene glycol dipelargonate as a complementary hydrophobic acceptor solvent,[25] and phospholipid membrane vesicles[26] as a more biologically relevant system.

### 1.3.4 Membrane–Water Partition Coefficients

Phospholipid vesicles have often been used as a model hydrophobic phase, of particular interest in modelling drug membrane effects. Different phospholipids have been used, but dimyristoyl phosphatidyl choline (DPMC) is commonly chosen. In order to measure partitioning, the alkyl chains need to be in the melted state, so the experimental temperature needs to be above the phase transition temperature of the membrane, which for DMPC is about 23 °C. Besides partitioning into the hydrophobic core of the membrane vesicles, ionisable compounds can partition in an interfacial way, as already mentioned for proxicromil, and which is particularly efficient for bases, where the positive charge results in ionic interactions with the negatively charged phosphates present in the phospholipid headgroups, while the hydrophobic part of the molecule can reach towards the hydrophobic membrane core.

Indeed, the partitioning of basic compounds into membrane vesicles becomes more enthalpically driven than structurally related neutral compounds, which are predominantly entropically driven as expected for hydrophobic partition.[26] This interfacial partition has been proposed to be the driving force for high tissue affinity of basic compounds, as shown by their high volumes of distribution (Vss)[27] and enhanced lung residency of basic respiratory drugs,[28] but this phenomenon may also in part drive the adaptive exchanges in membrane structure seen as phospholipidosis.[29] A recent review indicates over 50 clinically used drugs have been shown to induce phospholipidosis.[30] Most of them are lipophilic basic drugs with median $\log P = 4.2$ and $pK_a = 9.2$.

Due to the interfacial partitioning dominant for charged drug molecules, membrane partitioning systems are useful in understanding membrane affinity.

### 1.3.5 Chromatographic Log *D* Measurement

The *n*-octanol–water partition system for quantifying hydrophobicity is limited by the solubilities of molecules in the water and *n*-octanol phases, and for hydrophobic molecules, the analytical precision of measuring concentration differences between often high concentrations in the *n*-octanol phase and very low concentrations in the water phase. In order to quantify hydrophobicity in a high-throughput manner, retention times under standard conditions on reverse-phase HPLC columns,[31–34] or *n*-octanol coated columns, have been used. These methods have achieved widespread popularity because they are high-throughput and permit a wide range of lipophilicities, beyond the scope of shake-flask methods, to be estimated using retention times on reverse-phase HPLC gradient systems.

Young and colleagues[35] have demonstrated the that chromatographic $\log D_{7.4}$ values provided improved correlations over *n*-octanol–water $\log D_{7.4}$ values with a number of key ADMET endpoints including solubility, permeability and CYP inhibition, especially for very hydrophobic molecules (although one might question why so many hydrophobic molecules were made in the first place). They also highlighted the additional and independent importance of aromatic ring count in a number of these endpoints. The property forecast index (PFI) was defined as the chromatographically determined $\log D_{7.4}$ plus the aromatic ring count. Aromatic ring count was found, independently of lipophilicity, to have a negative influence on a number of developability parameters, including CYP inhibition, hERG inhibition, solubility and selectivity. PFI values were better at distinguishing the top 100 marketed oral drugs in 2009 from GSK development candidates 2001–2009 than $\log D_{7.4}$ alone. The guidance for three key properties for development of oral drugs which emerged from this study is dose ≤100 mg, FaSSIF solubility ≥100 μg $mL^{-1}$ and PFI ≤6.[81] FaSSIF solubility is a biorelevant solubility measure in fasted state simulated intestinal fluid.[36] As an indication that the control of physicochemical properties can mitigate unforeseen risks, Fournier and colleagues also found that the intrinsic property forecast index was related to phototoxicity.[37]

In summary, many different partitioning systems have been used to experimentally quantify hydrophobicity, and each system has its strengths and weaknesses. What is most important to the medicinal chemist is applying an experimental method to quantify hydrophobicity, to calibrate predictions for the next compound to be synthesised, so that this property can be controlled in the design of new molecules, as it is the fundamental compound quality indicator.

### 1.3.6 Calculating Log *P* and Log $D_{7.4}$

Probably the best known $\log P$ calculator, often acknowledged as the "gold standard", is the clog*P* algorithm. It was developed at Pomona College[38] and is available through their own software package and also the DAYLIGHT cheminformatics system.[39,40] This empirically derived calculator uses a fragment-based approach to estimate $\log P$ based on the 2-D graph of the molecule. The program fragments the molecule into polar fragments and isolating carbons (an isolating carbon is one which is not doubly or triply bonded to a polar fragment). The fragmental constants were estimated from known molecules in the measured $\log P$ database. Where the fragment is unknown, it can be estimated, historically this resulted in a "missing fragment" error. The additive approach includes correction terms to account for neighbourhood interactions of polar atoms and groups (which reduces their overall hydrophilicity due to the interaction of their hydration shells), intramolecular hydrogen bonding and electronic effects.

A simpler but widely used $\log P$ algorithm proposed by Ghose and Crippen[41] uses atom-based functions. Many different $\log P$ calculators have been proposed and are in common use, mostly being variants on the fragmental and atomic fundamental methods. The performance of over 20 algorithms, on two public databases and the Pfizer database of 95 809 measurements, has been evaluated.[42] While many methods produced reasonable results on the public database, few were successful predicting a Pfizer internal dataset. It is in the nature of empirical models that they do well on compounds similar to those on the which the model was trained (*e.g.* public data), but can do worse on unseen data, or more dissimilar compounds (such as the Pfizer internal database). A simple equation, based on the number of carbon atoms and number of heteroatoms, out-performed many methods:

$$\log P = 1.46(+/-0.02) + 0.11n_{\text{carbons}} - 0.11(+/-0.001)n_{\text{heteroatoms}} \quad (1.5)$$

Many pharmaceutical companies, with their own internal measured $\log P/\log D_{7.4}$ databases, use QSAR approaches to either "tune" the published methods, by having them as input descriptors to a multivariate QSAR model, or calculate $\log P/D_{7.4}$ directly from QSAR models trained on their internal measurement databases using their favourite molecular descriptors.

For medicinal chemists the important question is "does the algorithm I use predict the lipophilicity of my chemical series with acceptable accuracy and precision?" Which method is most suitable may differ from project to project according to the chemistry being pursued. For this reason, experimental determination is necessary. However, even if $\log P$ cannot be calculated with accuracy, it can still be used within a series, as pairwise differences in lipophilicity within a series are often well predicted, even if the absolute value is incorrectly estimated. For example, within a chemical series, when structural changes are being made remote from the ionising centre, the ionisation constants are often unchanged. Correlations between measured $\log D_{7.4}$ and calculated $\log P$ values can then use used to guide further compound optimisation. In a series of dual β2/D2 receptor agonists, different subseries gave different correlation lines between calculated $\log P$ and measured $\log D$, (largely due to differences in the basic $pK_a$ of each subseries), but within each series the calculations and measurements were well correlated,[43] Figure 1.4.

If automatically updating QSAR models are used to guide your project, any systematic errors in the predictions should be resolved as representatives from your series are measured and their values enter the $\log P$ model. One of the authors (AD) has spent many years calculating $\log D$, measuring $\log D$ and updating local models for projects with the latest measurements – so projects had available the most accurate and precise predictions to aid the decision on which compound to make next.

A number of free $\log P$ calculators are available. The very useful structure–activity tool Datawarrior contains a $\log P$ calculator,[44] as does the SWISS ADME[45] and the MedChem Toolkit iPad app.[46]

Free $\log D_{7.4}$ calculators are rarer. In order to calculate $\log D_{7.4}$ from $\log P$, the ionisation constants of the molecule must also be calculated. The commercial Physchem suite from ACDLabs has implemented a fully integrated package for calculating $\log P$, $pK_a$ and $\log D$,[47] and ADMETLAB[48] has a $\log D_{7.4}$ calculator. QSAR methods have been used to estimate $\log D_{7.4}$ directly from chemical structure[49] without the need to calculate $\log P$ and $pK_a$ separately.

## 1.4 Ionisation Constants

The ionisation constant of a compound is given by the following equation and quantified as an equilibrium constant $K_a$:

$$\left(K_a = \frac{[H^+][A^-]}{[AH]}\right) \quad \% \text{ ionised} = \frac{100}{1 + 10^{(pK_a - pH)}} \tag{1.6}$$

Since biological membranes only efficiently support the passive partition of neutral molecules, the ionisation state of a molecule is an important property. The strength of drug–receptor interactions such as charged-reinforced hydrogen bonding and salt bridges also implicitly depend upon the ionisation constant. Formulation of salts, and solubility, also critically depend on the ionisation constants.

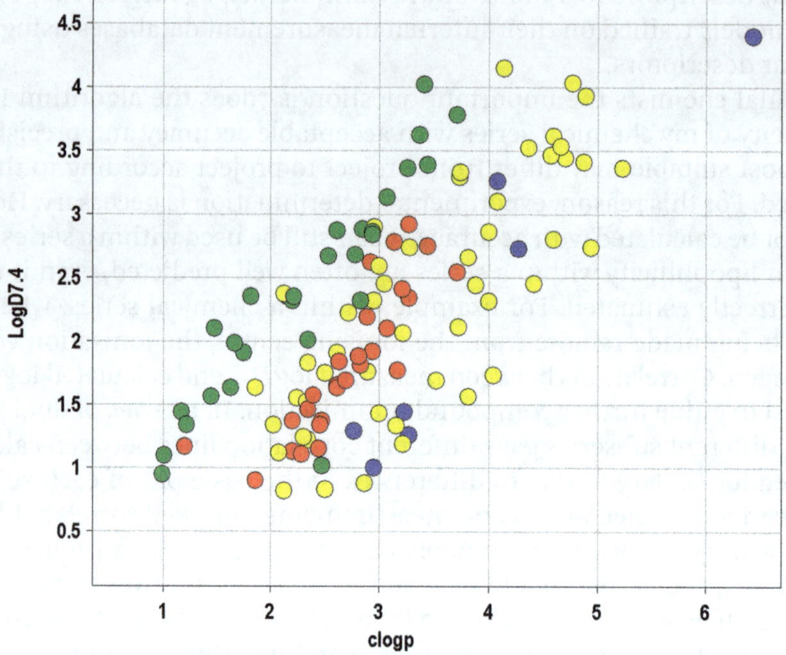


**Figure 1.4** Plot of clog*P* *vs.* log$D_{7.4}$ for a series of dual D2/b2 agonists colour-coded by substructure green circles X = $SO_2$, Y = $CH_2$; red circles X = $CH_2$, Y = $SO_2$; blue circles X = ($CH_2$), Y = $CH_2SO_2$; yellow circles all other compounds in the series.

The ionisation constant, $K_a$ is normally recorded as the negative logarithm of the ionisation constant, the p$K_a$, with most drugs with ionisable centres having p$K_a$ values in the range 2–12. The p$K_a$ is the pH at which the compound in solution is 50% ionised.

### 1.4.1 Measuring Ionisation Constants

Ionisation constants can be measured by a number of methods, including potentiometric titration, spectrophotometrically or by NMR. The determination of ionisation constants is not trivial, not being amenable to high throughput, and in the cases of potentiometric titration and NMR, requiring a large amount of material. Fortunately, p$K_a$s for most ionisable functional groups can be estimated by well-established linear free–energy relationships.

### 1.4.2 Calculating Ionisation Constants

In the 1930s, quantitative structure reactivity relationships (QSARs) defined the field of physical organic chemistry, through the work of Hammett,[50] Brønsted and Pederson, and others.[51] Hammett showed that the effect of meta- and para-substituents attached to a benzene ring on reaction rate or position of the chemical equilibrium in which the reaction centre participates, is determined by the electronic effect of the substituent. Different reactions may have different sensitivities to the substituent effect. Hammett defined an experimentally based descriptor $\sigma$, using the ionisation of benzoic acids as the calibrating reaction, and $\sigma_{\mathrm{m}}$ or $\sigma_{\mathrm{p}}$ represented the difference in p$K_{\mathrm{a}}$ between the meta- or para-substituted benzoic acids and unsubstituted benzoic acid itself. The sensitivity of a particular reaction to the electronic effect of a substituent was described by $\rho$, the slope of the correlation between the logarithm of the equilibrium ($K$) or rate constant ($k$) for that reaction and the sigma values, eqn (1.1):

$$\log k = \rho\sigma + \text{constant} \tag{1.7}$$

In Hammett's initial publication he tabulated $\sigma$ values for 31 substituents, and linear energy correlations for 39 reactions. While Hammett's observations were empirical, he recognised that they may indicate a common underlying physics-based explanation, relating to electron attraction or repulsion by inductive and resonance effects.

In the 1950s Taft extended Hammett's work to define a sigma scale for aliphatic systems.[52] Taft used the acid- and base-catalysed hydrolysis of esters as the calibrating reaction. He proposed that as the acid- and base-catalysed hydrolysis of esters 2 proceed through a very similar tetrahedral transition-state structure, and under identical conditions, both reactions would experience similar steric influences. As the base-catalysed reaction went from a neutral ground state to a negatively charged transition state, it would be more sensitive to electronic effects of substituents than the acid-catalysed hydrolysis reaction, which moves from a positively charged ground state (rapid pre-protonation of the ester carbonyl) to a similarly positively charged transition state. Therefore, the acid-catalysed hydrolysis of esters would be less sensitive to the electronic effect of substituents, while remaining sensitive to their size. On the other hand, base-catalysed hydrolysis would be sensitive to both size and electronic effects. Taft was therefore able to also define a new a steric substituent constant scale, termed Es. Taft gave the symbol $\sigma^*$ to the electronic effect of the aliphatic substituent. The sensitivity of a particular reaction to the electronic and steric effects of a substituent were described by $\rho^*$ and $\delta$, respectively, the regression coefficients from the correlation between the logarithm of the equilibrium ($K$) or rate constant ($k$) for that reaction and the $\sigma^*$ and Es values of the substituents, eqn (1.2):

$$\log(k-\mathrm{R}/k-\mathrm{Me}) = \rho^*\sigma^* + d{\cdot}\mathrm{Es} + \text{constant} \tag{1.8}$$

In the 1960s Swain and Lupton went on to factor the two effects into their Field & Resonance (F & R) scales for aromatic substituents,[53] building on the earlier proposal by Hammett.

Using tabulated $\sigma/\sigma^*$ values and $\rho$ values for different ionising centres, the p$K_{\mathrm{a}}$s of most ionising centres can be calculated where measurements are absent. When the author (AD) started work in the pharmaceutical industry, he spent many hours manually calculating p$K_a$s using tabulations of Hammett and Taft equations, and the book by Perrin "p$K_a$ Prediction of Organic Acids and Bases" was considered a bible.[54] Nowadays, expert systems such as ACDLabs can calculate p$K_a$s by applying these empirical relationships. The software uses a set of Hammett equations, and an internal database of $\sigma$-values, together with complex structural perception to identify the electronic environment of the ionising centre. But p$K_a$s can also be calculated using the physics-based approaches of computational chemistry,[55] and increasingly using machine learning algorithms[56] including some open-source packages.[57]

### 1.4.3 Manipulating p$K_a$ in Medicinal Chemistry Strategy

Manipulating p$K_a$ is an important strategy in drug design, to optimise potency through direct drug–receptor interactions, manipulation of overall physical properties such as $\log D_{7.4}$, improving solubility by introduction of an ionising centre, controlling other pharmacokinetic properties such as lung retention[28] and modulating off-target activities. For example, reduction of p$K_a$ of basic amines can successfully reduce unwanted hERG activity.[58]

In a classic example, p$K_a$ was shown to be a major controller of antibacterial activity of sulphanilamide drugs showing a biphasic dependence on potency, Figure 1.5. From p$K_a$ 7–3, potency decreases since only the neutral form of the compound can transport into the cell (pH partition hypothesis). From p$K_a$ 7–11, potency decreases since the

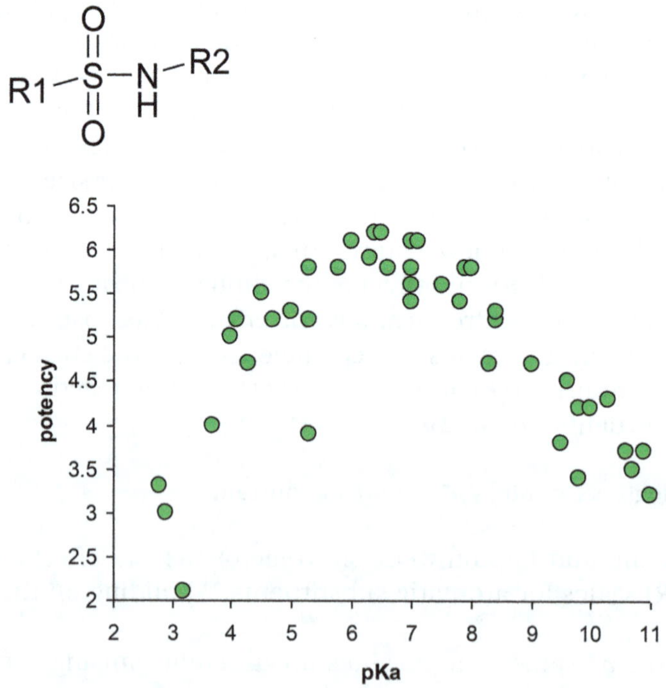


**Figure 1.5** Plot of antibacterial potency *vs.* p$K_a$ for a series of sulphanilamide antibiotics.

active species is the anion and its concentration decreases as the p$K_a$ increases, providing an optimal activity at around p$K_a$ 7.[59]

Ionisation constants are sensitive to conformational and stereoelectronic effects which are not always well predicted. For example, Muller showed that antiperiplanar sigma effects have a strong influence on p$K_a$ values of 4-fluoropiperidines, while 3-fluoropiperidines are subject to dipolar effects depending on axial or equatorial substitution,[60] Figure 1.6. Even in alicyclic systems such stereoelectronic effects can be significant,[61] and for this reason one should not rely on calculations alone, but measurements can highlight important effects where fine control of p$K_a$ is required.

In a comprehensive recent review by Walters,[62] the role of charge type and p$K_a$ control in medicinal chemistry programs effectively demonstrates how important p$K_a$ control can be in optimising efficacy, safety, CNS penetration and tissue distribution. For example, p$K_a$ manipulation was critical in the design of a series of geldanamycin HSP90 inhibitors. Many weakly basic anticancer agents accumulate extensively in the acidic lysosomes through ion trapping, reducing their activity, since anticancer drug targets are often localised in the cell cytosol or nucleus. Some cancer cells have defective acidification of lysosomes, which causes a redistribution of trapped drugs from the lysosomes to the cytosol. Such differences in drug localisation between normal and cancer cells can be exploited to improve cancer-cell selectivity. Control of the p$K_a$ of geldanamycin analogues to around 8.1 had the maximum degree of selectivity for HL-60 leukemic cells *vs.* normal human fibroblasts,[63] Figure 1.7.

In a second cited example, lowering the p$K_a$ of a lipophilic basic Met inhibitor, GEN-203 (*N*-ethyl-3-fluoro-4-aminopiperidine), through the introduction of an additional fluorine in the 3-position of the aminopiperidine, led to a decreased volume of distribution of the compound in mouse by approximately 4-fold (from 3.6 to 0.99 L $kg^{-1}$), while maintaining cell potency and *in vivo* efficacy against the target kinase, Figure 1.8. Compared to GEN-203, GEN-890 had reduced liver and bone-marrow toxicity in mice, Table 1.3.[64]

Reduction in p$K_a$ and/or log$P$ of a series of H1-antihistamines (for insomnia) through the introduction of a difluoroethyl side chain lowered the pKa of a guanidine-based 2-amino dihydroquinazoline 5-$HT_{5a}$ antagonist (from 9.9 to 8.9) and resulted in a significantly improved brain-to-plasma ratio, enhancing the pharmacological utility of these compounds.[65]

As we have previously mentioned, converting bases to zwitterions has been a successful strategy in producing non-sedating antihistamines. The incorporation of a carboxylic acid within a series of basic renin inhibitors to make them zwitterionic led to improved off-target profiles (CYP3A4 time-dependent inhibition and hERG affinity) relative to analogous non-zwitterionic inhibitors.[66]

## 1.5 Hydrogen Bonding

Hydrogen bonds are key drug–receptor interactions driving enthalpic binding, but also a key means of manipulating bulk physicochemical properties. It would be thought that increasing hydrogen bond strength would directly contribute to increased affinity

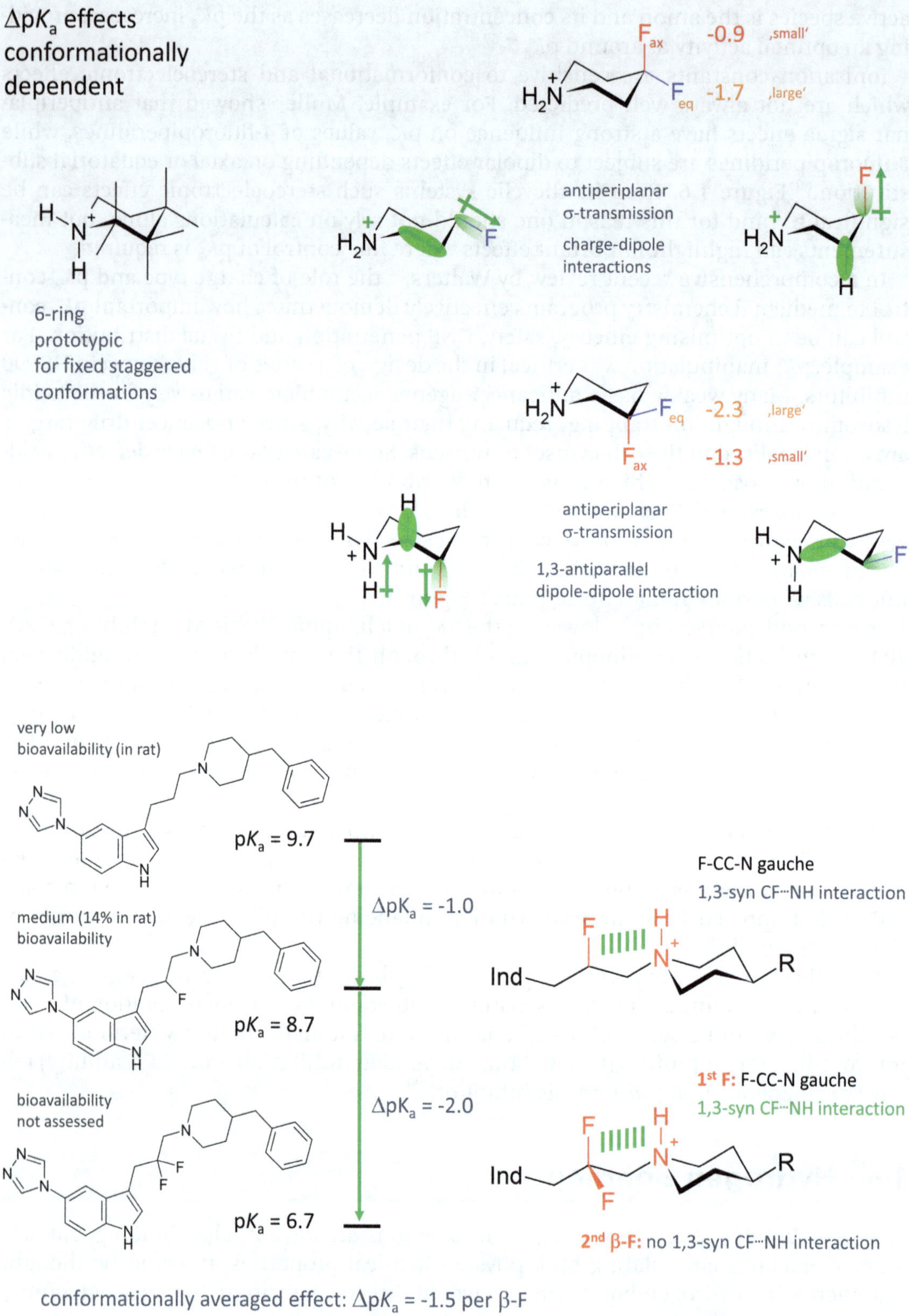


**Figure 1.6** Examples of conformational effects on p$K_a$s.

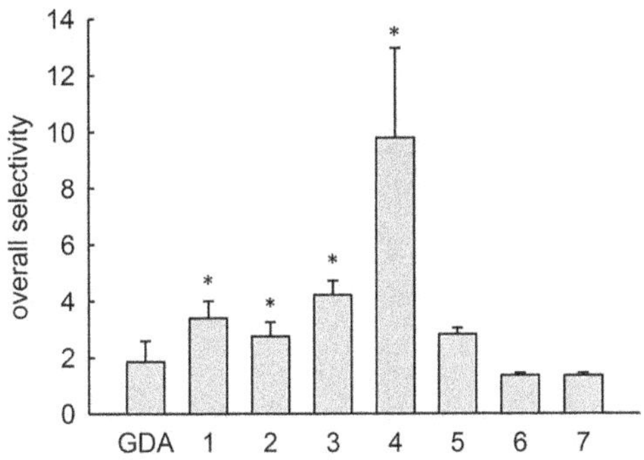


**Figure 1.7** Overall selectivity of HL-60 leukemic cells *vs.* normal human fibroblasts represents the $IC_{50}$ for a derivative in normal human fibroblasts divided by the value obtained in HL60 human leukemic cells. Bars represent mean ±s.d. ($n$ = 3); *, $p < 0.05$ compared to GDA. Reproduced from ref. 63 with permission from American Chemical Society, Copyright 2020.

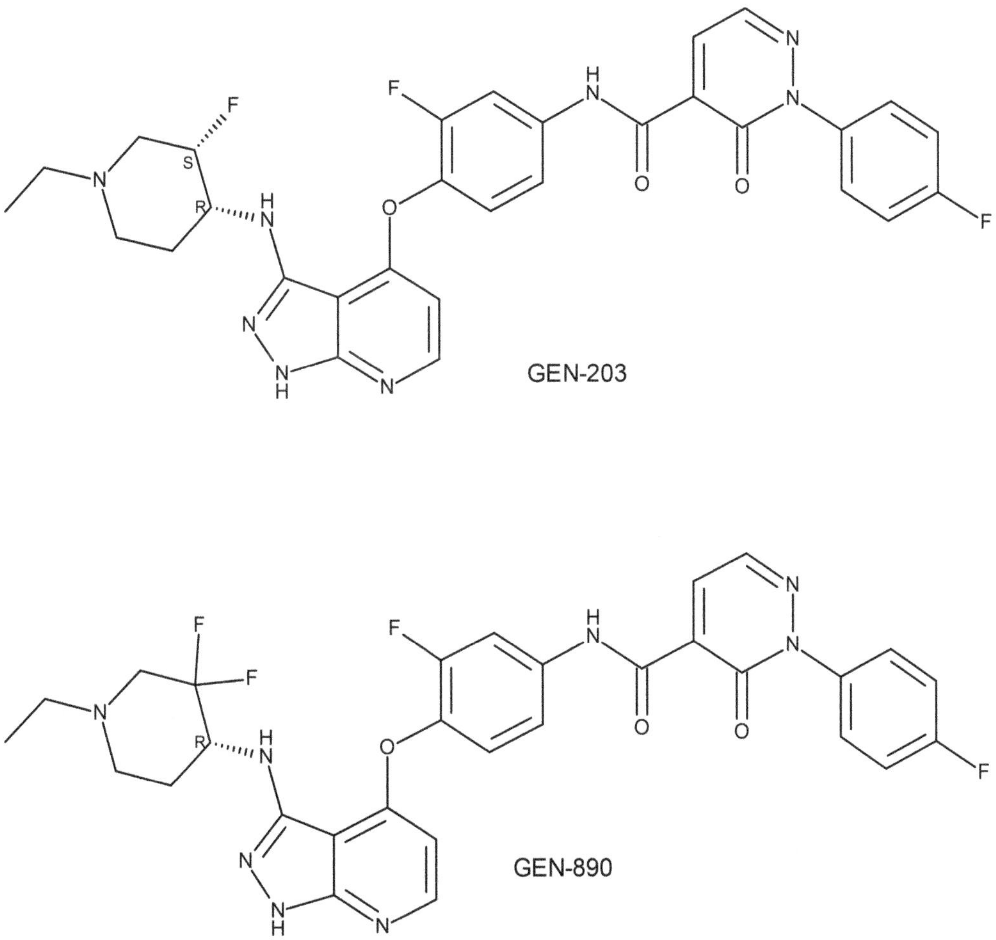


**Figure 1.8** Optimisation of MET inhibitor GEN-203 to GEN-890 by p$K_a$ manipulation resulted in lower volumes of distribution and reduced liver and bone-marrow toxicity in mice.[64]

**Table 1.3** The seven derivatives of geldinamycin with different weak base modifications at the 17-position with reported p$K_a$ and HSP90 affinity. Reproduced from ref 63, https://doi.org/10.1371/journal.pone.0049366, under the terms of the Creative Commons Attribution 4.0 International license, https://creativecommons.org/licenses/by/4.0/.

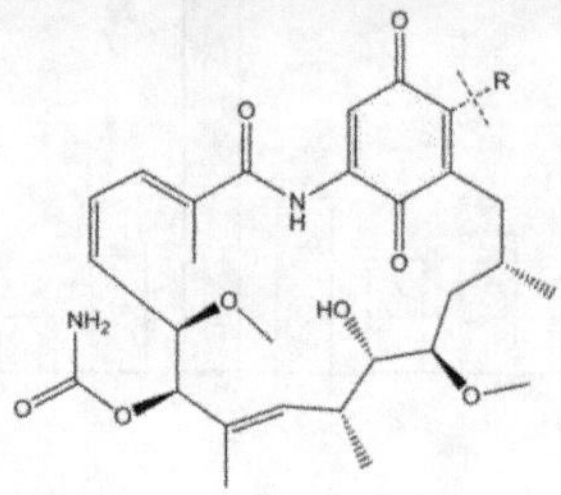

| Compound | R | p$K_a$ | rHsp90 affinity $K_i$ (nM) |
|---|---|---|---|
| GDA | 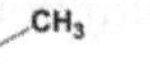 | NA | 117.8 |
| 1 | 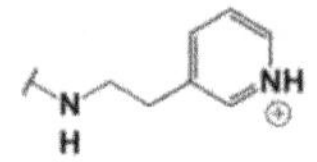 | 5.8 | 42.1 |
| 2 | 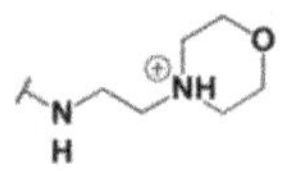 | 6.5 | 102.5 |
| 3 | 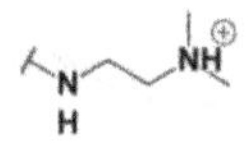 | 7.8 | 33.7 |
| 4 | 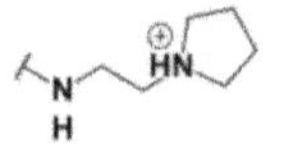 | 8.1 | 34.5 |
| 5 | 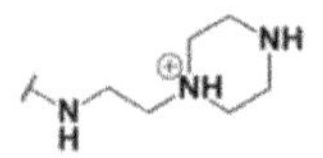 | 9.9 | 203.5 |
| 6 | 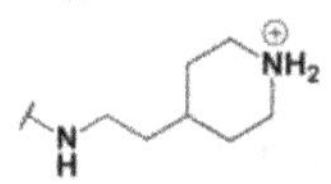 | 10.5 | 53.8 |
| 7 | 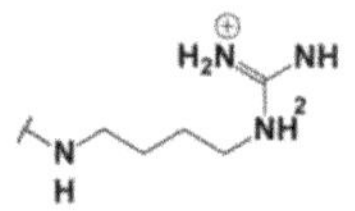 | 12.4 | 250.3 |

in drug–receptor interactions dependent upon hydrogen bonds and be an easy way to optimise interactions at the ligand target interface. Indeed, different functional groups have intrinsically different hydrogen bonding abilities, and various hydrogen bonding scales have been derived, usually through measuring the free energy of hydrogen bond formation of donors with a fixed reference acceptor or acceptors with a fixed donor in non-hydrogen bonding solvents.[67] But these parameters have found few applications in medicinal chemistry projects. The $\Delta \log P$ scales, whereby the difference between the $\log P$ in two different solvent systems, often *n*-octanol–water and alkane–water, appear to encode for hydrogen bonding capacity of a solute and its uptake into the brain,[68] and $\Delta \log P$ measurements have recently been proposed as a way of describing intramolecular hydrogen bonding.[69]

Maybe one of the reasons why the intrinsic hydrogen bonding ability is less important in drug–receptor interactions is because it is an exchange process. Hydrogen bonds that the solute makes to water molecules in the solvent are broken and exchanged for new hydrogen bonds in the receptor cavity. Increasing the hydrogen binding ability of a functional group may favour the formation of the new bond, say in the active site of a protein, but disfavour the breaking of other hydrogen bonds, say to bulk water, Figure 1.9.

The overall benefit gained by the exchange may be difficult to predict. Hydrogen bond counts are, however, widely used and, in particular, the number of hydrogen bond donors appears to be a very important compound quality metric, as it appears to have a large impact on permeability and brain penetration. In marketed oral drugs there is a wider tolerated number of hydrogen bond acceptors as it is the primary means of manipulating $\log P$ and balancing hydrophobicity. In contrast, the number of hydrogen bond donors appears more strictly "controlled". The reasons for this are not well understood, but desolvating a hydrogen bond donor may be more difficult than desolvating a hydrogen bond acceptor. In addition, the choice of *n*-octanol–water as the standard system for describing hydrophobicity may overly favour the partitioning of donors compared to the centre of a lipid bilayer, due to the high solubility of water in *n*-octanol itself, and the different nature of dissolved water *versus* bulk water. This would explain why $\Delta \log P$ is such a good surrogate for hydrogen bond donor count in modelling blood–brain barrier permeability. For whatever reason, it is very clear that controlling the number of hydrogen bond donors while balancing hydrophobicity, by manipulating

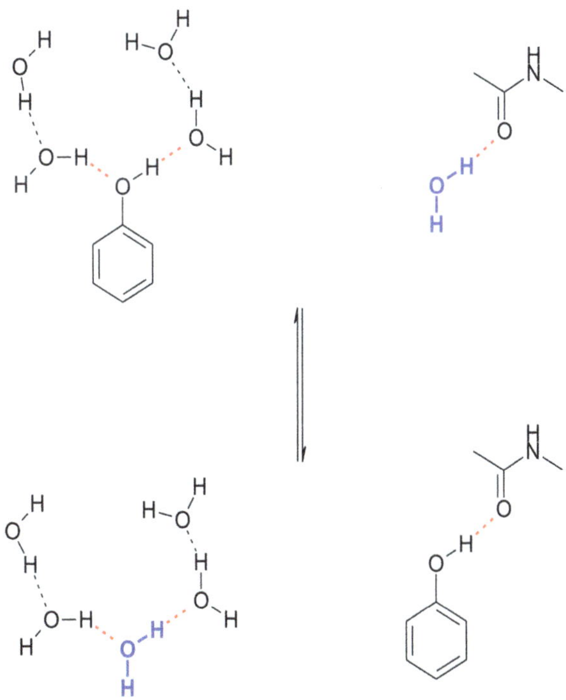

**Figure 1.9** Formation of a hydrogen bond in a drug–receptor interaction is an exchange process.

the hydrophobic groups and hydrogen bond acceptor count and polar surface area, is a fundamental design strategy in medicinal chemistry.

### 1.5.1 Polar Surface Area

The total polar surface area descriptor is a means of quantifying the overall number of polar hydrogen bonding groups contained in the molecule. It has been suggested that for CNS drugs the PSA should be below 90 Å,[2,70] while it can be somewhat higher for systemically restricted oral drugs.[71] A PSA <60 $Å^2$ has been reported to be desirable to ensure complete absorption.[72] Polar surface area is a key part of Pfizer's central nervous system (CNS) multi-parameter optimisation (MPO) algorithm for identifying drugs with greater probability of success in testing hypotheses in the clinic.[73,74] Their MPO uses several key physicochemical properties, Table 1.4.

This analysis indicates that higher CNS MPO desirability scores enhance the odds of identifying compounds with drug-like ADME and safety attributes, such as high passive permeability, low *P*-gp liability, low clearance and high cellular viability.

The PSA metric does not discriminate between polar surface contributed by donors and acceptors. As described above, controlling hydrogen bond donor surface area is much more critical than controlling hydrogen bond acceptor surface area, and therefore minimising hydrogen bond donors while manipulating hydrogen bond acceptors to control overall log*P* is a more nuanced medicinal chemistry strategy.

### 1.5.2 Quantifying the Contribution of a Hydrogen Bond

The authors' favourite paper quantifying the contribution of hydrogen bond to drug–receptor interactions comes from the systematic study of enzyme kinetics with site-directed mutation of the enzyme tyrosyl transfer RNA synthase. Of eleven possible hydrogen bonds identified from crystal structure tyrosyl-RNA synthase and tyrosyl adenylate, eight are from side chains that could be mutated. After mutation, the change in free energy of activation was determined from the measurement of $k_{cat}/K_m$. The loss of a charged-reinforced hydrogen bond was found to be worth an approximately 1000-fold decrease in binding, while loss of a neutral hydrogen bond was found to be worth only 2.5–15-fold,[75] Figure 1.10.

Equally elegant and comprehensive studies of the interaction of vancomycin and ristocetin antibiotics with small peptides came to similar conclusions.[76] While the benefit

**Table 1.4** The CNS MPO properties, functions, weighting value range and parameter ranges.

| Properties | Transformation | Weight | Most desirable range ($T0 = 1.0$) | Less desirable range ($T0 = 0.0$) |
|---|---|---|---|---|
| clog*P* | Monotonic decreasing | 1.0 | $\text{clog}P \leq 3.0$ | $\text{clog}P > 5.0$ |
| clog*D* | Monotonic decreasing | 1.0 | $\text{clog}D \leq 2$ | $\text{clog}D > 4$ |
| MW | Monotonic decreasing | 1.0 | MW ≤ 360 | MW > 500 |
| TPSA | Hump function | 1.0 | 40 < TPSA ≤ 90 | TPSA ≤ 20; TPSA > 120 |
| HBD | Monotonic decreasing | 1.0 | HBD ≤ 0.5 | HBD > 3.5 |
| p$K_a$ | Monotonic decreasing | 1.0 | p$K_a \leq 8.0$ | p$K_a > 10.0$ |

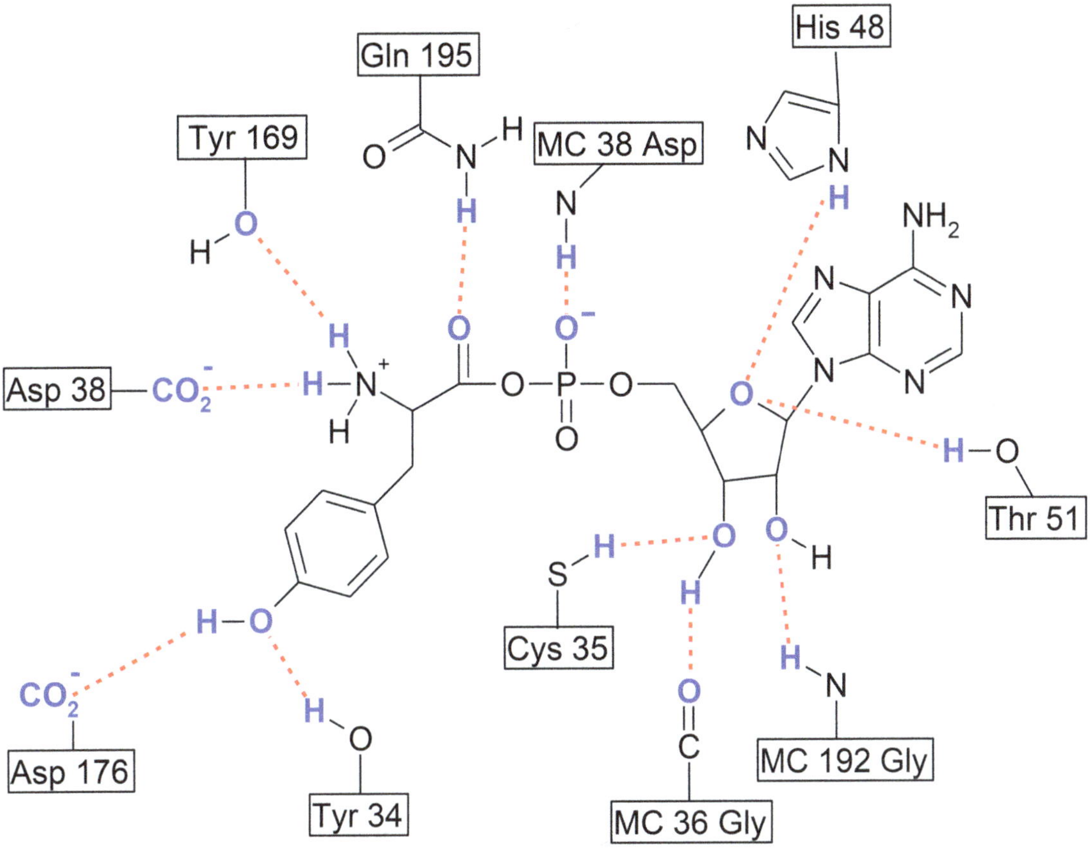


| Mutation A ⟶ B | $\Delta G^{\ddagger}_{B}$-$\Delta G^{\ddagger}_{A}$ (kJ mol$^{-1}$) |
|---|---|
| Tyr 34 to Phe 34 | 2.18 |
| Cys 35 to Gly 35 | 4.77 |
| His 48 to Gly 48 | 4.02 |
| Cys 51 to Ala 51 | 1.97 |
| Asn 48 to Gly 48 | 3.22 |
| Tyr 169 to Phe 169 | 15.56 |
| Gln 195 to Gly 195 | 18.79 |

**Figure 1.10** Site-directed mutation in the enzyme tyrosyl transfer RNA synthase of 8 of 11 possible hydrogen bonds identified from crystal structure tyrosyl-RNA synthase and tyrosyl adenylate, and their effect on free energy of activation. Adapted from ref. 75 with permission from Springer Nature, Copyright 1985.

in forming a neutral hydrogen bond may be small as hydrogen bonding is an exchange process, the penalty in not forming one in a protein active site may be large. This brings us to the much-pondered question, is it good to displace an active-site water or not? While it may be entropically favourable to displace a water molecule from a protein active site back to the bulk phase, it may be enthalpically favourable or unfavourable.

While no definitive literature exists on the subject, rules of thumb suggest one should consider the hydrogen bonding environment around the water molecule, and whether the water molecule is a happy or unhappy water. If it is already forming four hydrogen bonds in the protein active site, it would appear it may be a structural water and hard to replace, as displacing it with a donor or acceptor will form fewer hydrogens bonds than were lost, destabilising the protein and costing free energy. If the water molecule is forming three hydrogen bonds, one may get more free energy gain by forming an additional hydrogen bond to it. If it is making only one or two hydrogen bonds to the protein, it may be an unhappy water, which can be mimicked by the hydrogen bonding group of the drug and it may be favourable to displace it.

## 1.6 Solubility

It is a truism that in order for a drug to act on its protein target it must be in solution. Therefore, adequate aqueous solubility is a critically important molecular property. For poorly soluble compounds, dissolution rate is also an important factor, although dissolution rate is likely highly correlated to the overall equilibrium solubility, in that poorly soluble compounds are likely slower to dissolve, as has been demonstrated for a series of substituted benzoic acid salts of benzylamine.[77] Modern formulation techniques can improve solubility and dissolution, as discussed in the Pharmaceutical Properties Chapter 21, but add complexity and time to the development process. Poorly soluble drug candidates spend up to two years longer in development compared with those without solubility problems.[78]

But what is sufficient solubility? Much is dependent upon the dose. A simple rule of thumb uses the dose (in mg) divided by the solubility (mg mL$^{-1}$) – a ratio of <500 mL, an estimate of the standing volume available in the GI tract, is preferable to obviate the need for special formulations.[78] The concept of maximal absorbable dose (MAD) is a more sophisticated ranking tool for potential drug candidates:[79]

$$\mathrm{MAD} = (S) \times (K_\mathrm{a}) \times (\mathrm{SIWV}) \times (\mathrm{SITT}) \tag{1.9}$$

where $S$ = solubility (mg mL$^{-1}$ at pH 6.5; $K_\mathrm{a}$ = *trans*-intestinal absorption rate constant (min$^{-1}$); SIWV = small intestinal water volume (approximately 250 mL for man) and SITT = small intestinal transit time (approximately 270 min for man).

Estimates for a 1 mg Kg$^{-1}$ dose gives a minimum acceptable solubility of 5, 50 and 500 µg mL$^{-1}$ for low, medium and highly permeable compounds, respectively.

The Biopharmaceutics Classification system (BCS) of novel chemical entities classifies drugs based on their permeability and solubility, Table 1.5.

The FDA has issued guidance allowing applications for biowaivers for BCS class 1 immediate release solid-dose oral drugs from the need for *in vivo* bioequivalence testing, as absorption is unlikely to be dependent upon dissolution and gastric emptying time.

**Table 1.5** The biopharmaceutics classification system.

| | |
|---|---|
| BCS class 1 high permeability high solubility | BCS class 2 high permeability low solubility |
| BCS class 3 low permeability high solubility | BCS class 4 low solubility low permeability |

A drug substance is classified as highly soluble if the highest single therapeutic dose is completely soluble in 250 millilitre (mL) or less of aqueous media over the pH range of 1.2–6.8 at 37 ± 1 °C.

The assessment of permeability should preferentially be based on the extent of absorption derived from absolute bioavailability or mass balance human pharmacokinetic studies. But permeability can be also assessed by validated and standardised *in vitro* methods using Caco-2 cells and the results discussed in the context of available data on human pharmacokinetics. If high permeability is inferred by means of an *in vitro* cell system, permeability independent of active transport should be proven, as if high permeability is not demonstrated, the drug substance is considered to have low permeability for BCS classification purposes.

For low solubility drugs the media in which solubility is measured can be critical in accurately predicting *in vivo* dissolution. Fasted state simulated intestinal fluid, (FaSSIF) simulates conditions in the proximal small intestine, and solubility measured in FaSSIF can more accurately model the likely behaviour of poorly soluble drugs *in vivo*. Measurement in fed state simulated gastric fluid can indicate whether the formulation should be taken before or after meals.[36]

Solubility may be even more important than permeability in driving drug absorption. Measurements of solubility cover a wider dynamic range than measures of permeability (Caco-2 permeability for example) and a high solubility may be enough to drive absorption for poorly permeable drugs. Poorly permeable but high solubility BCS class 3 drugs such as cimetidine, amoxycillin and atenolol can show high and rapid absorption if the dissolution rate is high and they behave as BSC class 1 drugs. Biowaivers can be granted for BCS class 3 drugs if all of the excipients are qualitatively the same and quantitatively similar (except for film coating or capsule shell excipients).[80]

### 1.6.1 Measurement of Solubility

The measurement of solubility, while superficially a simple experiment, has many pitfalls and caveats. The experimentally determined solubility is dependent upon buffer choice, ionic strength, temperature, pH, supersaturation, the starting solid-state form and its history and impurities, amongst other factors.[81] Many experimental protocols try to measure thermodynamic equilibrium, but for some compounds this can take extended periods of time. The solubility is often measured at a particular pH, often pH 7.4 and in a particular buffer, at a fixed time point (4 h) although the solubility of the neutral form can be measured, in which case this is known as the intrinsic solubility.

Dissolution rate is an even more involved experiment. In order to control as many of the potential sources of variability as possible, intrinsic dissolution rate requires a compressed spinning disc of the solid to control surface area and fluid flow across the surface,[82,83] which requires large amounts of drug.

In order to generate solubility on a large number of compounds, solubility from a stock DMSO solution injected into a buffer, after suitable equilibration, can be measured. Solubility is determined from the turbidity threshold, or quantitated spectrophotometrically or by HPLC, after filtration of undissolved drug. In a validation study at AstraZeneca the measured solubilities of 200 compounds showed a good correlation with a gold-standard manual method measured from solid with an average fold deviation of 3-fold.[84] Some compounds showed much larger differences. It was noted that the authors did not expect a perfect correlation within the replicate error of each other's measurements, as they had changed the solid state form.

Solubility is often measured in pH 7.4 buffered aqueous solution, but as already mentioned, for pharmaceutical applications, dissolution into real or simulated intestinal fluid, under fasted (FaSSIF) or fed (FeSSIF) conditions can be used better model to model *in vivo* drug dissolution.[36]

### 1.6.2 Calculating Solubility

Solubility is difficult to measure accurately and precisely and more difficult to predict. Most solubility calculators use empirical QSAR equations based on literature data or in-house datasets. Their predictiveness for an individual chemical series should always be tested.

The Yalkowsky General Solubility Equation,[85] which is not in fact a QSAR model, but a physically derived equation, contains a negative coefficient for $\log P$ and melting point (mpt), as dissolution would require the breaking of crystal packing interactions and the disruption of water structure by the hydrophobic nature of the drug.

$$\log S = -\log P - 0.01\ \text{mpt} + 1.2 \quad (1.10)$$

Few QSAR models, nor indeed the Yalkowsky GSE for solubility, do better than an average error of +/−0.9 log units over a range of diverse drug-like chemistries, a range so wide as to be of limited utility in optimising solubility for most projects. But within local project series, solubility may be better predicted. The controlling influence of lipophilicity and the fact that many other ADMET properties depend upon $\log P$, means the best way to control solubility is to control lipophilicity. Other molecular strategies involve breaking up the crystal packing by introducing 3-D character into the drug molecule, and more pharmaceutical approaches such as changing the counter ion for salts, or forming co-crystals, as described in the Pharmaceutical Properties Chapter 21. Some of this thinking drives interest in another compound quality metric, $F\text{sp}^3$ (the fraction of carbon atoms that are $\text{sp}^3$ hybridised).[86] Increasing $F\text{sp}^3$ was found to correlate with decreased melting point (lower crystal packing forces) and increased solubility, in accord with the Yalkowsky general solubility equation.

Young *et al.* reported on the detrimental effect that aromatic rings can have on solubility, above and beyond that due to their $\log P$.[35] Molecular weight had no effect on solubility.[87] As aromatic ring count correlates inversely with $F\text{sp}^3$,[88] one can appreciate that both aromatic ring count and $F\text{sp}^3$ point to an independent contribution of crystal packing forces being important for solubility over and above their contribution to hydrophobicity.

## 1.7 The Rule of Five

The rule of five (Ro5), formulated by Lipinksi in 1997,[89] has become a central part of medicinal chemistry lore. Before the late 1980s, drug discovery relied on chemical starting points from natural products, follower drugs and classical medicinal chemistry design, and depended strongly on *in vivo* screening. The requirement for aqueous solubility sufficient for *in vivo* activity acted as a natural limiter on medicinal chemistry optimisation. However, around 1990 the situation changed. The advent of HTS, combinatorial chemistry and advances in molecular biology enabled the screening of 100 000s of compounds in *in vitro* assays, finding many more and diverse start points for projects than had previously been possible. But along with the advantages came compromises. Compounds were no longer solubilised in water but in DMSO, enabling the screening at high concentrations to find micromolar hits, sometimes exceeding their thermodynamic aqueous solubilities. The focus of drug optimisation became *in vitro* screening, and combinatorial screening libraries increased molecular weight and lipophilicity, since this appeared to increase the chances of finding sufficiently potent hits in the HTS campaigns.

Scientists at Pfizer were the first to realise that HTS was adversely affecting the physicochemical property distribution of their whole compound library. Leads were getting bigger and more lipophilic, and medicinal chemistry optimisation led to further drift in undesirable physicochemical properties, notably poor solubility and permeability.

In a bid to define guidelines for chemical synthesis, an aspirational library was chosen on the assumption it would represent a physicochemical property space consistent with success, with compound progression to Phase II as a selection filter. The hypothesis was that compounds with poorer physicochemical properties would have been weeded out by preclinical and Phase I safety evaluation, and that properties of resulting Phase II compounds would define a "holy grail" profile for early drug discovery. Considering the target audience of medicinal chemists, Lipinski and co-workers chose pragmatic descriptors known to be important for solubility and permeability, molecular weight, log*P* and hydrogen binding descriptors. For a calculated log*P* value they applied both the Moriguchi (Mlog*P*) method, which did not suffer the missing fragment problem of the then gold standard clog*P*, as well as clog*P* itself. For hydrogen bonding, donor and acceptor counts using sums of OH + NH groups and O + N atoms respectively, were unambiguous and did remarkably well compared to quantitative measures such as the Abraham solvatochromic or Raevsky C scales. In a similar manner to setting a confidence internal on an $IC_{50}$ from an *in vitro* assay, they chose "cutoffs" so that 90% of the Phase II compounds had parameters within the calculated range. Hence the rule of 5 was born.

The Ro5 states that poor solubility or permeability are judged as more likely when:

MW > 500
clog*P* > 5 or Mlog*P* > 4.15
N + O count > 10
NH + OH count > 5

The Ro5 was proposed to be violated when two or more of these criteria are not met. Compound classes, such as some natural products, known to be substrates for transporters, were recognised as being exceptions to the rule. The Lipinski paper has become a medicinal chemistry classic defining the whole genre of drug-like properties and compound quality metrics, stimulating a massive literature on these topics.

However, HTS identifies hits or leads rather than drugs. As medicinal chemistry optimisation appears most often to add mass and sometimes lipophilicity, ideally screening libraries for HTS should be smaller and less lipophilic than drugs, in fact more lead-like.[90,91] Further, the molecular complexity of larger molecules was suggested to preclude the chances of finding efficient leads, providing yet further justification for HTS collections being more lead-like.[92] An analysis[92] of historical lead drug-pairs previously compiled by Sneader[93] highlighted the increase in molecular weight between leads and drugs by an average of 42 daltons, which has also been proposed to be the answer to the ultimate question of life, the universe and everything.[94]

A more recent analysis of physical property changes seen in successful hit-to-candidate optimisations from the 2016–2017 literature shows a large average increase in molecular weight of 85, but this was accompanied by no average change in clog*P*, suggesting that control of lipophilicity is being widely pursued in contemporary drug discovery.[95] When starting points are already advanced literature leads, the changes in physicochemical properties are likely to be smaller or non-existent, as seen in the development of follow-on compounds from first-in-class drugs.[96]

One approach to overcome the hard cut-off approach of the Ro5 metrics is to use a desirability function approach as defined in the "quantitative estimate of drug-likeness" (QED), which scores molecules on a continuous scale, in the same way as the CNS MPO discussed above. QED is derived from the sum of desirability functions for eight different molecular properties that are based on their distributions in a curated historical set of >700 drugs.[97] A number of drugs that fail Lipinski criteria have QED scores that overlap with drugs that pass the criteria.

### 1.7.1 Beyond the Rule of Five

Medicinal chemists continually debate whether the rule of 5 and drug-like and lead-like thinking should fundamentally underpin medicinal chemistry strategy or if they overly constrain it, and studies of "beyond the rule of five" (bRo5) compounds and drugs have become popular and influential. Many of these papers are directly or indirectly critical of the "rule of five", often highlighting sets of approved drug compounds that "violate" the rules.[98–102] A consistent subset of these publications focuses in particular on antibiotic and other anti-infective compounds, despite the fact that Lipinski *et al.* explicitly stated that orally active antibiotic, fungicide and antiparasitic compounds fell outside the "rule of five space". Reports that potential antiparasitic drugs were being cast aside or deprioritised because they failed two of more of the "rules" so concerned the original Ro5 authors that a recent position piece was published, pointing out the salient facts and recommending the use of less stringent criteria for compounds progression in an area that is significantly under-funded.[103]

AbbVie analysed the property space of all compounds in their preclinical DMPK database that violated Lipinski's Ro5 ($n$ = 1116) by virtue of failing >1 rule.[104] Many such bRo5 molecules had poor *in vitro* permeability, which was ascribed to technical issues such as poor solubility and adherence to laboratory apparatus.[104] AbbVie scientists therefore decided to directly screen bRo5 compounds for their bioavailability *in vivo* in rats. A surprising observation was that the upper quartile bioavailability value found was 27% – *i.e. one quarter of the bRo5 compounds tested had bioavailability >25%.* This shows bioavailability can be achieved in bRo5 space across a range of structures, which is of course unexpected based on the Ro5 teaching. The AbbVie research found, contrary to preconceptions, that in order for bRo5 compounds to demonstrate acceptable oral absorption, they must nevertheless have the right balance of physicochemical properties endemic to successful oral drugs, namely, optimal lipophilicity, a low number of aromatic rings (echoing the importance of aromatic ring count highlighted in GSK's PFI metric) and a low number of rotatable bonds. They developed a multiparametric mnemonic, AB-MPS, combining the physicochemical properties most closely correlated with an increased probability of higher oral bioavailability in bRo5 space:

$$\text{AB-MPS} = \text{abs}(\text{clog}D\text{-}3) + \text{NRB} + \text{NAR} \tag{1.11}$$

Values of AB-MPS < 14 were associated with higher bioavailability.[104] Determination of experimental polar surface area[105] (EPSA) may be a useful tool for predicting acceptable permeability for bRo5 chemical series with high TPSA values. EPSA, a relative polarity profile derived by supercritical fluid chromatography (SFC) retention, may more adequately describe the formation of intramolecular hydrogen bonds, which some bRo5 compounds exploit to hide their polarity (hydrophobic collapse or their chameleonic efficiency) in non-polar milieu and hence facilitating membrane permeability.[106] The rotatable bond influence in AB-MPS is large and probably captures bioavailable bRo5 macrocyclic compounds, where intramolecular hydrophobic interactions and H-bonding are facilitated by the macrocyclic structure having restricted rotatable bonds, as notably demonstrated by the permeability of the immunosuppressive drug cyclosporine and its analogues.[107]

Orally available compounds can exist on the edge of Ro5 space and beyond, but may have some compromises. The emergence of proteolysis targeting chimeras (PROTACs) as a new drug modality has the potential to rival or surpass CRISPR/cas9 as a therapeutic modality in targeted protein degradation. PROTACs, having inherently high molecular weight (mostly >700), which comprise the template structure binding to the protein of interest, a linker moiety and an E3 ligase warhead, are forcing chemists, whether sceptics or fans of Ro5, to seek opportunities in bRo5 space.[108] Those PROTACs based on the VHL E3 ligase warhead have less favourable Ro5 properties than those based on cereblon E3 ligase ligands. This is largely irrespective of the protein ligand of interest and linker and is probably due to increased hydrogen bond donor count. In a series of cereblon-based PROTACS, bioavailability in the rat of >30% was seen in 1/3 of compounds tested, in comparison with molecules in conventional chemical space, where 2/3 had >30% bioavailability.[109] These bioavailable PROTACS required high chrom log$D$ values of 5–7. VHL-based PROTACS had <5% bioavailability in this study. While oral absorption may be compromised in the VHL class, the catalytic nature of the PROTAC mechanism of action may negate the need for 24 hour target coverage required of typical reversible non-covalent small-molecule antagonists,[110] and we are now seeing the first PROTAC molecules reaching clinical stages of drug development.

Many authors have examined changes in drug and discovery compound physicochemical properties over time.[91,111,112] The four Ro5 properties differ in that molecular weight and hydrogen bond acceptor counts are increasing significantly over time, whereas hydrogen bond donor count and lipophilicity remain near constant. It is fair to say the 90% cut-off values used for the Ro5 properties depend on the time frame chosen, leading some to argue that the notion of drug-likeness is intrinsically flawed.[111] However, those properties most resistant to change – particularly lipophilicity and hydrogen bond donor count – are arguably the most important to control in drug discovery programs.

## 1.8 Ligand Efficiency Metrics

Following the focus on drug-like and lead-like physical properties, medicinal chemists have tried to define further measures using *in vitro* potency, against which optimisation pathways can be quantified. A number of efficiency metrics[113] have been defined, which seek to quantify the physicochemical property "cost" of achieving potency. Some selected ligand efficiency metrics are shown below:

$$\text{LE} = (-2.303(\text{RT/HA})) \times \log K_\text{d} \quad (1.12)$$

$$\text{LE} = (p\text{IC}_{50} \times 1.37)/\text{HA} \quad (1.13)$$

$$\text{BEI} = (p\text{IC}_{50} \times 1000)/\text{MW} \quad (1.14)$$

$$\text{LLE} = p\text{IC}_{50} - \log P \text{ or } \log D \quad (1.15)$$

$$\text{LLEAT} = ((\text{LLE/HA}) \times 1.37) + 0.111 \quad (1.16)$$

$$\text{LELP} = \log P/\text{LE} \quad (1.17)$$

The most widely applied measures are ligand efficiency (LE)[116] and lipophilic ligand efficiency (LLE).[114] Both measures have useful features, as well as some compromises, which are summarised in Table 1.6.

**Table 1.6** Summary of pros and cons of application of ligand efficiency metrics.

| LE (ligand efficiency) | LLE (lipophilic ligand efficiency) |
|---|---|
| **Pros:**<br>• Useful for hit selection & FBDD<br>• Assess changes in optimisation | **Pros:**<br>• Plausible thermodynamic basis<br>• Link to specificity<br>• Mostly increases in optimisations (potency↑ & log *P*↕) |
| **Cons:**<br>• Treats all atoms similarly<br>• Reduces non-linearly as size increases<br>• Lacks firm thermodynamic basis<br>• Increases and decreases ~equally in optimisations (potency↑ & MW↑) | **Cons:**<br>• LLE dependence on low clog *P*/*D* risks poor permeability<br>• Log *P* ~ 0–3 optimal for ADMET<br>• Need for experimental log *P*/*D* |
| **No ideal values:**<br>• Absolute value unimportant<br>• Target & chemistry dependent<br>• *Change* in optimisation is important | **Values as high as possible (ideally >5):**<br>• Target & chemistry dependent<br>• *Change* in optimisation is important |

Ligand efficiency (LE) was first proposed as a method for comparing hit molecules from a screen according to their average binding energy per atom,[115] and a way of quantifying the "bang for your buck".[116] LE applies the principles of Occam's razor – every atom should contribute. With a drug having to balance so many factors to reach the clinic (potency, selectivity, ADMET properties, solubility, formulation and solid–state properties, *etc.*), carrying molecular features which do not clearly make a contribution, or are not specifically designed in for a reason, can build in unnecessary risks. Many medicinal chemistry programs, in particular those derived from fragment hits, focus on maintaining the implicit efficiency of a core scaffold or fragment as they are optimised towards leads and drugs. Fragment-based drug discovery (FBDD) has embraced the use of LE; indeed, FBDD has become a successful hit generation capability that truly embraces the lead-like concept[90,117] to facilitate successful multiparameter optimisation to clinical candidates. The fact that starting fragments, often having only mM affinity, retain the same binding pose once decorated with further substitution to reach nM potency drug candidates speaks to the efficiency of binding of the original fragment. In a cross-industry comparison on a target-by-target basis, Astex, a specialist fragment-based drug discovery organisation, had lower molecular weights, log*P* and rotatable bonds in patented molecules on the same shared targets compared to peer pharmaceutical companies.[118]

A plot of fragment–lead pairs from all publications in 2015–2019[119] shows that efficient fragments tend to yield efficient leads. However, the spread in the correlation shows that less efficient fragments can still yield highly efficient leads, if properly optimised, Figure 1.11. Hence it was proposed that LE should not be the sole driver of selection, but rather a guide for optimisation, although it may be difficult to find highly ligand-efficient leads from less ligand-efficient fragments. As the authors highlight, extremely high fragment-ligand efficiencies are difficult to maintain during optimisation. This stems from the fact that LE values decline as molecular size increases.[120]

LE has been criticised as a metric.[121,122] However, attempting to quantify how effectively an increase in molecular size translates to affinity gain over the course of hit to lead to candidate optimisation is a valid objective. This is captured by plots of potency *vs.* size (as well as other properties), which are highly useful and necessary tools for all drug discovery programs. Such plots can be used to track changes in LE that occur during optimisation, the absolute values of LE being less important. While LE is not a perfect metric, this does not mean it lacks utility.[123]

Optimising potency is very strong primary driver for drug discovery projects, as potency is broadly correlated to dose, and lower dose drugs have improved compliance, are cheaper, and tend to be more selective and carry fewer toxicological liabilities. With hydrophobicity being such a strong driver of potency for targets as well as off-targets (receptor active sites tend to be more hydrophobic than protein surfaces or bulk solvent) and ADMET properties, optimising potency in a chemical series by increasing hydrophobicity introduces a myriad of liabilities. For these reasons increasing lipophilic ligand efficiency (LLE)[114] was proposed as a key driver in optimisation. Essentially increasing LLE – the difference between *p*(activity) and log*P* or log*D* – is linked

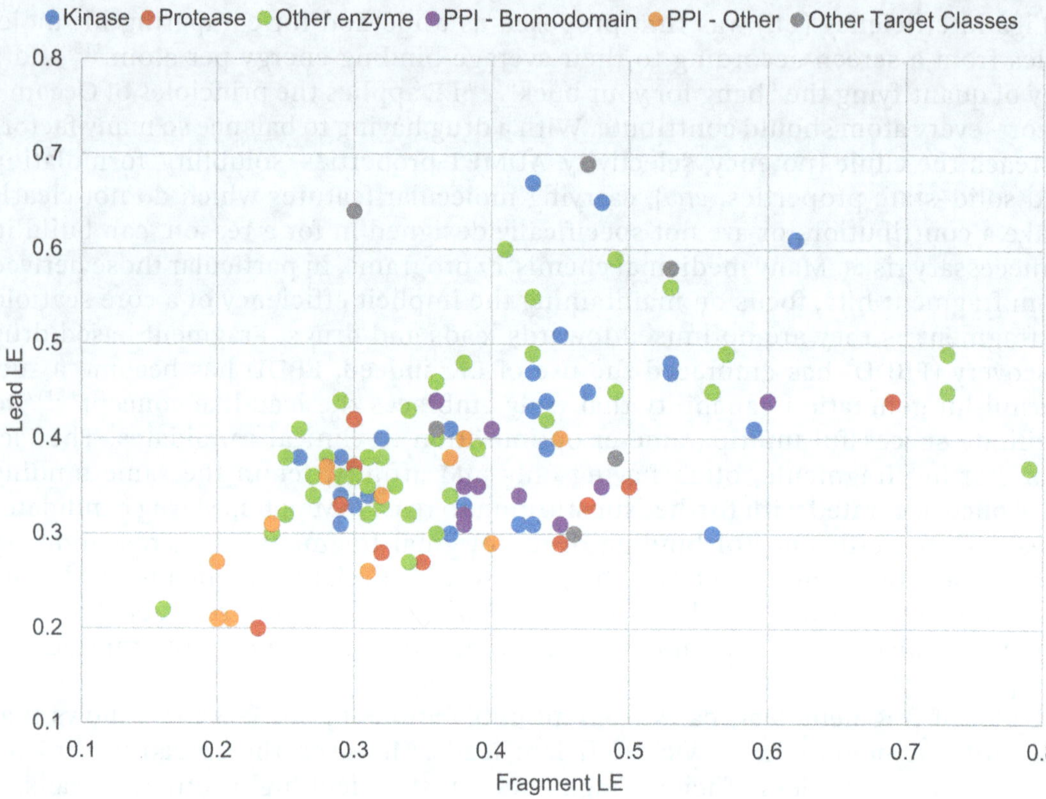


**Figure 1.11** Plot of lead LE *vs.* fragment LE for fragment–lead pairs from all publications in 2015–2019. Reproduced from ref. 119 with permission from American Chemical Society, Copyright 2020.

to increasing specificity for the target *versus* non-specific lipid binding and therefore it has a plausible thermodynamic basis:[124]

$$[\text{Drug}]_{\text{Target}} \underset{}{\overset{k_d}{\rightleftharpoons}} [\text{Drug}]_{\text{Water/pH7.4}} \underset{}{\overset{P\text{ or }D}{\rightleftharpoons}} [\text{Drug}]_{1\text{-Octanol}}$$

LLE tends to increase during optimisation and LLE values in candidates should be as high as possible. This is reflected by the mean values of LLE of >4 found in drugs.[125]

The "conundrum of drug discovery",[126] Figure 1.12, captures the essence of the LLE concept. Moving up and down the diagonal of this graph, a line of constant LLE, should in general be avoided in medicinal chemistry programs. Three strategies can be adopted: (a) increasing potency and LLE while lowering log *P* through finding a new drug–receptor polar interaction – this is in general the preferred way to go; (b) to lower log *P* and increase LLE without increasing potency, for example by finding polar substituents that are tolerated by extending from the binding site to bulk solvent; and (c) finally, if LLE values are already high enough, potency can be traded to obtain ADMET improvements. It should be noted that while LLE can be increased by lowering log *P*, if log *P* is <0, permeability may suffer. An optimal log *P* range of ~0–3 can be targeted,[22] but the actual log *P* value required in a candidate will ultimately depend on the multiparameter

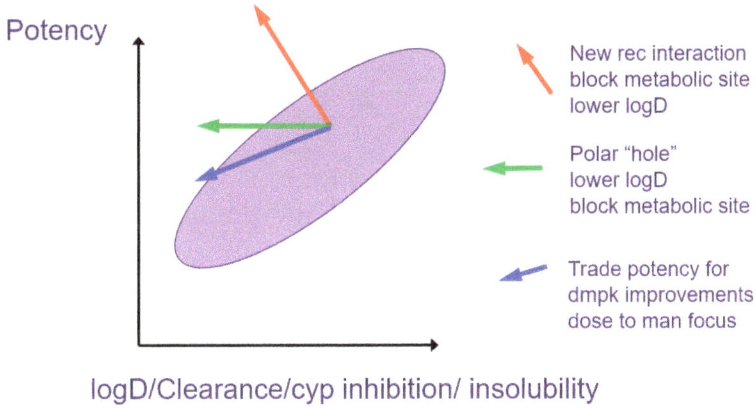


**Figure 1.12** The drug discovery conundrum - increasing potency can often be achieved by increasing lipophilicity but also many ADMET properties are worsened. Optimising compounds for improved potency while controlling hydrophobicity is a fundamental med-chem design strategy quantified by the LLE metric, increasing LLE would be moving toward the top left of this graph in the direction of the red and green arrows - lines of equal LLE would be diagonal lines on this plot parallel to the ellipse.[126]

optimisation compromises that are usually needed,[127] the chemical class pursued and the nature of the drug target ligand binding site.

Multiple analyses of changes to LLE in optimisations from the recent literature have been reviewed, providing strong support for the application of this metric in drug discovery programs.[128–132] LLE is improved in optimisation across multiple target classes, irrespective of whether it was addressed deliberately in the discovery phase, or not. Rather than relying solely on the Darwinian selection pressures for compound progression imposed by the discovery assay cascade, addressing the potency/lipophilicity balance rationally from the outset is recommended as a powerful strategy to help streamline compound design choices. Indeed, a survey of literature optimisations from 2014 revealed that when authors considered lipophilicity, log*P* was significantly reduced and LLE increased, *vs.* those that did not.[130]

An example showing successful optimisation trajectories from HTS hits to candidates acting at the CCR5 chemokine receptor is shown in Figure 1.13. In the discovery of both maraviroc and AZD5672, the project teams employed optimisation of physiochemical properties, to achieve good DMPK properties and to overcome hERG inhibition. LLE is markedly improved as shown by the movement to the top left of the potency *vs.* clog*P* plot. While molecular weight and HA count increased, LE nevertheless was also increased in these examples. Across a larger set of 60 lead-to-drug pairs, LLE was increased by 2 units on average, whereas average LE did not change, *i.e.* LE increases or decreases equally.[128]

It is evident from Figure 1.13 that the optimised CCR5 candidate drugs possess both LE and LLE values which are bettered by few other ligands for this target. This observation appears to be a general, if not exclusive trend, as shown in Figure 1.14.[125] Compared

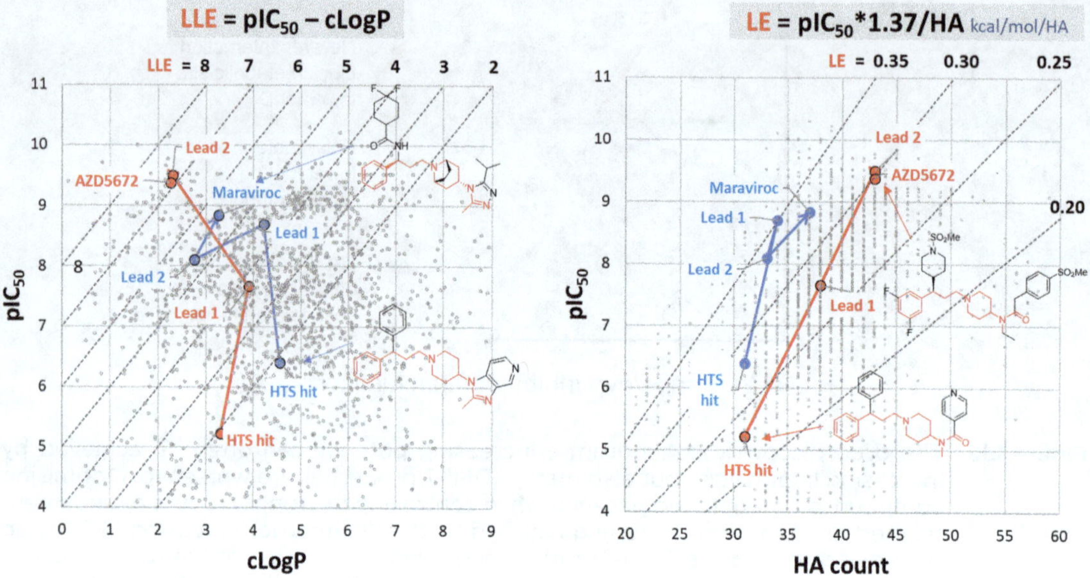


**Figure 1.13** Example of the optimisation trajectories of candidate drugs using potency *vs.* property plots, contoured by LE and LLE values, for compounds acting at the CCR5 receptor.[129] The background data are compounds with CCR5 potencies from CHEMBL ($n$ = 1875). Adapted from ref. 129 with permission from American Chemical Society, Copyright 2018.

to the median LE and LLE values of compounds acting at the drug's target, 96% of the drugs have improved LE or LLE, or both.[125] In this study, drugs approved in 2010–2020 had greater potency, but were equally likely to possess either higher or lower values of molecular weight, lipophilicity, hydrogen bond donors or acceptors, or aromatic ring count, in comparison with the median values of compounds acting at their targets. Thus, the most commonly used simple physicochemical properties, including the Ro5 and QED, failed to differentiate newer drugs from non-drugs on a target basis. In addition to LE and LLE, 2010–2020 drugs were distinguished from their target compounds by having increased numbers of stereocentres, and those that were carboaromatic (but not heteroaromatic) had reduced aromatic ring count and lipophilicity relative to their target compounds.[125]

## 1.9 Compound Quality and Drug-likeness

As medicinal chemists, our goal is to make drugs and to design "drug-like" compounds. We want to discover molecules that engage with chosen molecular targets at an acceptable dose, that can be delivered safely to patients by the chosen delivery route to treat unmet medical need. How well a compound matches this "drug-like" profile is the true measure of compound quality. In this sense, physicochemical properties are surrogates for true drug-likeness.

Drug-likeness applies to all therapeutic modalities: small-molecule drugs (oral, injectable, inhaled and topical); peptides; nucleic acids, oligonucleotides and antisense

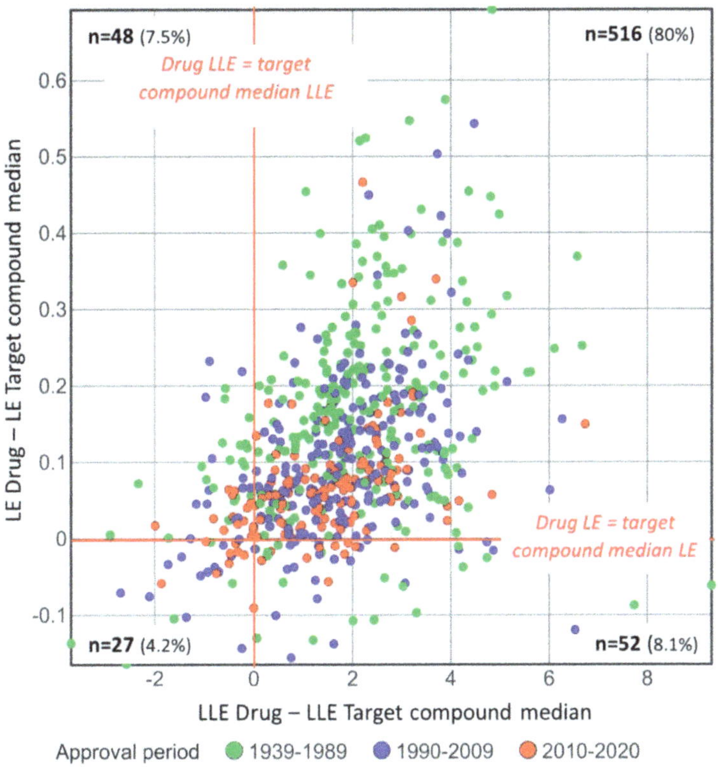


**Figure 1.14** Differentiation of drugs from their published target compounds using a combination of the differences in LE and LLE between the drug and the median values of published compounds acting at the drug's target of action. The population of drugs in each quadrant is shown. A total of 643 drugs are shown, acting at 194 targets, split by three time periods of drug approval. The differences seen for drugs in the three approval periods reflect increases in their size, and to a lesser extent, lipophilicity.[125] Adapted from ref. 125 with permission from American Chemical Society, Copyright

therapeutics; protein hormones, therapeutic antibodies and antibody-drug conjugates; vaccines and other protein scaffolds; non-protein biologics; sugars and sugar derivatives; lipids and lipopeptides; metals and metal prodrugs; modified differentiated cells and stem cell therapies; modified bacteria; vaccines and microbiome-based therapies. Drug-likeness is therefore a difficult, perhaps impossible, term to define, especially, as noted from a regulatory perspective "drug" is not an intrinsic property of medicines. The "drug" attribute is conferred by a regulatory agency such as the US Food and Drug Administration (FDA), based on available evidence at the time of the New Drug Application (NDA). Because scientific evidence requirements vary from country to country, the "drug" attribute is not only time-dependent (marketing approval can be bestowed, and later withdrawn), but also geographically based (not all drugs are approved in all countries).[133] It follows that compound quality is an equally difficult term to pin down. Within each modality class and target profile, however, a compound quality space can be defined. For much of this chapter we have referred only to small-molecule drugs, and for the most part, oral drugs. The physicochemical parameters we have discussed are important for binding to drug targets and are surrogates for the key experimental compound quality ADMET measures of permeability, metabolic clearance and solubility.

A candidate drug is the result of many years of a drug discovery campaign and the synthesis of hundreds or thousands of compounds, each of which we hoped could be "the one". Overall, the success rate of candidate drugs reaching the market is low (~1–5%). Spotting "the one that can make it" is a great challenge and the research and guidance summarised in this chapter, and book, is about increasing the chances of designing and selecting "the one". A quality compound needs to possess biological properties of specificity for on-target potency *vs.* off-targets, it needs to engage the target *in vivo* to produce a therapeutic benefit with a suitable safety margin. Known risks can be frontloaded into discovery testing cascades, and the major attributes of a quality small-molecule compound are:

- Potent (<10 nM *vs.* primary target)
- Selective (>100 × selective *vs.* other targets based on maximal exposure levels)
- Not a victim or perpetrator of drug–drug interactions (not a CYP inhibitor or inducer nor to interact with any significant other drug transporter that could affect the exposure of co-administered drugs)
- Pharmacokinetic profile suitable for exposure and therapeutic efficacy *via* the chosen dose route and frequency
- Soluble and formulatable
- Scalable synthetic route.

Some risks are hard to define and are not absolutes. For example, are nitro groups toxic liabilities or can they be acceptable in oral drugs? Certainly marketed drugs can contain nitro groups, but are a risk for reactive metabolism and have become abhorrent to most medicinal chemists. Likewise, some but not all aromatic amines can be genotoxic, and these can be screened out preclinically. Tables of molecular alerts containing unwanted or undesirable functionality such as AZFILTERS[134] have been published based on the experiences (and often biases) of medicinal chemists.

Metrics such LE and LLE discussed above, try to capture properties that may or may not be explicit in a candidate drug profile and could mitigate risks beyond poor permeability and solubility (as was the focus for Ro5), but also may more broadly improve chances of successful progression through clinical development.

## 1.10 Conclusions

Having a clear view on medicinal chemistry design strategies has never been more important. Control of physical properties such as hydrophobicity, ionisation and hydrogen bond donors, and the efficient use of chemical structure so that every atom plays an important part (the known knowns) can provide a framework to help mitigate later failure (the unknown unknowns). But these are guidelines, and candidate drugs most often contain project-specific compromises or sit in niches. For example: natural products have been optimised by evolution, and PROTACS and covalent drugs have different PK-PD requirements than non-covalent reversible drugs; different delivery routes allow different property ranges; and different diseases accept different safety compromises. We can aspire as Picasso did to "Learn the Rules Like a Pro, So You Can Break Them Like an Artist." As we partner with artificial intelligence (AI) and powerful machine learning algorithms for augmented drug design – and autonomous drug design by AI is now widely discussed – we should remember that machines are good at learning rules, but it takes a human to break them and demonstrate the true art of medicinal chemistry.

## 1.11 Hints and Tips

While the number of compound quality metrics and associated guidance keeps increasing, and we have made no attempt here to be comprehensive, we believe that medicinal chemistry strategy in relation to physical property control, particularly for oral drugs, is clear:

Optimise potency which results in lower dose.

Control $\log P$ – between 0 and 3 is ideal.

Where the compound series has an ionisable centre, you can manipulate $\log D$ by $pK_a$ modulation and $\log P$ modulation. Beware of lowering $\log D_{7.4}$ by modulation of $pK_a$, $\log P$ modulation should always be the focus.

LLE ≥5 is a good target value for a drug candidate. 96% of drugs possess LE or LLE, or both, greater than the average published compound acting at the drug's target.

Control the number of hydrogen bond donors: 0–2 will aid in cell penetration, absorption and CNS permeability.

Control aromatic ring count (especially phenyl rings), ideally ≤3.

Balance hydrophobicity by adjusting numbers of polar hydrogen bond acceptors.

Target aqueous solubility >100 micromolar in pH 7.4 buffer; if necessary use physiologically relevant assays such as FaSSIF solubility.

Acids and bases can help with solubility and bulk physical properties, but avoid extremes of $pK_a$ and avoid the addition of more than acid or basic groups if oral absorption is required.

Zwitterions can limit CNS penetration and still maintain oral absorption by passive and active processes.

Use calculations to guide compound design but validate with measurements to improve the accuracy of physical chemical control.

Never apply any rules literally – rules are merely guidelines – and the extremes of physical properties are not out of bounds, but carry additional risks and compromises.

## Key References

The original "Rule of Five" paper by Lipinski and co-workers remains a "must" read:

Experimental and computational approaches to estimate solubility and permeability in drug discovery and development settings C. A. Lipinski, F. Lombardo, B. W. Dominy and P. J. Feeney, *Adv. Drug Delivery Rev.*, 1997, **23**(1–3), 3–25.

Contemporary perspectives on the "Rule of Five":

C. P. Tinworth and R. J. Young, Facts, Patterns, and Principles in Drug Discovery: Appraising the Rule of 5 with Measured Physicochemical Data, *J. Med. Chem.*, 2020, **18**, 10091–10108.
D. A. DeGoey, H. J. Chen, P. B. Cox and M. D. Wendt, Beyond the Rule of 5: Lessons Learned from Abbvie's Drugs and Compound Collection, *J. Med. Chem.*, 2018, **61**, 2636–2651.

The origin of the lead-like concept:

The design of leadlike combinatorial libraries. S. J. Teague, A. M. Davis, P. D. Leeson and T. Oprea, *Angew. Chem., Int. Ed.*, 1999, **38**(24), 3743–3748.
Molecular Complexity and Its Impact on the Probability of Finding Leads for Drug Discovery, M. M. Hann, A. R. Leach and G. Harper, *J. Chem. Inf. Comp. Sci.*, 2001, **41**(3), 856–864.

Applications of efficiency metrics:

T. W. Johnson, R. A. Gallego and M. P. Edwards, Lipophilic Efficiency as an Important Metric in Drug Design, *J. Med. Chem.*, 2018, **61**, 6401–6420.
R. J. Young and P. D Leeson. Mapping the Efficiency and Physicochemical Trajectories of Successful Optimizations, *J. Med. Chem.*, 2018, **61**, 6421–6467.

## References


1. http://www.iupac.org/reports/1997/6905vanderwaterbeemd/index.html.
2. S. J. Gill and I. Wadso, *Proc. Natl. Acad. Sci. U. S. A.*, 1976, 73(9), 2955.
3. H. S. Frank and M. W. Evans, *J. Chem. Phys.*, 1945, **13**(11), 507.
4. T. P. Silverstein, *J. Chem. Educ.*, 1998, 75(1), 116.
5. A. M. Petros, J. R. Luly, H. Liang and S. W. Fesik, *J. Am. Chem. Soc.*, 1993, **115**(22), 9920.
6. L. David, M. Wenlock, P. Barton and A. Ritzen, *ChemMedChem*, 2021, **16**, 2669.
7. A. R. Fersht, in *Enzyme Structure and Mechanism*, W H Freeman, New York, 2nd edn, 1984, pp. 305–306.
8. V. N. Dorovskaya, S. D. Varfolomeyev, N. F. Kazanskaya, A. A. Klyosov and K. Martinek, *FEBS Lett.*, 1972, 23, 122.
9. J. Lang, *Chem. Eng. Data*, 2012, **57**, 2221.
10. C. Hansch, P. P. Maloney, T. Fujita and R. M. Muir, *Nature*, 1962, **194**, 178.
11. For a more detailed description of the emergence of this very first QSAR equation see T. Fujiita, *J. Comput.-Aided Mol. Des.*, 2011, **25**, 509.
12. J. Albert and J. Leo, *Chem. Rev.*, 1993, **93**(4), 1281.
13. M. C. Wenlock, T. Potter, P. Barton and R. P. Austin, *J. Biomol. Screening*, 2011, **16**(3), 348.
14. R. P. Austin, P. Barton, A. M. Davis, C. N. Manners and M. C. Stansfield, *J. Pharm. Sci.*, 1998, **87**(5), 599.
15. D. Quintanar-Guerrero, E. Alle´mann, H. Fessi and E. Doelker, *Pharm. Res.*, 1997, **14**, 119.
16. K. Gustavii, *Acta Pharm. Suec.*, 1967, **4**, 233.
17. K. Mazak and B. Noszal, *ChemMedChem*, 2020, **15**(13), 1102.
18. X. Ming, B. M. Knight and D. R. Thakker, *Mol. Pharm.*, 2011, **8**(5), 1677.
19. C. Chen, *Curr. Med. Chem.*, 2008, **15**(21), 2173.
20. S. M. R. Camargo, N. Vuille-dit-Bille, L. Mariotta, T. Ramadan, K. Huggel, D. Singer, O. Götze and F. Verrey, *J. Pharmacol. Exp. Ther.*, 2014, **351**(1), 114.
21. F. Haddad, M. Sawalha, Y. Khawaja, A. Najjar and R. Karaman, *Molecules*, 2018, **23**(1), 40/1–40/17.

22. M. J. Waring, *Expert Opin. Drug Discovery*, 2010, **5**, 235.
23. H. Meyer, *Naunyn-Schmiedebergs Arch. Exp. Pathol. Pharmakol.*, 1899, **42**, 109–118.
24. E. Overton, *Studien ¸ber die Narkose, zugleich ein Beitragzur allgemeinen Pharmakologie*, G. Fischer, Jena, 1901; English translation by R. L. Lipnick, Studies on Narcosis, Charles Ernest Overton, Chapman and Hall, London, 1991.
25. D. E. Leahy, P. J. Taylor and A. R. Wait, *Quant. Struct.-Act. Relat.*, 1989, **8**(1), 17.
26. R. P. Austin, P. Barton, A. M. Davis, R. F. Fessey and M. C. Wenlock, *Pharm. Res.*, 2005, **22**(10), 1649.
27. P. Barton, A. M. Davis, D. J. McCarthy and P. J. H. Webborn, *J. Pharm. Sci.*, 1997, **86**, 1034.
28. A. E. Cooper, D. Ferguson and K. Grime, *Curr. Drug Metab.*, 2012, **13**(4), 457.
29. M. Muehlbacher, P. Tripal, F. Roas and J. Kornhuber, *ChemMedChem*, 2012, **7**(11), 1925–1934, S1925/1-S1925/8.
30. B. Breiden and K. Sandhoff, *Biol. Chem.*, 2019, **401**(1), 31.
31. K. L. Valko, *J. Pharm. Biomed. Anal.*, 2016, **130**, 35.
32. K. Valko, C. Bevan and D. Reynolds, *Anal. Chem.*, 1997, **69**(11), 2022.
33. C. F. Poole and S. N. Atapattu, *J. Chromatogr. A*, 2020, **1626**, 461427.
34. K. Valko, *Physicochemical and Biomimetic Properties in Drug Discovery: Chromatographic Techniques for Lead Optimization*, John Wiley & Sons, Inc., Hoboken, NJ, 2014.
35. R. J. Young, D. V. S. Green, C. N. Luscombe and A. P. Hill, *Drug Discovery Today*, 2011, **16**(17/18), 822.
36. E. Galia, E. Nicolaides, D. Horter, R. Lobenberg, C. Reppas and J. B. Dressman, *Pharm. Res.*, 1998, **15**(5), 698.
37. J.-F. Fournie, C. Bouix-Peter, D. Duvert, A.-P. Luzy and G. Ouvry, *J. Med. Chem.*, 2018, **61**(7), 3231–3236.
38. A. J. Leo, *Chem. Rev.*, 1993, **93**, 1281.
39. http://www.biobyte.com/index.html.
40. http://www.daylight.com/.
41. A. K. Ghose and G. M. Crippen, *J. Chem. Inf. Comput. Sci.*, 1987, **27**, 21.
42. R. Mannhold, G. I. Poda, C. Ostermann and I. V. Tetko, *J. Pharm. Sci.*, 2009, **98**, 862.
43. R. P. Austin, P. Barton, R. V. Bonnert, R. C. Brown, P. A. Cage, D. R. Cheshire, A. M. Davis, I. G. Dougall, F. Ince and G. Pairaudeau, *et al.*, *J. Med. Chem.*, 2003, **46**(15), 3210.
44. https://openmolecules.org/datawarrior/index.html.
45. A. Daina, O. Michielin and V. Zoete, *Sci. Rep.*, 2017, **7**, 42717.
46. https://apps.apple.com/gb/app/medicinal-chemistry-toolkit/id910073742.
47. http://www.acdlabs.com/.
48. G. Xiong, Z. Wu, J. Yi, L. Fu, Z. Yang, C. Hsieh, M. Yin, X. Zeng, C. Wu, A. Lu, X. Chen, T. Hou and D. Cao, *Nucleic Acids Res.*, 2021, **49**, W5.
49. P. Bruneau and N. R. McElroy, *J. Chem. Inf. Model.*, 2006, **46**(3), 1379.
50. L. P. Hammett, *J. Am. Chem. Soc.*, 1937, **59**, 96.
51. J. N. Bronsted and K. Pedersen, *Phys. Chem.*, 1924, **108**, 185.
52. R. W. Taft, *J. Am. Chem. Soc.*, 1952, **74**, 2729, R. W. Taft, *J. Am. Chem. Soc.*, 1952, **74**, 3120, R. W. Taft, *J. Am. Chem. Soc.*, 1953, **75**, 4538.
53. C. G. Swain and E. C. Lupton Jr, *J. Am. Chem. Soc.*, 1968, **90**, 4328.
54. D. D. Perrin, B. Dempsey and E. P. Sergeant, *pKa Prediction for Organic Acids and Bases*, Springer 1981.
55. A. D. Bochevarov, M. A. Watson, J. R. Greenwood and D. M. Philipp, *J. Chem. Theory Comput.*, 2016, **12**(12), 6001.
56. F. Milletti, L. Storchi, G. Sforna and G. Cruciani, *J. Chem. Inf. Model.*, 2007, **47**(6), 2172.
57. K. Mansouri, N. F. Cariello, A. Korotcov, V. Tkachenko, C. M. Grulke, C. S. Sprankle, D. Allen, W. M. Casey, N. C. Kleinstreuer and A. J. Williams, *J. Cheminf.*, 2019, **11**, 60.
58. C. Jamieson, *J. Med. Chem.*, 2006, **49**, 5029.
59. C. Silipo and A. Vittoria, *Il Farmaco; Edizione Scientifica*, 1979, **34**, 858.
60. M. Morgenthaler, E. Schweizer, A. Hoffmann-Roder, F. Benini, R.E. Martin, G. Jaeschke, J. Schneidre, F. Diederich, M. Kansy, K. Muller, *ChemMedChem*, 2007, **2**, 1100.
61. M. B. van Niel, *et al.*, *J. Med. Chem.*, 1999, **42**, 2087.
62. P. S. Charifson and W. P. Walters, *J. Med. Chem.*, 2014, **57**, 9701.
63. R. A. Ndolo, Y. Luan, S. Duan, M. L. Forrest and J. P. Krise, *PLoS One*, 2012, **7**, e49366.
64. D. Diaz, K. A. Ford, D. P. Hartley, E. B. Harstad, G. R. Cain, K. Achilles-Poon, T. Nguyen, J. Peng, Z. Zheng, M. Merchant, D. P. Sutherlin, J. J. Gaudino, R. Kaus, S. C. Lewin-Koh, E. F. Choo, B. M. Liederer and D. M. Dambach, *Toxicol. Appl. Pharmacol.*, 2013, **266**, 86.
65. J.-U. Peters, T. Lübbers, A. Alanine, S. Kolczewski, F. Blasco and L. Steward, *Bioorg. Med. Chem. Lett.*, 2008, **18**, 262.

66. R. Aspiotis, A. Chen, E. Cauchon, D. Dubé, J.-P. Falgueyret, S. Gagné, M. Gallant, E. Grimm, R. Houle, H. Juteau, P. Lacombe, S. Laliberté, J.-F. Lévesque, D. MacDonald, D. McKay, M. D. Percival, P. Roy, S. M. Soisson and T. Wu, *Bioorg. Med. Chem. Lett.*, 2011, **21**, 2430.
67. M. H. Abraham, P. L. Grellier, D. V. Prior, R. W. Taft, J. J. Morris, P. J. Taylor, C. Laurence, M. Berthelot and R. M. Doherty, *J. Am. Chem. Soc.*, 1988, **110**(25), 8534.
68. M. H. Abraham, W. E. Acree Jr, A. J. Leo, D. Hoekman and J. E. Cavanaugh, *J. Pharm. Sci.*, 2010, **99**, 2492.
69. M. Shalaeva, G. Caron, Y. A. Abramov, T. N. O'Connell, M. S. Plummer, G. Yalamanchi, K. A. Farley, G. H. Goetz, L. Philippe and M. J. Shapiro, *J. Med. Chem.*, 2013, **56**(12), 4870.
70. H. van de Waterbeemd, G. Camenisch, G. G. Folkers, J. R. Chretien, O. A. Raevsky and A. J. Oleg, *Drug Target*, 1999, **6**, 151.
71. H. van de Waterbeemd, in *Methods for Assessing Oral Drug Absorption*, ed. J. Dressman, Dekker, New York, 2000, p. 31.
72. K. Palm, P. Stenberg, K. Luthman and P. Artursson, *Pharm. Res.*, 1997, **14**, 568.
73. T. T. Wager, X. Hou, P. R. Verhoest and A. Villalobos, *ACS Chem. Neurosci.*, 2010, **1**, 435.
74. T. T. Wager, X. Hou, P. R. Verhoest and A. Villalobos, *ACS Chem. Neurosci.*, 2016, **7**(6), 767.
75. A. R. Fersht, J.-P. Shi, J. Knill-Jones, D. M. Lowe, A. J. Wilkinson, D. M. Blow, P. Brick, P. Carter, M. M. Y. Waye and G. Winter, *Nature (London, U. K.)*, 1985, **314**(6008), 235.
76. D. H. Williams, M. S. Searle, J. P. Mackay, U. Gerhard and R. A. Maplestone, *Proc. Natl. Acad. Sci. U. S. A.*, 1993, **90**(4), 1172.
77. H. Parshad, K. Frydenvang, T. Liljefors and C. S. Larsen, *Int. J. Pharm.*, 2002, **237**, 193.
78. M. K. Bayliss, J. Butler, P. L. Feldman, D. V. Green, P. D. Leeson, M. R. Palovich and A. J. Taylor, *Drug Discovery Today*, 2016, **21**, 1719.
79. K. Johnson and A. Swindell, *Pharm. Res.*, 1996, **13**, 1795.
80. https://www.fda.gov/media/148472/download.
81. S. B. Murdande, M. J. Pikal, R. M. Shanker and R. H. Bogner, *Pharm. Dev. Technol.*, 2011, **16**(3), 187.
82. L. X. Yu, A. S. Carlin, G. L. Amidon. and A. S. Hussain, *Int. J. Pharm.*, 2004, **270**(1–2), 221.
83. A. Teleki, O. Nylander and C. A. S. Bergstrom, *Pharmaceutics*, 2020, **12**(6), 493.
84. N. Colclough, A. Hunter, P. W. Kenny, R. S. Kittlety, L. Lobedan, K. Y. Tam and M. A. Timms, *Bioorg. Med. Chem.*, 2008, **16**, 6611.
85. N. Jain and S. H. Yalkowsky, *J. Pharm. Sci.*, 2001, **90**(2), 234.
86. F. Lovering, J. Bikker and C. Humblet, *J. Med. Chem.*, 2009, **52**(21), 6752.
87. C. P. Tinworth and R. J. Young, *J. Med. Chem.*, 2020, **18**, 10091.
88. T. J. Ritchie and S. J. Macdonald, *J. Med. Chem.*, 2014, **57**, 7206.
89. C. A. Lipinski, F. Lombardo, B. W. Dominy and P. J. Feeney, *Adv. Drug Delivery Rev.*, 1997, **23**(1–3), 3.
90. S. J. Teague, A. M. Davis, P. D. Leeson and T. Oprea, *Angew. Chem., Int. Ed.*, 1999, **38**(24), 3743.
91. P. D. Leeson and A. M. Davis, *J. Med. Chem.*, 2004, **47**(25), 6338.
92. M. M. Hann, A. R. Leach and G. Harper, *J. Chem. Inf. Comput. Sci.*, 2001, **41**(3), 856.
93. *Drug Prototypes and Their Exploitation by Walter Sneader* (University of Strathclyde), John Wiley, Chichester, UK, 1996, xii + 788 pp. ISBN 0-471-94847-0.
94. D. Adams, *The Hitchhiker's Guide to the Galaxy*. Random House, 2007.
95. D. G. Brown and J. Boström, *J. Med. Chem.*, 2018, **61**, 9442.
96. F. Giordanetto, J. Boström and C. Tyrchan, *Drug Discovery Today*, 2011, **16**, 722.
97. G. R. Bickerton, G. V. Paolini, J. Besnard, S. Muresan and A. L. Hopkins, *Nat. Chem.*, 2012, **4**, 90.
98. G. Kuminek, F. Cao, A. Bahia de Oliveira da Rocha, S. Goncalves Cardoso and N. Rodriguez-Hornedo, *Adv. Drug Delivery Rev.*, 2016, **101**, 143.
99. P. Matsson, B. C. Doak, B. Over and J. Kihlberg, *Adv. Drug Delivery Rev.*, 2016, **101**, 42.
100. C. A. S. Bergstrom, W. N. Charman and C. J. H. Porter, *Adv. Drug Delivery Rev.*, 2016, **101**, 6.
101. B. C. Doak, J. Zheng, D. Dobritzsch and J. Kihlberg, *J. Med. Chem.*, 2016, **59**(6), 2312.
102. C. R. W. Guimaraes, A. M. Mathiowetz, M. Shalaeva, G. Goetz and S. Liras, *J. Chem. Inf. Model.*, 2012, **52**(4), 882.
103. J. H. McKerrow and C. A. Lipinski, *Int. J. Parasitology: Drugs Drug Resist.*, 2017, **7**, 248.
104. D. A. DeGoey, H. J. Chen, P. B. Cox and M. D. Wendt, *J. Med. Chem.*, 2018, **61**, 2636.
105. G. H. Goetz, W. Farrell, M. Shalaeva, S. Sciabola, D. Anderson, J. Yan, L. Philippe and M. J. Shapiro, *J. Med. Chem.*, 2014, **57**(7), 2920.
106. S. R. Sebastiano, B. C. Doak, M. Backlund, V. Poongavanam, B. Over, G. Ermondi, G. Caron, P. Matsson and J. Kihlberg, *J. Med. Chem.*, 2018, **61**, 4189.
107. K. M. Corbett, L. Ford, D. B. Warren, C. W. Pouton and D. K. Chalmers, *J. Med. Chem.*, 2021, **64**, 13131.

108. S. D. Edmondson, B. Yang and C. Fallan, *Bioorg. Med. Chem. Lett.*, 2019, **29**(13), 1555.
109. A. Pike, B. Williamson, S. Harlfinger, S. Martin and D. F. McGinnity, *Drug Discovery Today*, 2020, **25**(10), 1793.
110. D. F. McGinnity, J. Collington, R. P. Austin and R. J. Riley, *Curr. Drug Metab.*, 2007, **8**(5), 463.
111. M. D. Shultz, *J. Med. Chem.*, 2019, **62**, 1701.
112. M. P. Gleeson, P. D. Leeson and H. v. d. Waterbeemd, Physicochemical Properties and Compound Quality, in *The Handbook of Medicinal Chemistry: Principles and Practice*, ed. Davis, A. and Ward, S. E., The Royal Society of Chemistry, 2015; pp. 1–31.
113. A. L. Hopkins, G. M. Keseru, P. D. Leeson, D. C. Rees and C. H. Reynolds, *Nat. Rev. Drug Discovery*, 2014, **13**, 105.
114. P. D. Leeson and B. Springthorpe, *Nat. Rev. Drug Discovery*, 2007, **6**, 881.
115. I. D. Kuntz, K. Chen, K. A. Sharp and P. A. Kollman, *Proc. Natl. Acad. Sci. U. S. A.*, 1999, **96**, 9997.
116. A. L. Hopkins, C. R. Groom and A. Alex, *Drug Discovery Today*, 2004, **9**(10), 430.
117. T. I. Oprea, A. M. Davis, S. J Teague and P. D. Leeson, *J. Chem. Inf. Comput. Sci.*, 2001, **41**(5), 1308.
118. P. D. Leeson and S. A. St-Gallay, *Nat. Rev. Drug Discovery*, 2011, **10**, 749.
119. W. Jahnke, D. A. Erlanson, I. J. P. de Esch, C. N. Johnson, P. N. Mortenson, Y. Ochi and T. Urushima, *J. Med. Chem.*, 2020, **63**, 15494.
120. C. H. Reynolds, B. A. Tounge and S. D. Bembenek, *J. Med. Chem.*, 2008, **51**, 2432.
121. P. W. Kenny, A. Leitao and C. Montanari, *J. Comput.-Aided Mol. Des.*, 2014, **28**(7), 699.
122. P. W. Kenny, Journal of cheminformatics (2019), **11**, 8.
123. C. W. Murray, D. A. Erlanson, A. L. Hopkins, G. M. Keseru, P. D. Leeson, D. C. Rees, C. H. Reynolds and N. J. Richmond, *ACS Med. Chem. Lett.*, 2014, **5**, 616.
124. M. D. Shultz, *Bioorg. Med. Chem. Lett.*, 2013, **23**(21), 5992.
125. P. D. Leeson, A. P. Bento, A. Gaulton, A. Hersey, E. J. Manners, C. J. Radoux and A. R. Leach, *J. Med. Chem.*, 2021, **64**(11), 7210.
126. A. M. Davis, J. Dixon, C. J. Logan and D. W. Payling, *Ernst Schering Res. Found. Workshop*, 2002, **37**, 1.
127. R. R. Miller, M. Madeira, H. B. Wood, W. M. Geissler, C. E. Raab and I. J. Martin, *J. Med. Chem.*, 2020, **63**, 12156.
128. E. Perola, *J. Med. Chem.*, 2010, **53**, 2986.
129. R. J. Young and P. D. Leeson, *J. Med. Chem.*, 2018, **61**, 6421.
130. P. D. Leeson and R. J. Young, *ACS Med. Chem. Lett.*, 2015, **6**(7), 722.
131. T. W. Johnson, R. A. Gallego and M. P. Edwards, *J. Med. Chem.*, 2018, **61**, 6401.
132. J. S. Scott and M. J. Waring, *Bioorg. Med. Chem.*, 2018, **26**, 3006.
133. O. Ursu, A. Rayan, A. Goldblum and T. I. Oprea, *Wiley Interdiscip. Rev.: Comput. Mol. Sci.*, 2011, **1**, 760.
134. J. G. Cumming, A. M. Davis, S. Muresan, M. Haeberlein and H. Chen, *Nat. Rev. Drug Discovery*, 2013, **12**(12), 948.

# 2 Synthesis in Medicinal Chemistry

Allan M. Jordan*[a] and Robert J. Young[b]

[a]Sygnature Discovery, BioCity, Nottingham, NG1 1GR, UK; [b]Blue Burgundy Ltd, Ampthill, Bedfordshire, MK45 2AD, UK
*E-mail: a.jordan@sygnaturediscovery.com

## 2.1 The State of the Art – Where are We, and How did We Get Here?

The art and *practice* of synthetic organic chemistry underpins the entire repertoire of medicinal chemistry. Whilst molecular design, physicochemical properties and biological activity are often at the forefront of medicinal chemistry design philosophies, if the "ideal" molecule cannot be synthesised and submitted for biological evaluation, then the design process becomes meaningless. The efficient and pragmatic reduction to practice of those ideas is fundamental to the design–make–test cycle and, in many cases, becomes the rate-limiting step in the evaluation of potential new medicines. As target molecules become increasingly complex and challenging, exploring both new molecular characteristics and emerging new therapeutic modalities, the contribution of synthetic chemistry is experiencing a resurgence of both interest and importance. In this chapter, we review the evolution of synthetic chemistry in drug discovery, charting the trends in synthetic practices. We consider how the daily activities of the drug discovery chemist have changed and the drivers behind these shifting patterns. We then consider recent trends within the industry, and where current and future advances may help in the delivery of more biologically relevant molecules. Finally, case studies will be used to illustrate the evolving and innovative landscape of synthetic medicinal chemistry and thoughts on the future directions of the field will be summarised.

The Handbook of Medicinal Chemistry: Principles and Practice, 2nd Edition
Edited by Simon E. Ward and Andrew M. Davis

Published by the Royal Society of Chemistry, www.rsc.org

### 2.1.1 The Evolving Landscape of Synthetic Medicinal Chemistry – Changes in Discovery Practices

Twenty years ago, molecules designed and synthesised by medicinal chemists were often structurally simple, relying on hydrophobic interactions for potency and, as a result, the compounds suffered from less-than-ideal physicochemical properties. A recent publication[1] anecdotally suggested that, amongst non-chemists in the industry, there was a belief that the molecules delivered into screening cascades largely consisted of compounds resulting from:

- An amide coupling reaction
- A metal-mediated aryl–aryl coupling reaction
- Four to six synthetic steps
- An avoidance of chirality

Furthermore, analyses of synthetic practices suggested that medicinal chemists tended to gravitate toward a limited set of key reactions. Whilst these reactions were powerful tools for the rapid construction of multiple analogues, their exploitation limited exploration to a constrained set of molecular architectures.[2]

These anecdotal observations prompted more detailed analyses of the reactions commonly employed by the medicinal chemist, in an effort to define what has come to be referred to as "the Medicinal Chemist's Toolbox", a lexicon of the tools and techniques most often used to prepare new molecules for biological evaluation. The first such study, published in 2011,[1] sought to challenge the preconceptions around limited synthetic methodology and highlight the creativity of the synthetic chemist. A review of the published outputs of selected major pharmaceutical organisations over a single year, as a representative snapshot of medicinal chemistry as a whole, made disappointing reading. The analysis surveyed the synthesis of over 3500 molecules and almost 140 publications and, in essence, confirmed the anecdotal observations previously noted. It indicated that synthesis in medicinal chemistry had become highly focussed upon a small set of key reaction types and largely ignored the complexity and depth of methodology available to the synthetic chemist. Applied methodology focussed primarily on the construction of planar heterocyclic scaffolds, which were decorated *via* amide formation and palladium-mediated biaryl couplings. The limited inclusion of saturation and chirality led to flat molecules with little shape or conformational flexibility, such as the "prototypical" compounds **1** and **2** (Figure 2.1).

Concerningly, such rigid, highly aromatic entities are reported to often carry with them problematic properties such as off-target promiscuity and poor solubility, effectively building in biological attributes that the medicinal chemist must later fight to overcome. Analysis of these physicochemical properties over time revealed that, whilst the synthetic chemist's productivity has increased significantly over the past fifty years, molecular quality[3] has declined significantly.[4] The average molecular weight and lipophilicity of molecules steadily increased over time, with concomitant decreases in saturation and chirality. Trends in these parameters, which are used to define compound quality, indicated that modern synthetic practices were furnishing molecules with

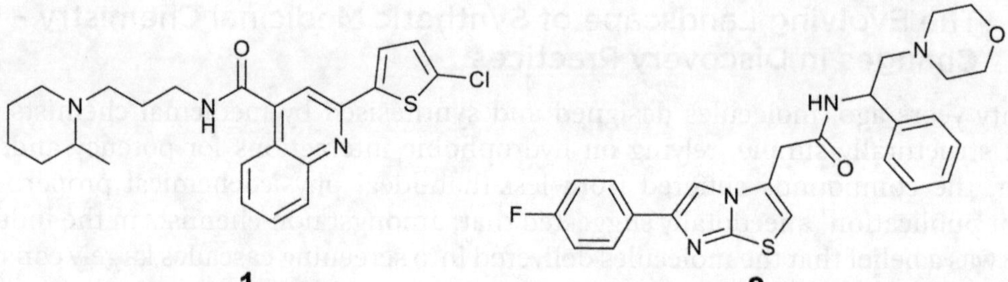

1 2

**Figure 2.1** Hypothetical "typical" medicinal chemistry compounds representative of the averaged data in ref. 1.

properties migrating further and further from those of approved orally bioavailable drugs.

Whilst this analysis examined molecular properties over time, the actual routes used for molecular construction were not assessed in detail and, until recently, the changing landscape of synthetic chemistry had not been examined. Extrapolating back over three decades, more detailed analysis suggests that the "simplification" and reductionist approach to synthetic chemistry is not a recent trend, with similar reaction types and frequencies in both datasets.[5] Whilst cross-coupling methodology was only becoming prevalent three decades ago, much of the common synthetic armoury has evolved little in the intervening time. However, it was shown that many of the "textbook" reactions taught at undergraduate level, such as the Wittig reaction, Friedel–Crafts acylation, diazotisation, olefin preparation and oxidation/reduction chemistries, have seen a significant decline in application in recent times.

There is evidence, therefore, that synthesis in medicinal chemistry has become decreasingly creative and complex since the prevalent practice shifted towards molecularly targeted agents, usually identified by *in vitro* screening. In the early post-war period of the 1950s, as medicinal chemistry was beginning to establish itself as a specific discipline in drug discovery, programmes were usually defined by the nature of the target under investigation and the natural ligands associated with that target.[6] The requirement to produce and modify complex natural products such as corticosteroids, opioids and beta-lactam antibiotics led to the development of complex and elegant synthetic pathways to allow the construction and modification of close analogues and a resurgence of research into new synthetic methodology to facilitate the construction of these more complex derivatives.

So, what changed? Why did the pursuit of natural products and natural product-like structures decline in favour of "blander" molecules with poorer physicochemical and biological properties?

In the 1980s, significant advances in molecular biology began to re-shape approaches to the discovery of new medicines and the investigation of new biological targets. The ability to clone, express and purify novel proteins allowed the large-scale production and investigation of emerging targets such as kinases and other disease-critical enzymes. Greater availability of isolated protein allowed a step-change in the evaluation of new molecules and their ability to interact with biologically relevant molecules. Such evaluations could be undertaken in simple, plate-based *in vitro* assays, and allowed a move away from complex, cell- or tissue-based phenotypic assays, at least for the earlier stages of drug discovery. This reductionist approach to biology significantly increased the throughput of compound evaluation and, in doing so, dramatically increased the demand for novel compounds to be evaluated. These advances ultimately resulted in the evolution of high-throughput screening (HTS) technologies and the ability to screen millions of compounds against many targets, in an effort to find the one "magic bullet" that inhibited the target of interest in a potent and selective manner. Chemistry, rather than biology, became the rate-limiting step in drug discovery.

To adapt to this challenge, the medicinal chemists turned to robust, reliable reaction types that could rapidly deliver families of analogues for testing, rather than considered, thoughtful and carefully designed bespoke derivatives. Speed and quantity became a key metric in synthetic chemistry, and the more traditional, holistic approach to drug-likeness and the likelihood of appropriate *in vivo* drug action was considered less and less. In retrospective analyses, this change in mindset, from quality to quantity, is often blamed on the advent of high-throughput screening (HTS), but the recent analyses already mentioned suggest that this reductionist approach was already becoming ingrained in drug discovery before the advent and ubiquitous adoption of HTS as a primary screening tool.[4]

Whilst perhaps not solely responsible, the advent of HTS methodology did lead to the rise in popularity of high-throughput and combinatorial chemistry, both within the pharmaceutical industry and within a new synthetic chemistry sector – the screening compound vendor. To satisfy this voracious appetite for compounds to screen, particularly from organisations new to the industry and therefore lacking established and diverse historical collections of compounds to draw upon, a new ecosystem of vendors evolved. These companies concentrated upon robust, reliable synthetic methodology to rapidly create extensive libraries of "drug-like" compounds, compliant with the oral bioavailability guidelines popularised at around the same time by Lipinski and co-workers.[7] To deliver significant chemical diversity in realistic timeframes, in order to meet these demands, it is unsurprising that reliance upon robust methodology became prevalent. In time, these compound libraries yielded preliminary hits in HTS and other screening methodologies and became the start-points for new medicinal chemistry programmes. In turn, exploration of these start-points demanded rapid access to related compounds, also synthesised using similar methodologies for expediency. This cycle of self-reinforcement has, over time, led to a dependence upon the relatively small number of chemistries described in the review literature (Figure 2.2).

### 2.1.2 Why Do We Use the Reactions We Use?

Given the lack of diversity in synthetic methods regularly employed in drug discovery, in contrast to the wide diversity of available synthetic methodology, it is worthwhile considering what defines a "good" reaction for the medicinal chemist, and why, particularly, certain reactions have become predominant in the pursuit of new medicines. Those reactions which are popular and prevalent in drug discovery

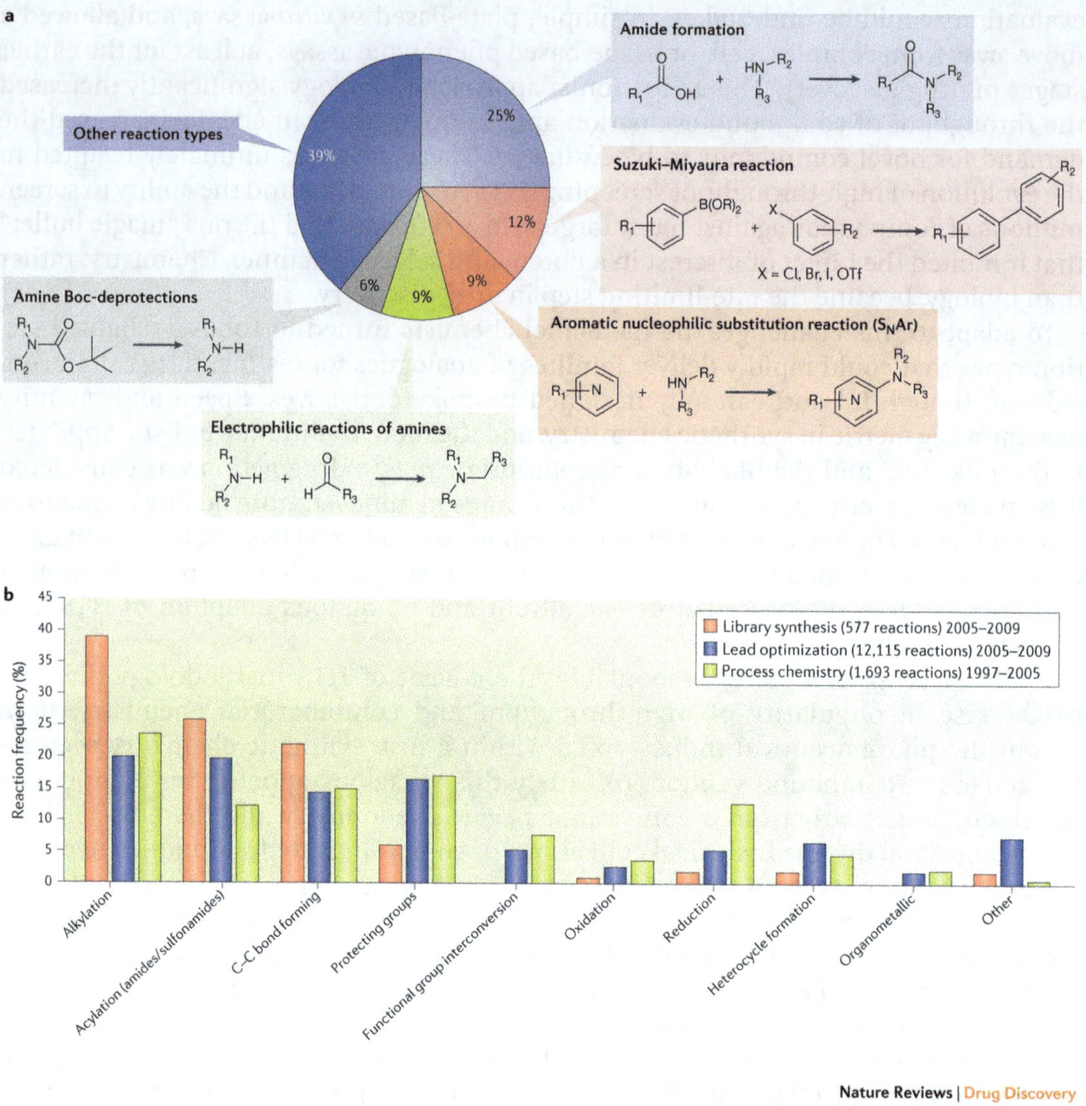


**Figure 2.2** Common chemical reactions in drug discovery and development showing (a) distributions of common reaction types frequently used in discovery and (b) comparisons of reaction frequencies in library synthesis, lead optimisation and process chemistry. Reproduced from ref. 3 with permission from Springer Nature, Copyright 2018.

laboratories are generally governed by a single unifying factor – expedience. In the early stages of a drug discovery project, each individual molecule has only limited specific value – whilst potency, stability, solubility and other factors critical to future success as a medicine have not been demonstrated, each molecule serves primarily to answer a simple structure–activity question. As this question may be answered by one or more alternate analogues, there is often perceived to be little benefit in striving to construct an elaborate and unique route to a specific analogue when an alternate, more easily accessible compound may suffice. As a project progresses, this value proposition per molecule changes as compounds are designed and prepared in a more thoughtful and specific fashion to tailor and fine-tune biological and physicochemical properties to deliver the "Goldilocks" molecule – the one that is "just right" for clinical evaluation.

In the earlier stages, then, reactions are prioritised toward those which reliably and repeatedly generate molecules with minimal failure rates, irrespective of the structure of the actual molecule of choice. New reactions face a high hurdle prior to widespread acceptance and demand a certain level of evidence of utility before becoming part of routine use. Generally, to be widely accepted into the "Medicinal Chemist's Toolbox", a novel reaction must satisfy certain key criteria:

i. Ready availability of reagents
ii. Functional group tolerance
iii. Reliability
iv. "Fit for purpose"

It is also helpful if these reactions do not rely on specialist equipment, have compelling literature precedent, and avoid risky or problematic reagents.[8] The importance and relevance of each of the factors above will be considered in turn.

### 2.1.2.1 Reagent Availability

At the outset of most new reaction development, it is evident that the availability of diverse reagents is unlikely to be in place, particularly if uncommon functionality is important to successful reactivity. Whilst palladium-mediated cross-couplings of boronic acids and esters became rapidly established as a powerful and robust synthetic technique, boronic acid derivatives were not commonplace in reagent catalogues. However, one of the significant features of this methodology was not just the utility of the reaction itself, but the accompanying ease of reagent preparation from common halogenated aromatic systems. This simple access to a diverse selection of reagents which could be prepared at will without significant impact on productivity quickly led to the adoption of these coupling techniques into mainstream synthetic planning and execution. As prevalence increased, reagent vendors were quick to react to both the demand for reagents and the ease of their production, which soon led to extensive and cheap access to many hundreds, if not thousands, of boronic acid and boronate ester precursors. Similarly, simple amine acylation remains highly popular for rapid investigation of structure–activity relationships given the commercial availability of many thousands of carboxylic acids, activated acids and related sulphonyl chlorides, isocyanates *etc.*, which can quickly yield families of related amides, esters, sulphonamides, carbamates and ureas for evaluation. Indeed, emerging novel reaction methodologies which employ commonly available functionality alongside factors such as long-term stability at room temperature, such as carboxylic acids, have significantly greater appeal to the community and as such increase their likelihood of widespread adoption.[9]

### 2.1.2.2 Tolerance of Functionality

Hit expansion, the first stage of most drug discovery projects, is the process of evaluating a putative molecule against a biological target and understanding how the interactions between the molecule and target may be improved. In this stage, various factors are investigated in parallel, to understand their impact on binding and potency. Compounds are prepared to investigate spatial arrangements of functionality, and the available space the molecule may be able to occupy. But also investigated are the nature of the interactions with the putative binding site and these investigations require the incorporation of a wide range of molecular functionality, such as acidic and basic groups, electron rich and deficient functionality, hydrogen bonding acceptors and donors *etc.* Ideally, all the functionalities will be installed at various positions around the core scaffold, and with a variety of orientations – *e.g.* amides, reverse amides and ureas. Whilst such groups are similar in many ways, they can offer widely differing biological activities and pharmacokinetic outcomes. Preparation of this diverse set of exploratory structures would require the utilisation of many building blocks, with considerable diversity of molecular properties, reactivity, and architecture.

Ideally, novel reaction methodology would be flexible enough to remain reliable in the presence of these very different reaction partners, permitting reactivity under conditions generally applicable for highly variable reactivity and solubility.[10] However, for many new reactions, utility is demonstrated only on a limited handful of new substrates, generally with apolar functionality, such as phenyl rings and small alkyl substituents.[11] Whilst these early demonstrations of methodology are understandable, a more comprehensive assessment of the functional group tolerance (or otherwise) of a novel method is critical to gaining wider acceptance and this process can require significant time and effort before a reaction becomes trustworthy. Moreover, until these tolerances are better known and can be accounted for, overall reaction outcomes tend to favour more lipophilic reaction products, with those reactions incorporating polar reagents and building blocks tending to be the ones most likely to fail. Given these reaction types are likely to be used to generate arrays or libraries of molecules for early SAR elaboration, such polarity-related failures skew the outcomes (and potential project start points) toward less favourable chemical space. Indeed, a recent review noted that without care and mitigation the resultant, high log*P* biased, compounds from such libraries may be anywhere from ten times to ten thousand times more lipophilic than would be desirable for a small molecule drug discovery programme.[12]

### 2.1.2.3 Reliability and Robustness

A widely applicable reaction will tend to be both reliable and robust. Reliability extends beyond functional group tolerance and suggests that reactivity is maintained across a variety of core templates, such that the reaction can be used to construct a variety of molecular architectures. Amide couplings, for example are reliable across a broad range of aliphatic and aromatic amines, largely irrespective of the other pendant functionality already present in those templates and precursor molecules. Further, the reaction is also generally robust, in that it is highly tolerant of minor variations of reaction condition, concentration, temperature *etc*. This tolerance of condition, especially when combined with mild, easily achievable conditions and absence of specialist techniques and equipment, often helps lead to rapid adoption of both reaction types and general methodologies. Contrast for example, the rapid adoption of microwave chemistry, where a single instrument could be applied to a wide variety of synthetic processes to improve productivity and permit reactions otherwise problematic, to the slower adoption of flow chemistry. Whilst flow chemistry is finally gaining a wider acceptance and adoption and can offer significant productivity and safety advantages in certain transformations, the requisite apparatus became available at a similar time to microwave devices but the necessity for specific optimisation on a reaction-by-reaction basis led to a much more gradual and case-specific adoption of the technology.

#### *2.1.2.4 "Fit for Purpose"*

Any reaction that delivers acceptable product yield could be defined as being "fit for purpose", however, this definition will change as a compound progresses through the drug discovery process. It may be that in the early stages of the project, simply delivering sufficient material to allow biological evaluation may be acceptable. However, when a particular derivative proves to be of interest, then a consideration of the longer-term suitability of the synthetic route becomes important, and inappropriate choices of methodology can significantly add to timelines later on in the project. Increasingly, factors such as scalability, purification methodology and atom efficiency are being considered at earlier stages to ensure that potentially beneficial molecules can be more easily transferred to scale up, initially to support *in vivo* evaluation of biological activity and eventually for the support of pre-clinical and clinical studies. For these reasons, there has been considerable recent effort in developing novel atom-efficient transformations which avoid toxic or troublesome reagents, environmentally damaging solvents and difficult purifications, to aid the transition from laboratory-scale synthesis to production on the multi-kilo (or greater) scale.

Similarly, greater thought is now often given not just to the specific reactions utilised, but also to the order in which the steps are undertaken. For example, prioritising metal-mediated couplings earlier in the synthesis, to reduce overall contamination in the final product, is a common tactic to reduce later purification difficulties and careful synthetic strategy can help alleviate unnecessary use of protecting groups and their inevitable deprotection. Such decisions, particularly around exothermic reactions, can also have dramatic effects upon safety.

### 2.1.3 We are Where we are – but Does it Matter?

Clearly, from the preceding discussion, synthesis lies at the heart of medicinal chemistry, but the inappropriate or metric-driven use of synthetic chemistry can have significant detrimental effects on our drug discovery projects, be it in facile production of potent molecules with poor physicochemical properties or the poor choice of reaction which slow latter development. Some prudent thought and synthetic expertise early in the process can make dramatic improvements in the overall success of these programmes, ultimately offering significant potential to deliver clinical success and patient benefit. Some areas for consideration, in the pursuit of these aims, are discussed in the following section.

## 2.2 How to Improve Molecules Through Synthesis

A recurring question for synthetic chemistry is "what kind of reactions or molecules are of interest or value for drug discovery programmes?", to which a correct answer might be that it depends on the target under investigation. The answer fits in correctly interpreting innovation – this is not the use of technology or methodology for their own sakes, but to consider the problem or issue being addressed and developing the most appropriate synthetic or biomimetic solution. To illustrate successful techniques and strategies where synthesis has impacted drug discovery, a number of case studies are used as examples in the following subsections.

### 2.2.1 Some Historic Examples where Synthesis Enabled Discovery

An historic example of the application of synthesis to meet an unmet medical need was the mobilisation of British academics in the 1950s to address the UK national need for cortisone.[13] This led to innovative solutions to address production requirements utilising bulk intermediates furnished from natural sources (Figure 2.3), within the machinations of international politics and industrial secrecy. Spin-offs from research in this area established Glaxo as a lead player in the corticosteroid field. Concurrently, work led by Carl Djerassi on the synthesis of cortisone from diosgenin found in Mexican wild yam roots was extended to the sex hormones estrone and estrodiol, followed by the synthesis of progesterones from strophanthidins (Figure 2.4), which established Syntex as a global leader in steroid hormone analogues, paving the way for oral contraceptives. This illustrates the impact of innovative synthetic or semi-synthetic solutions to address supply issues and the power of diversification around an endogenous structure.

More recently, synthetic innovations were key to delivering efficacy with the anti-viral nucleoside analogues sofosbuvir (an efficacious element of hepatitis C treatments) and remdesivir (developed for Ebola virus infections but since repurposed in the treatment of SARS-CoV-2 infection in Covid-19 cases, Figure 2.5). Sofosbuvir is a uridine analogue

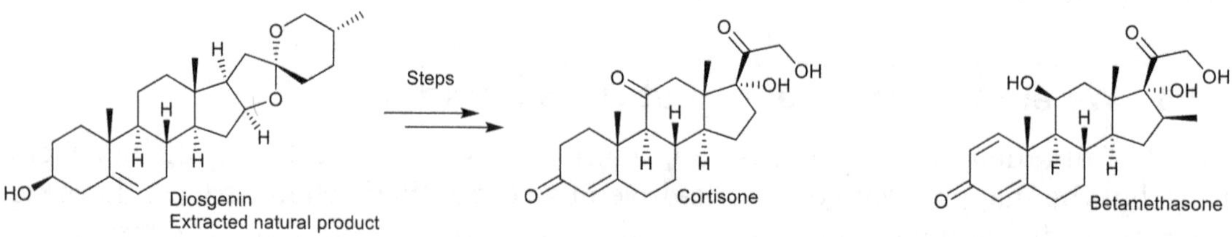


**Figure 2.3** Diosgenin, a key element towards the sustainable production of cortisone, the pioneering synthetic glucocorticoid; betamethasone – a semi-synthetic next generation glucocorticoid that helped establish Glaxo in the field.

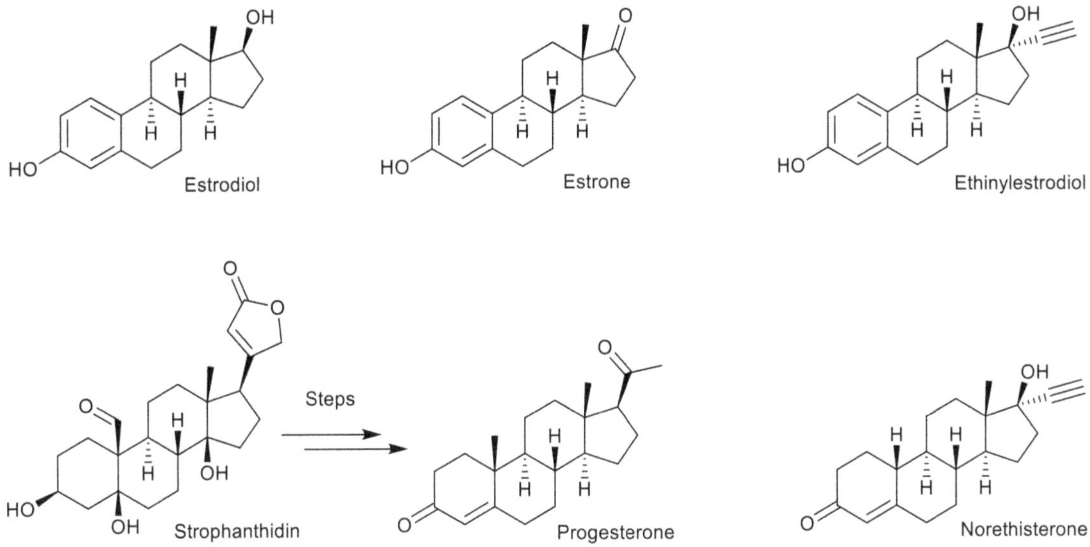


**Figure 2.4** The structures of estrodiol, estrone and ethinylestrodiol (an early synthetic estrogen used in the contraceptive pill) derived from diosgenin process. Modification of extracted stropanthidin aglycone led to synthetic progesterones used in combination with estrogens.

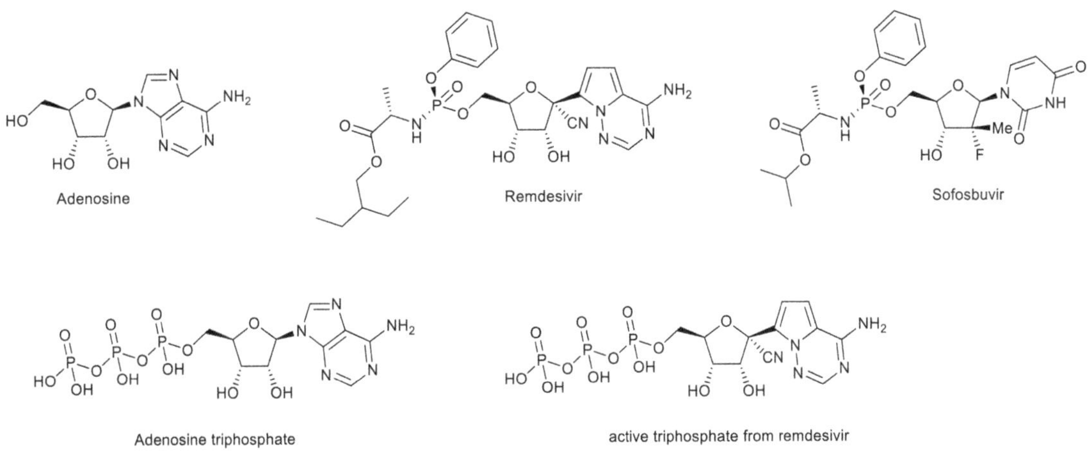


**Figure 2.5** Adenosine and its triphosphate, with the antiviral prodrugs remdesivir and sofosbuvir with the active triphosphate form of remdesivir.

with a synthetically modified ribose ring (methylation and fluorination at the 2′ position – see Section 2.2.2) and incorporates a ProTide (= PROdrug + nucleotide)-phosphoramidate ester on the 5′-hydroxyl that is an effective prodrug of the nucleotide. ProTides were designed and developed in the McGuigan group at Cardiff University and provided an elegant solution to the issue of delivering nucleotides to the site of action in virus-infected cells (Figure 2.6). The phosphorylation of nucleosides is often a barrier to achieving anti-viral activity and phosphorylation to yield the monophosphate/

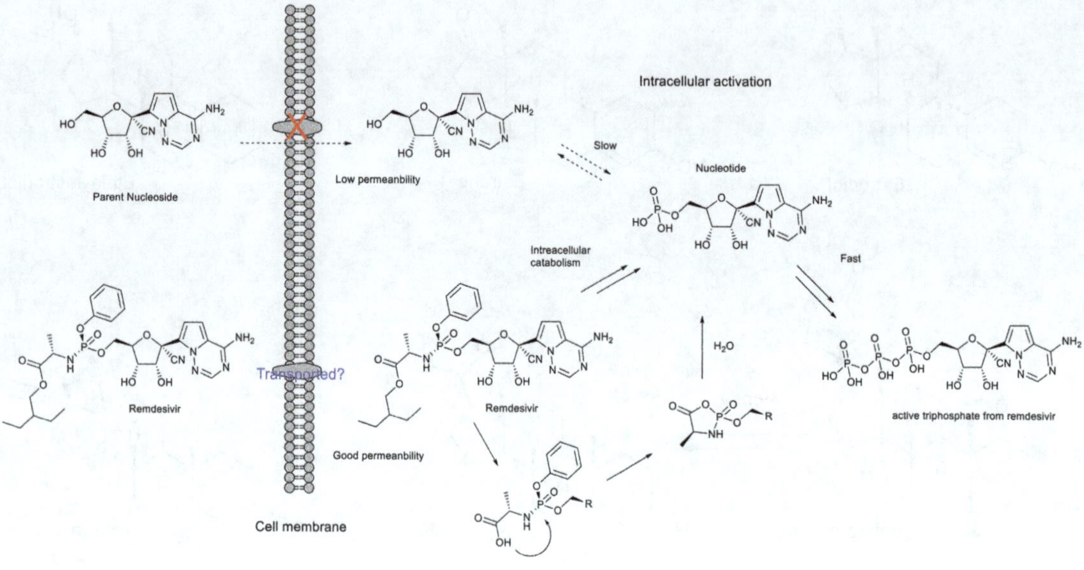


**Figure 2.6** The chemistry of ProTide prodrugs, exemplified by the intracellular processing of remdesivir, providing a solution to both cell permeability and nucleotide formation.

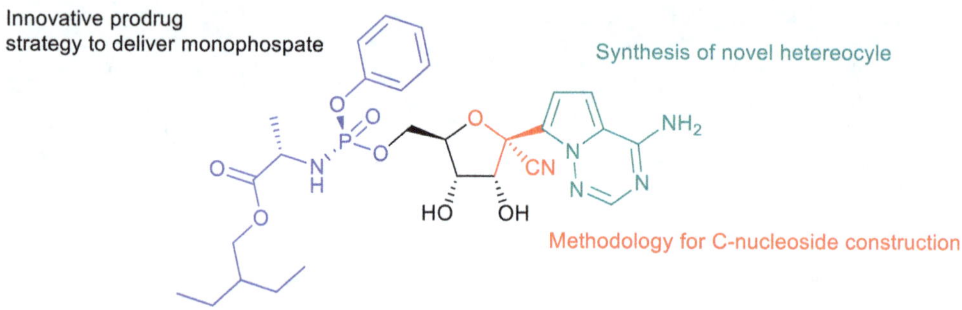


**Figure 2.7** Synthetic innovations combined to enable efficacy with remdesivir.

nucleotide is often a rate-limiting step in the bioactivation of nucleoside analogues, preventing formation of the nucleoside triphosphate necessary for activity. Remdesivir, like sofosbuvir, also features a ProTide motif, plus a unique chiral ribose mimetic *C*-linked to an uncommon heterocycle (see Section 2.2.2) to mimic adenosine, this *C*-linkage enhancing stability to purine nucleoside phosphorylase enzymes. Metabolism and phosphorylation of remdesivir ultimately delivers the active triphosphate, which mimics adenosine triphosphate, in the intracellular environment (Figure 2.6). In these exemplars, synthetic chemists have successfully delivered complex molecules to answer challenging biological problems, whilst continuing synthetic work delivers new opportunities to explore new analogues and address synthetic challenges in nucleoside chemistry (Figure 2.7).[14] Similarly, in the development of zidovudine (AZT™), the first licenced medicine to treat HIV, a major issue was the limited availability of thymidine (historically, supplies were extracted from herring sperm!), a need addressed by

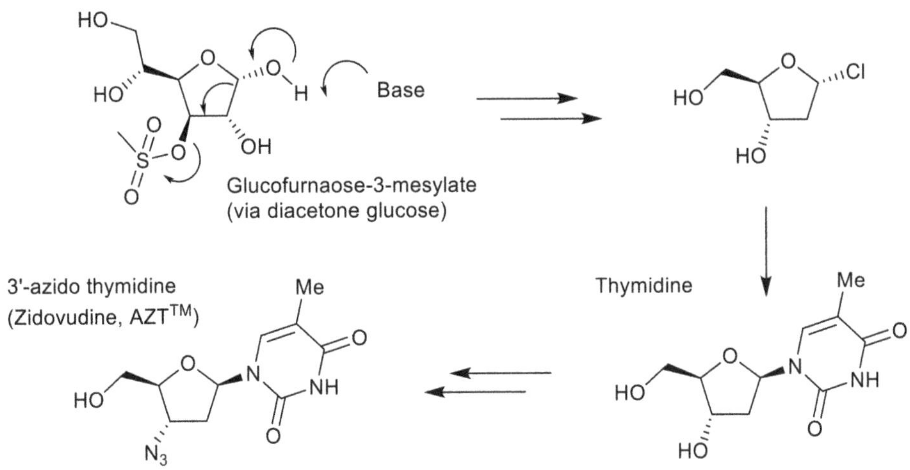


**Scheme 2.1** Outline of the large-scale synthesis of thymidine used as an intermediate for the synthesis of zidovudine.

chemistry from glucose *via* the α-chloro deoxyriboside (Scheme 2.1). Such examples highlight the pivotal role of innovative and creative synthetic chemistry in the evolution of drug discovery, a role which has perhaps been unfairly downplayed in recent times.

The following sections look in detail at some other themes where synthetic innovation has proved enabling in drug discovery and has directly led to the development of improved therapeutics, whilst recognising that further opportunities exist to expand the efficiency and throughput of techniques and generality of reactions.

### 2.2.2 Four Strategies to Improve Molecules: Methylation, Hydroxylation, Fluorination and Heterocycles

The headline changes of this subsection are four established means of improving the physicochemical profile of experimental molecules.[15] As such, all are worthy of consideration in the optimisation of new bioactive molecules, in combination with principles that increase the proportion of $sp^3$-hybridised centres and/or decrease the number of aromatic rings in experimental structures (Table 2.1).

i. *Methylation*, unlike the following three modifications, will generally increase the lipophilicity of a molecule, but can have a profound impact on conformation and binding interactions, thus modulating activity and properties. The effect of a "magic methyl" is an often-encountered concept,[16] sometimes improving activity by orders of magnitude, blocking unwanted off-target effects, or influencing intra- or intermolecular interactions to impact solubility and DMPK outcomes, and methods are emerging for late-stage installation.[17]
ii. Increasingly, the role of *fluorine* in conformational control is impacting drug discovery, well beyond its utility as a metabolism blocker in aromatic systems.[18] In particular, the impact of adding a fluorine atom on an aliphatic carbon reduces intrinsic lipophilicity, strongly modulates the p$K_a$ of any neighbouring charged

**Table 2.1** Examples of four strategies that can profoundly influence medicinal chemistry outcomes with single-atom changes.[3]

**i. Methylation**[27]

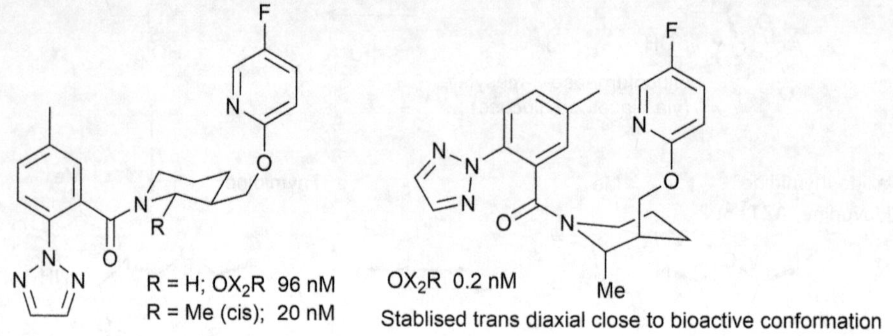


**ii. Fluorination**[28]

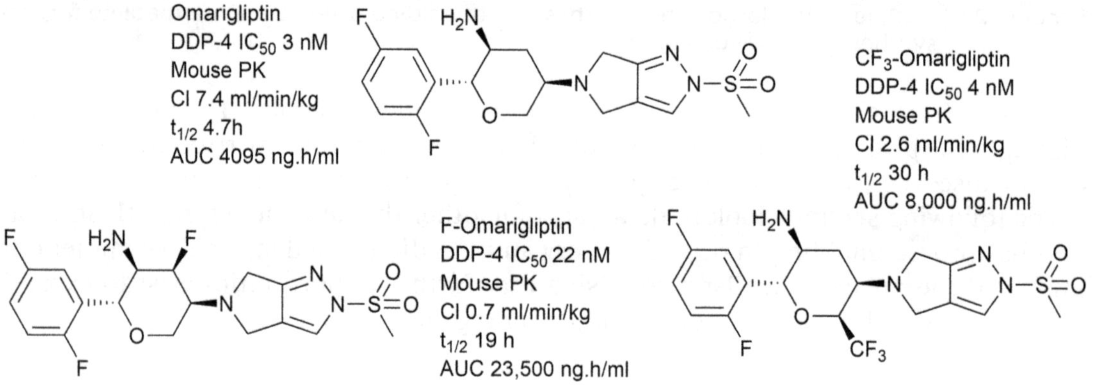


**iii. Hydroxylation**[29]

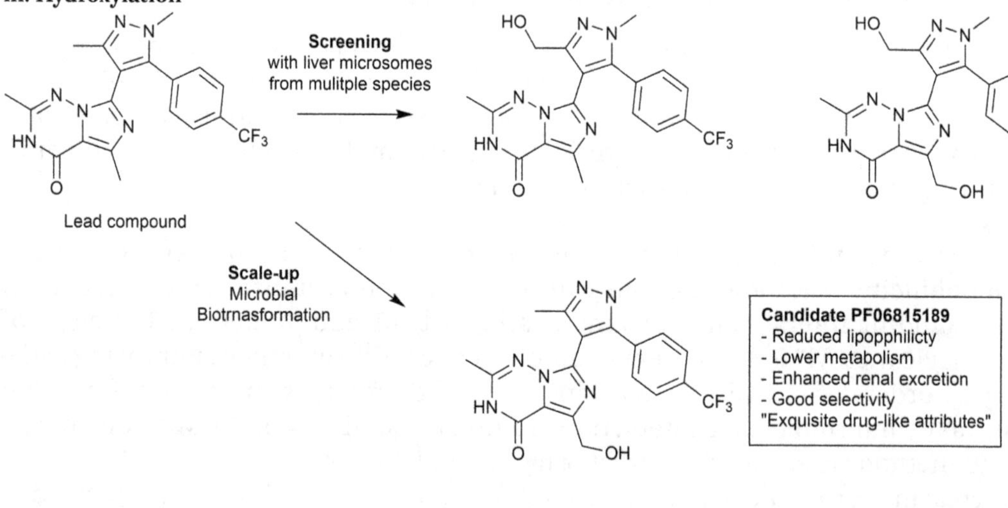

Table 2.1 *(continued)*

**iv. Necessary nitrogens**[30]

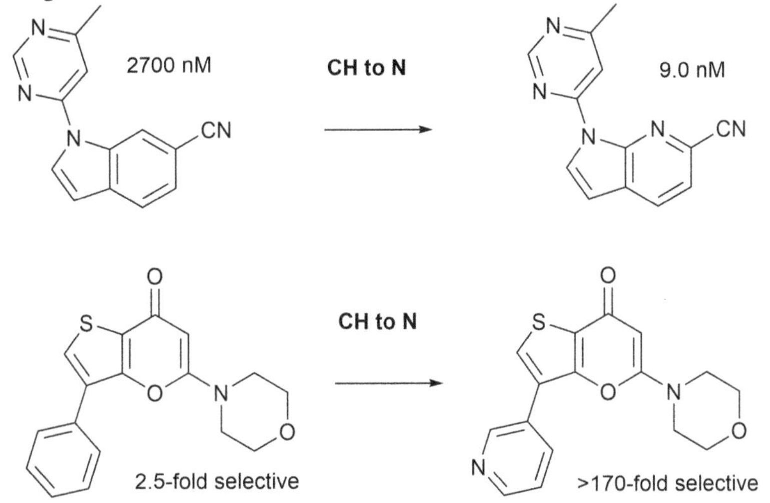


centres and there is a strong preference for it to stabilise a conformation where it is gauche to heteroatoms on neighbouring carbon centres.[19]

iii. *Hydroxyl groups* are ubiquitous in nature and common in drug structures;[20] they profoundly reduce lipophilicity and can form important intra- and intermolecular hydrogen bonds.

iv. *Heterocyclic replacements or necessary nitrogens*: nearly all drug molecules contain at least one ring structure, be it aromatic, semi-saturated or aliphatic and the most important variants on these themes incorporate one or more heteroatoms in a heterocyclic structure.[21] Such features are important on many levels,[22] including synthetic accessibility, ligand mimicking, making necessary interactions/hydrogen bonds, conformational influences, and property modulation.[23] Heteroaromatic chemistry, often furnishing biomimetic structures, is seemingly out of fashion, yet many potential structures remain unexplored,[24] so new and efficient syntheses and flexible derivatisation protocols remain highly attractive for discovery programmes. Indeed, if an aromatic ring needs to be incorporated in a structure, it is often best to make it a heterocyclic one that will generally reduce lipophilicity. In recent years, moves to reduce aromatic ring counts, the "escape from flatland", whilst minimising flexibility (rotatable bond count) encouraged new thinking and synthetic methodology to access necessarily chiral functionalised molecules and imaginative spirocyclic variants.[25,26]

### 2.2.3 Better Late-stage Functionalisation

Modern drug discovery is often based on screening hits that are derived from somewhat prosaic transformations. This often imposes a barrier to the pursuit of more synthetically complex molecules, natural products or natural-product-like skeletons that cannot be rapidly synthesised in iterative steps from readily available building blocks. This limited

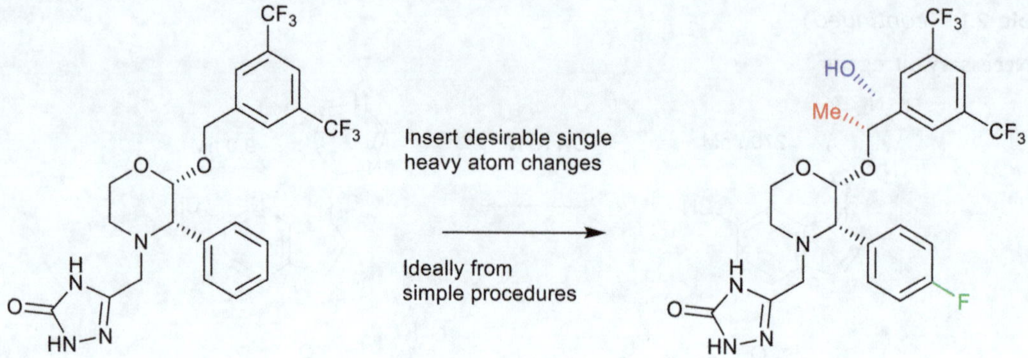


**Scheme 2.2** Examples and aspirations for late-stage functionalisation summarised in recent reviews.[31]

mindset could be expanded through exploitation of the developing range of late-stage functionalisation reactions (Scheme 2.2).[31] Such methodology allows facile exploration of three of the tactics suggested in Section 2.2.2, namely alkylation, hydroxylation and fluorination of hit structures, which can be accomplished using synthetic/biosynthetic and hybrids of these methodologies.[32] These methods not only diversify structures for SAR studies but can also improve physicochemical properties. Additionally, insight into sites of metabolism and/or a means of synthesising metabolites can prove invaluable, whilst sometimes identifying a means of circumventing the problem with a novel derivative. The use of such derivatisation circumvents the need to repeat entire synthetic routes to introduce variations on common synthetic intermediates. Further innovation in this area will undoubtedly enable more complex regio- and stereochemical control and improve access to these important changes with lesser impact on synthetic routes and timelines. However, the aspirational interconversion of carbocyclic ring structures into heterocycles remains significantly more difficult, so their introduction requires enhanced synthetic planning and/or modelling from the start. Of course, more modular or convergent syntheses offer more flexible opportunities to induce the suggested and other variations into the structures being optimised, but such optimisations will be necessarily constrained to the frequently used reactions and the ubiquitous motifs they produce.

New technologies that enable methodologies based on combinations of photoredox catalysis,[33] transition metal catalysis, radical chemistry and redox-[34]/electrochemistry[35] are starting to expand the toolbox for additional late-stage functionalisations and offer novel structural diversity (Figure 2.8). Examples are emerging where combinations of synthetic methods are used in conjunction with HPLC purification and microscale analysis techniques to diversify structures providing micrograms of products that are sufficient for primary testing (Figure 2.9).

### 2.2.4 Biotransformations

The employment of biotransformations in drug discovery is often not a reaction of first choice, but in many cases such methods are exploited in the manufacture of the active pharmaceutical ingredients. Yet, historically, many drugs (such as β-lactam

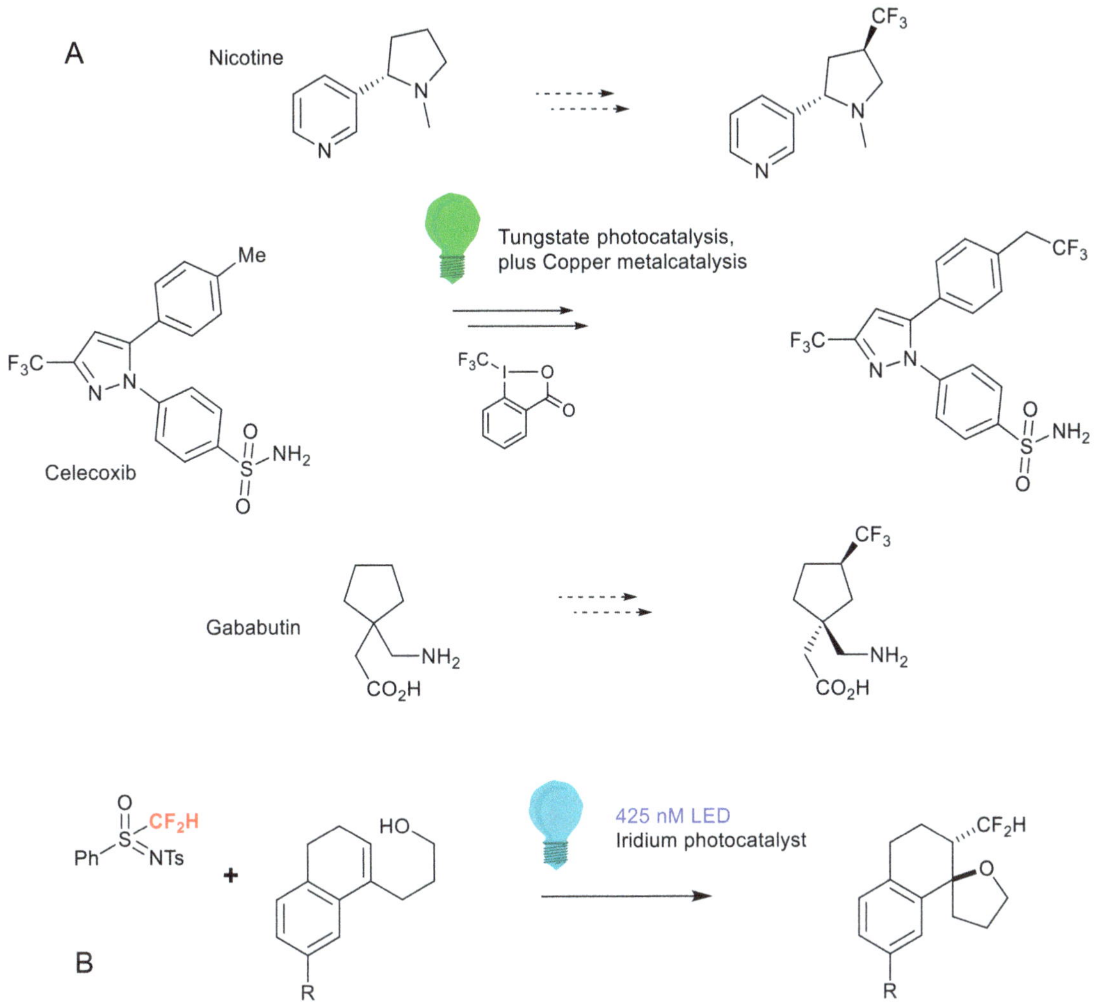


**Figure 2.8** Examples of (A) late-stage lead diversification methods of drug molecules using photoredox chemistry[36] and (B) access to novel structures *via* photocatalysis.[37]

antibiotics, steroids, alkaloids) are the products of natural processes or are semi-synthetic derivatives of natural products. For example, the anti-HIV carbocyclic nucleoside abacavir is manufactured with an enzyme-mediated biotransformation as the key step in the chiral opening of Vince lactam (Figure 2.10), whilst the production of the anti-influenza neuraminidase inhibitor zanamivir utilises enzyme-mediated production of neuraminic acid (Figure 2.11). Interestingly, the Vince lactam process illustrates the value of such intermediates, with its incorporation into the DPP-IV inhibitor melogliptin, a drug used in diabetes and the influenza neuraminidase inhibitor peramivir.

The use of microbial and liver microsome preparations to derivatise advanced molecules by oxidation is an increasingly used diversification technique, as illustrated by the formation of the hydroxylated analogue of the JAK inhibitor ruxolitinib Figure 2.12.[39]

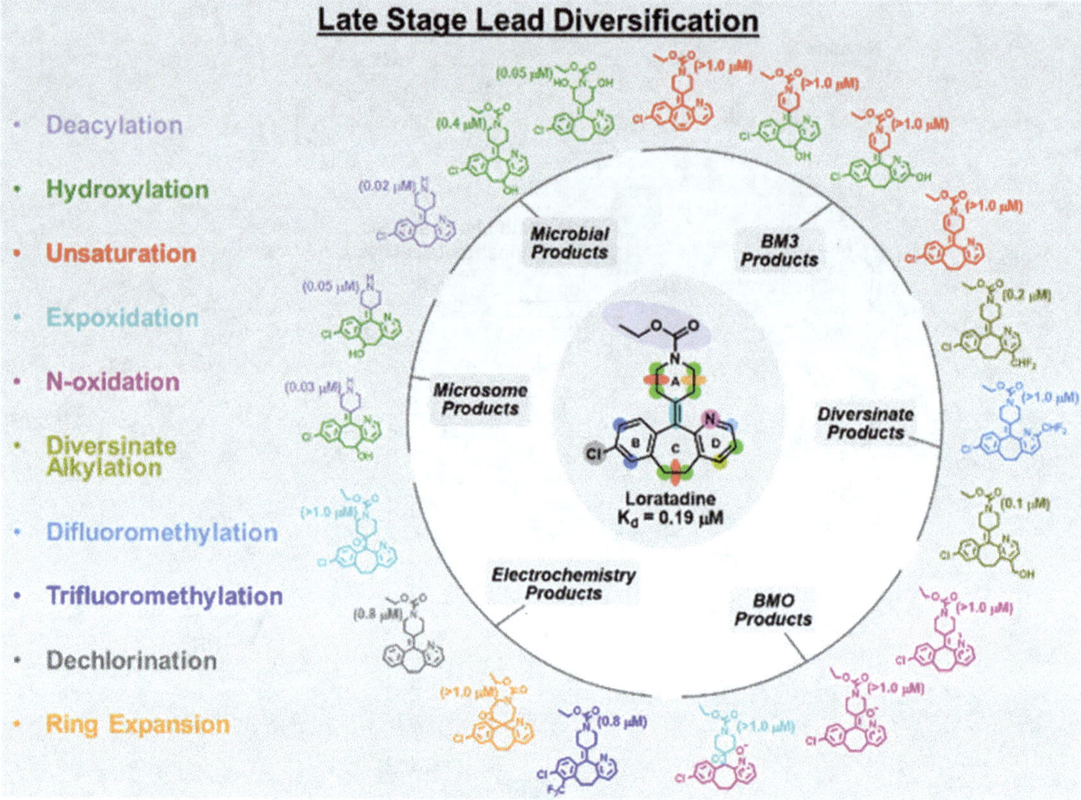


**Figure 2.9** A contemporary state of the art late-stage derivatisation of the antihistamine medicine loratadine. State of the art HPLC purification and characterisation methods (LCMS/NMR) on a nanomolar scale provided sufficient material for preliminary biological evaluation.[38] Reproduced from ref. 38 with permission from American Chemical Society, Copyright 2020.

An ultimate green aspiration could be the engineering of bacteria, yeasts or other single cell systems to produce drug substances or advanced intermediates to enhance the early stages of discovery.[40] Such a technique was developed to address the commercial production needs for paclitaxel. Taxol was first isolated from the bark of the Pacific yew tree in 1966 as part of an effort to characterise potential therapeutics derived from natural sources.[41] Its structure was confirmed in 1971,[42] but supply of the drug remained problematic for many years.

The first two total syntheses were published simultaneously in 1994,[43–45] but the precursor known as 10-deacetylbaccatin III (10-DAB-III) could be isolated in a more sustainable fashion from the needles of the European Yew,[46] leading to more commercially viable semi-synthetic processes (Figure 2.13).[47,48]

More recently, bespoke fermentation routes to key precursor molecules have been developed and optimised for flow chemistry to provide multi-gram quantities (Figure 2.14).[49] Moreover, it was proposed that paclitaxel itself might be obtained directly from plant cell culture. Whilst initially dismissed as unfeasible, the entire

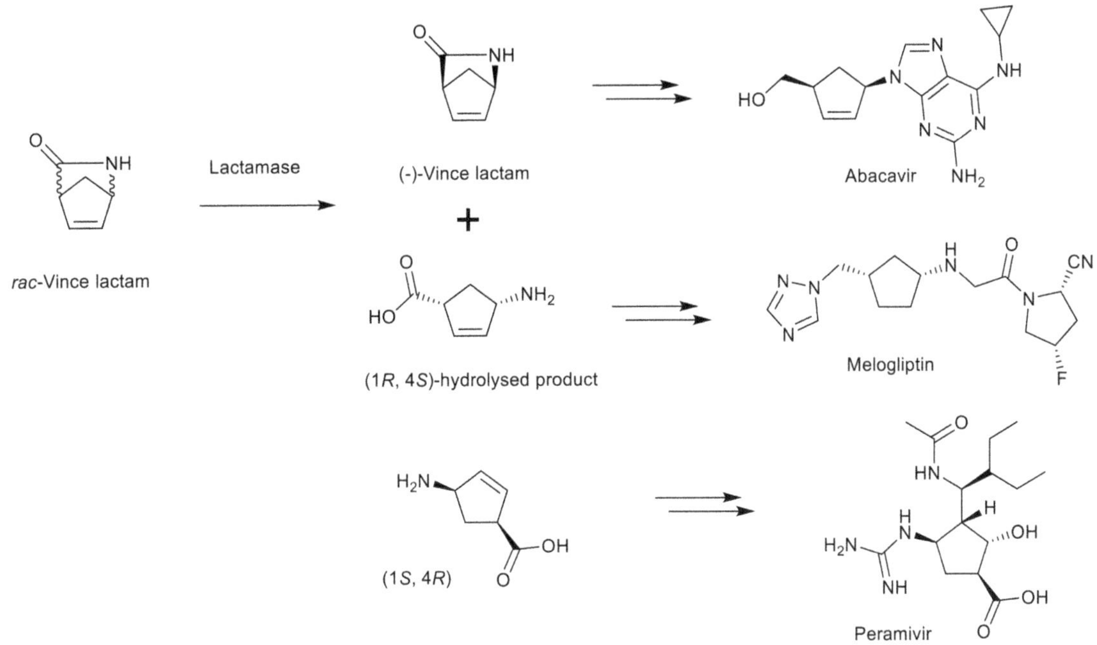


**Figure 2.10** Employment of lactamase enzymes to furnish homo chiral intermediates used in the commercial synthesis of the anti-HIV nucleoside abacavir, a route to the DPP-IV inhibitor melogliptin and the anti-influenza drug peramivir.

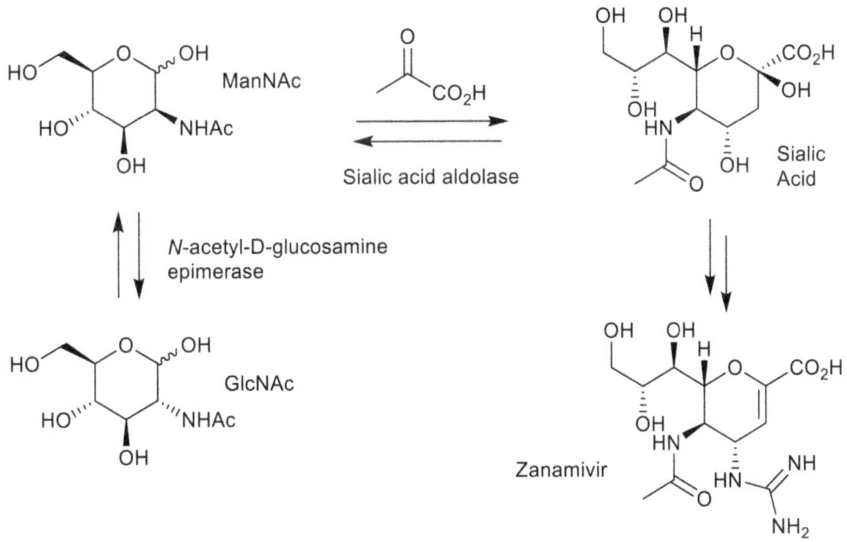


**Figure 2.11** Exploitation of enzymatic reactions in the commercial production of sialic acid, the key intermediate towards the production of the anti-influenza drug zanamivir. An enzymatic epimerisation of more readily available *N*-acetyl glucosamine (GlcNAc) is epimerised to the mannosamine substrate for the aldolase that incorporates pyruvic acid in the backward sense of this usually degrative enzyme.

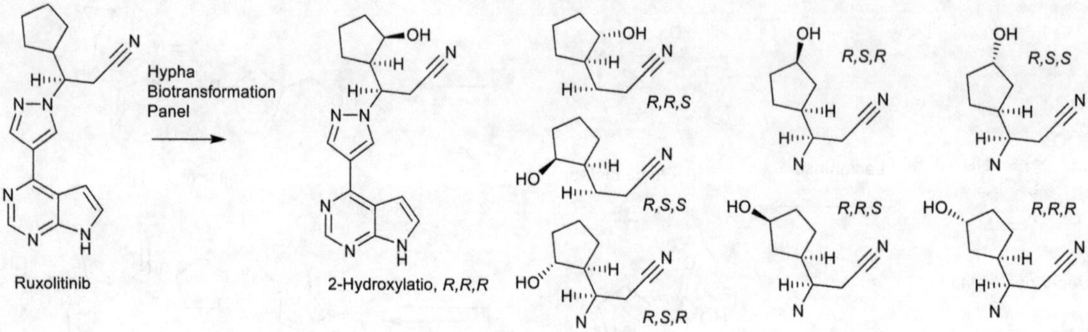


**Figure 2.12** Microbial oxidation in the diversification process leading to the isolation of all four diastereomers of monohydroxylation products of ruxolitinib in the cyclopentyl ring.[39]

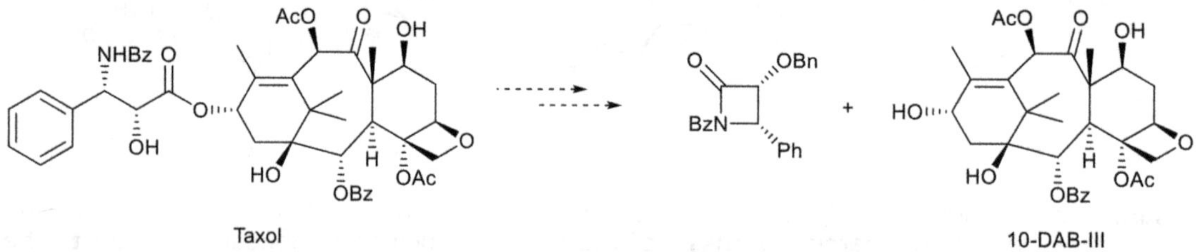


**Figure 2.13** Taxol™ (paclitaxel) and semi-synthetic precursor molecules.

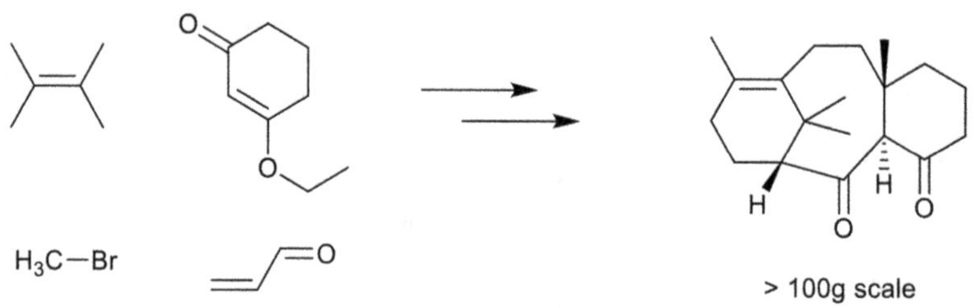


**Figure 2.14** Biomimetic route to paclitaxel precursors.

commercial supply of paclitaxel is now delivered *via* the plant cell culture of Chinese yew cells.[50,51]

Whilst these particular plant culture methods are specifically optimised and utilised for paclitaxel production, they suggest that similar approaches might allow the supply of other complex natural products or structurally diverse and complex starting materials. Future developments could furnish discovery teams with many more natural lead structures and offer alternative late-stage functionalisation strategies.[52] More widely, the use of enzymes in aqueous environments makes them compatible with DNA-encoding (as discussed below) and their limited use in library formation thus far is perhaps surprising.[53]

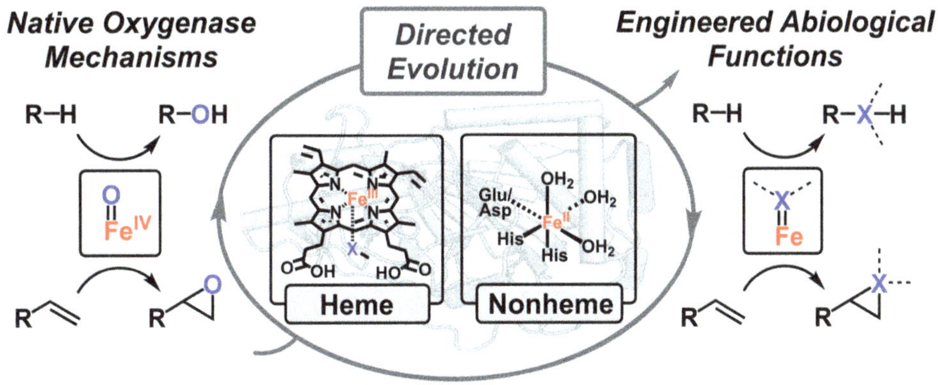


**Figure 2.15** Example of directed evolution enabling an expanded synthetic repertoire for iron-dependent oxygenases, whereby X can be O, C, B, N or Si, opening up a number of derivatisation options. Reproduced from ref. 54 with permission from American Chemical Society, Copyright 2020.

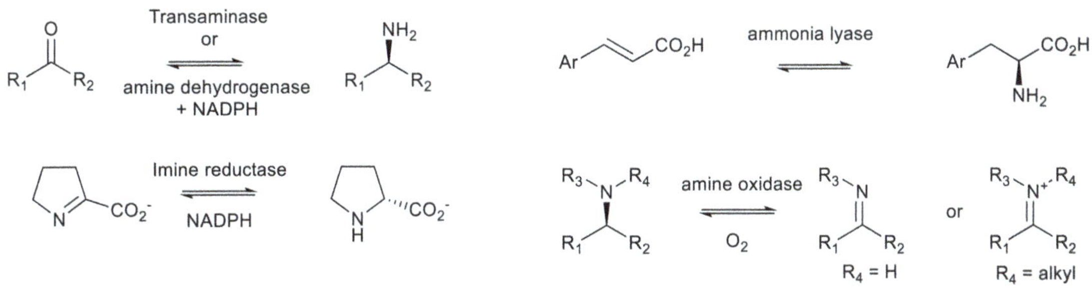


**Scheme 2.3** Examples of enzymatic methods to deliver chiral amines and amino acids.

A rapidly developing area within the biotransformation field is that of directed enzyme evolution, for which Frances Arnold was awarded the 2018 Nobel prize. By engineering the peptide structure of enzymes, new substrate specificities and even function can be introduced, such as the repertoire of iron-dependant oxygenases modified by the Arnold group, summarised in Figure 2.15.[54]

The production of chiral esters, amides and especially amines can be achieved with numerous enzymatic methods summarised in Scheme 2.3. In a neat extension of such methodology, the Turner group utilised a number of designed and engineered monoamine oxidases to deliver chiral amine building blocks and bioactive alkaloids based on the accumulation of the desired enantiomer as its antipode is consumed by the enzyme and the imine chemically reduced *in situ* (Scheme 2.4).[55]

## 2.2.5 Water-based Chemistry

The environmental impact of synthesis, in terms of the sourcing of raw materials solvents and reagents, their potential toxicity or contribution to carbon balance is coming under increased scrutiny. In these contexts, the use of water as a solvent is a very green

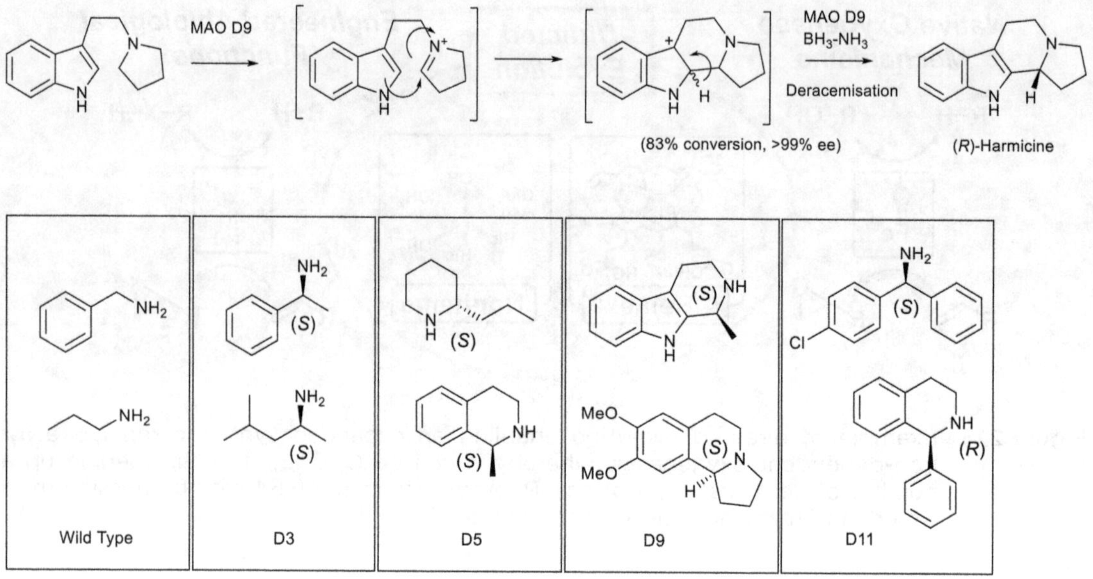


**Scheme 2.4** Enzyme-enabled synthesis and deracemisation that enabled the delivery of the alkaloid (R)-harmicine and valuable chiral building blocks for drug discovery and commercial synthesis.

option and is surprisingly useful for many transformations (beyond those described in Section 2.2.3). Tolerance of water is a prerequisite in the construction of DNA-encoded libraries,[56] to ensure fidelity and stability of the growing DNA "barcode" that is attached after each stage of the iterative construction of the split and mixed library.[57] Nonetheless, conditions to enable the classical combinatorial reactions of acylation, reductive amination, cross coupling and $S_NAr$ have delivered highly populated libraries limited in size only by the availability of building blocks. However, as this screening methodology has become more prevalent, the diversity of chemistries exploited "on-DNA" have increased and better design of the libraries, with custom building blocks and scaffolds, will enhance the impact of this powerful technology. Such improvements have already delivered compounds into the clinic, such as the RIP-1 kinase inhibitor GSK772 (Figure 2.16).

## 2.2.6 Mimicking Nature

Understanding the pharmacology and pharmacokinetics of xenobiotics is the crux of many drug discovery programmes. Modern practices furnish molecules that are often structurally dissimilar to the motifs encountered in natural products or the endogenous substances that broker the process the drug is designed to modulate. However, an analysis by Waldmann and co-workers suggests that the repertoire of distinct fragments in nature is somewhat more limited than has generally been imagined, reflecting a finite range of biosynthetic building blocks (Figure 2.17).[58] As such, employing or closely mimicking such structures, that have evolved to promote bioactivity, is a highly

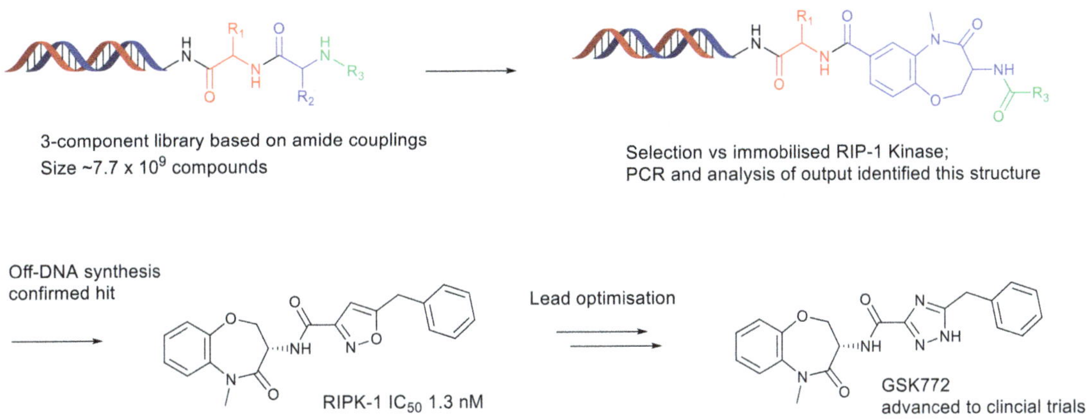


**Figure 2.16** The discovery of GSK772 using DNA-encoded library technology.

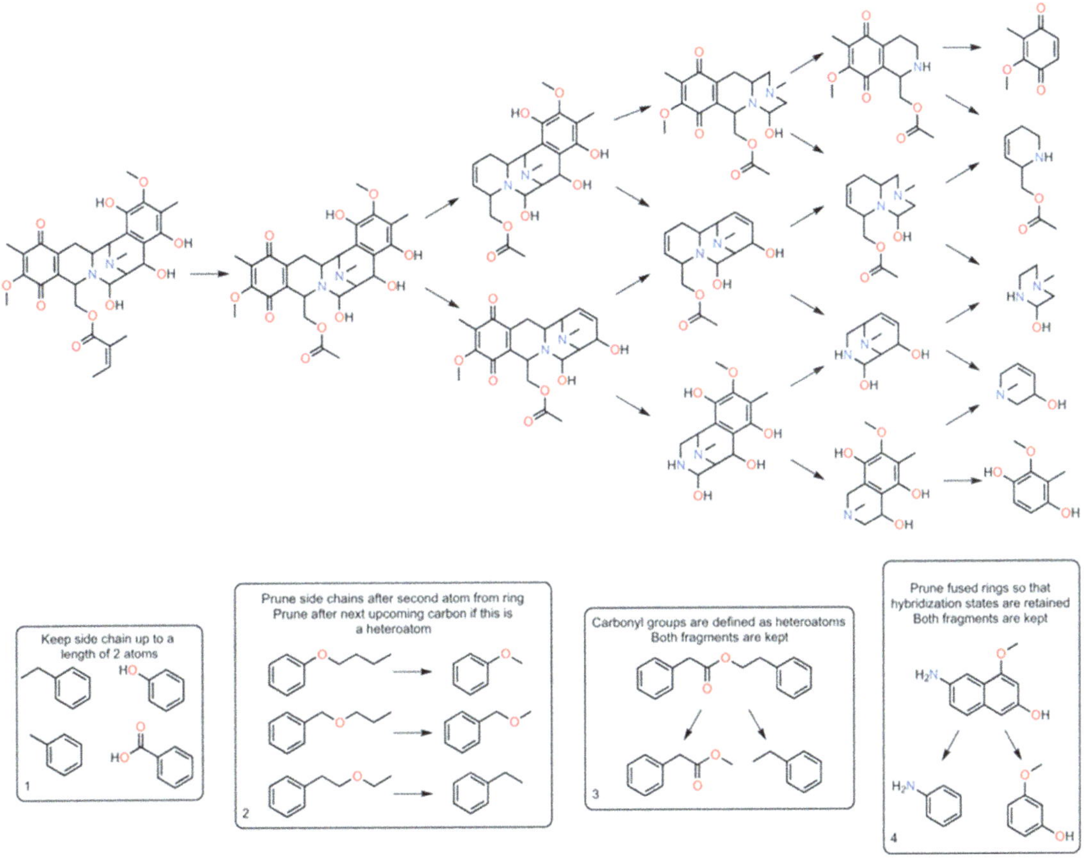


**Figure 2.17** Fragmentation of renieramycin by Waldmann *et al.*, used as an illustration of the finite variety of motifs in natural products. Reproduced from ref. 58 with permission from Springer Nature, Copyright 2013.

rational approach to drug discovery. It has further been suggested that all oral drugs bear some similarity to an exogenous natural product.[59,60]

A logical extension of this thinking would be that drugs most closely resembling endogenous or exogenous natural substances have the best chance of achieving pharmacological effects. There is evidence to suggest that the solute carriers that enable the passage of molecules through cell membranes[61] evolved to enable the concentration of beneficial xenobiotics within cells, so such compounds or their mimics may be reasonable starting points for drug discovery. Nature is replete with complex, chiral structures, not the flat and rigid polyaromatics we instinctively err toward constructing; indeed, non-fused biaryl structures, the ubiquitous products of cross coupling reactions, are exceedingly rare in nature. Whilst this proposed mechanism for uptake by carriers positively discriminates for natural structures, evolution has furnished complementary metabolism processes, which co-exist to remove xenobiotics through their modification by oxidative and conjugative processes to facilitate their removal. The lipophilicity–activity profiles of these processes are complementary for optimum permeation and peak cytochrome P450 oxidation;[62] lipophilicity modulation and/or strategic hydroxylation are therefore logical medicinal chemistry strategies, designed to work with nature in these contexts, not against it. Optimisation processes in drug discovery are frequently driven by compromises that enable the best balance of properties and physiological behaviour in molecules. Our contemporary understanding and established principles seek to parameterise the size, shape and lipophilicity of molecules; these will clearly be enhanced by better appreciation of what has evolved in nature and what human physiology has evolved to achieve.

#### 2.2.6.1 Natural Product Structures as Inspirations for Synthesis

The basis of most chemical methodology was the identification of methods to meet the challenges posed in the synthesis of complex natural products. Natural products and their semi-synthetic analogues have a rich history in drug discovery, and analyses support the prevalence of their substructures in drug molecules.[63] Accordingly, it would seem to be logical to populate screening libraries with molecules that have enhanced natural-product-like characteristics (such as higher content of $sp^3$-hydridised carbons)[64,65] and their utility demonstrated, particularly for novel/difficult targets.[66] The term pseudonatural products, coined by Waldmann,[67] was illustrated by such variations summarised in Figure 2.18.

As interest grows in motifs and linkers with increased $sp^3$ character, bicyclic and spirocyclic structures (Figure 2.19) have come to the fore with their multiple beneficial impacts on the properties and activities of molecules,[68] in addition to their broadening patentability with novel connectivities.[69] The reduced flexibility of the structures enables precise spacer design with control of both distance and geometry with their use as isosteric replacements (see Section 2.2.7).

#### 2.2.6.2 Diversity-oriented Synthesis

In the quest for more attractive properties in screening compounds, various strategies and initiatives are utilising imaginative syntheses to generate pertinent and well-designed

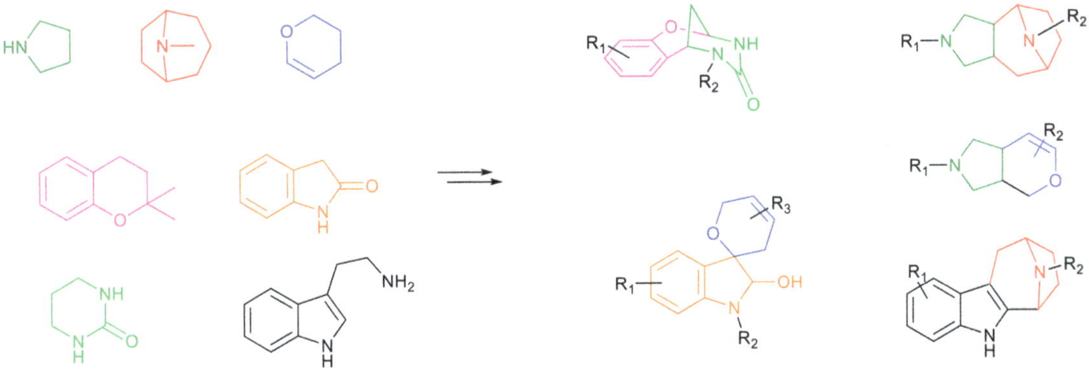

**Figure 2.18** Examples of composite variations on natural product structures termed "pseudo-natural" products.

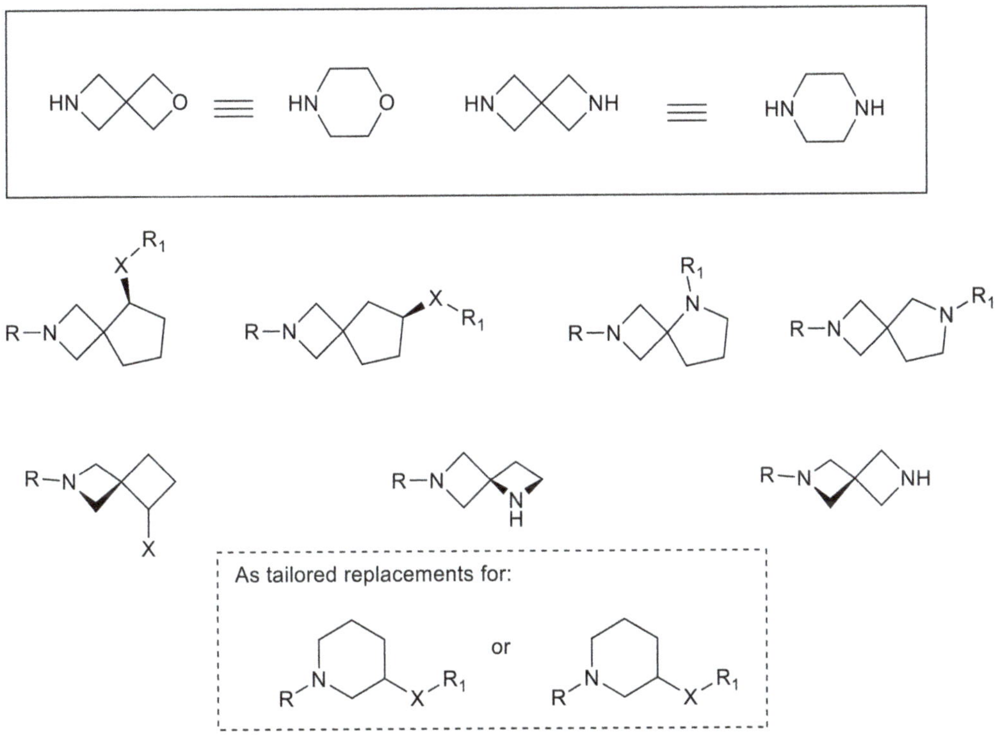


**Figure 2.19** Examples of spirocyclic and bicyclic structures, pseudonatural product analogues, that enhance structural diversity and $sp^3$ content of experimental molecules, whilst enabling control of conformation, space filling and geometry.

molecules. So-called diversity-oriented synthesis[70,71] exploits complementary reaction pathways that are designed to efficiently synthesise a variety of compounds from common starting points and intermediates, a technique extended to natural-product-derived substrates.[72] The concept of lead-likeness[73] (compounds being rather smaller and less lipophilic than average drug molecules, clog$P \leq 3.0$, MW $\leq 350$) influences thinking and

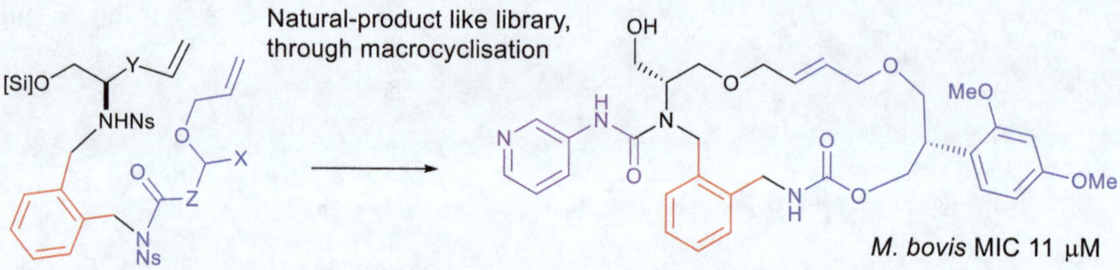


**Figure 2.20** Example of a chemical lead discovered from a natural-product-inspired combinatorial library produced through a macrocyclisation strategy.

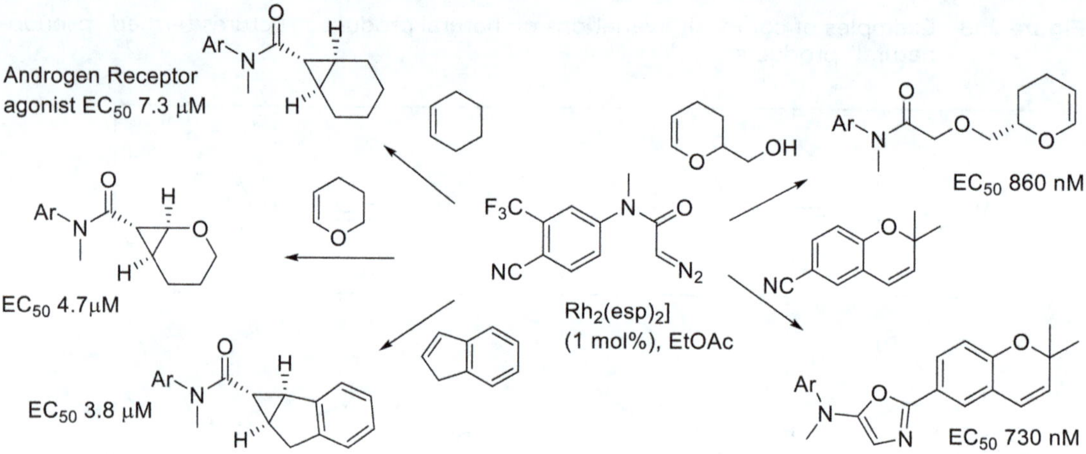


**Figure 2.21** Activity-directed synthesis, whereby inherent promiscuity of reactions is exploited to generate diverse structures, from which hits can be deconvoluted by synthesis.

the concept of lead-oriented synthesis[74] was formulated in recognition of observations that efficient syntheses tend to work best for more lipophilic compounds in multiple/automated synthesis efforts. A consortium of European academic groups, in partnership with industry, established the European Lead Factory[75,76] with the aim of developing new methodology to deliver sets of novel molecules with lead-like and/or less planar character.[77] The impact of this initiative is illustrated by a hit with anti-tuberculosis activity from a series of natural-product-inspired macrocycles (Figure 2.20).

An intriguing extension of this concept is activity-directed synthesis,[78] which utilises reactions deliberately chosen to have multiple potential outcomes, in conjunction with iterative screening to inform on which combinations produce activity, prior to hit confirmation. The utility of this technique is exemplified by the discovery of androgen receptors from a known fragment, using the inherent promiscuity of carbenoid chemistry[79] (Figure 2.21).

### 2.2.6.3 Biomimetic Synthesis

The previous sections exemplify how synthetic strategies that furnish natural products, or their semi-synthetic analogues, have been used to deliver many bioactive molecules.

In future, designer drugs or late-stage intermediates arising from engineered cells may be an aspiration for environmentally sustainable production. Likewise, imaginative use of existing synthetic methodology offers opportunities to furnish such molecules using iterative, divergent or complementary processes. This is illustrated by the automated assembly-line synthesis[80] of bioactive natural products and their analogues using methodology that mimics the biosynthesis of polypropionate-containing molecules.[81] The exploitation of synthetic cascade methodology[82] (Figure 2.22), successfully furnished all four diastereomers of $\Delta^9$-tetrahydrocannabinols from common reagents and catalysts (Figure 2.23); these isomers each displayed distinct pharmacological properties.[83]

Exploiting natural sources as feedstocks for chemical manipulation in this manner to deliver drug molecules offers significant future potential for a sustainable source of complex molecules. Pioneering research has delivered modified pacidamycin antibiotics from such processes, termed GenoChemetics (Scheme 2.5).[84] "Directing evolution" is a term coined for research in modified organisms where their survival is dependent on the presence of a necessary modulatory compound that can be deconvoluted as a hit structure (Figure 2.24).[85]

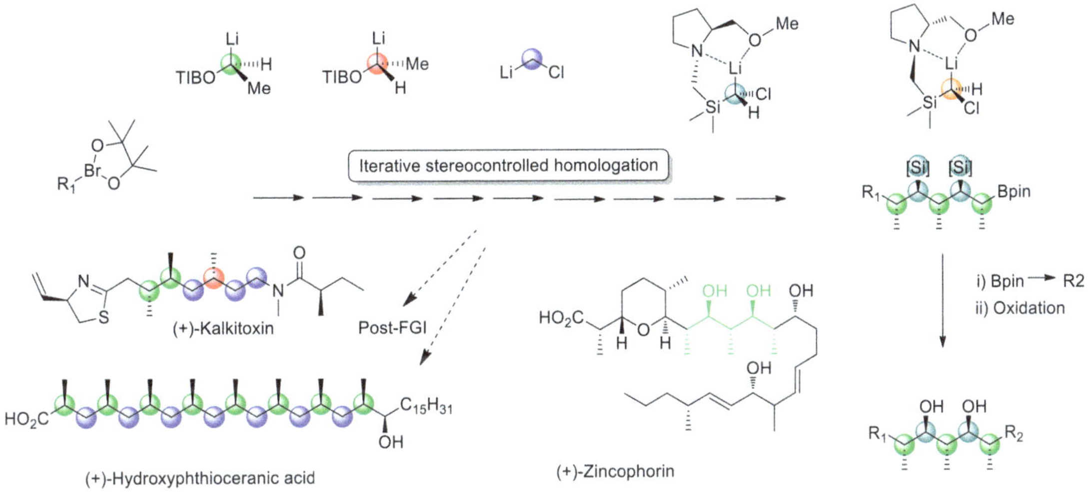


**Figure 2.22** Examples of biomimetic automated assembly line synthesis applied to the synthesis of natural products.

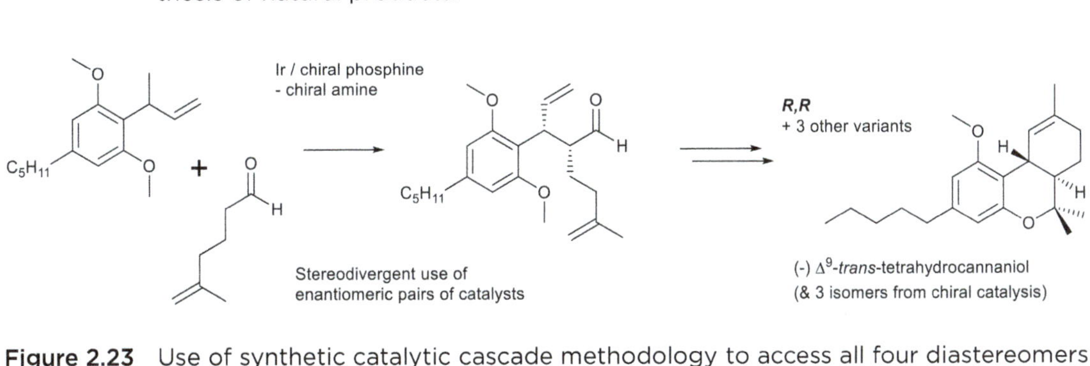


**Figure 2.23** Use of synthetic catalytic cascade methodology to access all four diastereomers of tetrahydrocannabinol, illustrating the power of synthesis in diversifying natural structures.

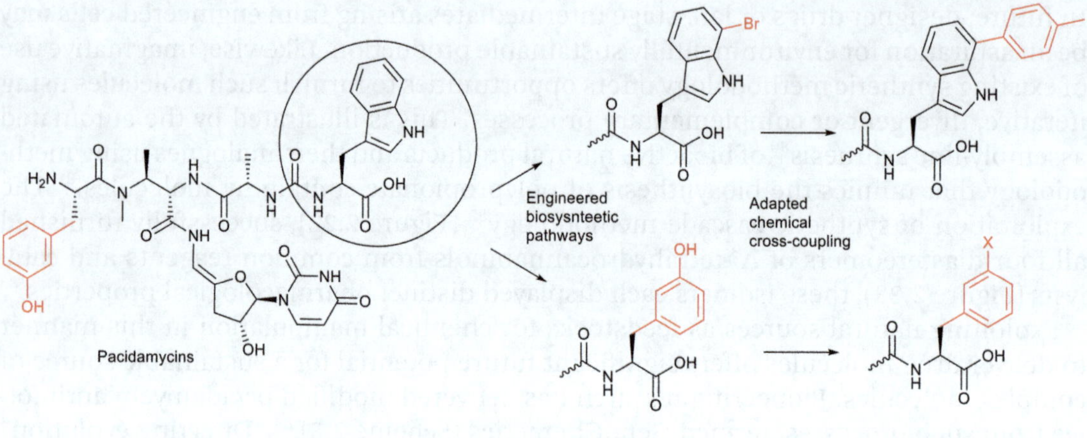


**Scheme 2.5** Using modified biosynthetic machinery in concert with synthesis to produce bioactive molecules related to pacidamycins.

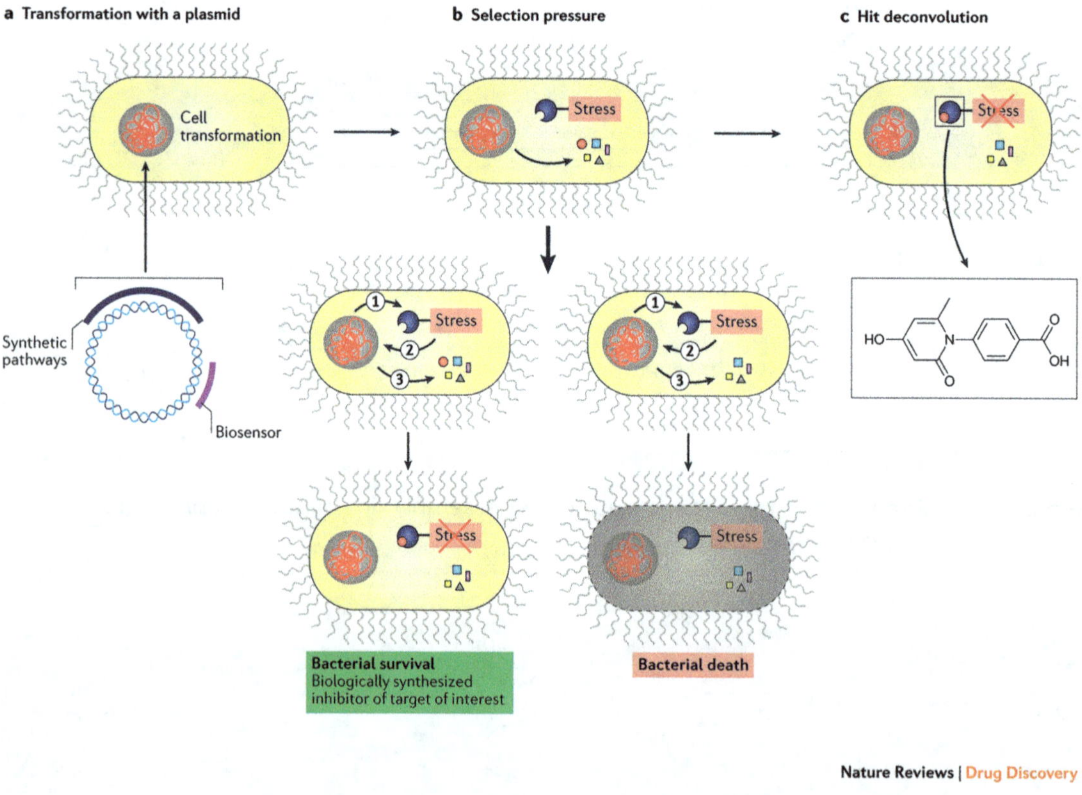


**Figure 2.24** The use of directed evolution as a screening method for synthetic or biosynthetic hits, summarizing the a) transformation, b) application of selection pressure, and c) hit deconvolution steps. Reproduced from ref. 85 with permission from Springer Nature Copyright 2017.

### 2.2.7 Isosteres

The essence of drug discovery is the mimicry of substrates, ligands and natural inhibitors of biologically relevant molecules to achieve a desirable biochemical outcome. A key element in that strategy is replacement of pertinent features of the mimicked molecules with isosteric motifs and connectivity, designed to maintain or modulate key interactions with an altered structural composition. The concepts of isosterism have deep roots in chemistry[86] and the simplest manifestation is an atom, or defined number of atoms, with the same number of valence electrons. Later, the term bioisostere was coined to recognise distinct structures that could elicit similar biological responses, despite different molecular architecture. The terminology used to describe various kinds of isosteres is summarised in Table 2.2.

Amides, ubiquitous motifs in biological molecules and notably the key linkage in polypeptides and proteins are the most mimicked linkages; Figure 2.25 illustrates variations on functionality and ring structures that act as isosteres of amide motifs and linkages.[87]

Similarly, increased interest in sulphoximines and other S=N–R variations on sulphones and sulphonamides are further examples of innovation to explore new chemical connectivities and their effect on biological properties (Figure 2.26).[88]

The incorporation of novel isosteric motifs may not only have profound biological implications but might also secure new intellectual property when such a change falls outside of the claims of existing patents or published work. The structures of the HIV integrase inhibitors dolutegravir and bictegravir (Figure 2.27) serve as an illustrative example where structural novelty was engendered in the bridged bicyclic moiety.

An area of considerable interest is the search for structural isosteres for the phenyl ring to improve the properties and increase the $sp^3$ character/shape of molecules. In this context, cubane and bicyclo[1.1.1]pentane (BCP) are exemplified in Figure 2.28, but many other bicyclic structures, enabled by synthetic imagination, have been utilised,

**Table 2.2** Classical and non-classical bioisosteres.

| | |
|---|---|
| **Classical bioisosteres** | |
| Monovalent bioisosteres | D and H<br>F and H<br>NH and OH<br>RSH and ROH<br>F, OH, $NH_2$ and $CH_3$<br>Cl, Br, SH and OH<br>C and Si |
| Bivalent bioisosteres<br>*two single bonds implicated* | C=C, C=N, C=O, C=S<br>$-CH_2-$, –NH–, –O–, –S–<br>RCOR′, RCONHR′, RCOOR′, RCOSR′ |
| Trivalent bioisosteres<br>*three bonds implicated* | $R_3CH$, $R_3N$<br>$R_4C$, $R_4Si$, $R_4N^+$<br>alkene, imine<br>–CH=CH–, –S–, –CH= and –N=C |
| **Non-classical bioisosteres** | |
| Subgroups<br>1. Cyclic and noncyclic isosteres<br>2. Exchangeable group isosteres | *Structurally distinct, often different atom count & exhibit different steric/electronic properties to the emulated functionality* |

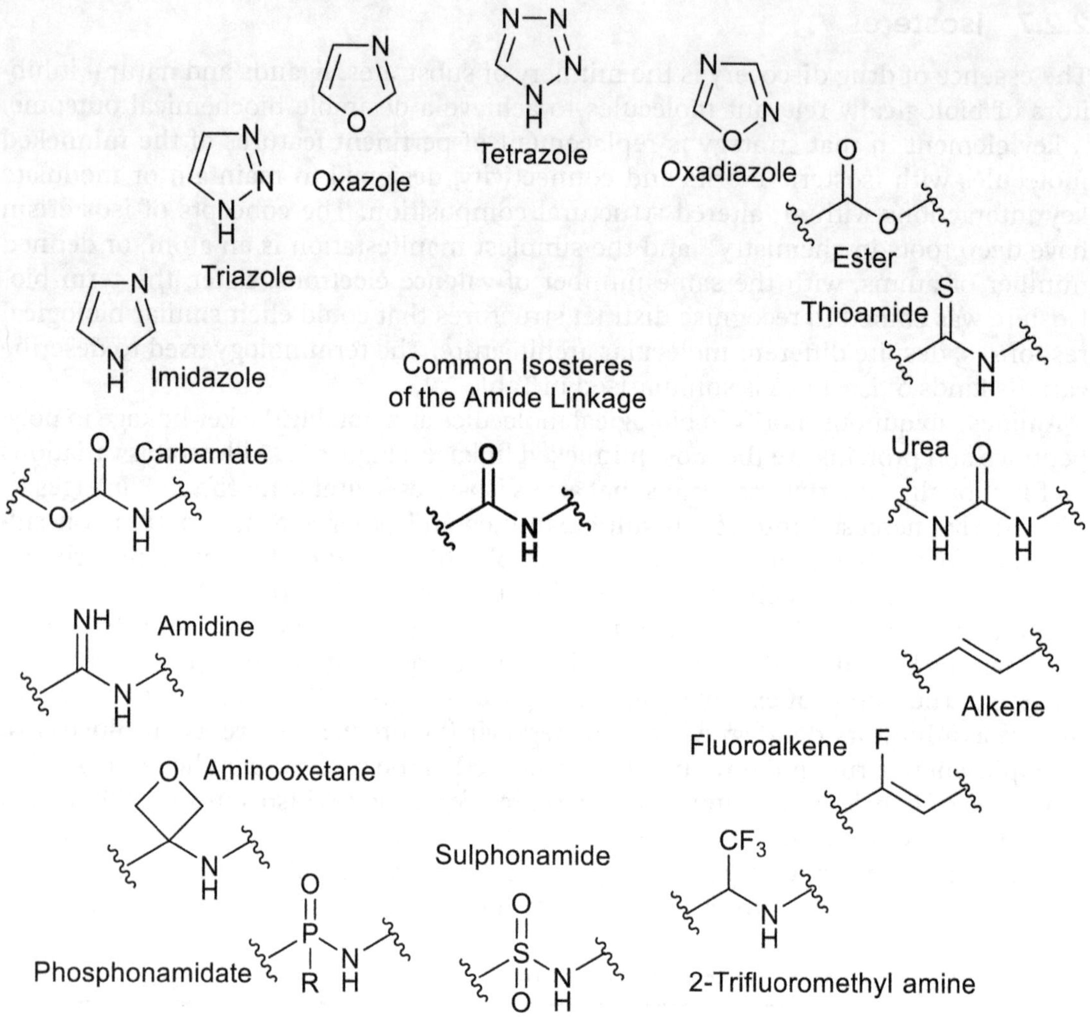


**Figure 2.25** Examples of structures used as amide isosteres in drug discovery.[87]

including adamantanes and *closo*-carborane analogues.[89] The increasing prevalence of sp$^3$-rich bicyclic and spirocyclic structures, see Section 2.2.6.1, should be considered as new developments in bioisosteres.

Opportunities exist with isosteres to profoundly influence the physical properties of analogues, often with retention of activity, illustrated by the scan of isosteres for the *tert*-butyl group of the endothelin receptor antagonist bostentan (Figure 2.29).[90]

## 2.2.8 Fragment-Based Drug Discovery (FBDD)

Advances in biophysical and structural techniques, coupled with structure-based design, paved the way for exploitation of fragment methodologies in the toolbox of drug discovery methods. Drugs and development candidates, such as vemurafenib[91] and venetoclax[92] were identified through this methodology, whilst "fragment thinking" has influenced discovery in terms of understanding ligand efficiency,[93] fragmentation

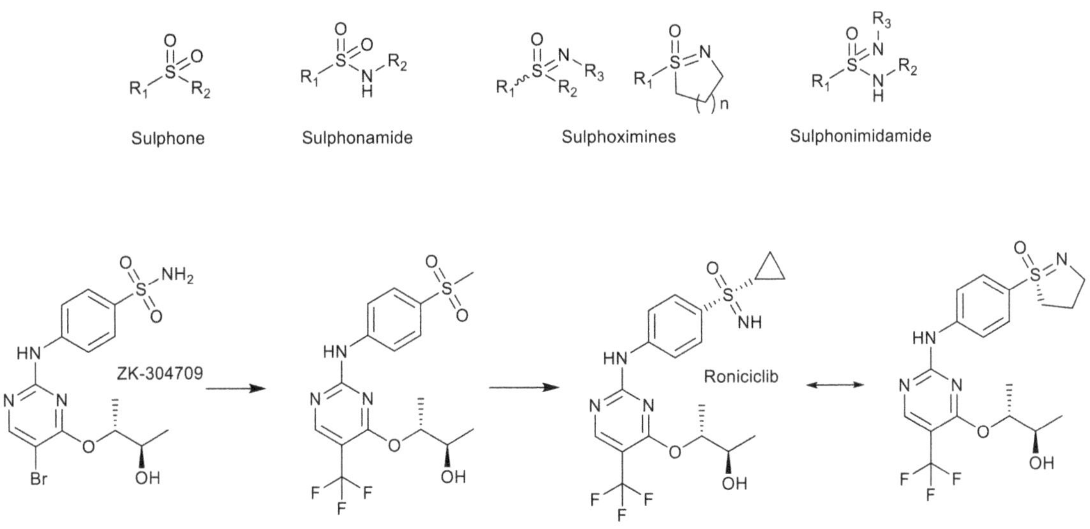


**Figure 2.26** A variety of functional groups containing sulphur, including configurationally stable sulphoximines, recently popularised isosteric groups exploited in the discovery of the pan-CDK inhibitor roniciclib to replace active sulphonamides and sulphones, with improved DMPK outcomes.

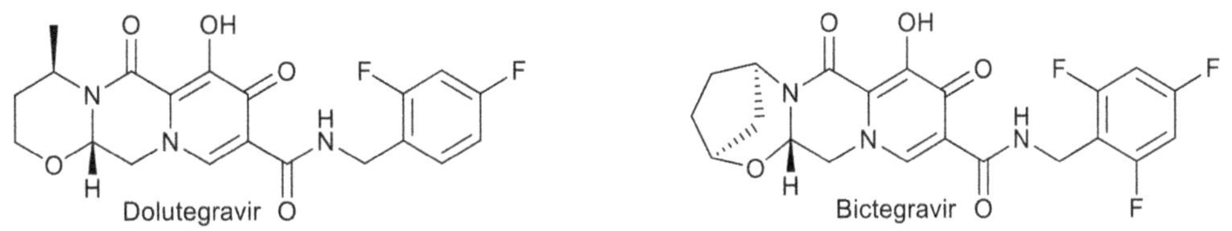


**Figure 2.27** The structures of marketed HIV integrase inhibitors dolutegravir and bictegravir.

of hits and growth vector optimisation. Imaginative synthesis plays a clear role in the growth and linking of fragments, to enable optimal connectivity, contacts and space filling, in a more focussed and deliberate manner than optimisation of HTS and DNA-encoded library hits (Table 2.3). The exploitation of small chiral monomers to grow fragment hits[94] is nicely showcased in the discovery of PF-06835919,[95] a clinical candidate for the treatment of metabolic disorders due to excessive fructose consumption, through the inhibition of ketohexokinase (Scheme 2.6).

Fragments are usually defined as compounds with roughly 10–17 heavy atoms (~130–250 Da), for which the "Rule of 3" was formulated to suggest MW ≤ 300, clog$P$ ≤ 3 and #HBA/#HBD ≤ 3 as guidelines for the compilation of fragment libraries. These molecules are designed to possess limited molecular complexity,[96] but, because they have numerous feasible binding modes, the chance of making a productive interaction is greatly increased. Practically, relatively small libraries (hundreds to one or two thousand compounds) are screened using various biophysical techniques (particularly X-ray crystallography, surface plasmon resonance and NMR spectroscopy) to detect weak interactions with biological targets at the necessary higher concentrations. Subsequently, these hits are then grown or linked, to increase interactions and potency,

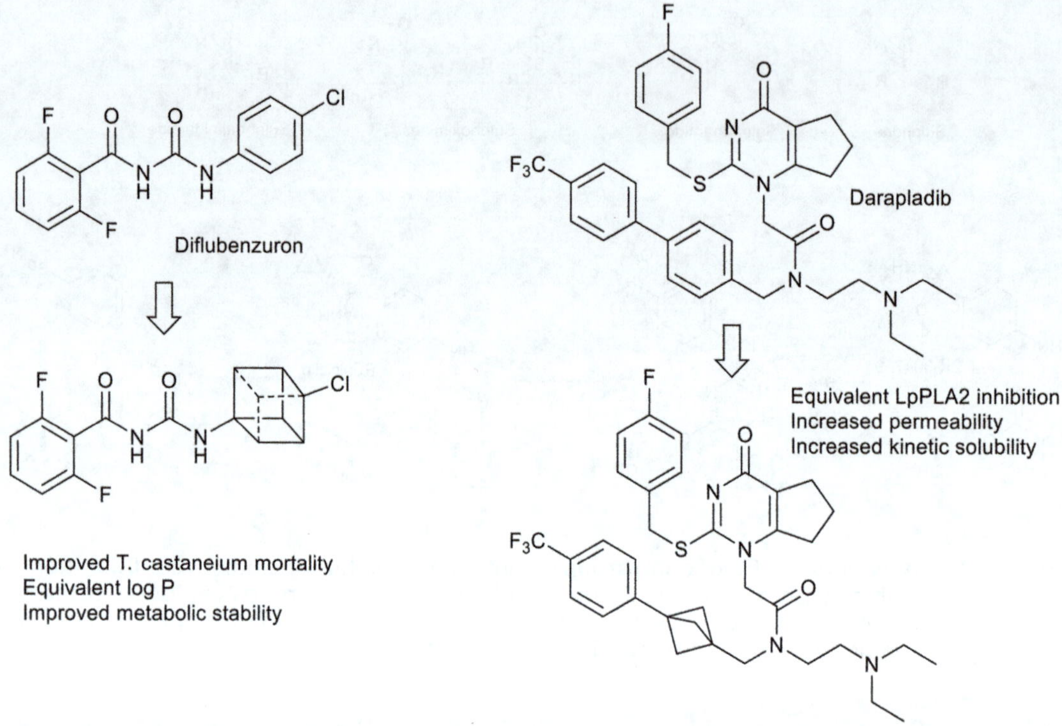


**Figure 2.28** Examples of the use of cubane and bicyclo[1.1.1]pentane (BCP) as isosteres for a phenyl ring.

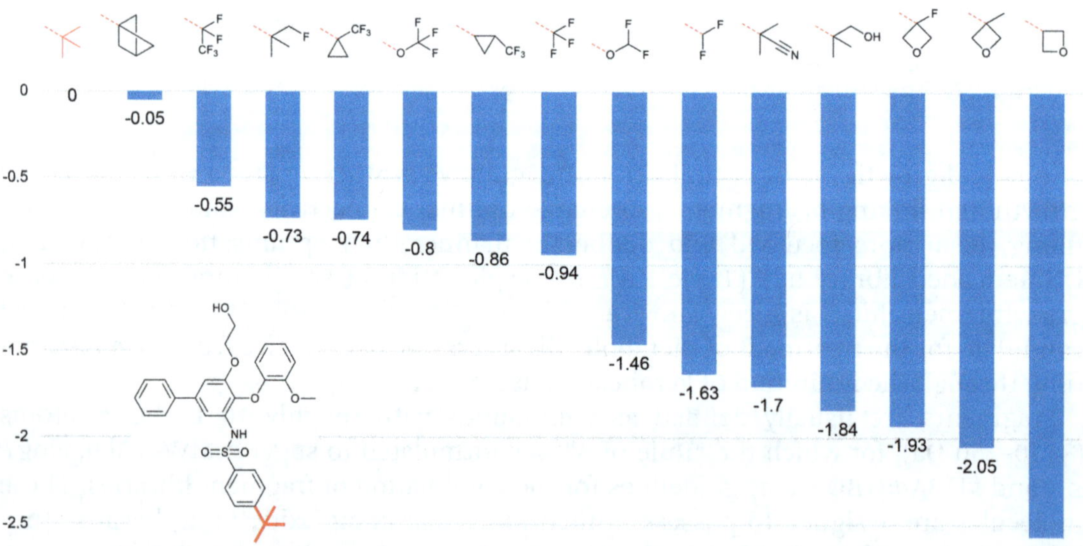


**Figure 2.29** Exploration of isosteres for the *tert*-butyl group of bosentan and their impact on the lipophilicity of the analogues; clog*P* data recalculated using Biobyte in ChemDraw Professional v16.

**Table 2.3** Comparison of the commonly employed hit-finding methods and how synthesis impacts upon them.

| | Fragments | High throughput (diversity) screening | DNA encoded library technology |
|---|---|---|---|
| Size (heavy = non-hydrogen, atoms) | 10–20 | 16–30 | 25 to 40+ |
| Numbers typically screened | $10^3$ | $10^5$ to $10^6$ | $10^9$ to $10^{12}$ |
| Infrastructure/ regent needs | Extensive protein & methodology support | Infrastructure & reagent supply to screen large numbers of compounds | Relatively low reagent needs: Polymerase chain reaction equipment to decode |
| Ability to enable diversity of exploration | Wide sampling of "chemical space" | Narrower sampling of chemical space | Diversity of space sampled limited despite numbers |
| Impact of synthesis | The most successful fragments often prosaic structures; innovation as fragments are grown, interest growing in chiral/more complex fragments | High throughput and combinatorial synthesis enable supply of large numbers; but costs, reaction logistics, purification and supply can limit quality | Innovation has impacted through the range of water-based chemistries and those that will not interfere with DNA functionality. Constrained by monomer availability |

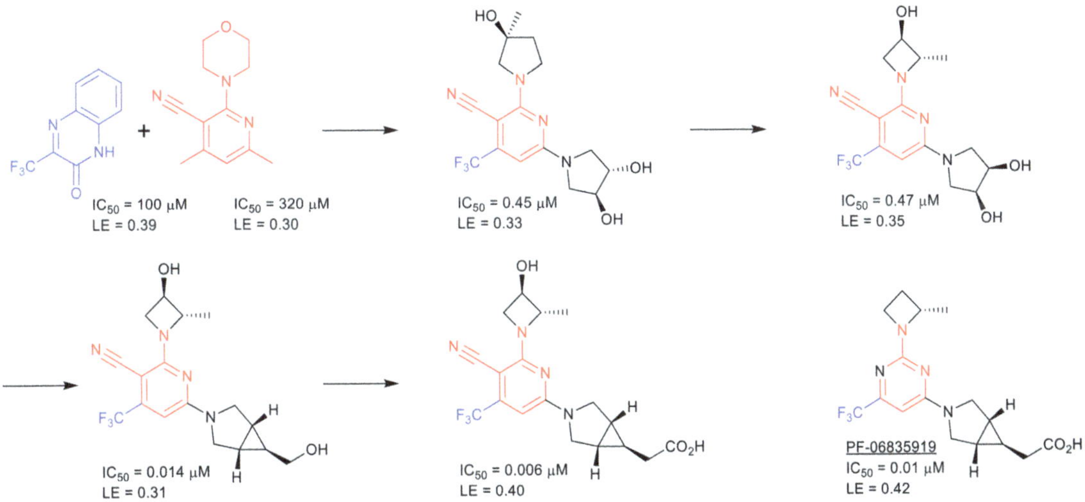


**Scheme 2.6** The developing structure and, ultimately, property-guided evolution of fragment hits into the development candidate PF-06835919, coloured to map the origins of key motifs in the structure.

typically guided by structural information. Fragment sets with increased three-dimensionality[97] and motifs from fragmented natural products have been targeted by synthesis.[98] However, data analysis indicated that less complex and flatter fragments had higher hit rates in fragment screens,[99] but the importance of imaginative synthesis is key to deliver more functionalised and/or asymmetric molecules to yield ligand-efficient structures maintaining good physical properties as the compounds are grown.[100] The important role and future opportunities for synthetic impact in FBDD were highlighted in a review[101] that summarised key common functionalisation strategies (Figure 2.30).

The importance of synthetic flexibility and tractability from fragment hits was highlighted by the introduction of a new term, "sociable" fragments, defined by published synthetic routes amenable to synthetic variations, which is demonstrated by the range of commercially available close analogues (Table 2.4). Opportunities exist to find new chemistries to transform unsociable examples or discover new flexible motifs with sociability in-built.

The utilisation of reactive fragments designed to make covalent interactions with target macromolecules is an area of increasing utility, whereby electrophilic fragments react with targeted or engineered residues, notably cysteines, in proteins of interest.[102] Fuelled by synthetic developments,[103] Cravatt and colleagues designed fragments with photoactivatable moieties (for example, diazirine-to-carbene transformation), coupled with an alkyne handle to enable addition of affinity or detection probes using *in situ* click chemistry (Figure 2.31). Such techniques enable a more generic chemical biology approach to target discovery,[104] termed Activity-Based Protein Profiling (ABPP), since

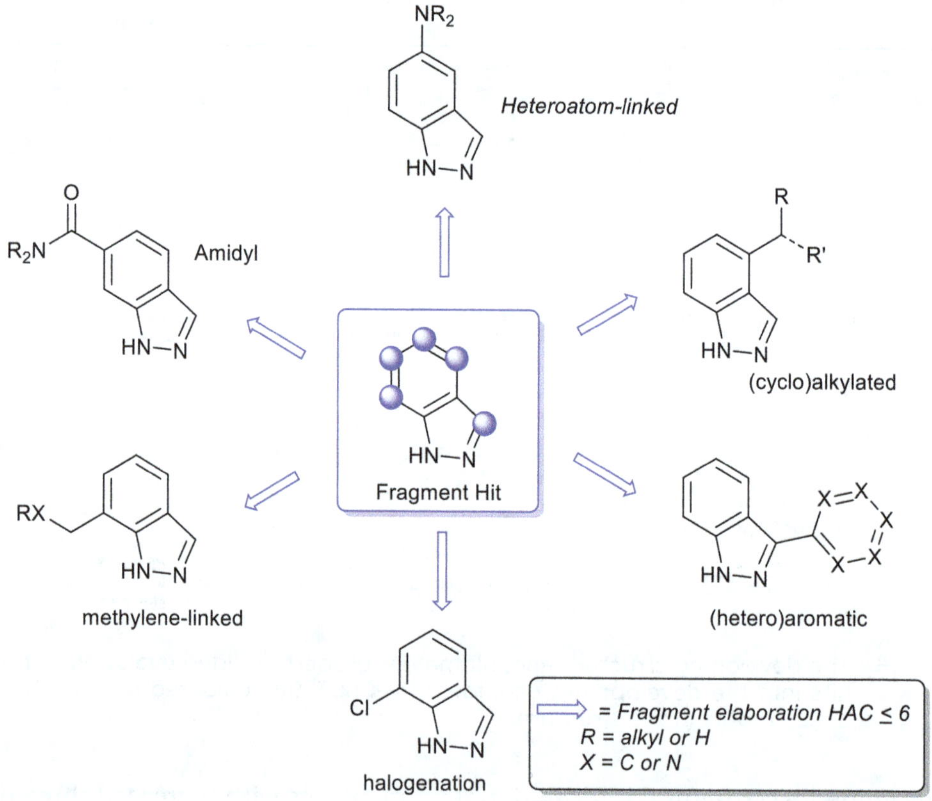


**Figure 2.30** Representative examples of common functional groups frequently added during fragment elaboration. HAC = number of non-hydrogen atoms (heavy atom count).[101]

**Table 2.4** Examples of fragment hits from Astex programmes and their designation as "Unsociable" or "Sociable" based on synthetic precedence and commercially available analogues.[101]

| Unsociable fragments | | | Sociable fragments | | |
|---|---|---|---|---|---|
| Structure | Published method | Commercially available close analogues | Structure | Published method | Commercially available close analogues |
| 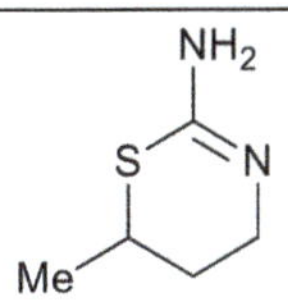 | No | <5 | 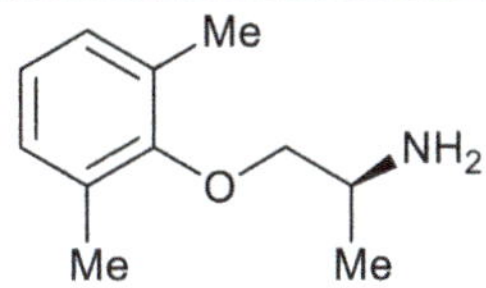 | Yes | >100 |
| 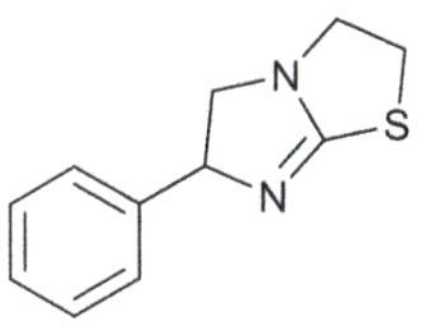 | Yes | <10 | 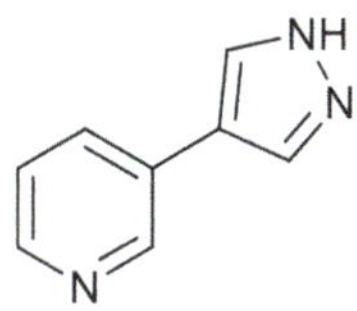 | Yes | >250 |
| 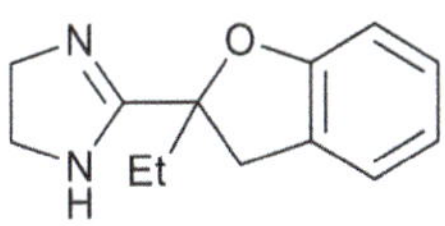 | Yes | <5 | 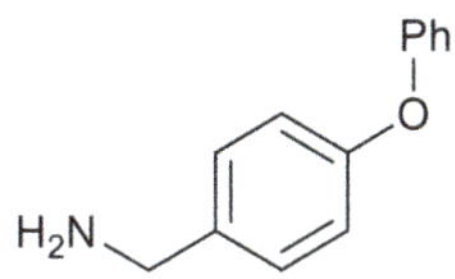 | Yes | >1000 |

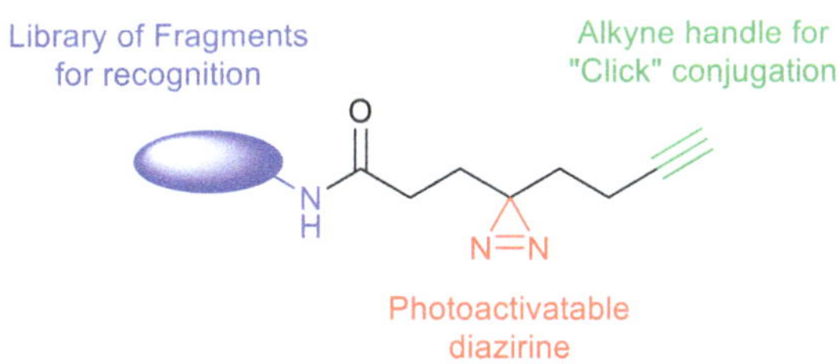


**Figure 2.31** Generic structure of the linking group utilised in fully functionalised fragment (FFF) libraries for the exploration of protein–ligand interactions using photoaffinity labelling and click chemistry to identify target proteins.

extended to whole-cell screening[105] and a Photoaffinity-Based Fragment-Screening Platform (PhABits) that are together being used to efficiently identify protein ligand interactions as starting points for discovery programmes.[106]

## 2.2.9 Avoiding Nuisance Compounds, PAINs and Potentially Reactive Species

In the risk-minimising culture of modern big Pharma, the identification and avoidance of substructures with potential liabilities can be a divisive issue.[107] Most medicinal chemists have favourite structures – some of these may be anathema to others; whist

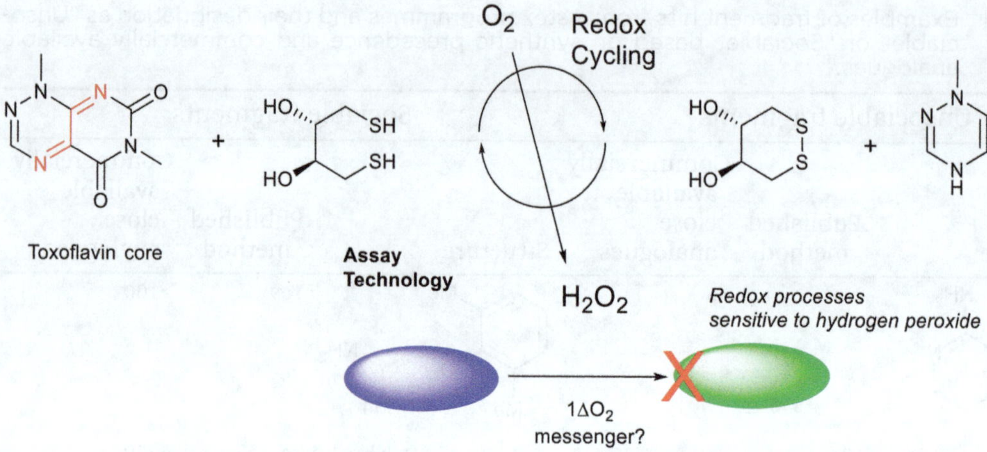


**Figure 2.32** Toxoflavin, as an example of a redox reactive heterocycle, that can produce hydrogen peroxide in an assay well, which interferes with energy transfer processes in the assay readout.

various substructures have known liabilities, known nuisance behaviour,[108] propensities for instability or to generate reactive metabolites that lead to toxicity. In various companies the incorporation of a nitro group would not be countenanced and/or is filtered out from screening collections, for fears over reactive metabolites, yet it is a feature of many successful medicines such as the blockbuster drug ranitidine. The extent/risk of metabolism or dose are just as important as substructures.[109] However, much effort is expended chasing false positives from screening campaigns and amongst the reasons for this are the interference of various structures with assay technology, be this due to colourimetric/fluorescence interference, aggregation or chemical interference.[110] Interference can occur when a compound is unstable or redox active and might produce hydrogen peroxide on prolonged storage or within an assay well, leading to protein denaturing or interference with electron transfer processes employed in the assay detection mechanisms (Figure 2.32, Table 2.5). These latter compounds are characterised as Pan Assay INterference compounds[111] (or PAINs) and publicity of these issues is resulting in increasing output quality, improving return on investment and saving time.[112] There is a note of caution when considering novel heterocyclic ring structures that might be able to participate in redox cycling or decompose to a reactive species; as such, the likely feasible number of unexplored structures may be rather smaller than predicted.[113]

## 2.3 Improving the Efficiency of Synthetic Medicinal Chemistry

In the preceding discussion, we have discussed how novel synthetic methodology has delivered dramatic impacts upon the ease with which molecules can be prepared, and the breadth of functionality that can now be readily incorporated. However, evolving

**Table 2.5** Some common motifs associated with Pan Assay Interference.

| Isothiazolones | Phenol-sulphonamides | Hydroxyphenyl hydrazones |
|---|---|---|
| 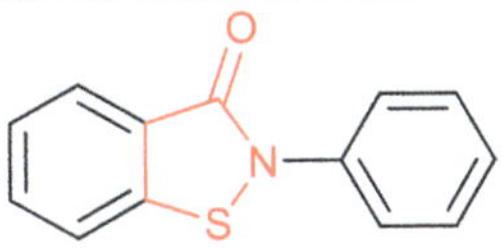 | 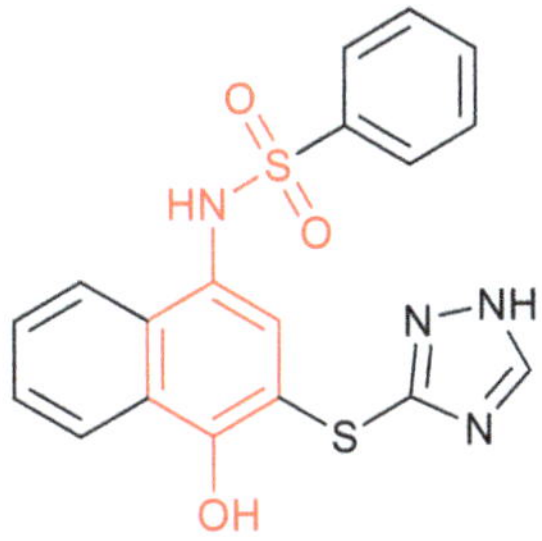 | 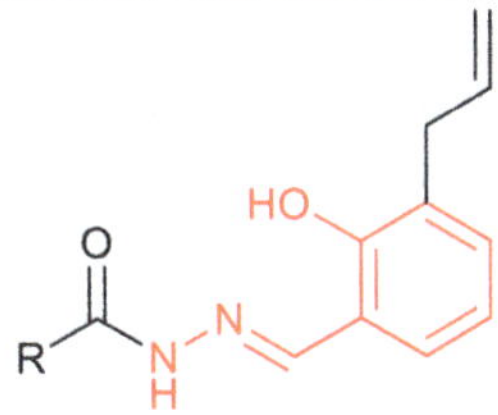 |
| Covalent modifiers, non-specific protein reactivity | Unstable, often reactive byproducts = redox cyclers, covalent modifiers | Covalent modifiers, metal complexers |
| **Ene-rhodanines** | **Benzofurazans** | **2-Amino-3-carbonyl-thiophenes** |
| 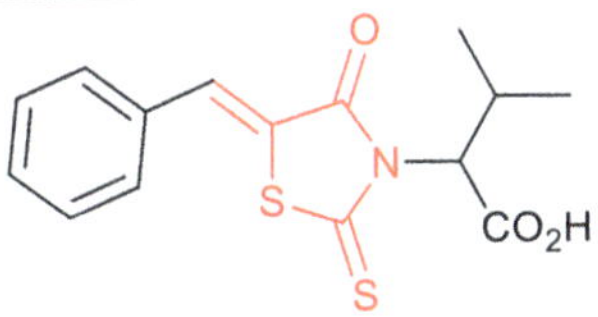 | 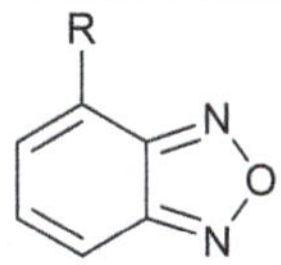 | 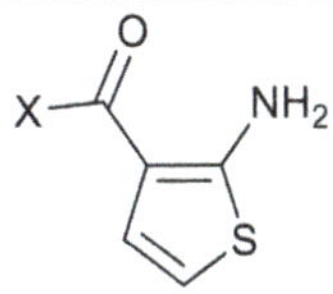 |
| Covalent modifiers, metal complexers | Unstable, biproducts = redox cyclers, | Promiscuous, non-specific and reactive |
| **Quinones and catechols** | **Curcumin (and enones)** | |
| 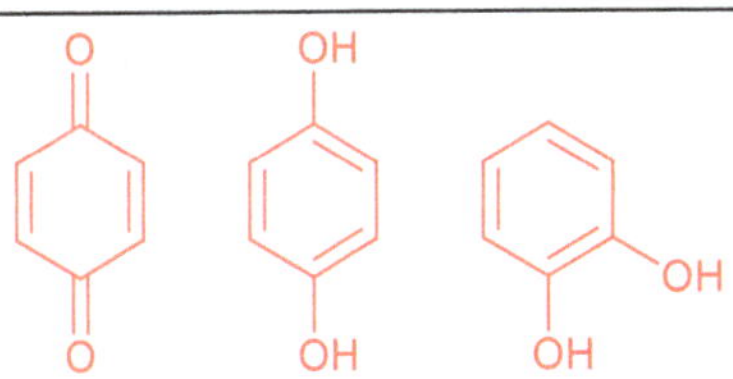 | 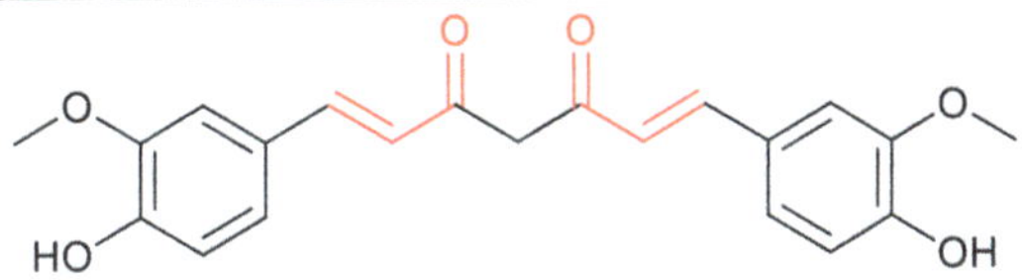 | |
| Redox cyclers, metal complexers, covalent modifiers | Covalent modifier, membrane disruptor | |

synthetic methodology has not been the only factor leading to improved bioactive molecules. Novel technologies, too, have delivered significant improvements in synthetic expediency and the ease with which complex molecules can be delivered into screening cascades. Advances in software, such as machine learning design algorithms and reaction planners, and hardware, such as flow chemistry platforms, have opened up new opportunities for the synthetic chemist, and a discussion on state-of-the-art synthesis in medicinal chemistry would be incomplete without consideration of the impacts and merits of these emerging technologies.

### 2.3.1 AI/Machine Learning in Synthesis Planning

Since the mid 1990s, synthetic chemists have grown increasingly accustomed to having facile desktop access to much of the published knowledge around organic synthesis. The widespread adoption of platforms such as REAXXYS[114] and SciFinder[115] have allowed the synthetic chemist to investigate potential routes to target molecules and investigate likely reaction conditions with prior precedent for success. With this ready accessibility comes a significant time saving in terms of literature searching and identification of appropriate synthetic options. However, such systems still require the expert knowledge of the chemist in order to sift through the myriad of options, to determine the "best" set of steps which are most likely to deliver success, given the specific arrangement of functionality and regiochemistry present in the target molecule. The intelligent automation of this process has become of significant interest in the past few years, as advances in machine learning algorithms and the systematic harvesting of the "rules" of synthesis have advanced. However, the concept is not a new one. Indeed, the first suggestion of automated reaction planning originated in Russia in the mid 1950s, even before the first demonstration of the integrated circuit. Vlédtus and Finn originally suggested an electronic tool that could, amongst other tasks, "*store…unlimited…chemical information*", "*search for classes of reactions…which a definite…compound can enter*" and "*search for ways of synthesising a given compound*".[116] Whilst the first two have been easier to deliver and form the core of the electronic chemistry data retrieval platforms, the latter goal has been significantly harder to achieve. Indeed, the scale of the problem is daunting. It has been estimated that, on average, there are around $3.5 \times 10^{28}$ potential reaction routes of 15 steps or less, all of which bring specific reactivity constrains, dependent upon the starting materials employed.[117] The first attempt to distil this complexity to a useable system came from the group of Corey and Wipke in the late 1960s, with the implementation of the OCSS design platform (Organic Chemical Simulation of Synthesis).[118] Like many later systems, OCSS attempted to distil organic synthesis into a systematic set of rules and guidelines which could be applied in a retrosynthetic fashion to a target molecule of choice. The platform, and many others since, suffered from a stepwise approach and, more importantly, an incomplete understanding of the complexities of organic synthesis.

More recently, advances in data processing and extraction of rules from the literature have permitted a more thorough understanding of this complexity, leading to systems capable of providing workable routes to a variety of molecules, from the drug-like small molecules found in typical medicinal chemistry projects, to complex total syntheses of natural products. Such systems are beginning to understand the limitations of certain reaction types and, importantly, where such reactions fail as well as where they may be successful.[119] Through the encapsulation of tens, if not hundreds or thousands, of reaction types, predictive power has increased dramatically and blind tests have demonstrated that workable routes to targets of interest can be delivered in a timely manner, with syntheses that are both sensible on paper and workable in the laboratory.[120] These systems, such as Synthia™ (formerly known as Chematica) offer the potential to expand the scope of reactions employed in the medicinal chemistry laboratory, by highlighting uncommon reaction types such as rearrangements and multi-component reactions which may not be at the forefront of the chemist's mind as obvious disconnections. However, the current systems are not without their drawbacks, and suffer from some potentially significant issues:

*Lack of awareness of failed reactions.* As many of these systems draw their entire knowledge base from the literature, they can only draw attention to that which has been reported. As authors and journals tend not to champion the reporting of failed reactions, systems may suggest a reaction is workable in the absence of knowledge to the contrary. To overcome this limitation, some larger pharmaceutical organisations are now re-training these expert systems on their own internal databases, harvesting knowledge on failed reactions from their electronic lab notebook records.[121]

*Incomplete datasets.* Again, the expert system is only as good as the data it derives its synthetic rules from. As a complete repository of all chemical knowledge does not exist, there may be useful transformations reported in the literature which are not captured and codified as a synthetic rule in such knowledge-based systems and therefore cannot be incorporated into synthetic planning.

*Intrinsic bias.* Whilst these expert systems can and do suggest truly innovative routes to new molecules, there is a significant potential to reinforce the biases of the chemists as reported in the literature. If not carefully implemented, these systems may prioritise methodology based on frequency of utilisation, *i.e.*, those most often used in the generation of large numbers of compounds, such as Pd-mediated couplings and amide formations. Quite naturally, such precedent is attractive, and the chemist may then select these familiar and well-exemplified routes based upon their robustness and wide reporting. In doing so, over time the utilisation of these reactions increases ever further, making them more likely to be suggested by latter generation of the AI systems, defeating their deployment in order to help us avoid over-reliance on certain reaction types.[122] Such self-reinforced bias may therefore reduce the desired creativity and power of the predictive systems unless the assessment and scoring of the resultant routes are made with such biases included in the rankings.

*Cost.* Given the tasks involved in creating these expert systems, it is unsurprising that access to the platforms comes with a significant potential cost. Whilst some platforms are open access and can be consulted *via* a simple web browser,[123] there may be some concerns around submitting commercially sensitive structures to a public access data system, in terms of confidentiality and IP protection. Does, for example, such a submission count as a public disclosure and thus preclude patent protection?

However, it is worthy of note that similar arguments were made against scientific database systems such as SciFinder and REAXXYS in their early iterations. Over time, such systems have become commonplace and it is not unreasonable to anticipate that similar access models will evolve in time. Notwithstanding the current limitations, it is becoming increasingly clear that these expert systems can now play a significant role in the prediction of likely routes to complex compounds of biological interest, potentially opening up significantly expanded areas of chemical space to the synthetic and medicinal chemist.

### 2.3.2 Automation and Linking to Reaction Planning

The advances in retrosynthetic planning software described above have led to a revival of the long-standing desire to fully automate medicinal and synthetic chemistry practices. Since the evolution of automated peptide synthesisers in the 1960s,[124,125] many attempts have been made to develop more flexible automated synthetic platforms that can process a variety of transformations, and not just amino acid deprotection and coupling steps. Extending this capability to encompass the breadth of chemistry transformations, reagents, conditions *etc.* has not been a trivial undertaking. In the 1990s and early 2000s, some notable progress toward automated and flexible synthesis was achieved with the development of integrated flow systems that could link multiple synthetic steps in series and deliver final compounds in a largely autonomous manner.[126,127] However, in order to synthesise an alternate molecule, the entire platform required bespoke re-configuration and these systems did not offer the level of flexibility required to truly deliver on their promise. Nonetheless, such systems could be configured, through selection of different reagent streams, to deliver small, focussed libraries of derivatives which could form the basis of hit expansion projects to support medicinal chemists.

More recently, significant improvements in automation and component interchangeability have led to more complex systems which can interpret standardised reaction protocols, re-configure the flow chemistry modules to suit specific reaction conditions, select variable reagent paths and, in doing so, deliver a range of bespoke libraries of compounds for screening, largely in the absence of human intervention.[128]

Improvements in microfluidic systems, coupled with such technologies, offer the advantage of miniaturisation, with further advantages over reaction heat flow and control and reagent cost minimisation to prepare extensive libraries of compounds for screening in an automated fashion.[129] Such systems have also been linked with parallel advances in microfluidics biological assay development.[130] Compounds exiting the synthetic flow path can therefore be immediately evaluated for their biological activity.

As such systems evolve, fully integrated and closed-loop design–make–test systems are starting to be developed, where computational or biological data are fed back to an automated design algorithm which then instructs the modular synthetic platform to prepare a further series of analogues for screening.[131–133] This iterative approach offers significant potential to dramatically increase the pace of obtaining structure–activity relationships and optimising compounds for biological activity. However, several technical issues remain to be solved before such systems are fully practicable:

- Whilst some standardised reaction protocols exist, these expert systems will need to be able to autonomously select the best generalised protocol to apply to the preparation of the proposed analogues. Whilst efforts are underway to extract such protocols from the patent and journal archives,[134,135] they are not yet comprehensive or fully robust.
- The configurable and modular synthetic systems are not yet able to effect all conceivable synthetic transformations. Again, significant efforts are underway to help incorporate structural diversity of scaffolds and peripheral functionality (including, for example, concise approaches to arrays of complex natural-product-like

functionality from commercially available building blocks),[136] the system must be able to distinguish what compounds it can, and cannot, prepare and adapt accordingly.
- Similarly, the automated reaction planning algorithms must also be encoded with the knowledge of what reaction types, conditions and purification techniques can, and cannot, be utilised, to enable the selection of the most facile reaction pathway.
- In-line biological assessment, at present, tends to be a single read-out which does not permit the multi-parametric optimisation of both potency, selectivity and pharmacokinetic profiles common to most medicinal chemistry projects. However, such systems could conceivably be linked to machine-learning based systems which draw upon matched-pairs analysis,[137] or internal databases to predict potential liabilities and incorporate suggested changes to improve overall selectivity or molecular properties,[138] not just intrinsic potency against the primary biological target.

Despite these present challenges, the advances made in this area suggest these fully integrated platforms are tantalisingly close to revolutionising the delivery of advanced leads for final medicinal chemistry problems. As such, these systems could be envisaged to reduce the value of the synthetic chemist. However, rather than a threat to the synthetic community, such systems will demand new synthetic methodology, optimised to be robust and of wide synthetic scope and which reveals new areas of chemical space, satisfying the factors for success described above. The systems will also require synthetic expertise to help develop and optimise the resultant compounds from these systems which, whilst accelerating the process to an advanced lead, are unlikely to deliver finalised, optimised molecules ready for clinical evaluation.

### 2.3.3 Synthetic Techniques and Technologies: Flow Chemistry

The fundamental procedure of organic synthesis is the controlled mixing of reagents to effect the combination and/or modification of one or more components in the reaction in a safe, effective and efficient manner. Traditionally, this is achieved in Quickfit™ glassware arranged to ensure controlled addition, stirring and temperature control, which by and large is a scalable process towards the reactor vessels employed in development and production. The advent of combinatorial chemistry advanced technologies to enable multiple parallel syntheses, with equipment capable of handling multiple reagents with distinct vessels or plate-based methods, often employing robotics or automation. An aspirational vision of a fully integrated robotic synthesis and purification platform coupled with biological and physicochemical screening (as described above) is proposed as one solution to reduce design–make–test cycle times, but would necessarily be limited by the availability and flexibility of applicable chemistries. The fashion for solid phase methods to deliver combinatorial products has evolved into the methodologies used for DNA encoded libraries. Other equipment enabling safer and more effective heating and cooling of reactions has seen widespread uptake; the techniques and automation with microwave heating of sealed vessels are highly impactful pieces of technology in discovery labs. Future opportunities are emerging with advances in such areas as photochemistry and electrochemistry, whilst new techniques and technologies with homogeneous and heterogenous catalysis will likely emerge.

Technologies utilising the mixing of reagents in continuous flow offer new opportunities in synthetic chemistry. The use of flow apparatus to enable safer and more controlled hydrogenation and hydrogenolysis reactions is now widespread; such control of conditions and minimisation of exposure to potentially hazardous/dangerous reagents or mixtures is an attractive feature of the technology. However, the use of flow apparatus in multiple parallel reactions is a typical example of misuse of technology advocated as innovation. The technology is exceptionally effective with highly optimised conditions, but often fails to transfer easily and directly to similar substrates, particularly when combinations of reagents require different conditions or monomers have differing solubilities (causing line blockages). Opportunities exist with flow reactors for the commercialisation of processes that were previously deemed too hazardous or risky, because of the enhanced control of conditions and limited volume and exposure of reactive intermediates. For example, the cooling power required to maintain the <1 litre volume of the flow reactor at low temperature is much less than is necessary for a 10 000 litre batch vessel!

A future vision would see developments in flow allied to other new technologies such as photochemistry and electrochemistry. Together, such approaches could reliably furnish high $sp^3$ content intermediates with novel architectures such as the example in Figure 2.33.[139] Incorporation of such novel architectures into library design (real or virtual), would allow facile translation of emerging reaction techniques from academic groups into medicinal chemistry laboratories to achieve true innovation, whereby the scalable flow methodology has been front loaded into the discovery process.

The significant potential for an integrated approach is illustrated by the commissioning of flow production plants with great success, which deliver considerable safety improvements and highly reproducible quality and yields. For example, Figure 2.34 shows the multi-stage continuous manufacturing rig commissioned to manufacture fluticasone propionate at GSK using a reworking of the existing batch process (Scheme 2.7) to deliver the drug substance in a more efficient and reproducible process with reduced environmental impact.[140]

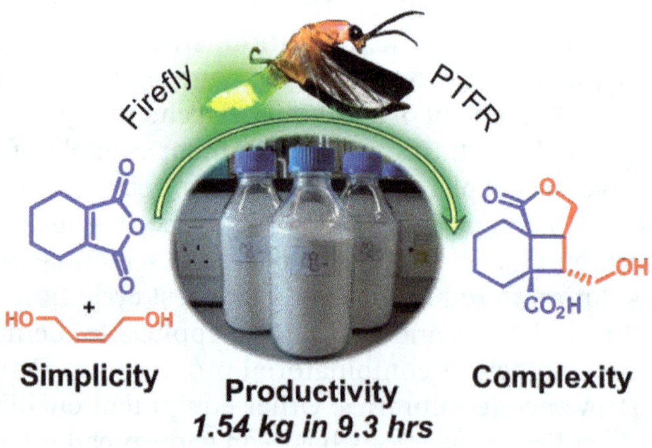


**Figure 2.33** An illustration of the potential for photochemical flow reactors to deliver complex structures suitable for divergent functionalisation in the generation of $sp^3$ rich and structurally diverse libraries. Reproduced from ref. 139 with permission from American Chemical Society, Copyright 2016.

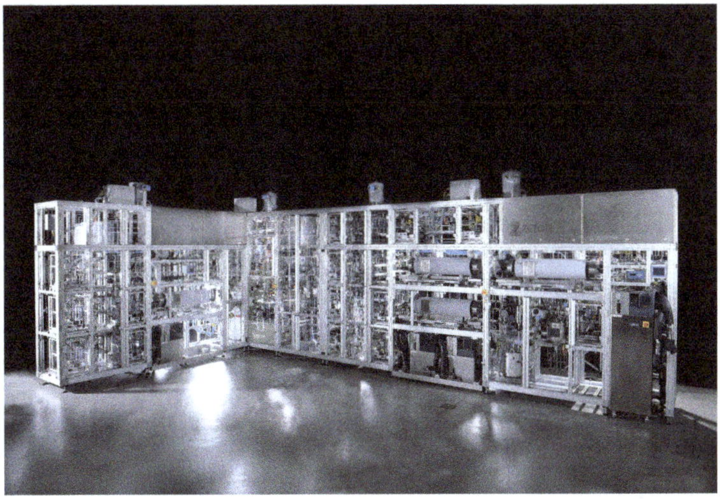

**Figure 2.34** The multi-stage continuous manufacturing rig for fluticasone propionate commissioned by GSK from Zeton, whom we thank for permission to use this photograph. Image Credit: © GSK.

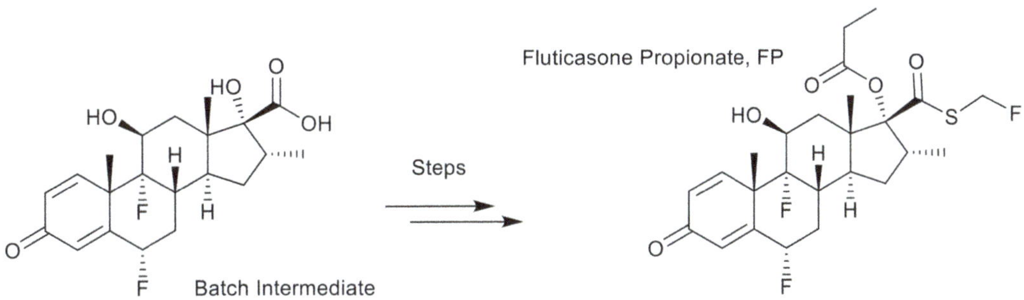


**Scheme 2.7** Batch process for fluticasone propionate, which has been reworked and modified for flow and to minimise environmental impact and enhance safety and reproducibility.

## 2.3.4 Purification Technologies and Compound Handling

A further rate-limiting step in drug discovery is the work-up, purification, characterisation and handling of the desired substance. In the early stages, the molecule is often the product of a sub-optimal, but fit for purpose, reaction that requires purification. Increasingly, technology impacts on these processes through automation and parallel handling, encompassing the extremes of miniaturisation and larger-scale systems. Typically, chromatographic purifications are employed on increasing scales from micro-/milligrams (mass-directed automatic preparative HPLC commonly used) to grams (often medium pressure semi-automated flash systems) and ultimately up to kilograms (commonly with extra-large columns on medium pressure systems). Developments in analytical techniques enable the direct scale-up of reverse-phase LCMS traces to medium pressure systems and direct mass spectral analysis from thin layer chromatography plates give rise to a further improvement in reaction monitoring and chromatography optimisation when the required product can be identified.

As drugs progress through the pipeline, increasing amounts are required and purification technology has enabled the exploitation of unoptimised, fit for purpose routes to deliver enough material for decision making studies. Clearly, better syntheses are more effective and efficient ways of achieving these aims, so joined up thinking through the process is impactful, contributing to a culture of expedient decision making. The time and cost of reworking synthetic routes can thus be recouped, which historically was often wasted in remaking quantities of compounds that failed.

The use of newer medium pressure and HPLC methods with more traditional silica chromatography is compared and contrasted in Table 2.6, whilst Table 2.7 illustrates the applicability of reverse-phase systems to more drug-like molecules and fragments.[141] This is an area of rapid technological developments in terms of the equipment, pumps, detectors and the column compositions and eluents, including variations on normal and reverse-phase silica columns, chiral columns with bespoke eluant compositions including supercritical fluids. Newer techniques such as Hydrophilic Interaction Liquid Chromatography and charge variants on the theme, complement older techniques (Figure

**Table 2.6** Comparison of preparative chromatography techniques.

| | Glass column flash | Medium pressure flash | HPLC |
|---|---|---|---|
| **Cost** | £ | ££ | £££££ |
| **Column container** | Glass | Plastic | Steel |
| **Pressure** | 1–2 bar | 3–10 bar | 100–200 bar |
| **Packing** | Self-packed loose silica (potential hazard) | Prepacked | Prepacked or specialised self-pack |
| **Normal phase** | Routine | Routine, quicker, scalable | Routine, little exploited |
| **Reverse phase** | Practically difficult | Yes, enhanced modified stationary phases increasingly available | Yes, many options available |
| **Gradient** | Difficult, stepped | Automated | Automated |
| **Detection/collection** | All fractions need to be analysed | UV/ELSD-driven automated collection | UV/ELSD/MS-driven automated collection |
| **Maintenance** | Very low | Low – robust systems operating at lower pressures | High – high pressures place demands on the system necessitating regular servicing and part replacement |
| **Routine scale** | Milligrams to 100 s of grams | Milligrams to kilograms | Milligrams to 10 s of grams |

**Table 2.7** Fragments, lead-like molecules and drug averages defined by their lipophilicity values: how these relate to the percentages of acetonitrile required to elute them by reverse-phase chromatography.

| Compound | log P (OW scale) | log D range (OW scale)[a] | Chrom log D[b] | C-18% MeCN to elute |
|---|---|---|---|---|
| Fragment | −0.5 to 2 | −3.5 to 2 | −1.5 to 4 | 6–70 |
| Lead-like | −1 to 3 | −4 to 3 | −2 to 5 | 0–81 |
| Average drug | 2.7 | −0.3 to 2.7[b] | 1.7–4.7[b] | 43–78[b] |

[a]Illustrative range assumes a 3 log shift on full ionisation for the given log *P*; some bases/acids can give a 4 log shift. For unionised compounds at a given pH, $\log D_{pH} = \log P$; Chrom $\log D_{pH} \approx$ OW $\log D_{pH} + 2$, where OW = *n*Octanol–water (aqueous buffer) *P*artition/*D*istribution.

[b]These figures are based on average log *P* of 2.7, the average OW $\log D_{pH7.4}$ of a drug is 0.8.

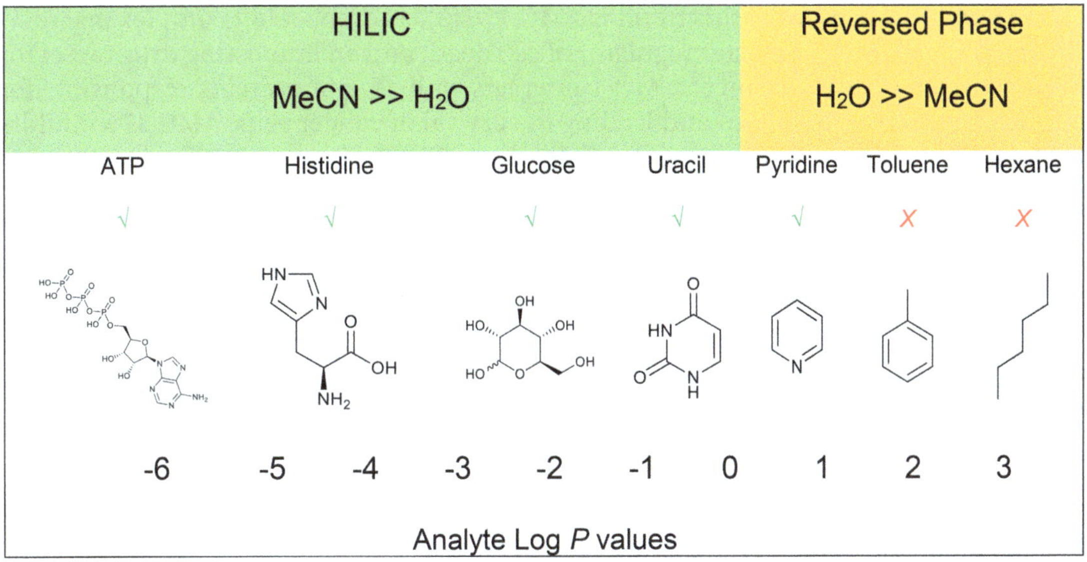


**Figure 2.35** Expanded range of molecular properties of molecules exemplifying the range of lipophilicities that can be purified by new partitioning chromatography techniques such as HILIC.

2.35). These expand the range of increasingly more prevalent, more polar molecules that can be purified, where traditional silica or reverse-phase methods would not be suitable.

## 2.4 Case Studies

At the outset of this chapter, the current state-of-the-art in synthesis was described, and assessment made of historical perspectives. This assessment painted a somewhat bleak picture of routine chemistries and rather unimaginative molecules as potential new therapeutics. However, synthetic determination and ambition remains a core component of drug discovery and has led to the progression of highly complex molecules into clinical evaluation and beyond. In contrast to the simple, prototypical molecules in Figure 2.1, the following examples discuss recent case studies from the medicinal chemistry literature where bespoke, exquisite syntheses have yielded highly active and complex molecules on scales appropriate for clinical supply. They serve as a timely reminder of the creativity of the synthetic chemist to overcome the challenges of drug discovery and the optimisation of drug molecules.

### 2.4.1 AMG-176

In certain areas of drug discovery, molecular complexity remains an important driver of biological activity and this is particularly true in the area of inhibitors of protein–protein interactions.[142,143] In these interactions, binding sites tend to be much larger, more open and often less featured than those found in the buried cavities exploited in enzymes or other drug targets. As such, the resultant molecules often tend to be elongated derivatives which exist in the "Beyond Rule of Five" physicochemical space.[144]

One notable exception to this trend is AMG-176 (**3**), a compact but complex macrocyclic inhibitor of Mcl-1, a master regulator of cell death and an interesting drug target for the treatment of various cancers. Mcl-1 interacts with several proteins responsible for cell death, sequestering them and leading to survival of cancer cells. AMG-176 inhibits these interactions, leading to cancer cell death.

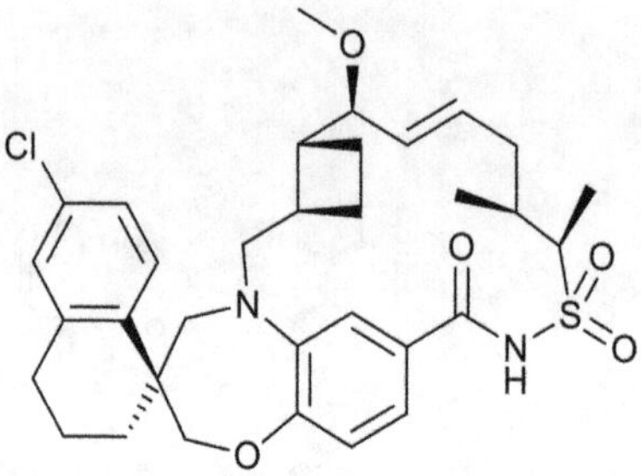

AMG-176 **3**

The medicinal chemistry design strategy leading to the discovery of AMG-176 is highly elegant,[145] but of equal elegance is the synthetic route devised to allow construction of the macrocycle and explore the SAR of many related derivatives, as described in Scheme 2.8. A convergent synthesis with some twenty linear steps in the longest pathway, the synthesis commences from a simple chlorodihdronaphthalinone **4** which is converted to the key *spiro*-benzoxazepine **6** following the selective monoacylation and desymmetrisation of dione **5** using Kang's catalyst.[146] A second desymmetrisation, this time using enzymatic deacylation,[147] generates the key chiral cyclobutyl intermediate **7** (four steps, 70% overall yield), which can be incorporated *via* reductive amination. A stereo-controlled vinylation of the resultant aldehyde establishes the final chiral centre in the left-hand side of the macrocyclic precursor. The right-hand side of the eventual macrocycle is then introduced using the chiral sulphonamide **8** (itself prepared in five steps with a 17% overall yield), allowing the key macrocyclisation step using a Hoyveda–Grubbs ring-closing metathesis.[148] Finally, O-methylation completes the synthesis of AMG-176 **3** in an overall reported yield of 10.4% for the longest sequence.[149] These yields equate to an average of 88% per step (or 85% average, including the synthesis of the key intermediates), to deliver an impressive 115 g of final material with six stereogenic centres.

### 2.4.2 E7130, C52-Halichondrin-B-amine

Natural products have been the mainstay of therapeutic agents for most of the history of medicines discovery but, for the most part, the complexity of these agents has precluded their widespread acceptance and production on a commercial scale. Whilst some natural products have seen commercial success after development of fermentation routes (such as the penicillins and cephalosporins)[150] or through semi-synthesis (such as the taxanes),[30] accessing these complex agents through total synthesis was usually considered to be too complex to facilitate clinical supply.

In an unprecedented commitment to the power of synthetic chemistry, Eisai recently entered into clinical trials with Halaven™ **9**, the mesylate salt of the wholly synthetic halichondrin derivative eribulin.[151] Arising from several years of collaboration with the

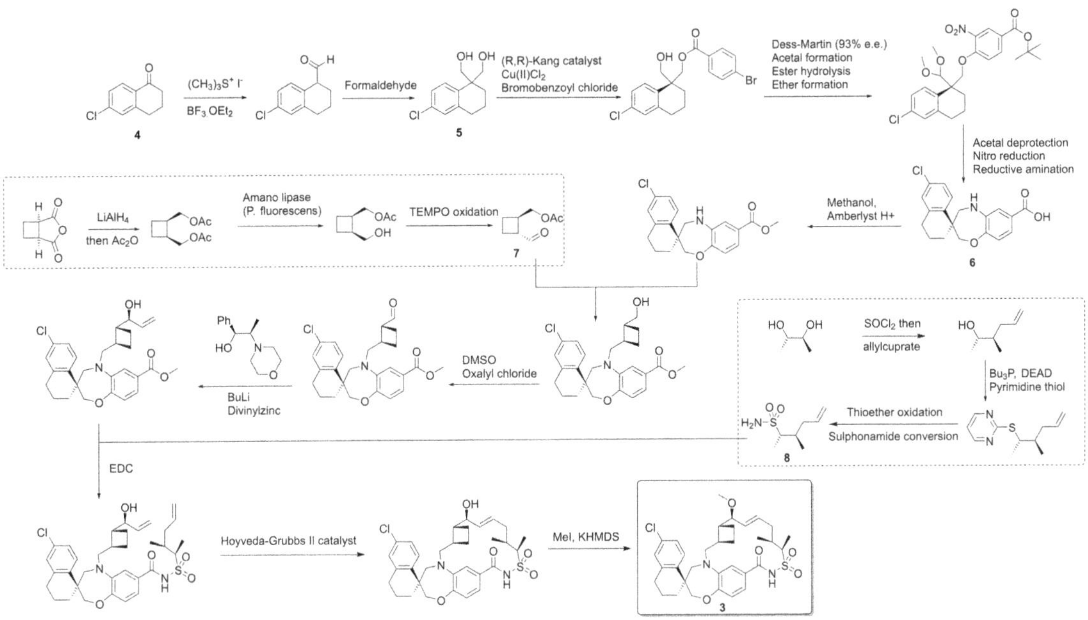

Scheme 2.8 Synthesis of AMG-176.

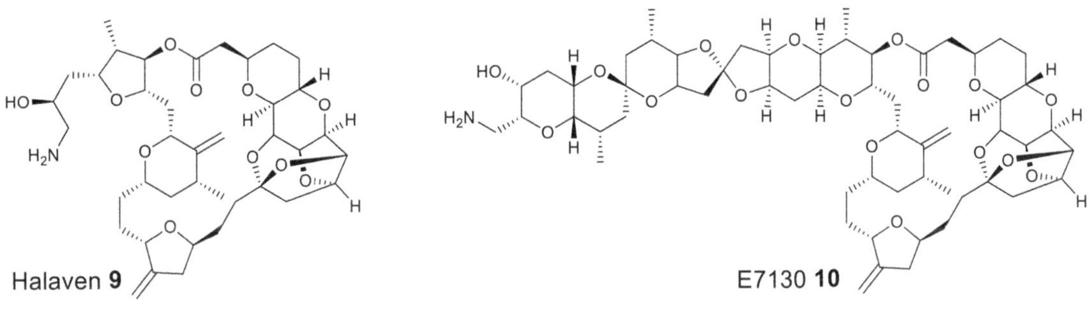

Figure 2.36 Halichondrin derivatives.

Kishi group, this molecule set a new standard for the complexity of molecules delivered into the clinic by synthesis. However, this bar was again raised by the entry into the clinic of the amino-halichondrin derivative E7130 **10** (Figure 2.36).

The key right-hand-side component of the compound is constructed in a convergent synthetic plan starting from D-gulonolactone **11** and D-galactal **12** (Scheme 2.9). D-Galactal is elaborated through key intermediate **13** to access, in a stereo-controlled manner, the upper tricyclic ether component of the halichondrin core, utilising a late-stage Cr-mediated allylation to introduce the tetrahydropyran-3-ene unit which forms the left-hand side of the primary macrocycle **14**.[152] In parallel, the D-gulonolactone **11** is elaborated through an ion-exchange-mediated acid/base cyclisation step to form the complex lower portion of the halichondrin core **15**. A Ni/Cr-mediated ring formation then joins the two component parts, followed by macrolactonisation to complete the synthesis of the main macrocyclic core **16**.[153]

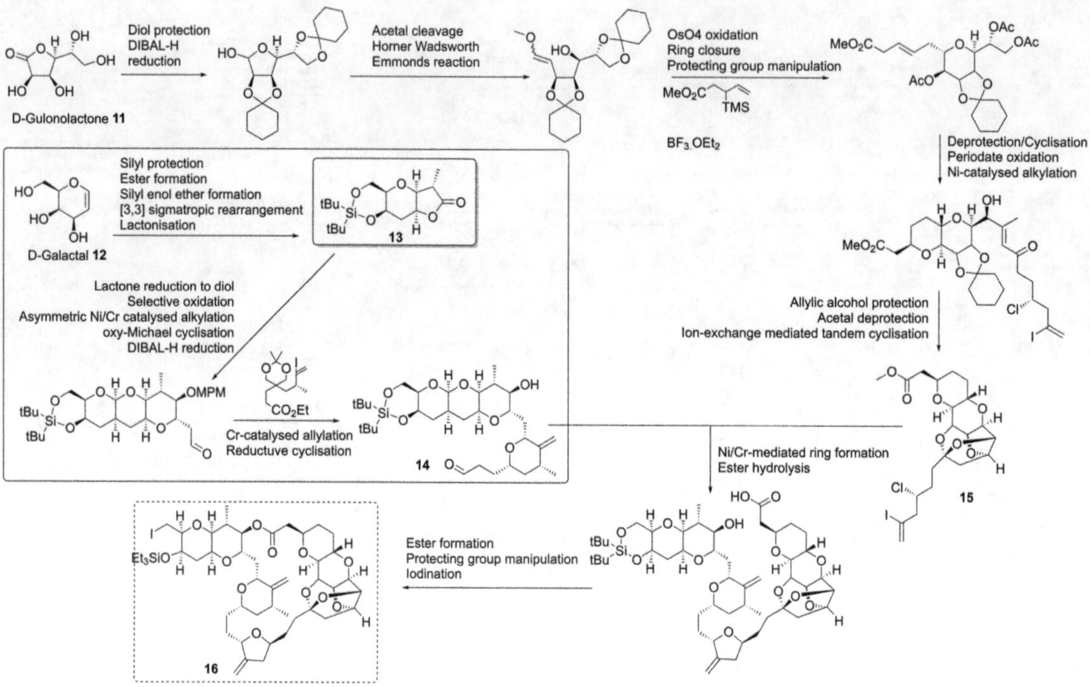

Scheme 2.9 Construction of the right-hand side of E7130.

With impressive efficiency of planning, the left-hand-side component of E7130 is also derived from the same key protected building block **13** from which the right-hand side originates (Scheme 2.10). After epimerisation, ring expansion and an oxy-Michael cyclisation to construct the spiropyran ring junction complete the key left-hand-side precursor **17**.[154] A Weix nickel-catalysed coupling of the resultant thioether appends the left-hand-side component to the previously prepared right-hand-side macrocycle **16**.[155] A further lactonisation step reveals the spiro-tetrahydrofuranyl moiety. Finally, deprotection and further functional group interconversions complete the synthetic journey, yielding 11.5 g of final material **10**.[156]

Overall, the synthesis comprises some 92 steps and the resultant molecule contains 31 stereo-controlled centres. The extreme potency of the molecule (with cellular cytotoxicity $IC_{50}$ values in the 0.01–0.1 nM range)[157] allows dosing at 25 μg $m^{-3}$ twice monthly, equating to roughly 100 μg per month per patient. As such, the delivered 11.5 g batch equates to some 115 000 clinical doses, or sufficient to treat almost 5000 patients for a year.

## 2.5 The Future? New Modalities and Synthetic Impact

What might be considered traditional small molecule medicinal chemistry could be seen as a declining practice; only a small proportion of the biggest selling medicines by value are now small molecules, overtaken by biological agents such as antibodies. However, the impact of small molecules on human health is still of vital importance when the number of prescriptions of both patented and generic medicines are considered,

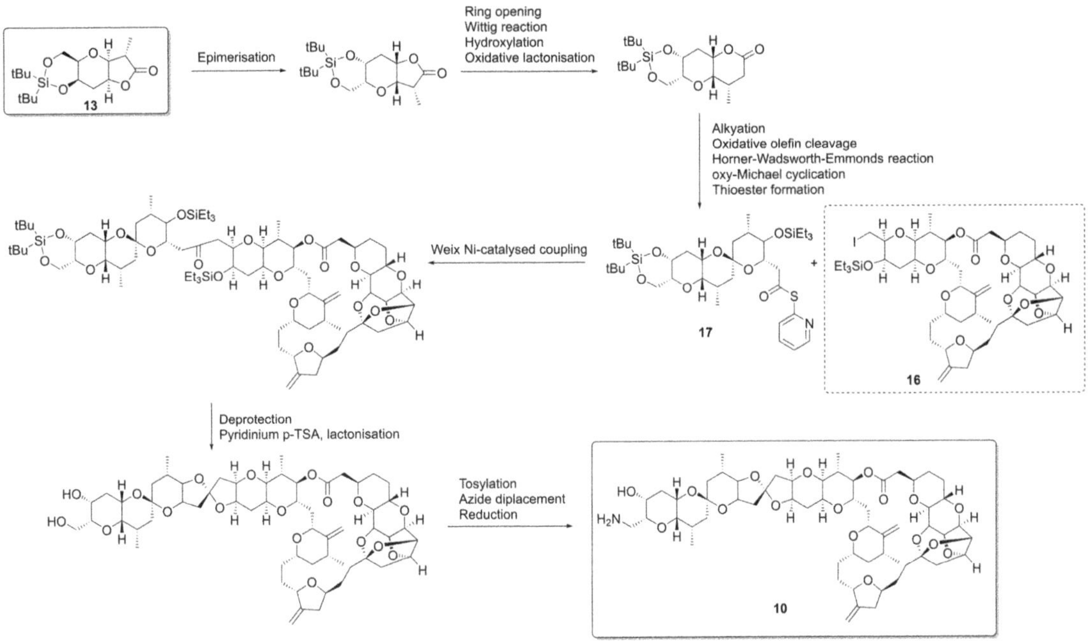


**Scheme 2.10** Synthesis of the E7130 left-hand side and completion of synthesis of E7130.

where small molecules by far outstrip the higher cost biologicals in terms of frequency of use and convenience in dosing and supply logistics. Looking toward the future, small molecules will continue to play a significant role in the delivery of novel and impactful therapeutics.

Of equal importance, synthetic chemistry also enables and enhances our understanding of novel biological mechanisms, through the delivery of potent, selective and robust chemical probe molecules, utilised in countless chemical biology experiments to confirm (or refute) the findings of genetic experiments.[158] In numerous cases, the complete removal of a protein though genetic engineering has a very different biological outcome to that of a small molecule inhibitor. The delivery a robust, credible chemical probe and the replication of the underlying biological hypothesis, marks a significant step forward in the progression of a medicinal chemistry project from hypothesis to marketed drug.[159] This crucial role of synthesis, to provide tools critical to target validation or invalidation, will remain a challenge for synthetic and medicinal chemists as new and more complex drug targets emerge from a deeper understanding of human biology.

In future, deeper therapeutic impact may well be achieved outside of traditional low molecular weight structures, as the properties and functions of macrocycles, chimeric molecules and other higher molecular weight molecules become better understood (Figure 2.37). The biological understanding and modulation of proteins was the focus for many years of drug discovery and new opportunities arise with stapled, cyclic and other peptide modifications to improve the pharmacology and pharmacokinetics of these agents and their mimetics. New opportunities for therapeutic intervention with nucleic acids (amenable to automated synthesis in the way that solid phase resins revolutionised protein work) and progress in the understanding of the structure and function of

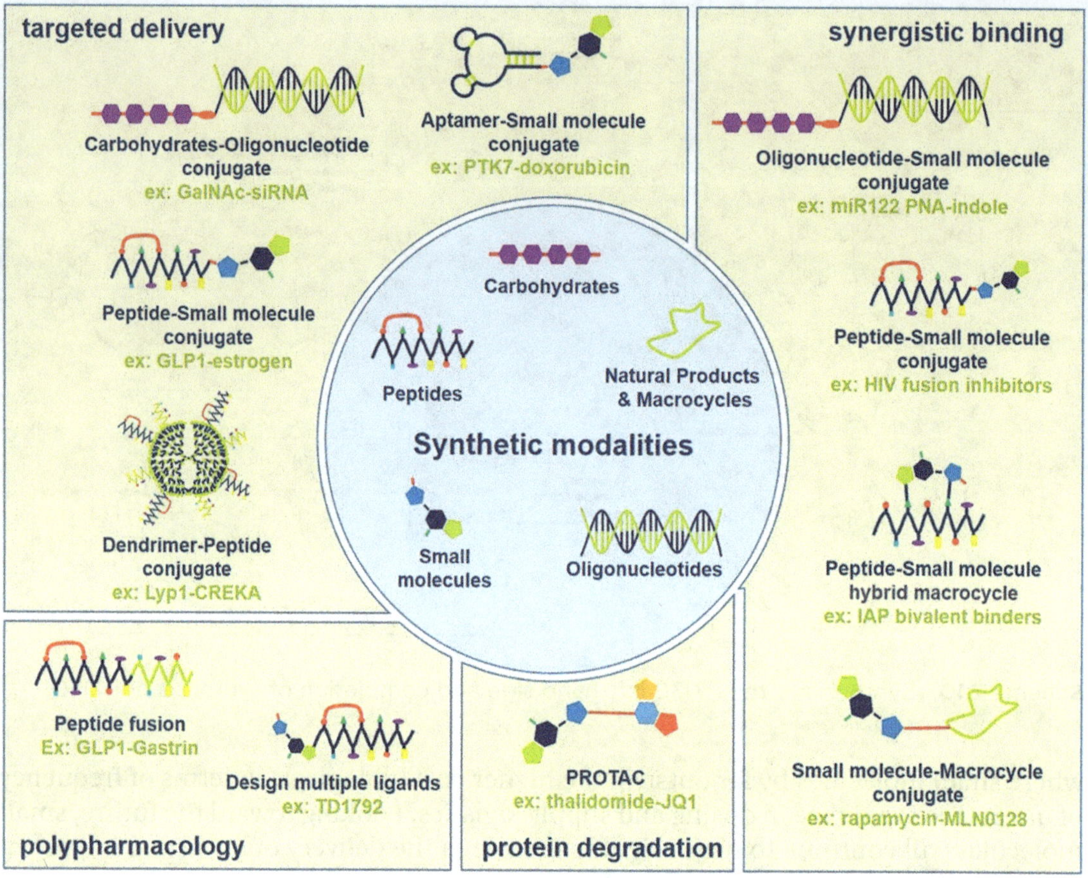


**Figure 2.37** New concepts in drug discovery exploiting hybrid approaches from traditional synthetic modalities to deliver novel therapeutics and modes of action.[160] Reproduced from ref. 160 with permission from John Wiley & Sons, Copyright © 2017 Wiley-VCH Verlag GmbH & Co. KGaA, Weinheim.

carbohydrates (wherein automated synthesis is now feasible chemically and developing further with biocatalysis) opens further avenues. Progress will undoubtedly be made with targeted hybrids of the various classes of small molecules, peptides, nucleic acids and oligosaccharides. After all, biological agents themselves are just rather bigger molecules which are defined, ultimately, by their chemistry and how they are synthesised, even if that might be by a biological system on a grand scale. Taken together, it is clear that synthetic chemistry remains vital to the progress and success of medicinal chemistry and will continue to have a major impact on drug discovery and human health for the foreseeable future.

## References

1. S. Roughley and A. Jordan, *J. Med. Chem.*, 2011, **54**, 3401.
2. A. Jordan and S. Roughley, *Drug Discovery Today*, 2009, **14**, 731.

3. J. Boström, D. Brown, R. Young and G. Keserü, *Nat. Rev. Drug Discovery*, 2018, **17**, 922.
4. W. Walters, J. Green, J. Weiss and M. Murko, *J. Med. Chem.*, 2011, **54**, 6405.
5. D. Brown and J. Boström, *J. Med. Chem.*, 2016, **59**, 4443.
6. D. Dias, S. Urban and U. Roessner, *Metabolites*, 2012, **2**, 303.
7. C. Lipinski, F. Lombardo, B. Dominy and P. Feeney, *Adv. Drug Delivery Rev.*, 2001, **46**, 3.
8. A. Tomberg and J. Boström, *Drug Discovery Today*, 2020, **25**, 2174.
9. F. Goldberg, J. Kettle, T. Kogej, M. Perry and N. Tompkinson, *Drug Discovery Today*, 2015, **20**, 11.
10. D. Blakemore, L. Castro, I. Churcher, D. Rees, A. Thomas, D. Wilson and A. Wood, *Nat. Chem.*, 2018, **10**, 383.
11. D. Foley, A. Nelson and S. Marsden, *Angew. Chem., Int. Ed.*, 2016, **55**, 13650.
12. T. Cooper, I. Campbell and S. MacDonald, *Angew. Chem., Int. Ed.*, 2010, **49**, 8082.
13. V. Quirke, *Stud. Hist. Philos. Biol. Biomed. Sci.*, 2005, **36**, 645–674.
14. M. Meanwell, S. M. Silverman, J. Lehmann, B. Adluri, Y. Wang, R. Cohen, L.-C. Campeau and R. Britton, *Science*, 2020, **369**, 725–730.
15. R. J. Young and P. D. Leeson, *J. Med. Chem.*, 2018, **61**, 6421–6467.
16. K. W. Kuntz, J. E. Campbell, H. Keilhack, R. M. Pollock, S. K. Knutson, M. Porter-Scott, V. M. Richon, C. J. Sneeringer, T. J. Wigle, C. J. Allain, C. R. Majer, M. P. Moyer, R. A. Copeland and R. Chesworth, *J. Med. Chem.*, 2016, **59**, 1556–1564.
17. D. Aynetdinova, M. C. Callens, H. B. Hicks, C. Y. X. Poh, B. D. A. Shennan, A. M. Boyd, Z. H. Lim, J. A. Leitch and D. J. Dixon, *Chem. Soc. Rev.*, 2021, **50**, 5517.
18. K. Muller, C. Faeh and F. Diederich, *Science*, 2007, **317**, 1881–1886.
19. E. P. Gillis, K. J. Eastman, M. D. Hill, D. J. Donnelly and N. A. Meanwell, *J. Med. Chem.*, 2015, **58**, 8315–8359.
20. J. Cramer, C. P. Sager and B. Ernst, *J. Med. Chem.*, 2019, **62**, 8915–8930.
21. A. P. Taylor, R. P. Robinson, Y. M. Fobian, D. C. Blakemore, L. H. Jones and O. Fadeyi, *Org. Biomol. Chem.*, 2016, **14**, 6611–6637.
22. T. Y. Zhang, in *Adv. Heterocycl. Chem.*, ed. E. F. V. Scriven and C. A. Ramsden, Academic Press, 2017, vol. 121, pp. 1–12.
23. J. Jampilek, *Molecules*, 2019, **24**, 3839.
24. W. R. Pitt, D. M. Parry, B. G. Perry and C. R. Groom, *J. Med. Chem.*, 2009, **52**, 2952–2963.
25. C. M. Marson, in *Adv. Heterocycl. Chem.*, ed. E. F. V. Scriven and C. A. Ramsden, Academic Press, 2017, vol. 121, pp. 13–33.
26. E. M. Carreira and T. C. Fessard, *Chem. Rev.*, 2014, **114**, 8257–8322.
27. P. J. Coleman, J. D. Schreier, C. D. Cox, M. J. Breslin, D. B. Whitman, M. J. Bogusky, G. B. McGaughey, R. A. Bednar, W. Lemaire, S. M. Doran, S. V. Fox, S. L. Garson, A. L. Gotter, C. M. Harrell, D. R. Reiss, T. D. Cabalu, D. Cui, T. Prueksaritanont, J. Stevens, P. L. Tannenbaum, R. G. Ball, J. Stellabott, S. D. Young, G. D. Hartman, C. J. Winrow and J. J. Renger, *ChemMedChem*, 2012, **7**, 415–424, 337.
28. C. Zhang, F. Ye, J. Wang, P. He, M. Lei, L. Huang, A. Huang, P. Tang, H. Lin, Y. Liao, Y. Liang, J. Ni and P. Yan, *J. Med. Chem.*, 2020, **63**, 7108–7126.
29. A. F. Stepan, T. P. Tran, C. J. Helal, M. S. Brown, C. Chang, R. E. O'Connor, M. De Vivo, S. D. Doran, E. L. Fisher, S. Jenkinson, D. Karanian, B. L. Kormos, R. Sharma, G. S. Walker, A. S. Wright, E. X. Yang, M. A. Brodney, T. T. Wager, P. R. Verhoest and R. S. Obach, *ACS Med. Chem. Lett.*, 2018, **9**, 68–72.
30. L. D. Pennington and D. T. Moustakas, *J. Med. Chem.*, 2017, **60**, 3552–3579.
31. T. Cernak, K. D. Dykstra, S. Tyagarajan, P. Vachal and S. W. Krska, *Chem. Soc. Rev.*, 2016, **45**, 546–576.
32. M. Moir, J. J. Danon, T. A. Reekie and M. Kassiou, *Expert Opin. Drug Discovery*, 2019, **14**, 1137–1149.
33. G. E. M. Crisenza and P. Melchiorre, *Nat. Commun.*, 2020, **11**, 803.
34. J. Liu, L. Lu, D. Wood and S. Lin, *ACS Cent. Sci.*, 2020, **6**, 1317–1340.
35. L. Gao and Y. Teng, *Future Med. Chem.*, 2016, **8**, 567–577.
36. P. J. Sarver, V. Bacauanu, D. M. Schultz, D. A. DiRocco, Y.-h. Lam, E. C. Sherer and D. W. C. MacMillan, *Nat. Chem.*, 2020, **12**, 459–467.
37. N. Noto, T. Koike and M. Akita, *J. Org. Chem.*, 2016, **81**, 7064–7071.
38. M. S. Lall, A. Bassyouni, J. Bradow, M. Brown, M. Bundesmann, J. Chen, G. Ciszewski, A. E. Hagen, D. Hyek, S. Jenkinson, B. Liu, R. S. Obach, S. Pan, U. Reilly, N. Sach, D. J. Smaltz, D. K. Spracklin, J. Starr, M. Wagenaar and G. S. Walker, *J. Med. Chem.*, 2020, **63**, 7268–7292.
39. J. Shanu-Wilson, L. Evans, S. Wrigley, J. Steele, J. Atherton and J. Boer, *ACS Med. Chem. Lett.*, 2020, **11**, 2087–2107.
40. J. C. Sadler, *ChemBioChem*, 2020, **21**, 3489.
41. M. Wani and S. Horwitz, *Anticancer Drugs*, 2014, **25**, 482.

42. M. Wani, H. Taylor, M. Wall, P. Coggan and A. McPhail, *J. Am. Chem. Soc.*, 1971, **93**, 2325.
43. R. Holton, C. Somoza, H. Kim, F. Liang, R. Beidiger, P. Boatman, M. Shindo, C. Smith, S. Kim, H. Nadizadeh, Y. Suzuki, C. Tao, S. Tang, P. Zhang, K. Murthi, L. Gentile and J. Liu, *J. Am. Chem. Soc.*, 1994, **116**, 1597.
44. R. Holton, H. Kim, C. S. F. Liang, R. Beidiger, P. Boatman, M. Shindo, C. Smith, S. Kim, H. Nadizadeh, Y. Suzuki, C. Tao, S. Tang, P. Zhang, K. Murthi, L. Gentile and J. Liu, *J. Am. Chem. Soc.*, 1994, **116**, 1599.
45. K. Nicolaou, Z. Yang, J. Lui, H. Ueno, P. Nantermet, R. Guy, C. Claibourne, J. Renaud, E. Couladouros, K. Paulvannen and E. Sorensen, *Nature*, 1994, **367**, 630.
46. J. Denis, A. Greene, D. Guenard, F. Guerittevoegelein, L. Mangatal and P. Potier, *J. Am. Chem. Soc.*, 1988, **110**, 5917.
47. I. Ojima, I. Habus, M. Zhao, M. Zucco, Y. Park, C. Sun and T. Brigaud, *Tetrahedron*, 1992, **48**, 6985.
48. R. Holton, *US patent*, 5015774, 1992.
49. S. Kratutsky, H. Jacobo, S. Tweedie, R. Krishnamoorthy and A. Filatov, *Org. Process Res. Dev.*, 2015, **19**, 284.
50. P. Mountford, *The Taxol Story – Development of a Green Synthesis via Plant Cell Fermentation*, Wiley-VCH, Weinheim, 2010.
51. T. Huang and K. McDonald, *Biochem. Eng. J.*, 2009, **45**, 168.
52. E. Romero, B. S. Jones, B. N. Hogg, A. Rue Casamajo, M. A. Hayes, S. L. Flitsch, N. J. Turner and C. Schnepel, *Angew. Chem., Int. Ed.*, 2021, **60**, 16824.
53. B. Thomas, X. Lu, W. R. Birmingham, K. Huang, P. Both, J. E. Reyes Martinez, R. J. Young, C. P. Davie and S. L. Flitsch, *ChemBioChem*, 2017, **18**, 858–863.
54. N. P. Dunham and F. H. Arnold, *ACS Catal.*, 2020, **10**, 12239–12255.
55. D. Ghislieri, A. P. Green, M. Pontini, S. C. Willies, I. Rowles, A. Frank, G. Grogan and N. J. Turner, *J. Am. Chem. Soc.*, 2013, **135**, 10863–10869.
56. R. A. Goodnow and C. P. Davie, in *Platform Technologies in Drug Discovery and Validation*, ed. R. A. Goodnow, Academic Press, 2017, vol. 50, pp. 1–15.
57. M. A. Clark, R. A. Acharya, C. C. Arico-Muendel, S. L. Belyanskaya, D. R. Benjamin, N. R. Carlson, P. A. Centrella, C. H. Chiu, S. P. Creaser, J. W. Cuozzo, C. P. Davie, Y. Ding, G. J. Franklin, K. D. Franzen, M. L. Gefter, S. P. Hale, N. J. Hansen, D. I. Israel, J. Jiang, M. J. Kavarana, M. S. Kelley, C. S. Kollmann, F. Li, K. Lind, S. Mataruse, P. F. Medeiros, J. A. Messer, P. Myers, H. O'Keefe, M. C. Oliff, C. E. Rise, A. L. Satz, S. R. Skinner, J. L. Svendsen, L. Tang, K. van Vloten, R. W. Wagner, G. Yao, B. Zhao and B. A. Morgan, *Nat. Chem. Biol.*, 2009, **5**, 647–654.
58. B. Over, S. Wetzel, C. Grutter, Y. Nakai, S. Renner, D. Rauh and H. Waldmann, *Nat. Chem.*, 2013, **5**, 21–28.
59. S. O'Hagan and D. B. Kell, *ADMET & DMPK*, 2017, **5**, 85–125.
60. S. O'Hagan, N. Swainston, J. Handl and D. B. Kell, *Metabolomics*, 2015, **11**, 323–339.
61. D. B. Kell, *Nat. Chem. Biol.*, 2020, **16**, 367–368.
62. R. J. Young, D. V. Green, C. N. Luscombe and A. P. Hill, *Drug Discovery Today*, 2011, **16**, 822–830.
63. E. Kellenberger, A. Hofmann and R. J. Quinn, *Nat. Prod. Rep.*, 2011, **28**, 1483–1492.
64. S. Wetzel, H. Lachance and H. Waldmann, in *Comprehensive Natural Products II*, ed. L. M. a. H.-W. Liu, Elsevier, Oxford, 2010, pp. 5–46.
65. H. Zaid, J. Raiyn, A. Nasser, B. Saad and A. Rayan, *Open Nutraceuticals J.*, 2010, **3**, 194–202.
66. J. W. Li and J. C. Vederas, *Science*, 2009, **325**, 161–165.
67. G. Karageorgis, D. J. Foley, L. Laraia and H. Waldmann, *Nat. Chem.*, 2020, **12**, 227–235.
68. E. M. Carreira and T. C. Fessard, *Chem. Rev.*, 2014, **114**, 8257–8322.
69. T. C. Fessard, K. Goncharenko, Q. Lefebvre and C. Salomé, *CHIMIA*, 2020, **74**, 803–807.
70. C. J. Gerry and S. L. Schreiber, *Nat. Rev. Drug Discovery*, 2018, **17**, 333–352.
71. M. Dow, M. Fisher, T. James, F. Marchetti and A. Nelson, *Org. Biomol. Chem.*, 2012, **10**, 17–28.
72. M. Pascolutti and R. J. Quinn, *Drug Discovery Today*, 2014, **19**, 215–221.
73. T. I. Oprea, A. M. Davis, S. J. Teague and P. D. Leeson, *J. Chem. Inf. Comput. Sci.*, 2001, **41**, 1308–1315.
74. R. Doveston, S. Marsden and A. Nelson, *Drug Discovery Today*, 2014, **19**, 813–819.
75. A. Karawajczyk, F. Giordanetto, J. Benningshof, D. Hamza, T. Kalliokoski, K. Pouwer, R. Morgentin, A. Nelson, G. Muller, A. Piechot and D. Tzalis, *Drug Discovery Today*, 2015, **20**, 1310–1316.
76. S. Y. Chow and A. Nelson, *J. Med. Chem.*, 2017, **60**, 3591–3593.
77. M. Dow, M. Fisher, T. James, F. Marchetti and A. Nelson, *Org. Biomol. Chem.*, 2012, **10**, 17–28.
78. G. Karageorgis, S. Liver and A. Nelson, *ChemMedChem*, 2020, **15**, 1776.
79. G. Karageorgis, M. Dow, A. Aimon, S. Warriner and A. Nelson, *Angew. Chem., Int. Ed.*, 2015, **54**, 13538–13544.

80. T. Bootwicha, J. M. Feilner, E. L. Myers and V. K. Aggarwal, *Nat. Chem.*, 2017, **9**, 896–902.
81. S. Balieu, G. E. Hallett, M. Burns, T. Bootwicha, J. Studley and V. K. Aggarwal, *J. Am. Chem. Soc.*, 2015, **137**, 4398–4403.
82. R. Ardkhean, D. F. Caputo, S. M. Morrow, H. Shi, Y. Xiong and E. A. Anderson, *Chem. Soc. Rev.*, 2016, **45**, 1557–1569.
83. M. A. Schafroth, G. Zuccarello, S. Krautwald, D. Sarlah and E. M. Carreira, *Angew. Chem., Int. Ed.*, 2014, **53**, 13898–13901.
84. S. V. Sharma, X. Tong, C. Pubill-Ulldemolins, C. Cartmell, E. J. A. Bogosyan, E. J. Rackham, E. Marelli, R. B. Hamed and R. J. M. Goss, *Nat. Commun.*, 2017, **8**, 229.
85. A. M. Davis, A. T. Plowright and E. Valeur, *Nat. Rev. Drug Discovery*, 2017, **16**, 681–698.
86. N. A. Meanwell, *J. Med. Chem.*, 2011, **54**, 2529–2591.
87. S. Kumari, A. V. Carmona, A. K. Tiwari and P. C. Trippier, *J. Med. Chem.*, 2020, **63**, 12290–12358.
88. P. Mäder and L. Kattner, *J. Med. Chem.*, 2020, **63**, 14243–14275.
89. E. G. Tse, S. D. Houston, C. M. Williams, G. P. Savage, L. M. Rendina, I. Hallyburton, M. Anderson, R. Sharma, G. S. Walker, R. S. Obach and M. H. Todd, *J. Med. Chem.*, 2020, **63**, 11585–11601.
90. M. V. Westphal, B. T. Wolfstädter, J.-M. Plancher, J. Gatfield and E. M. Carreira, *ChemMedChem*, 2015, **10**, 461–469.
91. J. Tsai, J. T. Lee, W. Wang, J. Zhang, H. Cho, S. Mamo, R. Bremer, S. Gillette, J. Kong, N. K. Haass, K. Sproesser, L. Li, K. S. Smalley, D. Fong, Y. L. Zhu, A. Marimuthu, H. Nguyen, B. Lam, J. Liu, I. Cheung, J. Rice, Y. Suzuki, C. Luu, C. Settachatgul, R. Shellooe, J. Cantwell, S. H. Kim, J. Schlessinger, K. Y. Zhang, B. L. West, B. Powell, G. Habets, C. Zhang, P. N. Ibrahim, P. Hirth, D. R. Artis, M. Herlyn and G. Bollag, *Proc. Natl. Acad. Sci. U. S. A.*, 2008, **105**, 3041–3046.
92. A. J. Souers, J. D. Leverson, E. R. Boghaert, S. L. Ackler, N. D. Catron, J. Chen, B. D. Dayton, H. Ding, S. H. Enschede, W. J. Fairbrother, D. C. Huang, S. G. Hymowitz, S. Jin, S. L. Khaw, P. J. Kovar, L. T. Lam, J. Lee, H. L. Maecker, K. C. Marsh, K. D. Mason, M. J. Mitten, P. M. Nimmer, A. Oleksijew, C. H. Park, C. M. Park, D. C. Phillips, A. W. Roberts, D. Sampath, J. F. Seymour, M. L. Smith, G. M. Sullivan, S. K. Tahir, C. Tse, M. D. Wendt, Y. Xiao, J. C. Xue, H. Zhang, R. A. Humerickhouse, S. H. Rosenberg and S. W. Elmore, *Nat. Med.*, 2013, **19**, 202–208.
93. A. L. Hopkins, G. M. Keseru, P. D. Leeson, D. C. Rees and C. H. Reynolds, *Nat. Rev. Drug Discovery*, 2014, **13**, 105–121.
94. K. Huard, K. Ahn, P. Amor, D. A. Beebe, K. A. Borzilleri, B. A. Chrunyk, S. B. Coffey, Y. Cong, E. L. Conn, J. S. Culp, M. S. Dowling, M. F. Gorgoglione, J. A. Gutierrez, J. D. Knafels, E. A. Lachapelle, J. Pandit, K. D. Parris, S. Perez, J. A. Pfefferkorn, D. A. Price, B. Raymer, T. T. Ross, A. Shavnya, A. C. Smith, T. A. Subashi, G. J. Tesz, B. A. Thuma, M. Tu, J. D. Weaver, Y. Weng, J. M. Withka, G. Xing and T. V. Magee, *J. Med. Chem.*, 2017, **60**, 7835–7849.
95. K. Futatsugi, A. C. Smith, M. Tu, B. Raymer, K. Ahn, S. B. Coffey, M. S. Dowling, D. P. Fernando, J. A. Gutierrez, K. Huard, J. Jasti, A. S. Kalgutkar, J. D. Knafels, J. Pandit, K. D. Parris, S. Perez, J. A. Pfefferkorn, D. A. Price, T. Ryder, A. Shavnya, I. A. Stock, A. S. Tsai, G. J. Tesz, B. A. Thuma, Y. Weng, H. M. Wisniewska, G. Xing, J. Zhou and T. V. Magee, *J. Med. Chem.*, 2020, **63**, 13546–13560.
96. M. M. Hann, A. R. Leach and G. Harper, *J. Chem. Inf. Comput. Sci.*, 2001, **41**, 856–864.
97. A. D. Morley, A. Pugliese, K. Birchall, J. Bower, P. Brennan, N. Brown, T. Chapman, M. Drysdale, I. H. Gilbert, S. Hoelder, A. Jordan, S. V. Ley, A. Merritt, D. Miller, M. E. Swarbrick and P. G. Wyatt, *Drug Discovery Today*, 2013, **18**, 1221–1227.
98. S. Rizzo, V. Wakchaure and H. Waldmann, in *Natural Products in Medicinal Chemistry*, Wiley-VCH Verlag GmbH & Co. KGaA, 2014, pp. 43–80.
99. R. J. Hall, P. N. Mortenson and C. W. Murray, *Prog. Biophys. Mol. Biol.*, 2014, **116**, 82–91.
100. G. G. Ferenczy and G. M. Keseru, *J. Med. Chem.*, 2013, **56**, 2478–2486.
101. J. D. St. Denis, R. J. Hall, C. W. Murray, T. D. Heightman and D. C. Rees, *RSC Med. Chem.*, 2021, **12**, 321–329.
102. E. Resnick, A. Bradley, J. Gan, A. Douangamath, T. Krojer, R. Sethi, P. P. Geurink, A. Aimon, G. Amitai, D. Bellini, J. Bennett, M. Fairhead, O. Fedorov, R. Gabizon, J. Gan, J. Guo, A. Plotnikov, N. Reznik, G. F. Ruda, L. Díaz-Sáez, V. M. Straub, T. Szommer, S. Velupillai, D. Zaidman, Y. Zhang, A. R. Coker, C. G. Dowson, H. M. Barr, C. Wang, K. V. M. Huber, P. E. Brennan, H. Ovaa, F. von Delft and N. London, *J. Am. Chem. Soc.*, 2019, **141**, 8951–8968.
103. D. S. Johnson, E. Weerapana and B. F. Cravatt, *Future Med. Chem.*, 2010, **2**, 949–964.
104. S. Niessen, M. M. Dix, S. Barbas, Z. E. Potter, S. Lu, O. Brodsky, S. Planken, D. Behenna, C. Almaden, K. S. Gajiwala, K. Ryan, R. Ferre, M. R. Lazear, M. M. Hayward, J. C. Kath and B. F. Cravatt, *Cell Chem. Biol.*, 2017, **24**, 1388–1400 e1387.

105. C. G. Parker, A. Galmozzi, Y. Wang, B. E. Correia, K. Sasaki, C. M. Joslyn, A. S. Kim, C. L. Cavallaro, R. M. Lawrence, S. R. Johnson, I. Narvaiza, E. Saez and B. F. Cravatt, *Cell*, 2017, **168**, 527–541 e529.
106. E. K. Grant, D. J. Fallon, M. M. Hann, K. G. M. Fantom, C. Quinn, F. Zappacosta, R. S. Annan, C.-w. Chung, P. Bamborough, D. P. Dixon, P. Stacey, D. House, V. K. Patel, N. C. O. Tomkinson and J. T. Bush, *Angew. Chem.*, 2020, **59**, 21096–21105.
107. Z.-Y. Yang, J.-H. He, A.-P. Lu, T.-J. Hou and D.-S. Cao, *Drug Discovery Today*, 2020, **25**, 657–667.
108. S. J. Chakravorty, J. Chan, M. N. Greenwood, I. Popa-Burke, K. S. Remlinger, S. D. Pickett, D. V. S. Green, M. C. Fillmore, T. W. Dean, J. I. Luengo and R. Macarron, *SLAS Discovery*, 2018, **23**, 532–545.
109. A. S. Kalgutkar, *J. Med. Chem.*, 2020, **63**, 6276–6302.
110. J. Sun, H. Zhong, K. Wang, N. Li and L. Chen, *Acta Pharm. Sin. B*, 2021, **11**, 3417.
111. J. B. Baell and G. A. Holloway, *J. Med. Chem.*, 2010, **53**, 2719–2740.
112. J. Baell and M. A. Walters, *Nature*, 2014, **513**, 481–483.
113. W. R. Pitt, D. M. Parry, B. G. Perry and C. R. Groom, *J. Med. Chem.*, 2009, **52**, 2952–2963.
114. www.reaxys.com/, retrieved 19 May 2020.
115. https://scifinder.cas.org/, retrieved 19 May 2020.
116. G. Vlédtus and V. Finn, *Inf. Storage Retr.*, 1963, **1**, 101.
117. S. S. Gajewska, T. Klucznic, P. Dittwald, M. Startek, M. Bajczeyk and B. Grzybowski, *Angew. Chem., Int. Ed.*, 2016, **55**, 5904.
118. E. Corey and W. Wipke, *Science*, 1969, **166**, 178.
119. T. Strubble, J. Alvarez, S. Brown, M. Chytil, J. Cisar, R. DesJarlais, O. Engkvist, S. Frank, D. Greve, D. Griffin, X. Hou, J. Johannes, C. Kreatsoulas, B. Lahue, M. Mathea, G. Mogk, C. Nicolaou, A. Palmer, D. Price, R. Robinson, S. Salentin, L. Xing, T. Jaakkola, W. Green, R. Barzilay, C. Coley and K. Jensen, *J. Med. Chem.*, 2020, **63**, 8667.
120. T. Badowski, K. Molga and B. Grzybowski, *Chem. Sci.*, 2019, **17**, 4640.
121. C. Christ, M. Zentgraf and J. Kriegl, *J. Chem. Inf. Model.*, 2012, **52**, 1745.
122. A. Jordan, *ACS Med. Chem. Lett.*, 2018, **9**, 1150.
123. https://beta.spaya.ai/, retrieved 19 May 2020.
124. R. Merrifield and J. Stewart, *Nature*, 1965, **207**, 522.
125. T. Chapman, *Nature*, 2003, **421**, 661.
126. D. Fitzpatrick, C. Battilocchio and S. Ley, *Org. Process Res. Dev.*, 2016, **20**, 386.
127. C. Battilocchio, L. Guetzoyan, C. Cervetto, L. Di Cesere Mannelli, D. Frattaroli, I. baxendale, G. Maura, A. Rossi, L. Sautebin, M. Biava, C. Ghelardini, M. Marcoli and S. Ley, *ACS Med. Chem. Lett.*, 2013, **4**, 704.
128. C. Coley, D. Thomas, J. Lummiss, J. Jaworski, C. Breen, V. Schultz, T. Hart, J. Fishman, L. Rogers, H. Gao, R. Hicklin, P. Plehiers, J. Byington, J. Piotti, W. Green, A. Hart, T. Jamison and K. Jensen, *Science*, 2019, **365**, eaax1566.
129. J. Hochlowski, P. Searle, N. Tu, J. Pan, S. Spanton and G. Djuric, *J. Flow Chem.*, 2011, **1**, 56.
130. P. Eribol, A. Uguz and K. Ulgen, *Biomicrofluidics*, 2016, **10**, 011502.
131. M. Reutlinger, T. Rodrigues, P. Schneider and G. Schneider, *Angew. Chem., Int. Ed.*, 2014, **53**, 582.
132. S. Wong Hawkes, M. Chapela and M. Montembault, *QSAR Comb. Sci.*, 2005, **24**, 712.
133. B. Desai, K. Dixon, E. Farrant, O. Feng, K. Gibson, W. van Hoorn, J. Mills, T. Morgan, D. Parry, M. Ramjee, C. Selway, G. Tarver, G. Whitlock and A. Wright, *J. Med. Chem.*, 2013, **56**, 3033.
134. D. Lowe, *Chemical Reactions from US Patents (1976-Sep2016)*, 2017, https://figshare.com/articles/Chemical_reactions_from_US_patents_1976-Sep2016, retrieved June 2020.
135. S. Steiner, J. Wolf, S. Glatzel, A. Andreou, J. Granda, G. Keenan, T. Hinkley, G. Aragon-Camarasa, P. Kitson, D. Angelone and L. Cronin, *Science*, 2019, **363**, eaav2211.
136. J. Li, S. Ballmer, E. Gillis, S. Fujii, M. Schmidt, A. Palazzolo, J. Lehmann, G. Morehouse and M. Burke, *Science*, 2015, **347**, 1221.
137. C. Krtamer, A. Ting, H. Zheng, J. Hert, T. Schindler, M. Stahl, G. Robb, J. Crawford, J. Blaney, S. Montague, A. Leach, A. Dosseter and E. Griffen, *J. Med. Chem.*, 2018, **61**, 3277.
138. E. Martin, V. Polyakov, X. Xhu, L. Tian, P. Mukherjee and X. Liu, *J. Chem. Inf. Model.*, 2019, **59**, 4450.
139. L. D. Elliott, M. Berry, B. Harji, D. Klauber, J. Leonard and K. I. Booker-Milburn, *Org. Process Res. Dev.*, 2016, **20**, 1806–1811.
140. https://www.americanpharmaceuticalreview.com/Featured-Articles/562258-Filing-a-Multi-stage-Continuous-Process-for-API/, accessed 01 December 2020.
141. A. N. Hobbs and R. J. Young, *Drug Discovery Today*, 2013, **18**, 148–154.
142. M. Arkin, Y. Tang and J. Wells, *Chem. Biol.*, 2014, **21**, 1102.
143. D. Scott, A. Bayly, C. Abell and J. Skidmore, *Nat. Rev. Drug Discovery*, 2018, **15**, 533.

144. B. Doak, B. Over, F. Giordanetto and J. Kihlberg, *J. Chem. Biol.*, 2014, **21**, 1115.
145. S. Caenepeel, S. Brown, B. Belmontes, G. Moody, K. Keegan, D. Chui, D. Whittington, X. Huang, L. Poppe, A. Cheng, M. Cardozo, J. Houze, Y. Li, B. Lucas, N. Paras, X. Wang, J. Taygerly, M. Vimolratana, M. Zancanella, L. Zhu, E. Cajulis, T. Osgood, J. Sun, L. Damon, R. Egan, P. Greninger, J. McClanaghan, J. Gong, D. Moujalled, G. Pomilio, P. Beltran, C. Benes, A. Roberts, D. Huang, A. Wei, J. Canon, A. Coxon and P. Hughes, *Cancer Discovery*, 2018, **8**, 1582.
146. J. Lee, Y. You and S. Kang, *J. Am. Chem. Soc.*, 2011, **133**, 1772.
147. U. Ader, D. Breitgoff, P. Klein, K. Laumen and M. Schneider, *Tetrahedron Lett.*, 1989, **30**, 1793.
148. S. Garber, J. Kingsbury, B. Gray and A. Hoveyda, *J. Am. Chem. Soc.*, 2000, **122**, 8168.
149. S. Brown, Y. Li, M. Lizarzaburu, B. Lucas, N. Paras, J. Taygerly, M. Vimolratana, X. Wang, M. Yu, M. Zancanella, L. Zhu, A. Gonzalez-Buenrostro and Z. Li, *US patent application*, US2017/0088560, 30 March 2017.
150. R. Elander, *Appl. Microbiol. Biotechnol.*, 2003, **61**, 385.
151. B. Austad, T. Calkins, C. Chase, F. Fang, T. Horstmann, Y. Hu, B. Lewis, X. Niu, T. Noland, J. Orr, M. Schnaderbeck, H. Zhang, N. Asakawa, N. Asai, H. Chiba, T. Hasebe, Y. Hoshino, H. Ishizuka, T. Kajima, A. Kayano, Y. Komatsu, M. Kubota, H. Kurada, M. Miyazawa, K. Tagami and T. Wanatabe, *Synlett*, 2013, **24**, 333.
152. C. Chen, K. Namba and Y. Kishi, *Org. Lett.*, 2009, **11**, 409.
153. K. Yahata, N. Ye, K. Iso, S. Naini, S. Yamashita, Y. Ai and Y. Kishi, *J. Org. Chem.*, 2017, **82**, 8792.
154. K. Yahata, N. Ye, K. Iso, Y. Ai, J. Lee and Y. Kishi, *J. Org. Chem.*, 2017, **82**, 8808.
155. K. Johnson, S. Biswas and D. Weix, *Chem. - Eur. J.*, 2016, **22**, 7399. Galactol synthesis: C. Chen, K. Namba and Y. Kishi, *Org. Lett.*, 2009, **11**, 409.
156. Y. Kishi, Y. Ai, N. Ye, Q. Wang, K. Yahata, K. Iso, S. Naini, S. Yamashita, J. Lee and I. Ohashi, *WO patent application*, WO2019010363, 10 January 2019.
157. S. Kawano, K. Ito, K. Kira, T. Abe, T. Agaki, M. Asano, K. Ito, Y. Sato, F. Matsuura, I. Ohashi, Y. Matsumoto, M. Isomura, T. Sasaki, T. Fukuyama, Y. MiyaShita, Y. Kaburagi, A. Yokoi, O. Asano, T. Owa and Y. Kishi, *Sci. Rep.*, 2019, **9**, 8656.
158. L. Jones and N. Gray, *MedChemComm*, 2014, **5**, 244–246 (and articles cited therein).
159. M. Bunnage, E. Piatnitski Checkler and L. Jones, *Nat. Chem. Biol.*, 2013, **9**, 195.
160. E. Valeur, S. M. Gueret, H. Adihou, R. Gopalakrishnan, M. Lemurell, H. Waldmann, T. N. Grossmann and A. T. Plowright, *Angew. Chem., Int. Ed. Engl.*, 2017, **56**, 10294.

# 3 Useful Computational Chemistry Tools for Medicinal Chemistry

Darren V. S. Green*[a] and Colin M. Edge[a]

[a]GlaxoSmithKline Medicines Research Centre, Gunnels Wood Road, Stevenage, Herts SG1 2NY, UK
*E-mail: Darren.vs.green@gsk.com

## 3.1 Physics-based *vs.* Empirical Models

> The underlying physical laws necessary for the mathematical theory of a large part of physics and the whole of chemistry are thus completely known, and the difficulty is only that the exact application of these laws leads to equations much too complicated to be soluble.
>
> P. A. M. Dirac[1]

Key to the application of computational chemistry to medicinal chemistry is the calculation of energy. Accurate calculation of absolute energies, for example, the change in free energy upon binding of a small molecule to a protein, remains an unfulfilled aspiration of computational chemists. Figure 3.1 Illustrates the complexity of ligand binding when expressed in free energy terms, involving changes in both enthalpy and entropy, and explains why it is that prediction of binding energy has been found to be so difficult.

This is a scientific Grand Challenge and it is therefore fortunate that components of the free energy of binding that are applicable to drug discovery, for example, the relative energies of molecular conformations, or tautomers in heterocyclic rings, are computationally tractable to a degree of accuracy that is useful in the design of new molecules.

The key difference between computational chemistry and QSAR modelling is in the atomistic level of detail that is modelled, with properties of molecules predicted from first principles study of the atoms that comprise them. This chapter will explore the

The Handbook of Medicinal Chemistry: Principles and Practice, 2nd Edition
Edited by Simon E. Ward and Andrew M. Davis

Published by the Royal Society of Chemistry, www.rsc.org

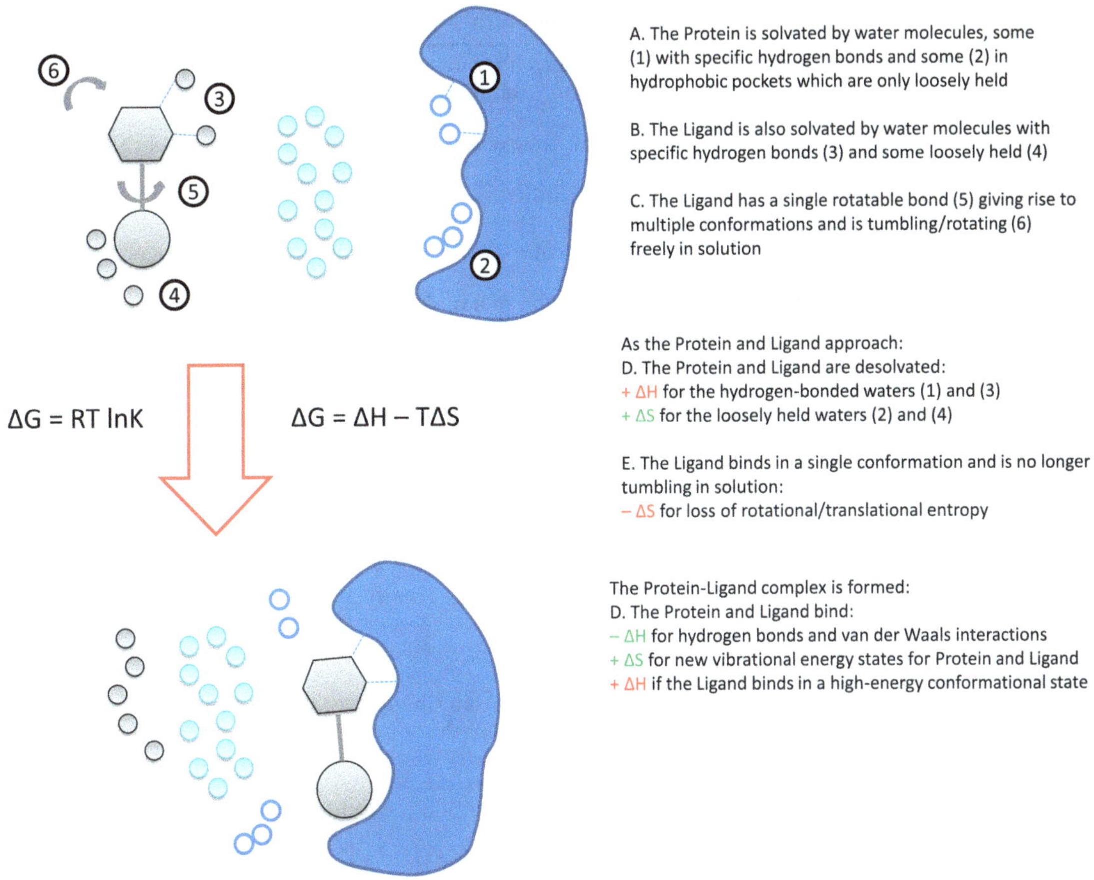


**Figure 3.1** The free energy of binding of a ligand to a protein comprises many components. Although enthalpic binding from direct molecular interactions receives most attention from chemists, the numerous entropic terms can come to dominate the energetics and these need to be considered with as much care.

various techniques available, outline the approximations which are made in order to enable the calculation and discuss what these might mean in real life application to medicinal chemistry problems (Table 3.1).

## 3.2 Molecular Mechanics and Molecular Orbital Theory

Central to all computational chemistry methods is the assumption that the Born–Oppenheimer approximation holds, that is, that the mass difference (a proton is 1836 times heavier than an electron) between nuclei and electrons is sufficient so that their motions can be considered separately.[29,30] This assumption then allows quantum mechanical methods to focus on the electronic state of the molecule, given a fixed position for the nuclei, whilst molecular mechanics may focus on the nuclear coordinates of a molecule in its ground electronic state.

Table 3.1 Key milestones in the development of computational chemistry as a discipline.

| | |
|---|---|
| 1924 | Lennard-Jones proposes the Lennard-Jones interatomic potential[2] |
| 1926 | Schrödinger develops the "wave equation" that mathematically describes the distribution of an electron through space[3] |
| 1928 | Mulliken develops a "molecular orbital" theory where electrons are assigned to orbitals across an entire molecule[4] |
| 1929 | Lennard-Jones introduces the linear combination of atomic orbitals approximation for the calculation of molecular orbitals[5] |
| 1930 | London explains van der Waals forces as due to the interacting fluctuating dipole moments between molecules[6] |
| 1938 | Coulson makes the first accurate calculation of a molecular orbital wave function with the hydrogen molecule[7] |
| 1946 | Westheimer publishes calculations on series of hindered biphenyls which demonstrate that observed molecular properties could be rationalised through the use of computed geometries and energies[8] |
| 1950 | Barton lays down the foundations of conformational analysis in a study of steroid chemistry[9] |
| 1956 | The first *ab initio* Hartree–Fock calculations on diatomic molecules |
| 1961 | Hendrickson publishes the first use of a computer for force field calculations in a study of ring conformations[10] |
| 1965 | The semi empirical method CNDO is published by Pople and co-workers[11] |
| 1965 | Wiberg employs a Steepest Descent algorithm for geometry optimisation with a molecular mechanics force field[12] |
| 1965 | The molecular structure drawing program ORTEP developed at Oak Ridge National Laboratory[13] |
| 1970 | Gaussian 70 made freely available *via* the Quantum Chemistry Program Exchange[14] (QCPE) |
| 1970 | The term "computational chemistry" first used to describe the new scientific discipline:[15] "It seems, therefore, that 'computational chemistry' can finally be more and more of a reality." |
| 1972 | Wiberg and Boyd describe the dihedral driver method for systematic conformational analysis[16] |
| 1973 | Cambridge Crystallographic Data Centre makes its 3D structure file widely available[17] |
| 1973 | N. L. Allinger describes the modelling of hydrocarbons with a new force field, MM1 [18] |
| 1975 | The first molecular dynamics simulation of a protein is published by Warshel and Levitt[19] |
| 1980 | The Carbo Index described for the quantitation of molecular similarity based on the 3D electron density distribution in molecules[20] |
| 1982 | Kuntz and co-workers lay down the foundations for the DOCK algorithm, the starting point for a multitude of researchers in the area of virtual screening[21] |
| 1983 | The Connolly Surface Algorithm enables real time visualisation of high-quality coloured molecular surfaces on desktop computers[22] |
| 1985 | GRID is published by Peter Goodford. A computational procedure for determining energetically favourable binding sites on biologically important macromolecules[23] |
| 1987 | Free Energy Perturbation predictions made for the potency of novel thermolysin inhibitors[24] |
| 1987 | The Concord automatic 3D structure generation program developed.[25] |
| 1993 | Zanamivir, an inhibitor of the influenza neuraminidase enzyme, is discovered with the assistance of GRID in one of the first examples of protein structure-based drug discovery[26] |
| 1997 | First geometry optimisation of a protein using semi-empirical quantum mechanics[27] |
| 2010 | The first millisecond simulation of a protein is performed using Anton, a computer designed specifically for high-speed molecular dynamics[28] |
| 2012 | The first example of successful automated molecular design using cheminformatics methods to generate molecular structures and QSAR models to select them for synthesis[149] |
| 2015 | The development of a industrialised version of the Free Energy Perturbation method[59] enables pharmaceutical researchers to predict relative free energies of binding a the speed and scale required to impact medicinal chemistry projects |
| 2020 | DeepMind's AlphaFold2 deep learning method predicts novel protein structures to near experimental accuracy in the CASP14 challenge[163] |

### 3.2.1 Quantum Mechanics

The key concept in molecular quantum mechanics is the wave function, most often denoted as $\Psi$. The wave function completely describes the properties of a quantum mechanical system and has a value at every point in space. The square of the wave function yields the electron density at that point, and integration of the electron density over a volume gives the probability of finding an electron in that volume. That the localisation of electron density is not fixed, but can be computed, is an important result from quantum mechanics, introducing concepts for molecular recognition such as partial atomic charges and polarisability.

All properties of the system (molecule, or collection of molecules) may be calculated by the application of various mathematical operators on the wave function (Figure 3.2).

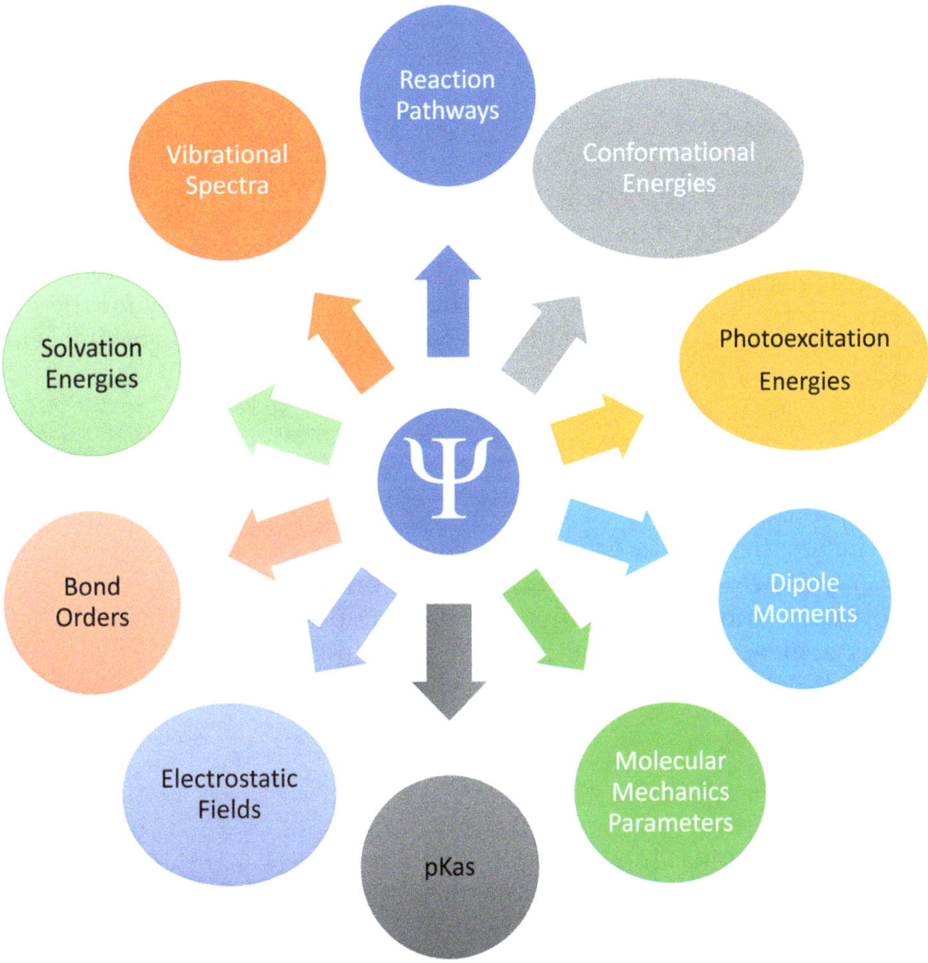


**Figure 3.2** The power and versatility of quantum mechanics. All molecular properties of interest to medicinal chemists can be computed from the wave function of a molecule.

The operator of most interest to us is the energy operator, or Hamiltonian $\hat{H}$, which gives rise to the familiar Schrödinger equation:

$$\hat{H}\Psi = E\Psi \tag{3.1}$$

Unfortunately it is not possible to analytically solve the Schrödinger equation for systems with more than one electron (the hydrogen atom). It can be argued that this fact spawned the discipline of what is now known as computational chemistry and the majority of the key milestones related to the 50+ year quest for accurate solutions. The most common technique used is the Hartree–Fock method, in which each electron is considered to move in a static field of all the other electrons. This is an iterative calculation which exploits the Variational Principle (the true energy of a system is always lower than that produced when the Hamiltonian is applied to an incorrect wave function). The wave function is first estimated and then iteratively modified to minimise the energy. In order to make the calculations tractable, the wave function itself is comprised of multiple molecular orbitals, $\psi$, each represented by a Linear Combination of Atomic Orbitals (LCAO) centred on each atom:

$$\psi = \sum_{i=1}^{n} c_i \varphi_i \tag{3.2}$$

Each atomic orbital $\varphi_i$ is modelled by mathematical functions designed to mimic the shape of s, p, d and f orbitals whilst being mathematically efficient (as solving the Schrödinger equation involves integrating across the overlap of these atomic orbitals). The most accurate atomic orbitals mimic those derived analytically for the hydrogen atom and are known as Slater-type Orbitals (STOs). The STO for a 1s orbital centred on an atom is given by:

$$\varnothing_{1s}^{SF} = \left(\frac{\zeta^3}{\pi}\right)^{1/2} e^{-\zeta r} \tag{3.3}$$

Where $\zeta$ is an exponent which varies according to the atom type, the larger the exponent the smaller the 1s orbital (for the hydrogen atom $\zeta = 1$, for the helium atom $\zeta = 1.69$). However, Hartree–Fock calculations involve computing the overlap between orbitals, and for STOs this is slow. The best combination of shape and efficiency is achieved by using multiple Gaussian-type Orbitals (GTOs) for each atomic orbital, chosen to provide a best fit to an STO. The form of an atom-centred GTO is:

$$\varnothing_{1s}^{GF} = \left(\frac{2\alpha}{\pi}\right)^{3/4} e^{-\alpha r^2} \tag{3.4}$$

As GTOs do not describe atomic orbitals well, particularly near the nucleus, normally it requires a combination of at least three of these functions to provide a reasonable representation (Figure 3.3).[31] The advantage of using GTOs is that the overlap of two Gaussians is itself a Gaussian, and this overlap can be computed very quickly. How many and what type of Gaussians are applied to each orbital are collectively referred to as a "basis set".

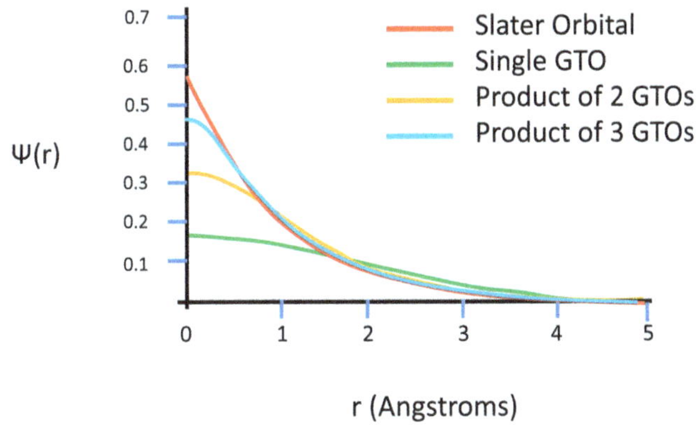


**Figure 3.3** In order to fit the mathematical form of a Slater-type Orbital (STO), which is a fine description of an atomic orbital, multiple Gaussian-type Orbitals must be combined. In this case three GTOs are used to produce a close match to a single STO.

There are many such basis sets to choose from, but the split-valence basis sets of Pople[32] have been the most successful at modelling the type of molecular systems of interest here. As most intermolecular interactions are dominated by the valence electrons, more attention is paid to those atomic orbitals than to the inner shell. Basis sets have their own nomenclature, for example the popular 6-31G** has the inner shell represented by a single basis function constructed from six GTOs, whilst the valence orbitals are represented by two basis functions, one of three GTOS and the other of just one. The "**" indicates that polarisation functions are added to both heavy (*i.e.*, d-type orbitals for C, N and O atoms) and hydrogen atoms (p-type orbitals), these functions allow the electron density on an atom to become anisotropic in response to, for example, a directional hydrogen bond. A "+" would indicate diffuse functions (larger s and p functions which tail off slowly as the distance from the nucleus increases) are added, for example in order to model charged species such as a carboxylate.

These approaches are sufficient to calculate many properties of interest to drug researchers – dipole moments, charge distributions, bond orders – and can be combined with optimisation algorithms to produce energy-minimised molecular conformations. A significant deficiency of so-called Restricted Hartree–Fock methods (RHF) is the neglect of electron correlation. As the RHF method considers the movement of an electron in an average, static, field of all the other electrons in the molecule it cannot model the observed behaviour that electrons tend to avoid each other where possible. There are many methods developed to overcome this, such as Møller–Plesset Perturbation Theory, which obtains a more accurate estimation of the true energy by writing the true eigenvalues as a power series of ever more complex wave functions, where the basic HF energy is given by the sum of the zeroth- and first-order energies. To improve on the HF energy, it is therefore necessary to add the second-order wave function, and this level of theory is referred to as MP2. MP2 includes the excitations obtained by promoting electrons into higher-energy orbitals. It is, however, computationally expensive and is therefore normally used as a single-point energy calculation, once the geometry of the molecule has been minimised using HF methods.

The time required for HF calculations scale at the rate of $N^3$ (where $N$ = number of electrons in the molecule) and therefore quickly consume available computing resources (even today). Therefore, techniques were developed which would allow quantum mechanical calculations whilst reducing the number of integral evaluations. Incorporation of experimental data and parameterisation are key to the success of such methods and give rise to the term "semi-empirical quantum mechanics" to describe them. For example, the energy of a carbon 1s orbital can be taken from experimental data rather than computed. The most successful methods focus on the reduction of calculations required for differential overlap, that is, the interaction between two orbitals centred on different atoms. The first method, CNDO (Complete Neglect of Differential Overlap) led to a variety of successive improvements (INDO, NDDO), with the most successful being the MNDO (Modified Neglect of Differential Overlap) methods. These neglect interactions between certain orbitals, based on atom and orbital type, but allow inclusion of, for example, the interaction of p orbitals in the C and O of a carbonyl bond. Although conjugation in such systems is therefore included in the model, the lack of a full inclusion of electron interactions across a conjugated bond does lead to lower estimates of, for example, rotational barriers in a molecule such as formamide. There are various forms of MNDO model in use, the most popular being AM1[33] and PM3[34] (or PM6). The difference between these is not in the level of theory used, but in the how the empirical parameters are derived. The advantage of these methods is that they scale well – modern codes scale linearly with the number of electrons in the system, whilst providing results which are competitive with moderate basis-set HF calculations (due to the inclusion of experimental and parameterisation, semi-empirical calculations also include some consideration of electron correlation).

In recent years, quantum mechanics practice has been heavily influenced by a third class of theoretical approach – Density Functional Theory (DFT). In contrast to HF theory, which is concerned with determination of the set of single electron wave functions (from which electron density distributions can be derived), DFT directly calculates the electron density distribution and the total electronic energy. Although the Thomas–Fermi model of 1920s heritage contained many of the key concepts, it was not until the 1960s that Hohenburg and Kohn[35] demonstrated that the ground-state energy and other properties of a system were uniquely defined by the electron density distribution. This finding gives rise to the language of DFT – the energy of the molecule is a unique *functional* of the electron density distribution. There are many advantages of DFT, in particular the explicit inclusion of electron correlation. Many of the methods used to implement DFT calculations are very similar to those used in HF theory, for example the iterative procedures to achieve self-consistency. Most of the difficulty in implementation resides in the derivation of the best mathematical function, and in this regard DFT resembles semi-empirical methods. For example, to compute the electron exchange and correlation contributions to the energy, it is necessary to estimate the electron density. The local density approximation (LDA) is based on a model of a uniform electron gas.

Chemists are most likely to encounter DFT as a hybrid calculation with HF methods which add a correlation term based on electron density to the electrostatic and configuration terms computed by HF. A popular combination is B3 LYP (Becke's three parameter functional[36] which combines HF and DFT terms for electron configuration; the Lee

Yang and Parr correlation functional[37]). These methods are implemented with traditional basis sets, and therefore a calculation will often be described as B3LYP/6-31G*. DFT allows the inclusion of electron correlation at a reasonable computational cost, scaling at ~$N^3$. However, for the purpose of drug discovery, DFT has some serious deficiencies. In particular, hydrogen bonds can be too short, and van der Waals interactions are poorly handled.[38] In contrast to HF theory, where the solution is to increase the level of theory and increase the basis set, DFT requires the empirical derivation of an improved functional (how the electron density is described mathematically, and specifically how the electron exchange and correlation energies are modelled). The M06 suite of functionals is widely employed,[39] due to their good performance where dispersion forces are important. The trade-off for this performance is that a different functional needs to be used depending on the problem to hand. It is wise to try several DFT methods and see which reproduce the desired chemistry.

### 3.2.2 Molecular Mechanics

The technique of molecular mechanics (MM) originated with the vibrational spectroscopy community, who determined the forces holding molecules together from knowledge of the molecular structure and the observed vibrational frequencies. In vibrational spectroscopy, electrons are not studied and are assumed to adopt an optimal distribution around the nuclei. Application of the Born–Oppenheimer approximation then allows the energy of the molecule to be defined in terms of the nuclear positions.

Due to its origins, the energy of the molecule in MM has contributions from bond stretches, angle stretches, out-of-plane bending and torsional energies, with additional terms to describe non-bonded terms for van der Waals and electrostatic interactions (Figure 3.4).

A common mathematical form for a simple MM method is:

$$E(r^N) = \sum_{\text{bonds}} \frac{ki}{2}(l_i - l_{i,0}) + \sum_{\text{angles}} \frac{ki}{2}(\theta_i - \theta_{i,0})^2 + \sum_{\text{torsions}} \frac{Vn}{2}(1 + \cos(n\omega - \gamma))$$
$$+ \sum_{i=1}^{N} \sum_{j=i+1}^{N} \left( 4\varepsilon_{ij} \left[ \left( \frac{\sigma_{ij}}{r_{ij}} \right)^{12} - \left( \frac{\sigma_{ij}}{r_{ij}} \right)^{6} \right] + \frac{q_i q_j}{4\pi\varepsilon_0 r_{ij}} \right) \quad (3.5)$$

where $r$ denotes the positions of a set of N atoms. The first term is the bond stretch of two bonded atoms, which increases as the bond length $l_i$ deviates from the reference value $l_0$, and in this implementation is modelled by a harmonic (symmetrical) potential, as described by Hooke's Law. Similarly, the second term describes the energies associated with deformation of a bond angle from its reference and again is modelled by a harmonic potential. The third, torsional, term describes how the energy changes as a bond rotates and this, necessarily a more complex term, comprises the cosine of the torsional angle. The final term is a composite function to describe the non-bonded interactions between atoms and in this instance uses a 6–12 Lennard–Jones potential for van der Waals energies and a simple Coulomb charge potential, modified by the dielectric constant, $\varepsilon$, of the environment (1 for a vacuum, 78.4 for water, approximately 2 for the interior of a protein).

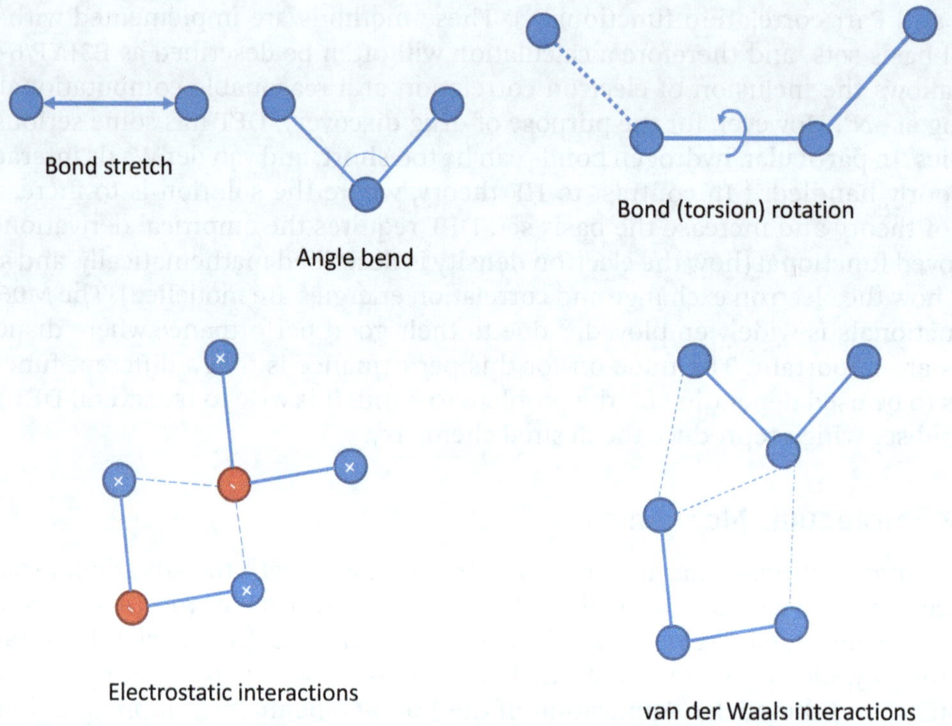


**Figure 3.4** The fundamental molecular motions and interactions encoded in a molecular mechanics force field.

The reference bond lengths, angles and torsional terms, van der Waals radii and atomic charges all need to be provided in order for a calculation to be performed. The combination of the mathematical energy function and the set of required parameters together define a force field. The first accurate and common purpose force field for hydrocarbons was Allinger's MM1.[18] Since then, ever more complex schemes have been invented, adding better bond stretch and angle terms and so-called cross-terms between them (for example, as a bond angle decreases, adjacent bonds stretch to minimise the 1,3 atomic interactions).

All force fields make use of atom typing. Typically each atom is defined by its hybridisation state (*e.g.* $sp^2$, $sp^3$), number or type of substituents (*e.g.* OH), formal charge (N+) and sometimes bond type (Namide). Parameters are then assigned to bonds between atom types to reproduce bond lengths, angles and torsions. A force field can therefore contain hundreds of parameters.

For applications in drug discovery, such as conformational analysis and protein–ligand interactions, the most important terms are the non-bonded interactions, which are also the most difficult to parameterise. There is a multitude of force fields available and it is not always easy to select the most appropriate for a molecule.[40] There is certainly no "universal" force field that reliably models all molecules. Unlike quantum mechanics, where a result can usually be improved by an increase in theory, poor behaviour with a MM force field is difficult to improve, as it is not easy to identify a single parameter as the "fault" and even harder to rebalance a force field after having made a change. It is most common to swap force fields completely in an attempt to get a better result, this particularly applies for applications in the condensed state (*e.g.* small molecule crystal) where specialist force fields such as COMPASS[41] are employed.

### 3.2.3 Electronic Distribution and Electrostatic Isopotentials

One of the most challenging set of parameters to derive are the Coulombic terms. The energy function itself is straightforward, but requires that there are charges for each atom. (This is an artificial fractional charge – "partial charge" – to represent the effect of the nuclear charge and the surrounding electron cloud.) Partial charges are one of the major deficiencies in the MM method. Quantum mechanics tells us that the charge distribution in an atom is anisotropic (uneven) – for example, the water molecule has two lone pairs (high electron density) and two hydrogen atoms (low electron density) arranged in a tetrahedral configuration. Many force fields, however, use a single charge centred on each atom, a "monopole".

There are a variety of methods for determining partial charges. Quantum mechanics calculations are now the method of choice, with the earliest method due to Mulliken,[42] who proposed that each atom receive half of the electron density where that was due to contributions from two atoms. However, this method neglects differences in electronegativity between atoms, and is also highly dependent on the basis set used. Other, more empirical, methods were developed, such as the widely adopted Gasteiger–Marsili method.[44] This is an iterative approach, based on electronegativities of atoms. Each atom is allocated a starting partial charge (based on atom types) which is then modified by the difference in electronegativities of the bonded atoms. As this is a pairwise comparison, these changes are iterated until the charges no longer change (the process has reached convergence). Once *ab initio* quantum mechanics calculations were sufficiently accessible, a new method came to dominate: fitting atomic charges to reflect the electrostatic potential of the molecule.

The valence bond model of molecules has been hugely successful. It allows an orderly depiction of molecules where electrons are assigned bond orders of whole numbers (single, double, triple), where formal charges are assigned to atoms (*e.g.* N+) and where chemical reactions occur by movements of whole electrons between bonds, rationalised by the drawing of curly arrows. None of this is real, of course, with only the complexity of the –quantum mechanical – truth preventing wholesale rejection of this over-simplified model of chemistry. However, if we wish to model molecular recognition, we are forced to abandon representations that are useful to human minds, and to adopt representations that are closer to what a molecule "sees and feels" of other molecules. The molecular electrostatic potential (MEP)[43] of a molecule can be calculated at any point in space, for example, at the location of a protein atom, even if the molecule is far away. As electrostatic forces are relatively long range, and are large at short range, the MEP of a molecule is an excellent description of how the molecule is "seen" by other molecules and the magnitude of the MEP at any point describes how forcefully its potential energy might be "felt" by another molecule. The MEP can be calculated from the wave function by placing a unit positive charge at a point in space and summing the coulombic

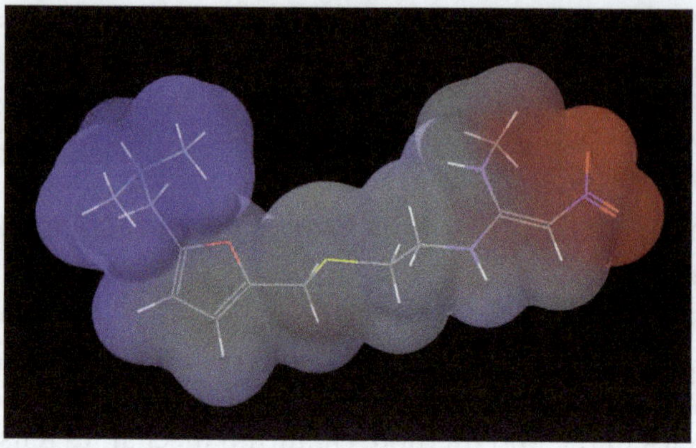

**Figure 3.5** The molecular electrostatic potential of Zantac mapped onto a surface of constant electron density.

interaction energies between it and the electrons and nuclei in the molecule. (Therefore, one can also calculate an MEP from a molecular mechanics force field). An MEP at a single point in space is not in itself particularly useful, therefore it is usual to calculate the MEP of a molecule on a surface, typically chosen close to the van der Waals radii of the atoms, or at constant electron density. This surface is an excellent visualisation of the molecule (Figure 3.5), but can also be used to derive accurate partial charges for a molecule for use with a force field, which by definition cannot pre-define partial charges for all possible molecules. In the standard CHELPG algorithm,[45] a regular grid of points are placed around the molecule, extending to 3 angstroms further than the van der Waals radii of atoms in the molecule. A set of atom-centred partial charges are derived using a procedure that minimises the error function (the difference between the electrostatic potential values from the quantum mechanics calculation and those produced by the partial charges) subject to a constraint that the partial charges sum to the total molecular charge.

### 3.2.4 3-Dimensional Molecular Similarity

If the molecular electrostatic potential is a good representation of how a protein sees a ligand, then two molecules with similar MEPs should share similar biological properties. The similarity between two MEPs can be defined using a form of cosine similarity, often known as the Carbo index:[20]

$$R_{AB} = \frac{\int P_A P_B dv}{\left(\int P_A^2 dv\right)^{1/2} \left(\int P_B^2 dv\right)^{1/2}} \tag{3.6}$$

$P$ denotes the MEP for molecule A or B integrated over the 3D space surrounding the two molecules. The potential, $P_r$ at a point $r$ for a molecule of $n$ atoms may be calculated directly from the electron density or from point charges:

$$P_r = \sum_{i=1}^{n} \frac{q_i}{(r - R_i)} \tag{3.7}$$

where $(r - R_i)$ is the distance from atom $i$ to the point $r$ in 3D space and $q_i$ is the partial charge on the atom. By assigning partial lipophilicity constants to atoms, a molecular lipophilic similarity can also be calculated in the same way.[46]

As computational chemistry makes common use of Gaussian functions to model electron distribution, it was realised that the Carbo index could be used to provide a measure of shape similarity, and this could be made fast enough for general use by use of atom-centred Gaussian functions to fit the curve of electron density against distance from the nucleus.[47] These methods are at the heart of most modern methods of computing 3D shape similarities such as the ROCS method.[48]

### 3.2.5 Energy Minimisation

Using a force field allows the calculation of the molecular energy for a particular set of nuclear positions. In the very first studies, these atomic positions were taken from physical molecular models.[49] In order to realise the full potential of the methods, it is necessary to be able to compute the atomic positions which give rise to the lowest potential energy. This is termed energy minimisation, and there are a variety of techniques employed. One of the simplest and earliest methods is that of Steepest Descents.[50] Think of the potential energy surface of a molecule as a hill with a ball on it. If we start halfway down the hill, the force on the ball (gravity) will point down the slope. The Steepest Descents Algorithm will move the ball parallel to the force on it, *i.e.*, straight down the hill. The algorithm does not know where the hill ends and therefore needs to know how far to move the ball downhill before recalculating the potential energy. The most common way of doing this is to use a fixed "step size". If we extend our analogy from a hill slope to a valley, there is now a more complex minimisation. Steepest Descents will "tack" down the valley (Figure 3.6) using a series of orthogonal steps. The fixed step size may not be the most efficient, but avoids overshooting the energy minimum at the bottom of the valley. A more efficient method is Conjugate Gradients,[51] which takes into account the previous step and the current forces on the ball, to produce a much better idea of the true nature of the potential energy surface and will minimise using fewer steps, and therefore fewer energy calculations. Even more complex minimisation methods are the so-called second derivative methods, which take into account not just the gradients (as in Conjugate Gradients), but the curvature of the energy surface. One popular method is the Newton–Raphson,[52] which will find the energy minimum for a quadratic function in one step.

The great benefits of MM over QM methods are the ability to directly incorporate experimental data on molecular structure (bond lengths, angles, torsions) and the sheer speed of the calculations which, with modern computers, allow studies on drug-like molecules in seconds. This speed allows the study of large molecules such as proteins, and the motion of molecules in time, an area of computational chemistry generally referred to as molecular simulation.

## 3.3 Molecular Simulation and Dynamics

Energy minimisation allows us to generate individual energy minima on the potential energy surface of a molecule. However, as the laws of thermodynamics tell us, properties of interest (binding energies, solvation energies, movement of a molecule

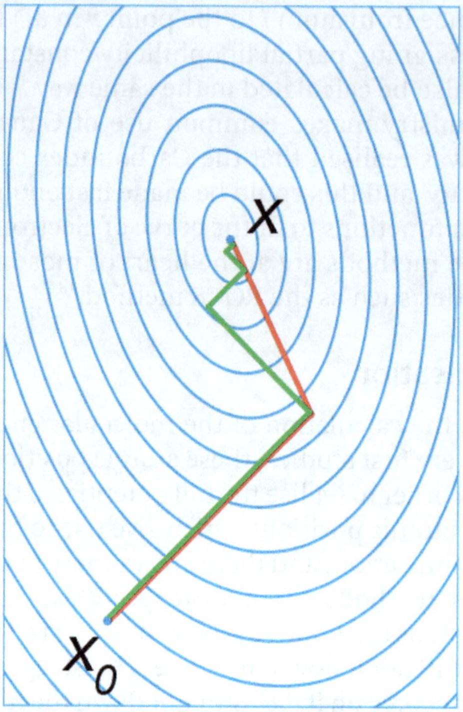


**Figure 3.6** A comparison of the convergence of a steepest descent algorithm (green) and the corresponding performance of the conjugate gradients method (in red) for minimizing a quadratic function associated with a given linear system. Conjugate gradient, assuming exact arithmetic, converges in at most $n$ steps where $n$ is the size of the matrix of the system (here $n$ = 2).

through a membrane *etc.*) are the product of all of the energy states in a system, including the vibrational and conformational energy minima. For a protein–ligand system, a full quantification of all the possible energy states of the system is infeasible. Techniques which sample the possible energy states in order to approximate the true ensemble of states are commonly referred to as molecular simulations. Simulations are also able to model time-dependent behaviour, providing a detailed representation of, for example, how a molecule changes conformation upon binding to a protein.

The first published simulation method, the Monte Carlo (MC) technique,[53] uses a random sampling of states of the system (for example, conformations) to build up a representative ensemble from which the properties (*e.g.*, binding energy) can be calculated. A new conformation is generated, for example by rotating a random torsional angle a random number of degrees. The energy of the conformer is calculated, and then accepted in to the ensemble of representative conformations according to a probability ($p$) which is modified by the energy ($E$) of the conformation:

$$p = e^{-E/kT} \tag{3.8}$$

Therefore, low-energy conformers have a much higher probability of being accepted into the ensemble of states than would a high-energy conformer, but these will have at least some representation in the model.

It was recognised that the equations of motion could be harnessed to describe the behaviour of a real system, and this begat the technique of molecular dynamics (MD).[54] In contrast to the sampling strategy of Monte Carlo methods, molecular dynamics is a deterministic method, which means that any future state of the system can be predicted from the current state. Given a starting configuration of a molecule, or collection of molecules, the forces on the atoms are determined, typically using a MM force field.[55] Newtonian mechanics are then applied to the system in order to move the atoms for a particular time. After each time step, the forces on the atoms are recalculated and combined with the current positions and velocities of the atoms to produce new atomic coordinates, directions and velocities. For typical molecular systems, bearing in mind how quickly non-bonded forces can change as atoms become close to each other (*e.g.* using the Lennard–Jones 6–12 potential), the time step between calculations must be very short – of the order of 1–10 femtoseconds ($10^{-15}$ to $10^{-14}$ s). In this way, molecular dynamics produces a trajectory which describes the change of molecular motion over time.

There are subtle theoretical differences between Monte Carlo and molecular dynamics methods. Monte Carlo is typically performed under conditions of constant number of atoms, volume and temperature ("NVT" or canonical ensemble) whilst molecular dynamics uses constant energy but not temperature ("NVE" or microcanonical ensemble). Therefore, the temperature in a MD simulation can be varied, and this is often exploited to put more energy in the system to allow, for example, high-energy conformational changes, to be seen in a shorter time than would usually be observed, so that the simulation would be possible using available computational resources. (CPU time is proportional to the number of time steps required for evaluation in the simulation.)

Both MC and MD methods require significant computing resources, as the number of configurations of a system, particularly for larger molecules, is extremely large and the number of non-bonded terms to be evaluated in the MM force field scales by the square of the number of atoms in the system. There are a number of common approximations applied in order to make the simulations feasible. A non-bonded cut-off is generally applied: the Lennard–Jones potential declines rapidly with distance (at 2.5 times the vdW radius, $\sigma$, the potential has just 1% of the value at $\sigma$). Electrostatic terms, in contrast, have a much longer range and generally require calculation up to at least 10 Å distance. It is also useful to keep a list of atom pairs which are included in the calculation – the non-bonded neighbour lists. This prevents the recalculation of interatomic distances on every atom pair in the system at every time step in the simulation. The neighbour lists are typically updated every 10–20 time steps.

Molecular simulations allow the study of conformational ensembles. As such they allow the inclusion of entropic contributions to calculations, where previously we have spoken only about enthalpic energies. However, particularly for MD, it is unlikely that the sampling of high-energy states is always comprehensive.

Simulations hold out the tantalising possibility of being able to predict the free energy of binding for a novel molecule to a protein. There are many reasons why this is not yet, and may never be, possible, but for a time it seemed that the computational community was on the brink of a revolution in how drug discovery was performed. Calculation of the absolute free energy of binding of a ligand to a protein is fraught with difficulty, and to compare calculated free energies for two different molecules would normally produce small differences from very large numbers, where any differences are swamped by the errors in the large numbers. The Free Energy Perturbation (FEP) method[24] uses a non-physical application of the thermodynamic energy cycle to compare the binding energies of two different ligands to the same protein (Figure 3.7). $\Delta G_1$ and $\Delta G_2$ are respectively the free energies of binding of Ligand 1 and Ligand 2 to the protein. As stated above, accurate calculation of this free energy may not be computationally feasible. The key to the method is to calculate the *relative* free energies between the systems. Because the value around a thermodynamic cycle must be zero, the difference in free energies of binding, $\Delta G_2 - \Delta G_1$ must equal $\Delta G_4 - \Delta G_3$. $\Delta G_3$ is the difference in free energy between the ligands in solution, and $\Delta G_4$ the free energy difference of the two ligand–receptor complexes, neither of which can be observed in the laboratory. However, the FEP method, being theoretical, can exploit the non-observable changes $\Delta G_3$ and $\Delta G_4$. The calculation starts with one of the ligands, x, and gradually changes it into the other ligand, y, *via* a gradual perturbation, $\lambda$, of the molecular mechanics parameters. For example, the van der Waals energy term in the calculation can be written as the sum of the contributions from the partial ligands x and y:

$$v_{ij}^{\mathrm{LJ}}(\lambda) = 4(1-\lambda)\varepsilon_{\mathrm{x}}(\alpha_{\mathrm{x}}^{\mathrm{LJ6-12}}) + 4\lambda\varepsilon_{\mathrm{y}}(\alpha_{\mathrm{y}}^{\mathrm{LJ6-12}})$$

Where $\alpha_{\mathrm{x}}^{\mathrm{LJ6-12}}$ is a modified Lennard–Jones 6–12 potential for ligand x, to ensure that the system behaves well as x disappears to nothing, *i.e.* the mutation from ligand x to ligand y is complete.

Initial FEP calculations were encouraging: relative free energies of binding could be calculated within experimental error for drug-like molecules. Unfortunately, further experience with the method served to highlight the many difficulties of simulating complex molecular interactions with simple force fields, approximate methods and insufficient computing resources.[56]

A semi-empirical alternative is the Linear Response Method,[57] which attempts to compute absolute free energies of binding from just two simulations, one for the ligand in solution and one for the protein–ligand complex. The electrostatic and van der Waals

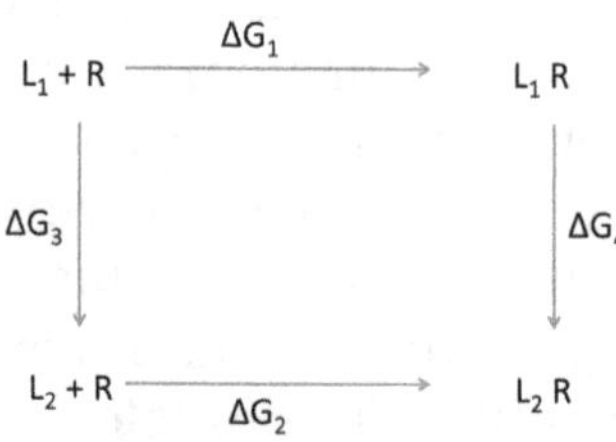


**Figure 3.7** The thermodynamic cycle for the binding energies of two protein–ligand complexes which is exploited by the Free Energy Perturbation method. By using the purely theoretical energy changes $\Delta G_3$ and $\Delta G_4$, the difference in free energies of binding between the ligands can be computed.

interaction energies from these simulations are then combined to produce an estimate of the free energy of binding:

$$\Delta G = \beta\left(\left\langle \gamma^{\mathrm{el}}_{\mathrm{ligand-protein}} \right\rangle - \left\langle \gamma^{\mathrm{el}}_{\mathrm{ligand-solvent}} \right\rangle\right) + \alpha\left(\left\langle \gamma^{\mathrm{vdw}}_{\mathrm{ligand-protein}} \right\rangle - \left\langle \gamma^{\mathrm{vdw}}_{\mathrm{ligand-solvent}} \right\rangle\right) \tag{3.9}$$

where β and α are parameters. Initially it had been hoped that some generic values of β and α could be derived from existing data, but it soon became clear that this is not the case.

Although many improvements have been published and new approaches invented, numerous experts doubt that the reliable, high throughput prediction of free energy of binding is a tractable problem for computational chemistry.[58] Nonetheless, the advent of an "industrialised" version of the FEP method, FEP+ from Schrödinger[59] has demonstrated that, for suitable systems, predictions can be made that are fit for medicinal chemistry design, with accuracies often within 1 kcal $mol^{-1}$. There are now examples of simulations which are able to predict absolute binding energies for pharmaceutical data sets. For example, Wan *et al.* describe simulations on a set of 16 bromodomain inhibitors[60] where the binding mode of the series was known through crystallography. The set was designed to represent the typical features of an industrial lead optimisation project, with a range of chemical functionality and binding affinities, but also to contain sets of closely related compounds with key SAR trends. Specifically, there are two growth vectors which cause a drop off in potency, a growth vector where substantial structural variation is tolerated and an enantiomeric pair where one isomer is significantly more potent than the other. The predicted binding free energies exhibit good Spearman correlations of 0.78–0.92 with the experimental data, and precisions between 0.2 and 1.71 kcal. With the expected growth in accessible computational power this is an area of science that will improve with time.

## 3.4 Modelling Solvation

The previous sections concentrate on the energy surface of a single molecule and many computational studies are conducted without consideration of the environment of the molecule – in the active site of an enzyme, in a membrane or in solution. Such studies are termed *in vacuo* or "gas phase" calculations. However, the environment of a molecule may have a profound effect on the energetics. For example, the preferred tautomer state of pyridone is reversed from gas phase to aqueous phase[61] (Figure 3.8).

In the gas phase, the internal hydrogen bond from the hydroxyl proton to the nitrogen lone pair stabilises that tautomer. However, in water, this coulombic attraction is screened by the dielectric, whilst in the keto-form, the resonance structure allows electrons to be drawn from the ring towards the electronegative oxygen, yielding a strong electrostatic interaction with the polar solvent, at the same time increasing the dipole of the molecule and hence adding further to the large solvation energy.

The intuitive method of modelling solvation is to include explicit solvent molecules in the calculation and immerse the ligand in a "water bath". This is the method of choice for modern simulation methods. However, inclusion of explicit solvent molecules is impractical for quantum mechanics calculations (remember the $N^4$ or $N^3$ scaling) and

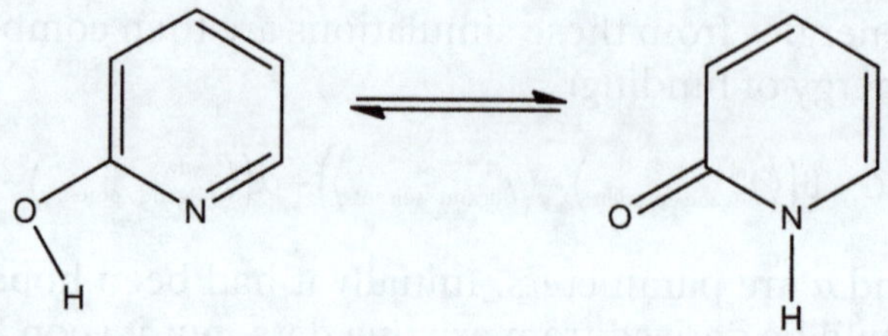

| | | |
|---|---|---|
| Gas phase relative energy | 0 kcal/mol | 0.5 kcal/mol |
| Aqueous phase relative energy | +4.1 kcal/mol | 0 kcal/mol |

**Figure 3.8** Solvent effects can have profound impacts on molecular structure. In the gas phase, and in non-polar solvents, the dominant form of 2-pyridone is the hydroxyl tautomer. However, in water, the large solvation energy of the keto tautomer makes it the dominant form.

| | TIP3P | ST2 |
|---|---|---|
| r(OH) | 0.9572Å | 1.0Å |
| HOH | 104.52° | 109.47° |
| q(O) | −0.834 | 0.0 |
| q(H) | 0.417 | 0.2375 |
| q(LP) | | −0.2375 |
| r(O-LP) | | 0.8Å |

**Figure 3.9** A comparison of two water models used in molecular simulations. The TIP3P was an early standard, even though it did not reflect the tetrahedral hydrogen binding preference of water. More recent models such as ST2 provide a more accurate representation, albeit at a higher computational cost.

even for molecular mechanics; the need to evaluate all the molecular interaction terms for each pair of water molecules adds significantly to the computation required. Hence, simplified models of water were sought, one of the most successful being Jorgensen's TIP3P (Figure 3.9) model.[62] This model has charges centred on the oxygen and both hydrogens. The water molecule is kept rigid during the simulation, and water–water van der Waals terms are computed *via* a single Lennard–Jones term centred on the oxygen of each molecule. In order to reproduce the properties of bulk water (effective dipole moment of 2.6 debyes), the atomic charges are large. The TIP3P model does not adequately describe the directionality of electron density on a water molecule, which is towards the oxygen lone pairs. There are more realistic models available, such as the ST2 system,[63] which uses a more realistic tetrahedral geometry with "lone pair" point charges on the oxygen atom, but the increased computational effort required to use these has meant that the simpler models are more likely to be used. These models have been proven very effective and can even be polarised by their environment by use of a fluctuating charge model.[64]

A simpler solution is to utilise classical reaction field theory.[65] Here, the solvent is considered as a bulk continuum and characterised by the dielectric constant. The solute model is considered as being embedded in a cavity within the solvent; in the simplest case, a spherical cavity is used. The solute charge distribution and dipole cause a reaction field in the solvent (as, for example, water molecules orientate to hydrogen bond with a carboxylic acid solvate) and the interaction of these fields produces the electrostatic energy of solvation. Such models, known as continuum solvation models, are simple to compute and surprisingly accurate for simple solutes. More sophisticated solutions involve the construction of more realistic cavity shapes by interlocking spheres,[66] or using an isoelectronic electron density surface to describe the shape of the cavity.[67] In these models, the solute molecular electrostatic potential is calculated at points on the surface, and these charges then represent the solvent reaction field which is used to compute electrostatic interactions with the solute. An alternate, but related, approach is the use of Poisson–Boltzmann methods,[68] which allow a better description of the ionic strength of the solvent and the change in dielectric from molecule to bulk solvent.

Other terms, such as the energy to create the cavity in the solvent, and van der Waals interactions, are generally computed in a much more approximate fashion, for example in the GBSA (Generalised Born Surface Area) method:[69]

$$\Delta G_{\text{sol}} = \Delta G_{\text{el}} + 7.2 \times \text{SA cal mol}^{-1}\,\text{Å}^{-2} \tag{3.10}$$

where the electrostatic term is calculated from a continuum solvent model and the other terms abstracted to a relationship with the Solvent Accessible Surface Area (SASA) of the solute. The surface area terms are important, as for non-polar molecules they model the observed behaviour that hydrophobic molecules prefer to minimise the amount of surface that interacts with water, preferring instead to self-associate or adopt appropriate conformations. Although still a contentious topic, this phenomenon, known as the hydrophobic effect,[70] is thought to be entropy driven (Figure 3.10).

This phenomenon is known to affect binding of ligands to proteins, increasing the affinity *via* non-specific binding. The majority of drug molecules are moderately lipophilic, exploiting the effect to help adhere to the target of choice, without incurring penalties associated with too much lipophilicity (poor solubility, low levels of absorption, promiscuous binding to other proteins, toxicity[71]). Recent studies with isothermal calorimetry confirm a relationship between lipophilicity and entropic binding energies,[72] whilst at the same time highlighting that our ability to decompose free energy contributions and use them in prospective design remains imperfect.[73]

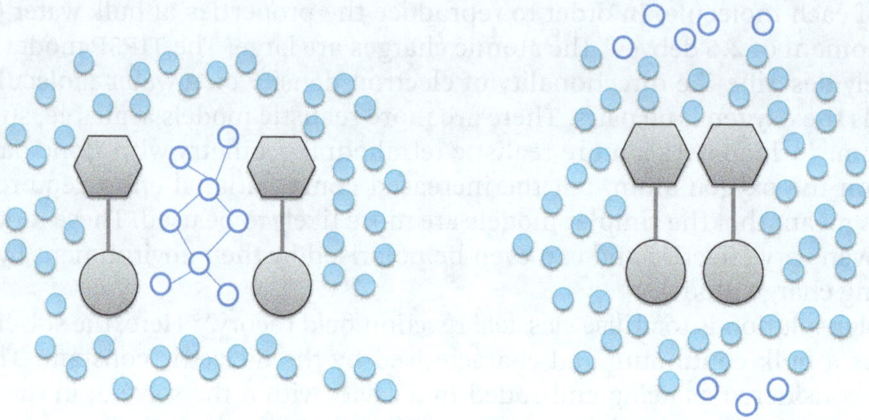

**Figure 3.10** A representation of the hydrophobic effect. Two organic molecules are dissolved in water. Between them is a water network that cannot hydrogen bond with the lipophilic molecules, and therefore adopts an ordered network of hydrogen bonds. As the two organic molecules come together, reducing the hydrophobic surface area exposed to the solvent, the ordered water molecules are released to bulk solvent, therefore increasing entropy, and lowering the free energy of the system.

Being entropic in nature, this effect is also very hard to model with the methods described here, the most successful methods being those based on measurements and QSAR techniques, for example the many log$P$ models that are available.[74]

## 3.5 Conformations, Conformational Energy and Drug Design

The biological and physicochemical properties of a molecule are determined to a large extent by the 3D structures, or conformations, which are accessible. The scientific field of conformational analysis can be said to have originated in a study by Barton,[9] who related the reactivity of substituted cyclohexanes to the equatorial or axial orientation of the ring substituents. Molecular mechanics calculations allowed theoreticians to take the principles of conformational analysis and reduce it to routine practice.[16] Conformational analysis necessitates a search for accessible conformations of a molecule. The preferred conformations can then be determined through calculation of relative energies of the accessible conformations. For simple molecules, a systematic search is facile: each rotatable bond is systematically rotated *via* a fixed amount (say, 30°) whilst the bond lengths and angles are kept constant. Energies may be computed at each point, or energy minimisation conducted starting at low energy conformers. The objective is to discover all the accessible conformations, which will lie at energy minima. Ideally, the global energy minimum will be determined, which will describe the dominant conformation. This systematic conformational data can be used to produce a map of the potential energy surface for a molecule. Possibly the most famous example of this type of analysis is the Ramachandran plot[75] for the alanine peptide, a model for the accessible conformations of amino acids in proteins (Figure 3.11).

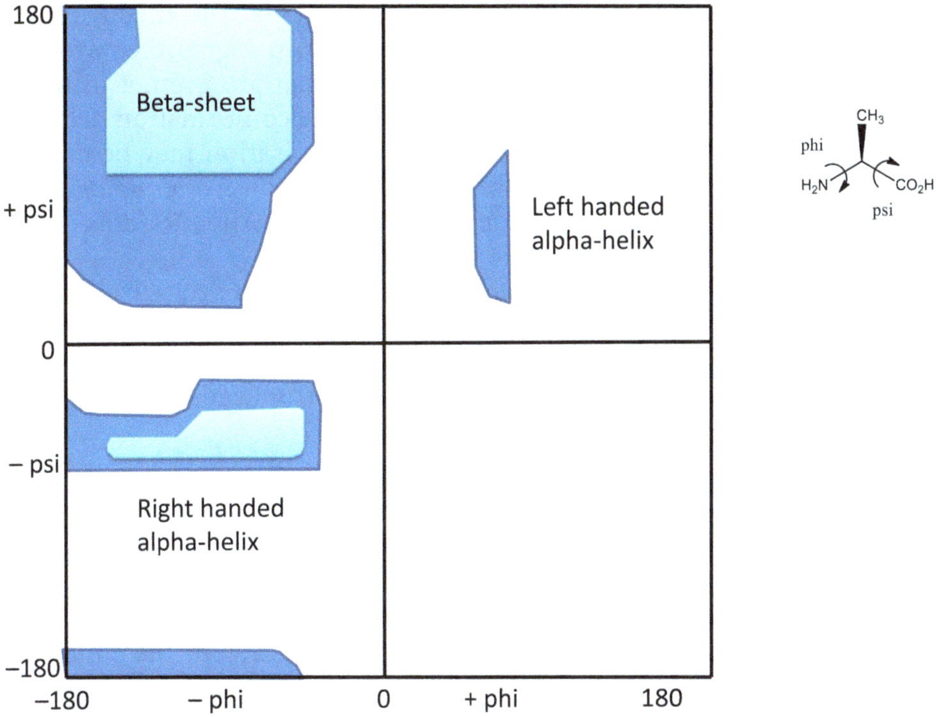


**Figure 3.11** The famous Ramachandran plot for peptides. The torsion angles phi and psi (shown here for the amino acid alanine) are systematically rotated and close contacts between atoms noted. Any combination of phi and psi which result in steric clashes are disallowed, and are responsible for all the white space in the graph. These regions are therefore not accessible to any amino acid except for glycine, which is unique in that it does not have a sidechain. The blue areas are those which can be accessed if the van der Waals radii are slightly reduced, and this allows the emergence of the left-handed helix region, which is sometimes observed in protein structures. The light blue areas are the low energy conformers, and correspond to the commonly observed beta-sheet and alpha-helix conformations.

Systematic searches become problematic when dealing with drug-size molecules, however, in that the number of conformations to be computed scales by $O^N$ where N is the number of rotatable bonds. For example, a small molecule with three rotational bonds, sampled at 30° intervals, has 1728 conformations. A molecule roughly twice the size (six rotatable bonds) would have 2.9 million conformations, and adding a single atom to that molecule could lead to 36 million conformations! At 1 second per conformer, the analysis would take over a year. Fortunately, search algorithms have been developed which reduce the size of the problem by avoiding unproductive areas of conformational space.[76] Search trees allow the early recognition of, say, a high-energy torsion, and then ignore all conformers in that branch of the search. As conformational analysis is such a fundamental technique, many other methods have been invented: fragment-based building,[77] random and Monte Carlo searches,[78] molecular dynamics/simulated annealing, genetic algorithms[79] and distance geometry.[80] This last method is useful in the generation of conformers which satisfy experimentally determined distance information, for example from NMR experiments. Distance geometry uses matrices of distances between atoms alongside rules from trigonometry to parse randomly generated conformations and weed out those that are geometrically impossible. Those that cannot be ruled out are refined until the conformation better satisfies the distance constraints and finally a force field minimisation may be employed on the smaller numbers of remaining conformers. Information from databases of small molecule crystal structures can also be used to generate experiment-derived rule-based conformer generators.[81]

Relative conformational energies are crucially important in drug discovery. A difference in energy of only 1.4 kcal $mol^{-1}$ results in a ratio of 1 : 10 in the populations of two conformers.

Returning to the relationships of Gibbs free energy introduced in Section 3.1, we can write:

$$\Delta H - T\Delta S = -2.3\ RT \log K$$

From this we can use conformational properties to increase the enthalpy of binding ($\Delta H$) or reduce the entropic penalty of binding ($\Delta S$). Both of these require us to use the technique of conformational constraints. If we are able to constrain a molecule to have a better geometric match of the functionality of the ligand with the complementary groups on the receptor, this will increase $\Delta H$. This requires much precision in design and is challenging even with protein structure data. A more forgiving approach is to increase the concentration of the binding conformation of the molecule in solution, which reduces the entropic penalty upon binding. Take a simple molecule with three accessible conformations arising from one rotatable, C–C bond.

We exploit the Boltzmann relationship between the number of states in a system and its entropy:

$$S = k \ln W$$

Comparing the change from a molecule with a freely rotating C–C bond ($W1$, 3 conformational states) with that where the C–C bond has been constrained ($W2$, 1 state), the change in entropy is:

$$\Delta S = R \ln (W1/W2)\ \text{kcal mol}^{-1}$$

$T\Delta S = RT \ln(1/3)$ kcal $mol^{-1}$ = −0.6 kcal $mol^{-1}$. This is a gain of ~4-fold in affinity, and is comparable to that gained from a strong hydrogen bond.[82]

Conformational constraints are a familiar tactic in small molecule drug discovery, offering predicable gains in affinity from small changes to molecules without requiring detailed understanding of the receptor site.

Figure 3.12 shows two successful examples of conformational constraints, one by use of a ring system to constrain the rotation about an important bond vector,[83] whilst the other example uses intramolecular hydrogen bonding to constrain the accessible conformations of the molecule.[84] Modern computational chemistry methods are quite capable of predicting the geometries and energetics of this type of system.

Figure 3.13 illustrates that it is quite possible for conformational constraints to fail if one has insufficient knowledge of the receptor environment or binding conformations

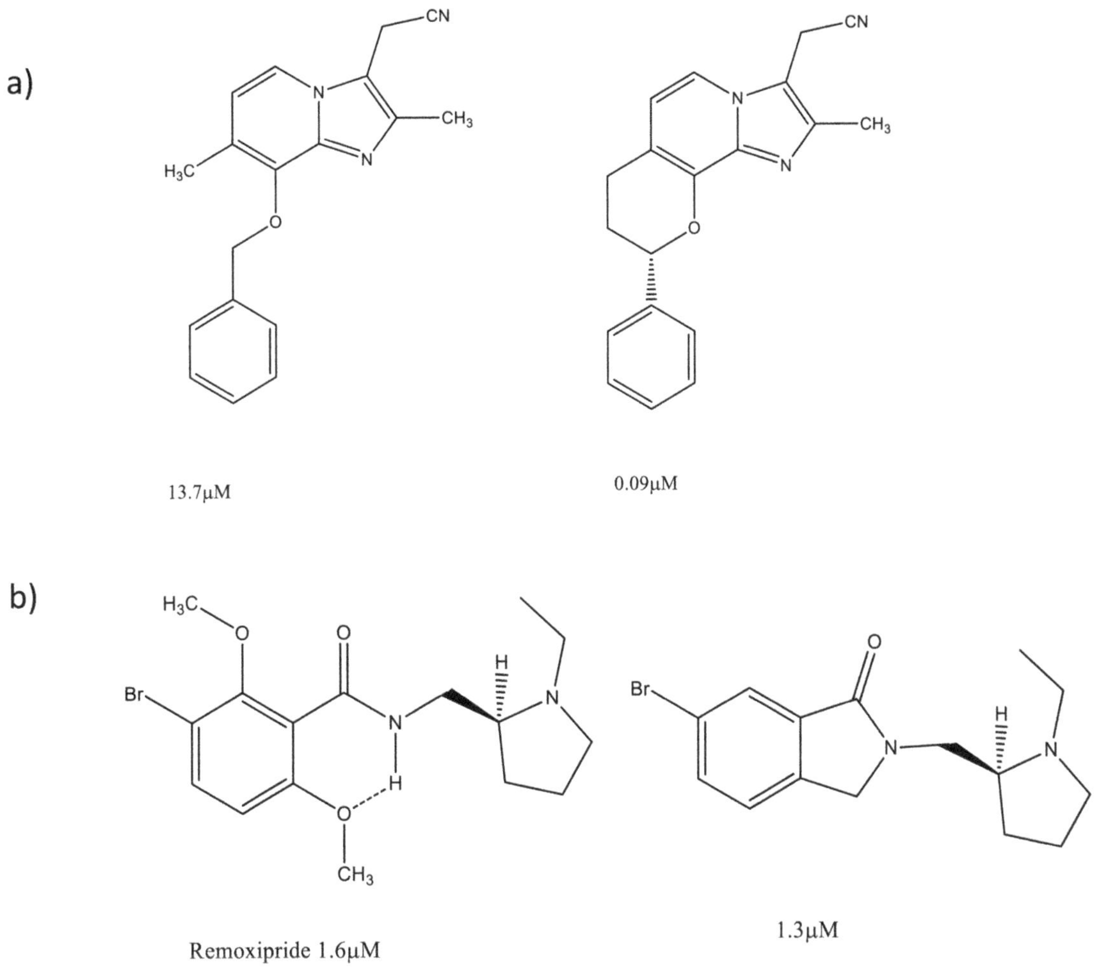


**Figure 3.12** (a) Shows the successful introduction of a conformational constraint in gastric H+/K+ ATPase inhibitors. (b) Is an example of the use of intramolecular hydrogen bonds to constrain a conformation in D2 receptor antagonists.

of the molecule. The small molecule crystal structure of baclofen was determined and used to design analogues which would lock the molecule into the observed low-energy conformation.[85] None of these were active, meaning that either the binding conformation of the molecule is different to that seen in the solid state, or that the atoms providing the conformational constraint may not be tolerated in the active site of the receptor.

## 3.6 Quantifying Molecular Interactions from Experimental Data

There is a significant body of experimental data that can be used instead of, in conjunction with or to train computational approaches. One of the most useful of these is the Cambridge Crystallographic Database (CSD) of small molecule crystal structures.[86] Starting from a straightforward repository of data, the Cambridge Crystallographic

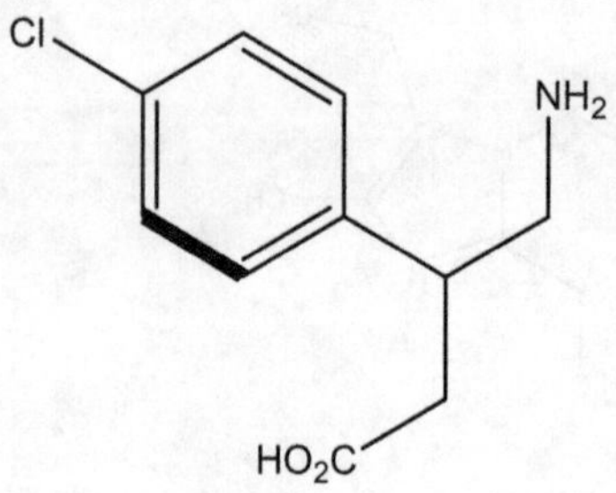


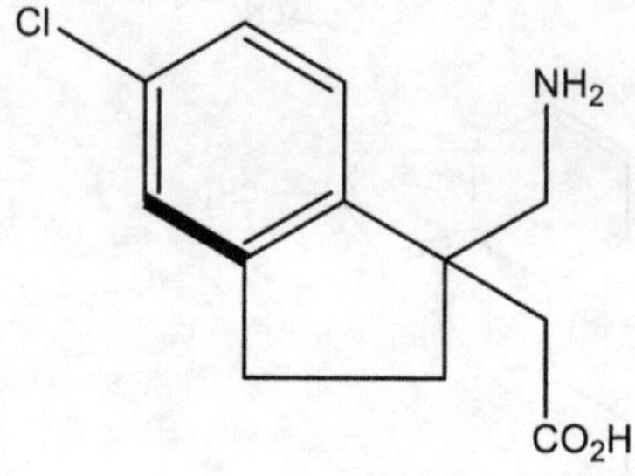


**Figure 3.13** An unsuccessful application of conformational constraints in GABAb receptor ligands.

Data Centre (CCDC) have developed a number of analysis tools which reveal a treasure trove of information about small molecule conformation and functional group interaction geometries.

IsoStar[87] is a tool that gives access to a library of the intermolecular interactions found within the CSD (and some from the Protein Data Bank (PDB)). Searches of the CSD have been carried out for over 12 000 particular intermolecular interactions. The data can be analysed by functional group, and a picture of how that group interacts with others can be displayed in various forms. For example, Figure 3.14 shows the interaction patterns of an ester group with any hydroxyl group (phenolic, aliphatic or water).

These plots can be reduced to a contour plot to reveal underlying distributions. In Figure 3.15 two contours have been computed to represent the density of observations per unit volume of space. This method clearly shows the preference of an ester to use the carbonyl to hydrogen bond, and the geometrical preference to have the hydrogen bond directed towards the oxygen lone pairs.

The CCDC data provides geometric preference and likelihood statistics, but the observational data does not provide insight into the strength of hydrogen bonds nor of the binding energy that might be afforded by making such interactions with the protein. For many years researchers relied on the elegant work of Abraham *et al.*[88] which yielded a set of standard hydrogen bond strengths for common organic functional groups and rings. It is also possible to use quantum mechanics calculations to produce such values for novel fragments, and to do so using quite straightforward methods such as computing the MEP.[89]

## 3.7 Docking and Scoring Functions

Perhaps the most familiar application of computational chemistry is that of structure-based design, where the crystal structure of the protein has been determined. Computational methods offer the possibility of virtual screening to discover leads in

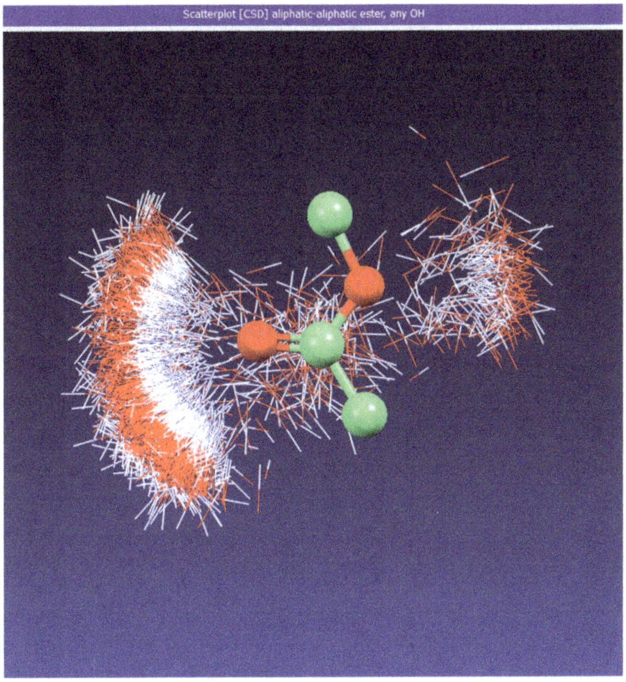


**Figure 3.14** Example output from IsoStar for an ester fragment interacting with hydroxyl groups.

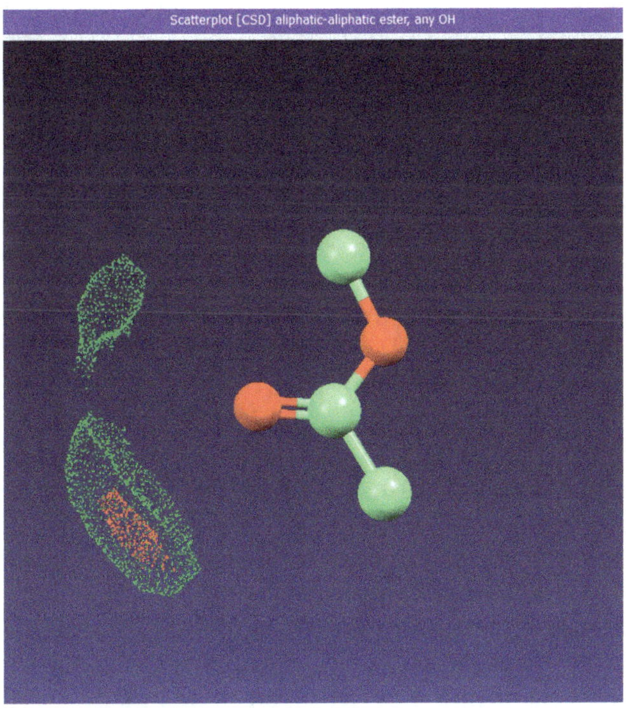


**Figure 3.15** The IsoStar output contoured according to the density of observations, illustrating how the ester fragment prefers to make hydrogen bonds with its p orbitals.

an existing collection of molecules, or to select from possible molecules which could be synthesised as part of a lead optimisation programme. It is useful to think of this problem in two parts, that of docking (generation of plausible poses of the ligand and protein) and scoring (selecting the correct binding mode and conformation for a single molecule and correctly ranking molecules against each other).

The generation of ligand poses within a protein is a similar problem to that of conformational analysis, with the added complexity that we must also take account of the orientation of the ligand to the protein. The two most common approaches may be categorised as systematic and random. A systematic search seeks to sample all the possible conformations and orientations of the molecule, but faces the same problems as for conformational analysis, multiplied by the fact that calculations are needed on every conformer to test the interaction with the protein. A common strategy, as employed by the popular methods Dock[21] and FlexX,[90] is to fragment the molecule and dock the largest or most rigid part of the molecule into the protein. Other parts of the molecule are grown onto the successfully docked fragments, until the whole set of plausible docking poses have been generated for the molecule. Alternative approaches often employ stochastic (random) methods to generate poses. The popular GOLD algorithm[91] uses a genetic algorithm, with the bond torsions encoded in the chromosome which is allowed to mutate and breed, with better scoring ("fitter") solutions being more likely to pass on their DNA to new poses. Monte Carlo approaches are also effective at exploring possible binding modes.

Plausible docking poses need to be compared to each other, and to those of other ligands, in order to perform a useful virtual screen. Even if the correct binding poses are produced, this cannot be used unless a scoring function can distinguish it from the other possibilities. Scoring functions are best categorised into three classes.[92] The first, and earliest, are the physics-based methods, using the first principles methods described in this chapter, typically using molecular mechanics force fields (although there are some studies using QM). The seminal GRID program[23] employs a molecular mechanics force field, which is used to calculate the potential energy of the protein at points on a grid thrown over the protein active site. GRID uses atom-type probes to generate interaction energy contours for visualisation, and the approach is readily adapted and used for whole molecules. AutoDock[93] employs the AMBER force field.[94] A problem with the use of force fields to score docking poses is the "hardness" of the Lennard–Jones 6–12 potential. A small error in positioning of a molecule in close proximity to the protein can result in very large repulsion energies, and therefore some methods such as G-Score[95] utilise a softer potential, for example an 8–4 term, which is more forgiving.

Pure force-field-based methods were not found to be satisfactory, and require significant compute time, and therefore empirical methods have emerged. These methods derive scoring functions which reproduce experimental data such as binding energies and observed binding geometries as extracted from the CCDC database. The LUDI scoring function[96] involves the number of hydrogen bonds made (which need to be of an orientation and geometry consistent with those observed in crystal structures), lipophilic contact surface and the number of rotatable bonds:

$$\log\frac{1}{Ki} = 1.4 \times ionichydrogenbonds + 0.83 \times neutralhydrogenbonds$$
$$+ 0.030 \times lipophiliccontactsurfacearea - 0.25 \times numberofrotatablebonds - 0.91$$

Subsequent empirical schemes utilised different methods to encode the non-bonded interactions, for example ChemScore[97] replaces the hydrophobic surface area with contacts between hydrophobic atom pairs, and the F-Score[90] adds a specific term for aromatic interactions. One advantage of empirical methods is the ability to add fitted terms for phenomena that are difficult to compute from first principles, for example entropic components (often based on the number of rotatable bonds) and desolvation energies.

The third category is knowledge-based scoring functions. These attempt to encode observed information from protein–ligand crystal structures in a way that can be employed to good effect on novel systems. Typically, this entails extraction of all pairs of atoms seen to interact in a crystal structure (for example, a ligand carbon atom in an aromatic ring contacting an aromatic carbon atom in the protein). The geometries and configurations of all examples of each atom pair are combined to define the optimal position, and allowable deviation for that type of interaction. A score for a docking pose is then the sum of all the atom-pair interactions. Examples of these methods are the Potential of Mean Force,[98] DrugScore[99] and SmoG.[100] A significant advantage of such methods is the speed by which they can be computed, however, like QSAR models, the predictions can be suspect when applied to molecular systems which are unlike those in the training set.

There are dozens of scoring functions in the literature, none of which can be relied on to work for every problem.[101] It is also difficult to predict when a particular method might work well. This problem gave rise to the development of consensus scoring schemes, whereby several scoring functions are employed at the same time and the results combined. Typically, a set of complementary scoring functions are chosen, for example the X-CSCORE[102] model uses force-field-based (GOLD, DOCK, FlexX), empirical (ChemScore) and knowledge-based (PMF) functions. The hope is that by combining the models, consistent high-performing docking poses will be raised to the top, and good molecules will be penalised less by a poor prediction in one method.

Although much intellectual firepower has been deployed in the quest for reliable docking and scoring methods, the problem remains stubbornly resistant to the best efforts of the computational community. The same issues that prevent reliable predictions of free energy changes with the most sophisticated computer models reappear, and are amplified, as we try to compare the properties of very diverse ligands. As a general rule of thumb, generation of plausible docking poses is less of a problem than having a scoring function that recognises the right answer when it has been found. Despite these problems, impressive results are possible if enough computational resources are devoted to a problem. Lyu *et al.*[103] took a large (170 million compounds) library of "tangible" molecules (molecules that a compound vendor believes they can synthesise, but have not yet done so) and used docking to select 50 and 589 compounds for interactions with AmpC β-lactamase (AmpC) and the D4 dopamine receptor, respectively. These molecules were synthesized, tested and novel hits discovered for both receptors. Five compounds were active from 1.3–400 mM at AmpC and 81 compounds revealed Ki values that ranged from 18.4 nM to 8.3 μM at the D4 dopamine receptor. These results suggest that virtual screening may be about to deliver significant benefits to the lead discovery process.

## 3.8 Cheminformatics

Wave functions or force fields are too cumbersome for some tasks in computational chemistry, where one only cares about the chemical connectivity of the structure. Wiswesser line notation was an early (1950s) system used by information scientists to encode molecules in short text strings[104] and therefore determine if two molecular structures were the same – the foundation of chemical registration systems. Researchers seeking to substructure search databases of chemical structures employed a different representation, the connection table.[105] The connection table was the standard structure representation format for many years, before line notations had a resurgence in popularity with the publication of the SMILES notation in the 1980s.[106] A molecule can be represented by more than one syntactically correct SMILES, and to compare them the string must be "canonicalised". Canonicalisation algorithms vary and are often proprietary, and so more recently, the International Chemical Identifier (InChI)[107] has been developed as a non-proprietary international standard to represent chemical structures. All of these structure formats have been used for the creation and indexing of huge chemical structures databases, which then enables search, either for whole molecules (structure matching) or for parts of molecules (substructure searching, SSS) (Figure 3.16). There are many applications for these searches: looking up information such as physical properties or assay results, finding examples with the same central ring or functional group, searching the literature, *etc.*, but there are limits. For instance, a very common task for a medicinal chemist is to think of similar structures – perhaps swapping an indole for a pyrrolopyrimidine. The power of line notation pattern representations is exemplified by the SMARTS language,[108] derived from SMILES, which allowed the user to define substructures with atom and bond patterns rather than fully defined substructures. For instance, one can specify definitions for Lipinski's hydrogen bond donors (where donors are defined as nitrogen or oxygen atoms that have at least one directly bonded hydrogen atom): [N,n,O;!H0] where N is an aliphatic nitrogen, n aromatic nitrogen, O an aliphatic oxygen and "!H0" means the atoms do not have zero Hydrogens attached, a more elegant way of defining atoms that could have one, two or three hydrogens. Recursive SMARTS allow very precise and powerful chemical definitions to be written, for example a definition of common acidic groups could be [$([OH][C,S,P]=O),$([nH]1nnnc1)], which covers carboxylic, sulfuric, phosphinic acids and tetrazole in a single expression. SMARTS patterns are particularly useful in refining lists of molecules – for instance in removing reactive molecules such as alkyl halides from screening sets or identifying reagents for a planned reaction. Another important use is to detect structures that do not obey "business rules" in a database – for instance, do we store nitro as a neutral (N(=O)(=O)) or charge-separated form ([N+](=O)([O−])? If we have both forms in our database, then a SSS might only return a portion of the available data. (The desirability of nitro groups in medicinal chemistry is another matter!)

SMARTS thus extends the SSS capabilities, but it results in a binary response – either a pattern matches or it does not. But for many applications, what we really need is a measure of molecular similarity.

Similarity has already been discussed in the form of the Carbo index for comparing electron density or electrostatic potential, but for chemical connectivity there was a need for something simpler and faster. A suitable metric would be more continuous, so that a list of molecules could be ranked in terms of similarity to a lead or to each other. In other words, a similarity or distance metric, where more similar molecules are closer together. Nikolova and Jaworska[109] have an intuitive classification of similarity methods into categories: similarity by constitution, by configuration, by property and by wave function (or what an entity contains, how it is shaped, what it does and what it is…). Most of these methods require a list of properties, fragments or distances that can be compared to another. When reduced to a list of 1s and 0s, this is a molecular binary fingerprint. The advantage of a binary string representation is very fast computer processing, using bit-string operations. Indeed, many of the first molecular fingerprints derived from the bit screens used in chemical database searching to reduce the number of possible matches in the database before starting more compute-expensive graph comparisons.[110] These have been augmented by fingerprints designed specifically for molecular similarity calculations.[111,112]

The commonest method of comparing fingerprints is the Jaccard similarity measure, more commonly known as the Tanimoto similarity measure. This is a simple but effective metric, being a ratio of the number of bits that are in common in two strings over the number of bits set in either string. The Tanimoto similarity between two equal length molecular fingerprints, $M$ and $N$, is

$$T(M,N)=\frac{\sum_i (M_i \cap N_i)}{\sum_i (M_i \cup N_i)}.$$

**Connection Table**

```
12 12  0  0  1  0        999 V2000
  0.7145  -0.4125   0.0000 C  0 0 0 0 0 0 0 0 0 0 0 0
 -0.0000   0.0000   0.0000 C  0 0 0 0 0 0 0 0 0 0 0 0
  0.0000   0.8250   0.0000 C  0 0 0 0 0 0 0 0 0 0 0 0
  0.7145   1.2375   0.0000 C  0 0 0 0 0 0 0 0 0 0 0 0
  1.4289   0.8250   0.0000 C  0 0 0 0 0 0 0 0 0 0 0 0
  1.4289  -0.0000   0.0000 C  0 0 0 0 0 0 0 0 0 0 0 0
  0.7145   2.0625   0.0000 C  0 0 0 0 0 0 0 0 0 0 0 0
  0.0000   2.4750   0.0000 C  0 0 1 0 0 0 0 0 0 0 0 0
  0.0000   3.3000   0.0000 C  0 0 0 0 0 0 0 0 0 0 0 0
 -0.7145   3.7125   0.0000 O  0 0 0 0 0 0 0 0 0 0 0 0
  0.7145   3.7125   0.0000 O  0 0 0 0 0 0 0 0 0 0 0 0
 -0.7145   2.0625   0.0000 N  0 0 0 0 0 0 0 0 0 0 0 0
 1  2  4  0  0  0  0
 2  3  4  0  0  0  0
 3  4  4  0  0  0  0
 4  5  4  0  0  0  0
 5  6  4  0  0  0  0
 1  6  4  0  0  0  0
 4  7  1  0  0  0  0
 8  7  1  0  0  0  0
 8  9  1  0  0  0  0
 9 10  2  0  0  0  0
 9 11  1  0  0  0  0
 8 12  1  6  0  0  0
```

**L-Phenylalanine**

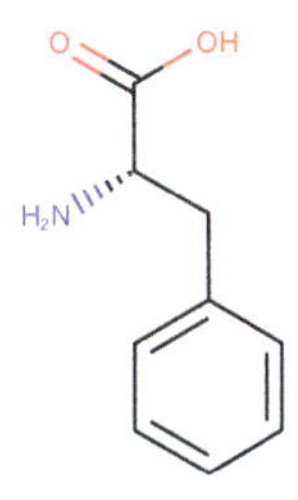


**WLN**

QVYZ1R

**SMILES**

c1ccc(cc1)C[C@@H](C(=O)O)N

**InChi**

InChI=1S/C9H11NO2/c10-8(9(11)12)6-7-4-2-1-3-5-7/h1-5,8H,6,10H2,(H,11,12)/t8-/m0/s1

**Figure 3.16** Connection table *vs.* WLN, SMILES and InCHI representations for L-phenylalanine.

This can be rewritten for fast bit-string operations (where & is bitwise AND):

$$T(M,N)=\frac{M\&N}{M\&M+N\&N-M\&N}$$

Tanimoto similarity has become a *de facto* standard in medicinal chemistry, although it can be difficult to interpret. A score of 1.0 shows that there is an exact match in the pattern of 1s and 0s in the bit-strings *M* and *N*. This often means that they represent the same molecule, as the bit-strings are identical, but that depends on the fingerprint. For instance, some do not distinguish between stereoisomers. Tanimoto scores of less than one are more problematic. Scores very close to one – above 0.85, say – have been suggested as indicating a zone of bioisosterism, *i.e.*, molecules giving similar biological activity about 80% of the time,[113] though later work by the same group suggested that there was only a 30% chance of any one molecule with that score being active![114] This sounds poor at first, but simple probability suggests that the chance of finding no hits in a set of 10 molecules would be $(70\%)^{10} = 2.8\%$. (The problem is usually one of cost instead – if one searched a typical database, where the number of active molecules is heavily outweighed by inactives, then the number of true positives would also be heavily outweighed by false positives.[115])

The ratio of bits in common to bits in total does not necessarily correlate with a chemist's idea of similarity, so lower scores do not provide a chemist-friendly metric, and it is difficult to say what (if anything) a score of 0.35 means in terms of chemistry. There are several reasons for this, not least the fact that we chemists do not agree with each other (or even ourselves!) about structures.[116] Very similar compounds can be at the boundary of an "activity cliff",[117] usually because of some inconvenient steric clash and quite different molecules can be equipotent, if a large part is solvent-exposed rather than involved in binding. This was all pointed out last century,[118] but the lure of "efficiency over efficacy" has ensured the continued use of bit-string comparison.

For many years, databases of chemical structures and the tools with which to manipulate them were the domain of specialist commercial software systems. In practice, industrial scientists often rely on the very fine toolkits produced and refined over many decades. However, in recent years the open source movement has delivered data and tools which have enabled a democratisation of the discipline and an increasingly sophisticated suite of accessible methods. The ChEMBL,[119] PubChem[120] and Chemspider[121] databases offer a broad range of published chemical structures alongside experimental biological and physicochemical data. These databases offer great service to the chemistry community and enable development of new methods and models by making large literature datasets available to all. Some care does need to be taken, as much of the extraction/curation is, by necessity, automated and of course literature is biased by successful experiments, with the "Journal of Inactive Molecules" yet to land a publishing deal. The GDB project of the Reymond group[122] seeks to enumerate all possible chemical structures, and databases of these enumerated structures, up to limited numbers of atoms, are made available. Millions of commercially available compounds can be accessed from online sources such as eMolecules,[123] Zinc,[124] Mcule[125] and Molport.[126] Increasingly, chemical companies are offering compounds that they could make, in addition to the ones they have already made, the most prominent examples being the Enamine Real Database.[127]

In order to read, search and manipulate these chemical structures, specialist tools are needed to create a digital model of the chemical structure which can be operated on. The popular RDKit[128] has an extensive suite of cheminformatics functions: property predictors, fingerprint and similarity calculation, clustering, SMARTS matching, *etc.*, all of which can be accessed *via* the Python scripting language.[129]

Once we have our molecular representation sorted out, we can start doing cheminformatics. A common task is building a descriptive statistical model. This could be as simple as looking at the location of a batch of data (*e.g.*, the median or mean) or at particular limit values (*e.g.*, pIC50 > 8). For instance, a mini-industry of identifying the limits of "drug-like chemical space" grew out of Lipinski's thoughtful but rarely read paper on bioavailability (not drug-likeness).[130]

A very common cheminformatics function is to curate and maintain the quality of HTS screening collections. An essential component of this is the development and use of substructure filters to remove undesirable compounds from a collection, or prevent them from coming in the first place. An extensive example are the Lilly "Rules for Identifying Potentially Reactive or Promiscuous Compounds",[131] a set of 275 rules, developed over an 18 year period. Reasons for rejection include reactivity (*e.g.*, acyl halides), interference with assay measurements (fluorescence, absorbance, quenching), activities that damage proteins (oxidizers, detergents), instability (*e.g.*, latent aldehydes), and lack of druggability (*e.g.*, compounds lacking both oxygen and nitrogen). The system uses the concept of "demerits", with a score of 100 sufficient to reject the compound. An example is provided by furan, with a matching SMARTS of o1cccc1 and a demerit value of 50, meaning that at least one other undesirable substructure would be needed to reject the compound.

When judging the "quality" of a molecular structure, it can be useful to combine molecular properties and substructure filters. It is difficult to decide what weight should be given to each property, and to avoid the trap of simple thresholds (*e.g.*, rejecting a molecule with a molecular weight of 501, but accepting one with 499). The QED score is an example of the use of a desirability function,[132] a method which allows the combination of a variety of data with optional weights and choice of mathematical functions to soften penalties at thresholds.

The simplest way to view diversity is *via* the concept of dissimilarity, which in turn could be defined as (1 – similarity) if using a similarity index such as the Tanimoto. A dissimilarity selection algorithm's aim is to select sets of compounds which are maximally similar to each other. The MaxMin algorithm is applied widely and has been subject of extensive evaluation.[133] For a set of compounds in a database, a lead molecule is selected and placed in the subset to be selected. The distance (in our case dissimilarity) is calculated between the selected subset and those remaining in the database. The molecule in the database with the maximum value of the minimum distance to any member of the existing subset is then selected for addition to the subset (*i.e.*, the maximal distance to the subset of near neighbours). In this way, a diverse set of molecules is built up one by one. Clustering[134] is an alternative to this, where a set of compounds are organised into chemically similar clusters, and then representative compounds picked from each cluster to form a set which is both diverse with respect to each other, and representative of the starting set of compounds as a whole. These methods can be applied to any of the fingerprint representations discussed above. Clustering methods have by and large replaced dissimilarity-based algorithms. Although hierarchical methods such as wards were identified as preferable,[134] it is common to see faster methods quoted. The widely used sphere exclusion clustering algorithm[135] deserves a detailed description. First, a "near neighbours" table is assembled which is a list of the molecules and the number of analogues they have, given a defined similarity threshold (the ubiquitous Tanimoto coefficient is most often applied, although there is some evidence that alternative coefficients may be superior). The table is ordered and, starting with the molecule with the most near neighbours, it and all the molecules within the defined similarity threshold to it are marked as belonging to the same cluster and removed from the set. Taking the remaining compounds, the molecule with the most near neighbours is selected, a new cluster created from it and molecules similar to it, and the whole process repeated until there are no molecules remaining. The algorithm is fast, intuitive and reliable.

Combinatorial chemistry, DNA encoded libraries and associated spin-off technologies for parallel synthesis, or simply higher-throughput synthesis, imparts some practical restrictions on a design. In a classic core template and R-group representation, the most common design is to select a number of reagents at each position that will fit to the synthetic equipment in use, be it 96-well "blocks" or more elaborate automation. The key restriction in design terms is that each reagent at R1 is coupled with every reagent at R2 and every reagent at R3. Therefore, an array with 10 reagents at each position yields $10 \times 10 \times 10 = 1000$ final molecules. Designing combinatorial libraries involves dealing with very large numbers of theoretical molecules, and an associated large number of possible solutions, for example there are $10^{26}$ ways of selecting $10 \times 10$ reagents from a $100 \times 100$ combinatorial library! Many elegant solutions have been developed to deal with this problem, in the main part utilising stochastic optimisation methods such as genetic algorithms.[136] The most sophisticated can design to multiple objectives and at the same time compare size and configuration of designs.

One of the most powerful cheminformatics techniques for structure–activity relationship (SAR) analysis and consequent molecular design is the concept of matched molecular pairs (MMPs).[137,138] By identifying every pair of molecules that differ only by a particular, well-defined, structural transformation in a database of measured properties and computing the corresponding change in property, we obtain an overview of the effect that structural change has upon the property and set an expectation for what will happen when that transformation is applied elsewhere. Pharmaceutical companies have rich databases which, when transformed into MMPs can guide chemists towards small changes to a molecule that, for example, might improve solubility whilst at the same time keeping low clearance (Figure 3.17). This concept has been extended to matched molecular series,[139] which allows legacy structure–activity relationships to be used to guide current lead optimisation projects.

Drug development pipelines are prone to attrition due to unexpected toxicities.[140] Even drugs that make it to the market may need to be withdrawn as they are prescribed to large patient populations and adverse drug reactions (ADRs) discovered.[141] Serious ADRs are subjected to investigative toxicology and ideally their adverse outcome pathway and molecular initiating event (MIE) elucidated.[142] For example, several drugs, such as the antihistamine terfenadine, have been withdrawn because they caused arrhythmias and death, which have been attributed to their off-target inhibition of the human *ether-à-go-go*-related gene potassium channel (hERG).[143] Anticipating these problems, thus allowing medicinal chemistry teams to dial out potential liabilities through

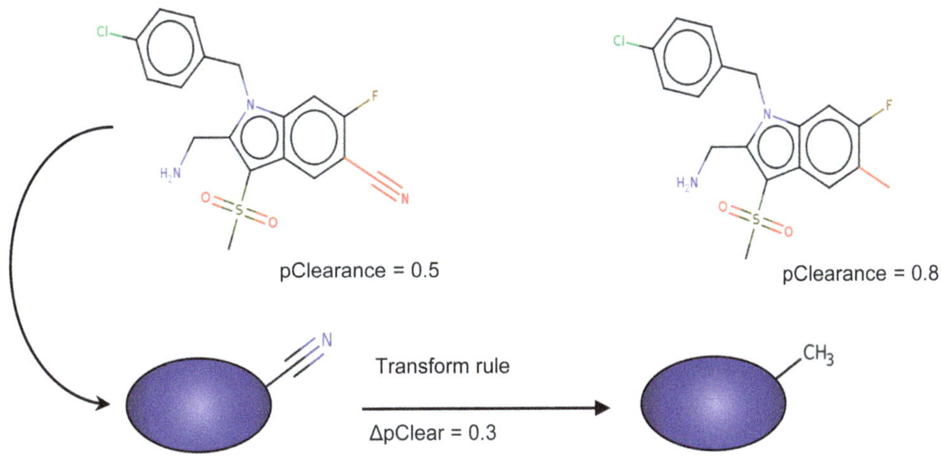


**Figure 3.17** An example of a matched molecular pair where the molecules are identical except for a single change (cyano → methyl). Differences in properties, in this case an *in vitro* clearance assay, may be ascribed to the small change and these can be aggregated across multiple examples to derive predictions and rules.

chemical structure changes in lead optimisation, would therefore be very impactful. A study by Lounkine *et al.*[144] demonstrated the effectiveness of a modified chemical structure similarity function to predict AERs. Predictions were made for 656 marketed drugs across 73 targets thought to be MIEs, creating a drug-target–AERs network. The system predicted that the abdominal pain side effect of the synthetic oestrogen chlorotrianisene is mediated through inhibition of the enzyme cyclooxygenase-1 enzyme, which was confirmed in laboratory assays.

Chemical similarity methods are commonly employed in lead discovery, for example to design high throughput screening (HTS) decks[145] and to follow up hits.[146] The methods may also be used to drive alternatives to full diversity screening, for example iterative screening,[147] where cost or experimental constraints limit the number of compounds that can be screened. In a large study, Pertusi *et al.*[148] compared a full HTS to an initial screen of 50 000 compounds followed up with a number of iterative selections made by 2D fingerprint similarity, 3D shape similarity and machine learning/QSAR models. Molecules were selected using a combination of these models, using a novel fusion score. Across 17 assays studied, this approach was able to identify 80% of the HTS hits, by sampling only 20% of the compounds in the HTS deck.

The power of modern cheminformatics methods is beginning to be demonstrated by pharmaceutical companies with large legacy datasets. The promise of automated molecular design using cheminformatics and machine learning has been demonstrated where good datasets are already available, (Figure 3.18).[149] Extension of this concept to situations where data is not so readily available is demonstrated by the BRADSHAW system[150] which employs cheminformatics, experimental design and machine learning approaches in tandem. The combination of large legacy data and modern cheminformatics enables the algorithms to learn from every project ever undertaken by a company (or published in the public domain). The effectiveness of these approaches

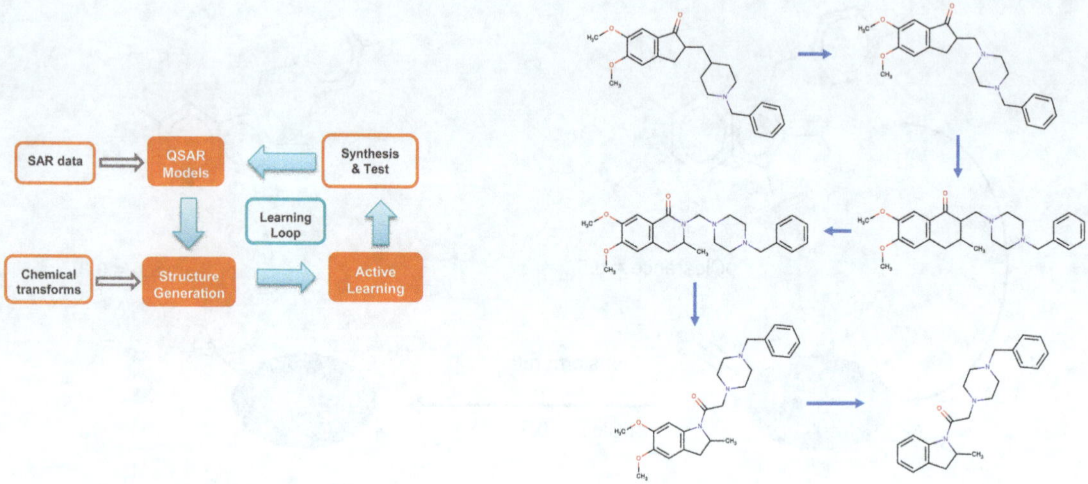


**Figure 3.18** The automated design process used (left) to optimise the off-target dopamine D4 activity of the marketed drug donepezil (dopamine D4 Ki 614 nM) into a selective dopamine D4 inverse agonist (dopamine D4 Ki 9 nM).

is demonstrated by Bush *et al.*[151] where a molecular generation algorithm, based on MMPs, passed the Turing Test[152] by producing ideas which experienced medicinal chemists could not distinguish from ideas from their fellow chemists.

## 3.9 Examples of Impactful Computational Chemistry on Drug Design

It is rare to see examples of computational design which are primarily responsible for a drug molecule. This is because drug discovery is a very difficult occupation, and although computational techniques might help with binding affinity or solubility, application to areas such as predictive toxicology is in its infancy.[153] In recent years, the proportion of drugs derived from protein-structure-based approaches has increased and therefore these have had computational input. One of the cleanest examples of computational impact is the neuraminidase inhibitor, Relenza. The introduction of the key 4-amino, and then 4-guanidine substituent was prompted by the use of the GRID program, which enabled the chemistry team to gain multiple orders of binding affinity whilst making only tens of molecules (Figure 3.19).[26]

A less successful example, but one which provides many excellent touch-points, is the work of Lam *et al.* on inhibitors of the HIV-1 Protease[154] (Figure 3.20). Starting from a linear peptide which was seen to bind to the protein *via* a water molecule, a 3D database search yielded some ideas that a six-membered ring could deliver a water mimetic in the right geometric orientation whilst at the same time positioning a key hydroxyl group to bind with the active site aspartic acid residues. Using knowledge from the peptide SAR, where two hydroxyls provide better binding affinity, a seven-membered ring was postulated. As a ketone has poor hydrogen bond strength, this was substituted for a

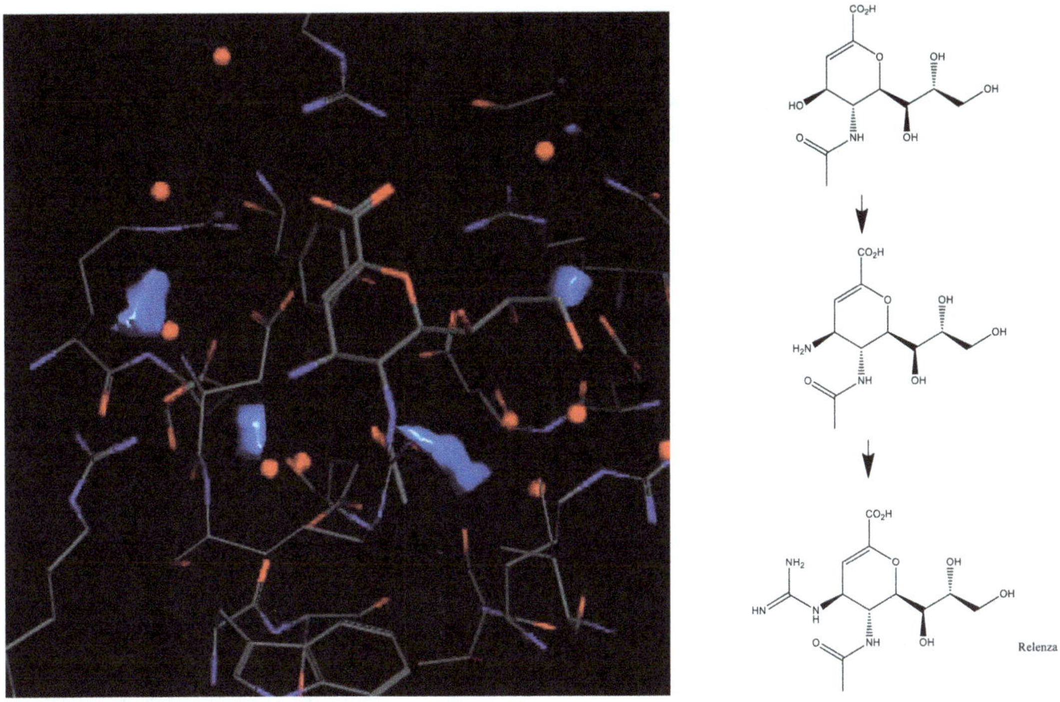


**Figure 3.19** The discovery of relenza. Starting with a crystal structure of the neuraminidase enzyme and a weak inhibitor, 2-deoxy-2,3-didehydro-*N*-acetylneuraminic acid (DANA), the GRID program was used to guide medicinal chemistry. First the 4-amino substituent was introduced, which increased affinity for the enzyme. The image shows the crystal structure of the 4-amino analogue, with the blue area directly below the amino group clearly indicating the predicted increase in potency with the introduction of a larger positively charged moiety. Following this prediction, the 4-guanidino group was one of several functional groups introduced and was found to be a potent inhibitor of the enzyme, yielding the anti-influenza drug relenza.[156]

urea. With the idea taking shape, the challenge was to predict the correct stereoisomers and substituents that would produce a low energy conformation of the ring and deliver all the substituents to the correct binding pockets. This was decided using computational approaches, and the resulting molecule synthesised. The team was successful in designing a non-peptidic ligand, and the subsequent protein–ligand crystal structure confirmed the predictivity of the design. However, the molecular structure and associated substituents is very lipophilic, which gave rise to insurmountable DMPK issues and the series did not deliver a drug (Figure 3.20).

An example of how molecular electrostatic potentials can be applied in lead optimisation is given by Bamford *et al.*[155] in the design of novel inhibitors of squalene synthase. The calculations were first used to aid interpretation of the structure–activity relationships in a series of carboxylic acid and methyl ester analogues, and then applied to aid design of heterocyclic isosteres of the methyl ester (Figure 3.21).

A fine example of the successful application of ligand-based modelling is the design of selective 5HT-1D agonists for the treatment of migraine by Glen *et al.*[156] The

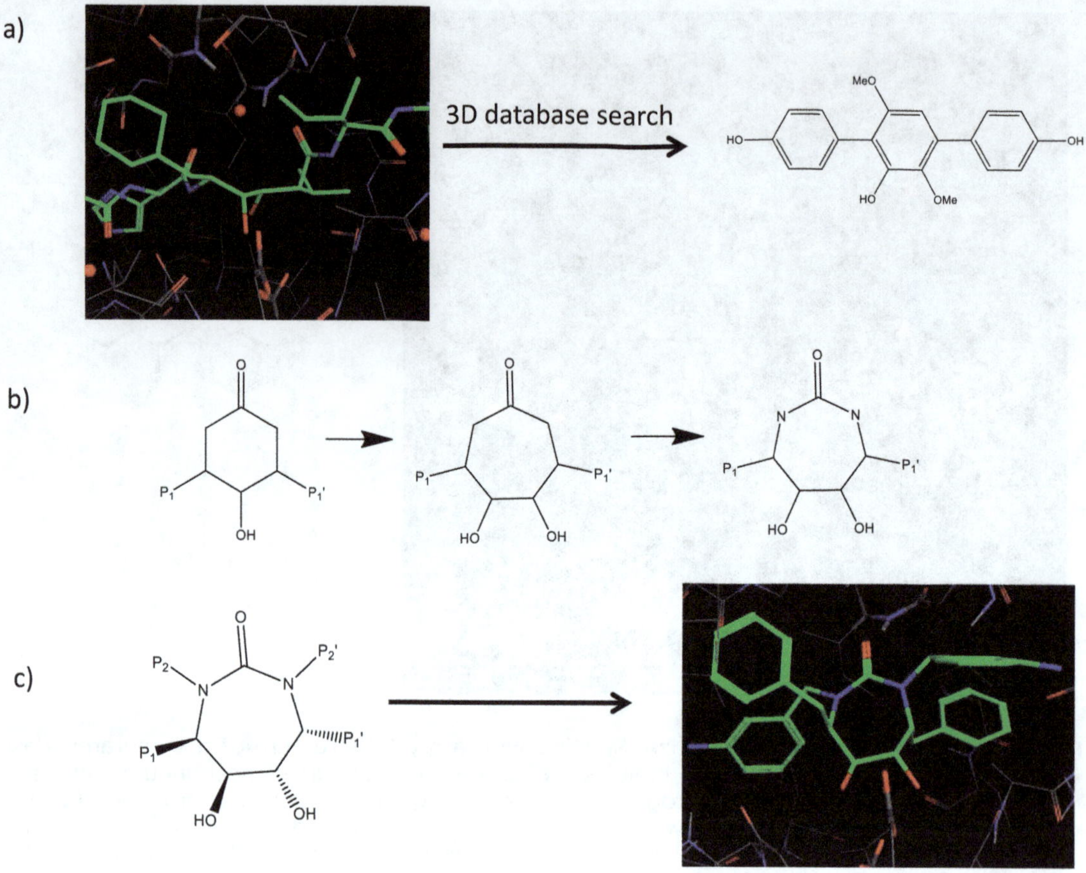


**Figure 3.20** The design of non-peptidic inhibitors of HIV protease. Starting from crystal structures of peptide inhibitors, a 3D database search was used to identify molecular architectures which could replace a key water molecule and position a hydroxyl group which was required to bind to the catalytic aspartic acids in the protein active site (shown in the first crystal structure image). This search yielded the tri-phenyl moiety shown in part a), which inspired the team to design a six-membered ring which might better position the functionality whilst incorporating some synthetic routes to add substituents which could interact with the protein's other recognition pockets. This initial idea was refined to a seven-membered ring (so as to incorporate two hydroxyl groups, known to be better inhibitors in the peptide analogues) and the ketone was replaced by a urea to incorporate a stronger hydrogen bonding group, and also to allow further points of diversification (shown in part b). Only then was "pure" computation invoked, to determine the precise stereochemistry required to fit the active site and position the key functional groups with a low-energy conformation of the ring template. The design can be seen to be correct in the second protein structure image, shown in part c).

conformationally restricted agonist methysergide was used to map the 3D positions of critical binding motifs, such as the basic amine, using the active analogue method.[157] By this method, a 3D pharmacophore was developed and used to screen potential ligands. The design process involved conformational analysis of potential ligands using molecular mechanics, with charges derived from AM1 semi-empirical calculations.

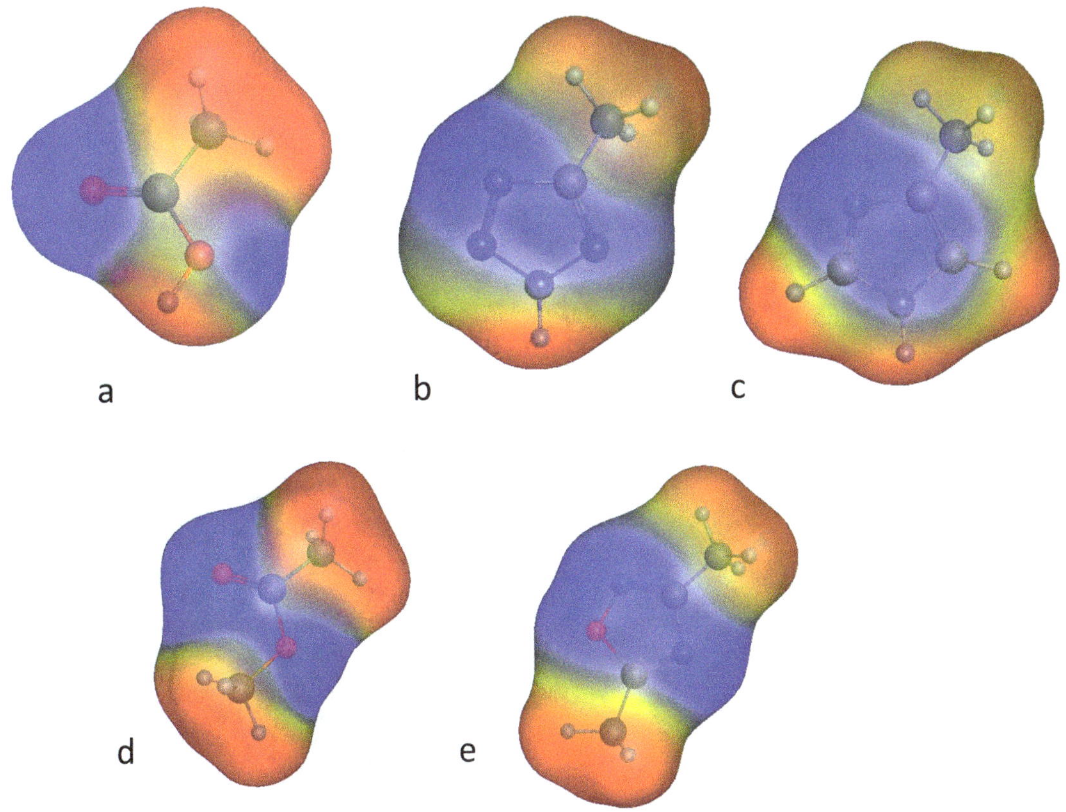


**Figure 3.21** The use of molecular electrostatic potential maps to design inhibitors of squalene synthase.[155] Analogues with a carboxylic acid (a) or tetrazole (b) substituent are more potent than the inactive imidazole (c). The MEP maps of (a) and (b) show a similar pattern of charge density which is not shared by (c), but is shared by the active methyl ester (d) and subsequently designed 3,5-dimethyl-1,2,4-oxadiazole (e).

Low-energy conformations found from the molecular mechanics calculations were then superimposed onto the 3D pharmacophore using constrained molecular mechanics minimisation with a simplex algorithm. There were concerns over potential intramolecular hydrogen bonds which might prevent adoption of the preferred conformation, and these were examined with molecular dynamics simulations. One of the key design criteria was selectivity for the 5HT-1D receptor over the related 5HT-2A, and therefore a "selectivity site" was computed by the differential volume occupied by ligands selective for 5HT-1D over 5HT-2A *vs.* those with no selectivity, and the volume added to the pharmacophore model. This computationally based design strategy yielded the drug zolmitriptan (Figure 3.22).

Finally, a case study which exemplifies current "structure-guided drug design" practice in the discovery of asunaprevir for the treatment of hepatitis C.[158] As with many antiviral protease projects, initial information is from peptide-derived inhibitors. Crystallography and SAR data showed the critical interaction of the C-terminal carboxyl group. In an effort to improve the binding affinity of a series of tripeptide inhibitors of

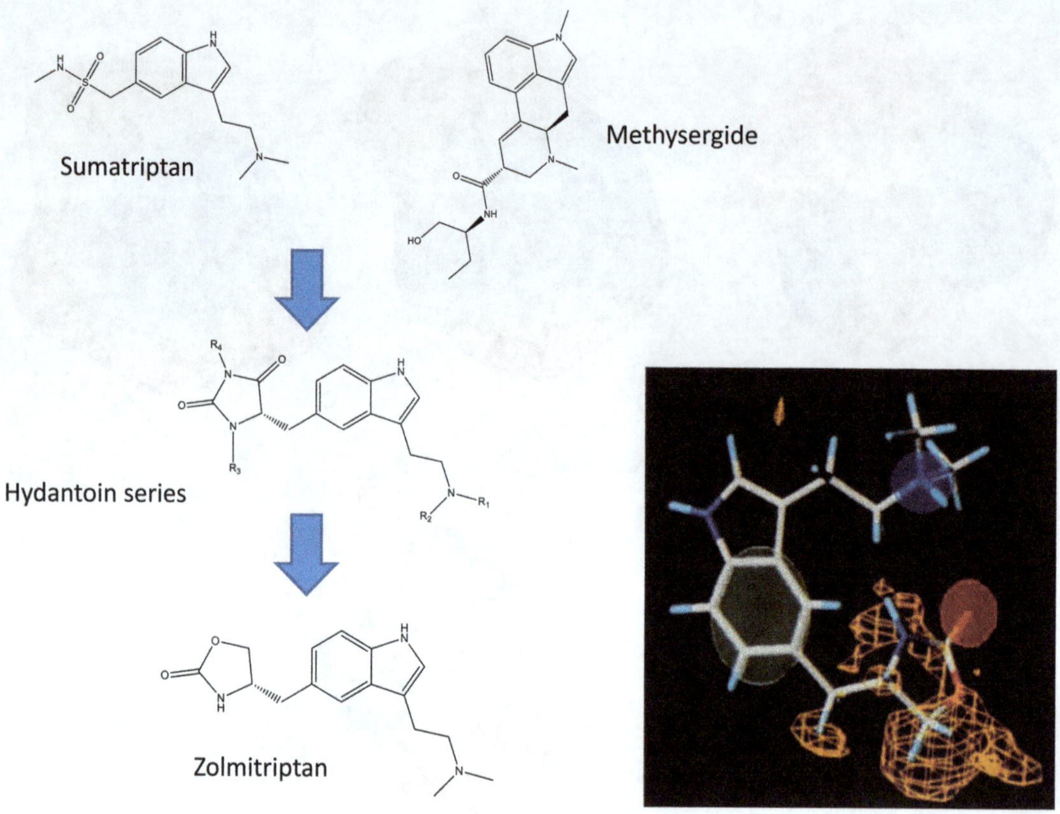


**Figure 3.22** The discovery of zolmitriptan employed rigorous molecular mechanics conformational analysis combined with a 3D pharmacophore. Known 5HT-1D agonists such as methysergide and sumatriptan were used to define a 3D pharmacophore and selectivity volume. A series of hydantoins were designed using systematic conformational analysis and superimposition onto the 3D model (shown for zolmitriptan). The molecular graphics image is adapted with permission from Glen *et al.*[156] Copyright 1995 American Chemical Society.

the NS3/4A enzyme, a ligand design strategy was pursued in which the essential interactions between the carboxylic acid group of the peptide and the catalytic site were maintained while projecting functionality into the S1′ pocket.[159] On the basis of modelling considerations, acylsulfonamides were proposed as a structural motif that could maintain the electrostatic interactions of the parent carboxylic acid while offering the potential to extend structural elements into the prime side of the enzyme and engage in favourable non-bonding interactions. Guided by modelling, the cyclopropyl substituent was quickly identified as optimal (Figure 3.23).

## 3.10 Hints and Tips

The application of computational chemistry to a drug design problem is not a simple matter of installing a software package and pressing some buttons. Nor is it a case of always running the most complex simulation available to you. What this chapter has

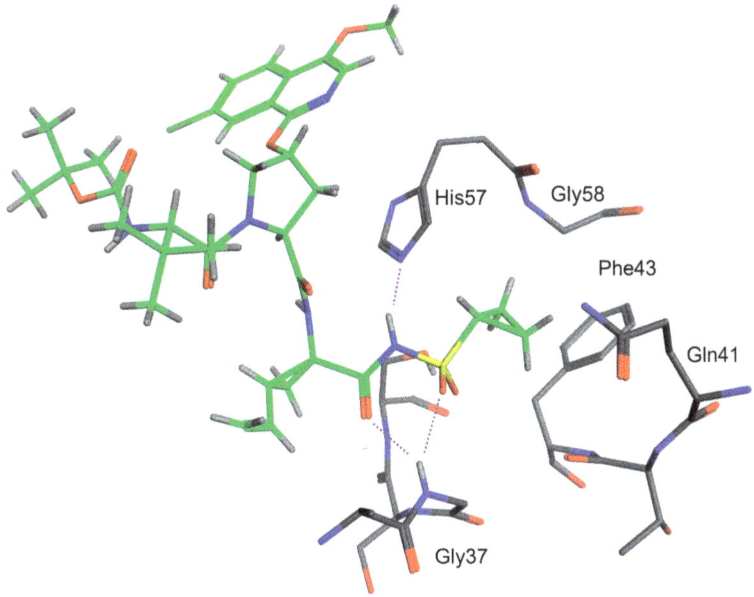


**Figure 3.23** The discovery of asunaprevir involved the replacement of a carboxylic acid group with an acylsulfonamide, which enabled placement of a cyclopropyl group in the S1′ pocket of the hepatitis C protease. Molecular modelling predicted the perfect fit and binding mode of the new functionality.

sought to impart is that computational chemistry involves approximations, and it is vitally important to have an appreciation of how those approximations impact the ability of a calculation to answer the question to hand. This advice extends to the consideration of when 3D methods should be employed, given the speed, accessibility and performance of modern cheminformatics methods. Nowhere is this more important than in the growing trend for virtual screening for hit discovery. It has long been known that 3D methods are not automatically superior to their 2D counterparts,[160] and ligand-based 3D methods are often employed in preference to docking models. With this in mind, one must always ask what the experiment must achieve, for example if you are happy to find molecules with the same overall topology but different scaffold, then a 2D "reduced graph" similarity[161] may provide a simple solution. If a dramatically new scaffolding is required then a 3D pharmacophore may be the method of choice, and if the search is for a new binding mode then a docking experiment is needed. If starting from public databases, use SMARTS queries to remove reactive and undesirable compounds and physicochemical properties to filter molecules before you start the calculations, otherwise you will spend a lot of CPU time (and money, if using cloud computing) finding things that you did not wish to find.

If a molecule has the potential to form an intramolecular hydrogen bond, then it is more useful to include solvation effects in the calculation than to use expensive electron correlation methods. On the other hand, if there is a potential for a ligand to be polarised by adjacent residues in an active site, it may be more useful to run quantum mechanics calculations than to use molecular dynamics simulations of the entire complex.

In particular with modern molecular graphics packages, it is important to remember that what you see on the screen is not real, it is a model. Proteins move, often in surprising ways. Hydrogens are only observed in very high-resolution crystal structures, most of the time they are assigned to a position by the crystallographer, as are many water molecules. Indeed, the use of crystallography data is not always as straightforward as it might seem.[162]

Always consider how solvation is treated in your system, especially when thinking of hydrogen bonding. Are you taking entropy into account, particularly if using flexible chains to bridge two apparently important binding motifs?

Hydrophobicity, being entropic in nature, is very hard to model with the physics-based methods, the most successful methods being those based on measurements and QSAR techniques, for example the clog*P* and alog*P* algorithms. However, molecular simulations are beginning to show value in understanding of the role of water in structure-based design and this is an area full of promise for the future. The physics-based methods and empirical-based methods therefore both have a complementary role in trying to understand drug–receptor interactions.

Finally, remember that internal ligand energies have the same contribution to the free energy of binding as do protein–ligand interaction energies. Always model the ligand in solution as well as in the protein.

## References


1. P. A. M. Dirac, *Proc. R. Soc. London*, 1929, **123**, 714.
2. J. E. Lennard-Jones, *Proc. R. Soc. London*, 1924, **106**, 463.
3. E. Schrödinger, *Ann. Phys.*, 1926, **79**, 361.
4. R. S. Mulliken, *Phys. Rev.*, 1928, **32**, 186.
5. J. E. Lennard-Jones, *Trans. Faraday Soc.*, 1929, **25**, 668.
6. R. Eisenschitz and F. London, *Z. Phys.*, 1930, **60**, 491.
7. C. Coulson, *Trans. Faraday Soc.*, 1938, **33**, 1479.
8. F. H. Westheimer and J. E. Mayer, *J. Chem. Phys.*, 1946, **14**, 733.
9. D. H. R. Barton, *Experimentia*, 1950, **6**, 316.
10. J. B. Henrickson, *J. Am. Chem. Soc.*, 1961, **83**, 4537.
11. J. A. Pople, D. P. Santry and G. A. Segal, *J. Chem. Phys.*, 1965, **43**, S129.
12. K. B. Wiberg, *J. Am. Chem. Soc.*, 1965, **87**, 1070.
13. C. K. Johnson, Oak Ridge National Laboratory Report no. ORNL-3794, 1965. See: http://www.ornl.gov/ortep/ortep.html.
14. W. J. Hehre, W. A. Lathan, R. Ditchfield, M. D. Newton and J. A. Pople, *Gaussian 70, Quantum Chemistry Program Exchange, Program No. 237*, 1970.
15. S. Fernbach and A. H. Taub, in *Computers and Their Role in the Physical Sciences*, ed. S. Fernbach and A. H. Taub, Gordon and Breach, New York, 1970, p. 539.
16. K. A. Wiberg and R. H. Boyd, *J. Am. Chem. Soc.*, 1972, **94**, 8426.
17. F. H. Allen, O. Kannard, W. D. S. Motherwell, W. G. Town and D. G. Watson, *J. Chem. Doc.*, 1973, **13**, 211.
18. N. L. Allinger, *J. Am. Chem. Soc.*, 1973, **95**, 3893.
19. M. Levitt and A. Warshel, *Nature*, 1975, **94**, 253.
20. R. Carbó, L. Leyda and M. Arnau, *Int. J. Quantum Chem.*, 1980, **17**, 1185.
21. T. D. Kuntz, J. M. Blaney, S. J. Oatley, R. Langridge and T. E. Ferrin, *J. Mol. Biol.*, 1982, **161**, 269.
22. M. L. Connolly, *J. Appl. Crystallogr.*, 1983, **16**, 548.
23. P. J. Goodford, *J. Med. Chem.*, 1985, **28**, 849.
24. P. A. Bash, U. C. Singh, F. K. Brown, R. Langridge and P. A. Kollman, *Science*, 1987, **235**, 574.
25. R. S. Pearlman, *Chem. Des. Auto. News*, 1987, **2**, 1.

26. M. von Itzstein, W.-Y. Wu, G. B. Kok, M. S. Pegg, J. C. Dyason, B. Jin, T. Van Phan, M. L. Smythe, H. F. White, S. W. Oliver, P. M. Colman, J. N. Varghese, D. M. Ryan, J. M. Woods, R. C. Bethell, V. J. Hotham, J. M. Cameron and C. R. Penn, *Nature*, 1993, **363**, 418.
27. J. J. P. Stewart, *J. Mol. Struct.: THEOCHEM*, 1997, **401**, 195.
28. D. E. Shaw, P. Maragakis, K. Lindorff-Larsen, S. Piana, R. O. Dror, M. P. Eastwood, J. A. Bank, J. M. Jumper, J. K. Salmon, Y. Shan and W. Wriggers, *Science*, 2010, **330**, 341. The author recommends two text books for students who wish to further understand the theoretical background to computational chemistry applications. The best general text is:
29. *Molecular Modelling: Principles and Applications*, ed. A. R. Leach, Pearson Education Ltd, Harlow, UK, 2nd edn, 2001.Quantum Mechanics demands its own text:
30. *Modern Quantum Chemistry: Introduction to Advanced Electronic Structure Theory*, ed. A. Szabo and N. S. Ostlund, McGraw-Hill, New York, 1st (Revised) Edition, 1989.
31. See "Gaussian Approximations to 1s SlaterType Orbitals" from the Wolfram Demonstrations Project: http://demonstrations.wolfram.com/GaussianApproximationsTo1sSlaterTypeOrbitals.
32. J. S. Binkley, J. A. Pople and W. J. Hehre, *J. Am. Chem. Soc.*, 1980, **102**, 939.
33. M. J. S. Dewar, E. G. Zoebisch, E. F. Healy and J. J. P. Stewart, *J. Am. Chem. Soc.*, 1985, **107**, 3902.
34. J. J. P. Stewart, *J. Comput. Chem.*, 1989, **10**, 221.
35. P. Hohenberg and W. Kohn, *Phys. Rev.*, 1964, **136**, B864.
36. A. D. Becke, *Phys. Rev. A*, 1988, **38**, 3098.
37. C. Lee, W. Yang and R. G. Parr, *Phys. Rev. B*, 1988, **37**, 785.
38. C. J. Cramer, in *Essentials of Computational Chemistry: Theories and Models*, John Wiley & Sons, 2013, ch. 8.
39. Y. Zhao and D. G. Truhlar, *Theor. Chem. Acc.*, 2008, **120**, 215.
40. T. Liljefors, K. Gundertofte, P. Norrby and I. Petterson, Molecular Mechanics and Comparison of Forcefields, in *Computational Medicinal Chemistry for Drug Discovery*, ed. P. Bultinck, H. De Winter, W. Langenaeker and J. P. Tollenare, CRC Press, 2003.
41. H. Sun, *J. Phys. Chem. B*, 1998, **102**, 7338.
42. R. S. Mulliken, *J. Chem. Phys.*, 1955, **23**, 1833.
43. J. Gasteiger and M. Marsili, *Tetrahedron*, 1980, **22**, 3219.
44. R. Bonaccorsi, A. Pullman, E. Scrocco and J. Tomasi, *Theor. Chim. Acta*, 1972, **24**, 51.
45. C. M. Brenerman and K. B. Wiberg, *J. Comput. Chem.*, 1990, **11**, 361.
46. P. Gaillard, P.-A. Carrupt, B. Testa and A. Boudon, *J. Comput.-Aided Mol. Des.*, 1994, **8**, 83.
47. A. C. Good and W. G. Richards, *J. Chem. Inf. Comput. Sci.*, 1993, **33**, 112.
48. A. Nicholls, G. B. McGaughey, R. P. Sheridan, A. C. Good, G. Warren, M. Mathieu, S. W. Muchmore, S. P. Brown, J. A. Grant, J. A. Haigh, N. Nevins, A. N. Jain and B. Kelley, *J. Med. Chem.*, 2010, **53**, 3862.
49. N. L. Allinger, *J. Am. Chem. Soc.*, 1959, **81**, 5727.
50. E. W. Weisstein, Method of Steepest Descent, From MathWorld--A Wolfram Web Resource. http://mathworld.wolfram.com/MethodofSteepestDescent.html.
51. R. Fletcher and C. M. Reeves, *Comput. J.*, 1964, **7**, 149.
52. E. W. Weisstein, Newton's Method, From MathWorld—A Wolfram Web Resource. http://mathworld.wolfram.com/NewtonsMethod.html.
53. N. Metropolis and S. Ulam, *J. Am. Stat. Assoc.*, 1949, **44**, 335.
54. B. J. Alder and T. E. Wainwright, *J. Chem. Phys.*, 1959, **31**, 459.
55. J. A. McCammon, B. R. Gelin and M. Karplus, *Nature*, 1977, **267**, 585.
56. P. Kollman, *Chem. Rev.*, 1993, **93**, 2395.
57. J. Åqvist, C. Medina and J. E. Samuelsson, *Protein Eng.*, 1994, **7**, 385.
58. J. Tirado-Rives and W. Jorgensen, *J. Med. Chem.*, 2006, **49**, 5880.
59. L. Wang, Y. Wu, Y. Deng, B. Kim, L. Pierce, G. Krilov, D. Lupyan, S. Robinson, M. K. Dahlgren, J. Greenwood, D. L. Romero, C. Masse, J. L. Knight, T. Steinbrecher, T. Beuming, W. Damm, E. Harder, W. Sherman, M. Brewer, R. Wester, M. Murcko, L. Frye, R. Farid, T. Lin, D. L. Mobley, W. L. Jorgensen, B. J. Berne, R. A. Friesner and R. Abel, *J. Am. Chem. Soc.*, 2015, **137**, 2695.
60. S. Wan, A. P. Bhati, S. J. Zasada, I. Wall, D. Green, P. Bamborough and P. V. Coveney, *J. Chem. Theory Comput.*, 2017, **13**, 784.
61. A. R. Katritzky, *Handbook of Heterocyclic Chemistry*, Pergamon, New York, 1985, pp. 47–50.
62. W. L. Jorgensen, J. Chandrasekhar, J. D. Madura, R. W. Impey and M. L. Klein, *J. Chem. Phys.*, 1983, **79**, 926.
63. F. H. Stillinger and A. Rahman, *J. Chem. Phys.*, 1974, **60**, 1545.
64. S. W. Rick, S. J. Stuart and B. J. Berne, *J. Chem. Phys.*, 1994, **101**, 6141.
65. L. Onsager, *J. Am. Chem. Soc.*, 1936, **58**, 1486.

66. S. Miertus, E. Scrocco and J. Tomasi, *Chem. Phys.*, 1981, **55**, 117.
67. M. Cossi, V. Barone, R. Cammi and J. Tomasi, *Chem. Phys. Lett.*, 1996, **255**, 327.
68. M. K. Gilson and B. Honig, *Proteins: Struct., Funct., Genet.*, 1988, **4**, 7.
69. W. C. Still, A. Tempczyk, R. C. Hawley and T. Hendrickson, *J. Am. Chem. Soc.*, 1990, **112**, 6127.
70. G. Nemethy and H. A. Scheraga, *J. Chem. Phys.*, 1962, **36**, 3382.
71. M. Waring, *Expert Opin. Drug Discovery*, 2010, **5**, 235.
72. A. Biela, F. Sielaff, F. Terwesten, A. Heine, T. Steinmetzer and G. Klebe, *J. Med. Chem.*, 2012, **55**, 6094.
73. A. Schön, N. Madani, A. B. Smith, J. M. Lalonde and E. Freire, *Chem. Biol. Drug Des.*, 2011, **77**, 161.
74. R. Mannhold, G. I. Poda, C. Ostermann and I. V. Tetko, *J. Pharm. Sci.*, 2009, **98**, 861.
75. G. N. Ramachandran, C. Ramakrishnan and V. Sasisekharan, *J. Mol. Biol.*, 1963, **7**, 95.
76. A. R. Leach, K. Prout and D. P. Dolata, *J. Chem. Inf. Comp. Sci.*, 1990, **30**, 316.
77. K. D. Gibson and H. A. Scheraga, *J. Comput. Chem.*, 1987, **8**, 826.
78. Z. Q. Li and H. A. Scheraga, *Proc. Natl. Acad. Sci. U. S. A.*, 1987, **84**, 6611.
79. R. S. Judson, W. P. Jaeger, A. M. Treasurywala and M. L. Peterson, *J. Comput. Chem.*, 1993, **14**, 1407.
80. G. M. Crippen and T. F. Havel, *Distance Geometry and Molecular Conformation*, Chemometrics Research Studies Series 15, John Wiley & Sons, New York, 1988.
81. C. R. Groom and F. H. Allen, *WIREs Comp. Mol. Sci.*, 2011, **1**, 368.
82. P. R. Andrews, D. J. Craik and J. L. Martin, *J. Med. Chem.*, 1984, **27**, 1648.
83. J. J. Kaminski, B. Wallmark, C. Briving and B. M. Andersson, *J. Med. Chem.*, 1991, **34**, 533.
84. C. G. Wermuth, in *The Practice of Medicinal Chemistry*, ed. C. G. Wermuth, Academic Press, London, 2nd edn, 2003, p. 219.
85. A. Mann, T. Boulanger, B. Brandau, F. Durant, G. Evrard, M. Heaulme, E. Desaulles and C. G. Wermuth, *J. Med. Chem.*, 1991, **34**, 1307.
86. F. H. Allen, *Acta Crystallogr.*, 2002, **B58**, 380.
87. I. J. Bruno, J. C. Cole, J. P. M. Lommerse, R. S. Rowland, R. Taylor and M. L. Verdonk, *J. Comput.-Aided Mol. Des.*, 1997, **11**, 525.
88. M. H. Abraham, P. P. Duce, D. V. Prior, D. G. Barratt, J. J. Morris and P. J. Taylor, *J. Chem. Soc., Perkin Trans. 2*, 1989, 1355.
89. J. A. Platts, *Phys. Chem. Chem. Phys.*, 2000, **2**, 973.
90. B. Kramer, M. Rarey and T. Lengauer, *Proteins: Struct., Funct., Bioinf.*, 1999, **37**, 228.
91. G. Jones, P. Willett, R. C. Glen, A. R. Leach and R. Taylor, *J. Mol. Biol.*, 1997, **267**, 727.
92. D. B. Kitchen, H. Decornez, J. R. Furr and J. Bajorath, *Nat. Rev. Drug Discovery*, 2004, **3**, 935.
93. D. S. Goodsell, G. M. Morris and A. J. Olson, *J. Mol. Recognit.*, 1996, **9**, 1.
94. P. A. Kollman, *J. Am. Chem. Soc.*, 1984, **106**, 795.
95. R. D. Clark, A. Strizhev, J. M. Leonard, J. F. Blake and J. B. Matthew, *J. Mol. Graphics Modell.*, 2002, **20**, 281.
96. H.-J. Böhm, *J. Comput.-Aided Mol. Des.*, 1994, **8**, 243.
97. M. D. Eldridge, C. W. Murray, T. R. Auton, G. V. Paolini and R. P. Mee, *J. Comput.-Aided Mol. Des.*, 1997, **11**, 425.
98. I. Muegge and Y. C. Martin, *J. Med. Chem.*, 1999, **42**, 791.
99. H. Gohlke, M. Hendlich and G. Klebe, *J. Mol. Biol.*, 2000, **295**, 337.
100. R. S. DeWitte and E. I. Shakhnovich, *J. Am. Chem. Soc.*, 1996, **118**, 11733.
101. G. L. Warren, C. W. Andrews, A.-M. Capelli, B. Clarke, J. LaLonde, M. H. Lambert, M. Lindvall, N. Nevins, S. F. Semus, S. Senger, G. Tedesco, I. D. Wall, J. M. Woolven, C. E. Peishoff and M. S. Head, *J. Med. Chem.*, 2006, **49**, 5912.
102. R. Wang, L. Lai and S. Wang, *J. Comput.-Aided Mol. Des.*, 2002, **16**, 11.
103. J. Lyu, S. Wang, T. E. Balius, I. Singh, A. Levit, Y. S. Moroz, M. J. O'Meara, T. Che, E. Algaa, K. Tolmachova, A. A. Tolmachev, B. K. Shoichet, B. L. Roth and J. J. Irwin, *Nature*, 2019, **566**, 224.
104. W. J. Wiswesser, *Chem. Eng. News*, 1952, **30**, 3523.
105. L. C. Ray and R. A. Kirsch, *Science*, 1957, **126**, 814.
106. D. Weininger, *J. Chem. Inf. Comput. Sci.*, 1988, **28**, 31.
107. S. R. Heller, A. McNaught, I. Pletnev, S. Stein and D. Tchekhovskoi, *J. Cheminf.*, 2015, **7**, 1.
108. Daylight Theory Manual, Daylight Chemical Information Systems Inc., Laguna Niguel, CA, https://www.daylight.com/dayhtml/doc/theory/theory.smarts.html.
109. N. Nikolova and J. Jaworska, *QSAR Comb. Sci.*, 2003, **22**, 1006.
110. P. Willett, *Similarity and Clustering in Chemical Information Systems*, Chemometrics Research Studies Press, Letchworth, UK, 1987.
111. R. E. Carhart, D. H. Smith and R. Venkataraghavan, *J. Chem. Inf. Comput. Sci.*, 1985, **25**, 64.
112. D. Rogers and M. Hahn, *J. Chem. Inf. Model.*, 2010, **50**, 742.

113. R. D. Brown and Y. C. Martin, *SAR QSAR Environ. Res.*, 1998, **8**, 23.
114. Y. C. Martin, J. L. Kofron and L. M. Traphagen, *J. Med. Chem.*, 2002, **45**, 4350.
115. S. Jasial, Y. Hu, M. Vogt and J. Bajorath, *F1000Research*, 2016, **5**, 591.
116. M. J. Lajiness, G. M. Maggiora and V. Shanmugasundaram, *J. Med. Chem.*, 2004, **47**, 4891.
117. X. Hu, Y. Hu, M. Vogt, D. Stumpfe and J. Bajorath, *J. Chem. Inf. Model.*, 2012, **52**, 1138.
118. D. R. Flower, *J. Chem. Inf. Comput. Sci.*, 1998, **38**, 379.
119. A. Gaulton, L. J. Bellis, A. P. Bento, J. Chambers, M. Davies, A. Hersey, Y. Light, S. McGlinchey, D. Michalovich, B. Al-Lazikani and J. P. Overington, *Nucleic Acids Res.*, 2012, **40**, 1100.
120. S. Kim, P. A. Thiessen, E. E. Bolton, J. Chen, G. Fu, A. Gindulyte, L. Han, J. He, S. He, B. A. Shoemaker, J. Wang, B. Yu, J. Zhang and S. H. Bryant, *Nucleic Acids Res.*, 2016, **44**, 1202.
121. H. E. Pence and A. Williams, *J. Chem. Educ.*, 2010, **87**, 1123.
122. L. Ruddigkeit, R. van Deursen, L. C. Blum and J.-L. Reymond, *J. Chem. Inf. Model.*, 2012, **52**, 2864.
123. Emolecules, San Diego CA, USA, https://www.emolecules.com/.
124. T. Sterling and J. J. Irwin, *J. Chem. Inf. Model.*, 2015, **55**, 2324.
125. Mcule Inc, Palo Alto CA, USA, https://mcule.com/database/.
126. Molport, SIA, Riga, Latvia, https://www.molport.com/.
127. A. N. Shivanyuk, S. V. Ryabukhin, A. V. Bogolyubsky, D. M. Mykytenko, A. A. Chupryna, W. Heilman, A. N. Kostyuk and A. A. Tolmachev, *Chim. Oggi*, 2007, **25**, 58.
128. RDKit, https://www.rdkit.org/.
129. Python, https://www.python.org/.
130. C. A. Lipinski, F. Lombardo, B. W. Dominy and P. J. Feeney, *Adv. Drug Delivery Rev.*, 1997, **23**, 3.
131. R. F. Bruns and I. A. Watson, *J. Med. Chem.*, 2012, **55**, 9763.
132. G. R. Bickerton, G. V. Paolini, J. Besnard, S. Muresan and A. L. Hopkins, *Nat. Chem.*, 2012, **4**, 90.
133. M. Ashton, J. Barnard, F. Casset, M. Charlton, G. Downs, D. Gorse, J. Holliday, R. Lahana and P. Willett, *Quant. Struct.-Act. Relat.*, 2002, **21**, 598.
134. G. M. Downs and J. M. Barnard, *Reviews in Computational Chemistry Volume 18*, John Wiley & Sons, Hoboken, New Jersey, 2002, p. 1.
135. R. Taylor, *J. Chem. Inf. Comput. Sci.*, 1995, **35**, 59.
136. D. V. S. Green and S. D. Pickett, *Mini-Rev. Med. Chem.*, 2004, **4**, 1067.
137. A. G. Leach, H. D. Jones, D. A. Cosgrove, P. W. Kenny, L. Ruston, P. MacFaul, J. M. Wood, N. Colclough and B. Law, *J. Med. Chem.*, 2006, **49**, 6672.
138. J. Hussain and C. Rea, *J. Chem. Inf. Model.*, 2010, **50**, 339.
139. N. M. O'Boyle, J. Boström, R. A. Sayle and A. Gill, *J. Med. Chem.*, 2014, **57**, 2704.
140. J. Arrowsmith, *Nat. Rev. Drug Discovery*, 2011, **10**, 328–329.
141. K. M. Giacomini, R. M. Krauss, D. M. Roden, M. Eichelbaum, M. R. Hayden and Y. Nakamura, *Nature*, 2007, **446**, 975.
142. G. T. Ankley, R. S. Bennett, R. J. Erickson, D. J. Hoff, M. W. Hornung, R. D. Johnson, D. R. Mount, J. W. Nichols, C. L. Russom, P. K. Schmieder, J. A. Serrrano, J. E. Tietge and D. L. Villeneuve, *Environ. Toxicol. Chem.*, 2010, **29**, 730.
143. M. E. Curran, I. Splawski, K. W. Timothy, G. M. Vincen, E. D. Green and M. T. Keating, *Cell*, 1995, **80**, 795.
144. E. Lounkine, M. J. Keiser, S. Whitebread, D. Mikhailov, J. Hamon, J. L. Jenkins, P. Lavan, E. Weber, A. K. Doak, S. Cote, B. K. Shoichet and L. Urban, *Nature*, 2012, **486**, 361.
145. G. Harper, S. D. Pickett and D. V. S. Green, *Comb. Chem. High Throughput Screening*, 2004, **7**, 63.
146. A. Alanine, M. Nettekoven, E. Roberts and A. W. Thomas, *Comb. Chem. High Throughput Screening*, 2003, **6**, 51.
147. D. K. Jones-Hertzog, P. Mukhopadhyay, C. E. Keefer and S. S. Young, *J. Pharmacol. Toxicol. Methods*, 1999, **42**, 207.
148. D. A. Pertusi, G. O'Donnell, M. F. Homsher, K. Solly, A. Patel, S. L. Stahler, D. Riley, M. F. Finley, E. N. Finger, G. C. Adam, J. Meng, D. J. Bell, P. D. Zuck, E. M. Hudak, M. J. Weber, J. E. Nothstein, L. Locco, C. Quinn, A. Amoss, B. Squadroni, M. Hartnett, M. Ra Heo, T. White, S. A. May, E. Boots, K. Roberts, P. Cocchiarella, A. Wolicki, A. Kreamer, P. S. Kutchukian, A. M. Wassermann, V. N. Uebele, M. Glick, A. Rusinko III and J. C. Culberson, *SLAS Discovery*, 2017, **22**, 995.
149. J. Besnard, G. F. Ruda, V. Setola, K. Abecassis, R. M. Rodriguiz, X. P. Huang, S. Norval, M. F. Sassano, A. I. Shin, L. A. Webster, F. R. Simeons, L. Stojanovski, A. Prat, N. G. Seidah, D. B. Constam, G. R. Bickerton, K. D. Read, W. C. Wetsel, I. H. Gilbert, B. L. Roth and A. L. Hopkins, *Nature*, 2012, **492**, 215.
150. D. V. S. Green, S. Pickett, C. Luscombe, S. Senger, D. Marcus, J. Meslamani, D. Brett, A. Powell and J. Masson, *J. Comput.-Aided Mol. Des.*, 2020, **34**, 747.

151. J. T. Bush, P. Pogany, S. D. Pickett, M. Barker, A. Baxter, S. Campos, A. W. J. Cooper, D. Hirst, G. Inglis, A. Nadin, V. K. Patel, D. Poole, J. Pritchard, Y. Washio, G. White and D. V. S. Green, *J. Med. Chem.*, 2020, **63**, 11964.
152. A. M. Turing, *Mind*, 1950, **49**, 433.
153. C. Merlot, *Drug Discovery Today*, 2010, **15**, 16.
154. P. Y. Lam, P. K. Jahdav, C. J. Eyermann, C. N. Hodge, Y. Ru, L. T. Bacheler, J. L. Meek, M. J. Otto, M. M. Rayner, Y. N. Wong, C.-H. Chang, P. C. Weber, D. A. Jackson, T. R. Sharpe and S. Erickson-Viitanen, *Science*, 1994, **263**, 380.
155. M. J. Bamford, C. Chan, A. P. Craven, B. W. Dymock, D. Green, R. A. Henson, B. E. Kirk, M. G. Lester, P. A. Procopiou, M. A. Snowden, S. J. Spooner, A. R. P. Srikantha, N. S. Watson and J. A. Widdowson, *J. Med. Chem.*, 1995, **38**, 3502.
156. R. C. Glen, G. R. Martin, A. P. Hill, R. M. Hyde, P. M. Woollard, J. A. Salmon, J. Buckingham and A. D. Robertson, *J. Med. Chem.*, 1995, **38**, 3566.
157. G. R. Marshall, C. D. Barry, H. E. Bosshard, R. A. Dammkoehler and D. A. Dunn, *The Conformational Parameter in Drug-Design: The Active Analogue Approach, Computer Assisted Drug Design: ACS Symposium Series 112*: American Chemical Society: Washington DC, 1979.
158. P. M. Scola, L.-Q. Sun, A. X. Wang, J. Chen, N. Sin, B. L. Venables, S.-Y. Sit, Y. Chen, A. Cocuzza, D. M. Bilder, S. V. D'Andrea, B. Zheng, P. Hewawasam, Y. Tu, J. Friborg, P. Falk, D. Hernandez, S. Levine, C. Chen, F. Yu, A. K. Sheaffer, G. Zhai, D. Barry, J. O. Knipe, Y.-H. Han, R. Schartman, M. Donoso, K. Mosure, M. W. Sinz, T. Zvyaga, A. C. Good, R. Rajamani, K. Kish, J. Tredup, H. E. Klei, Q. Gao, L. Mueller, R. J. Colonno, D. M. Grasela, S. P. Adams, J. Loy, P. C. Levesque, H. Sun, H. Shi, L. Sun, W. Warner, D. Li, J. Zhu, N. A. Meanwell and F. McPhee, *J. Med. Chem.*, 2014, **57**, 1730.
159. P. M. Scola, A. X. Wang, A. C. Good, L.-Q. Sun, K. D. Combrink, J. A. Campbell, J. Chen, Y. Tu, N. Sin, B. L. Venables, S.-Y. Sit, Y. Chen, A. Cocuzza, D. M. Bilder, S. D'Andrea, B. Zheng, P. Hewawasam, M. Ding, J. Thuring, J. Li, D. Hernandez, F. Yu, P. Falk, G. Zhai, A. K. Sheaffer, C. Chen, M. S. Lee, D. Barry, J. O. Knipe, W. Li, Y.-H. Han, S. Jenkins, C. Gesenberg, Q. Gao, M. W. Sinz, Ke. S. Santone, T. Zvyaga, R. Rajamani, H. E. Klei, R. J. Colonno, De. M. Grasela, E. Hughes, Ca. Chien, S. Adams, P. C. Levesque, D. Li, J. Zhu, N. A. Meanwell and F. McPhee, *J. Med. Chem.*, 2014, **57**, 1708.
160. V. Venkatraman, V. I. Perez-Nueno, L. Mavridis and D. W. Ritchie, *J. Chem. Inf. Model.*, 2010, **50**, 12.
161. G. Harper, G. S. Bravi, S. D. Pickett, J. Hussain and D. V. S. Green, *J. Chem. Inf. Comput. Sci.*, 2004, **44**, 2145.
162. A. M. Davis, S. J. Teague and G. J. Kleywegt, *Angew. Chem., Int. Ed.*, 2003, **42**, 2718.
163. 14th Community Wide Experiment on the Critical Assessment of Techniques for Protein Structure Prediction, https://www.predictioncenter.org/cadsp14/index.cgi.

# 4 Structure-based Design for Medicinal Chemists

Jeff Blaney*[a] and Andrew M. Davis[b]

[a]Small Molecule Drug Discovery, Genentech, 1 DNA Way, South San Francisco, CA 94080, USA; [b]Hit Discovery, Discovery Sciences, R&D, AstraZeneca, Cambridge, UK
*E-mail: blaney.jeff@gene.com, andy.davis@astrazeneca.com

## 4.1 Introduction

Medicinal chemistry is the most expensive part of pre-clinical research.[1] Hit-to-lead optimization to a clinical development candidate is an iterative, empirical process that frequently requires the design, synthesis, and testing of several thousand compounds by large research teams during several years. Identifying the best compounds as early as possible through efficient selection and optimization is critical. Understanding structure–activity relationships (SAR) and multi-parameter optimization is the key to designing new analogs with better properties. Structure-based design uses high-resolution X-ray crystallographic or cryo-electron microscopy (cryo-EM) structures and models of analog series members bound to the target protein to interpret SAR and help create new, testable design hypotheses.

Structure-based design is an essential part of medicinal chemistry. The availability of experimental structures for many drug discovery targets and improvements in molecular modeling software makes it practical for medicinal chemists to do their own modeling and design. The amazing rapid advances in cryo-EM over the last several years are the most exciting and dramatic advance for structure-based design since the previous edition of this book. Those advances have enabled structure determination of membrane proteins and large protein complexes. Structure-based design is used during hit identification, hit-to-lead optimization, and late-stage optimization. Its most obvious applications are for improving potency and selectivity, but it can also help guide

The Handbook of Medicinal Chemistry: Principles and Practice, 2nd Edition
Edited by Simon E. Ward and Andrew M. Davis

Published by the Royal Society of Chemistry, www.rsc.org

later-stage optimization of pharmacokinetic, toxicity, solubility, or other challenges by modeling small molecule scaffold or substituent changes which are likely to retain activity.

We will focus on how we've seen structure-based design performed during many medicinal chemistry projects in industry. Structure-based design relies most critically on a solid understanding of physical organic chemistry, especially conformational analysis and intra- and intermolecular interactions. Iterative determination of X-ray co-crystal or cryo-EM structures, accurate biophysical, biochemical, and cell-based assays to measure binding affinity and cellular activity, expert use of molecular modeling software, structure and physical property databases, plus associated data-mining and analysis software are all critical parts of structure-based design. The most successful approaches focus on iterative, hypothesis-based designs by expert scientists driven by computer modeling.[2] The review by Bissantz, Kuhn, and Stahl[3] and the book chapters by Klebe[4,5] are excellent additional sources to learn about structure-based design. *De novo* design of new small molecules without a previously known ligand is still rarely attempted and rarely successful.

## 4.2 History

Beddell *et al.* designed small molecules from scratch (*de novo* design) to bind to an allosteric site on hemoglobin in the first structure-based design publication in 1976.[6,7] They performed this impressive feat of *de novo* design with wire Kendrew models of hemoglobin's crystal structure! This is particularly amazing given how difficult it still is to design today with high-resolution structures, vastly improved modeling tools, and much greater knowledge of protein–ligand interactions. Enthusiasm for *de novo* design peaked during the 1980s and early 1990s. However, *de novo* design was not reliable: most designs were inactive. We learned that it is relatively easy to design a molecule that appears to fit into a binding site; the challenge is recognizing which apparently complementary molecules actually bind to their target and to rank-order their affinities: this is the "scoring" problem. Predicting protein–ligand binding affinity has proven to be incredibly difficult. We still cannot routinely predict relative free energies of binding reliably and accurately enough to drive design and synthesis during hit-to-lead optimization. This is the crux problem of structure-based design and remains an area of active research. "Generative design" approaches use machine learning to tackle *de novo* design.[8] They suffer the same "scoring" problem as previous approaches. Their most successful application has been in "fast follower" analog design, where they can take advantage of prior SAR and knowledge of the target.[9]

The first protein–ligand docking paper was published in 1982.[10] Docking predicts the pose (the ligand's orientation in the binding site and its conformation) and relative affinity of compounds selected from a database of available or virtual small molecules. Many docking programs have been developed since then, but they all struggle to predict affinity (scoring).[11–15] Docking has had modest success until recently with virtual screening, providing hits in the low μM ($IC_{50}$, $K_i$, $K_d$, *etc.*) affinity range, especially if guided with prior SAR knowledge of active molecules.[16,17] More recent very large-scale docking has had surprising success in virtual screening and is becoming an established "best practice."[18,19] Docking is more successful at predicting poses than predicting affinity. It is commonly used to qualitatively test whether a proposed molecule binds as designed. Shape- and feature-based methods are often competitive with docking for virtual screening.[20,21] This is surprising since these methods usually ignore the protein and only include the ligand: this suggests there is more *exploitable* knowledge in the bound ligand structure than in the protein site. Swann *et al.* developed a shape/feature protocol focused solely on pose prediction that can provide a more reliable result when co-crystal structures of similar analogs are available during a hit-to-lead optimization project.[22]

## 4.3 Protein Structures for Structure-based Design

### 4.3.1 Experimentally Determined Structures

Structure-based design uses high-resolution X-ray co-crystal or cryo-EM structures, or computationally predicted models of protein–ligand complexes to interpret structure–activity relationships (SAR) and enable scientists to design new molecules. NMR structures are not commonly used; indeed only 360 NMR structures were deposited in the Protein Data Bank in 2021, compared to 9269 from X-ray and 2953 from cryo-EM. X-ray crystal and cryo-EM structures for most non-membrane proteins and many membrane proteins are frequently accessible with sufficiently high resolution (≤2.5 Å) to enable design. G-protein-coupled receptor (GPCR) structure determination accelerated dramatically during the last decade, first due to breakthroughs in protein engineering and crystallization, and then due to cryo-EM.[23–25] More membrane protein structures have been determined by cryo-EM since 2019 than by X-ray. By the end of 2020, 455 GPCR structures from 82 different receptors were available.

A well-supported project can deliver structures in one to three weeks from request in many cases, which is fast enough to drive iterative design.

Structure-based design can begin with publicly available structures of relevant structures with similar ligands in the Protein Data Bank (PDB, www.rcsb.org).[26] Bespoke structures determined on the desired target of interest with robust iterative follow-up for analog structures are preferred and usually essential for success. This requires a robust crystallographic or cryo-EM system. X-ray complexes are usually determined by soaking pre-formed protein crystals in a solution containing the small molecule inhibitor. Co-crystallization is sometimes required and can be practical if the crystals grow quickly enough. Teague and Davis reviewed issues and recommendations in interpreting protein crystal structures for use in structure-based design.[27,28] Virtual screening (VS) can often provide new hits from previously available structures. Hit-to-lead optimization requires consistent, iterative feedback of new experimental structures determined with inhibitors you have designed and synthesized complexed with your protein.

Cryo-EM has been available since the 1980s, but until recently its resolution was far too low to enable structure-based design. Major advances in detectors, automation, and computational methods have brought cryo-EM to the levels of resolution comparable to X-ray crystallography and therefore suitable for structure-based design.[29,30] The 2017 Nobel Prize for Chemistry was awarded to Jacques Dubochet, Joachim Frank, and Richard Henderson for developing cryo-EM for high-resolution structure determination of biomolecules in solution.[31] The technique does not rely on the production of diffracting single crystals, as required by X-ray crystallography, which becomes increasingly difficult for larger proteins, membrane proteins, and large protein complexes. Instead, cryo-EM captures many 2D images of individual protein particles illuminated with an electron beam frozen in a thin ice film in different orientations, and the computational merging of these images to generate a three-dimensional structure.

Cryo-EM can provide atomic resolution structures at high resolution,[32] especially for membrane-bound proteins that had previously been extremely challenging or completely intractable for X-ray crystallography. These structures have enabled many more structure-based projects, but do not significantly change how to interpret the structures for design. Protein crystal structures typically contain about 40–60% solvent by volume, mostly water. Cryo-EM structures are flash-frozen from solution, are more highly solvated, and arguably more representative of solution structures. In the cryo-EM technique, proteins can be seen in multiple conformations, unlike X-ray crystallography in which only a single average structure is determined.

"An X-ray crystal structure is one crystallographer's subjective interpretation of an observed electron-density map expressed in terms of an atomic model."[28] The same is true of cryo-EM structures. Interpretation bias becomes less of a factor at higher resolutions below about 1.5 Å. Below we recommend how to use X-ray crystal structures for design. Cryo-EM structures should be treated similarly, viewing the experimental density maps to understand which parts of the model have the highest confidence. Cryo-EM structure resolution is heterogenous across the image and may have different resolutions across different parts of a protein. Cryo-EM resolutions are not directly comparable to X-ray crystal structure resolutions. The state of the art for estimating confidence across different parts of a cryo-EM structure is still advancing, so it's even more important to collaborate with the structural biologist who determined the structure. Garcia-Nafria and Tate[33] compared GPCR structure determination by X-ray crystallography and cryo-EM in 2021; their conclusions generalize to other classes of proteins.

### 4.3.2 Limitations of the Use of X-ray Crystal and Cryo-EM Structures

Teague, Davis, and co-workers reviewed the use, interpretation, and limitations of X-ray structures.[27,28,34,35] While the structural biologist does their best to fit the atomic structure into the observed electron density map, the atomic model will have regions of more or less confidence, depending upon the quality of the observed density in that region. But a chemist might interpret the atomic coordinates as if they are at perfect resolution, irrespective of the quality of the original density. The ambiguities within the model may be at the level of atoms, residues, or even whole regions of the protein, and without forewarning, these ambiguities can misguide design hypotheses. Examination of the atomic model together with its density minimises the ambiguities, but does not remove them. Common ambiguities include the positions of N and O atoms in the sidechains of glutamine and asparagine, as they are isoelectronic, and even the position of nitrogens and carbons in histidines, imidazoles, and pyridines can be ambiguous. Waters are particularly difficult. Unless at high resolution (typically ≤ 2.5 Å), the presence of a water molecule in a structure cannot be determined with certainty, and it becomes quite a subjective matter whether a feature in the electron density map is a water molecule or noise. Further, as hydrogen atoms cannot normally be seen in X-ray structures, the orientation of water molecules and their hydrogen bonds, or indeed any hydrogen involved in a hydrogen bond, are only inferred from calculations, unless neutron diffraction is used. Very high-resolution cryo-EM can directly observe waters, including their hydrogens.[29,30] Any small molecule also present within the protein structure poses different problems for the structural biologist. The experimental density usually lacks sufficient information to completely determine the atomic positions, so a molecular mechanics force field is used to help refine both protein and small molecule atoms. If appropriate terms are lacking or wrong for the small molecule, the fit of these atoms into observed electron density may be wrong.

A very recent survey of the rotatable bond geometry of drug-like ligands has been reported for high-resolution (<1.1 Å) and medium-resolution (2.4–2.8 Å) crystallographic protein–ligand complexes.[36] About 37% of the high-resolution ligands fit the electron density perfectly with single occupancy, as did 38% of the medium-resolution ligands. Somewhat surprisingly, 35% of the high-resolution set were found not to fit the electron density perfectly, despite these being high-quality structures. A possible explanation for these cases is that the ligand can adopt multiple binding conformations, and the single refined conformation is necessarily a compromise that gives the best refinement statistics for single occupancy. The review concludes that multiple conformer ligand binding is an under-recognized phenomenon in structure-based drug design and that there is a need for more robust crystallographic refinement methods to better handle such cases.

Finally, the degree of flexibility of the protein is often underestimated, and the assumption of a rigid receptor may limit the design space that can be explored. Multiple structures determined with different ligands can often reveal different protein and binding site conformations. A recent examination of the differences between co-crystallisation and soaking to obtain co-crystal structures highlighted that for flexible proteins and larger ligands, co-crystallization captures more reliably the correct binding pose and induced protein adaptations.[37] Collaborate closely with your structural biologist, so the uncertainties in the structure are considered within your design hypotheses.

Garcia-Nafria and Tate provide examples of intermolecular protein contacts in crystals that can affect protein conformation, especially at flexible loops on the surface.[33] Cryo-EM structures are flash-frozen in solution and do not have such crystallographic artifacts. These problems are less common in crystals of soluble proteins, but can impact ligand binding if the binding site is near a protein–protein contact: check that your protein–ligand binding site is not at a protein–protein contact in the crystal.

### 4.3.3 Predicting Protein Structures: AlphaFold and RoseTTAFold

Due to major advances in AI and machine learning, three-dimensional structures of proteins can in many cases now be predicted from their primary sequence, provided they have at least 30 homologous sequences.[38] In 2020, in the 14th Community Wide

Experiment on the Critical Assessment of Techniques for Protein Structure Prediction (CASP), AlphaFold 2 achieved accuracy comparable in many cases to experimental structures.[39] AlphaFold 2 [40,41] is a publicly available database of the whole human proteome predicted directly from sequence. AlphaFold 2 and RoseTTAFold[42,43] made major advances in the state of the art for computational protein structure prediction of individual proteins and protein–protein complexes.[44,45] Both methods predict structures for many proteins with reasonable accuracy, and in some cases, extremely high accuracy. Most structures may not be directly useful for structure-based design since they are apo structures and do not necessarily predict the structure of the binding site for a protein–ligand complex accurately.[46] Molecular dynamics simulations may eventually enable protein–ligand complex prediction and the identification of cryptic or allosteric binding sites, but these simulations require massive compute resource and are still rare.[47,48] Machine learning approaches have recently been developed to predict cryptic sites, with reasonable accuracy.[49] Predicting the structure of a specific target protein from the crystal structure of a highly similar protein (homology modeling), where the sequence identity is ≥30%, can provide structures that are helpful to generate hypotheses. Experimental structures of relevant ligands bound to the target protein are much more valuable.

## 4.4 Theory and Practice of Structure-based Design

### 4.4.1 Visualizing Shape Complementarity

Focus design on shape complementarity between the binding site and ligand first. Molecular graphics programs provide a variety of display options. The clearest way to view and interpret protein–ligand interactions is to display the stick model (bonds) of the ligand and the protein binding site, along with the transparent solvent-accessible surface[50] (also called the "interaction surface") of the binding site, for example by selecting all protein atoms within ≤10 Å of any ligand atom. The solvent-accessible surface is calculated 1.4 Å beyond the van der Waals surface of the protein. (1.4 Å is the radius of a water molecule if it is treated as a sphere, slightly smaller than the radius of carbon, nitrogen, and oxygen.) The resulting smooth surface touches ligand atoms if they are in van der Waals contact. Ligand atoms intersect the surface if they make a hydrogen bond or ionic interaction; otherwise, intersection indicates a steric clash. If you observe this in a X-ray or cryo-EM structure, inspect the experimental density map and consult with your structural biologist to determine whether the structure needs additional refinement. If you observe this in a model, the ligand is unlikely to bind as modeled unless either it or the site change conformation. The shape and size of unfilled pockets and larger regions in the site is much easier to see with this solvent-accessible surface than with the more familiar Connolly molecular surface.[50] Non-planar ligand features provide opportunities to improve solubility[51] and new vectors for design: solvent-accessible surfaces make it easier to spot where non-planar groups can fit. Figures 4.1 and 4.2 compare the solvent-accessible and Connolly surfaces of a chymotrypsin–inhibitor complex. The solvent-accessible surface makes chymotrypsin's specificity for aromatic

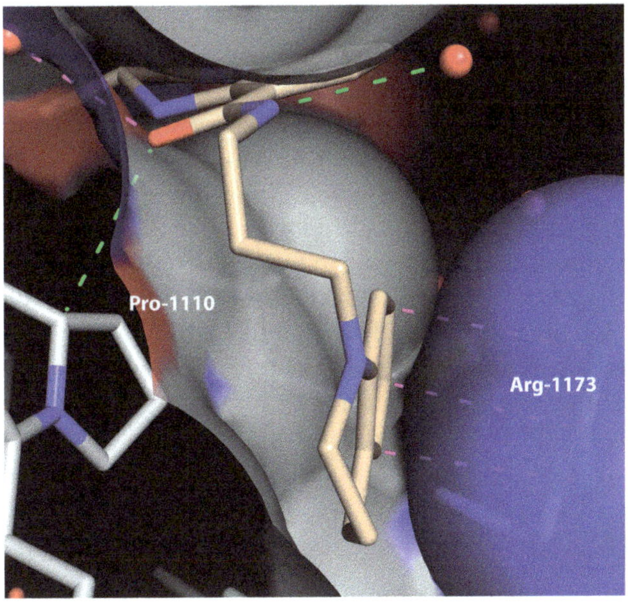


**Figure 4.1** Solvent-accessible or interaction surface of a chymotrypsin-inhibitor complex (PDB 3VGC). The protein solvent-accessible surface is color-coded by simple properties: carbon (hydrophobic) = gray, hydrogen bond acceptor = pink, hydrogen bond donor = cyan, Asp/Glu negatively charged sidechain oxygens = red, Arg/Lys/His positively charged sidechain nitrogens = blue, Cys/Met sulfur = yellow. Divalent sulfur attached to an aromatic ring is "invisible" from a log*P* perspective (log*P* $PhSCH_3$ = 2.74, log*P* $PhCH_3$ = 2.73), but it is hydrophilic in an alkyl chain (log*P* $CH_3CH_2SCH_3$ = 1.54, log*P* $CH_3CH_2CH_3$ = 2.36[52]). All molecular graphics were done with PyMOL.[53]

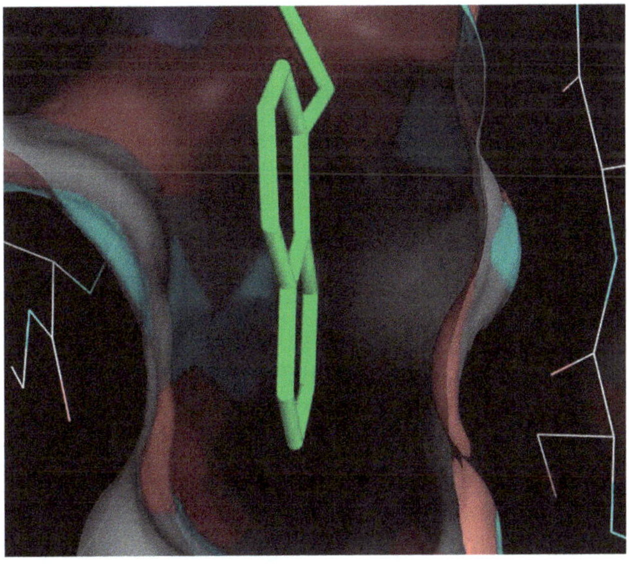

**Figure 4.2** Connolly molecular surface of the same chymotrypsin-inhibitor complex.

rings much more obvious. The Connolly surface is displayed at the actual surface of the protein, so that viewing the complementarity of a ligand in the site also requires displaying the surface of the ligand (or an unusually good three-dimensional imagination). Displaying both surfaces is straightforward in molecular modeling software, but interpreting the fit of the two complicated, three-dimensional surfaces is much more difficult than simply comparing the protein solvent-accessible surface with the stick model of the ligand.

We previously recommended visualization techniques and emphasized the importance of 3D stereoscopic display technology. 3D stereoscopic display was very helpful for many designers, but is no longer commercially available. Virtual reality (VR) hardware and software is beginning to fill this gap through lower cost, head-mounted displays such as Oculus 2, enabled with software such as Nanome.[54,56,57] VR enables collaboration for multiple users in different sites and is already impacting molecular design. Many users find its visualization more intuitive and easier to understand than 3D stereoscopic display.

### 4.4.2 What Drives Binding?

Gas-phase non-covalent association is driven by polar and electrostatic interactions; van der Waals interactions are weak. The situation reverses in water, where hydrophobic interactions drive protein folding and intermolecular interactions. Fersht *et al.*[58] used site-directed mutagenesis to show that, in general, binding is driven by shape complementarity and hydrophobicity, while polar interactions drive specificity. Water is 55.5 M and dominates all aspects of aqueous non-covalent binding. Water is an excellent hydrogen-bond donor and acceptor: a free small molecule and unbound protein site are well solvated prior to binding. Water must be removed from the ligand and protein during binding. The desolvation penalty incurred by a highly polar substituent, such as a hydroxyl group, may cost more than the energy of its interaction in the protein–ligand complex. Polar interactions only improve potency if they improve upon the interactions between the free ligand and water, and the protein binding site and water: it's difficult to form better interactions than water.

Why is predicting protein–ligand affinity so hard? The relationship between the Gibbs free energy and the binding constant shows that each ten-fold change in potency is only a 1.4 kcal $mol^{-1}$ (5.9 kJ $mol^{-1}$) change in binding free energy:

$$\Delta G = \Delta H - T\Delta S$$

$$\Delta G = -2.3RT\log K = -1.4\log K$$

Small changes in binding energy cause exponential changes in binding affinity. A medicinal chemist may be thrilled to improve potency by two-fold (0.4 kcal $mol^{-1}$, 1.7 kJ $mol^{-1}$), but the current practical computational predictive accuracy in the best cases, for closely related analogs, is ~10-fold (1.4 kcal $mol^{-1}$, 5.9 kJ $mol^{-1}$). Affinity does not correlate with the number of hydrogen bonds formed, the buried surface area of hydrophobic interactions, or many other simple first- and second-order terms. X-ray crystallography and cryo-EM structures provide high-resolution models of how molecules interact, but can't label interactions by their relative importance. For example, a shorter protein–ligand hydrogen bond doesn't necessarily provide higher affinity.

### 4.4.3 Favorable and Unfavorable Waters and Water Networks

We present a very brief overview of the very complex and incompletely understood role of water in protein–ligand interactions. Our understanding of water, how to simulate and predict its effects in protein–ligand interactions is still advancing and remains an area of active research. We highly recommend a recent excellent, comprehensive review from a medicinal chemistry/structure-based design perspective by Spyrakis *et al.*,[59] who summarize the state-of-the-art knowledge of water structure, thermodynamics, experimental and computational studies, and computational tools for predicting favorable and unfavorable waters, and case studies.

Some parts of a binding site are not optimal for binding water and waters in these regions will be easy to displace. Some waters are also tightly bound and very difficult to displace. A common problem is to decide whether to design a compound to interact with a bound water molecule or to displace the water. Crystallographic B-factors indicate the relative level of order and disorder for atoms and are sometimes mistakenly interpreted as a surrogate for water affinity, such that waters with low B-factors are deemed to bind more tightly and therefore are harder to displace. Well-ordered waters may be trapped in an energetically suboptimal orientation and displaceable. For example, most kinase inhibitors bind to the kinase "hinge" with one to three hydrogen bonds, and most kinase fragment hits bind to the hinge. Why do small molecules bind so frequently to the hinge? Computational analysis suggests that the waters which hydrogen-bond to the hinge in the apo protein are thermodynamically unstable: they are trapped by the hydrophobic floor and roof of the planar binding site and cannot make their full set of possible hydrogen bonds,[60] so they are easily displaced by a ligand with the appropriate shape and hydrogen-bond donor and acceptor geometry.

Computational methods for predicting whether to interact with, displace, avoid, or bridge bound waters in a binding site are frequently used for design and SAR analysis. This is an incredibly complex problem, with many different computational approaches.[61–65] These include ViewContacts,[66] WaterMap,[60,67,68] 3D-RISM,[69] SZMAP,[70] HINT,[71] and WaterFlap.[72] Each have different methodologies, strengths, and weaknesses; a recent comparative analysis of several of them on two different protein families showed that each method could identify crystallographically observed water molecules, but found little correlation with affinity changes due to displaced waters.[73] Another comparative analysis found that WaterMap was somewhat more accurate at predicting SAR on three different proteins than other methods.[74] Spyrakis *et al.*[59] noted that WaterFlap and HINT showed high accuracy in predicting water locations and displacement propensity. There are few prospective design studies and it is unclear which method is the best. Indeed, it is very difficult to test their relative accuracy beyond predicting experimentally observed water locations. These methods are best used as a qualitative tool to interpret SAR and generate design hypotheses.

SAR combined with very high-resolution crystallography and careful calorimetry is helping to us understand the complexity of enthalpy–entropy compensation in protein–ligand binding.[75–78] These studies highlight the role of ligand–water interactions to either stabilize or de-stabilize water networks in a binding site. Much protein–ligand SAR may actually be due to ligand substituent changes perturbing water networks.

Krimmer *et al.*[76] performed an elegant, tour-de-force SAR study on a congeneric series of thermolysin inhibitors at the hydrophobic S2′ subsite, with substituents ranging from methyl to phenethyl (Figure 4.3). Previous work showed that thermolysin is unusually rigid, with very little conformational variability, and diffracts to very high resolution. Increasing affinity was associated with a better-ordered water network next to the surface of the protein–ligand complex, which suggested an unusual strategy to improve affinity: design different non-polar substituents to impose different shapes on the solvent-exposed surface to attempt to improve the surface water network. They modeled the structure of the water network around each designed analog with MD simulations, ranking their designs by the completeness and quality of the network. They synthesized and characterized five analogs with isothermal microcalorimetry (ITC), surface plasmon resonance (SPR), and determined their high-resolution co-crystal structures (1.16–1.38 Å). The analog predicted by MD to form the most complete water network had the highest affinity by ITC, about a 50-fold enhancement (8.7 kJ $mol^{-1}$, 2.1 kcal $mol^{-1}$) over the parent compound with R = $CH_3$ (Figures 4.4–4.6).

The solvent-accessible protein surface is gray. The substituent R is green. Red spheres show X-ray crystallographic waters in the first hydration shell around the inhibitor. Blue spheres show more distal, less structured waters.

Their interpretation is that the more optimized, tight surface water network binds the inhibitor tighter to the protein. Their MD simulations did not require prior knowledge

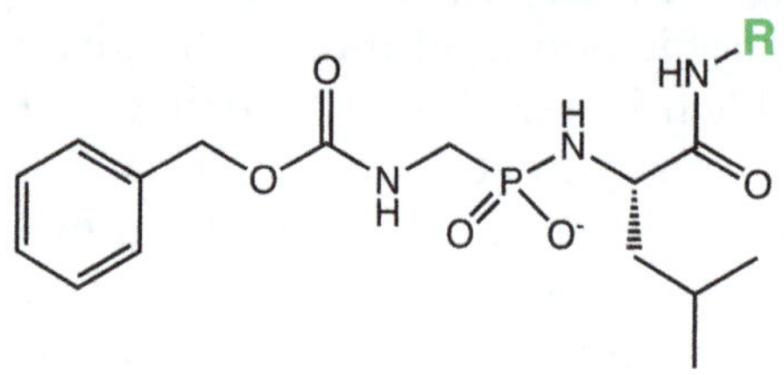

Figure 4.3 Thermolysin inhibitors.[76]

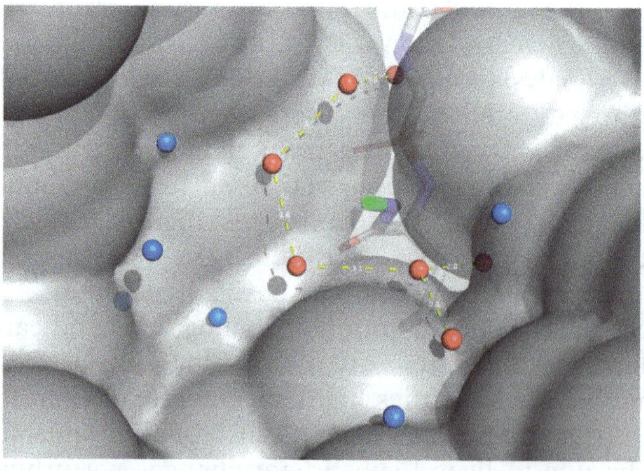

Figure 4.4 Thermolysin complex with parent compound **1** (PDB 3T73), R = $CH_3$.

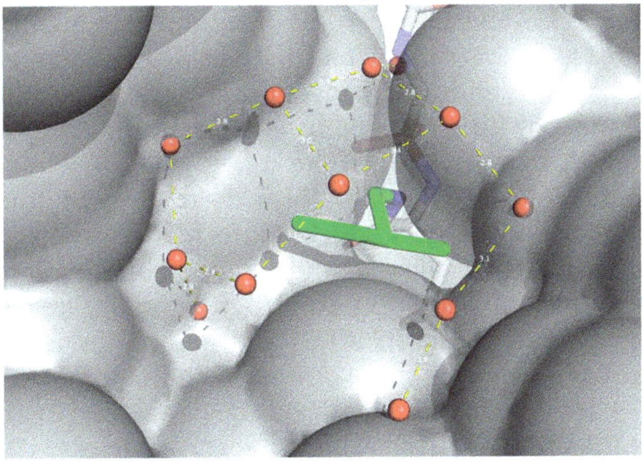

**Figure 4.5** Thermolysin complex (PDB 4MZN) with higher affinity analog **2**, R = 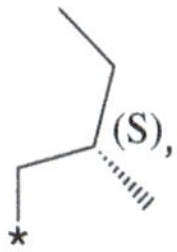, with well-defined water network.ITC $\Delta(\Delta G)$ Analog 1 → 2 = 7 kJ $mol^{-1}$ (1.7 kcal $mol^{-1}$)

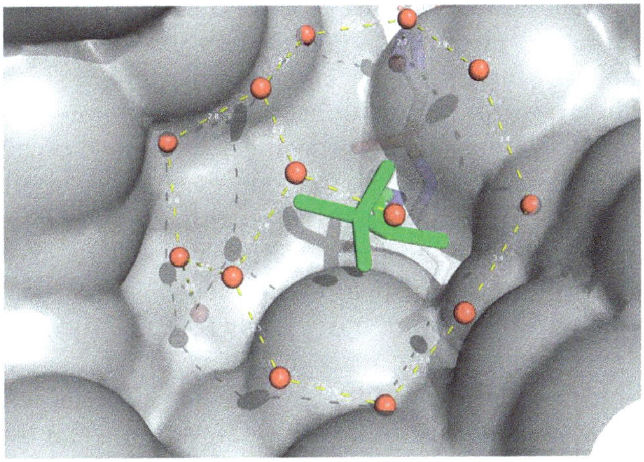

**Figure 4.6** Thermolysin complex (PDB 5JS3) with highest affinity analog **3**, R = 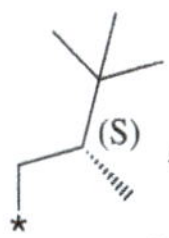, with complete water network.ITC $\Delta(\Delta G)$ Analog 1 → 3 = 8.7 kJ $mol^{-1}$ (2.1 kcal $mol^{-1}$)

about experimental water positions and showed remarkable agreement with the experimental electron density for the waters, suggesting this approach might be possible for lead optimization with more typical resolutions <2.5 Å.

## 4.4.4 Protein Flexibility

Proteins are flexible and their binding sites may change conformation in response to different small molecule ligands, other interacting proteins, temperature, pH, and ionic strength. Ligand binding modes can change dramatically due to changes in crystal conditions. For example, co-crystal structures of trypsin with an inhibitor containing a weakly basic pyridine (p$K_a$ = 7.5) were determined in two different crystal forms, at pH 7 and 8. The inhibitor binds with its pyridyl group in the S1 specificity pocket in one crystal form, but completely flips over end-for-end in the other crystal form and places its neutral chloronaphthyl group in the S1 pocket.[79]

A single X-ray crystal structure of a protein with an empty binding site (apo form) is not necessarily a good model for a bound conformation; the active or binding site may change conformation when a ligand binds. Flipped binding modes can occur with very weakly bound fragments ($K_i$ > 100 μM) or tightly bound larger inhibitors ($K_i$ <10 nM). Rather than interpret such observations as evidence of unstable binding leading to confusing SAR, consider viewing these different binding modes as separate starting points for new series designs. In structure-based design, series membership should be viewed as a combination of the chemical series (scaffold) along with its binding mode. For example, adding a group to a ligand to fill a pocket in the site can lock in a binding mode, prevent subsequent flipping, and differentiate one binding mode from the other.

### 4.4.5 Enthalpy–Entropy Compensation

Biochemical, biophysical, and cell biology assays measure a ligand's $K_i$, $K_d$, or $IC_{50}$ to estimate the Gibbs free energy of binding. Computational chemistry approaches usually estimate enthalpies of binding. X-ray crystal and cryo-EM structures tell us about structure, but provide no information about binding enthalpies or free energies. The observation of an interaction tells us nothing about its impact on affinity.

Biophysical experiments can factor the free energy changes upon binding into their enthalpic and entropic contributions. In principle this provides a greater level of detail for structure-based design, although there are few prospective case studies. Freire *et al.* analyzed a number of well-known structure-based lead-drug optimizations and suggested enthalpy-driven binders are more likely to make drugs.[80–82] This prompted the study of enthalpy–entropy within drug discovery programs and suggested a paradigm of selecting enthalpic-driven binders as far back as the lead selection phase. This has proven to be an overly simplistic view.[83] It is still unclear how to use enthalpy–entropy data to help drive iterative, structure-based drug design due to the complexity of enthalpy–entropy compensation.

The simple concept that hydrophobic binding is driven by entropy, and that polar interactions such as hydrogen bonds are enthalpic contributors to binding, is not supported by an increasing number of studies.[84,85] There are examples of entropically driven hydrogen bonds, and enthalpically driven hydrophobic interactions. The cooperative nature of drug–ligand binding resulting in enthalpy–entropy compensation complicates the original concept.

Klebe used isothermal calorimetry together with X-ray crystallography to analyze the structure–activity relationships of a series of thrombin inhibitors.[86] Confusingly, cyclopropyl and cyclohexyl analogs, while very similar in $\Delta G$, showed completely opposite behavior in $\Delta H$ and $\Delta S$. The cyclopentyl analog's binding was more entropically driven, while the cyclohexyl analog's binding was enthalpically driven. The differences in $\Delta H$

and $\Delta S$ were large, but resulted in nearly identical overall free energy of binding for the two compounds, which only differed by one methylene group. On close examination of the X-ray crystal structures, the cyclohexyl showed well-resolved density and the cyclopentyl was disordered. While a retrospective rationalization can always be made, this level of subtlety is impossible to predict with our current level of understanding of drug–receptor interactions. Klebe also studied the binding of a set of congeneric inhibitors of thermolysin.[84] Through the series, H, methyl, iso-propyl, *n*-propyl, sec-butyl, i-butyl, and benzyl, the binding became increasingly entropic, although with substantial enthalpic compensation, so overall across the series the change in Gibbs free energy was small, compared to substantial changes in entropy or enthalpy. The changes in thermodynamic signatures were rationalized with changes observed in high-resolution X-ray structures. As they highlighted, the analyses worked at the limit of accuracy in current protein crystallography, and required considerations of details not usually considered in computational chemistry, simply because we are not aware of their importance in protein–ligand structure–activity relationships.

### 4.4.6 Electrostatics

Detailed electrostatics inside a binding site are poorly understood. The local dielectric constant inside a protein binding site is believed to vary from 2–4, and must increase to bulk water's dielectric (80) outside of the protein.[87] Mutagenesis experiments by Fersht *et al.* showed that the p$K_a$ of sidechains in binding sites could vary over 1 p$K_a$ unit due to perturbations over 10 Å away,[88] which suggests that charged groups at similar distances from a bound ligand could also influence its binding and selectivity. Long-range electrostatics are clearly significant, but are seldom deliberately exploited in structure-based design, where we typically focus on simpler direct and water-mediated protein–ligand contacts. Electrostatics can dramatically impact affinity and selectivity due to their strength and long-range effects. Some binding sites favor a charged group in a general location, despite having no direct, first-shell interactions: the electrostatic potential due to long-range effects is sufficiently strong to require a charged group. Phosphoglycerate dehydrogenase[89] is an excellent example.

SAR revealing long-range electrostatic effects is usually empirically observed and explained later. Predictive computational approaches have been developed. They are well worth exploring, since these effects are not easily recognized through qualitative modeling relying on visual analysis, even with expert designers. Tidor described an elegant approach to design inhibitors that includes long-range electrostatics.[90–92] Free energy perturbation (FEP) and related methods are newer approaches that also explicitly include long-range electrostatics, rather than implicitly with a continuum solvation model.[93,94] Why does the classic "fluorine walk" work sometimes? Fluorine causes the maximum electronic perturbation with minimal steric change and can empirically probe the local dielectric environment in a binding site. A FEP-based method was developed specifically for the "fluorine walk," with good results in a retrospective analysis.[95]

### 4.4.7 Small Molecules Bind in Their Lowest Energy, Preferred Conformations

Small molecules rarely bind to proteins outside of their preferred minimum energy conformations. Early work argued that a significant number of bound ligand conformations in the PDB were high energy, in some cases, higher than the total free energy of binding. (The total free energy of binding of a protein–ligand complex is 1.4 × p$K_i$, for example, a complex with a $K_i$ = 1 nM has a free energy of binding of 1.4 × 9 = 13.6 kcal $mol^{-1}$ or 56.9 kJ $mol^{-1}$). These studies suffered from ligand refinement errors in PDB X-ray crystal structures,[96] molecular mechanics force field issues, and other problems. More recent work with higher resolution, higher quality co-crystal structures and more careful computational analysis concludes that most ligands bind in one of their preferred, low-energy conformations, if not their minimum energy conformation.[36,97,98] A protein dissipates strain energy through small changes across its many degrees of freedom much more easily than for the ligand to adopt an unfavorable conformation by straining its few rotatable bonds.

Brameld *et al.* provide an excellent survey of preferred conformational preferences for small molecule linkers and groups encountered in medicinal chemistry.[99] "Soft," low-energy torsion barriers are important, for example, anisoles ($ArOCH_2X$) and anilines (ArNHX) prefer coplanar conformations, while alkylaryls ($ArCH_2X$) prefer a perpendicular conformation (Figure 4.7).

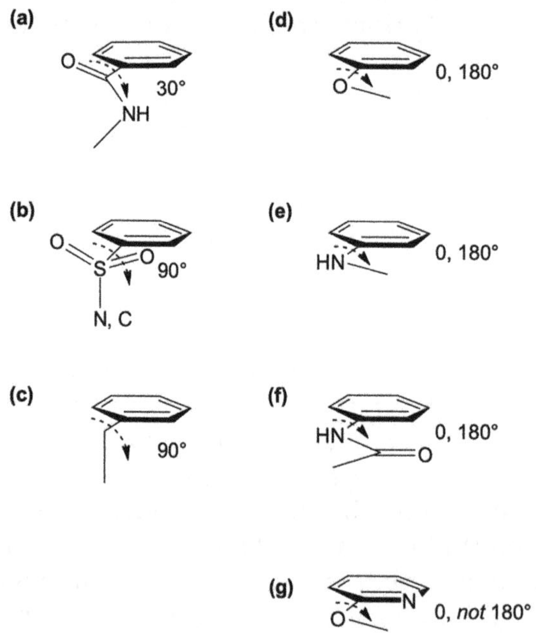


**Figure 4.7** The most frequently observed torsions[99] in the CSD and PDB for (a) benzamides, (b) arylsulfonamides and arylsulfones, (c) arylalkyls, (d) anisoles, (e) anilines, (f) anilides, and (g) 2-alkoxypyridines, which have a very strong preference for a co-planar torsion with the alkyl group *syn* to the pyridine N, so that the pyridine N and alkoxy O lone pairs are *anti*.

These preferences must be considered and exploited when designing linkers between aryl rings; small deviations are seldom observed and cost binding free energy. Linker atoms control both distance and direction. There are also subtle, but critical geometric differences between the substituent vectors coming off of different five-member heterocycles. Replacing carbon, nitrogen, or oxygen with sulfur obviously alters the ring geometry and orientation of substituent exit vectors, but the various C, N, O heterocycles are typically presumed to be isosteric, with similar substituent vector orientations. Salonen *et al.*[55] probed the SAR of Factor Xa inhibitors in the S1 pocket by comparing three heterocycle linkers in inhibitor **1** (Figure 4.8): 3,5-disubstituted isoxazole **1a**, 2,4-disubstituted oxazole **1b**, and 2,5-disubstituted oxazole **1c**. Oxazoles **1b** (146 nM $K_i$) and **1c** (1620 nM $K_i$) were much less potent inhibitors than isoxazole **1a** (9 nM $K_i$). X-ray co-crystal structures determined at 1.25–1.33 Å resolution revealed that the oxazoles **1b** and **1c** flipped over 180° relative to the isoxazole **1a**. Searching the Cambridge Structural Database (CSD) showed surprising differences between the substituent vectors in these three heterocycles (Figure 4.8). The 15- to 180-fold lower activity of **1b** and **1c** is likely due to a combination of the different steric requirements (due to the different exit vector angles) of the oxazoles *vs.* the parent isoxazole, different preferred conformations of the heterocycle linker relative to the main inhibitor scaffold, and also their different dipole vectors. **1a**, **1b**, and **1c** stack face-to-face against peptide bonds lining

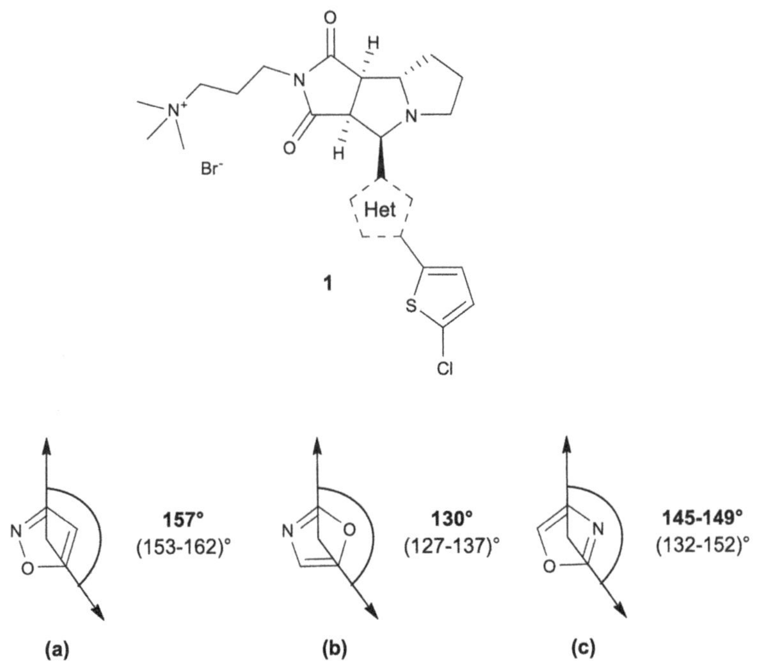


**Figure 4.8** CSD search results from Salonen *et al.*[55] for the angle between the two substituent vectors of isoxazole **1a**, and oxazoles **1b** and **1c** in Factor Xa inhibitor **1**. The most frequently observed angles are shown in **bold** and the range of angles is shown in parentheses. These angular preferences are reproduced by MOE[69] with the MMF94 force field.[171,172]

the Factor Xa S1 pocket. Harder *et al.*[102] studied the face-to-face packing of aromatic heterocycles to peptide bonds and concluded the optimal interacting dipole vectors should be antiparallel, consistent with the improved activity of **1b** *vs.* **1c**.

### 4.4.8 Preferred and Competitive Protein–Ligand Interactions

The Protein Data Bank[26] had about 185 000 structures in December 2021, with 143 468 from X-ray, 11 850 from NMR, and 6416 from electron microscopy, of which about 70 000 are protein–ligand complexes. The growth rate is accelerating. The Cambridge Structural Database (CSD)[100] reached 1 million small molecule crystal structures in 2019.[101] It grows by about 55 000 molecules per year (average since 2015), with many high-quality structures that are relevant for medicinal chemistry.

The PDB and CSD crystal structure databases have been studied extensively to understand the geometric preferences of non-covalent interactions[3,66,102–109] and small molecule conformational preferences.[99,110–112] Protein crystal structures typically contain about 40–60% solvent by volume (mostly water), while small molecule crystal structures are dry (some are solvates, with one to a few molecules of solvent per organic molecule). Small molecule crystal "packing forces" were previously believed to induce conformational strain on small molecules, but recent analysis of the much larger PDB and CSD databases shows that such cases are rare:[113,114] the CSD does in fact provide a reference set of preferred small molecule conformations (in particular, preferred torsion angles) that are relevant for structure-based design.[110,111] However, the small molecule X-ray crystal structure conformation is typically only one of many possible preferred conformations and is unlikely to represent the conformation bound to a drug target. We highlight below the most important recent analyses and their application to structure-based design.

The structure-based design review from Bissantz, Kuhn, and Stahl provides detailed examples with preferred geometries for the common classes of protein–ligand interactions: hydrogen bonds OH–O=C, OH–N(=)–, NH–O=C, NH–N(=)–, halogen bonds, multipolar interactions C=O–amide, C–F–O=C (peptide backbone), cation–Pi, hydrophobic contacts, aromatic face-to-face, aromatic edge-to-face, aromatic ring face-to-face with amide, and sulfur–aryl.[3] Kuhn *et al.* took this qualitative study another step to develop "ViewContacts," a software tool to annotate protein–ligand complexes with each of these interaction types which also provides qualitative scoring to highlight favorable and unfavorable interactions (Figures 4.9 and 4.10).[66]

Neutral hydrogen bond distances range from 2.7–3.2 Å, while charged hydrogen bonds with carboxylates range from 2.6–3.0 Å. The hydrogen bond angle for the donor–hydrogen–acceptor is most frequently observed >150°, with the hydrogen bond oriented to approach the lone pair of the acceptor. Sulfonamide and sulfone oxygens are weak hydrogen bond acceptors and prefer to orient their hydrogen bonds linearly along the S=O bond. Hydrogen bonds to acceptors in aromatic rings or carbonyl groups lie within 30° of the plane of the aromatic ring or carbonyl group. Aromatic hydrogens (ArH) in aromatic rings with electron-withdrawing groups or in aromatic heterocycles are weak hydrogen bond donors; ArH hydrogen bonds are frequently observed between kinase inhibitors and one of the kinase hinge backbone carbonyl oxygens. ArH hydrogen bond

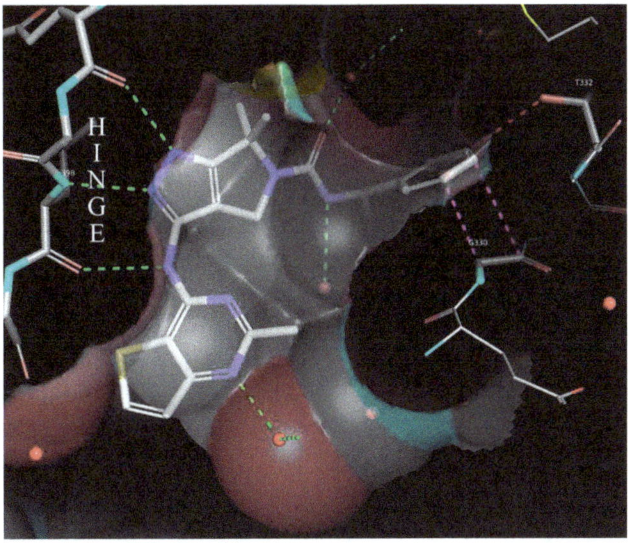


**Figure 4.9** PAK4 kinase–inhibitor complex (PDB 2X4Z) interactions highlighted by ViewContacts:[66] three hydrogen bonds (green) between the kinase hinge and an inhibitor, an aromatic face-to-face interaction (magenta) with the peptide backbone, and a probable repulsive interaction (red) between a phenyl ring and the hydroxyl of Thr-332.

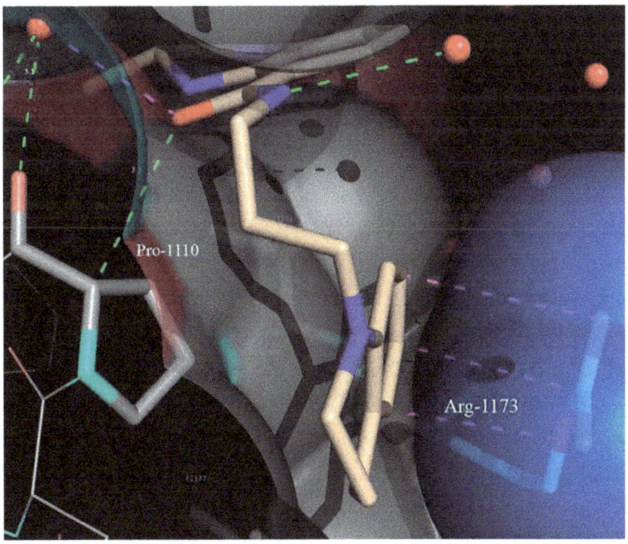


**Figure 4.10** Bromodomain CREBBP–inhibitor complex (PDB 4NYW) interactions highlighted by ViewContacts[66] show a hydrogen bond (green) between the inhibitor's amide carbonyl oxygen and the alpha carbon proton of Pro-1110, and an aromatic face-to-face interaction (magenta) with the guanidinium group of Arg-1173.

lengths vary from about 3.1–3.6 Å. The hydrogen on the alpha carbon of the peptide backbone can also be a weak hydrogen bond donor (Figure 4.10).

Halogen bonds occur between aromatic chlorine, bromine, and iodine substituents in aromatic rings with electron-withdrawing groups, and a carbonyl oxygen from the protein backbone, Asn, Gln, Asp, or Glu sidechains. Halogen bonds are counterintuitive: instead of the halogen behaving as though it has a partial negative charge, it acts as a surrogate hydrogen-bond donor. This is due to the "sigma-hole" at the end of the bond between the aromatic carbon and the halogen, which creates a partial positive charge on the halogen for on–axis interactions.[115] Increasing the electron-withdrawing power of substituents on the halogen's aromatic ring (*i.e.*, increasing their Hammett sigma constant) enhances the halogen bond. The halogen–oxygen distance is much shorter than the normal van der Waals contact distance and becomes progressively shorter as the halogen gets larger. The preferred halogen bond C–X–O angle is linear. Halogen bond interaction strengths also increase with the size of the halogen. Halogen bonds are frequently observed, but very challenging to design. Hardegger *et al.* designed halogen bonds for inhibitors of MEK1 kinase and cathepsin L, where they compared ArX interacting with a backbone carbonyl oxygen for X = H, F, Cl, Br, and I.[116] Halogen bonds for Cl, Br, and I improved $IC_{50}$ relative to H by 2–13-fold, 7–24-fold, and 26–45-fold for MEK1 and cathepsin L, respectively. Fluorine does not form halogen bonds, but can interact orthogonally with the carbonyl carbons of amides, where the C–F bond is oriented perpendicular to the plane of the amide bond and oriented such that the F contacts the carbonyl carbon with a range of 3.0–3.7 Å. This orthogonal dipolar C–F–C=O interaction can contribute several-fold to binding affinity. Aromatic rings and peptide bonds pack against each other with T-shaped, edge-to-face or parallel-displaced, face-to-face interactions (Figure 4.9).[102,106] Aromatic rings also make face-to-face interactions with the guanidinium group of arginine (Figure 4.10).

Kuhn *et al.* adapted a new, more precise "Line-of-Sight" analysis developed by Taylor for the CSD[117] to identify the most significant *competitive* and *non-competitive* protein–ligand interactions in the PDB in three recent publications.[107–109] Non-competitive interactions are outcompeted by more statistically preferred interactions. Non-competitive interactions are not necessarily repulsive, but indicate that there are better ligand options to interact with the binding site in the same region. This is a complementary, and more likely meaningful distinction than previous approaches that focus on classifying interactions as favorable and unfavorable.

The key point of Line-of-Sight analysis is to determine which interactions can be improved by differentiating observed close contacts from those that are most likely to stabilize or destabilize binding. Line-of-Sight analysis ranks interactions between specific atom types by the ratio of their observed frequency to their frequency expected at random, based on their exposed surface areas. This eliminates nearest-neighbor or "bystander" interactions to focus on the most statistically significant interactions.

Their analysis supports previously identified interactions, identifies some previously unrecognized interactions, and challenges others that were believed to be important. They provide further support for ArX–O=C directional halogen bonds for X = Cl, Br, and I, with competitive interactions from 0–40° and a strong preference at 0–10° for Cl. They also show that F does not form halogen bonds.

We include only a few examples here (Figures 4.11–4.23) from their comprehensive analysis.

Guanidinium–nitrile interactions are strongly competitive, with either an in-plane hydrogen bond or above-the-plane cation-dipole geometry, as shown in Figures 4.16 and 4.17.

Tosstorff *et al.*[107] describe non-obvious competitive and non-competitive amide–heterocycle stacking examples with pyridine and pyrimidine, and also pyridine and pyrimidine interacting with amide carbonyl O. Many more examples are available in their paper and its supplementary information.

Truly repulsive protein–ligand interactions are rare. Some are due to crystallographic errors and can be diagnosed by comparing the molecular model with the electron density map. But others are correct and reveal opportunities to improve affinity. Uncompetitive

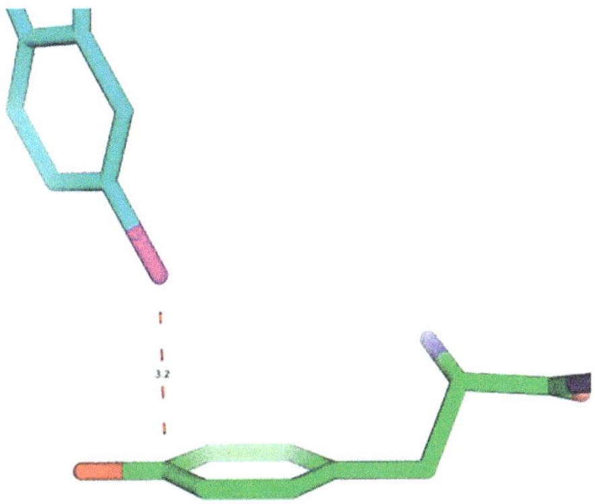

**Figure 4.11** PDB (3Q3K) ArX-aromatic C halogen bonds are competitive interactions, where the ArX halogen points towards the aryl carbon from above the plane of the aryl ring.

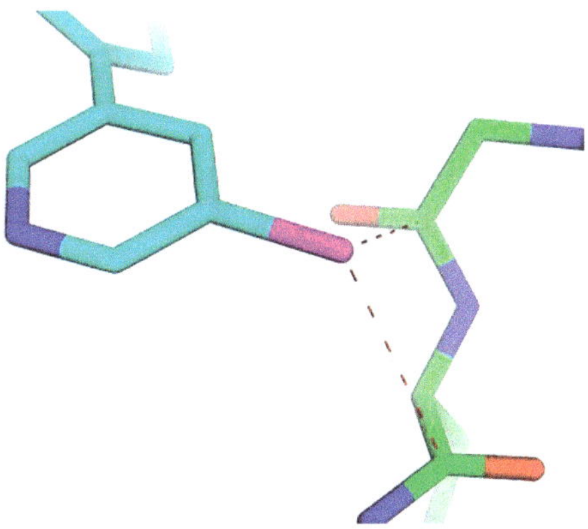

**Figure 4.12** PDB (4DJX) Highly competitive ArCl interactions with peptide amide groups position the Ar–Cl bond parallel to the carbonyl plane or orthogonal to the amide plane.

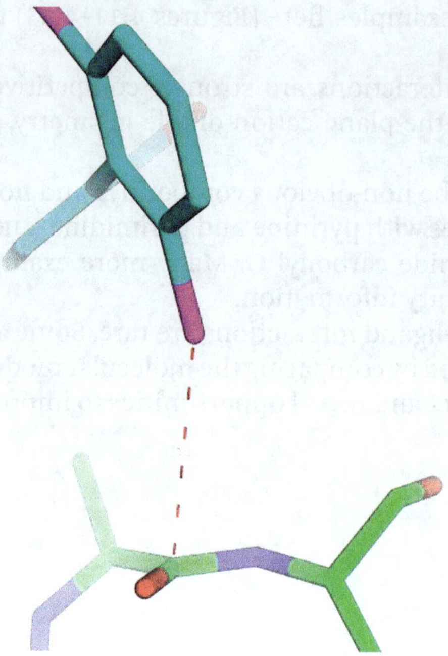

**Figure 4.13** PDB (5IA3) Orthogonal Ar–Cl interaction with amide plane.

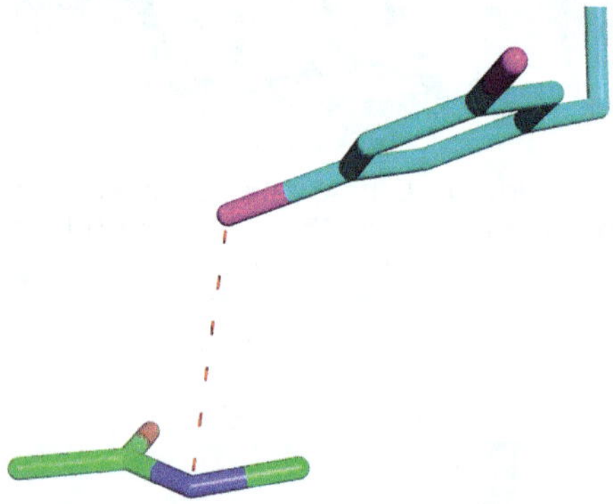

**Figure 4.14** PDB (4WX6) A less competitive (but still competitive) out-of-plane Ar–Cl–amide geometry.

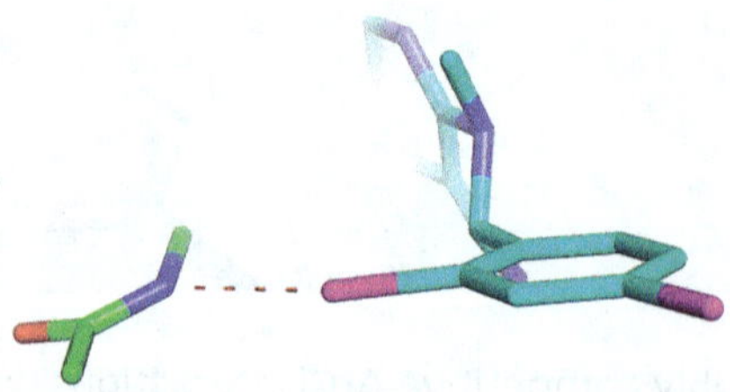

**Figure 4.15** PDB (5AL3) ArCl–amide nitrogen interactions are non-competitive in-plane.

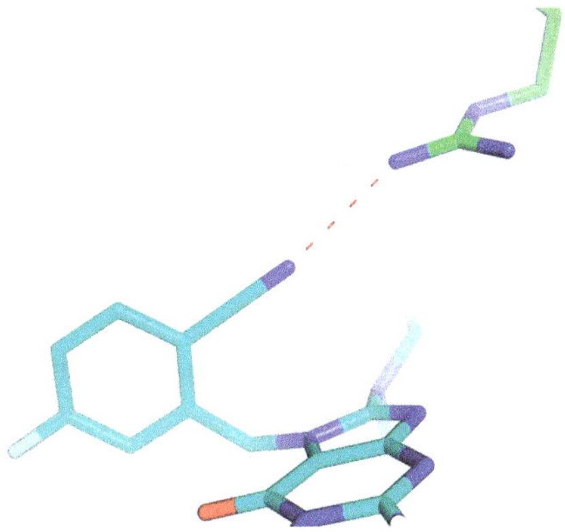

**Figure 4.16** PDB (5I7U) in-plane, short 3.0 Å Ar-CN-Arg guanidinium hydrogen bond in DPP-4. CN is 15- to 80-fold more potent than the shorter CF3 or F groups, respectively.

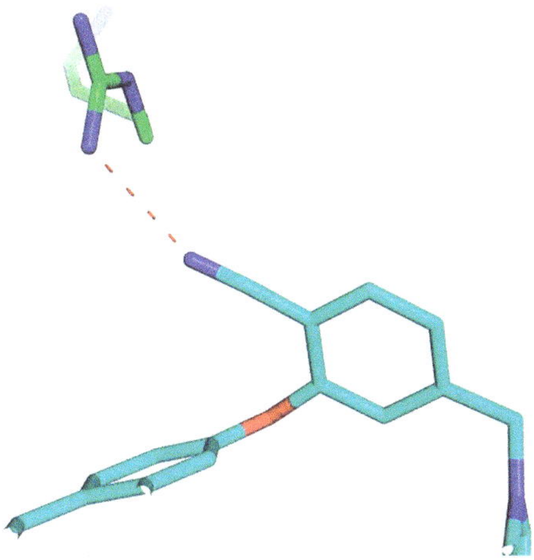

**Figure 4.17** PDB (1LD7) above-the-plane, short 3 Å cation-dipole interaction in farnesyltransferase.

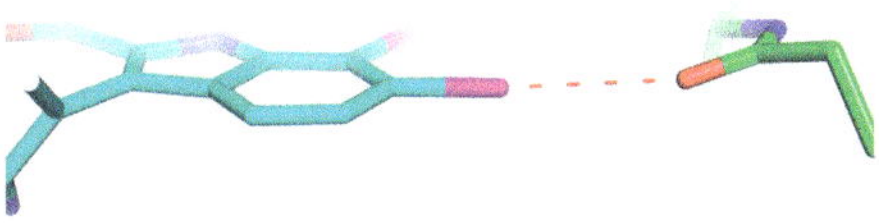

**Figure 4.18** PDB (2VAG) Non-competitive in-plane halogen bond.

protein–ligand interactions are less common than competitive interactions and also provide important clues to improve affinity or selectivity.

A comparison of Ar–Cl–O=C halogen bond geometries clarifies the distinction between non-competitive and unfavorable: the in-plane, *bona fide* halogen bond shown below (Figure 4.18) is classified as non-competitive, while the out-of-plane halogen bond (Figure 4.19) is competitive. The in-plane halogen bond with Ar–Cl

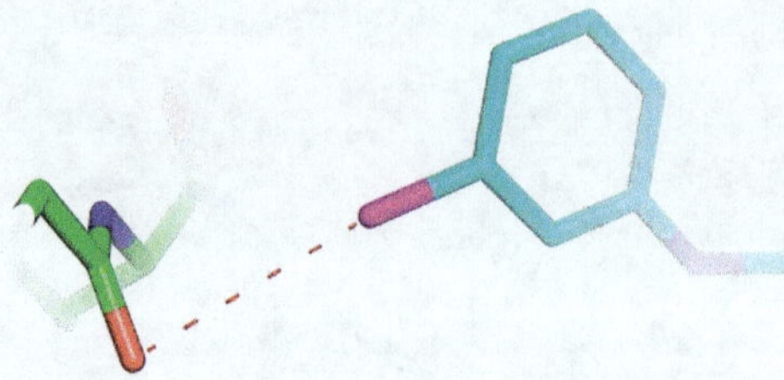

**Figure 4.19** PDB (2IZU) Competitive out-of-plane halogen bond.

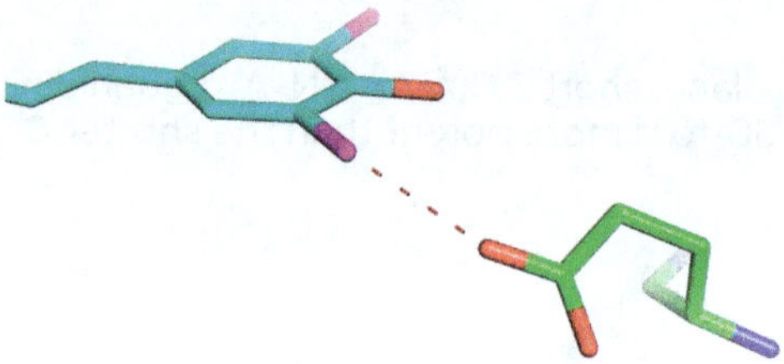

**Figure 4.20** PDB (6MHI) non-competitive Ar–Cl-carboxylate interaction.

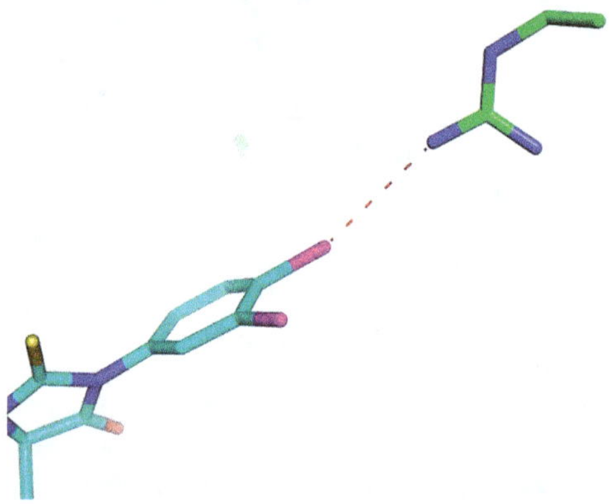

**Figure 4.21** PDB (3V4A) non-competitive Ar–Cl–Arg guanidine.

is out-competed by hydrogen bond donors, which is why the interaction is non-competitive. However, in-plane Ar–Cl–O=C halogen bonds can be favorable and improve affinity; Ar–Br and Ar–I have higher competitive interaction scores and usually improve affinity more.

Tosstorff *et al.*[108] highlight aromatic chlorine interacting with Asp/Glu carboxylates, Arg guanidines, and Lys amine sidechains as among the most non-competitive interactions, shown in Figures 4.20 and 4.21.

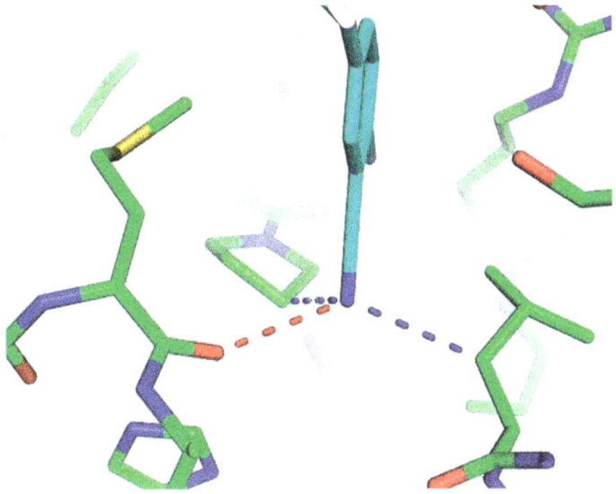

**Figure 4.22** HCV polymerase (PDB 6W4G) complex. The CN analog makes two weakly competitive interactions (blue) and one very poor non-competitive interaction (red).

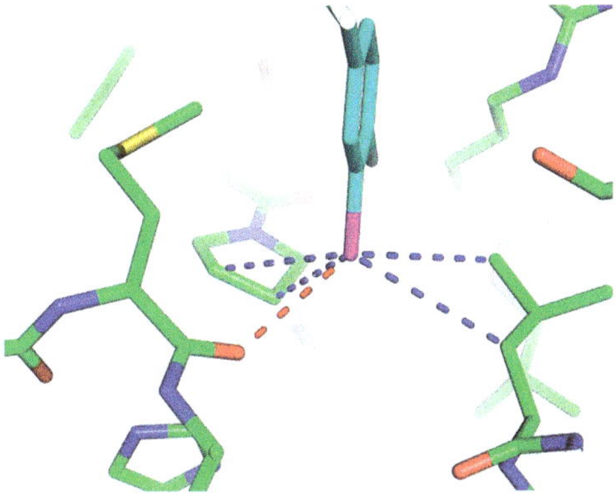

**Figure 4.23** HCV polymerase (PDB 3D5M) complex. The Cl analog picks up an additional competitive interaction and is 100 times more potent in a biochemical assay.

They describe three SAR case studies where replacing a non-competitive interaction with a more competitive interaction improved affinity or selectivity. An example for HCV polymerase inhibitors shows how subtle interaction differences can cause large affinity changes (Figures 4.22 and 4.23).

Tosstorff *et al.* used this analysis to post-process and improve docking scores for virtual screening. They developed[107] and described an interactive, visualization tool in MOE[69] to annotate protein–ligand complexes with competitive/non-competitive interaction scores in real-time.

Molecular mechanics and dynamics rely on empirical, parameterized force fields. Current force fields are remarkably good, but cannot reproduce or predict many of the subtle competitive and non-competitive interactions identified in the three "Line-of-Sight" papers or with ViewContacts. Force field methods are also frequently inaccurate for predicting preferred torsion angles in small molecules, as we note in the next section. We highly recommend using these qualitative tools for design and analysis along with force field methods.

## 4.5 Ligand-induced Conformational Change

Proteins can be highly flexible and can adapt to the ligand that is binding. It is unclear whether proteins actually open up new "cryptic" sites or binding site pockets in response to a ligand or whether these sites continually appear, disappear, and change as the protein samples many energetically similar metastable states. This distinction doesn't matter for structure-based design, which requires observation of a new pocket or site from structural biology. But it does have implications for predicting conformational change within a known binding site, or cryptic and allosteric sites. If ligand-induced conformational change actually requires the ligand to induce the conformation, MD simulations will not be able to predict it without the appropriate ligand present during the simulation. Recent long time-scale MD simulations show that the latter is possible.[47,48]

Teague and Davis[35] highlighted a number of examples where such protein movement provided new opportunities for medicinal chemistry design to improve potency, selectivity, and generate new intellectual property as the pocket and hence pharmacophore had changed. These changes may manifest to the chemist as unusual SAR, and without structural information can be overlooked as not fitting the binding paradigm. But the observation of induced changes can be a powerful stimulus to a medicinal chemistry program, and in a structurally enabled program, chemists should be on the lookout for unusual SAR that can be investigated by structure-based design.

In a program to discover orally available, selective inhibitors of iNOS (inducible nitric oxide synthase), most of the known inhibitors contained a basic amidine mimicking the guanidine of the substrate arginine, which binds over the active-site heme forming a salt bridge with an invariant glutamate residue, Glu-377. The three NOS isoforms have highly conserved binding sites and very similar structures, so gaining selectivity for iNOS was likely to prove difficult.

AstraZeneca scientists followed several chemical series containing an arginine guanidine mimic, either an amidine or aminopyridine (Figure 4.24).[118,119] The program was supported by iterative crystallography, with over 70 co-crystal structures determined. Potent inhibitors were synthesized, but all suffered from poor pharmacokinetics. Chemists optimized potency by growing into the iNOS pocket, building in hydrophobicity and attempting to make new polar interactions, for example by interacting with residues important for binding the arginine substrate. Potency was improved and 10 nM $IC_{50}$ iNOS inhibitors became common. Computational chemistry was able to rule out medicinal chemistry designs that didn't fit the active site, but was rarely able to confidently predict potency. Detailed structural investigations driven by a close dialog between medicinal chemists, crystallographers, and computational chemists were critically important in unraveling SAR and guiding design hypotheses. As the iNOS active-site pocket was filled, SAR began to identify iNOS inhibitors with selectivity over the highly similar isozymes, nNOS and eNOS (Figure 4.24). X-ray structures showed that selective inhibitors displaced an invariant glutamine residue, Gln-263, and opened a new pocket (Figure 4.25).

Gln-263, although common to all three NOS isoforms, proved a valuable source of selectivity.[118,119] Gln-263 adopts a different conformation with bulky inhibitors, which

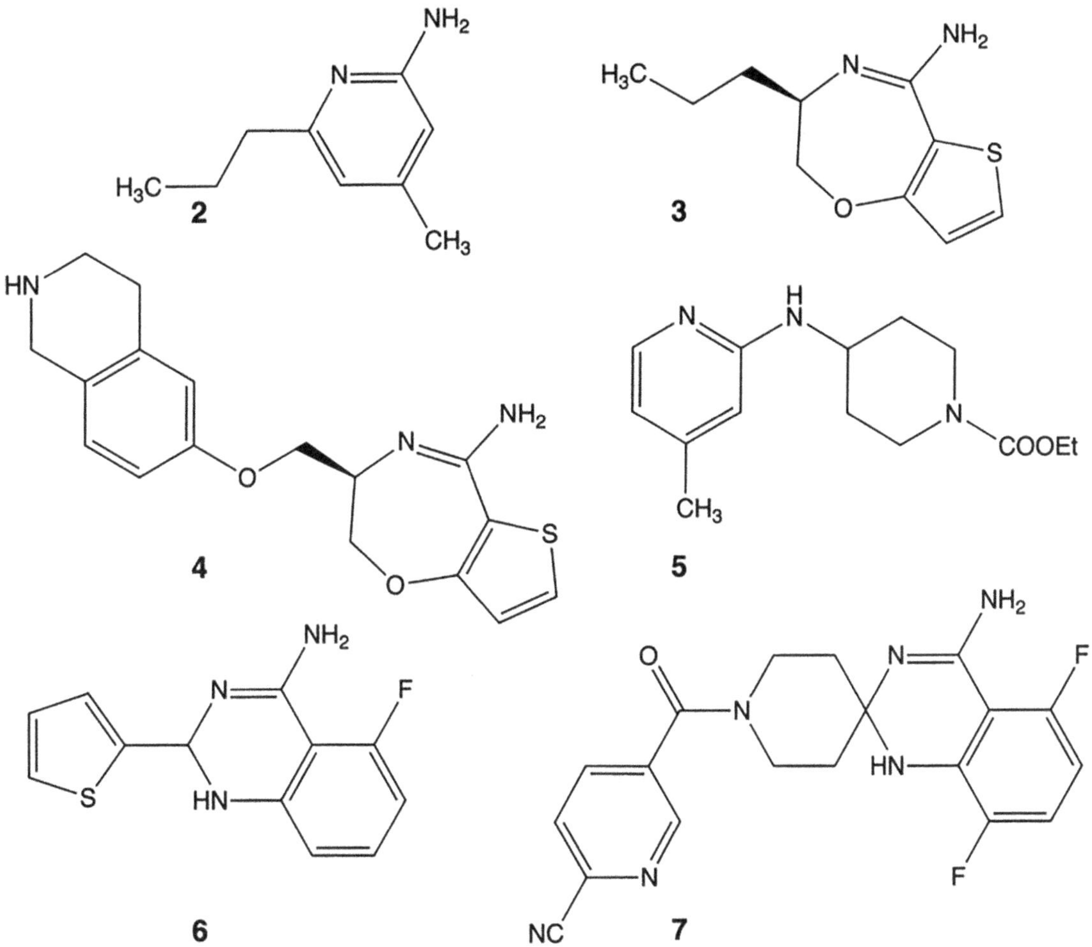

| | iNOS $IC_{50}$ (μM) | Selectivity eNOS/iNOS | Selectivity nNOS/iNOS | PDB |
|---|---|---|---|---|
| 2 | 0.015 | 2.3 | 1.5 | 3E6N |
| 3 | 0.04 | 5 | 1.2 | 3EAH |
| 4 | 0.4 | 125 | 2.5 | 3EBF |
| 5 | 0.35 | 166 | 57 | 3E7G |
| 6 | 0.01 | 250 | 100 | 3E7I |
| 7 | 0.035 | >2860 | 23 | 3E7T |

**Figure 4.24** Part of the iNOS inhibitor series studied by AstraZeneca, their iNOS $IC_{50}$s, selectivity *vs.* eNOS and nNOS, and PDB codes for their X-ray co-crystal structures.[118]

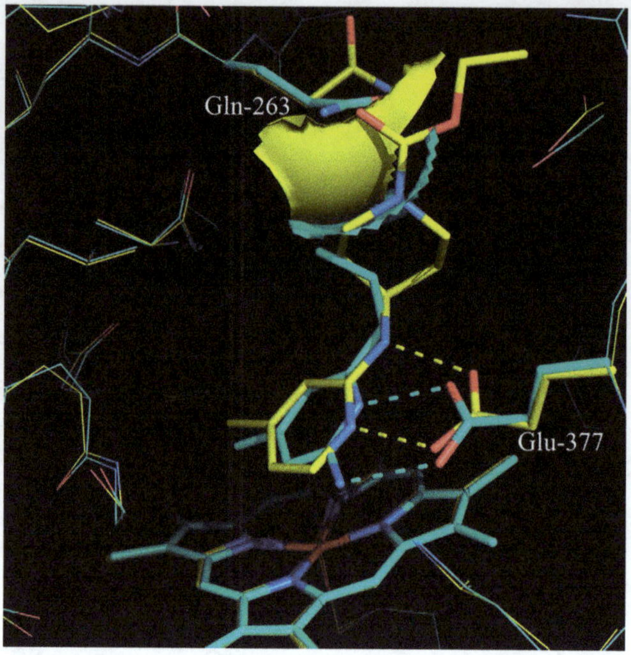


**Figure 4.25** Non-selective aminopyridine **2** (cyan, PDB 3E6N, mouse iNOS) makes a charged, bidentate interaction (dashed cyan lines) between its amidine and Glu-377. The 2-aminopyridine of a selective analog, **5** (yellow, PDB 3E7G, human iNOS), flips over 180°, but still makes a similar bidentate interaction (dashed yellow lines) with Glu-377. The *N*-carboxyethylpiperidine group of **5** displaces Gln-263, which rotates its sidechain to a different conformation and opens a new pocket, shown by comparing the solvent-accessible surfaces of the sidechains of the two Gln-263 conformers.

opens a new iNOS selectivity pocket. This only occurs in iNOS, due to second and third shell differences in the sidechains in the other NOS isoforms. Some conformations introduced n/e NOS selectivity, but at the expense of some iNOS activity, while other glutamine conformations increased iNOS potency while increasing selectivity over n/e NOS. Selectivity through perturbation of the invariant glutamine residue proved to be a very valuable design learning, and the "Gln pocket" became design dogma. Even with potent and selective inhibitors, pharmacokinetic limitations prevented further optimization of many of the amidine or amino pyridine series. A different starting point was required.

The project team had been aware of a number of published non-basic iNOS inhibitors,[120] for example compound **8** (Figures 4.26 and 4.27), but all were weak (>10 μM $IC_{50}$), did not contain the bidentate donor–acceptor interaction with Glu-377, and were therefore considered non-specific inhibitors as they did not fit the project SAR dogma. They were overlooked for many months, but out of desperation for a new starting point the team decided to use iterative X-ray crystallography capability to explore the surprising SAR of these weak inhibitors. The new X-ray crystal structures

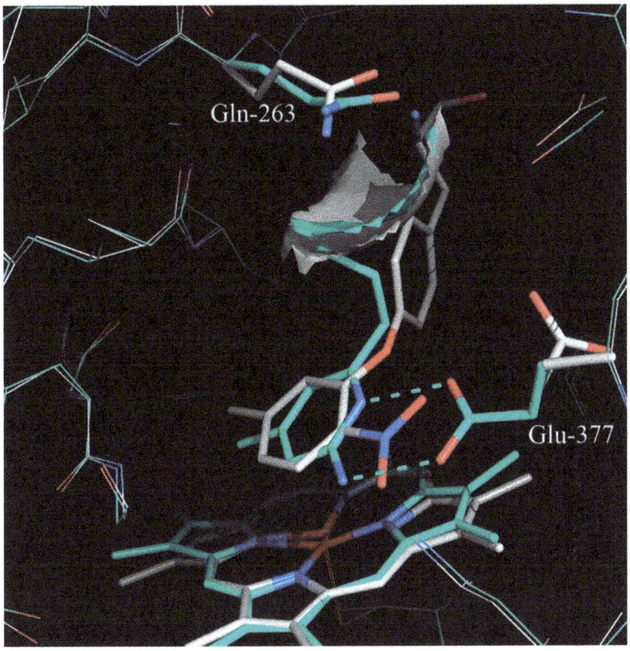


**Figure 4.26** The X-ray co-crystal structure of compound **8** (white) in mouse iNOS reveals that it stacks its neutral aromatic ring over the heme,[119] similar to the basic amidine **2** (cyan, PDB 3E6N, mouse iNOS),[118] and displaces Glu-377 from its position observed with amidines. The solvent-accessible surfaces of the sidechains of Gln-263 are similar. Both compounds have little selectivity.

were an eye-opener.[119] They showed that the non-basic inhibitors all bound over the heme, and instead of forming an interaction with the active site glutamate residue, displaced it, Figure 4.26.

This was a turning point for the project. These inhibitors were no longer dismissed as weak non-specific start points, but considered a priority opportunity for a new series. Design progressed through a sequence of hybrid structures using previously learned SAR, starting with the neutral heme binder, displacing the glutamate, reaching for arginine's amino acid binding site initially with a zwitterion, building into the glutamine pocket for selectivity, and replacing the zwitterionic amino acid with a basic group to improve cell permeability, Figures 4.27 and 4.28.

The iNOS project suggests a general strategy ("anchored plasticity") for designing selective inhibitors of a target with highly similar isoforms (*e.g.*, kinases), where the majority of direct protein–ligand (first shell) contacts are identical across the different isoforms: look for variations in sequence and structure outside of the pocket, in the second or third shells, that could be exploited by pushing against the site in those directions. The second and third shell differences in the NOS isoforms are fairly subtle and were not obvious at the outset of the project; they were revealed by pushing on the site with bulky inhibitors.

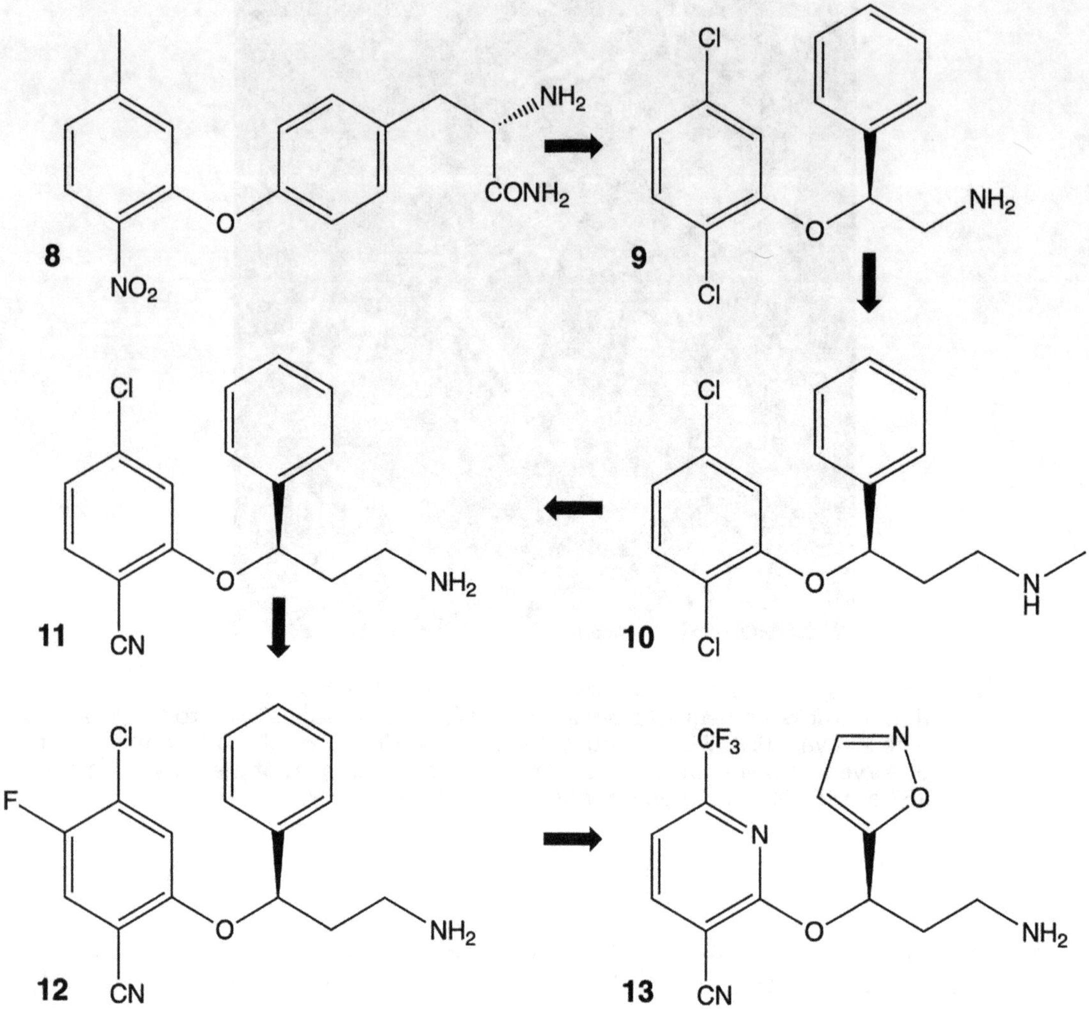

| | iNOS $IC_{50}$(μM) | Selectivity eNOS/iNOS | Selectivity nNOS/iNOS | PDB |
|---|---|---|---|---|
| **8** | 1.2 | | | |
| **9** | 1.9 | >533 | 52 | |
| **10** | 0.022 | >4500 | 210 | |
| **11** | 0.004 | $>10^4$ | >270 | 2Y37 |
| **12** | 0.006 | $>10^4$ | 35 | |
| **13** | 0.005 | $>10^4$ | 1.3 | |

**Figure 4.27** iNOS inhibitor selectivity progression.

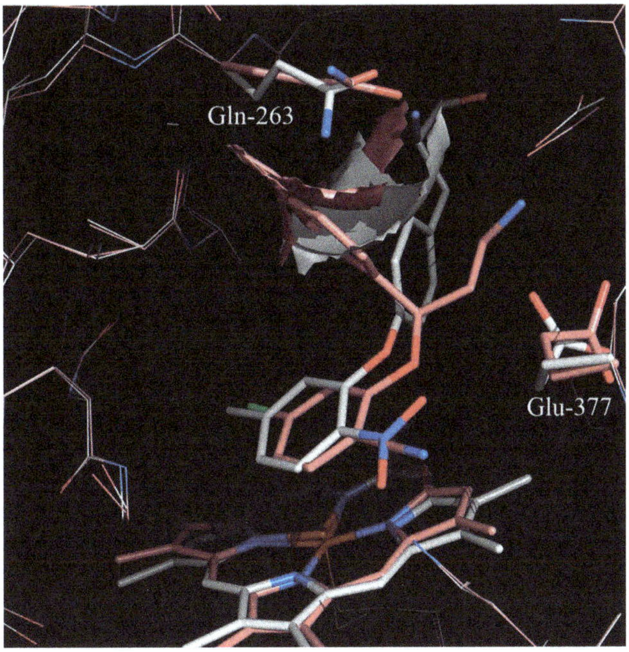


**Figure 4.28** X-ray co-crystal structures of poorly selective compound **8** (white) and highly selective compound **11** (pink, PDB 2Y37) in mouse iNOS, showing the different Gln-263 residue positions influenced by the Gln-pocket substituent.[75] Solvent-accessible surfaces for the sidechain of Gln-263 highlight the extra volume opened up by compound **11**.

## 4.5.1 Hypothesis-based Design

Structure-based design is done by proposing hypotheses based on observed SAR, structures of relevant series with the target and related proteins, database searches and analysis, and modeling. A typical hypothesis would be to improve potency by modifying a known ligand to fill a pocket or make a specific interaction. We use X-ray crystallography or cryo-EM structures, biochemical, and biophysical assays to test the hypothesis: did the compound bind as expected and achieve its structural design goal? If so, did it actually improve potency, selectivity, or other desired outcomes? Do unexpectedly active or inactive compounds bind like their close analogs?

Interactive 3D modeling sessions with project teams are a valuable part of compound design and idea generation: structure-based design in a medicinal chemistry project is very complex and benefits from the combined knowledge and ideas from different scientists. Indeed, the huge increase in experimental structures in the PDB and CSD have increased our empirical knowledge of favorable and unfavorable interactions to the point where it's increasingly important to guide expert design with both empirical tools derived from these data[66,107] and also physics-based modeling tools. Many ideas are proposed in an interactive 3D project design meeting and should be modeled and prioritized quickly.[121]

We recommend the following guidelines for approaching a structure-based design program. To begin, review all available high-quality co-crystal structures for your target protein and highly similar proteins: any observed binding site conformation is a viable target for inhibitor design. Look for conserved features in structures, including bound or computationally predicted waters that may differentiate the target from off-targets. Search the CSD and PDB for molecules that make similar interactions to those observed in your co-crystal structures or models; matches in these databases can provide valuable clues to how to improve existing interactions and also identify similar groups that might also fit your site. Crossminer,[122] from the CSD, is an excellent software tool for searching the CSD. We use Crossminer to search for interactions similar to those observed in co-crystal structures of protein–ligand complexes during structure-based design projects; these searches can provide ideas for how to optimize the ligand. Shape-based methods[21,123] find molecules with similar shape to bound ligands and can also provide good ideas for "scaffold-hopping": swapping cores or other features of lead molecules to identify new compounds with improved properties.

As your design–synthesize–test cycle begins, consider each new design as a probe to interrogate the protein: a well-designed molecule will provide useful feedback, even if it is less potent than its reference analog. Each design should test a specific hypothesis, for example, to fill a pocket, stabilize a conformation, or make a hydrogen bond. Designs should also test protein flexibility by pushing into pockets to learn whether they can expand. Long timescale (millisecond) molecular dynamics simulations are beginning to access significant conformational change,[124–126] but it is still not practical to predict conformational change of a protein in response to ligand binding. An X-ray co-crystal or cryo-EM structure can determine whether the structural design objective was met. Structure-based design considerations are part of the medicinal chemistry multiparameter optimization process and need to be balanced against the many other terms covered in Chapter 20 on Lead Optimization.

Hydrogen bonds and polar interactions do not necessarily improve binding free energy, but they are critical for specificity. Hydrogen-bond donor/acceptor mismatches are not tolerated and will cost substantial binding free energy; you might be able to exploit a mismatch with a related off-target protein to increase selectivity. Burying a polar group in a hydrophobic region or *vice versa* will also hurt binding. Compounds that are ionized at physiological pH are likely to reduce membrane permeability, so it's usually best to minimize the overall charge of the small molecule to zero or one, avoid strong acids and bases (p$K_a$s <3 or >10, respectively), and to focus on using neutral substituents (or at least those with p$K_a$ close to 7.4) to interact with charged sidechains on the protein. Where part of your ligand points to solvent, this may be a good region to incorporate a solubilizing group, while not compromising potency.

Surprising changes in SAR are occasionally observed at the solvent front, where ligand atoms contact protein atoms in a highly exposed area. Such interactions usually have little effect on affinity, presumably due to being highly solvated and flexible. We previously summarized Krimmer *et al.*'s work[76] on thermolysin inhibitor water networks at the surface of the active site. Two different groups independently discovered a strong enzyme–inhibitor interaction at the surface of hepatitis C viral polymerase (HCVp). Antonysamy *et al.* optimized a weak 14 μM $K_d$ fragment screening hit with small libraries using parallel synthesis to a 0.46 μM $K_d$ lead compound.[127] The most potent members of the series had a tertiary amide that bound through a face-to-face interaction between the plane of the amide and the imidazole of His-475 on the protein's surface (Figure 4.29). The His ND1 forms a hydrogen-bond to the OH of the adjacent Ser-476, such that the five atoms of the imidazole and the Ser CB-OG are coplanar. This His-475/Ser-476 interaction is rigid and conserved across the many co-crystal structures determined during this project. This interaction appears to have been responsible for improving $K_d$ by 30–70-fold. Li *et al.* also discovered a similar face-to-face interaction with an aromatic, fused ring heterocycle from a different chemical series binding at the same site.[128]

As the structure–activity relationships within a chemical series develop, and confidence in the understanding gained from the structural information grows, compounds whose biological data appear as outliers within SAR should ideally be followed up by crystallography. These outliers can sometimes identify new binding poses that could lead to improved designs.

Affinity does not correlate with the number of hydrogen bonds. The goal is to identify which observed or potential hydrogen bonds are most important and try to optimize them. Individual protein–ligand hydrogen bonds contribute zero to about 3 kcal $mol^{-1}$ (13 kJ $mol^{-1}$) to binding free energy.[129] Quantitative prediction of hydrogen bonding

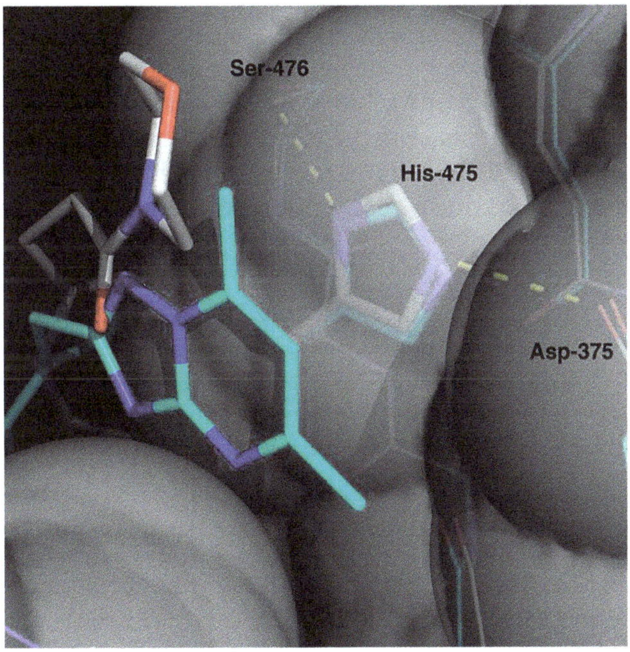


**Figure 4.29** The white HCVp inhibitor's tertiary amide[127] makes a face-to-face interaction with His-475 on the surface of HCVp (PDB 3CJ5). The cyan inhibitor's aromatic heterocycle[128] makes a similar face-to-face interaction (PDB 3FRZ). Dashed yellow lines indicate hydrogen bonds between His-475, the adjacent Ser-476, and the backbone carbonyl oxygen of Asp-375. The solvent-accessible surface of the protein is light gray.

strength is still extremely difficult; empirical rules based on geometry and network coordination through software such as ViewContacts[66] and the new Line-of-Sight analysis[107] provide qualitative help. What other clues can we use to design and optimize hydrogen bonding? Bissantz *et al.* suggested that hydrogen bonding is energetically asymmetric: binding site donors are more important to target than acceptors.[3] This is based on affinity data from several protein–ligand systems showing that not satisfying a protein donor costs more than ignoring an acceptor. It is further supported by analysis of PDB kinase–inhibitor complexes which show a strong preference for satisfying the kinase hinge's central backbone NH with an acceptor, while many inhibitors ignore one of the hinge's backbone carbonyl oxygens, leaving it desolvated. This is also qualitatively consistent with the asymmetry of Lipinski's "Rule of 5," which allows up to ten acceptors, but only five donors.

Laurence *et al.* developed the experimental p*K*(BHX) scale to measure the relative strengths of over 1100 different hydrogen bond acceptors (HBA).[130] This is the most self-consistent and comprehensive database available of relative hydrogen bond acceptor strengths. It is an excellent reference for choosing HBA groups in structure-based design. Bissantz *et al.* found a good agreement between p*K*(BHX) acceptor strength and the frequency of hydrogen bonds to OH groups in the CSD.[3] Hydrogen bond accepting ability does not correlate with proton basicity. HBA strengths tend to decrease in the order amides/sulfoxides/pyridines/*N*-methylimidazoles > ketones > esters/alcohols > sulfones/sulfonamides/ethers, but there are large variations depending on cyclization and substituents. Some of the p*K*(BHX) results seem counter-intuitive. For example, sulfonamide and sulfones are very hydrophilic based on their $\pi$ values and might also seem similar to amides and ketones, but they are weak hydrogen-bond acceptors on the p*K*(BHX) scale. This is consistent with the observation that only about 30% of the sulfonamides in the CSD or PDB form hydrogen bonds, but 75–80% of them are in close contact with an aliphatic carbon.[3] Green and Popelier published a quantum chemical approach to calculate p*K*(BHX) which should be practical to predict values for those groups missing from the database.[131]

Look for potential long-range electrostatic effects beyond the first-order interactions that you see at the binding site surface: most binding sites will have several charged residues within 10 Å of the ligand that are likely to influence its binding and SAR. We recommended exploring recent computational methods to predict these effects,[93–95] since these effects are not easily recognized through qualitative modeling relying on visual analysis.

### 4.5.2 Predicting Affinity: Free Energy Perturbation

Free energy perturbation (FEP) simulation methods were developed in the 1980s. They have finally become practical after decades of research in molecular mechanics force fields, methodology, and due to massive increases in computational power. FEP methodology, ease of use, range of applicability, and accuracy have improved during the last several years. Increased access to large-scale, relatively cheap, parallel computing power has dramatically improved turnaround time such that a complete predictive simulation can be completed in about one day, wall-clock time, after the simulation has been enabled and validated.

Several recent reviews provide excellent, detailed, and comprehensive overviews of FEP theory, methodology, practice, and limitations for drug discovery.[132–135] FEP software is now available from commercial and academic sources. However, accurate prediction of relative protein–ligand affinities is still extremely challenging, with good success in some cases. It is difficult to predict in advance which protein targets and which chemical series will work well.

Wang *et al.*[132] demonstrated the broad range of FEP applicability in 2015 through retrospective analyses of over 200 ligands and 10 targets, including two prospective kinase projects. For IRAK4, 22 compounds were chosen for synthesis out of 195 calculated with FEP. Of the 22 compounds, 15 were predicted to have $pK_i \le 8$; 14 of these predictions were correct. The other 7 compounds were predicted to have $pK_i > 8$; 5 were correct. The average error between predicted and experimental affinity for the 22 compounds was 1.1 kcal $mol^{-1}$ ($pK_i$ error 0.8). The results were similar for the second kinase target, TYK2.

Schrödinger added several key improvements to FEP+, their version of FEP, since the Wang *et al.* 2015 review,[132] including scaffold-hopping[136] and changes in net ligand charge. Scaffold-hopping transformations include ring opening/closing, ring fusion, and ring contraction/expansion. Other recent retrospective examples include predicting selectivity[93] and fragment hit elaboration.[137]

Schindler *et al.*[138] published an excellent, comprehensive study from Merck KGaA, Darmstadt, Germany in 2020 of FEP+ on in-house drug discovery targets. They describe their FEP+ workflow for industrial drug discovery, with caveats and recommended best practices. They evaluated 28 targets for FEP feasibility, performed validation studies on 18 targets and 44 chemical series, and progressed 14 targets and 25 chemical series to prospective calculations. They performed over 35 000 individual FEP+ calculations, yielding valid predictions for over 6000 compounds. Over 400 of those were synthesized and tested. They achieved good accuracy (RMSE <1.3 kcal $mol^{-1}$) for 14 targets and 21 chemical series.

They made several important observations. FEP+ gave poor results when starting with homology models on three separate projects. They had mixed experience relying on a docked structure binding mode to initiate FEP+. They performed retrospective validation studies across at least 10 known ligands per series per target. They found that a stringent validation accuracy threshold of RMSE <1.3 kcal $mol^{-1}$ was required to provide good blind prediction accuracy of RMSE <2 kcal $mol^{-1}$. New validation studies were required when shifting to a new chemical series or new co-crystal structures. For almost every new series, they had to re-parameterize some torsion potentials. FEP+ performed better in ranking compounds than other typical computational scoring methods. FEP+ also performed better than null hypothesis models such as correlation with molecular weight and $\log P$. Prediction accuracy varied across protein targets and between chemical series on the same target.

FEP is limited to small ligand perturbations up to about 10 non-hydrogen atoms. Exciting new work suggests that predicting absolute free energies of binding may become practical.[139,140] It is too early to know whether current absolute free energy methods are reliable and general enough. This is the "holy grail" of computational structure-based design, since it would enable the prediction of affinity for *de novo*-designed compounds without requiring a closely related reference analog.

FEP use is growing in industrial drug discovery, but is not yet routinely applied in most projects. It requires a highly expert and trained user, and considerable time and effort to set up and validate the computational protocol for each new protein site and chemical series. We typically predict which molecules to synthesize next empirically, guided by observations of preferred non-covalent interactions and supplemented with simpler computational methods. In those cases where FEP has been validated to be robust relative to known structures and SAR, we test our designs with FEP. The current practical computational blind predictive accuracy is within ±10-fold (2.8 kcal $mol^{-1}$, 10.8 kJ $mol^{-1}$) for closely related analogs in a protein binding site whose conformationally flexibility is limited to sidechain motions with little mainchain motion.

### 4.5.3 Test the Quality of a Design with Ligand Strain Energy, MD, and Docking

Structure-based design software enables medicinal chemists to design and model new compounds manually or with docking. Energy minimization provides a first approximation to test whether the design is feasible. It does not sufficiently test whether the minimized structure is in a metastable local minimum, whether the designed pose is the most likely pose, and whether the bound ligand conformation is a preferred conformation. Further analysis of preferred small molecule torsion angles, small molecule strain energy, docking, and short MD simulations can diagnose unstable poses and strained ligand conformations.

Excellent empirical tools are available to compare modeled ligand torsions with preferred torsions; significant deviations from preferred torsions should be avoided.[110,111,141] These methods compare torsional angle distributions observed from high-quality structures in the CSD and PDB with those in the modeled ligand.

Ligand strain energy is the energetic difference between the ligand's preferred solution conformations and its bound conformation. This is extremely difficult, if not impossible, to calculate accurately, but qualitative estimates are useful to eliminate designs which require a strained ligand conformation. New computational tools estimate the difference in strain enthalpy between the receptor-bound conformation and the ligand's preferred solution conformations.

Lee *et al.*[142] developed a molecular mechanics-based approach to estimate ligand strain energy which is fast and qualitatively helpful. Gu *et al.* included ligand strain energy as part of their large-scale docking virtual screening workflow.[143]

Sellers *et al.*[144] demonstrated that molecular mechanics is unreliable for calculating preferred bond rotation (torsion) angle minima and their barrier heights for some torsions encountered in drug-like molecules. Incorrect calculated torsion minima lead to a qualitatively wrong choice of preferred conformations and is the more serious of the two errors. Quantum mechanical methods are required for accurate prediction. Tong and Zhao, and Rai *et al.* reached the same conclusion.[98,145] It is difficult for experienced modelers to predict which molecules require quantum mechanical analysis. Quantum mechanics-based torsion or strain analysis is too slow for practical use in structure-based design. Rai *et al.* developed TorsionNet, a much faster machine learning method trained on a large dataset with quantum mechanical torsion calculations.[146]

TorsionNet's accuracy is reported to be comparable to the quantum mechanically derived values in the training set. TorsionNet should be fast enough to support structure-based design work. Calculated strain energies above an empirical threshold of ~4 kcal $mol^{-1}$ indicate that the ligand is unlikely to bind. These qualitative estimates can be used to rule out unfavorable ligand designs.

Alternate docking poses should be generated and compared with the desired design pose to identify whether the designed pose is at least among the most favorable calculated poses; this is a very qualitative test due to the inaccuracies of docking scoring functions. Stable, favorable designs should be in a deep local minimum relative to other poses.[147]

Short molecular dynamics (MD) simulations of ~10 ns can test the stability of an energy-minimized ligand design. Metastable, unfavorable designs will drift away from their designed, minimized starting point during the short MD simulation. This basic concept has been extended to dynamic undocking, which has been shown to provide an orthogonal, complementary test to other protein–ligand assessment tools.[148] Dynamic undocking evaluates structural, rather than thermodynamic, stability and was shown to improve virtual screening success. It is likely that it will be a useful qualitative test to assess manually created designs.

### 4.5.4 Large-scale Virtual Screening

Shoichet *et al.* demonstrated surprising improvements with very large-scale virtual screening (VS) by docking up to 500 million synthesis-on-demand, drug-like compounds.[46] This work, and a new approach that uses an iterative scaffold-synthon docking approach to access extremely large virtual libraries of ~11 billion compounds,[149] greatly improve our ability to find new hits. This work also used VS for initial hit-to-lead optimization, by following up the most promising docking hits.

Why does large-scale VS work so much better than recent VS of <1 million compounds, since the methods and scoring functions haven't changed significantly? The likely answer is that the final step usually relies on human experts reviewing the top few hundred to 1000 scoring VS hits, regardless of the size of the VS library. Shoichet *et al.* found that hit rates improve probabilistically with better docking scores. The scoring functions are not accurate enough to rank-order compounds, but they are better than random. Pushing orders of magnitude more VS compounds through the same process, but still selecting only ~1000 at the end, forces the "cream to rise to the top" to provide higher hit rates than we've seen before. This suggests that computational scoring of a large number of lead optimization designs may also achieve higher success rates.

### 4.5.5 Visual Docking Pose Assessment and Human Expertise

Docking and virtual screening functions are insufficient to rank-order compounds, but are clearly better than random. Virtual screening and docking therefore usually rely on human triage of the top computationally scored poses for a few hundred to 1000 compounds for the final step. Guidelines for how to do this are rarely mentioned in virtual screening and docking papers, so we can expect that human triage performance will vary depending on who performs the triage. All of the many concepts and factors we summarized in previous sections need to be considered when rank-ordering compounds from VS or manually designed compounds using modeling software. Recent papers[46,149] and another docking study from SAMPL4[150] showed that human triage outperformed a purely computational approach. Another recent study performed a challenge on three different proteins to recognize native from incorrect decoy poses.[19] In two out of three cases, a majority of participants selected the native pose. In the third case, the incorrect pose was selected by a slight majority, where "less experienced scientists (fewer than five years of experience) were selecting the correct pose more frequently than the more experienced scientist". Human bias from more experienced scientists influenced their choice based on knowledge of similar proteins. The conclusion of all these studies is that triage performed by a group of structure-based design experts will usually improve performance relative to a purely computational approach. Group expertise can compensate for individual biases and gaps in knowledge. We also recommend that a similar group review and prioritize structure-based designs before proceeding to synthesis.

### 4.5.6 Covalent Inhibitor Design

Covalent and reversible covalent inhibitor warhead design is highly empirical and can be assisted with new computational approaches.[151] For example Wei and colleagues developed a protocol called Cov_FB3D, which applies the principle of *de novo* fragment-based drug design to the design of covalent inhibitors and also incorporated a synthetic accessibility score.[152] A test of the protocol against the crystal structures of 15 covalent complexes consisting of BTK inhibitors, KRAS inhibitors, EGFR inhibitors, EphB1 inhibitors, MAGL inhibitors, and MAPK inhibitors revealed that most of these inhibitors could be *de novo* reproduced from the fragments by Cov_FB3D. A novel human ALDOA inhibitor (T1) with potent inhibitory activity (0.34 ± 0.03 μM) and greater synthetic accessibility was successfully *de novo* designed by this protocol.

Cysteine is the most frequently targeted sidechain for covalent inhibition, but not all cysteines are sufficiently reactive. Harris *et al.* described a promising computational approach to predict cysteine reactivity that may help prioritize cysteines for covalent inhibitor design.[153] Lysine is typically less reactive than cysteine, but has been successfully attacked in selective covalent inhibition with aryl sulfonyl fluorides using a covalent docking approach.[154]

CovalentInDB is a comprehensive database facilitating the discovery of covalent inhibitors, and contains over 4500 covalent inhibitors (including 68 approved drugs) with 57 different reactive warheads for 280 protein targets.[155] The crystal structures of some of the proteins bound with a covalent inhibitor are provided to visualize the protein–ligand interactions around the binding site. Each covalent inhibitor is annotated with the structure, warhead, experimental bioactivity, physicochemical properties, *etc.* Moreover, CovalentInDB provides the covalent reaction mechanism and the corresponding experimental verification methods for each inhibitor for its target. High-quality datasets are downloadable for users to evaluate and develop computational methods for covalent drug design.[155]

Protein arginine methyltransferase 6 (PRMT6) plays important roles in several biological processes associated with multiple cancers. Although there are several known reversible PRMT6 inhibitors, covalent PRMT6 inhibitors had not been reported. Aligning protein sequences of multiple PRMTs, PRMT6 was the only one with a cysteine residue (Cys-50) in the substrate-binding site. Analysis of the co-crystal structure of PRMT6 with the non-covalent inhibitor MS023 showed that the distance between the Cys-50 thiol and the meta-position of the MS023 phenyl ring was 4.9 Å, suitable for introducing an acrylamide group as a Michael acceptor to form a covalent bond (Figure 4.30). Compound **4** (Figure 4.31) did not covalently modify other closely related PRMTs, potently inhibited PRMT6 in biochemical ($K_i$ 16 nM) and cellular assays ($IC_{50}$ 1.3 mM), and was selective for PRMT6 over other methyltransferases.[156,157]

## 4.6 Future Directions

Structure-based design is now a mature field. We have seen hundreds of good examples since the writing of the first edition of this handbook. Browsing any medicinal chemistry journal will uncover yet more fascinating and instructive examples.

Structural information continues to inspire new medicinal chemistry design using the techniques herein described with the sheer unexpectedness of some of the binding sites and poses revealed. As the old saying goes, a picture is worth a thousand words. Structure-based design is guiding and inspiring ideas in new areas of medicinal chemistry such as optimizing hits from DNA encoded libraries (DEL), and proteolysis targeting chimera (PROTAC) degrader design. Cryo-EM is increasing the opportunities for rational design for targets that were previously limited to homology models.

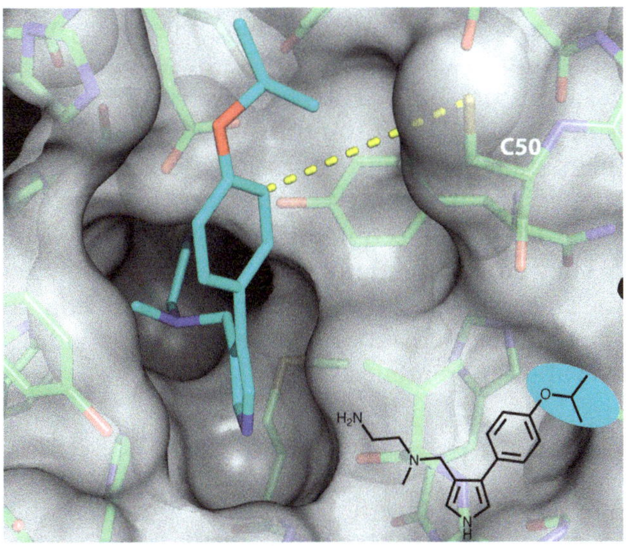


**Figure 4.30** PRMT6 (green bonds, light gray molecular surface) complex with non-covalent inhibitor MS023 (cyan). Dashed yellow line indicates design vector to react with Cys-50.

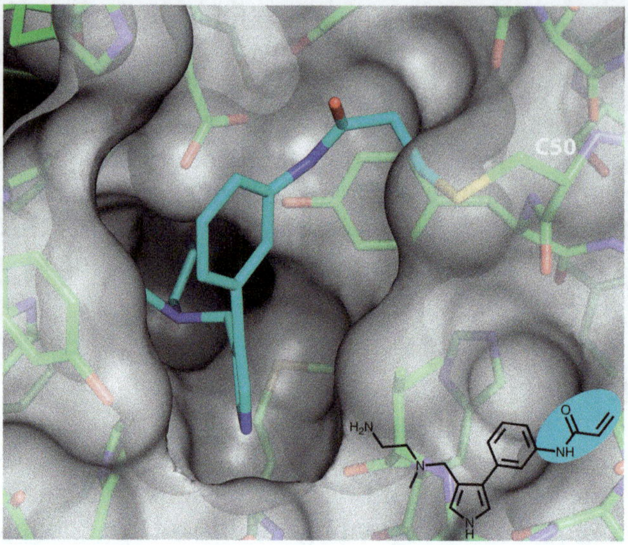


**Figure 4.31** PRMT6 (green bonds, light gray molecular surface) complex with covalent inhibitor compound **4** (cyan).

## 4.6.1 DNA Encoded Libraries

DNA encoded libraries (DEL) enable searching through libraries containing billions of molecules for compounds that bind to the target protein, agnostic to functional activity or perceived druggable binding sites. DEL chemistry has advanced dramatically to where it can frequently deliver good-quality hits.[158] Hence cryptic binding pockets or induced pockets can be found that can form the basis of medicinal chemistry campaigns for inhibitors, activators, or PROTAC ligands. A DNA encoded library screen for novel Bruton's tyrosine kinase (BTK) inhibitors from a library of over 110 million compounds with multiple parallel selection conditions found hits enriched only at high concentrations of BTK competitive with ATP, and also hits enriched at both high and low concentrations of BTK but not competitive with ATP.[159] A compound representing the latter profile showed low nanomolar potency in biochemical and cellular BTK assays. Analysis of the co-crystal structure of the most potent compound demonstrated a novel binding mode that revealed a new pocket in BTK, providing new opportunities for the design of novel and differentiated BTK inhibitors.

## 4.6.2 DEL and Machine Learning

Google and X-Chem built a target-specific scoring function by training a machine learning (ML) model on DEL data to predict affinity. They used the ML scoring function to perform large-scale VS, resulting in unusually high hit rates with some novel and potent compounds.[160] This is an exciting new approach which we expect to become more common for virtual screening and, perhaps, for lead optimization. DEL coupled with X-ray crystallography or cryo-EM is a powerful tool for finding new binding sites or new binding poses.

### 4.6.3 PROTAC Degraders and Molecular Glues

A successful PROTAC (proteolysis targeting chimera) must not only recruit two proteins to be in close proximity, but also align them so the ubiquitination of the target protein of interest (POI) can occur. PROTAC design is largely empirical, relying on choosing E-3 ligase and POI warheads, selecting vectors from each warhead to link chains of different geometries, lengths, and physical properties, and then testing for functional POI degradation. Structural information of such ternary complexes is starting to supplement the empiricism with rational design insights.

The X-ray crystal structure of the ternary complex of the VHL-based BRD4 PROTAC, MZ1, with the E-3 ligase VHL elongin B, elongin A, and its target, the second bromodomain (BD2) of the BET protein, Brd4, revealed that two vectors within MZ1's U-shaped conformation could enable a cross-linked design to create a macrocycle (Figure 4.32, cyan).[161] This is classic medicinal chemical strategy, to lock an inhibitor conformation in its receptor-bound state, aiming to reduce conformational entropy and thereby improve affinity for the ternary complex, and hopefully improved degradation.

Several factors need to be considered for linker design, including ensuring that all linker torsions are close to their preferred minima, that the resulting macrocycle's

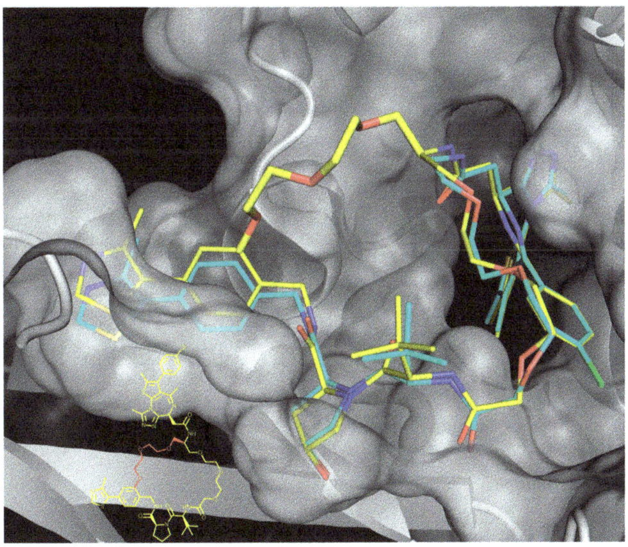

**Figure 4.32** The X-ray structure of PROTAC MZ1(PDB 5T35, cyan) in complex with VHL and BRD4 inspired the macrocycle design of the macroPROTAC (PDB, 6SIS, yellow). The chemical structure of MZ1 is shown in the inset with the macroPROTAC linker in red.

minimum energy conformation matches the original target conformation, that all linker contacts with the protein are favorable, and, of course, synthetic feasibility. The authors evaluated two different vectors from the pro-chiral carbon alpha to the amide nitrogen (Figure 4.32) to design the linker attachment so that its preferred conformation would be similar to MZ1's conformation in the ternary complex. They analyzed the torsions of model compounds *N*-ethylacetamide and *N*-isopropylacetamide with a DFT quantum mechanical method to identify the preferred linker attachment. They simulated different lengths of PEG linkers with MD to identify those that were most stable during the course of a ~200 ns simulation.

The design hypothesis for the macroPROTAC was validated by further X-ray crystallography (Figure 4.32, yellow). Biophysical studies revealed enhanced selectivity between the second and the first bromodomains of BET proteins, but a 12-fold loss of binary binding affinity for Brd4. However, the macroPROTAC-1 had cellular activity comparable to MZ1. While this study validates the macrocyclization strategy, it also leaves room for possible improvement: the conformation of the aryl ether linkage is close to perpendicular, rather than its preferred torsion of co-planar. That could have been addressed by adding a methyl *ortho* to the phenolic oxygen or replacing the phenolic oxygen with a carbon. Either of those approaches would have been more synthetically challenging.

The development of FAK PROTAC degraders based on FAK ligand VS-4718/PND-1186 (FAK pIC50 8.3) and the Von-Hippel Lindau (VHL) E3-ligase ligand VHL-021 involved empirical linker length and chemotype variations.[173] These resulted in a variety of functional degraders showing cooperativity. However, consistent with the complex SAR commonly seen with PROTACs, there was no simple correlation between linker length, $K_d$, or cooperativity. The most potent degradation was obtained with the unusually short acetamide linker of GSK215, and this compound was selected for further investigation. A 2.2 Å structure was determined by X-ray crystallography to understand the structural determinants of the high cooperativity observed in engagement of FAK and VHL-ElonginC-ElonginB (VCB) by GSK215 (Figure 4.33).

The high ternary complex cooperativity induced by GSK215 was due to many interactions between FAK and VHL that occur at both ends of the PROTAC molecule. As expected, the FAK binding moiety of the PROTAC was completely enclosed by the FAK protein. However, beyond the FAK ligand binding site, the VHL and FAK proteins make many non-cognate, direct protein–protein interactions. While the structure was not used in prospective design in this paper, this work highlighted the importance of thoroughly surveying linker length and rigidity in PROTAC design, and the effect small modifications can have on cooperativity and DC50.

### 4.6.4 Cryo-EM

Cryo-EM may hold even more promise than X-ray for imaging PROTAC and heterobifunctional molecules in their ternary complexes due to its suitability to large flexible complexes over X-ray crystallography.

The anticancer drug indisulam is a fascinating molecule, inhibiting cell proliferation by causing RBM39 degradation through inducing proximity of RBM39 to DCAF15 E3-ligase. Hence, it models a targeted protein degrader mechanism without having the

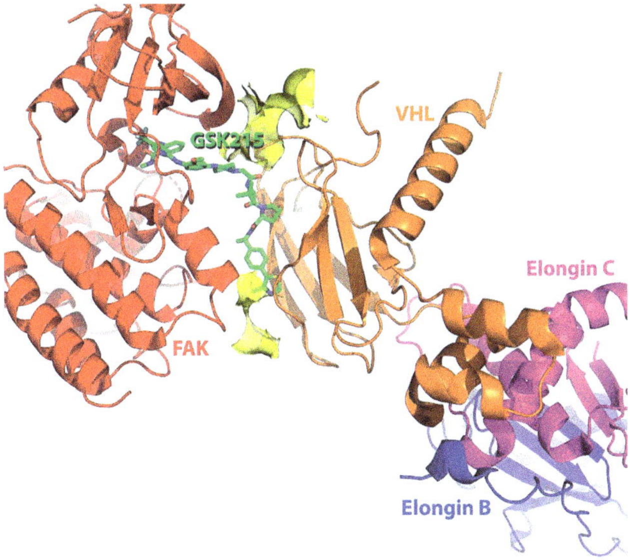


**Figure 4.33** FAK-GSK215-VCB complex (PDB 7PI4). The yellow solvent-accessible surface highlights protein–protein interaction contacts between FAK and VHL.

chemical complexity of a PROTAC molecule. It was unclear whether indisulam acted allosterically by binding DCAF15 or RBM39 to bring about a conformational change that enhances DCAF15-RBM39 interaction, whether indisulam stabilizes a weak DCAF15-RBM39 interaction, or whether indisulam acts as a "molecular glue" to enhance RBM39 binding to DCAF15. To further understand its mode of action, the indisulam structure was determined in complex with E3-ligase components DDB1, DDA1, and DCAF15 by X-ray crystallography (2.3 Å resolution) and cryo-EM (3.5 Å resolution), recruiting part of neosubstrate RBM39 (PDB: 6SJ7 EMD-10213).[162] The X-ray and cryo-EM structures are very similar, with a main chain RMSD of 1.2 Å. The indisulam pose and binding pocket differ slightly. The structure revealed that indisulam is indeed a "molecular glue" (Figures 4.34 and 4.35). It sits in a well-defined pocket formed by DCAF15 and coordinates several direct and water-mediated interactions with both RBM39 and DCAF15. There is also a series of direct protein–protein interactions between DCAF15 and RBM39. These DCAF15-RBM39 interactions are insufficient to enable binding on their own, as interaction in the absence of indisulam could not be detected. It is therefore unlikely that indisulam binds to a site pre-formed by RBM39 and DCAF15. Indisulam failed to bind RBM39 alone but does bind the DCAF15-DDB1-DDA1 complex with weak affinity (~17 μM). However, it binds more tightly in the presence of RBM39 (187 nM). This ~100-fold binding affinity enhancement likely comes from the additional direct and water-mediated polar contacts made between RBM39 and indisulam, along with the series of non-polar interactions emerging from the apparent structural complementarity between DCAF15 and RBM39. Overall, the data suggests that an indisulam-DCAF15 interaction precedes association with RBM39, whose recruitment in turn stabilizes indisulam binding. Medicinal chemists hope the structural insights

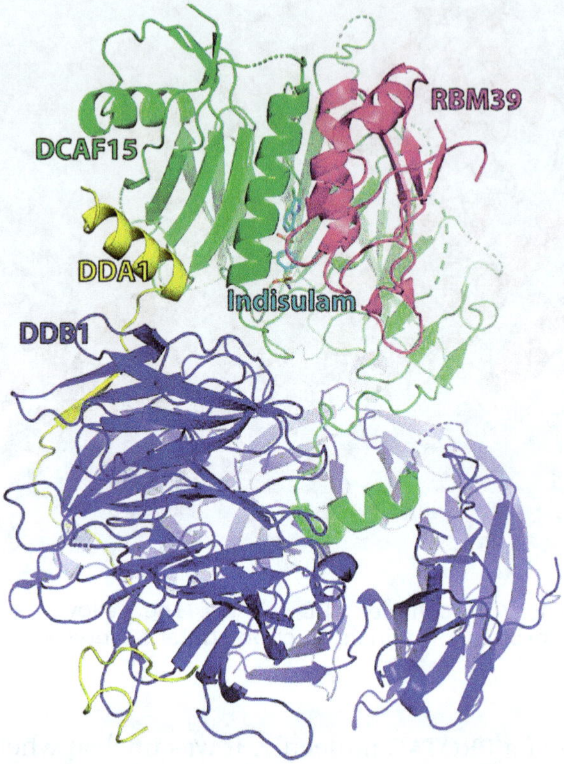


**Figure 4.34** Indisulam complex with DCAF15-DDB1-DDA1-RBM39 (PDB 6SJ7).

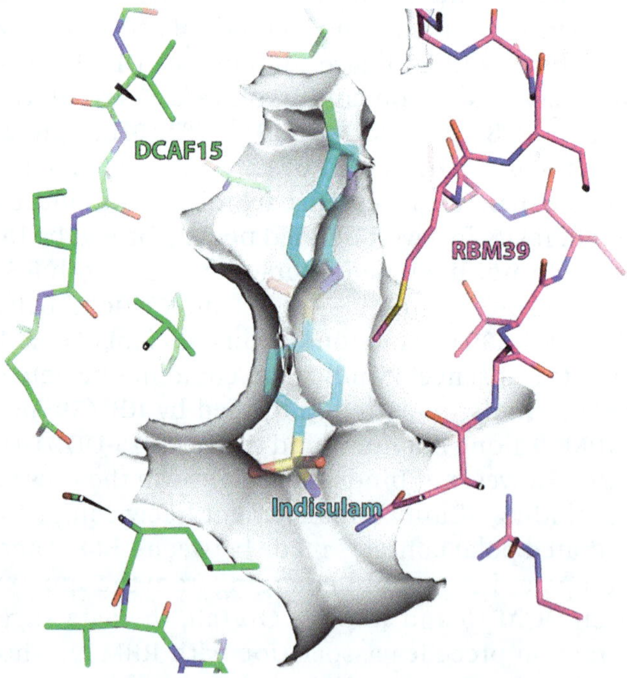


**Figure 4.35** Indisulam is completely buried in the DCAF15-RBM39 protein–protein interface (light gray solvent-accessible surface).

will enable them to exploit the mode of action of indisulam as a platform for novel DCAF15-based molecular glue degraders. However, while the indisulam structure is revealing, it also highlights the incredibly subtle complexity of its mode of action which may be challenging to prospectively exploit to recruit other proteins for degradation from this scaffold.

TRPA1 is an ion channel, expressed on sensory nerves that innervate the respiratory tract. TRPA1 senses oxidative stress and can be activated by a whole range of endogenous and exogenous stimuli irritants leading to coughing and parasympathetic reflex (bronchospasm and mucus production). These activities can be inhibited by selective blockers and hence TRPA1 antagonists have generated broad interest in the pharmaceutical industry for the treatment of respiratory diseases. Multiple antagonist classes have been reported in the literature with a wide range of structural diversity. Cryo-EM structures are now revealing the binding sites for these chemical series, illuminating new opportunities for optimisation, scaffold hopping, and medicinal chemistry design. The group at Genentech[163] found that their lead series, proline sulfonamide and hypoxanthine-based antagonists, bind at two distinct binding sites, a membrane-exposed proline sulfonamide transmembrane site and an intracellular hypoxanthine site near the membrane interface. A retrospective look at the discovery program revealed how the different binding sites, and their location relative to the cell membrane, influenced the optimization trajectories and overall drug profiles of each antagonist class.

### 4.6.5 Machine Learning (ML)

It is inevitable that the explosion in ML/AI will have a growing impact on structure-based drug design. We will likely see the greatest impact by combining physics-based models with ML, such as approaches inspired by ANI.[164] ANI calculates small molecule enthalpies with near quantum mechanics accuracy, but at much faster speed closer to molecular mechanics. Recent methods related to ANI include TorsionNet ligand strain energy analysis[146] and hybrid ML/molecular mechanics protein–ligand models.[165,166] Schrödinger developed active-learning FEP+ to calculate near-FEP+ quality results at very high speed with a ML model.[167]

## 4.7 Summary

Many marketed drugs can trace a key moment in their discovery to a design decision driven by a structure-based approach. For example, structure-guided drug design underpins kinase drug discovery and the FDA has approved 71 small molecule kinase inhibitors (May 2021),[168] a number that has more than doubled since 2015. A recent review[169] highlights the structure-guided drug design impacts on drugs from other target classes since 2015, including darolutamide and apalutamide targeting the androgen receptor for prostate cancer, talazoparib targeting poly(ADP-ribose) polymerase-PARP for advanced breast cancer with germline BRCA mutations, vaborbactam targeting β-lactamase, venetoclax, a BH3 mimetic targeting the anti-apoptotic protein Bcl-2 for the treatment of chronic lymphocytic leukaemia, small lymphocytic lymphoma, or acute myeloid leukaemia, lifitegrast targeting the integrin LFA-1 for dry eye, grazoprevir targeting HCV NS3/4a protease for the treatment of hepatitis C, to name a few examples. With the advent of cryo-EM, even more protein targets are amenable to structure-based design, and as small molecule drug design approaches RNA[170] as a target, opportunities exist there too.

In the 45 years since it began, structure-based drug design is still qualitative and driven by human scientific expertise. Steadily advancing computational methods improve our ability to propose new molecules and not just weed out obviously poor molecules. We are reaching the stage of "augmented design," where computational approaches propose new molecules to be reviewed by human experts. However, many surprises are revealed by experiment through SAR, structural biology, microcalorimetry, SPR, and other biophysical methods. We are still learning how to model and predict protein–ligand interactions and small molecule conformations and their properties. Protein–ligand structures are now frequently available for most drug discovery projects and can be determined quickly enough to keep pace with medicinal chemists. However, frequently does not imply *routinely*: the many steps required to generate a protein–ligand structure are still very demanding and expensive in most cases. X-ray and, increasingly, cryo-EM structures help us interpret SAR and stimulate new design hypotheses in the minds of drug discovery scientists. Structure-based design is an integral part of drug discovery. Medicinal chemists are now fully involved in structure-based design, along with computational chemists, structural biologists, and other project team members.

## 4.8 Hints and Tips

The best design tool is a human expert who carefully analyzes the SAR information and visualizes protein–ligand complexes in 3D, looking for opportunities to improve the ligand's affinity, selectivity, and properties.

The transparent solvent-accessible surface of the binding site provides the simplest and most interpretable visualization to identify unfilled pockets, unsatisfied interactions, suboptimal interactions, and strained conformations.

Use computational tools such as ViewContacts and Line-of-Sight analysis to annotate the protein–ligand complex to identify non-obvious suboptimal interactions and suggest better ones.

Always compare the experimental X-ray or cryo-EM density to the protein–ligand model to see the limits of the model. Collaborate with your structural biologist to interpret and possibly exploit those limits.

Check that your protein–ligand binding site is not at a protein–protein contact in the crystal.

Focus design on shape complementarity between the binding site and ligand first and polar interactions second.

Polar interactions only improve potency if they improve upon the interactions between the free ligand and water, and the protein binding site and water: it's difficult to form better interactions than water. However, well-placed polar interactions can make very large differences.

Try at least one of the many available tools to identify which site waters are good candidates to displace, and consider "empty" space where the experimental structure did not resolve waters, too.

Ensure that protein hydrogen bond donors make good hydrogen bonds with ligand acceptors or water: satisfying protein donors is usually more important than satisfying acceptors.

Flipped binding modes can occur between similar small molecules, whether they are weakly or tightly bound. Treat these different binding modes as separate starting points for the design of a new series: series membership should be viewed as a combination of the chemical series along with its binding mode.

Consult the p*K*(BHX) table to rank-order relative hydrogen bond acceptor strengths for groups to model into your binding site.

Each design should test a specific hypothesis. Most successful structure-based design is iterative, based on previous X-ray co-crystal structures and SAR, plus modeling to test the feasibility of a hypothesis.

Designs should occasionally attempt to push into protein pockets to learn whether they can expand.

Compounds that are unexpectedly active or inactive should be prime candidates for structure determination: outliers sometimes contain surprises that lead to new designs.

The CSD and PDB databases provide excellent sources of data for preferred conformations and interactions. Ensure your bound ligand conformation is close to a preferred low-energy conformation using computational methods to search for the lowest energy conformations, by comparison with molecules with similar torsion types in the CSD, and with newly available strain energy methods.

Small molecules rarely bind to proteins outside of their low-energy conformations. A protein dissipates strain energy through small changes across its many degrees of freedom much more easily than for the ligand to adopt an unfavorable conformation by straining its few rotatable bonds.

Minimize the overall charge of the small molecule to zero or one, avoid strong acids and bases ($pK_a$s $<3$ or $>10$, respectively), and use neutral substituents (or at least those with $pK_a$ close to 7.4) to interact with charged sidechains on the protein.

Binding selectivity between protein isoforms can come not only from sequence differences within the binding site, but also from charge and steric differences further away.

## Key References

The review by Bissantz, Kuhn, and Stahl, and book chapters by Klebe are excellent additional sources to learn about structure-based design

C. Bissantz, B. Kuhn and M. Stahl, *J. Med. Chem.*, 2010, 53, 5061–5084.

G. Klebe, in *Drug Design: Methodology, Concepts and Mode-of-Action*, Springer-Verlag, Berlin Heidelberg, Editon edn., 2013, pp. 61–88.

G. Klebe, in *Drug Design: Methodology, Concepts, and Mode-of-Action*, Springer-Verlag, Berlin Heidelberg, Edition edn., 2013, pp. 429–447.

The keynote reviews by Teague Davis and Kleywegt highlight lessons and limitations in the use of X-ray structures in drug design:

A. Davis, S. Teague and G. Kleywegt, *Angew. Chem., Int. Ed.*, 2003, **42** (24), 2718–2736.
A. Davis, S. St-Gallay and G. Kleywegt, *Drug Discovery Today*, 2008, **13**, 831.

These are the key papers about preferred protein–ligand interactions, preferred small molecule conformations, and hydrogen bond acceptors:

K. A. Brameld, B. Kuhn, D. C. Reuter and M. Stahl, *J. Chem. Inf. Model.*, 2008, **48**, 1–24.
C. Laurence, K. A. Brameld, J. Graton, J.-Y. Le Questel and E. Renault, *J. Med. Chem.*, 2009, **52**, 4073–4086.
B. Kuhn, J. E. Fuchs, M. Reutlinger, M. Stahl and N. R. Taylor, *J. Chem. Inf. Model.*, 2011, **51**, 3180.
A. Tosstorff, J. C. Cole, R. Bartelt and B. Kuhn, *ChemMedChem*, 2021, **16**, 3428.

## References


1. S. M. Paul, D. S. Mytelka, C. T. Dunwiddie, C. C. Persinger, B. H. Munos, S. R. Lindborg and A. L. Schacht, *Nat. Rev. Drug Discovery*, 2010, **9**, 203.
2. J. Blaney, *J. Comput.-Aided Mol. Des.*, 2012, **26**, 13–14.
3. C. Bissantz, B. Kuhn and M. Stahl, *J. Med. Chem.*, 2010, **53**, 5061–5084.
4. G. Klebe, in *Drug Design: Methodology, Concepts and Mode-of-Action*, Springer-Verlag, Berlin Heidelberg, Editon edn, 2013, pp. 61–88.
5. G. Klebe, in *Drug Design: Methodology, Concepts, and Mode-of-Action*, Springer-Verlag, Berlin Heidelberg, Editon edn, 2013, pp. 429–447.
6. C. R. Beddell, P. J. Goodford, F. E. Norrington, S. Wilkinson and R. Wootton, *Br. J. Pharmacol.*, 1976, **57**, 201–209.
7. C. R. Beddell, P. J. Goodford, G. Kneen, R. D. White, S. Wilkinson and R. Wootton, *Br. J. Pharmacol.*, 1984, **82**, 397–407.
8. J. Meyers, B. Fabian and N. Brown, *Drug Discovery Today*, 2021, **26**, 2707.
9. A. Zhavoronkov, Y. A. Ivanenkov, A. Aliper, M. S. Veselov, V. A. Aladinskiy, A. V. Aladinskaya, V. A. Terentiev, D. A. Polykovskiy, M. D. Kuznetsov, A. Asadulaev, Y. Volkov, A. Zholus, R. R. Shayakhmetov, A. Zhebrak, L. I. Minaeva, B. A. Zagribelnyy, L. H. Lee, R. Soll, D. Madge, L. Xing, T. Guo and A. Aspuru-Guzik, *Nat. Biotechnol.*, 2019, **37**, 1038.
10. I. D. Kuntz, J. M. Blaney, S. J. Oatley, R. Langridge and T. E. Ferrin, *J. Mol. Biol.*, 1982, **161**, 269–288.
11. J. B. Cross, D. C. Thompson, B. K. Rai, J. C. Baber, K. Y. Fan, Y. Hu and C. Humblet, *J. Chem. Inf. Model.*, 2009, **49**, 1455–1474.
12. N. Moitessier, P. Englebienne, D. Lee, J. Lawandi and C. R. Corbeil, *Br. J. Pharmacol.*, 2008, **153** Suppl. 1, S7–S26.
13. I. J. Enyedy and W. J. Egan, *J. Comput.-Aided Mol. Des.*, 2008, **22**, 161–168.
14. G. B. McGaughey, R. P. Sheridan, C. I. Bayly, J. C. Culberson, C. Kreatsoulas, S. Lindsley, V. Maiorov, J.-F. Truchon and W. D. Cornell, *J. Chem. Inf. Model.*, 2007, **47**, 1504–1519.
15. G. L. Warren, C. W. Andrews, A.-M. Capelli, B. Clarke, J. LaLonde, M. H. Lambert, M. Lindvall, N. Nevins, S. F. Semus, S. Senger, G. Tedesco, I. D. Wall, J. M. Woolven, C. E. Peishoff and M. S. Head, *J. Med. Chem.*, 2006, **49**, 5912–5931.
16. P. Kolb, R. S. Ferreira, J. J. Irwin and B. K. Shoichet, *Curr. Opin. Biotechnol.*, 2009, **20**, 429–436.
17. A. R. Leach, B. K. Shoichet and C. E. Peishoff, *J. Med. Chem.*, 2006, **49**, 5851–5855.
18. B. J. Bender, S. Gahbauer, A. Luttens, J. Lyu, C. M. Webb, R. M. Stein, E. A. Fink, T. E. Balius, J. Carlsson, J. J. Irwin and B. K. Shoichet, *Nat. Protoc.*, 2021, **16**, 4799–4832.
19. A. Fischer, M. Smiesko, M. Sellner and M. A. Lill, *J. Med. Chem.*, 2021, **64**, 2489.

20. G. B. McGaughey, R. P. Sheridan, C. I. Bayly, J. C. Culberson, C. Kreatsoulas, S. Lindsley, V. Maiorov, J.-F. Truchon and W. D. Cornell, *J. Chem. Inf. Model.*, 2007, **47**, 1504–1519.
21. A. Nicholls, G. B. McGaughey, R. P. Sheridan, A. C. Good, G. Warren, M. Mathieu, S. W. Muchmore, S. P. Brown, J. A. Grant, J. A. Haigh, N. Nevins, A. N. Jain and B. Kelley, *J. Med. Chem.*, 2010, **53**, 3862–3886.
22. S. L. Swann, S. P. Brown, S. W. Muchmore, H. Patel, P. Merta, J. Locklear and P. J. Hajduk, *J. Med. Chem.*, 2011, **54**, 1223–1232.
23. D. Yang, Q. Zhou, V. Labroska, S. Qin, S. Darbalaei, Y. Wu, E. Yuliantie, L. Xie, H. Tao, J. Cheng, Q. Liu, S. Zhao, W. Shui, Y. Jiang and M. W. Wang, *Signal Transduction Targeted Ther.*, 2021, **6**, 7.
24. A. J. Kooistra, S. Mordalski, G. Pandy-Szekeres, M. Esguerra, A. Mamyrbekov, C. Munk, G. M. Keseru and D. E. Gloriam, *Nucleic Acids Res.*, 2021, **49**, D335.
25. M. Congreve, C. de Graaf, N. A. Swain and C. G. Tate, *Cell*, 2020, **181**, 81.
26. H. M. Berman, J. Westbrook, Z. Feng, G. Gilliland, T. N. Bhat, H. Weissig, I. N. Shindyalov and P. E. Bourne, The Protein Data Bank, *Nucleic Acids Res.*, 2000, **28**, 235–242.
27. A. Davis, S. Teague and G. Kleywegt, *Angew. Chem., Int. Ed.*, 2003, **42**(24), 2718.
28. A. Davis, S. St-Gallay and G. Kleywegt, *Drug Discovery Today*, 2008, **13**, 831.
29. J. H. Van Drie and L. Tong, *Bioorg. Med. Chem. Lett.*, 2020, **30**, 127524.
30. T. Nakane, A. Kotecha, A. Sente, G. McMullan, S. Masiulis, P. Brown, I. T. Grigoras, L. Malinauskaite, T. Malinauskas, J. Miehling, T. Uchanski, L. Yu, D. Karia, E. V. Pechnikova, E. de Jong, J. Keizer, M. Bischoff, J. McCormack, P. Tiemeijer, S. W. Hardwick, D. Y. Chirgadze, G. Murshudov, A. R. Aricescu and S. H. W. Scheres, *Nature*, 2020, **587**, 152.
31. https://www.nobelprize.org/prizes/chemistry/2017/summary/.
32. T. M. de Oliveira, L. van Beek, F. Shilliday, J. É. Debreczeni and C. Phillips, Cryo-EM, *SLAS Discovery*, 2021, **26**(1), 17–31.
33. J. Garcia-Nafria and C. G. Tate, *Biochem. Soc. Trans.*, 2021, **49**, 2345.
34. S. Teague, *Nat. Rev. Drug Discovery*, 2003, **2**, 527.
35. A. M. Davis and S. J. Teague, *Angew. Chem., Int. Ed.*, 1999, **38**, 736–749.
36. J. W. Liebeschuetz, *J. Med. Chem.*, 2021, **64**(11), 7533–7543.
37. B. Wienen-Schmidt, M. Oebbeke, K. Ngo, A. Heine and G. Klebe, *ChemMedChem*, 2021, **16**(1), 292–300.
38. M. Baek and D. Baker, *Nat. Methods*, 2022, **19**, 11.
39. A. Kryshtafovych, T. Schwede, M. Topf, K. Fidelis and J. Moult, *Proteins: Struct., Funct., Bioinf.*, 2021, **89**(12), 1607–1617.
40. https://www.alphafold.ebi.ac.uk/
41. M. Varadi, S. Anyango, M. Deshpande, S. Nair, C. Natassia, G. Yordanova, D. Yuan, O. Stroe, G. Wood and G. Kleywegt, *et al.*, *Nucleic Acids Res.*, 2021, D439–D444.
42. https://robetta.bakerlab.org/
43. M. Baek, F. DiMaio, I. Anishchenko, J. Dauparas, S. Ovchinnikov, G.-R. Lee, J. Wang, Q. Cong, L. N. Kinch and R. D. Schaeffer, *et al.*, *Science*, 2021, **373**(6557), 871–876.
44. I. R. Humphreys, J. Pei, M. Baek, A. Krishnakumar, I. Anishchenko, S. Ovchinnikov, J. Zhang, T. J. Ness, S. Banjade, S. R. Bagde, V. G. Stancheva, X. H. Li, K. Liu, Z. Zheng, D. J. Barrero, U. Roy, J. Kuper, I. S. Fernandez, B. Szakal, D. Branzei, J. Rizo, C. Kisker, E. C. Greene, S. Biggins, S. Keeney, E. A. Miller, J. C. Fromme, T. L. Hendrickson, Q. Cong and D. Baker, *Science*, 2021, **374**, eabm4805.
45. R. Evans, M. O'Neill, A. Pritzel, N. Antropova, A. Senior, T. Green, A. Žídek, R. Bates, S. Blackwell, J. Yim, O. Ronneberger, S. Bodenstein, M. Zielinski, A. Bridgland, A. Potapenko, A. Cowie, K. Tunyasuvunakool, R. Jain, E. Clancy, P. Kohli, J. Jumper and D. Hassabis, bioRxiv 2021.10.04.463034, doi: https://doi.org/10.1101/2021.10.04.463034.
46. A. Alon, J. Lyu, J. M. Braz, T. A. Tummino, V. Craik, M. J. O'Meara, C. M. Webb, D. S. Radchenko, Y. S. Moroz, X. P. Huang, Y. Liu, B. L. Roth, J. J. Irwin, A. I. Basbaum, B. K. Shoichet and A. C. Kruse, *Nature*, 2021, **600**, 759.
47. Y. Shan, V. P. Mysore, A. E. Leffler, E. T. Kim, S. Sagawa and D. E. Shaw, *PLoS Comput Biol.*, 2022, **18**(3), e1009817.
48. A. Kuzmanic, G. R. Bowman, J. Juarez-Jimenez, J. Michel and F. L. Gervasio, *Acc. Chem. Res.*, 2020, **53**, 654.
49. P. Cimermancic, P. Weinkam, T. J. Rettenmaier, L. Bichmann, D. A. Keedy, R. A. Woldeyes, D. Schneidman-Duhovny, O. N. Demerdash, J. C. Mitchell, J. A. Wells, J. S. Fraser and A. Sali, *J. Mol. Biol.*, 2016, **428**, 709.
50. M. L. Connolly, *Science*, 1983, **221**, 709–713.
51. F. Lovering, J. Bikker and C. Humblet, *J. Med. Chem.*, 2009, **52**, 6752–6756.

52. C. Hansch, A. Leo and D. Hoekman, *Exploring QSAR: Hydrophobic, Electronic, and Steric Constants*, American Chemical Society, Washington, D.C., 1995.
53. Schrödinger, L. L. C., *The PyMOL Molecular Graphics System, Version 2.0*, 2022.
54. A. Zhavoronkov, B. Zagribelnyy, A. Zhebrak, V. Aladinskiy, V. Terentiev, Q. Vanhaelen, D. S. Bezrukov, D. Polykovskiy, R. Shayakhmetov, A. Filimonov, M. Bishop, S. McCloskey, E. Leija, D. Bright, K. Funakawa, Y. Lin, S. Huang, H. Liao, A. Aliper and Y. Ivanenkov ChemRxiv, DOI: 10.26434/chemrxiv.12301457.v1.2020.
55. L. M. Salonen, M. C. Holland, P. S. J. Kaib, W. Haap, J. Benz, J.-L. Mary, O. Kuster, W. B. Schweizer, D. W. Banner and F. Diederich, *Chem. –Eur. J.*, 2012, **18**, 213.
56. T. Qin, M. Cook and M. Courtney, *J. Chem. Educ.*, 2020, **98**, 521.
57. L. J. Kingsley, V. Brunet, G. Lelais, S. McCloskey, K. Milliken, E. Leija, S. R. Fuhs, K. Wang, E. Zhou and G. Spraggon, *J. Mol. Graphics Modell.*, 2019, **89**, 234.
58. A. R. Fersht, J. P. Shi, J. Knill-Jones, D. M. Lowe, A. J. Wilkinson, D. M. Blow, P. Brick, P. Carter, M. M. Waye and G. Winter, *Nature*, 1985, **314**, 235–238.
59. F. Spyrakis, M. H. Ahmed, A. S. Bayden, P. Cozzini, A. Mozzarelli and G. E. Kellogg, *J. Med. Chem.*, 2017, **60**, 6781.
60. D. D. Robinson, W. Sherman and R. Farid, *ChemMedChem*, 2010, **5**, 618–627.
61. D. L. Mobley and M. K. Gilson, *Annu. Rev. Biophys.*, 2017, **46**, 531.
62. D. Cappel, W. Sherman and T. Beuming, *Curr. Top. Med. Chem.*, 2017, **17**, 2586.
63. S. W. Jung, M. Kim, S. Ramsey, T. Kurtzman and A. E. Cho, *Sci. Rep.*, 2018, **8**, 10400.
64. T. E. Balius, M. Fischer, R. M. Stein, T. B. Adler, C. N. Nguyen, A. Cruz, M. K. Gilson, T. Kurtzman and B. K. Shoichet, *Proc. Natl. Acad. Sci. U. S. A.*, 2017, **114**, E6839.
65. R. M. Cooke, A. J. Brown, F. H. Marshall and J. S. Mason, *Drug Discovery Today*, 2015, **20**, 1355.
66. B. Kuhn, J. E. Fuchs, M. Reutlinger, M. Stahl and N. R. Taylor, *J. Chem. Inf. Model.*, 2011, **51**, 3180.
67. T. Young, R. Abel, B. Kim, B. J. Berne and R. A. Friesner, *Proc. Natl. Acad. Sci. U. S. A.*, 2007, **104**, 808–813.
68. R. Abel, T. Young, R. Farid, B. J. Berne and R. A. Friesner, *J. Am. Chem. Soc.*, 2008, **130**, 2817–2831.
69. Chemical Computing Group Inc., *Molecular Operating Environment (MOE)*, Montreal, QC, Canada, 2013.
70. OpenEye Scientific Software, Santa Fe, NM, Editon edn., 2013.
71. A. Amadasi, J. A. Surface, F. Spyrakis, P. Cozzini, A. Mozzarelli and G. E. Kellogg, *J. Med. Chem.*, 2008, **51**, 1063.
72. M. Baroni, G. Cruciani, S. Sciabola, F. Perruccio and J. S. Mason, *J. Chem. Inf. Model.*, 2007, **47**, 279.
73. E. Nittinger, P. Gibbons, C. Eigenbrot, D. R. Davies, B. Maurer, C. L. Yu, J. R. Kiefer, A. Kuglstatter, J. Murray, D. F. Ortwine, Y. Tang and V. Tsui, *J. Comput.-Aided Mol. Des.*, 2019, **33**, 307.
74. D. Bucher, P. Stouten and N. Triballeau, *J. Chem. Inf. Model.*, 2018, **58**, 692.
75. B. Breiten, M. R. Lockett, W. Sherman, S. Fujita, M. Al-Sayah, H. Lange, C. M. Bowers, A. Heroux, G. Krilov and G. M. Whitesides, *J. Am. Chem. Soc.*, 2013, **135**, 15579.
76. S. G. Krimmer, J. Cramer, M. Betz, V. Fridh, R. Karlsson, A. Heine and G. Klebe, *J. Med. Chem.*, 2016, **59**, 10530.
77. M. Betz, T. Wulsdorf, S. G. Krimmer and G. Klebe, *J. Chem. Inf. Model.*, 2016, **56**, 223.
78. S. G. Krimmer, M. Betz, A. Heine and G. Klebe, *ChemMedChem*, 2014, **9**, 833.
79. M. T. Stubbs, S. Reyda, F. Dullweber, M. Möller, G. Klebe, D. Dorsch, W. W. K. R. Mederski and H. Wurziger, *Chembiochem*, 2002, **3**, 246–249.
80. E. Freire, *Drug Discovery Today*, 2008, **13**, 869–874.
81. E. Freire, *Chem. Biol. Drug Des.*, 2009, **74**, 468–472.
82. J. E. Ladbury, G. Klebe and E. Freire, *Nat. Rev. Drug Discovery*, 2010, **9**, 23–27.
83. G. Klebe, *Drug Discovery Today*, 2019, **24**, 943.
84. A. Biela, N. N. Nasief, M. Betz, A. Heine, D. Hangauer and G. Klebe, *Angew. Chem., Int. Ed.*, 2013, **52**, 1822.
85. P. W. Snyder, J. Mecinovic, D. T. Moustakas, S. W. Thomas 3rd, M. Harder, E. T. Mack, M. R. Lockett, A. Heroux, W. Sherman and G. M. Whitesides, *Proc. Natl. Acad. Sci. U. S. A.*, 2011, **108**, 17889.
86. C. Gerlach, M. Smolinski, H. Steuber, C. A. Sotriffer, A. Heine, D. G. Hangauer and G. Klebe, *Angew. Chem., Int. Ed.*, 2007, **46**, 8511–8514.
87. P. Kukic, D. Farrell, L. P. McIntosh, B. García-Moreno E, K. S. Jensen, Z. Toleikis, K. Teilum and J. E. Nielsen, *J. Am. Chem. Soc.*, 2013, **135**, 16968–16976.
88. A. J. Russell and A. R. Fersht, *Nature*, 1987, **328**, 496–500.
89. H. Weinstabl, M. Treu, J. Rinnenthal, S. K. Zahn, P. Ettmayer, G. Bader, G. Dahmann, D. Kessler, K. Rumpel, N. Mischerikow, F. Savarese, T. Gerstberger, M. Mayer, A. Zoephel, R. Schnitzer, W.

Sommergruber, P. Martinelli, H. Arnhof, B. Peric-Simov, K. S. Hofbauer, G. Garavel, Y. Scherbantin, S. Mitzner, T. N. Fett, G. Scholz, J. Bruchhaus, M. Burkard, R. Kousek, T. Ciftci, B. Sharps, A. Schrenk, C. Harrer, D. Haering, B. Wolkerstorfer, X. Zhang, X. Lv, A. Du, D. Li, Y. Li, J. Quant, M. Pearson and D. B. McConnell, *J. Med. Chem.*, 2019, **62**, 7976.

90. K. A. Armstrong, B. Tidor and A. C. Cheng, *J. Med. Chem.*, 2006, **49**, 2470.
91. Y. Shen, M. K. Gilson and B. Tidor, *J. Chem. Theory Comput.*, 2012, **8**, 4580.
92. D. J. Huggins, W. Sherman and B. Tidor, *J. Med. Chem.*, 2012, 1424–1444.
93. K. Albanese, J. D. Chodera, A. Volkamer, S. Keng, R. Abel and L. Wang, *J. Chem. Inf. Model.*, 2020, **60**, 6211.
94. A. D. Wade and D. J. Huggins, *J. Chem. Theory Comput.*, 2019, **15**, 6504.
95. A. D. Wade, A. Rizzi, Y. Wang and D. J. Huggins, *J. Chem. Inf. Model.*, 2019, **59**, 2776.
96. G. L. Warren, T. D. Do, B. P. Kelley, A. Nicholls and S. D. Warren, *Drug Discovery Today*, 2012, 1270–1281.
97. J. Liebeschuetz, J. Hennemann, T. Olsson and C. R. Groom, *J. Comput.-Aided Mol. Des.*, 2012, **26**, 169–183.
98. J. Tong and S. Zhao, *J. Chem. Inf. Model.*, 2021, **61**, 1180.
99. K. A. Brameld, B. Kuhn, D. C. Reuter and M. Stahl, *J. Chem. Inf. Model.*, 2008, **48**, 1–24.
100. F. H. Allen, *Acta Crystallogr., Sect. B: Struct. Sci.*, 2002, **58**, 380.
101. R. Taylor and P. A. Wood, *Chem. Rev.*, 2019, **119**, 9427.
102. M. Harder, B. Kuhn and F. Diederich, *ChemMedChem*, 2013, **8**, 397.
103. E. A. Meyer, R. K. Castellano and F. Diederich, *Angew. Chem., Int. Ed.*, 2003, **42**, 1210.
104. K. Müller, C. Faeh and F. Diederich, *Science*, 2007, **317**, 1881.
105. R. Paulini, K. Müller and F. Diederich, *Angew. Chem., Int. Ed.*, 2005, **44**, 1788.
106. L. M. Salonen, M. Ellermann and F. Diederich, *Angew. Chem., Int. Ed.*, 2011, **50**, 4808.
107. A. Tosstorff, J. C. Cole, R. Bartelt and B. Kuhn, *ChemMedChem*, 2021, **16**, 3428.
108. A. Tosstorff, J. C. Cole, R. Taylor, S. F. Harris and B. Kuhn, *J. Chem. Inf. Model.*, 2020, **60**, 6595.
109. B. Kuhn, E. Gilberg, R. Taylor, J. Cole and O. Korb, *J. Med. Chem.*, 2019, **62**, 10441.
110. W. Guba, A. Meyder, M. Rarey and J. Hert, *J. Chem. Inf. Model.*, 2016, **56**, 1.
111. C. Schärfer, T. Schulz-Gasch, H.-C. Ehrlich, W. Guba, M. Rarey and M. Stahl, *J. Med. Chem.*, 2013, **56**, 2016.
112. S. J. Cottrell, T. S. G. Olsson, R. Taylor, J. C. Cole and J. W. Liebeschuetz, *J. Chem. Inf. Model.*, 2012, **52**, 956.
113. S. E. Wright, M. J. Bryant and A. J. Cruz-Cabeza, *CrystEngComm*, 2020, **22**, 7217.
114. A. J. Cruz-Cabeza, J. W. Liebeschuetz and F. H. Allen, *CrystEngComm*, 2012, **14**, 6797.
115. R. Wilcken, M. O. Zimmermann, A. Lange, A. C. Joerger and F. M. Boeckler, *J. Med. Chem.*, 2013, **56**, 1363.
116. L. A. Hardegger, B. Kuhn, B. Spinnler, L. Anselm, R. Ecabert, M. Stihle, B. Gsell, R. Thoma, J. Diez, J. Benz, J.-M. Plancher, G. Hartmann, Y. Isshiki, K. Morikami, N. Shimma, W. Haap, D. W. Banner and F. Diederich, *ChemMedChem*, 2011, **6**, 2048.
117. R. Taylor, *CrystEngComm*, 2014, **16**, 6852.
118. E. D. Garcin, A. S. Arvai, R. J. Rosenfeld, M. D. Kroeger, B. R. Crane, G. Andersson, G. Andrews, P. J. Hamley, P. R. Mallinder, D. J. Nicholls, S. A. St-Gallay, A. C. Tinker, N. P. Gensmantel, A. Mete, D. R. Cheshire, S. Connolly, D. J. Stuehr, A. Aberg, A. V. Wallace, J. A. Tainer and E. D. Getzoff, *Nat. Chem. Biol.*, 2008, **4**, 700.
119. D. R. Cheshire, A. Aberg, G. M. K. Andersson, G. Andrews, H. G. Beaton, T. N. Birkinshaw, N. Boughton-Smith, S. Connolly, T. R. Cook, A. Cooper, S. L. Cooper, D. Cox, J. Dixon, N. Gensmantel, P. J. Hamley, R. Harrison, P. Hartopp, H. Käck, P. D. Leeson, T. Luker, A. Mete, I. Millichip, D. J. Nicholls, A. D. Pimm, S. A. St-Gallay and A. V. Wallace, *Bioorg. Med. Chem. Lett.*, 2011, **21**, 2468.
120. M. Cowart, E. A. Kowaluk, J. F. Daanen, K. L. Kohlhaas, K. M. Alexander, F. L. Wagenaar and J. F. Kerwin, *J. Med. Chem.*, 1998, **41**, 2636.
121. B. Kuhn, W. Haap, U. Obst-Sander, C. Kramer and M. Stahl, *ChemMedChem*, 2021, **16**, 2760.
122. O. Korb, B. Kuhn, J. Hert, N. Taylor, J. Cole, C. Groom and M. Stahl, *J. Med. Chem.*, 2016, **59**, 4257.
123. J. A. Grant, M. A. Gallardo and B. T. Pickup, *J. Comput. Chem.*, 1996, **17**, 1653.
124. A. C. Pan, D. W. Borhani, R. O. Dror and D. E. Shaw, *Drug Discovery Today*, 2013, **18**, 667–673.
125. S. Piana, K. Lindorff-Larsen and D. E. Shaw, *Proc. Natl. Acad. Sci. U. S. A.*, 2012, **109**, 17845–17850.
126. Y. Shan, E. T. Kim, M. P. Eastwood, R. O. Dror, M. A. Seeliger and D. E. Shaw, *J. Am. Chem. Soc.*, 2011, **133**, 9181–9183.
127. S. S. Antonysamy, B. Aubol, J. Blaney, M. F. Browner, A. M. Giannetti, S. F. Harris, N. Hebert, J. Hendle, S. Hopkins, E. Jefferson, C. Kissinger, V. Leveque, D. Marciano, E. McGee, I. Nájera, B. Nolan, M. Tomimoto, E. Torres and T. Wright, *Bioorg. Med. Chem. Lett.*, 2008, **18**, 2990–2995.

128. H. Li, J. Tatlock, A. Linton, J. Gonzalez, T. Jewell, L. Patel, S. Ludlum, M. Drowns, S. V. Rahavendran, H. Skor, R. Hunter, S. T. Shi, K. J. Herlihy, H. Parge, M. Hickey, X. Yu, F. Chau, J. Nonomiya and C. Lewis, *J. Med. Chem.*, 2009, **52**(5), 1255.
129. M. A. Williams and J. E. Ladbury, *Methods Princ. Med. Chem.*, 2003, **19**, 137–161.
130. C. Laurence, K. A. Brameld, J. Graton, J.-Y. Le Questel and E. Renault, *J. Med. Chem.*, 2009, **52**, 4073–4086.
131. A. J. Green and P. L. A. Popelier, *J. Chem. Inf. Model.*, 2014, **54**, 553.
132. L. Wang, Y. Wu, Y. Deng, B. Kim, L. Pierce, G. Krilov, D. Lupyan, S. Robinson, M. K. Dahlgren, J. Greenwood, D. L. Romero, C. Masse, J. L. Knight, T. Steinbrecher, T. Beuming, W. Damm, E. Harder, W. Sherman, M. Brewer, R. Wester, M. Murcko, L. Frye, R. Farid, T. Lin, D. L. Mobley, W. L. Jorgensen, B. J. Berne, R. A. Friesner and R. Abel, *J. Am. Chem. Soc.*, 2015, **137**, 2695.
133. T. S. Lee, B. K. Allen, T. J. Giese, Z. Guo, P. Li, C. Lin, T. D. McGee Jr, D. A. Pearlman, B. K. Radak, Y. Tao, H. C. Tsai, H. Xu, W. Sherman and D. M. York, *J. Chem. Inf. Model.*, 2020, **60**, 5595.
134. Z. Cournia, B. Allen and W. Sherman, *J. Chem. Inf. Model.*, 2017, **57**, 2911.
135. R. Abel, S. Mondal, C. Masse, J. Greenwood, G. Harriman, M. A. Ashwell, S. Bhat, R. Wester, L. Frye, R. Kapeller and R. A. Friesner, *Curr. Opin. Struct. Biol.*, 2017, **43**, 38.
136. L. Wang, Y. Deng, Y. Wu, B. Kim, D. N. LeBard, D. Wandschneider, M. Beachy, R. A. Friesner and R. Abel, *J. Chem. Theory Comput.*, 2017, **13**, 42.
137. T. B. Steinbrecher, M. Dahlgren, D. Cappel, T. Lin, L. Wang, G. Krilov, R. Abel, R. Friesner and W. Sherman, *J. Chem. Inf. Model.*, 2015, **55**, 2411.
138. C. E. M. Schindler, H. Baumann, A. Blum, D. Bose, H. P. Buchstaller, L. Burgdorf, D. Cappel, E. Chekler, P. Czodrowski, D. Dorsch, M. K. I. Eguida, B. Follows, T. Fuchss, U. Gradler, J. Gunera, T. Johnson, C. Jorand Lebrun, S. Karra, M. Klein, T. Knehans, L. Koetzner, M. Krier, M. Leiendecker, B. Leuthner, L. Li, I. Mochalkin, D. Musil, C. Neagu, F. Rippmann, K. Schiemann, R. Schulz, T. Steinbrecher, E. M. Tanzer, A. Unzue Lopez, A. Viacava Follis, A. Wegener and D. Kuhn, *J. Chem. Inf. Model.*, 2020, **60**, 5457.
139. Z. Li, Y. Huang, Y. Wu, J. Chen, D. Wu, C. G. Zhan and H. B. Luo, *J. Med. Chem.*, 2019, **62**, 2099.
140. G. Heinzelmann and M. K. Gilson, *Sci. Rep.*, 2021, **11**, 1116.
141. I. J. Bruno, J. C. Cole, M. Kessler, J. Luo, W. D. S. Motherwell, L. H. Purkis, B. R. Smith, R. Taylor, R. I. Cooper, S. E. Harris and A. G. Orpen, *J. Chem. Inf. Comput. Sci.*, 2004, **44**, 2133.
142. M. L. Lee, I. Aliagas, J. A. Feng, T. Gabriel, T. J. O'Donnell, B. D. Sellers, B. Wiswedel and A. Gobbi, *J. Cheminf.*, 2017, **9**, 38.
143. S. Gu, M. S. Smith, Y. Yang, J. J. Irwin and B. K. Shoichet, *J. Chem. Inf. Model.*, 2021, **61**, 4331.
144. B. D. Sellers, N. C. James and A. Gobbi, *J. Chem. Inf. Model.*, 2017, **57**, 1265.
145. B. K. Rai, V. Sresht, Q. Yang, R. Unwalla, M. Tu, A. M. Mathiowetz and G. A. Bakken, *J. Chem. Inf. Model.*, 2019, **59**, 4195.
146. B. Rai, V. Sresht, Q. Yang, R. J. Unwalla, M. Tu, A. M. Mathiowetz, and G. A. Bakken, *J. Chem. Inf. Model.*, 2022, **62**, 785–800.
147. P. A. Rejto and G. M. Verkhivker, *Proc. Natl. Acad. Sci. U. S. A.*, 1996, **93**, 8945.
148. S. Ruiz-Carmona, P. Schmidtke, F. J. Luque, L. Baker, N. Matassova, B. Davis, S. Roughley, J. Murray, R. Hubbard and X. Barril, *Nat. Chem.*, 2017, **9**, 201.
149. A. Sadybekov, A. V. Sadybekov, Y. Liu, C. Iliopoulos-Tsoutsouvas, X. P. Huang, J. Pickett, B. Houser, N. Patel, N. K. Tran, F. Tong, N. Zvonok, M. K. Jain, O. Savych, D. S. Radchenko, S. P. Nikas, N. A. Petasis, Y. S. Moroz, B. L. Roth, A. Makriyannis and V. Katritch, *Nature*, 2022, **601**, 452–459.
150. A. L. Perryman, D. N. Santiago, S. Forli, D. Santos-Martins and A. J. Olson, Virtual screening with AutoDock Vina and the common pharmacophore engine of a low diversity library of fragments and hits against the three allosteric sites of HIV integrase: Participation in the SAMPL4 protein–ligand binding challenge, *J. Comput.-Aided Mol. Des.*, 2014, **28**, 429–441.
151. R. Lonsdale and R. A. Ward, *Chem. Soc. Rev.*, 2018, **47**, 3816.
152. L. Wei, W. Wen, L. Rao, Y. Huang, M. Lei, K. Liu, S. Hu, R. Song, Y. Ren and J. Wan, *J. Chem. Inf. Model.*, 2020, **60**(9), 4388–4402.
153. R. C. Harris, R. Liu and J. Shen, *J. Chem. Theory Comput.*, 2020, **16**, 3689.
154. X. Wan, T. Yang, A. Cuesta, X. Pang, T. E. Balius, J. J. Irwin, B. K. Shoichet and J. Taunton, *J. Am. Chem. Soc.*, 2020, **142**, 4960.
155. H. Du, J. Gao, G. Weng, J. Ding, X. Chai, J. Pang, Y. Kang, D. Li, D. Cao and T. Hou, *Nucleic Acids Res.*, 2021, **49**(D1), D1122–D1129.
156. Y. Shen, F. Li, M. M. Szewczyk, L. Halabelian, K. S. Park, I. Chau, A. Dong, H. Zeng, H. Chen, F. Meng, D. Barsyte-Lovejoy, C. H. Arrowsmith, P. J. Brown, J. Liu, M. Vedadi and J. Jin, *J. Med. Chem.*, 2020, **63**, 5477.

157. G. Du, S. Rao, D. Gurbani, N. J. Henning, J. Jiang, J. Che, A. Yang, S. B. Ficarro, J. A. Marto and A. J. Aguirre, *et al.*, *J. Med. Chem.*, 2020, **63**(4), 1624–1641.
158. A. Gironda-Martínez, E. J. Donckele, F. Samain and D. Neri, *ACS Pharmacol. Transl. Sci.*, 2021, **4**, 1265.
159. J. W. Cuozzo, P. A. Centrella, D. Gikunju, S. Habeshian, C. D. Hupp, A. D. Keefe, E. A. Sigel, H. H. Soutter, H. A. Thomson and Y. Zhang, *et al.*, *ChemBioChem*, 2017, **18**(9), 864–887.
160. K. McCloskey, E. A. Sigel, S. Kearnes, L. Xue, X. Tian, D. Moccia, D. Gikunju, S. Bazzaz, B. Chan, M. A. Clark, J. W. Cuozzo, M. A. Guie, J. P. Guilinger, C. Huguet, C. D. Hupp, A. D. Keefe, C. J. Mulhern, Y. Zhang and P. Riley, *J. Med. Chem.*, 2020, **63**, 8857.
161. A. Testa, S. J. Hughes, X. Lucas, J. E. Wright and A. Ciulli, *Angew. Chem., Int. Ed.*, 2020, **59**(4), 1727–1734.
162. D. E. Bussiere, L. Xie and H. Srinivas, *et al.*, *Nat. Chem. Biol.*, 2020, **16**, 15–23.
163. E. Villemure, J. A. Terrett, R. Larouche-Gauthier, M. Déry, H. Chen, R. M. Reese, S. D. Shields, J. Chen, S. Magnuson and M. Volgraf, *ACS Med. Chem. Lett.*, 2021, **12**(8), 1230–1237.
164. S. Smith, O. Isayev and A. E. Roitberg, *Chem. Sci.*, 2017, **8**, 3192.
165. S. J. Lahey and C. N. Rowley, *Chem. Sci.*, 2020, **11**, 2362.
166. D. A. Rufa, H. E. Bruce Macdonald, J. Fass, M. Wieder, P. B. Grinaway, A. E. Roitberg, O. Isayev and J. D. Chodera, bioRxiv, 2020, 2020.07.29.227959.
167. K. D. Konze, P. H. Bos, M. K. Dahlgren, K. Leswing, I. Tubert-Brohman, A. Bortolato, B. Robbason, R. Abel and S. Bhat, *J. Chem. Inf. Model.*, 2019, **59**, 3782.
168. M. M. Attwood, D. Fabbro and A. V. Sokolov, *et al.*, *Nat. Rev. Drug Discovery*, 2021, **20**, 839–861.
169. V. T. Sabe, T. Ntombela, L. A. Jhamba, G. E. M. Maguire, T. Govender, T. Naicker and H. G. Kruger, *Eur. J. Med. Chem.*, 2021, **224**, 113705.
170. J. Manigrasso, M. Marcia and M. De Vivo, *Chem*, 2021, 7(11), 2965–2988.
171. T. A. Halgren, *J. Comput. Chem.*, 1999, **20**, 730.
172. T. A. Halgren, *J. Comput. Chem.*, 1996, **17**, 490.
173. R. P. Law, J. Nunes, C. W. Chung, M. Bantscheff, K. Buda, H. Dai, J. P. Evans, A. Flinders, D. Klimaszewska, A. J. Lewis, M. Muelbaier, P. Scott-Stevens, P. Stacey, C. J. Tame, G. F. Watt, N. Zinn, M. A. Queisser, J. D. Harling and A. B. Benowitz, *Angew. Chem.*, 2021, **60**, 23327–23334.

# 5 Fragment-based Ligand Discovery (FBLD)

Roderick E. Hubbard( 0000-0002-8233-7461)*[a,b]

[a]YSBL, University of York, Heslington, York, YO10 5DD, UK; [b]Vernalis (R&D) Ltd, Granta Park, Abington, Cambridge, CB21 6GB, UK
*E-mail: roderick.hubbard@york.ac.uk

## 5.1 Introduction

The starting point for small molecule drug discovery programs is to identify initial "hit" compounds that bind to the target and which have the potential for optimisation to clinical candidates with the desired therapeutic effect. For many organisations, the preferred way of identifying such compounds has conventionally been by screening large numbers (often millions) of compounds in some cellular, biochemical, or target binding assay (High Throughput Screening, HTS). Usually, these compounds are of molecular weight 300 to 450 Da and selected to have appropriate drug-like[1–3] or lead-like[4,5] properties. There are two major issues with such approaches. The first is that these initial hits usually need substantial and often challenging modification to introduce the required properties. The second is that HTS often generates no tractable hits, particularly for new target classes. Even with many millions of compounds, HTS only samples a very small fraction of available chemical space and the collection is usually dominated by compounds from previous drug discovery campaigns.[6]

The essential feature of fragment-based methods is that drug discovery begins with screening of a relatively small library (typically 1000s) of compounds of low molecular weight (average 190 Da) that are more likely to bind because they fit into the binding site.[7] The fragment hits are then evolved, usually guided by the structure of the compounds bound to the therapeutic target, to larger lead compounds which can then be optimised by conventional medicinal chemistry methods. There have been great advances in the methods of fragment-based ligand discovery over the past 25 years, and

The Handbook of Medicinal Chemistry: Principles and Practice, 2nd Edition
Edited by Simon E. Ward and Andrew M. Davis

Published by the Royal Society of Chemistry, www.rsc.org

there are now many compounds in the clinic (summarised in ref. 8) and several fragment-derived drugs have now been approved and are on the market.[9–12]

This chapter provides an overview of the current practise of fragment-based ligand discovery (see also previous reviews[13–20]). The emphasis is on practical aspects of the methods. Although there are some examples of fragments binding to other targets (such as nucleic acids[21]), the methods have been mostly applied to protein targets, which will be the focus of this discussion. In addition, a section describing some of the history of the evolution of fragment-based discovery is included.

## 5.2 The General Features of FBLD

Figure 5.1 is a summary of the general approach to fragment-based discovery that has been developed at Vernalis over the past 20 years.[19,22] Most practitioners have a similar approach: a fragment library is screened, usually by a biophysical method. Information about fragments is combined with other hits from virtual or experimental screening of conventional libraries (such as by HTS or screening of DNA-encoded libraries, DEL) and from the literature. The binding of the various hits is usually validated by one or more orthogonal biophysical methods while attempts are made to determine a structure, preferably by X-ray crystallography, but if necessary, using NMR and other methods to generate models of ligand binding.

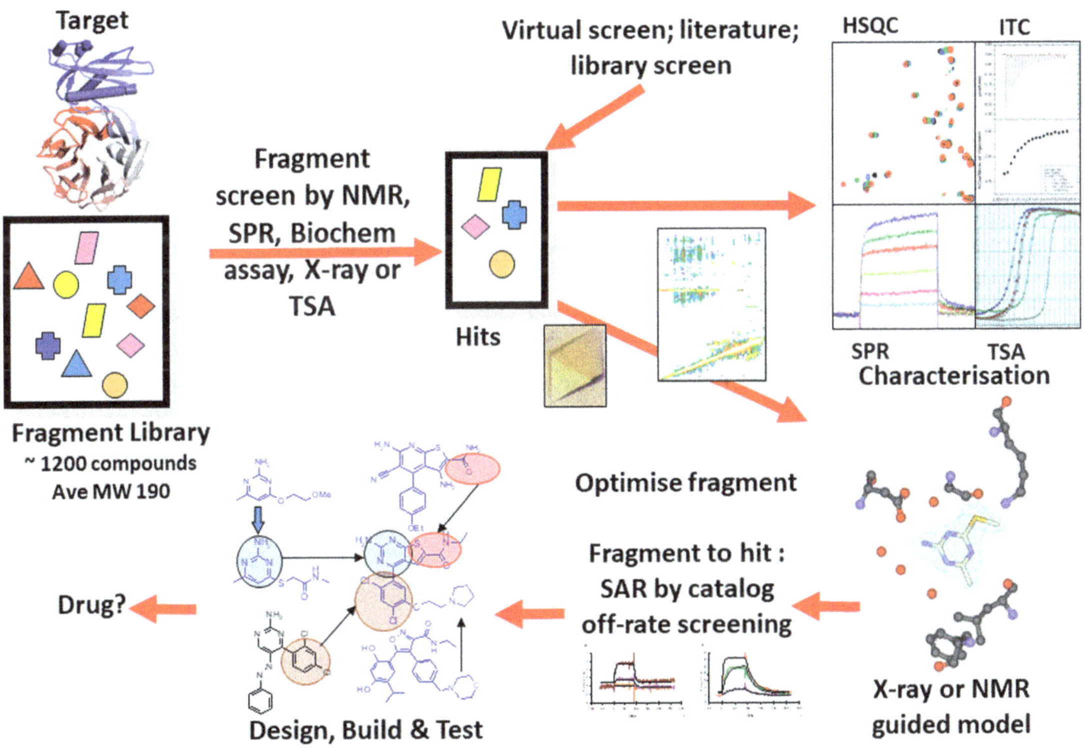


Figure 5.1 A schematic representation of the overall fragment-based drug discovery process at Vernalis. See text for details.

Finding fragments that bind to most binding sites on most targets is relatively straightforward: the challenge is knowing what to do with the fragments – both in choosing which fragments to progress and how to evolve them to compounds which can be advanced like any other compound in lead optimisation. An important first step is to optimise the fragment core itself, exploring SAR by purchase (often called SAR by catalogue) or limited synthesis to test binding hypotheses and to identify the key vectors for optimisation. There are two key characteristics that fragments bring to the fragment to hit to lead optimisation process. The first is that for most targets, fragment screening provides choice in the number and diversity of chemical starting points. The second is that the medicinal chemist has a small start point; with careful design, this gives opportunities for developing highly efficient, lower molecular weight lead compounds while optimising the required drug-like properties.

The following five sections summarise the key features of these different steps.

## 5.3 Fragment Library

The main difference between a fragment and any other hit compound in drug discovery is that fragments are typically in the molecular weight range of 110–240 Da and bind with a low affinity to the target. The low affinity means that sensitive methods are needed (discussed later) to detect such weak binding. Both the screening technology and the method for growing the fragments need to be considered in designing the library. Many different properties can be used to select compounds for a fragment library, but the most important criteria are the size, measured as heavy atom count (non-hydrogen atoms) or molecular weight and solubility.

First, a comment on the molecular weight of the compounds in the fragment library. A key feature of fragment screening is that a small number of compounds samples a potentially huge chemical space – *i.e.* a small fragment is representative of many more compounds that can incorporate or be inspired by that fragment. The scaling of the chemical space with number of heavy atoms is nicely illustrated by the work of Reymond. His group has developed algorithms to enumerate the compounds that can be generated using standard chemical protocols and which fit within what can be termed drug-like space.[23,24] Although there are many approximations in the analysis, the main message is that chemical space increases approximately 8.3-fold for the addition of each heavy atom. This means that a library of 1000 fragments of molecular weight 190 is equivalent to $10^7$ compounds of molecular weight 280 and $10^{18}$ compounds of molecular weight 450. This emphasises the need to keep the fragments within a library as small as possible, while still having sufficient mass and functionality to register in an assay.[7] For these reasons, it is usual to think of fragments as less than 250 Da (about 18 heavy atoms) and calling compounds between 250 to 350 Da scaffolds.

As with any screening approach, the number of compounds in the library can have an impact on success. The hope is that a small fragment library is sufficiently diverse to identify some of the chemical motifs that can bind. The hits will not be optimal, but rapid expansion around the initial fragment hits will improve the interactions and affinity. One striking example of the impact of the number of compounds in a library is the screen of a 11 000 member fragment library against the enzyme COMT.[25] Only three hits were found, the most useful of which was a pyrazole – but there were many other pyrazoles in the library that were not identified as a hit.

The quality of the hits obtained from a fragment screen depend on the quality of the compounds in the library. There has been a considerable literature on library design.[26–34] Most practitioners have adopted a similar approach, which is summarised in Figure 5.2. The available compounds (either commercially available or from the

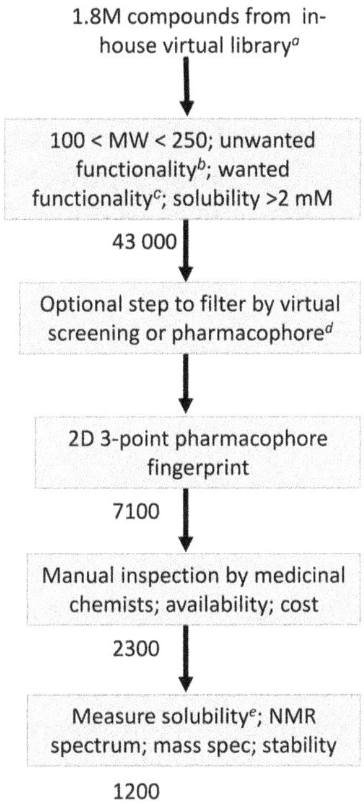


**Figure 5.2** A typical workflow to design a fragment library. The numbers are the number of compounds which remain to be considered and are taken from a fragment design protocol followed at Vernalis in 2003.[29]

[a]The database of available compounds rCAT.[173]

[b]SMARTs strings were used to remove compounds that had:

- Four aliphatic carbons except if also contains X–C–CC–X, X–C–C–X, X–C–X with X = O or N
- Any atom different from H, C, N, O, F, Cl, S
- -SH, S–S, O–O, S–Cl, N-halogen; Sugars
- Conjugated system: R=C–C=O, with R different from O, N, or S or aromatic cycle
- (C=O)-halogen, O–(C=O)-halogen, $SO_2$-halogen, N=C=O, N=C=S, N–C(=S)–N
- Acyclic C(=O)–S, acyclic C(=S)–O, acyclic N=C=N
- Anhydride, aziridine, epoxide, ortho ester, nitroso
- Quaternary amines, methylene, isonitrile
- Acetals, thioacetal, N–C–O acetals, nitro group
- >1 chlorine atom.

[c]SMARTs strings were used to accept compounds that had:

- R-COOMe, R-COOH; R-NHMe, R-N$(Me)_2$, R-$NH_2$
- R-CONHMe, R-CON$(Me)_2$, R-$CONH_2$; R-$SO_2$NHMe, S-$SO_2$N$(Me)_2$, R-$SO_2NH_2$
- R-OMe, R-OH; R-Sme; ≥1 ring system.

[d]This filter was not included for the example numbers used here.

[e]For NMR screening (see later), the compounds are stored at 200 mM in $d_6$-DMSO and need to be soluble aqueous at 500 μM; the requirements differ for other methods of screening.

corporate collection) are filtered to identify compounds with the desired molecular weight, excluding those that contain functional groups that are predicted to be toxic or reactive and excluding compounds that do not have identified sites for synthetic elaboration. This step also includes a filter on predicted solubility. Some libraries have an additional step, selecting compounds predicted to be suitable for a particular target class, either through requiring a particular pharmacophore or through virtual screening. The remaining set of compounds is then usually assessed on some measure of chemical diversity – in the case of the Vernalis fragment library, we have used the three-point 2D pharmacophore method. The final selection of compounds usually involves a manual inspection step, where medicinal chemists triage the list of compounds to identify the chemotypes that they feel could be progressed. The involvement of medicinal chemists in library design encourages take-up of the hits once they are identified, particularly important in larger organisations.[30,35] The compounds are then purchased and checked for purity and solubility.

The maintenance and curation of a fragment library takes considerable effort. The fragments are screened at relatively high concentrations (100s of μM for most biophysical screens; many mM for crystallographic soaks), so the solubility and purity of the compounds needs to be regularly checked, particularly when the libraries are maintained in high concentration stock solutions. This is not only to ensure that the compounds are still in solution, but also to check for aggregation or stability issues. A small percentage of some contaminants can have a marked effect in a high concentration assay. The physicochemical requirements of a library are a major factor that constrains the contents of a fragment library, in particular the solubility which is usually linked to the lipophilicity (see the discussion in Section 5.4.6).

There have been continued developments in recent years, much of which have not been published. The trend has been to maintain different libraries for use with different screening platforms, with differing requirements for properties, in particular solubility in the different buffer conditions and concentrations used. In many larger organisations, this can be a library of 10 000–20 000 compounds with molecular weight up to 300 Da for use in high concentration screening, a library of 1000–2000 compounds of average molecular weight of 200 Da for use in biophysical screening (such as NMR or SPR, see later) and a library of a few hundred smaller compounds with high solubility for use in crystallographic screening (Section 5.4.6) or for second site screening in the SAR by NMR approach (details in Section 5.8.3, with examples of application in Figures 5.7–5.9).

At Vernalis, the primary screening library is assessed and updated every 6–12 months. Compounds are removed if they show lack of solubility or stability, or when stocks are depleted and the compound is no longer available. In addition, fragments that have proven particularly difficult to progress or demonstrated liabilities (metabolic *etc.*) are removed to make way for new fragments. All compounds synthesised within the company that meet the general criteria for fragments are considered for inclusion; in addition, novel scaffolds are often synthesised based on ideas from the literature or understanding of a particular target class. The overall size of the primary screening library used across all screening methods is maintained between 1100 and 1500 compounds – mainly because of the overhead of library QC and maintenance, with a crystallographic screening library of 200 or so compounds of lower molecular weight and higher solubility (discussed in more detail in Section 5.4.4).

There are a number of published variations on these general principles. The first of these are libraries that have been constructed to include particular elements to aid the screening method. Dalvit *et al.*[36–38] are enthusiastic proponents of using $^{19}F$ as a probe and many groups have explored $^{19}F$ fragment libraries;[39,40] the main advantage is that the $^{19}F$ nucleus is particularly sensitive in the NMR experiment and also the isotope is 100% abundant. This markedly increases the sensitivity compared to $^{1}H$ NMR spectra, such that as low as 5 μM fragment is required, dramatically reducing the solubility constraint. One of the early proponents of structure-based design, the company SGX, designed a library containing Br atoms as electron dense atoms to aid identification in crystallographic screening;[41] one group went as far as designing a paired set of libraries where a fragment with a Br could be used for crystallographic screening with a non-Br fragment available for other assays. An issue with both approaches is that the atom introduced as a probe can itself be important for interaction, complicating the pathway to fragment optimisation.

A second variation is to enrich the fragment library with fragments derived from known drugs (so-called privileged scaffolds) or to use virtual screening or a pharmacophore (as described above) for a particular target class. Usually, these approaches will increase the hit rate, but by definition, are not providing any new insights into the chemotypes which will interact with the target. For these reasons, most practitioners aim for the library to be generic and suitable for most targets.[26,29–31]

A final variation to note is to construct a fragment library that is representative of the available compounds. This could be through analysis of the available compounds[27] or so-called "poised" fragments[2] from which there are established routes to synthesise compounds based on the fragments. This type of approach ensures there are near neighbours of fragments available for rapid generation of SAR.

There has recently been some discussion about how important it is for drug molecules to include $sp^3$ carbon atoms, giving a more three dimensional shape.[42] Such considerations have also led to the proposal that 3D fragments may also be important, particularly for some of the new target classes (protein–protein interactions, carbohydrate processing proteins). Although there have been a number of academic projects developing synthesis of interestingly shaped compounds (such as ref. 43–46) and commercial suppliers have generated libraries from their inventory (including many natural product inspired compounds) there remains much debate on the value of such compounds. Such compounds tend to be more complex (and larger) than "flat" fragments, so more compounds will be needed to cover equivalent chemical space. In addition, although interestingly shaped hits can be found for some targets, synthesis of analogues with (usually) quite complex stereochemistry is synthetically challenging.

A concern expressed by some is that many drug discovery campaigns will begin from screening the same fragment library and so the same fragment hits will be considered. Anecdotally, there is remarkably little overlap in the exact chemical structures selected to be in different fragment libraries – it appears that there is enough diversity in the commercially available compounds less than 250 Da that the chance of choosing exactly the same fragment for a particular chemotype is quite low. However, it is the case that rather similar fragments are found by different project teams; what is important is the optimisation of the fragments. This is the difficult part of fragment-based discovery and where real discovery is made. Two examples are described elsewhere in this chapter. The first is the compounds now on the market from Plexxikon (see Figure 5.7) where the same azaindole fragment led to very different inhibitors of two kinases.[47,48] The second is the analysis of various Hsp90 projects[49] in Section 5.10, where very similar fragments were identified by different companies which optimised to distinct candidate compounds.

## 5.4 Fragment Screening Approaches

For a simple binding event of a ligand (L) to a protein (P), the equilibrium can be represented as shown in eqn (5.1).

$$\begin{aligned}
&(\mathrm{a})\mathrm{PL}_{(\mathrm{aq})} \underset{k_{\mathrm{on}}}{\overset{k_{\mathrm{off}}}{\rightleftharpoons}} \mathrm{P}_{(\mathrm{aq})} + \mathrm{L}_{(\mathrm{aq})} \\
&(\mathrm{b})K_{\mathrm{D}} = \frac{k_{\mathrm{off}}}{k_{\mathrm{on}}} = \frac{[\mathrm{P}_{(\mathrm{aq})}][\mathrm{L}_{(\mathrm{aq})}]}{[\mathrm{PL}_{(\mathrm{aq})}]} \\
&(\mathrm{c})\Delta G^{\circ} = \Delta H^{\circ} - T\Delta S^{\circ} = -RT\ln K_{\mathrm{D}}
\end{aligned} \qquad (5.1)$$

For the simple equilibrium in eqn (5.1a), the dissociation constant ($K_D$) is the ratio of the off rate ($k_{off}$) divided by the on rate ($k_{on}$), as shown in eqn (5.1b). $K_D$ is related to the standard Gibbs free energy ($\Delta G^\circ$) and the enthalpy ($\Delta H^\circ$) and entropy ($\Delta S^\circ$) of binding as shown in eqn (5.1c) at temperature ($T$); $R$ is the molar gas constant.

There are now many examples where small fragments that bind to a target with a dissociation constant in the mM range can be progressed to lead compounds. The need to detect binding at such low affinity has inspired the development of many techniques for screening fragments. These have relied not only on the development of more sensitive equipment, but also an increased understanding of how to set up and validate the assays and the limitations and advantages of the different methods.

Figure 5.3 summarises the range of affinities which are usually accessible by these techniques, based on experience at Vernalis.[19] The following is a brief summary of the main characteristics and considerations for each of the screening approaches.

### 5.4.1 Protein-observed NMR

This is the screening method, named "SAR by NMR" developed at Abbott, used in the first published fragment-based discovery project[50] and many of the subsequent fragment campaigns at that company.[51,52] The strategy is described in more detail in Section 5.8.3. The main NMR pulse sequence used is known as HSQC (Heteronuclear Single Quantum Coherence) which is a 2D NMR experiment, most often where transfer of signal between $^{1}$H and $^{15}$N in the isotopically labelled protein results in a spectrum where each amide yields a peak; the position of each peak depends on the local chemical environment and is sensitive to ligand binding (see typical spectrum in the top

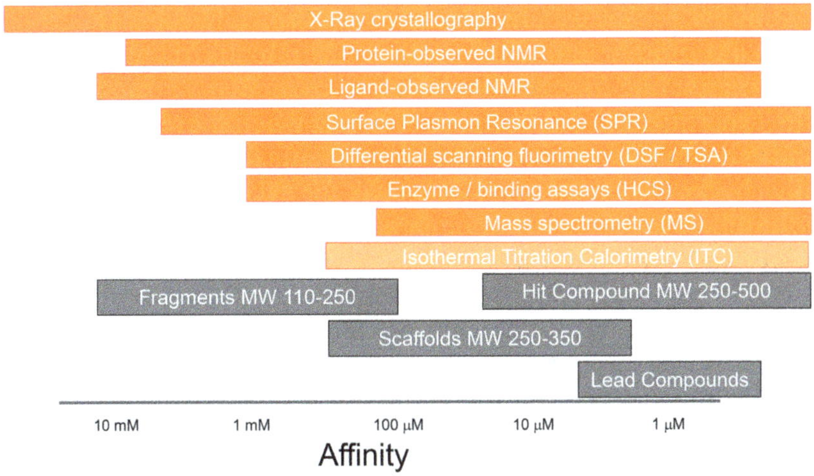


**Figure 5.3** A schematic representation of the sensitivity range of the different techniques presented in the text for detecting binding of compounds to protein targets. The affinity scale is for the dissociation constant for the equilibrium PL = P + L. For all techniques, there will be exceptions to these sensitivity limits; the diagram summarises the general experience in most projects, presuming that all components are soluble and do not interfere with the detection method.

right panel of Figure 5.1). Although more sophisticated NMR experiments are possible for larger proteins, the usual limitation is for proteins less than 35 kDa (otherwise the peaks are too broad due to the slower tumbling time). Usually, the experiments are performed with protein at a concentration of 20–50 μM to give sufficient signal. This solubility requirement increases the amount of protein needed for screening; as it is the protein that is being observed, this also makes screening with mixtures more complicated (see ligand-observed NMR below). The dynamic range of HSQC measurements is quite broad, mainly limited by compound solubility. Hits (that is some change) can be seen for compounds up to mM in affinity.

There has been limited use of the method for screening of fragments at other organisations; to some extent, this is because of the patent that Abbott gained on some of the methods, but mainly because of the limitations outlined above. However, protein-observed NMR is used more widely for characterising fragment binding. An advantage of the method is that it can identify fragments that bind to alternate regions of the protein – this would be seen in a different pattern of amide shifts in the HSQC spectrum.[53]

## 5.4.2 Ligand-observed NMR

This is regarded by many as the most robust of the biophysical screening methods, because of the dynamic range of the assay (hits can be identified with $K_D$ between 100 nM and 10 mM), there is no need for labelling of the protein (as it is the ligand that is observed), there is no limit on the size of the protein being studied and there is quality control within each experiment – the NMR signals report that the ligand is intact and in solution and that the protein is still folded and in solution.

Figure 5.4 summarises the experimental design. Typically, these experiments are performed with 10 µM protein and with mixtures of up to 10 fragments at 500 µM each; as long as there is not one fragment which has a particularly strong residence time on the target, the experiment should be able to detect when more than one fragment in a mixture binds to the target. The selection of fragments for each mixture is not too onerous – the only checks are that there is one peak for each fragment in the mixture that is distinctive and that the fragments do not associate with each other in the mixture. A number of different NMR experiments are used with the most widely applied being Saturation Transfer Difference.[54] In this experiment, the protein sample is irradiated at the chemical shift of the protons of the hydrophobic core; this radiation is transferred to any ligand which touches the protein during the timescale of the experiment, which is measured as the difference seen in the 1D spectrum recorded for the ligand. Additional experiments that are used by some are water-logsy[55] (which involves transfer of radiation from solvent molecules) and Carr–Purcell–Meiboom–Gill[56] (CPMG, measuring differential relaxation of the ligand in solution and bound). Each of these experiments have a different physical basis, so a hit in all three of the experiments is more reliable. The general experience at Vernalis is that a hit in all three NMR experiments has a 70% success rate in giving a crystal structure, falling to 40% if only a hit in two of the experiments and rarely if a hit in only one experiment. The main limitation for detection is the solubility of the ligand; at Vernalis (see Figure 20.5 in ref. 19), fragments have been reliably identified between 100 nM and 5 mM binding. The high concentration of fragments needed to observe such low affinity binding can sometimes result in non-specific

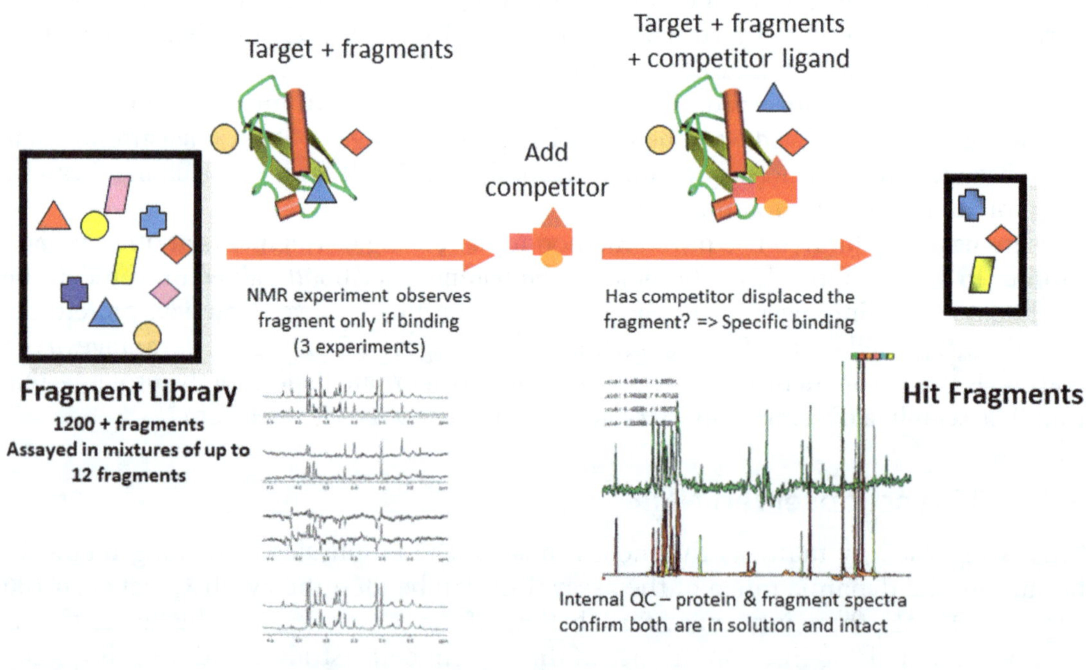


**Figure 5.4** A schematic representation of fragment screening by competitive ligand-observed NMR spectroscopy. See text for details.

binding. To control for this, a competitive step is used where a known ligand (which can be a peptide or a tool compound) is added and the spectra reacquired to see if the signal disappears.

Such a competitive experiment identifies fragments whose binding is effected by such a competitor ligand and so, in principle, would identify a true allosteric site as well. However, many alternate, cryptic sites (sometimes functional, often not) elsewhere on the protein active site can only be probed if the experiment is constructed to look for them. For example, the primary active site can be blocked by incubation with a high concentration of a known tight binding (*i.e.* slow kinetics) inhibitor during screening.

A variation of the ligand-observed NMR screening is the proprietary Target Immobilised NMR Screen (TINS) method. Here, the protein is immobilised on a column and ligands flowed past.[57–59]

### 5.4.3 Technologies that Sense Binding to Labelled Protein Through Change in Optical Properties

A number of instruments have been developed that are capable of measuring the interaction of small, low affinity fragments binding to protein. All of them require the protein to be modified in some way – either immobilised onto a surface or labelled with a fluorophore.

The most established and widely used is Surface Plasmon Resonance (SPR). The experiment is based on immobilising one component (either protein or ligand) on a surface; the change in properties of an optical beam shining on this surface reflects the mass of what is attached. It is then possible to observe the change in mass as the binding partner is flowed over the surface. SPR is capable of measuring both the thermodynamics and kinetics of binding and will be described in a little detail.

There are two main configurations: direct mode and indirect mode.

Figure 5.5 is a sketch of the direct binding mode which provides the most information on the kinetics of binding (see eqn (5.1)). The protein is immobilised to the surface and the ligand flowed over. As the ligand binds, there is a change in the response of the detector; the on rate or $k_{\text{on}}$ for binding can be calculated from this initial slope. When

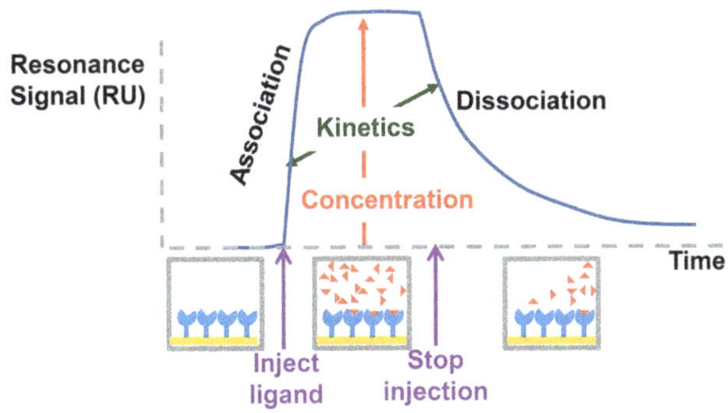


**Figure 5.5** A schematic representation of Surface Plasmon Resonance (SPR). See text for details.

the ligand is no longer injected over the surface, the ligand dissociates from the surface and the off rate or $k_{off}$ can be measured from the resulting change in the response. For most targets, the fragments bind with a low affinity, with rapid on and off rates, so it is not possible to make a great deal from the kinetics (see the SPR trace in the panel at the top right of Figure 5.1). However, the off rate is usually what changes as a ligand is optimised. SPR can thus be an effective way of detecting progress in compound optimisation.[60,61] In addition, slow off-rate compounds can be of great benefit in some therapeutic indications (such as oncology), as a long half-life on the target (or residence time) can be associated with increased efficacy.[62]

In indirect mode, a good ligand is immobilised to the surface, usually through an extended linker which needs careful design so as not to impede binding to the protein. The protein is then injected over the surface. As the protein binds, there is a large change in signal – inclusion of a high concentration of a fragment that binds to the protein will prevent binding. In this case, it is not possible to directly measure kinetics of binding but binding affinities can be extracted.

This technique has been available for many decades following the introduction of the first instrument (the initial manufacturer/trade name is Biacore). Although more sensitive equipment now allows weak fragment binding to be observed, the major advances have come with experience in the attachment methods, in the software that analyses the response traces, and importantly, a wider understanding of how to validate the binding and how to recognise when there are anomalies.[63–66] It is now generally found that fragment hits of 120 Da can be seen; although some practitioners have pushed the limit on affinity into the mM range, most find that it is challenging to reliably measure fragments binding with an affinity worse than 500 μM, mainly for reasons of solubility and interference with the chip surface and equivalent failures. A recent entry that has similar characteristics is a machine from Creoptix[67] which uses different physics (Grating Couple Interferometry, GCI) to monitor interactions. Another variant is biolayer interferometry (BLI – as used in ref. 68), where the protein is immobilised to the outside of a glass capillary – a change in molecular weight is detected by changes in light shone down the centre of the capillary.

There are a variety of attachment strategies for these sensor techniques. Kits are available that biotinylate free lysine residues on the surface of the protein[69] or use direct amine coupling reactions. There are protocols for establishing the best conditions, but this can result in a surface where the protein is randomly oriented; in addition, it is not possible to regenerate the surface once it has been used with a tight binding compound (and they can be quite expensive consumables). A more robust alternative is to couple *via* a specifically introduced tag at either the N or C terminus of the protein. One, long established option is to use the histidine tag usually attached to most over-expressed proteins for purification purposes, which can be immobilised to a $Ni^{2+}$ surface. The standard hexa-his tag can be too weak to give a stable chip surface (the protein leaches off) but a double his tag[70] can provide a stable surface which has the advantage that it can be cleared to regenerate the rather expensive chips for different proteins. Another more recent innovation is to introduce an Avitag[71] (GLNDIFEAQKIEWHE) sequence at the N or C terminus of the protein. This can be specifically biotinylated on the lysine by the enzyme BirA biotin ligase, either post-expression or through co-expression. This has proven very successful and generation of such Avitag constructs is now regularly included in the exploratory phases of projects.

All these methods (SPR, GCI, BLI) claim to be "label-free" – but are actually labelling the protein with an instrument. Some other recent methods label the protein with a fluorophore and then monitor some change in the properties when compounds bind. One example is MicroScale Thermophoresis (MST, from the company, Nanotemper[72,73]) which measures the change when a ligand binds in the diffusion rate of a labelled protein back into a region of the solution that has been ablated by a laser. Another recent innovation is second harmonic generation (SHG, from the company originally called Biodesy, now Bluelight Therapeutics[74]). Here, the protein is also labelled with a fluorophore but also anchored to a lipid bilayer – the optics measure changes in the orientation of the fluorophore to the membrane on binding of ligand. These techniques give valuable information on binding of large ligands to proteins; there are varying experiences of using these methods for fragment screening.

### 5.4.4 Thermal Shift Analysis (TSA) or Differential Scanning Fluorimetry

In this method, a solution containing the target protein and the possible ligand or fragment is slowly heated up in the presence of a fluorescent dye. As the protein unfolds, there is a change in fluorescence as the dye binds to the hydrophobic surfaces; a change in the so-called melting temperature (or $T_m$) indicates that the ligand has bound and stabilised the protein. The top right panel of Figure 5.1 shows some representative traces.

The method was initially developed for screening of compound libraries[75] and very powerfully applied to select ligands which could increase the chance of crystallisation[76] or improving the stability of proteins.[77] For such ligands (usually better than a $K_D$ of 1 μM) the method is reasonably robust as the ligands will tend to provide a clear stabilisation of the protein. A number of groups (particularly academics) have exploited the technique for fragment screening. As documented by many (*e.g.* ref. 78), there are challenges in recognising the very small $T_m$ shift seen for fragments. Because such small molecules give little stabilisation of the protein (if any) there can be many false negatives if TSA is used as the primary screening method.[19,78]

The main advantage of the technique is the relatively small amount of protein material required for screening and that standard laboratory equipment (such as a PCR machine) can be used.

### 5.4.5 Biochemical Assay

This category includes any assay that depends on a readout of enzyme activity or any assay where a spectrophotometric readout (such as fluorescence or UV/visible light) monitors binding or the displacement of a labelled ligand. The advent and investment in High Throughput Screening (HTS) has stimulated the development of a range of robust screening approaches and platforms for measuring such activity or binding. The main issues for such assays for screening fragments are their detection limits and their sensitivity to the high concentrations needed to observe such low affinity binding; this has led to a wide literature on the origins of frequent hitter compounds and false positives.[79,80] For some classes of target (such as kinases), such assays are reasonably robust, particularly where the binding site being inhibited has a good ligandable shape and chemistry. In such cases, it is possible to screen a fragment library with reasonable confidence and minimal false positives and negatives. However, for some targets, the assays either lack sufficient sensitivity or are susceptible to interference (*e.g.* fluorescence). This is illustrated in one study[19] which summarises experience with fragment screening for a number of different targets. Validated hits identified by NMR screening and for which crystal structures are available were assessed for binding in the relevant wet assay. Whereas the false negatives in the wet assay were minimal for kinases and ATPases, there were some targets for which very few of the fragment hits would have been identified if only a wet assay had been used (see Figure 20.4 in ref. 19).

### 5.4.6 Crystallography

An early emphasis in fragment-based methods was to use X-ray crystallography to identify fragment hits (see the discussion in Section 5.8). To some extent, this was because many of the early adopters and adapters of the methods had a strong background in structural biology and crystallography, but the main advantages are that an immediate picture is obtained of how the fragment is binding and it is possible to obtain discrete structures for very weak ligand binding. However, the main challenge is whether the protein crystal is suitable, that is whether the crystal will withstand soaking in high concentrations of ligands and still diffract and whether crystal packing makes it difficult for low affinity ligands to readily soak into the binding site. The latter constraint emphasises that observing a ligand binding from a crystal soaking experiment is as much about kinetics as thermodynamics. It can take a number of attempts (varying soaking time, temperature *etc.*) before a structure of a complex is obtained.

Generating a suitable crystal system for ligand soaking can be a real challenge. Sometimes, modifications to the protein construct and/or crystallisation conditions will generate a suitable crystal form; however, requiring this can limit the types of projects for which fragment screening can be performed. In addition, as many protein crystals are formed with protein produced from truncated or mutated constructs, the cryptic sites are not always natural or functional. However, there are a number of examples where soaking into a crystal identifies unexpected cryptic (occasionally allosteric) binding sites on the protein (see discussion below in Section 5.6 and examples[81–83]).

Notwithstanding these caveats, a crystal structure of a fragment bound to the target protein validates fragment binding and provides important information to aid the design of improved compounds.

Using X-ray crystallography to screen a fragment library takes considerable effort in crystal mounting, soaking, data collection and subsequent refinement of the structures. Recent years have seen the development of impressive facilities such as XChem[84–86] at the Diamond synchrotron which have harnessed robotics and innovative software to streamline the process, such that a whole fragment library can be screened and the data analysed within a week. This still requires a suitable crystal form for the protein of interest (robust, accessible binding site). The approach can also support rapid hit and lead optimisation[87] where crude reaction mixtures are soaked directly into suitable crystals.

Obtaining a structure of a fragment soaked into a crystal gives no indication of the affinity of binding, beyond noting what concentration was used for soaking. It can, however, highlight accessible sites on the protein in the crystal which are attractive to chemical matter. Early work (see Section 5.8.2 on MSCS) established the principles which have received renewed attention recently. The Fraglites[88] approach soaks crystals with a library of halogen containing small fragments where the anomalous scattering from the halogen aids crystal structure solution. Minifrags[89] are fragments with between five and seven heavy atoms which can probe binding sites in a protein crystal for hot-spots. Both approaches can assess ligandability of a protein (see Section 5.6) and provide ideas for interactions that can be exploited in fragment and hit evolution.

### 5.4.7 Mass Spectrometry

There have been great advances in mass spectrometry instrumentation for detection and characterisation of non-covalent complexes and this has delivered real insight into the composition of multi-protein assemblies (*e.g.* ref. 90) and have been successfully used in detecting protein–ligand binding when the ligand binds with affinities better than 100 μM (*e.g.* ref. 21). However, this is not an appropriate range for fragment screening, although the technique has found application when there is covalent fragment binding[91] and such as the tethering approaches of Sunesis.[92]

### 5.4.8 Isothermal Titration Calorimetry (ITC)

This technique is based on measuring the heat (enthalpy in eqn (5.1b)) that is taken up or released on binding of a ligand to a protein. There are two main limitations to the dynamic range of affinities that can be monitored – the amount of heat that is released and the solubility of one or other of the protein or ligand. The usual configuration is to inject small amounts of a concentrated solution of the ligand into a sample of protein; if the ligand is poorly soluble and the protein very soluble, then the protein can be injected into the ligand sample. The instrument compares the heat difference between the cell containing the protein (or ligand) and a blank sample; this is recorded as spikes of heat; the total heat is obtained from integrating under that curve. As increasing amounts of ligand and protein bind, so the amount of heat reduces, and a sigmoidal curve such as seen in the top right panel of Figure 5.1 is observed. The concentration at which equilibrium is achieved allows the equilibrium constant to be calculated; it is then possible to calculate the entropy change on binding.

The detection limit is generally for a $K_D$ in the 500 μM to 5 nM range; however, the main limitation is the amount of protein required to generate sufficient heat. This means the method has limited application to fragment screening but is a reliable method for validating fragment hits and subsequent optimisation of compounds.

### 5.4.9 Virtual Screening

Although there have been great advances in both the methods and computational power available for molecular calculations, it remains a challenge to predict the pose and affinity for a compound binding to a protein.[93] Some successes for computational fragment screening have been reported where the binding site is highly ligand efficient (such as a Class A GPCR[94] or a well-studied enzyme active site[95]). However, in general, the calculations are confounded by two features of fragments. First, the fragments bind quite weakly, so the (usually) empirical energy calculations cannot correctly identify when a significant interaction is made. Second, the size of the compounds mean that there are fewer steric clashes with the binding site (which is a major filter in molecular docking), so many different binding poses of similar energy can be adopted by a fragment.

### 5.4.10 Other Ideas and Approaches

The success and investment in fragment-based discovery has coincided with recognition of the importance of compound properties in lead optimisation. Taken together, these have encouraged the development of a number of other technologies for detecting and characterising protein–ligand interactions. Some of these methods are proprietary, such as the fluorescence-based interferometry method from the company Evotec[96] and the capillary electrophoresis methods from the company Selcia.[97] A method developed by an academic group in Sweden – Weak Affinity Chromatography or WAC[98] has been commercialised by Carna Biosciences. In this technique, the protein is attached to a silica gel and loaded onto a chromatography column; a mixture of fragments is flowed over the column. The retention time reflects the binding to the protein and the ligand can be identified if the column is connected to a mass spectrometer. As with any immobilisation technique, the main challenge is to fix the protein to the support, while retaining its folding and binding integrity.

### 5.4.11 Validating Fragment Hits – Comparing Methods

It is important to validate any fragment hits found in a screening campaign. Although the false positive rate for some targets (such as kinases) is relatively low for well-conducted, competitive binding screens, it is useful to remove any false hits before investing too much time and resource. Validation is crucial for more challenging targets – such as protein–protein interaction targets – where the screening techniques can report incorrectly for all sorts of reasons.

There has been some debate (and reports) of the differences between the biophysical techniques both in hit rates and the nature of the hits.[99,100] In principle all the methods should give the same results, provided that the conditions are equivalent. However, it is the case that the sensitivity between the methods varies and in particular the differences in buffer conditions required for the different assays may have a differential effect on compound solubility or aggregation, or on the binding affinity itself.

## 5.5 Fragment Hit Rates

### 5.5.1 Hits *vs.* Non-hits

For the Vernalis fragment library, 35% of the library is a hit against at least one target, whereas 65% of the library has not yet been a hit against any target. To date, it has not been possible to find any combination of physico-chemical or other properties that differentiates a hit from a non-hit sufficiently to be used as a criteria for removal of that class of compounds from the library. An analysis of hit rates and properties[26] showed that the hits are slightly more hydrophobic (higher lipophilicity, calculated as Slog$P$[101]) than non-hits, with slightly fewer rotatable bonds and more rings. However, these differences are subtle. The description of the Pfizer library design process[30] included a preliminary report on hit rates for the first library of 2592 fragments (so-called GFI-I) screened against 13 different targets by STD-NMR. Of the 2593 fragments, 766 hit at least one target, with only 1 fragment hitting all 13 targets – about 30%. The hit rates reported by AstraZeneca for an earlier fragment library are between 0.2% for a protein–protein interaction to 6% for a well-defined serine protease active site. However, these results are more difficult to compare, as a number of different screening strategies from high concentration screening to ligand-observed NMR were used.[31] To emphasise points made elsewhere, the hit rate from a fragment screen will depend on the size of the compounds, the solubility and aggregation propensity of the fragments under the conditions of the screen, the nature of the target, but also critically on the sensitivity of the method used for screening and the criteria for a hit.

### 5.5.2 Hits for Different Types of Target

The Vernalis analysis[26] also found slight variation in the nature of the hits found for conventional targets such as kinases compared to the hits found for protein–protein interaction (PPI) targets which tend to have larger, flatter and more hydrophobic binding cavities. The hits for PPIs were of higher molecular weight, with more rotatable bonds and rings compared to those for other targets.

### 5.5.3 Membrane-bound Proteins

The therapeutic targets for many current drugs are membrane-bound proteins, such as G-protein coupled receptors (GPCRs) and ion channels. The major difficulty in applying biophysical methods of fragment screening to these classes of protein is preparing the large amounts of purified and stable protein that are required. For GPCRs, these problems have been overcome for some systems through either introducing stabilising mutations,[102–104] introducing a stabilising protein into the internal loop between two helices[105,106] or for non-covalent stabilisation such as using nanobodies.[107] The main driver for this protein engineering was to provide protein for crystallographic structure determination, but it has also provided the material for fragment screening[102–104] and there has been (unpublished) progress in preparing high concentrations of native receptors in liposome preparations, which can be subjected to fragment screening by

SPR, or performing a high concentration screen in a functional assay, such as patch clamp for an ion channel. However, many of these receptors have fragment-sized natural ligands and very highly ligand-efficient binding sites, which means that the hit rates in a fragment screen can be very high.

## 5.6 Fragments for Chemical Biology – Target and Mechanism Assessment and Discovery

Fragments have increasingly been used as chemical tools to probe biological systems. The libraries of very low molecular weight fragments, such as Fraglites[88] and Minifrags[89] for crystallographic screening, can be used to search for binding sites on proteins, and facilities such as XChem (see Section 5.4.6) have allowed wider access to crystallographic fragment screening to probe binding sites.[108] The proposal that fragments can be used to assess the "druggability"[109] (perhaps more properly, "ligandability") of a protein was recognised early on,[28,110,111] and has been developed by some as an early indicator of how successful a drug discovery campaign could be for a target[112,113] or to prioritise targets to study.[114] This emphasises the idea that fragments assess the available chemical space for binding to a target; for one example (Hsp90) the central binding features of all the published inhibitors were represented by just 5 of the more than 40 fragment hits.[49]

As well as assessing ligandability of a known active or binding site, fragments can also highlight other sites on a protein where chemical matter could interact. A retrospective analysis by Astex[115] of the data generated in a crystallographic fragment screen of 24 proteins, identified a number of additional binding sites. This is similar to what has been seen by others, soaking crystals with different solvents[116,117] and the identification of the components of the crystallisation liquor in many structures. The difficulty is knowing how functionally relevant these sites are. Most crystal structures are determined for individual protein domains, and the "additional" sites may reflect interactions with missing domains. It can take some work to demonstrate functional relevance of a novel site to know whether it is "allosteric" or "cryptic", requiring evolution of the fragment hit into a compound with sufficient potency to register in a functional assay. Two striking examples of where such "novel" sites can be relevant are: (1) discovery of fragments that bind to a novel site between the protease and helicase domain of NS3 from heptatitis C,[81] stabilising the inactive form and (2) discovery of an allosteric site on the enzyme, FPPS.[118]

There are two other interesting applications of fragments in chemical biology. The first is an impressive approach in which fragments are synthesised with a photoactivatable tag – soaking cells with the library followed by a light flash links a fragment that binds to a protein site – which can identify novel targets in the cell.[119] The second idea is to use fragments to identify compounds that activate enzymes.[120] This could be an interesting, though yet little explored strategy for drug discovery. A therapeutic effect could be achieved by only small increases in an enzyme activity, in contrast to the high affinity usually required for enzyme inhibition. For other applications, such as industrial enzymes, an approach could be to covalently link (*via* a native or introduced cysteine) the fragment to enhance activity.[121]

## 5.7 Determining Structures of Fragments Bound

X-ray crystallography is the most information-rich method for providing a detailed picture of how a fragment is binding to a target. In some organisations, a fragment does not qualify as a true "hit" to be considered for progression until a crystal structure of the target is obtained with the fragment bound. Although other structural information (such as from NMR[122] or from molecular docking) can provide enough information, the details of solvent and protein conformation provided by an X-ray structure gives a more robust framework for designing modifications to evolve the fragment. There are some caveats on the detailed interpretation of the structures – nearly all structures are determined from crystals immersed in cryoprotectant and frozen at liquid nitrogen temperature to protect against damage from the X-ray beam. In addition, sometimes crystal packing can affect the detail of the protein conformation.

There are two ways of obtaining a protein–ligand crystal structure – either soaking or co-crystallisation. Co-crystallisation can be resource consuming – the crystallisation conditions may vary from ligand to ligand and it can take time and protein to identify new conditions for each ligand. In general, soaking provides the same structures (though there are exceptions, where the ligand can induce a conformational change). In most projects, the approach is to do soaking for speed, with occasional co-crystallisation attempts to cross-check the structures.

There are variants in the soaking protocols. The ligand can be added to the crystallisation solution or added to the cryoprotectant. For some crystals, it is not possible to obtain an apo structure (that is unliganded); one approach is to generate crystals with a moderately weak ligand binding (an example would be ADP-PNP binding to a kinase) and then soak out the ligand with the fragment solution which then binds, an approach used for the kinase PDPK1.[123]

In general, determining the structure of individual complexes by NMR is very time consuming – both in the time taken to collect the various NMR spectra, but also in assigning the spectra. Except for the SAR by NMR approaches of Abbott (see Figures 5.7–5.9), all of the successful fragment optimisation campaigns have relied on X-ray crystal structures. What has been successful is to use a surrogate – for example, the initial fragments and hits that led to the drug Vemurafenib (see Figure 5.15) that targets the kinase, Braf, were characterised in crystal structures of Pim1 and then FGFR kinase. Such a surrogate approach can provide the necessary structural guidance for fragment and hit optimisation. A crystal structure is only a model and this approach can be successful as long as the rationale from the structures in the surrogate correlate with the inhibitory data generated in wet assays. A more extreme example of a surrogate is where the binding site residues of a related protein which forms crystals are mutated to be those of the target of interest. A striking example is for LRRK2, where extensive efforts by many groups have failed to generate crystal structures of the kinase domain. Ten-point mutations were introduced into the readily crystallised enzyme Chk1 to transform the ATP binding site of this kinase to be similar to that of LRRK2. Structures of fragments, hits and lead compounds bound of this ten-point surrogate guided the optimisation of potent, brain-penetrant LRRK2 inhibitors.[124]

The past few years has seen a revolution in detector and electron gun technology used for electron cryo-microscopy (commonly called Cryo-EM), with an explosion in reports of structures of large proteins (and complexes) from reconstruction of images of cryo-cooled samples without the need for crystals. These structures have transformed our structural understanding of many biological processes. Current methods are generating structures with resolutions in the 2 Å range for samples down to 80 kDa in size. The main limitations are sample preparation (retaining sample integrity in the molecule-thin grids needed for microscopy) and the time taken to collect and process the huge amounts of image data. However, there are prospects in the near future for the use of the method for structure-based and fragment-based discovery.[125]

## 5.8 The Evolution of the Ideas and Methods – a Historical Perspective

As with most areas of science, it is possible to track the emergence over time of the main results that underpin current practice. The following is a selective discussion of the origin of some of the underlying principles and early applications of fragment-based methods, see also ref. 126.

### 5.8.1 Some Early Ideas

Most discussions of fragment-based discovery begin with the papers from Jencks.[127] He reminded the community that for the simple equilibrium describing the dissociation of a protein–ligand complex (eqn (5.1)), the Gibbs free energy relationship means that a doubling of the energy of interaction between protein and ligand will square the binding constant, $K_D$.

This means that if two functional groups each bind with a 1 mM $K_D$ (equivalent to −17 kJmol$^{-1}$) then a molecule containing both groups making the same strength of interaction will have a binding energy of −34 kJ mol$^{-1}$, equivalent to a $K_D$ of 1 μM. The Jencks paper also discusses how the binding of one group will overcome the rotational and translational entropy for the interaction, so any subsequent interactions are contributing to binding affinity alone.

The notion of different functional groups making a distinct contribution to binding was explored by Andrews in 1984.[128] In this paper, he performed a simple analysis of the average energy of interaction that is achieved by a particular functional group. This paper was to a large extent ignored on first publication; it was not until the mid-2000s that the ideas of functional group efficiency[129] were formalised and more widely accepted.

One of the central features of many fragment screening campaigns is the determination of large numbers of crystal structures of the fragments and subsequent evolved hits binding to the protein. Perhaps the first recorded example of multiple crystal structures with potential ligands bound was the work by Perutz and Abraham[130] who looked at the structure of haemoglobin with various compounds such as bezafibrate bound, to understand the structural basis of their potential to affect the conformation of the protein and be used as anti-sickling agents.

### 5.8.2 The Emergence of *De Novo* Structure-based Design

During the 1980s and early 1990s, computational chemists developed a series of ideas on how to exploit the structure of a protein to identify potential interaction sites for ligands. The first widely used example was the Grid program.[131] Here, a virtual grid of points is placed over the binding site of interest and a simple energy of interaction (van der Waals and electrostatic) computed for a particular probe – say a methyl group or a water molecule. The resulting grid of points can then be contoured to generate a very graphical representation of the regions of the binding site which would favour such an interaction. An early demonstration of the simplicity and power of this approach was the optimisation of the sialic acid analogue, Neu5Ac2en for binding to the influenza enzyme neuraminidase, to introduce a guanidinium group, guided by Grid calculations.[132] The resulting compound became zanamivir, marketed by GSK as Relenza. Further examples of such computational mapping approaches were the programs MCSS (Multiple Copy Simultaneous Search[133]) – where molecular dynamics calculations identify binding poses (that is a conformation, position and orientation) for larger functional groups such as acetamide or benzene – and LUDI[134] – which used the pattern of functional group interactions seen in small molecule structures to predict hot spots for binding on the surface of a protein. Together, these computational approaches reinforced the idea that there are discrete binding sites for small functional groups on the surface of proteins.

The development of the MSCS approach (Multiple Solvent Crystal Structures) by Ringe[135] was the first attempt to map the binding site of a protein experimentally and was extended by others in the 1990s to a range of solvents, and used to investigate the concentration dependence of binding.[116,117] These structures emphasised that the binding sites of proteins have evolved to be chemically attractive and that discrete binding poses can be observed even for very weak binding molecules.

As well as identifying functional group binding sites, the computational community also developed a number of different program that attempted to link the observed or computed functional groups together – examples include the Caveat approach,[136] Hook (Eisen *et al.*, 1994)[192] and the linking components in LUDI.[134] Although intellectually attractive and computationally elegant, these approaches did not gain widespread acceptance. The approaches can generate many millions of possible molecules and the main issue (which in many respects remains today) is the inability to accurately predict the energy of interaction of an evolved molecule. In addition, the programs would often generate compounds that were synthetically intractable. Ironically, the maturing of fragment-based discovery has generated many thousands of crystal structures of fragments bound to a protein – a rich dataset on which these computational approaches could be revisited and refined.

### 5.8.3 The Emergence of Fragment-based Discovery

The first published example of the successful use of fragment-based methods to generate potent lead compounds is the pioneering work of the Abbott group in the mid-1990s. The first paper[50] coined the phrase "SAR by NMR" and described the discovery of nanomolar inhibitors of the FK506 binding protein. The approach relies on NMR spectroscopy for detecting fragment binding (using HSQC measurements, see above) and for determining the structure of protein–fragment complexes. Five separate stages can be identified, as sketched out in Figure 5.6(a). (Screen 1) a library of fragments (in Abbott's case, up to 10 000 of average molecular weight 210) is screened for binding to the target by HSQC NMR; (Optimise 1) selected hits are optimised for binding by

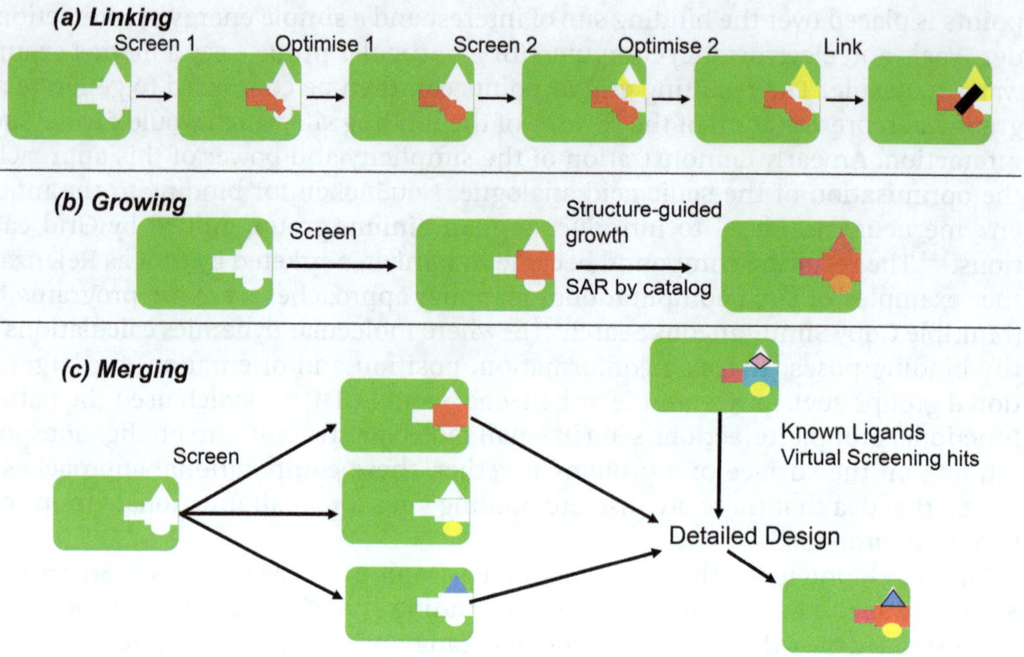


**Figure 5.6** A schematic representation of the different strategies for fragment evolution: (a) linking, (b) growing and (c) merging.

limited chemistry; (Screen 2) a second screen is performed of the protein with the optimised fragment bound, usually with smaller molecular weight fragments; (Optimise 2) this second fragment is then optimised for binding to the target. The structure(s) of the target with the fragment(s) bound is determined by NMR and this information used to guide (Linking) the linking of the fragments together to give higher affinity hits.

This initial paper on FK506 inhibitor discovery was followed by further work from this group, including stromelysin,[137] E2 from papilloma virus,[138] urokinase[139] and metalloproteases.[140] However, there were few reports of successful application of this same SAR by NMR approach from other organisations; this perhaps reflects the challenge of organising the appropriate medicinal chemistry resource around the biophysical methods, ensuring that such low affinity starting points are exploited by what can be quite challenging chemistry. In addition, there were not many targets where this strategy of linking multi-site fragments was appropriate. As well as NMR, Abbott were the first (and sometimes forgotten) proponents of the use of X-ray crystallography for screening of fragments; the work of Nienaber *et al.*[141] established the approach which many others then went on to exploit.

The late 1990s saw variations of the methods developed in various large pharma, such as the work at Roche[142] on crystallographic screening – the so called Needles approach exemplified on DNA gyrase. However, the most significant growth in development and use of the methods, as well as increasingly vigorous campaigning for the approach, came from within the small, structure-based discovery companies such as Astex, Vernalis, SGX and Plexxikon that were established in the late 1990s and early 2000s. The core rationale for these companies was to build medicinal chemistry around a structure-based platform. Fragments (or in the case of Plexxikon, scaffolds focussed on a particular chemogenomic space[143,144]) provided a way for these smaller companies to obtain the initial hits without the investment in multi-million member compound libraries and the automation required for HTS. Some of the important method developments and examples from the early days of these companies were:

- Development of high throughput crystallography for screening and structure determination. Astex focussed on developing a crystal system suitable for soaking of fragment mixtures and have invested heavily in developing the crystallographic and data analysis tools to analyse the resulting structures.[145,146] SGX (and also a company called Syrrx[147–149]) developed and exploited high throughput crystallisation coupled with dedicated synchrotron beamlines.
- Development of fragment libraries – Vernalis published one of the first detailed descriptions of how to select fragments for a library.[29] Astex developed some ideas on the characteristics of compounds that were hits in fragment screens and coined the phrase "rule of 3"[150,151] which was a useful marketing tool in establishing the field.[152] These early analyses of the characteristics of fragments helped to guide further library design.[26,153,154] A later perspective from Astex,[150] redefined this rule more as a guideline – as useful current fragment libraries contain smaller compounds with an average molecular weight closer to 180 Da.

### 5.8.4 What's in a Name?

Practitioners have used various terms to label fragment-based approaches. When applied to pharmaceutical discovery of therapeutic agents, the term "lead" discovery is appropriate. Fragments can make a significant contribution in the early stages of discovery of the lead compound, but a compound is not a drug until after successful completion of Phase II clinical trials (demonstrating an effect on disease in patients). Progression from lead to drug mainly rests on conventional medicinal chemistry and pharmacology and has little to do with fragment-based methods. In recent years, the methods have increasingly been applied in the sphere of chemical biology (see Section 5.6) – hence the use of the word "ligand" in the title of this chapter.

### 5.8.5 Some Important Underpinning Concepts

An important early concept for fragments comes from the discussion of molecular complexity by Hann and co-workers.[7] They argued that a compound needs to be of a certain size (and complexity – that is number of features capable of interaction) to bind to a target, but if it gets too large then it is more likely to have features that prevent it from binding. A second important concept which has had a major impact on medicinal chemistry in general, and fragment evolution in particular, is that of ligand efficiency,[155] which built on some earlier ideas about the maximal affinity attainable by ligands.[156] These ideas have merged with others from retrospective analyses of the properties of successful drug-like compounds[157–159] to give a whole raft of different efficiency metrics.[160] There is a danger that these metrics can be applied too rigorously – for example, an early fragment may have much potential once optimised, but low ligand efficiency to begin with. However, they do provide a useful monitor of compound properties to advise the chemist/modeller and a useful metric with which to persuade the fragment sceptic that these low affinity starting points are efficient.

## 5.9 Fragment Evolution

Quite a lot of time (and space) has been used in this article describing the design of fragment libraries and the methods for detecting fragment binding. However, it is relatively straightforward to find fragment hits for most sites on most protein targets. The real challenge is deciding which fragments to choose for optimisation and evolving those fragments to effective hits and leads. There have been a number of reviews of published fragment-based evolution.[161–163]

Figure 5.6 is a schematic summary of the three main approaches to fragment evolution. The initial ideas were to identify fragments binding to different sites on a protein and link them together – SAR by NMR, as discussed above. Although there are some striking examples from the Abbott group, there are few other examples of fragment linking from other groups (some examples are ref. 164 and 165). Most examples in the literature are of fragment growing – where the structure of the initial fragment guides the addition of functional groups to achieve the required affinity and selectivity. Fragment merging is where information is used from a number of different sources (fragments, virtual screening, literature compounds) to design new scaffolds.

Figures 5.7 to 5.19 provide a summary of a set of fragment evolution stories, chosen to reflect these different approaches. The captions to the individual examples include notes on some of the lessons that can be learnt. A more general comment is on ligand efficiency. As discussed above, this idea plays an important role in fragment and lead optimisation. The calculation keeps the design focussed on achieving the maximal potency possible with the addition of heavy atoms. This principle is nicely illustrated in the Chk1 example (Figure 5.11) where the fall in ligand efficiency highlighted that a particular modification was not optimal – and could be corrected. The CDK2 example (Figure 5.12) emphasises another aspect of fragment evolution: if the ligand efficiency is kept as high as possible during the early optimisation, then some of that efficiency can be “spent” in making modifications to improve drug-like potency and efficacy (Figures 5.10, 5.13 and 5.14).

A great deal of time and resource is required in the purification of each compound during optimisation to then generate a solution of known concentration for the compound activity to be measured. An innovation which can remove the need for these steps is so-called Off-Rate Screening (ORS) where a crude reaction mixture is directly assessed. In most cases, an increase in affinity comes about through a change in $k_{off}$ (off-rate). As can be seen from eqn (5.1), this is a first-order rate constant which is independent of concentration. This means that a slowing in off-rate (measured for example by SPR) will be seen for a compound of higher affinity if there is some product generated in the reaction. This has been exploited by a number of groups.[60,61] The approach can be further extended with high throughput crystallography, where the crystal can select a higher affinity product.[87,166]

## 5.10 Fragments and Chemical Space

An early concern in fragment-based discovery was whether selecting hits from such a small library would lead to problems in issues with IP for the optimised compounds. This fear has not been realised. There is some evidence that certain targets are attractive for certain scaffolds,[99,167] and it is clear that some companies have very similar fragments in their libraries. This becomes apparent when comparing fragment and other drug discovery campaigns from different companies. The example in Figure 5.15 shows how an azaindole led to multiple clinical candidates for different targets. This can also hold for the same target. A detailed analysis has been carried out for Hsp90 projects[168] – this analysis also emphasises the point that a fragment screen can quite effectively assess the accessible chemical space for a target. The first fragment screen on this target in 2002 identified 17 hits from a ligand-observed screen of a library of 729 fragments.[169] An analysis in 2011 of Hsp90 showed that just five of the fragments recapitulate the key features of the published lead and candidate compounds. In some cases, very similar fragments had been chosen for evolution by different companies; although there are sometimes some echoes of one company's compound in another, all of the compounds have achieved sufficient novelty (Figures 5.16–5.19).

## 5.11 Concluding Remarks

This article has covered most of the practical aspects of fragment-based discovery. It will hopefully be useful in introducing the ideas and methods, with some practical examples of methods of fragment library design, screening and fragment evolution.

Those new to the area should consider a general mantra for any new technology or method. When assessing a new technique, there are three variables to consider – the technology, the experience of the practitioner and the target it is being applied to. It is useful in any assessment if there is only one variable – inexpert application or inappropriate target is not a fair assessment of a new technology. This applies to fragment-based discovery overall, as well as the different components, such as the fragment library, screening methods and approach to fragment evolution. The key is to gain a depth of experience with a particular approach, to understand how to recognise and deal with artefacts, to understand in detail the principles on which the techniques depend and to think carefully about effective positive and negative controls.

There are many opportunities for future development of the methods and their effective integration with medicinal chemistry. In this concluding section, I consider some of them.

It is clear from the examples presented here, that most of the published examples of successful fragment-based discovery campaigns are for "conventional" targets, such as kinases, where there are well-defined binding sites and where structure-based design can rapidly progress fragments to leads. Although other screening methods such as HTS or DEL will identify many hit compounds, the advantage that fragments bring is in identifying novel scaffolds and binding motifs that can be exploited to give selectivity, novel IP, and most importantly, choice in the lead optimisation process. The main challenge in effective use of fragment-based methods on such targets within established organisations is to persuade the medicinal chemist that starting from such a small starting point can be successful, rather than trying to fix the issues with a large hit. The opportunity in large organisations is using the fragments alongside HTS and DEL (see for example Figure 5.20).[170] The fragment hits can give insights into the important motifs and interactions that can be made and either suggest scaffold replacements or how to deconstruct the screening hit into constituent parts.

There is real potential for fragments to provide starting points against "non-conventional" targets, such as protein–protein interactions, large multi-subunit complexes or intrinsically disordered proteins; the challenge here is that although it is relatively straightforward to find fragment hits against such targets, it can take time (a number of years) and commitment to progress these fragments to suitable leads or even respectable hit compounds. There are still relatively few examples of success against such targets, but what there is[122,171] demonstrate that extreme care needs to be taken in evolving the fragments to hits – not only because of the difficulty of establishing robust models of how the fragments bind, but also because there are often issues with the assays for such targets that take some time to resolve.

In conclusion – the main advantage of fragment-based discovery is that the methods give the medicinal chemist choice. They provide a large choice of starting points, the opportunity to start small and grow carefully to do "good" medicinal chemistry, and they provide starting points for targets for which more conventional screening approaches fail. An important message is that fragment-based discovery is not necessarily any faster – most projects spend some time exploring fragment SAR before embarking on optimisation chemistry. But the evidence suggests that the fragment-based methods can deliver a better quality of compounds and a higher chance of success in reaching clinical candidates.

## 5.12 Hints and Tips

- Fragments are small (molecular weight <250 Da, optimally around 170 Da) compounds that have suitable physicochemical properties for high concentration screening. The crucial property of a fragment is low molecular weight – the size of chemical space increases by 8× per heavy atom added, so the smaller the compounds the greater the chemical space sampled when screening.
- Most methods for detecting fragment binding require high concentration screening; this means that most fragment libraries consist of highly soluble compounds.
- It is vital that the fragment library is regularly curated to check for aggregation, solubility or decomposition; this will save a lot of time and effort chasing false positives in screening.
- Most practitioners find that a fragment library of around 1000 low molecular weight fragments is sufficient to provide hits for most targets – it is resource intensive to curate much larger libraries. Key is to maintain a chemically diverse library.
- The most widely applicable and robust method for fragment screening is ligand-observed NMR; for proteins below 30 kDa which can be over-expressed in bacteria, protein-observed NMR (HSQC) is the gold standard for detecting and characterising fragment binding. If sufficient protein is not available for NMR experiments, then SPR is a good general-purpose screening method. Key is gaining experience and expertise in the method, so that anomalies can be identified, and the screening library optimised for that technique.
- Most successful fragment-to-lead campaigns involve structure-guided growth of the fragment.
- As fragment methods are increasingly deployed, there are opportunities for using the fragment hits to dissect key features and improve hits from other screening paradigms such as HTS and DEL.

## Key References

- The very first publication on fragment based discovery from Abbott.[50]
- A review of the first 20 years of fragment-based discovery.[16]
- Volume 493 of *Methods in Enzymology*: there are many papers from key practitioners in the field, with good commentaries on the methods and reviews. For example ref. 19.

## Acknowledgements

I thank all at Vernalis and York who have made such important contributions to the development of my ideas about fragment-based drug discovery. For this article, I particularly value the enthusiasm and input to discussions from Ben Davis and James Murray and the analysis from Ijen Chen on fragment hit rates.

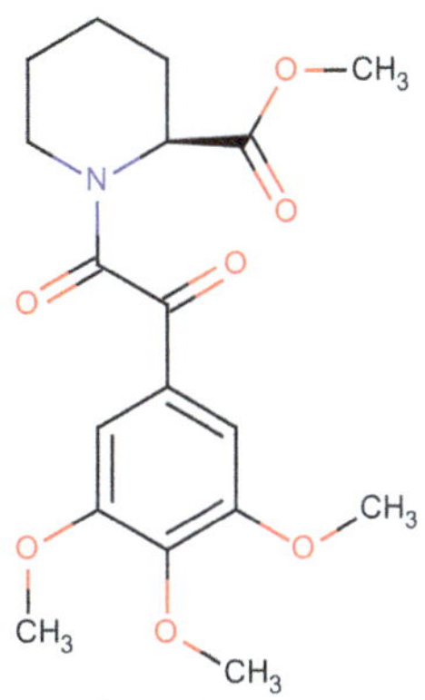

**1** 2 μM
Fragment in site 1

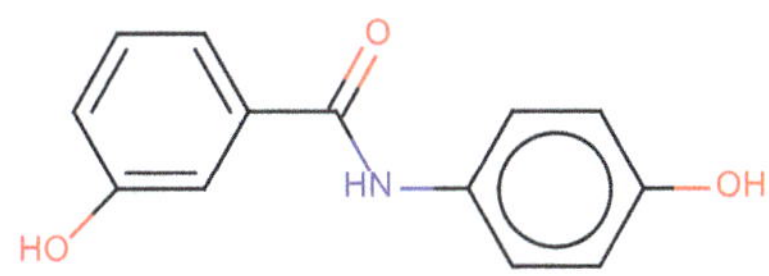

**2** 100 μM
Fragment in site 2

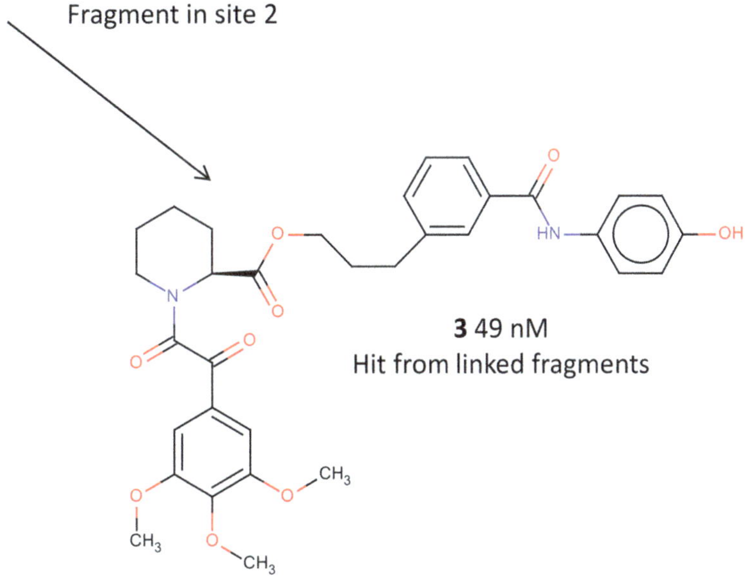

**3** 49 nM
Hit from linked fragments

**Figure 5.7** SAR by NMR: FKBP.[50] Compound **1** was identified by HSQC NMR from a screen of a fragment library as binding to an $^{15}$N-labelled sample of the protein FKBP. A subsequent screen by HSQC NMR of FKBP with a library of fragments in the presence of compound **1** identified compound **2** binding to an alternate site. Structures determined by NMR identified the appropriate vectors for linking the two fragments and compound **3** was identified as one of the more potent hits. The activity numbers are the reported $K_D$ from the NMR HSQC titrations.

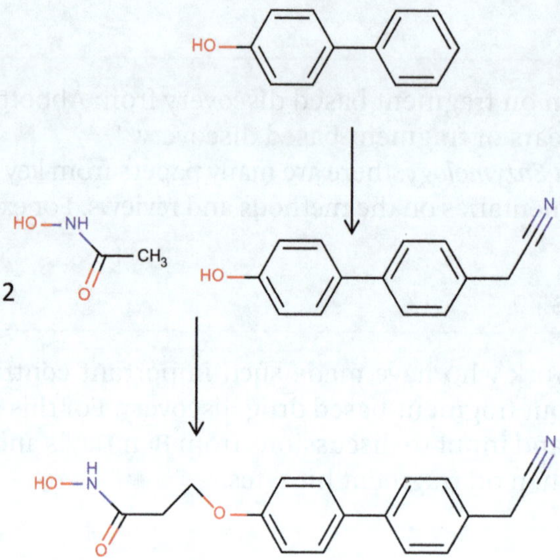

**4** 0.3 mM
Fragment in site 1

**6** 7 mM
Fragment in site 2

**5** 0.02 mM
Optimised Fragment in site 1

**7** 25 nM
Hit from linked fragments

**Figure 5.8** SAR by NMR: Stromelysin.[137] Compound **4** was identified by HSQC NMR from a screen of a fragment library as binding to an $^{15}N$-labelled sample of the metalloprotease, stromelysin. Subsequent optimisation led to compound **5**; a subsequent screen by HSQC NMR of stromelysin with a library of smaller fragments in the presence of compound **5** identified compound **6** binding to an alternate site. Structures determined by NMR identified the appropriate vectors for linking the two fragments and compound **7** was identified as one of the more potent hits.

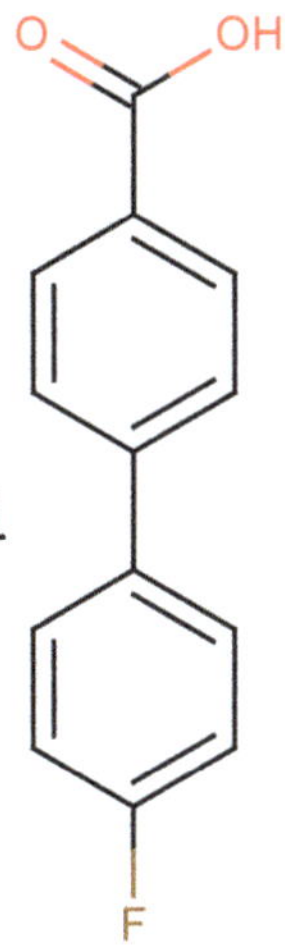

**8** $K_D$ 0.3 mM
Fragment in site 1

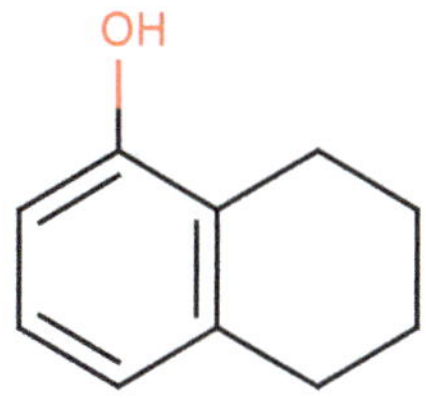

**9** $K_D$ 4.3 mM
Fragment in site 2

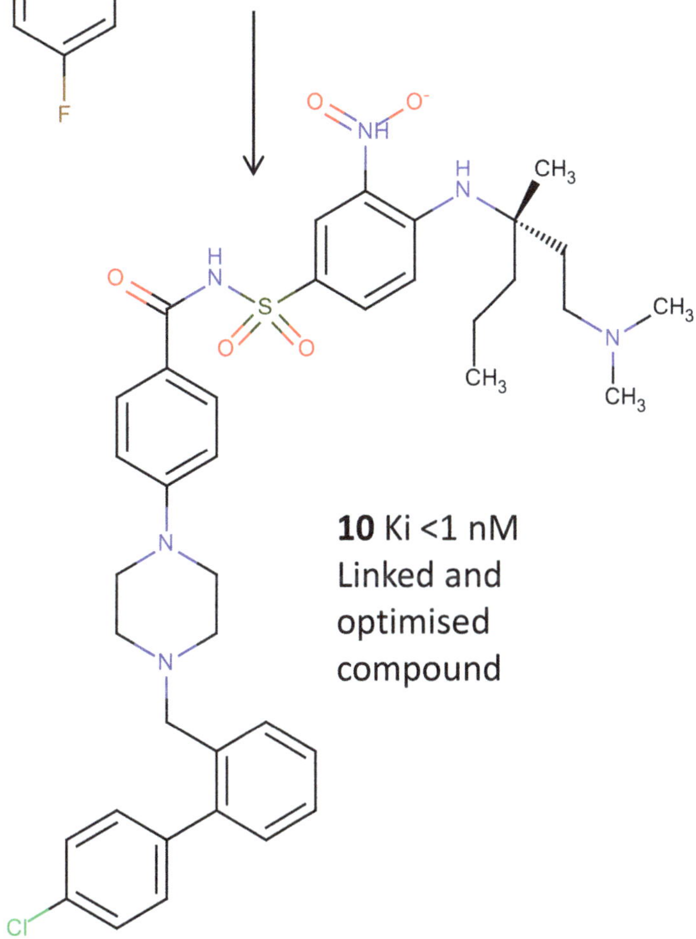

**10** Ki <1 nM
Linked and optimised compound

**Figure 5.9** SAR by NMR: Bcl-2/Bcl-$x_L$.[9,173,174] Compound **8** was identified by HSQC NMR from a screen of a fragment library as binding to an $^{15}$N-labelled sample of the pro-apoptotic protein, Bcl-$x_L$. A subsequent screen by HSQC NMR of Bcl-$x_L$ with a library of smaller fragments in the presence of compound **8** identified compound **9** binding to an alternate site. A combination of NMR structure determination and substantial chemistry effort led to the clinical candidate, ABT737, compound **10**, which *(continued)*

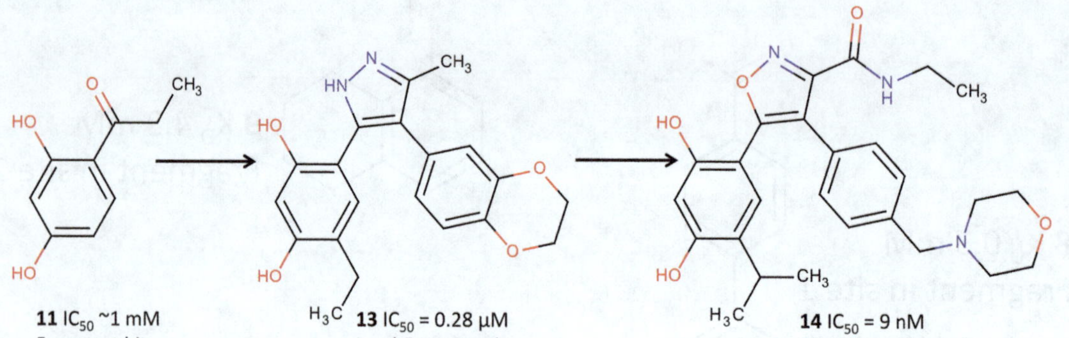

**11** $IC_{50}$ ~1 mM
Fragment hit

**13** $IC_{50}$ = 0.28 μM
Lead Compound

**14** $IC_{50}$ = 9 nM
Clinical candidate

**12**
Competitor PU3

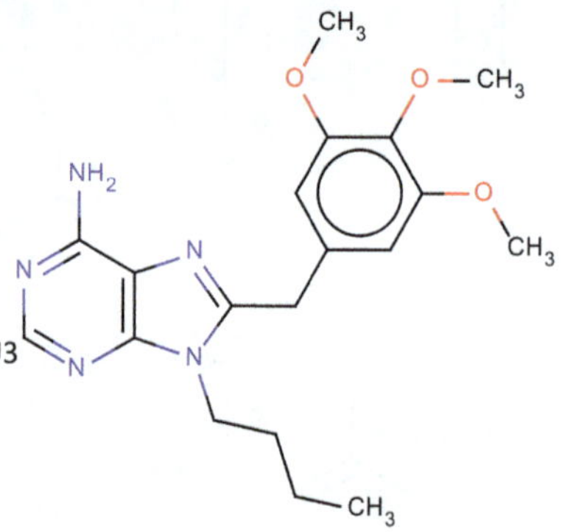

**Figure 5.10** SAR by Catalogue: HSP90.[169,176–179] Compound **11** was identified from a fragment library by ligand-observed NMR as competing with PU3[180] (compound **12**) for binding to the N-terminal domain of the molecular chaperone, HSP90. The resorcinol sub-structure was used to search a database of commercially available compounds;[172] the resulting compounds were assessed by computational docking for fit into the binding site. Compound **13** was identified as a sub-micromolar hit; this compound was also found by a medium throughput screen and by virtual screening. Subsequent structure-based optimisation led to the compound **14** (AUY922) which entered numerous Phase II trials for various cancers. The activity numbers are the reported $IC_{50}$ values from fluorescence polarisation measurements made for displacing a fluorescein-labelled resorcinol-pyrazole.[181]

**Figure 5.9** *(continued)* was further optimised (for compound properties) to ABT263[175] and then to introduce selectivity for Bcl-2 over Bcl-$x_L$ in the compound ABT199,[9] the drug venetoclax, which is now treating patients with various cancers. The $K_D$ values were the reported from an HSQC titration; the $K_i$ value estimated from inhibition of BH3 domain binding in a wet assay. The projects summarised in Figures 5.7 and 5.8 are striking examples of linking two fragments where the initial fragments are very clearly present in the linked compounds. In the Bcl-2 example of Figure 5.9, there has been substantial evolution and movement of the fragments in their respective binding sites. However, the fragment methods provided starting points for chemistry which were not obtained from high throughput screening. Although considerable chemistry effort (and time) is needed to generate leads against such targets, the fragments at least provide a starting point.

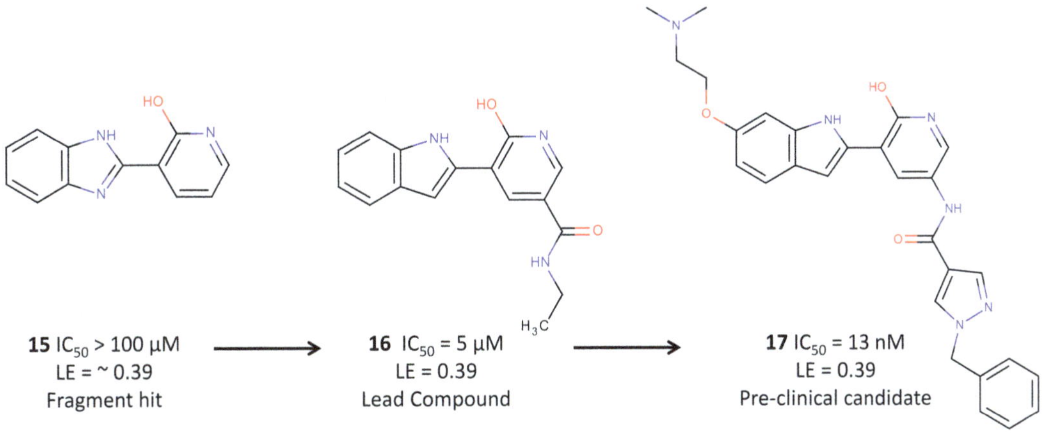

**15** $IC_{50}$ > 100 µM
LE = ~ 0.39
Fragment hit

**16** $IC_{50}$ = 5 µM
LE = 0.39
Lead Compound

**17** $IC_{50}$ = 13 nM
LE = 0.39
Pre-clinical candidate

**Figure 5.11** Fragment growth: Chk-1.[182] Compound **15** was identified from a fragment library as inhibiting the enzyme activity of the kinase, Chk-1. The crystal structure of the fragment bound to the ATP pocket of Chk-1 identified suitable vectors for growth - addition of the amide to give compound **16** gave an improvement in affinity while maintaining ligand efficiency. Subsequent optimisation led to compound **17**, which retains the ligand efficiency. Earlier analogues of compound **17** had a reversed amide; the affinity was 200 µM with a ligand efficiency of 0.33. Analysis of the crystal structure identified sub-optimal hydrogen bonding to the solvent, which was corrected in compound **17**. The activity numbers are the $IC_{50}$ values from an activity assay for Chk-1 which monitors the ATP-driven phosphorylation of a Chk-1 substrate.

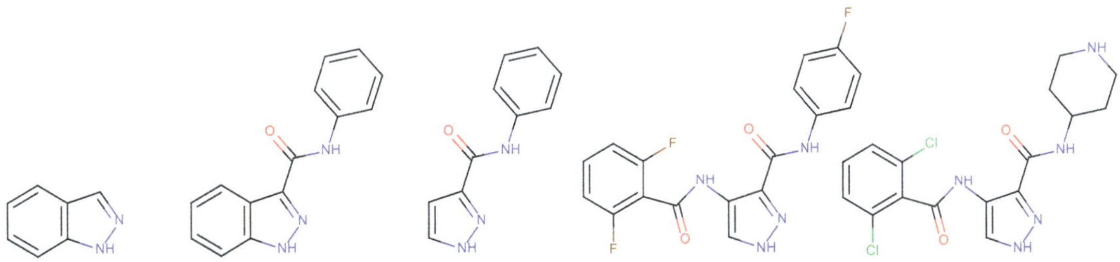

**18** $IC_{50}$ 185 µM
LE = 0.57
Initial fragment

**19** $IC_{50}$ 3 µM
LE = 0.42

**20** $IC_{50}$ 97 µM
LE = 0.39

**21** $IC_{50}$ 0.003 µM
LE = 0.45

**22** $IC_{50}$ 0.047 µM
LE = 0.40
Clinical candidate

**Figure 5.12** Fragment growth: CDK inhibitor.[183] Compound **18** was identified from an X-ray crystallographic screen of a fragment library as binding to CDK2. Iterative, detailed structure-based design led to compounds **19** to **21** in which the crystal structures of the growing compounds was used to identify regions of the compound for modification and addition. The final compound **22** is AT7519, assessed in clinical trials as a therapy for solid tumours. The activity numbers are from a kinase activity assay. As discussed in the text, the high ligand efficiency achieved for compound **21** provided opportunities to tune the properties in compound **22** by "spending" some of that ligand efficiency.

**23** $K_D$ 550 µM, LE = 0.37, Initial fragment → **24** $K_D$ 15 µM, LE = 0.39 → **25** $K_D$ 200 µM, $K_i$ >500µM, LE = 0.39 → **26** Ki 3.7 µM, LE = 0.45 → **27** Ki 2 nM, LE = 0.48

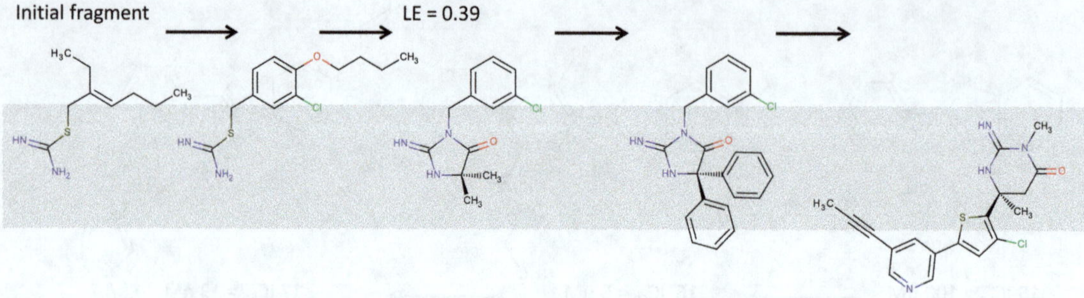

**Figure 5.13** Fragment growth: BACE1 inhibitor.[184] Compound **23** was identified as binding to BACE1 from an HSQC NMR screen of a fragment library. Based on this, 204 close analogues were synthesised from which compound **24** was identified, which was co-crystallised with BACE1. The structure led to the design of the iminohydantoin scaffold (compound **25**) which presented vectors into substrate recognition pockets; subsequent structure-based design led to compound **26**, which has the right balance of physico-chemical properties for *in vivo* efficacy. The grey square in the background emphasises the development of the core of this series. $K_D$ values were from NMR HSQC titrations, $K_i$ values from an activity assay. This project demonstrated the importance of taking time to identify and optimise the initial scaffold and the need for careful and persistent structure-guided chemistry.

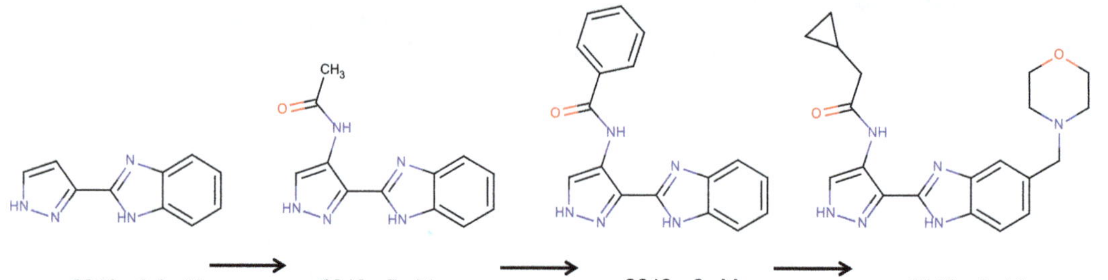

**28** $IC_{50}$ 0.9 µM, LE = 0.59, CDK2 = 28 µM, Initial fragment → **29** $IC_{50}$ 7 nM, LE = 0.54, CDK2 = 1µM → **30** $IC_{50}$ 6 nM, LE = 0.49, CDK2 = 52nM → **31** $IC_{50}$ 3 nM, LE = 0.41, CDK2 = 510nM

**Figure 5.14** Fragment growth: Aurora inhibitor.[185] Compound **28** was initially identified from an X-ray crystallographic screen of a fragment library as binding to CDK2 with an affinity of 28 µM; it was subsequently found to be a highly efficient inhibitor of Aurora A. This practise is variously called target hopping or chemogenomics, where a library of compounds which has some affinity for a class of proteins can be used as a starting point for generation of selective inhibitors for specific members of the family (see also Figure 5.15, where an azaindole fragment was used for three different kinases). Iterative, detailed structure-based design led to compounds **29** to **31** in which the crystal structures of the growing compounds were used to identify regions of the compound for modification and addition. Of particular concern with this series was selectivity; as with the CDK2 example above, the high ligand efficiency of compound **29** has been "spent" to improve the selectivity (and other physicochemical properties). The final compound **31** is AT9283, assessed in clinical trials as a therapy for solid tumours and haematological malignancies. The activity numbers are from a kinase activity assay.

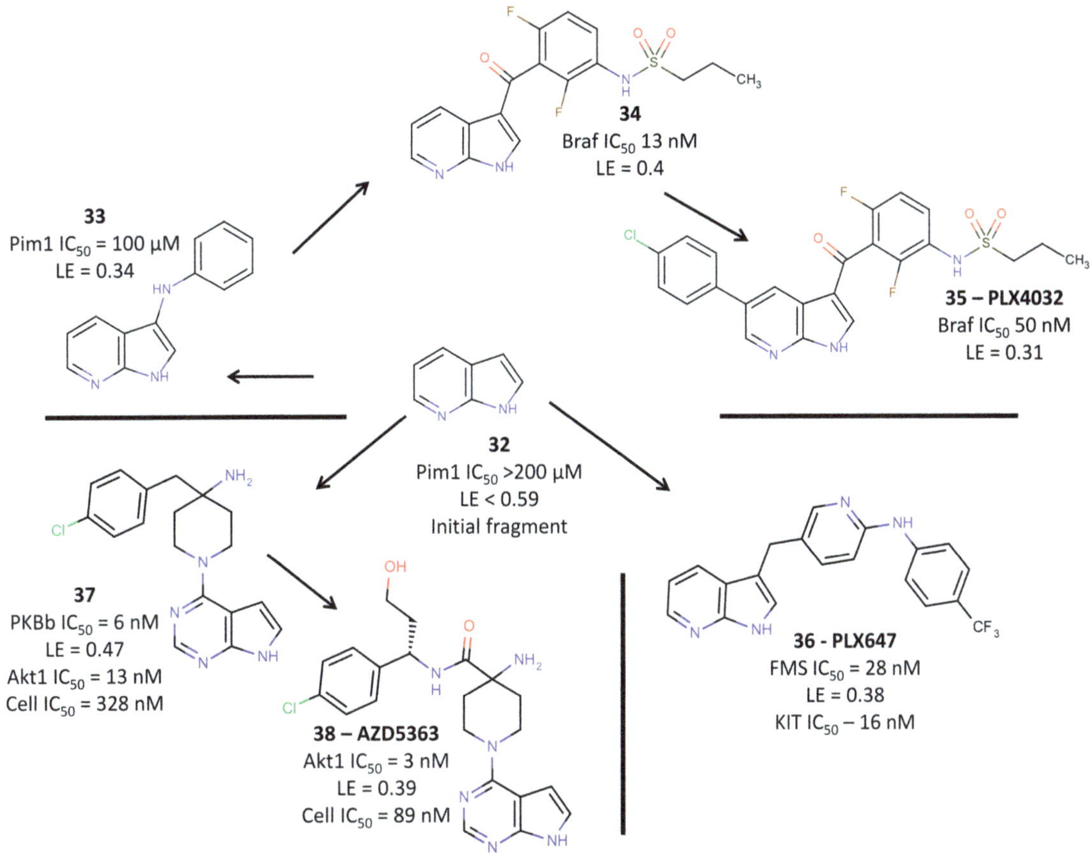


**Figure 5.15** Fragment growth: 7-azaindole providing inhibitors of Braf kinase,[10,48] Akt,[186,187] and a dual inhibitor of FMS and Kit kinases.[47] Compound **32** was initially identified by biochemical screening and confirmed by X-ray crystallography as binding to the kinase Pim1 and early structure-guided optimisation gave compound **33** and the compound **34** (PLX4720). This design was based on binding to first Pim1 and then Fgfr1 kinase, both of which were more readily crystallised. Eventually, structures of Braf were generated, leading to compound **35** now on the market as vemurafenib for the treatment of mutant-Braf-driven melanoma. Although the activity on the enzyme (and the targeted mutant Braf with V600E) is modest, it shows remarkable selectivity in cellular and *in vivo* models. The activity numbers are the reported activity from a kinase activity assay. Fragment **32** was also the starting point for the same Plexikkon group to identify a marketed dual inhibitor of FMS and Kit kinase, **36**; the same fragment was elaborated by Astex and Institute of Cancer Research[186] initially focussed on optimising to **37** as an inhibitor of PKB, which AstraZeneca subsequently optimised to the clinical candidate **38** (AZD5363)[187] for Akt kinase.

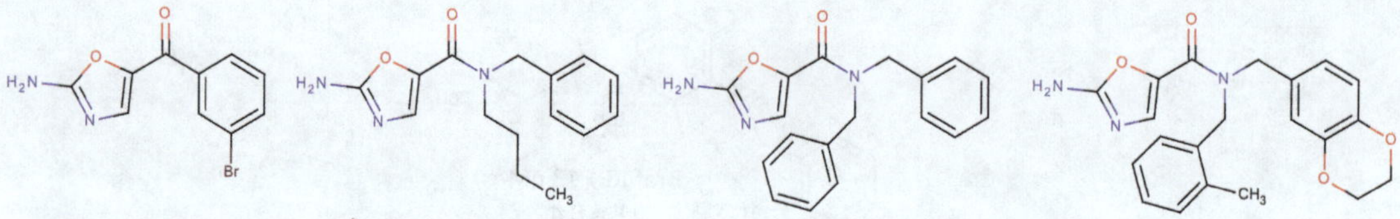

**39** $IC_{50}$ 21.5 µM, LE < 0.40, Initial fragment → **40** $IC_{50}$ 1 µM, LE = 0.41 → **41** $IC_{50}$ 125 nM, LE = 0.41 → **42** $IC_{50}$ 7 nM, LE = 0.40

**Figure 5.16** Fragment growth: Biotin carboxylase.[188] The initial fragment **39** was identified by biochemical screening of a library of 5200 fragments with validation by STD NMR. The crystal structure bound to biotin carboxylase identified potential regions for optimisation and led to the redesigned amide-containing template **40**. Subsequent structure-guided growth led to **41** and then **42**. Additional hit series were also generated for this target by merging features of fragments and also merging fragments with functional groups identified from hit compounds discovered by virtual screening. The activity numbers are the reported $IC_{50}$ from an activity assay for acetyl-CoA carboxylase (biotin carboxylase is a subunit of this enzyme). See also a recent review on fragment-based discovery for antibacterial targets.[13]

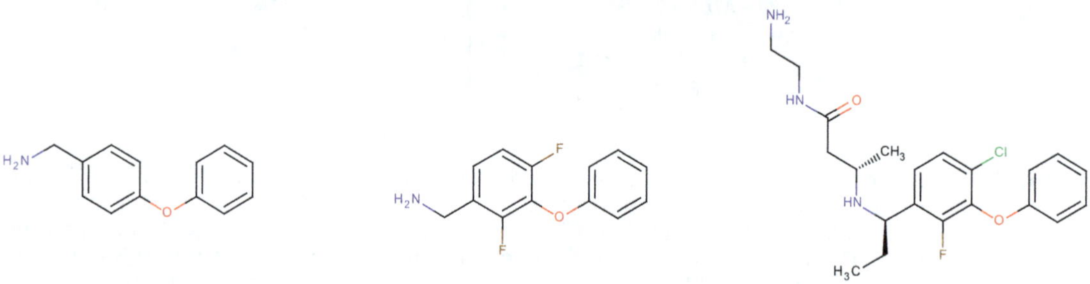

**43** $IC_{50}$ ~500 µM, LE < 0.30, Initial fragment → **44** $K_D$ 20 µM, LE = 0.38 → **45** $K_D$ 22 nM, LE = 0.39

**Figure 5.17** Fragment growth: HCV protease/helicase.[81] Crystals of the HCV protease/helicase were screened by X-ray crystallography; a novel, pre-existing cavity was identified at the interface between the two domains, into which fragments such as **43** bound. Such compounds stabilise the inactivated conformation of the protein; the functional significance of this allosteric effector was realised early on in optimisation of the compounds. The initial fragment was optimised to compound **44** before structure-guided growth led to compound **45**; this inhibits the virus *in vivo*. The activity numbers are the reported $IC_{50}$ from a protease FRET based assay; $K_D$ was measured by ITC.

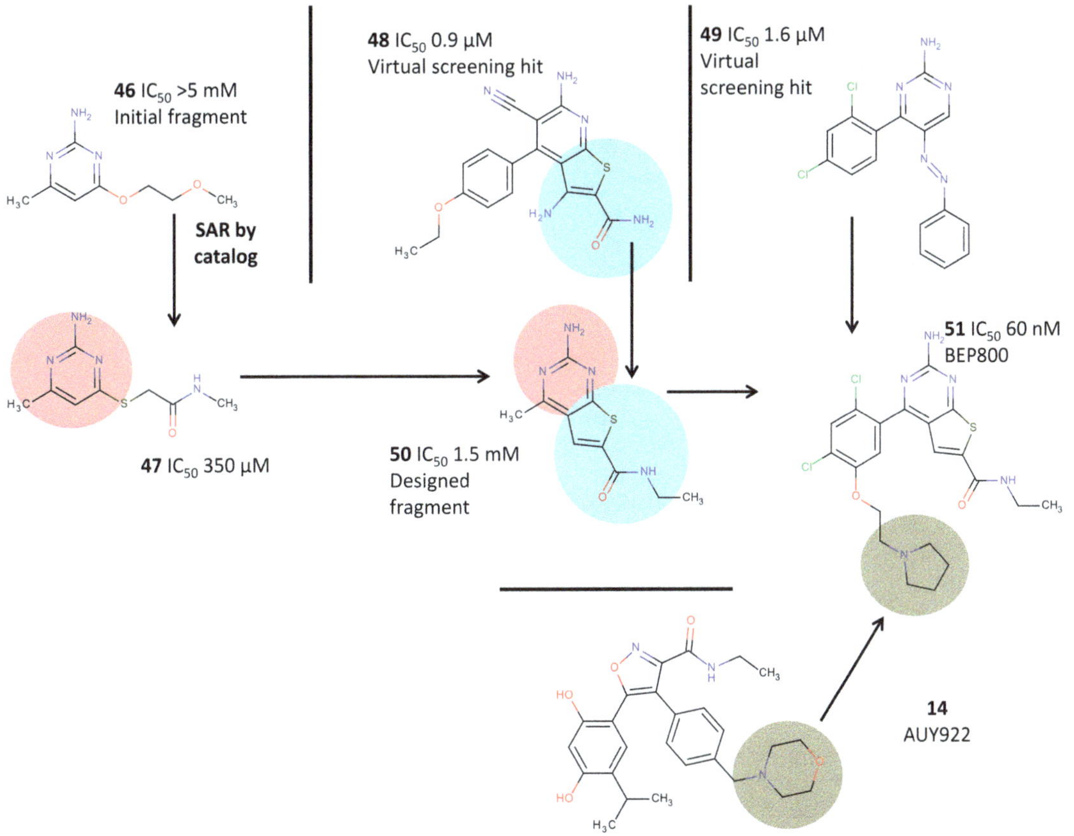


**Figure 5.18** Merging fragments and other hits: Hsp90.[169,189] Compound **46** was one of the 17 fragments identified as binding competitively with PU3[190] (compound **12**) by ligand-observed NMR screening of the N-terminus of HSP90 with the initial Vernalis fragment library of 729 compounds[29] (SeeDs1) in 2002; subsequent SAR by catalogue (guided by the crystal structure) led to compound **47**. Compounds **48** and **49** were identified by virtual screening of the ATPase site of the N-terminus of HSP90. When these hits were initially considered, there was a concern that the thioether of **47** has potential metabolic liabilities; in addition, the cyano moiety of **48** was making unfavourable interactions with the binding site. The crystal structures of these various compounds bound to HSP90 suggested the design of the fragment **50**; this was synthesised and, although relatively weakly binding, the crystal structure showed it bound as predicted. Subsequent structure-guided evolution of **51** was rapid, with incorporation of the dichloro-benzene suggested by **52** and the incorporation of a solubiliser at the position suggested by **14**, AUY922 (Figure 5.10). The resulting compound **51** (BEP800) is orally bioavailable and shows efficacy in tumour regression models. The activity numbers are the reported $IC_{50}$ from a fluorescence polarisation assay.[181] This example illustrates the power of combination of compound properties understood from multiple crystal structures; it also emphasises that the weaker binding fragments should be considered – the decision of which fragment to evolve is a balance of synthetic opportunity, the vectors that are available and the physico-chemical properties of the resulting compounds. Another example of fragment merging from Vernalis is for the kinase, PDPK1.[123] Another example of designing a fragment using multiple crystal structures of different chemotypes is the work at Vertex on Itk kinase inhibitors.[191]

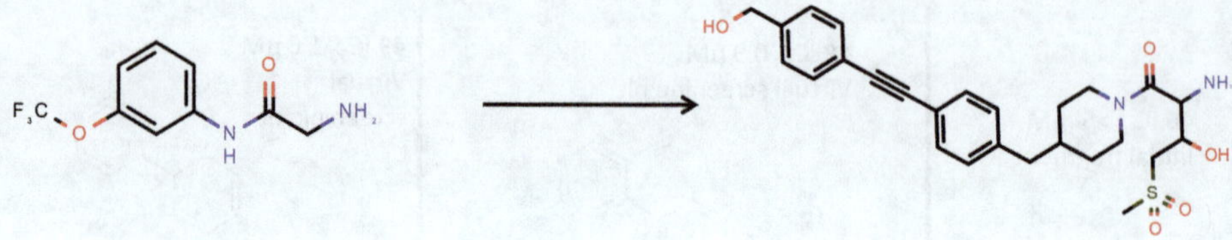

**52**
Fragment
*Pa*LpxC $IC_{50}$ = 40 µM
LE = 0.37

**53**
*Pa*LpxC $IC_{50}$ 6 nM
LE = 0.33

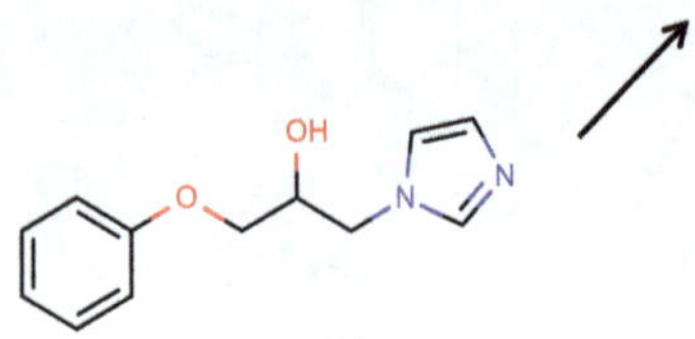

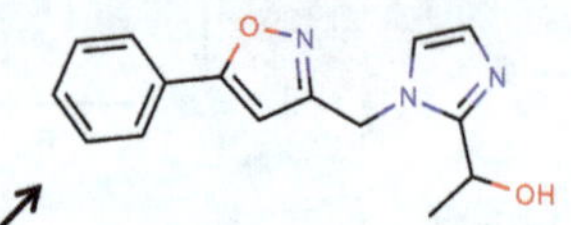

**55**
*Pa*LpxC $IC_{50}$ 125 nM
LE = 0.47

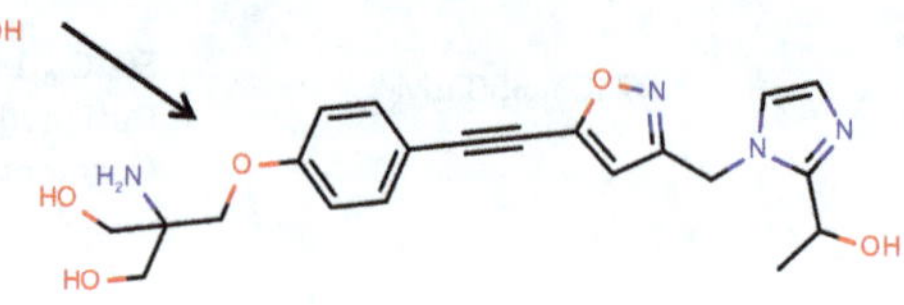

**54**
Fragment
*Pa*LpxC $IC_{50}$ = 40 µM
LE = 0.37

**56**
*Pa*LpxC $IC_{50}$ 20 nM
LE = 0.35
*Pa* MIC = 8 µg/ml

**Figure 5.19** Novel metal-chelating motifs from fragments: LpxC. The zinc metalloenzyme LpxC catalyses a critical step in biosynthesis of the bacterial cell wall. Many inhibitors had been developed which contained a hydroxamate group to chelate the zinc – which also binds to other metalloproteases, causing off-target toxicity. A ligand-observed NMR screen identified zinc-binding fragments including a glycine (**52**) and an imidazole (**54**) motif. Structure-guided design generated **53** for the glycine series, which showed antibacterial activity. Addition of 2-hydroxy to the imidazole improved the affinity and selectivity of zinc chelation and introduction of the isoxazole in **55** picked up additional selective interactions in the binding site. Further optimisation for interactions and compound properties led to **56**, which showed antibacterial activity (Pa = *Pseudomonas aeruginosa*). $IC_{50}$ values are for a functional assay measuring breakdown of a lipopolysaccharide substrate.

**58**
Fragment
$IC_{50}$ = 62 µM
LE = 0.36

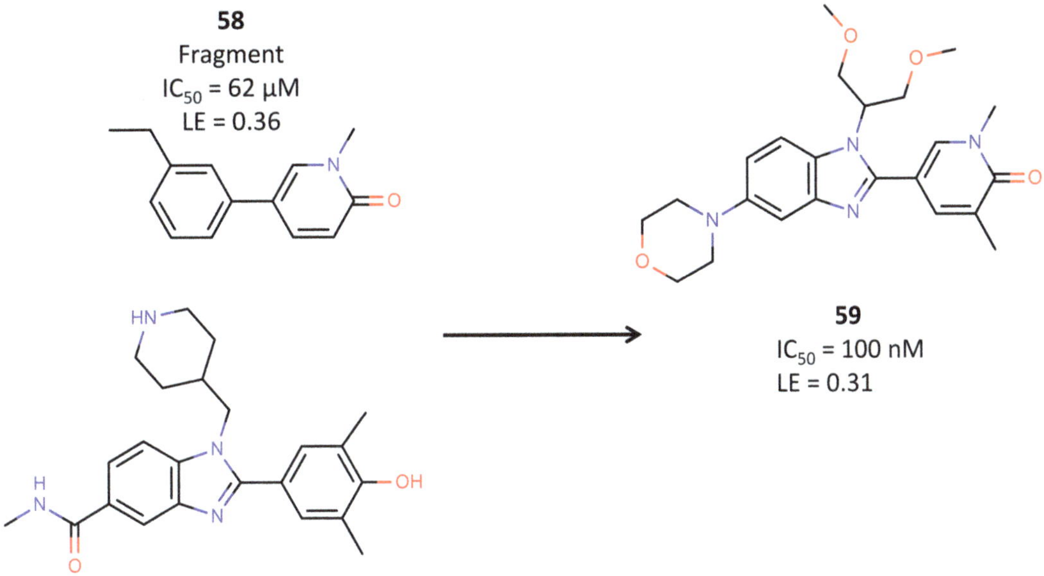

**57**
DEL hit
$IC_{50}$ = 11 µM
LE = 0.27

**59**
$IC_{50}$ = 100 nM
LE = 0.31

**Figure 5.20** Combining fragments with DNA-encoded libraries: bromodomain inhibition.[170] A screen of a 117 million DEL against the bromodomain BRD4, identified **57**, which has poor ADME properties. A previous fragment screen had identified **58**; crystal structures showed that the *N*-methyl pyridone of **58** binds in the same acetyl-lysine binding pocket as the dimethyl, hydroxy phenyl moiety of **57** which led to design of compounds that were optimised to **59**, which is orally active *in vivo.* $IC_{50}$ values are for a FRET assay measuring displacement of a known BET inhibitor.

## References


1. A. Ajay, W. P. Walters and M. A. Murcko, *J. Med. Chem.*, 1998, **41**, 3314–3324.
2. O. B. Cox, T. Krojer, P. Collins, O. Monteiro, R. Talon, A. Bradley, O. Fedorov, J. Amin, B. D. Marsden, J. Spencer, F. von Delft and P. E. Brennan, *Chem. Sci.*, 2016, **7**, 2322–2330.
3. S. Sreeramulu, C. Richter, T. Kuehn, K. Azzaoui, M. J. J. Blommers, R. Del Conte, M. Fragai, N. Trieloff, P. Schmieder, M. Nazaré, E. Specker, V. Ivanov, H. Oschkinat, L. Banci and H. Schwalbe, *J. Biomol. NMR*, 2020, **74**, 555–563.
4. S. J. Teague, A. M. Davis, P. D. Leeson and T. Oprea, *Angew. Chem., Int. Ed.*, 1999, **38**, 3743–3748.
5. M. M. Hann and T. I. Oprea, *Curr. Opin. Chem. Biol.*, 2004, **8**, 255–263.
6. R. Macarron, *Drug Discovery Today*, 2006, **11**, 277–279.
7. M. M. Hann, A. R. Leach and G. Harper, *J. Chem. Inf. Comput. Sci.*, 2001, **41**, 856–864.
8. D. A. Erlanson, http://practicalfragments.blogspot.com/2020/03/fragments-in-clinic-2020-edition.html, 2020.

9. A. J. Souers, J. D. Leverson, E. R. Boghaert, S. L. Ackler, N. D. Catron, J. Chen, B. D. Dayton, H. Ding, S. H. Enschede, W. J. Fairbrother, D. C. Huang, S. G. Hymowitz, S. Jin, S. L. Khaw, P. J. Kovar, L. T. Lam, J. Lee, H. L. Maecker, K. C. Marsh, K. D. Mason, M. J. Mitten, P. M. Nimmer, A. Oleksijew, C. H. Park, C. M. Park, D. C. Phillips, A. W. Roberts, D. Sampath, J. F. Seymour, M. L. Smith, G. M. Sullivan, S. K. Tahir, C. Tse, M. D. Wendt, Y. Xiao, J. C. Xue, H. Zhang, R. A. Humerickhouse, S. H. Rosenberg and S. W. Elmore, *Nat. Med.*, 2013, **19**, 202–208.
10. G. Bollag, J. Tsai, J. Zhang, C. Zhang, P. Ibrahim, K. Nolop and P. Hirth, *Nat. Rev. Drug Discovery*, 2012, **11**, 873–886.
11. T. P. S. Perera, E. Jovcheva, L. Mevellec, J. Vialard, D. De Lange, T. Verhulst, C. Paulussen, K. Van De Ven, P. King, E. Freyne, D. C. Rees, M. Squires, G. Saxty, M. Page, C. W. Murray, R. Gilissen, G. Ward, N. T. Thompson, D. R. Newell, N. Cheng, L. Xie, J. Yang, S. J. Platero, J. D. Karkera, C. Moy, P. Angibaud, S. Laquerre and M. V. Lorenzi, *Mol. Cancer Ther.*, 2017, **16**, 1010–1020.
12. W. D. Tap, Z. A. Wainberg, S. P. Anthony, P. N. Ibrahim, C. Zhang, J. H. Healey, B. Chmielowski, A. P. Staddon, A. L. Cohn, G. I. Shapiro, V. L. Keedy, A. S. Singh, I. Puzanov, E. L. Kwak, A. J. Wagner, D. D. Von Hoff, G. J. Weiss, R. K. Ramanathan, J. Zhang, G. Habets, Y. Zhang, E. A. Burton, G. Visor, L. Sanftner, P. Severson, H. Nguyen, M. J. Kim, A. Marimuthu, G. Tsang, R. Shellooe, C. Gee, B. L. West, P. Hirth, K. Nolop, M. van de Rijn, H. H. Hsu, C. Peterfy, P. S. Lin, S. Tong-Starksen and G. Bollag, *N. Engl. J. Med.*, 2015, **373**, 428–437.
13. B. Lamoree and R. E. Hubbard, *SLAS Discovery*, 2018, **23**, 495–510.
14. B. Lamoree and R. E. Hubbard, *Essays Biochem.*, 2017, **61**, 453–464.
15. R. E. Hubbard, *Fragment-based Drug Discovery Lessons and Outlook*, in ed. D. A. Erlanson and W. Jahnke, Wiley, 2016, DOI: 10.1002/9783527683604.ch01, pp. 1–36.
16. D. A. Erlanson, S. W. Fesik, R. E. Hubbard, W. Jahnke and H. Jhoti, *Nat. Rev. Drug Discovery*, 2016, **15**, 605–619.
17. R. E. Hubbard, *Fragm.-Based Drug Discovery*, 2015, 126–152.
18. R. E. Hubbard, in *The Handbook of Medicinal Chemistry: Principles and Practice*, The Royal Society of Chemistry, 2015, pp. 122–153, DOI: 10.1039/9781782621836-00122.
19. R. E. Hubbard and J. B. Murray, *Methods Enzymol.*, 2011, **493**, 509–531.
20. J. Osborne, S. Panova, M. Rapti, T. Urushima and H. Jhoti, *Biochem. Soc. Trans.*, 2020, **48**, 271–280.
21. P. P. Seth, A. Miyaji, E. A. Jefferson, K. A. Sannes-Lowery, S. A. Osgood, S. S. Propp, R. Ranken, C. Massire, R. Sampath, D. J. Ecker, E. E. Swayze and R. H. Griffey, *J. Med. Chem.*, 2005, **48**, 7099–7102.
22. R. E. Hubbard, B. Davis, I. Chen and M. J. Drysdale, *Curr. Top. Med. Chem.*, 2007, **7**, 1568–1581.
23. J.-L. Reymond, *Acc. Chem. Res.*, 2015, **48**, 722–730.
24. T. Fink and J. L. Reymond, *J. Chem. Inf. Model.*, 2007, **47**, 342–353.
25. M. Lanier, G. Ambrus, D. C. Cole, R. Davenport, J. Ellery, R. Fosbeary, A. J. Jennings, A. Kadotani, Y. Kamada, R. Kamran, S.-I. Matsumoto, A. Mizukami, S. Okubo, K. Okada, K. Saikatendu, L. Walsh, H. Wu and M. S. Hixon, *J. Med. Chem.*, 2014, **57**, 5459–5463.
26. I. J. Chen and R. E. Hubbard, *J. Comput.-Aided Mol. Des.*, 2009, **23**, 603–620.
27. M. N. Schulz, J. Landstrom, K. Bright and R. E. Hubbard, *J. Comput.-Aided Mol. Des.*, 2011, **25**, 611–620.
28. R. E. Hubbard, I. Chen and B. Davis, *Curr. Opin. Drug Discovery Dev.*, 2007, **10**, 289–297.
29. N. Baurin, F. Aboul-Ela, X. Barril, B. Davis, M. Drysdale, B. Dymock, H. Finch, C. Fromont, C. Richardson, H. Simmonite and R. E. Hubbard, *J. Chem. Inf. Comput. Sci.*, 2004, **44**, 2157–2166.
30. W. F. Lau, J. M. Withka, D. Hepworth, T. V. Magee, Y. J. Du, G. A. Bakken, M. D. Miller, Z. S. Hendsch, V. Thanabal, S. A. Kolodziej, L. Xing, Q. Hu, L. S. Narasimhan, R. Love, M. E. Charlton, S. Hughes, W. P. van Hoorn and J. E. Mills, *J. Comput.-Aided Mol. Des.*, 2011, **25**, 621–636.
31. J. S. Albert, N. Blomberg, A. L. Breeze, A. J. Brown, J. N. Burrows, P. D. Edwards, R. H. Folmer, S. Geschwindner, E. J. Griffen, P. W. Kenny, T. Nowak, L. L. Olsson, H. Sanganee and A. B. Shapiro, *Curr. Top. Med. Chem.*, 2007, **7**, 1600–1629.
32. B. C. Doak, C. J. Morton, J. S. Simpson and M. J. Scanlon, *Aust. J. Chem.*, 2013, **66**, 8.
33. G. M. Keseru, D. A. Erlanson, G. G. Ferenczy, M. M. Hann, C. W. Murray and S. D. Pickett, *J. Med. Chem.*, 2016, **59**, 8189–8206.
34. C. L. Francis, P. W. Kenny, O. Dolezal, S. Saubern, M. Kruger, G. P. Savage, T. S. Peat and J. H. Ryan, *Aust. J. Chem.*, 2013, **66**, 1473–1482.
35. P. S. Kutchukian, S. S. So, C. Fischer and C. L. Waller, *Methods Mol. Biol.*, 2015, **1289**, 43–53.
36. C. Dalvit and A. Vulpetti, *Magn. Reson. Chem.*, 2012, **50**, 592–597.
37. A. Vulpetti and C. Dalvit, *Drug Discovery Today*, 2012, **17**, 890–897.
38. C. Dalvit, N. Mongelli, G. Papeo, P. Giordano, M. Veronesi, D. Moskau and R. Kummerle, *J. Am. Chem. Soc.*, 2005, **127**, 13380–13385.

39. A. Lingel, A. Vulpetti, T. Reinsperger, A. Proudfoot, R. Denay, A. Frommlet, C. Henry, U. Hommel, A. D. Gossert, B. Luy and A. O. Frank, *Angew. Chem., Int. Ed.*, 2020, **59**, 14809.
40. R. S. Norton, E. W. Leung, I. R. Chandrashekaran and C. A. MacRaild, *Molecules*, 2016, **21**, 860.
41. J. Blaney, V. Nienaber and S. K. Burley, in *Fragment-based Approaches in Drug Discovery*, ed. W. Jahnke and D. A. Erlanson, 2006.
42. F. Lovering, J. Bikker and C. Humblet, *J. Med. Chem.*, 2009, **52**, 6752–6756.
43. P. O'Brien, T. D. Downes, S. P. Jones, H. F. Klein, M. C. Wheldon, M. Atobe, P. S. Bond, J. D. Firth, N. S. Chan, L. Waddelove, R. E. Hubbard, D. C. Blakemore, C. De Fusco, S. D. Roughley, L. R. Vidler, M. A. Whatton, A. J.-A. Woolford and G. L. Wrigley, *Chem. – Eur. J.*, 2020, **26**, 8969–8975.
44. M. Luthy, M. C. Wheldon, C. Haji-Cheteh, M. Atobe, P. S. Bond, P. O'Brien, R. E. Hubbard and I. J. Fairlamb, *Bioorg. Med. Chem.*, 2015, **23**, 2680–2694.
45. A. R. Hanby, N. S. Troelsen, T. J. Osberger, S. L. Kidd, K. T. Mortensen and D. R. Spring, *Chem. Commun.*, 2020, **56**, 2280–2283.
46. R. Zhang, P. J. McIntyre, P. M. Collins, D. J. Foley, C. Arter, F. von Delft, R. Bayliss, S. Warriner and A. Nelson, *Chemistry*, 2019, **25**, 6831–6839.
47. C. Zhang, P. N. Ibrahim, J. Zhang, E. A. Burton, G. Habets, Y. Zhang, B. Powell, B. L. West, B. Matusow, G. Tsang, R. Shellooe, H. Carias, H. Nguyen, A. Marimuthu, K. Y. Zhang, A. Oh, R. Bremer, C. R. Hurt, D. R. Artis, G. Wu, M. Nespi, W. Spevak, P. Lin, K. Nolop, P. Hirth, G. H. Tesch and G. Bollag, *Proc. Natl. Acad. Sci. U. S. A.*, 2013, **110**, 5689–5694.
48. J. Tsai, J. T. Lee, W. Wang, J. Zhang, H. Cho, S. Mamo, R. Bremer, S. Gillette, J. Kong, N. K. Haass, K. Sproesser, L. Li, K. S. Smalley, D. Fong, Y. L. Zhu, A. Marimuthu, H. Nguyen, B. Lam, J. Liu, I. Cheung, J. Rice, Y. Suzuki, C. Luu, C. Settachatgul, R. Shellooe, J. Cantwell, S. H. Kim, J. Schlessinger, K. Y. Zhang, B. L. West, B. Powell, G. Habets, C. Zhang, P. N. Ibrahim, P. Hirth, D. R. Artis, M. Herlyn and G. Bollag, *Proc. Natl. Acad. Sci. U. S. A.*, 2008, **105**, 3041–3046.
49. S. D. Roughley and R. E. Hubbard, *J. Med. Chem.*, 2011, **54**, 3989–4005.
50. S. B. Shuker, P. J. Hajduk, R. P. Meadows and S. W. Fesik, *Science*, 1996, **274**, 1531–1534.
51. P. J. Hajduk and J. Greer, *Nat. Rev. Drug Discovery*, 2007, **6**, 211–219.
52. P. J. Hajduk, *Mol. Interventions*, 2006, **6**, 266–272.
53. W. Jahnke, R. M. Grotzfeld, X. Pelle, A. Strauss, G. Fendrich, S. W. Cowan-Jacob, S. Cotesta, D. Fabbro, P. Furet, J. Mestan and A. L. Marzinzik, *J. Am. Chem. Soc.*, 2010, **132**, 7043–7048.
54. M. Mayer and B. Meyer, *Angew. Chem., Int. Ed.*, 1999, **38**, 1784–1788.
55. C. Dalvit, P. Pevarello, M. Tatò, M. Veronesi, A. Vulpetti and M. Sundström, *J. Biomol. NMR*, 2000, **18**, 65–68.
56. S. Meiboom and D. Gill, *Rev. Sci. Instrum.*, 1958, **29**, 688–691.
57. M. Kobayashi, K. Retra, F. Figaroa, J. G. Hollander, E. Ab, R. J. Heetebrij, H. Irth and G. Siegal, *J. Biomol. Screening*, 2010, **15**, 978–989.
58. G. Siegal and J. G. Hollander, *Curr. Top. Med. Chem.*, 2009, **9**, 1736–1745.
59. S. Vanwetswinkel, R. J. Heetebrij, J. van Duynhoven, J. G. Hollander, D. V. Filippov, P. J. Hajduk and G. Siegal, *Chem. Biol.*, 2005, **12**, 207–216.
60. P. A. Brough, L. Baker, S. Bedford, K. Brown, S. Chavda, V. Chell, J. D'Alessandro, N. G. Davies, B. Davis, L. Le Strat, A. T. Macias, D. Maddox, P. C. Mahon, A. J. Massey, N. Matassova, S. McKenna, J. W. Meissner, J. D. Moore, J. B. Murray, C. J. Northfield, C. Parry, R. Parsons, S. D. Roughley, T. Shaw, H. Simmonite, S. Stokes, A. Surgenor, E. Stefaniak, A. Robertson, Y. Wang, P. Webb, N. Whitehead and M. Wood, *J. Med. Chem.*, 2017, **60**, 2271–2286.
61. J. B. Murray, S. D. Roughley, N. Matassova and P. A. Brough, *J. Med. Chem.*, 2014, **57**, 2845–2850.
62. R. A. Copeland, D. L. Pompliano and T. D. Meek, *Nat. Rev. Drug Discovery*, 2006, **5**, 730–739.
63. A. M. Giannetti, in *Fragment-Based Drug Design: Tools, Practical Approaches, and Examples*, ed. L. C. Kuo, 2011, vol. 493, pp. 169–218.
64. R. L. Rich, G. A. Papalia, P. J. Flynn, J. Furneisen, J. Quinn, J. S. Klein, P. S. Katsamba, M. B. Waddell, M. Scott, J. Thompson, J. Berlier, S. Corry, M. Baltzinger, G. Zeder-Lutzi, A. Schoenemann, A. Clabbers, S. Wieckowski, M. M. Murphy, P. Page, T. E. Ryan, J. Duffner, T. Ganguly, J. Corbin, S. Gautam, G. Anderluh, A. Bavdek, D. Reichmann, S. P. Yadav, E. Hommema, E. Pol, A. Drake, S. Klakamp, T. Chapman, D. Kernaghan, K. Miller, J. Schuman, K. Lindquist, K. Herlihy, M. B. Murphy, R. Bohnsack, B. Andrien, P. Brandani, D. Terwey, R. Millican, R. J. Darling, L. Wang, Q. Carter, J. Dotzlaf, J. Lopez-Sagaseta, I. Campbell, P. Torreri, S. Hoos, P. England, Y. Liu, Y. Abdiche, D. Malashock, A. Pinkerton, M. Wong, E. Lafer, C. Hinck, K. Thompson, C. Di Primo, A. Joyce, J. Brooks, F. Torta, A. B. B. Hagel, J. Krarup, J. Pass, M. Ferreira, S. Shikov, M. Mikolajczyk, Y. Abe, G. Barbato, A. M. Giannetti, G. Krishnamoorthy, B. Beusink, D. Satpaev, T. Tsang, E. Fang, J. Partridge, S. Brohawn, J. Horn, O. Pritsch, G. Obal, S. Nilapwar, B. Busby, G. Gutierrez-Sanchez, R. Das Gupta, S. Canepa, K. Witte, Z. Nikolovska-Coleska, Y. H.

Cho, R. D'Agata, K. Schlick, R. Calvert, E. M. Munoz, M. J. Hernaiz, T. Bravman, M. Dines, M. H. Yang, A. Puskas, E. Boni, J. J. Li, M. Wear, A. Grinberg, J. Baardsnes, O. Dolezal, M. Gainey, H. Anderson, J. L. Peng, M. Lewis, P. Spies, Q. Trinh, S. Bibikov, J. Raymond, M. Yousef, V. Chandrasekaran, Y. G. Feng, A. Emerick, S. Mundodo, R. Guimaraes, K. McGirr, Y. J. Li, H. Hughes, H. Mantz, R. Skrabana, M. Witmer, J. Ballard, L. Martin, P. Skladal, G. Korza, I. Laird-Offringa, C. S. Lee, A. Khadir, F. Podlaski, P. Neuner, J. Rothacker, A. Rafique, N. Dankbar, P. Kainz, E. Gedig, M. Vuyisich, C. Boozer, N. Ly, M. Toews, A. Uren, O. Kalyuzhniy, K. Lewis, E. Chomey, B. J. Pak and D. G. Myszka, *Anal. Biochem.*, 2009, **386**, 194–216.

65. M. Elinder, M. Geitmann, T. Gossas, P. Kallblad, J. Winquist, H. Nordstrom, M. Hamalainen and U. H. Danielson, *J. Biomol. Screening*, 2011, **16**, 15–25.
66. U. H. Danielson, *Curr. Top. Med. Chem.*, 2009, **9**, 1725–1735.
67. P. Kozma, F. Kehl, E. Ehrentreich-Förster, C. Stamm and F. F. Bier, *Biosens. Bioelectron.*, 2014, **58**, 287–307.
68. A. Chaikuad, E. M. Tacconi, J. Zimmer, Y. Liang, N. S. Gray, M. Tarsounas and S. Knapp, *Nat. Chem. Biol.*, 2014, **10**, 853–860.
69. G. Papalia and D. Myszka, *Anal. Biochem.*, 2010, **403**, 30–35.
70. M. Fischer, A. P. Leech and R. E. Hubbard, *Anal. Chem.*, 2011, **83**, 1800–1807.
71. M. Fairhead and M. Howarth, *Methods Mol. Biol.*, 2015, **1266**, 171–184.
72. M. Jerabek-Willemsen, T. André, R. Wanner, H. M. Roth, S. Duhr, P. Baaske and D. Breitsprecher, *J. Mol. Struct.*, 2014, **1077**, 101–113.
73. P. Linke, K. Amaning, M. Maschberger, F. Vallee, V. Steier, P. Baaske, S. Duhr, D. Breitsprecher and A. Rak, *J. Biomol. Screening*, 2016, **21**, 414–421.
74. T. A. Young, B. Moree, M. T. Butko, B. Clancy, M. Geck Do, T. Gheyi, J. Strelow, J. J. Carrillo and J. Salafsky, *Methods Enzymol.*, 2018, **610**, 167–190.
75. J. K. Kranz and C. Schalk-Hihi, *Methods Enzymol.*, 2011, **493**, 277–298.
76. F. H. Niesen, H. Berglund and M. Vedadi, *Nat. Protoc.*, 2007, **2**, 2212–2221.
77. M. Vedadi, F. H. Niesen, A. Allali-Hassani, O. Y. Fedorov, P. J. Finerty Jr., G. A. Wasney, R. Yeung, C. Arrowsmith, L. J. Ball, H. Berglund, R. Hui, B. D. Marsden, P. Nordlund, M. Sundstrom, J. Weigelt and A. M. Edwards, *Proc. Natl. Acad. Sci. U. S. A.*, 2006, **103**, 15835–15840.
78. M. N. Schulz, J. Landstrom and R. E. Hubbard, *Anal. Biochem.*, 2013, **433**, 43–47.
79. K. Babaoglu, A. Simeonov, J. J. Irwin, M. E. Nelson, B. Feng, C. J. Thomas, L. Cancian, M. P. Costi, D. A. Maltby, A. Jadhav, J. Inglese, C. P. Austin and B. K. Shoichet, *J. Med. Chem.*, 2008, **51**, 2502–2511.
80. K. E. Coan and B. K. Shoichet, *J. Am. Chem. Soc.*, 2008, **130**, 9606–9612.
81. S. M. Saalau-Bethell, A. J. Woodhead, G. Chessari, M. G. Carr, J. Coyle, B. Graham, S. D. Hiscock, C. W. Murray, P. Pathuri, S. J. Rich, C. J. Richardson, P. A. Williams and H. Jhoti, *Nat. Chem. Biol.*, 2012, **8**, 920–925.
82. J. D. Bauman, D. Patel, C. Dharia, M. W. Fromer, S. Ahmed, Y. Frenkel, R. S. Vijayan, J. T. Eck, W. C. Ho, K. Das, A. J. Shatkin and E. Arnold, *J. Med. Chem.*, 2013, **56**, 2738–2746.
83. A. L. Perryman, Q. Zhang, H. H. Soutter, R. Rosenfeld, D. E. McRee, A. J. Olson, J. E. Elder and C. D. Stout, *Chem. Biol. Drug Des.*, 2010, **75**, 257–268.
84. P. M. Collins, A. Douangamath, R. Talon, A. Dias, J. Brandão-Neto, T. Krojer and F. von Delft, *Methods Enzymol*, 2018, **610**, 251–264.
85. N. M. Pearce, T. Krojer, A. R. Bradley, P. Collins, R. P. Nowak, R. Talon, B. D. Marsden, S. Kelm, J. Shi, C. M. Deane and F. von Delft, *Nat. Commun.*, 2017, **8**, 15123.
86. T. Krojer, R. Talon, N. Pearce, P. Collins, A. Douangamath, J. Brandao-Neto, A. Dias, B. Marsden and F. von Delft, *Acta Crystallogr., Sect. D: Struct. Biol.*, 2017, **73**, 267–278.
87. L. M. Baker, A. Aimon, J. B. Murray, A. E. Surgenor, N. Matassova, S. D. Roughley, P. M. Collins, T. Krojer, F. von Delft and R. E. Hubbard, *Commun. Chem.*, 2020, **3**, 122.
88. D. J. Wood, J. D. Lopez-Fernandez, L. E. Knight, I. Al-Khawaldeh, C. Gai, S. Lin, M. P. Martin, D. C. Miller, C. Cano, J. A. Endicott, I. R. Hardcastle, M. E. M. Noble and M. J. Waring, *J. Med. Chem.*, 2019, **62**, 3741–3752.
89. M. O'Reilly, A. Cleasby, T. G. Davies, R. J. Hall, R. F. Ludlow, C. W. Murray, D. Tisi and H. Jhoti, *Drug Discovery Today*, 2019, **24**, 1081–1086.
90. S. E. Rollauer, M. J. Tarry, J. E. Graham, M. Jaaskelainen, F. Jaeger, S. Johnson, M. Krehenbrink, S.-M. Liu, M. J. Lukey, J. Marcoux, M. A. McDowell, F. Rodriguez, P. Roversi, P. J. Stansfeld, C. V. Robinson, M. S. P. Sansom, T. Palmer, M. Hogbom, B. C. Berks and S. M. Lea, *Nature*, 2012, **492**, 210–214.
91. M. K. Ameriks, S. D. Bembenek, M. T. Burdett, I. C. Choong, J. P. Edwards, D. Gebauer, Y. Gu, L. Karlsson, H. E. Purkey, B. L. Staker, S. Q. Sun, R. L. Thurmond and J. A. Zhu, *Bioorg. Med. Chem. Lett.*, 2010, **20**, 4060–4064.
92. D. A. Erlanson, J. A. Wells and A. C. Braisted, *Annu. Rev. Biophys. Biomol. Struct.*, 2004, **33**, 199–223.

93. M. M. Rachman, X. Barril and R. E. Hubbard, *Curr. Opin. Pharmacol.*, 2018, **42**, 34–39.
94. E. P. Istyastono, A. J. Kooistra, H. F. Vischer, M. Kuijer, L. Roumen, S. Nijmeijer, R. A. Smits, I. J. P. de Esch, R. Leurs and C. de Graaf, *MedChemComm*, 2015, **6**, 1003–1017.
95. A. Rudling, R. Gustafsson, I. Almlöf, E. Homan, M. Scobie, U. Warpman Berglund, T. Helleday, P. Stenmark and J. Carlsson, *J. Med. Chem.*, 2017, **60**, 8160–8169.
96. T. Hesterkamp, J. Barker, A. Davenport and M. Whittaker, *Curr. Top. Med. Chem.*, 2007, **7**, 1582–1591.
97. C. Austin, S. N. Pettit, S. K. Magnolo, J. Sanvoisin, W. Chen, S. P. Wood, L. D. Freeman, R. J. Pengelly and D. E. Hughes, *J. Biomol. Screening*, 2012, **17**, 868–876.
98. E. Meiby, H. Simmonite, L. le Strat, B. Davis, N. Matassova, J. D. Moore, M. Mrosek, J. Murray, R. E. Hubbard and S. Ohlson, *Anal. Chem.*, 2013, **85**, 6756–6766.
99. P. S. Kutchukian, A. M. Wassermann, M. K. Lindvall, S. K. Wright, J. Ottl, J. Jacob, C. Scheufler, A. Marzinzik, N. Brooijmans and M. Glick, *J. Biomol. Screening*, 2015, **20**, 588–596.
100. J. Schiebel, N. Radeva, H. Koster, A. Metz, T. Krotzky, M. Kuhnert, W. E. Diederich, A. Heine, L. Neumann, C. Atmanene, D. Roecklin, V. Vivat-Hannah, J. P. Renaud, R. Meinecke, N. Schlinck, A. Sitte, F. Popp, M. Zeeb and G. Klebe, *ChemMedChem*, 2015, **10**, 1511–1521.
101. S. A. Wildman and G. M. Crippen, *J. Chem. Inf. Comput. Sci.*, 1999, **39**, 868–873.
102. J. A. Christopher, J. Brown, A. S. Dore, J. C. Errey, M. Koglin, F. H. Marshall, D. G. Myszka, R. L. Rich, C. G. Tate, B. Tehan, T. Warne and M. Congreve, *J. Med. Chem.*, 2013, **56**, 3446–3455.
103. S. P. Andrews, G. A. Brown and J. A. Christopher, *ChemMedChem*, 2014, **9**, 256–275.
104. J. A. Christopher, S. J. Aves, K. A. Bennett, A. S. Dore, J. C. Errey, A. Jazayeri, F. H. Marshall, K. Okrasa, M. J. Serrano-Vega, B. G. Tehan, G. R. Wiggin and M. Congreve, *J. Med. Chem.*, 2015, **58**, 6653–6664.
105. D. M. Rosenbaum, V. Cherezov, M. A. Hanson, S. G. Rasmussen, F. S. Thian, T. S. Kobilka, H. J. Choi, X. J. Yao, W. I. Weis, R. C. Stevens and B. K. Kobilka, *Science*, 2007, **318**, 1266–1273.
106. V. P. Jaakola, M. T. Griffith, M. A. Hanson, V. Cherezov, E. Y. Chien, J. R. Lane, A. P. Ijzerman and R. C. Stevens, *Science*, 2008, **322**, 1211–1217.
107. E. Pardon, T. Laeremans, S. Triest, S. G. F. Rasmussen, A. Wohlkönig, A. Ruf, S. Muyldermans, W. G. J. Hol, B. K. Kobilka and J. Steyaert, *Nat. Protoc.*, 2014, **9**, 674.
108. S. E. Thomas, P. Collins, R. H. James, V. Mendes, S. Charoensutthivarakul, C. Radoux, C. Abell, A. G. Coyne, R. A. Floto, F. von Delft and T. L. Blundell, *Philos. Trans. R. Soc., A*, 2019, **377**, 20180422.
109. T. A. Halgren, *J. Chem. Inf. Model.*, 2009, **49**, 377–389.
110. P. J. Hajduk, J. R. Huth and C. Tse, *Drug Discovery Today*, 2005, **10**, 1675–1682.
111. P. J. Hajduk, J. R. Huth and S. W. Fesik, *J. Med. Chem.*, 2005, **48**, 2518–2525.
112. M. Chilton, B. Clennell, F. Edfeldt and S. Geschwindner, *J. Med. Chem.*, 2017, **60**, 4923–4931.
113. F. N. Edfeldt, R. H. Folmer and A. L. Breeze, *Drug Discovery Today*, 2011, **16**, 284–287.
114. P. Canning, K. Birchall, C. A. Kettleborough, A. Merritt and P. J. Coombs, *Drug Discovery Today*, 2020, **22**, 2030–2037.
115. R. F. Ludlow, M. L. Verdonk, H. K. Saini, I. J. Tickle and H. Jhoti, *Proc. Natl. Acad. Sci. U. S. A.*, 2015, **112**, 15910–15915.
116. A. C. English, C. R. Groom and R. E. Hubbard, *Protein Eng.*, 2001, **14**, 47–59.
117. A. C. English, S. H. Done, L. S. Caves, C. R. Groom and R. E. Hubbard, *Proteins*, 1999, **37**, 628–640.
118. A. L. Marzinzik, R. Amstutz, G. Bold, E. Bourgier, S. Cotesta, J. F. Glickman, M. Gotte, C. Henry, S. Lehmann, J. C. Hartwieg, S. Ofner, X. Pelle, T. P. Roddy, J. M. Rondeau, F. Stauffer, S. J. Stout, A. Widmer, J. Zimmermann, T. Zoller and W. Jahnke, *ChemMedChem*, 2015, **10**, 1884–1891.
119. C. G. Parker, A. Galmozzi, Y. Wang, B. E. Correia, K. Sasaki, C. M. Joslyn, A. S. Kim, C. L. Cavallaro, R. M. Lawrence, S. R. Johnson, I. Narvaiza, E. Saez and B. F. Cravatt, *Cell*, 2017, **168**, 527–541 e529.
120. J. F. Darby, J. Landstrom, C. Roth, Y. He, G. J. Davies and R. E. Hubbard, *Angew. Chem., Int. Ed.*, 2014, **53**, 13419–13423.
121. J. F. Darby, M. Atobe, J. Firth, P. Bond, P. A. O'Brien, G. J. Davies and R. E. Hubbard, *Chem. Sci.*, 2017, **8**, 7772–7779.
122. J. B. Murray, J. Davidson, I. Chen, B. Davis, P. Dokurno, C. J. Graham, R. Harris, A. Jordan, N. Matassova, C. Pedder, S. Ray, S. D. Roughley, J. Smith, C. Walmsley, Y. Wang, N. Whitehead, D. S. Williamson, P. Casara, T. Le Diguarher, J. Hickman, J. Stark, A. Kotschy, O. Geneste and R. E. Hubbard, *ACS Omega*, 2019, **4**, 8892–8906.
123. R. E. Hubbard, *J. Synchrotron Radiat.*, 2008, **15**, 227–230.
124. D. S. Williamson, G. P. Smith, P. Acheson-Dossang, S. T. Bedford, V. Chell, I. J. Chen, J. C. A. Daechsel, Z. Daniels, L. David, P. Dokurno, M. Hentzer, M. C. Herzig, R. E. Hubbard, J. D. Moore, J. B. Murray, S. Newland, S. C. Ray, T. Shaw, A. E. Surgenor, L. Terry, K. Thirstrup, Y. Wang and K. V. Christensen, *J. Med. Chem.*, 2017, **60**, 8945–8962.

125. M. Saur, M. J. Hartshorn, J. Dong, J. Reeks, G. Bunkoczi, H. Jhoti and P. A. Williams, *Drug Discovery Today*, 2020, **25**, 485–490.
126. G. Chessari and A. J. Woodhead, *Drug Discovery Today*, 2009, **14**, 668–675.
127. W. P. Jencks, *Proc. Natl. Acad. Sci. U. S. A.*, 1981, **78**, 4046–4050.
128. P. R. Andrews, D. J. Craik and J. L. Martin, *J. Med. Chem.*, 1984, **27**, 1648–1657.
129. G. Saxty, S. J. Woodhead, V. Berdini, T. G. Davies, M. L. Verdonk, P. G. Wyatt, R. G. Boyle, D. Barford, R. Downham, M. D. Garrett and R. A. Carr, *J. Med. Chem.*, 2007, **50**, 2293–2296.
130. D. J. Abraham, M. F. Perutz and S. E. Phillips, *Proc. Natl. Acad. Sci. U. S. A.*, 1983, **80**, 324–328.
131. P. J. Goodford, *J. Med. Chem.*, 1985, **28**, 849–857.
132. M. Vonitzstein, W. Y. Wu, G. B. Kok, M. S. Pegg, J. C. Dyason, B. Jin, T. V. Phan, M. L. Smythe, H. F. White, S. W. Oliver, P. M. Colman, J. N. Varghese, D. M. Ryan, J. M. Woods, R. C. Bethell, V. J. Hotham, J. M. Cameron and C. R. Penn, *Nature*, 1993, **363**, 418–423.
133. A. Miranker and M. Karplus, *Proteins*, 1991, **11**, 29–34.
134. H. J. Bohm, *J. Comput.-Aided Mol. Des.*, 1992, **6**, 61–78.
135. K. N. Allen, C. R. Bellamacina, X. C. Ding, C. J. Jeffery, C. Mattos, G. A. Petsko and D. Ringe, *J. Phys. Chem.*, 1996, **100**, 2605–2611.
136. P. A. Bartlett, G. T. Shea, S. Waterman and S. J. Telfer, *Abstr. Pap., Am. Chem. Soc.*, 1991, **202**, 44-COMP.
137. E. T. Olejniczak, P. J. Hajduk, P. A. Marcotte, D. G. Nettesheim, R. P. Meadows, R. Edalji, T. F. Holzman and S. W. Fesik, *J. Am. Chem. Soc.*, 1997, **119**, 5828–5832.
138. P. J. Hajduk, J. Dinges, G. F. Miknis, M. Merlock, T. Middleton, D. J. Kempf, D. A. Egan, K. A. Walter, T. S. Robins, S. B. Shuker, T. F. Holzman and S. W. Fesik, *J. Med. Chem.*, 1997, **40**, 3144–3150.
139. P. J. Hajduk, S. Boyd, D. Nettesheim, V. Nienaber, J. Severin, R. Smith, D. Davidson, T. Rockway and S. W. Fesik, *J. Med. Chem.*, 2000, **43**, 3862–3866.
140. S. W. Fesik, P. J. Hajduk, G. Sheppard, E. T. Olejniczak, D. G. Nettesheim, R. P. Meadows, P. A. Marcotte, S. B. Shuker, D. H. Steinman, G. M. Carrera, J. Severin, K. Walter, H. Smith, E. Gubbins, R. Simmer, T. F. Holzman, D. W. Morgan, S. K. Davidsen and J. B. Summers, *Abstr. Pap., Am. Chem. Soc.*, 1997, **214**, 109-MEDI.
141. V. L. Nienaber, P. L. Richardson, V. Klighofer, J. J. Bouska, V. L. Giranda and J. Greer, *Nat. Biotechnol.*, 2000, **18**, 1105–1108.
142. H. J. Boehm, M. Boehringer, D. Bur, H. Gmuender, W. Huber, W. Klaus, D. Kostrewa, H. Kuehne, T. Luebbers, N. Meunier-Keller and F. Mueller, *J. Med. Chem.*, 2000, **43**, 2664–2674.
143. D. R. Artis, J. J. Lin, C. Zhang, W. Wang, U. Mehra, M. Perreault, D. Erbe, H. I. Krupka, B. P. England, J. Arnold, A. N. Plotnikov, A. Marimuthu, H. Nguyen, S. Will, M. Signaevsky, J. Kral, J. Cantwell, C. Settachatgull, D. S. Yan, D. Fong, A. Oh, S. Shi, P. Womack, B. Powell, G. Habets, B. L. West, K. Y. Zhang, M. V. Milburn, G. P. Vlasuk, K. P. Hirth, K. Nolop, G. Bollag, P. N. Ibrahim and J. F. Tobin, *Proc. Natl. Acad. Sci. U. S. A.*, 2009, **106**, 262–267.
144. G. L. Card, L. Blasdel, B. P. England, C. Zhang, Y. Suzuki, S. Gillette, D. Fong, P. N. Ibrahim, D. R. Artis, G. Bollag, M. V. Milburn, S. H. Kim, J. Schlessinger and K. Y. Zhang, *Nat. Biotechnol.*, 2005, **23**, 201–207.
145. W. T. Mooij, M. J. Hartshorn, I. J. Tickle, A. J. Sharff, M. L. Verdonk and H. Jhoti, *ChemMedChem*, 2006, **1**, 827–838.
146. T. L. Blundell, H. Jhoti and C. Abell, *Nat. Rev. Drug Discovery*, 2002, **1**, 45–54.
147. P. Kuhn, K. Wilson, M. G. Patch and R. C. Stevens, *Curr. Opin. Chem. Biol.*, 2002, **6**, 704–710.
148. Z. Zhang, N. K. Sauter, H. van den Bedem, G. Snell and A. M. Deacon, *J. Appl. Crystallogr.*, 2006, **39**, 112–119.
149. D. Hosfield, J. Palan, M. Hilgers, D. Scheibe, D. E. McRee and R. C. Stevens, *J. Struct. Biol.*, 2003, **142**, 207–217.
150. H. Jhoti, G. Williams, D. C. Rees and C. W. Murray, *Nat. Rev. Drug Discovery*, 2013, **12**, 644.
151. M. Congreve, R. Carr, C. Murray and H. Jhoti, *Drug Discovery Today*, 2003, **8**, 876–877.
152. H. Koster, T. Craan, S. Brass, C. Herhaus, M. Zentgraf, L. Neumann, A. Heine and G. Klebe, *J. Med. Chem.*, 2011, **54**, 7784–7796.
153. P. J. Hajduk, M. Bures, J. Praestgaard and S. W. Fesik, *J. Med. Chem.*, 2000, **43**, 3443–3447.
154. P. J. Hajduk, *J. Med. Chem.*, 2006, **49**, 6972–6976.
155. A. L. Hopkins, C. R. Groom and A. Alex, *Drug Discovery Today*, 2004, **9**, 430–431.
156. I. D. Kuntz, K. Chen, K. A. Sharp and P. A. Kollman, *Proc. Natl. Acad. Sci. U. S. A.*, 1999, **96**, 9997–10002.
157. J. R. Empfield and P. D. Leeson, *IDrugs*, 2010, **13**, 869–873.
158. P. D. Leeson and B. Springthorpe, *Nat. Rev. Drug Discovery*, 2007, **6**, 881–890.
159. A. P. Hill and R. J. Young, *Drug Discovery Today*, 2010, **15**, 648–655.
160. M. D. Shultz, *Bioorg. Med. Chem. Lett.*, 2013, **23**, 5980–5991.

161. G. G. Ferenczy and G. M. Keseru, *J. Med. Chem.*, 2013, **56**, 2478–2486.
162. D. A. Erlanson, *Curr. Opin. Biotechnol.*, 2006, **17**, 643–652.
163. M. N. Schulz and R. E. Hubbard, *Curr. Opin. Pharmacol.*, 2009, **9**, 615–621.
164. J. J. Barker, O. Barker, S. M. Courtney, M. Gardiner, T. Hesterkamp, O. Ichihara, O. Mather, C. A. Montalbetti, A. Muller, M. Varasi, M. Whittaker and C. J. Yarnold, *ChemMedChem*, 2010, **5**, 1697–1700.
165. N. Howard, C. Abell, W. Blakemore, G. Chessari, M. Congreve, S. Howard, H. Jhoti, C. W. Murray, L. C. Seavers and R. L. van Montfort, *J. Med. Chem.*, 2006, **49**, 1346–1355.
166. M. R. Bentley, O. V. Ilyichova, G. Wang, M. L. Williams, G. Sharma, W. S. Alwan, R. L. Whitehouse, B. Mohanty, P. J. Scammells, B. Heras, J. L. Martin, M. Totsika, B. Capuano, B. C. Doak and M. J. Scanlon, *J. Med. Chem.*, 2020, **63**, 6863–6875.
167. P. J. Hajduk, M. Bures, J. Praestgaard and S. W. Fesik, *J. Med. Chem.*, 2000, **43**, 3443–3447.
168. S. D. Roughley and R. E. Hubbard, *J. Med. Chem.*, 2011, **54**, 3989–4005.
169. S. Roughley, L. Wright, P. Brough, A. Massey and R. E. Hubbard, *Top. Curr. Chem.*, 2012, **317**, 61–82.
170. C. R. Wellaway, D. Amans, P. Bamborough, H. Barnett, R. A. Bit, J. A. Brown, N. R. Carlson, C.-w. Chung, A. W. J. Cooper, P. D. Craggs, R. P. Davis, T. W. Dean, J. P. Evans, L. Gordon, I. L. Harada, D. J. Hirst, P. G. Humphreys, K. L. Jones, A. J. Lewis, M. J. Lindon, D. Lugo, M. Mahmood, S. McCleary, P. Medeiros, D. J. Mitchell, M. O'Sullivan, A. Le Gall, V. K. Patel, C. Patten, D. L. Poole, R. R. Shah, J. E. Smith, K. A. J. Stafford, P. J. Thomas, M. Vimal, I. D. Wall, R. J. Watson, N. Wellaway, G. Yao and R. K. Prinjha, *J. Med. Chem.*, 2020, **63**, 714–746.
171. Z. Szlavik, L. Ondi, M. Csekei, A. Paczal, Z. B. Szabo, G. Radics, J. Murray, J. Davidson, I. Chen, B. Davis, R. E. Hubbard, C. Pedder, P. Dokurno, A. Surgenor, J. Smith, A. Robertson, G. LeToumelin-Braizat, N. Cauquil, M. Zarka, D. Demarles, F. Perron-Sierra, A. Claperon, F. Colland, O. Geneste and A. Kotschy, *J. Med. Chem.*, 2019, **62**, 6913–6924.
172. N. Baurin, R. Baker, C. Richardson, I. Chen, N. Foloppe, A. Potter, A. Jordan, S. Roughley, M. Parratt, P. Greaney, D. Morley and R. E. Hubbard, *J. Chem. Inf. Comput. Sci.*, 2004, **44**, 643–651.
173. T. Oltersdorf, S. W. Elmore, A. R. Shoemaker, R. C. Armstrong, D. J. Augeri, B. A. Belli, M. Bruncko, T. L. Deckwerth, J. Dinges, P. J. Hajduk, M. K. Joseph, S. Kitada, S. J. Korsmeyer, A. R. Kunzer, A. Letai, C. Li, M. J. Mitten, D. G. Nettesheim, S. Ng, P. M. Nimmer, J. M. O'Connor, A. Oleksijew, A. M. Petros, J. C. Reed, W. Shen, S. K. Tahir, C. B. Thompson, K. J. Tomaselli, B. Wang, M. D. Wendt, H. Zhang, S. W. Fesik and S. H. Rosenberg, *Nature*, 2005, **435**, 677–681.
174. A. M. Petros, J. Dinges, D. J. Augeri, S. A. Baumeister, D. A. Betebenner, M. G. Bures, S. W. Elmore, P. J. Hajduk, M. K. Joseph, S. K. Landis, D. G. Nettesheim, S. H. Rosenberg, W. Shen, S. Thomas, X. Wang, I. Zanze, H. Zhang and S. W. Fesik, *J. Med. Chem.*, 2005, **49**, 656–663.
175. C. Tse, A. R. Shoemaker, J. Adickes, M. G. Anderson, J. Chen, S. Jin, E. F. Johnson, K. C. Marsh, M. J. Mitten, P. Nimmer, L. Roberts, S. K. Tahir, Y. Xiao, X. Yang, H. Zhang, S. Fesik, S. H. Rosenberg and S. W. Elmore, *Cancer Res.*, 2008, **68**, 3421–3428.
176. X. Barril, P. Brough, M. Drysdale, R. E. Hubbard, A. Massey, A. Surgenor and L. Wright, *Bioorg. Med. Chem. Lett.*, 2005, **15**, 5187–5191.
177. P. A. Brough, W. Aherne, X. Barril, J. Borgognoni, K. Boxall, J. E. Cansfield, K. M. Cheung, I. Collins, N. G. Davies, M. J. Drysdale, B. Dymock, S. A. Eccles, H. Finch, A. Fink, A. Hayes, R. Howes, R. E. Hubbard, K. James, A. M. Jordan, A. Lockie, V. Martins, A. Massey, T. P. Matthews, E. McDonald, C. J. Northfield, L. H. Pearl, C. Prodromou, S. Ray, F. I. Raynaud, S. D. Roughley, S. Y. Sharp, A. Surgenor, D. L. Walmsley, P. Webb, M. Wood, P. Workman and L. Wright, *J. Med. Chem.*, 2008, **51**, 196–218.
178. B. W. Dymock, X. Barril, P. A. Brough, J. E. Cansfield, A. Massey, E. McDonald, R. E. Hubbard, A. Surgenor, S. D. Roughley, P. Webb, P. Workman, L. Wright and M. J. Drysdale, *J. Med. Chem.*, 2005, **48**, 4212–4215.
179. S. A. Eccles, A. Massey, F. I. Raynaud, S. Y. Sharp, G. Box, M. Valenti, L. Patterson, A. de Haven Brandon, S. Gowan, F. Boxall, W. Aherne, M. Rowlands, A. Hayes, V. Martins, F. Urban, K. Boxall, C. Prodromou, L. Pearl, K. James, T. P. Matthews, K. M. Cheung, A. Kalusa, K. Jones, E. McDonald, X. Barril, P. A. Brough, J. E. Cansfield, B. Dymock, M. J. Drysdale, H. Finch, R. Howes, R. E. Hubbard, A. Surgenor, P. Webb, M. Wood, L. Wright and P. Workman, *Cancer Res.*, 2008, **68**, 2850–2860.
180. L. Wright, X. Barril, B. Dymock, L. Sheridan, A. Surgenor, M. Beswick, M. Drysdale, A. Collier, A. Massey, N. Davies, A. Fink, C. Fromont, W. Aherne, K. Boxall, S. Sharp, P. Workman and R. E. Hubbard, *Chem. Biol.*, 2004, **11**, 775–785.
181. R. Howes, X. Barril, B. W. Dymock, K. Grant, C. J. Northfield, A. G. Robertson, A. Surgenor, J. Wayne, L. Wright, K. James, T. Matthews, K. M. Cheung, E. McDonald, P. Workman and M. J. Drysdale, *Anal. Biochem.*, 2006, **350**, 202–213.

182. A. J. Massey, S. Stokes, H. Browne, N. Foloppe, A. Fiumana, S. Scrace, M. Fallowfield, S. Bedford, P. Webb, L. Baker, M. Christie, M. J. Drysdale and M. Wood, *Oncotarget*, 2015, **6**, 35797–35812.
183. P. G. Wyatt, A. J. Woodhead, V. Berdini, J. A. Boulstridge, M. G. Carr, D. M. Cross, D. J. Davis, L. A. Devine, T. R. Early, R. E. Feltell, E. J. Lewis, R. L. McMenamin, E. F. Navarro, M. A. O'Brien, M. O'Reilly, M. Reule, G. Saxty, L. C. Seavers, D. M. Smith, M. S. Squires, G. Trewartha, M. T. Walker and A. J. Woolford, *J. Med. Chem.*, 2008, **51**, 4986–4999.
184. Z. Zhu, Z. Y. Sun, Y. Ye, J. Voigt, C. Strickland, E. M. Smith, J. Cumming, L. Wang, J. Wong, Y. S. Wang, D. F. Wyss, X. Chen, R. Kuvelkar, M. E. Kennedy, L. Favreau, E. Parker, B. A. McKittrick, A. Stamford, M. Czarniecki, W. Greenlee and J. C. Hunter, *J. Med. Chem.*, 2010, **53**, 951–965.
185. S. Howard, V. Berdini, J. A. Boulstridge, M. G. Carr, D. M. Cross, J. Curry, L. A. Devine, T. R. Early, L. Fazal, A. L. Gill, M. Heathcote, S. Maman, J. E. Matthews, R. L. McMenamin, E. F. Navarro, M. A. O'Brien, M. O'Reilly, D. C. Rees, M. Reule, D. Tisi, G. Williams, M. Vinkovic and P. G. Wyatt, *J. Med. Chem.*, 2009, **52**, 379–388.
186. J. J. Caldwell, T. G. Davies, A. Donald, T. McHardy, M. G. Rowlands, G. W. Aherne, L. K. Hunter, K. Taylor, R. Ruddle, F. I. Raynaud, M. Verdonk, P. Workman, M. D. Garrett and I. Collins, *J. Med. Chem.*, 2008, **51**, 2147–2157.
187. M. Addie, P. Ballard, D. Buttar, C. Crafter, G. Currie, B. R. Davies, J. Debreczeni, H. Dry, P. Dudley, R. Greenwood, P. D. Johnson, J. G. Kettle, C. Lane, G. Lamont, A. Leach, R. W. A. Luke, J. Morris, D. Ogilvie, K. Page, M. Pass, S. Pearson and L. Ruston, *J. Med. Chem.*, 2013, **56**, 2059–2073.
188. I. Mochalkin, J. R. Miller, L. Narasimhan, V. Thanabal, P. Erdman, P. B. Cox, J. V. Prasad, S. Lightle, M. D. Huband and C. K. Stover, *ACS Chem. Biol.*, 2009, **4**, 473–483.
189. P. A. Brough, X. Barril, J. Borgognoni, P. Chene, N. G. Davies, B. Davis, M. J. Drysdale, B. Dymock, S. A. Eccles, C. Garcia-Echeverria, C. Fromont, A. Hayes, R. E. Hubbard, A. M. Jordan, M. R. Jensen, A. Massey, A. Merrett, A. Padfield, R. Parsons, T. Radimerski, F. I. Raynaud, A. Robertson, S. D. Roughley, J. Schoepfer, H. Simmonite, S. Y. Sharp, A. Surgenor, M. Valenti, S. Walls, P. Webb, M. Wood, P. Workman and L. Wright, *J. Med. Chem.*, 2009, **52**, 4794–4809.
190. B. Dymock, X. Barril, M. Beswick, A. Collier, N. Davies, M. Drysdale, A. Fink, C. Fromont, R. E. Hubbard, A. Massey, A. Surgenor and L. Wright, *Bioorg. Med. Chem. Lett.*, 2004, **14**, 325–328.
191. J. D. Charrier, A. Miller, D. P. Kay, G. Brenchley, H. C. Twin, P. N. Collier, S. Ramaya, S. B. Keily, S. J. Durrant, R. M. Knegtel, A. J. Tanner, K. Brown, A. P. Curnock and J. M. Jimenez, *J. Med. Chem.*, 2011, **54**, 2341–2350.
192. M. B. Eisen, D. C. Wiley, M. Karplus and R. E. Hubbard, *Proteins*, 1994, **19**, 199–221.

# 6 Machine Learning in Drug Design

Ola Engkvist*[a], Lewis H. Mervin[b], Hongming Chen[c] and Ting Ran[c]

[a]Molecular AI, Discovery Sciences, R&D, AstraZeneca, Gothenburg, Sweden; [b]Molecular AI, Discovery Sciences, R&D, AstraZeneca, Cambridge, UK; [c]Bioland Laboratory (Guangzhou Regenarative Medicine and Health-Guangdong Laboratory), Guangzhou, China
*E-mail: Ola.Engkvist@astrazeneca.com

## 6.1 Introduction

Machine learning (ML) applications in drug design have now been available for more than two decades. Recently an increased use of deep learning (DL) methods have been witnessed. DL has gained huge success in a wide range of applications such as computer games, speech recognition, computer vision, natural language processing, and self driving cars, among others.[1] DL is penetrating into many aspects of our everyday life. In the Gartner-selected top ten technology trends of 2018, DL-represented AI technologies were ranked at the top position.[2]

Deep learning is a subset of machine learning methods, most often based on artificial neural networks (ANN). An ANN is a collection of nodes called artificial "neurons," inspired by the highly interconnected structure of neurons in a biological brain for processing data. In an ANN, the neurons are organised as an input layer, where data is input, one or more hidden layers where data is processed, and an output layer where the results are presented. Each "neuron" acts like the synapses in a biological brain, and can transmit a signal to other neurons. A "neuron" that receives a signal from a connected neuron can process it and can signal to neurons connected to it. The "signal" at a connection is a number, and the output of each neuron is computed by an often non-linear transformation of the sum of its inputs. In the training phase, weightings in the summing process are adjusted iteratively. Training continues until the output layer responses closely match the input layer values. Once the model is trained, it can be used to predict by inputting new values at the input layer. It is the highly interconnected nature of the network, and the weighted summing of non-linear transformed data that

The Handbook of Medicinal Chemistry: Principles and Practice, 2nd Edition
Edited by Simon E. Ward and Andrew M. Davis

Published by the Royal Society of Chemistry, www.rsc.org

give ANNs their power to model data. The "deep" in deep learning refers to the number of hidden layers through which the input data is transformed.

The origin of the AI and deep learning story is surprisingly quite old. William McCulloch and Walter Pitts published A Logical Calculus of the Ideas Immanent in Nervous Activity in 1943,[3] in which they outlined the first computational model of a neural network. This paper served as the blueprint for the first ANNs. The increased use of DL in the last decade has taken advantage of a rapid increase of available data, development of computer hardware such the graphics processing unit (GPU) and invention of new algorithms such as deep neural networks.

The application of DL in drug discovery has also quickly developed in the last few years.[4,243] The ever increasing volume of chemical and biological data in combination with increased automation technology have promoted further use of ML and DL algorithms. Accurate prediction of various biological and ADMET (Adsorption, Distribution, Metabolism, Excretion Toxicology) end points is a key application of ML algorithms in drug design and numerous DL algorithms have been proposed for building predictive models.[5] Bioactivity predictions including *in silico* protein target deconvolution is a computational technique for identifying protein–ligand interactions utilizing bioactivity data (ligand–target pairs) from experiments. ML/DL algorithms are a natural choice for addressing the target deconvolution problem computationally. Generative modeling for molecular *de novo* drug design is another novel area where DL is applied, and to a certain extent it can be regarded as a revolution compared to the traditional method of structure generation. Also areas like synthesis prediction and retrosynthesis planning have made significant progress due to DL, performing better or on par with traditional rule-based methods. Recent applications of ML/DL technologies in the above-mentioned cheminformatics research areas are summarized in this chapter. Remaining challenges and potential directions of future development of DL in drug discovery are also discussed to some extent.

## 6.2 Development of Deep Generative Models for Molecular Structure Generation

### 6.2.1 The Emergence of Deep Generative Models

One of the most exciting developments for DL technology is the use of so-called generative models for *de novo* drug design.[6] Many *de novo* drug design methodologies have been reported previously in the literature.[7–13] For structure-based *de novo* design methods, molecules are grown or assembled based on the predefined reaction rules and fragment libraries to achieve matches on either geometric shape or the electrostatic field between ligand and protein binding pocket.[7,8] For ligand-based methods in general, a virtual compound library is first enumerated, and the search for suitable molecules in the library is carried out through various scoring functions. The enumeration of virtual libraries is usually performed using predefined reaction rules and commercially available building blocks.[9] Another type of approach is to use transformation rules based on the experience of medicinal chemists to transform the query structure into target molecules. Besnard *et al.* reported on the use of transformation rules to design new active molecules against dopamine receptors.[10] The commonality of these methods is that enumeration based on predefined rules is a prerequisite for generating structures. One limitation for these rule-based methods is that the size of the searchable virtual library space ($10^{10}$–$10^{12}$ molecules) is much smaller than that of the commonly recognized drug-like chemical space (about $10^{60}$ molecules). Genetic algorithms are also used as a non-enumerable method for structure generation,[11] but the problem with this type of method is the lack of prior knowledge to describe drug-like molecules, resulting in low drug-likeness as well as poor synthesis feasibility of the generated structures. There are also approaches called inverse QSAR (quantitative structure and activity relationship) methods for molecule design. These methods aim to use the structure–activity relationship model to map out the chemical space satisfying certain constraints to generate molecular structures.[12,13] However, the bottleneck encountered by these methods is that it is difficult to find molecular descriptors that can be used not only to construct a structure–activity relationship model but that can also be easily mapped back to molecular structures.

The generative model based on deep learning represents a paradigm shift in the domain of structure generation, which is completely data-driven and does not depend on any predefined rules. It can learn the underlying probability distribution of structure description from a large amount of molecular structure data, in effect "learning" the medicinal chemistry rules of compound design, and can therefore theoretically search in the entire drug-like space, hence generating more novel structures beyond those explicitly contained within the definition of the original virtual library.

### 6.2.2 SMILES-based Generative Models

At present, DL generation models are mainly divided into two types depending on whether the structure is described by SMILES language[14] or based on a molecular graph. Figure 6.1 summarizes several major generative model architectures. Figure 6.1a, b, and c belong to the SMILES generative model, and Figure 6.1d belongs to the molecular graph generative model.

The SMILES (Simplified Molecular Input Line Entry System) language is a common way to characterize molecular structures[14] (online tutorial: https://www.daylight.com/meetings/summerschool98/course/dave/smiles-intro.html). It is essentially a one-dimensional sequence of characters and numbers arranged according to a specific grammar.[15] Each atom is represented by a letter, for example carbon, nitrogen, and oxygen are represented by C, O, and N, and the environment represented by upper case for aliphatic and lower case for aromatic. Single bonds are implicit, with double bonds represented by = and triple bonds by #. Rings are represented by labelling the joining atoms by a number, sidechains are placed in brackets. So, for example, benzamide is a ring of six aromatic carbons with an amide sidechain and one SMILES representation is c1ccccc1C(=O)N. It can be written in other ways depending on which atom is chosen as the startpoint, so C=O(N)c1ccccc1 is also an equally valid SMILES representation for benzamide. But grammar rules within the SMILES language can define a unique SMILES representation for any molecule, The SMILES sequence can be converted into a

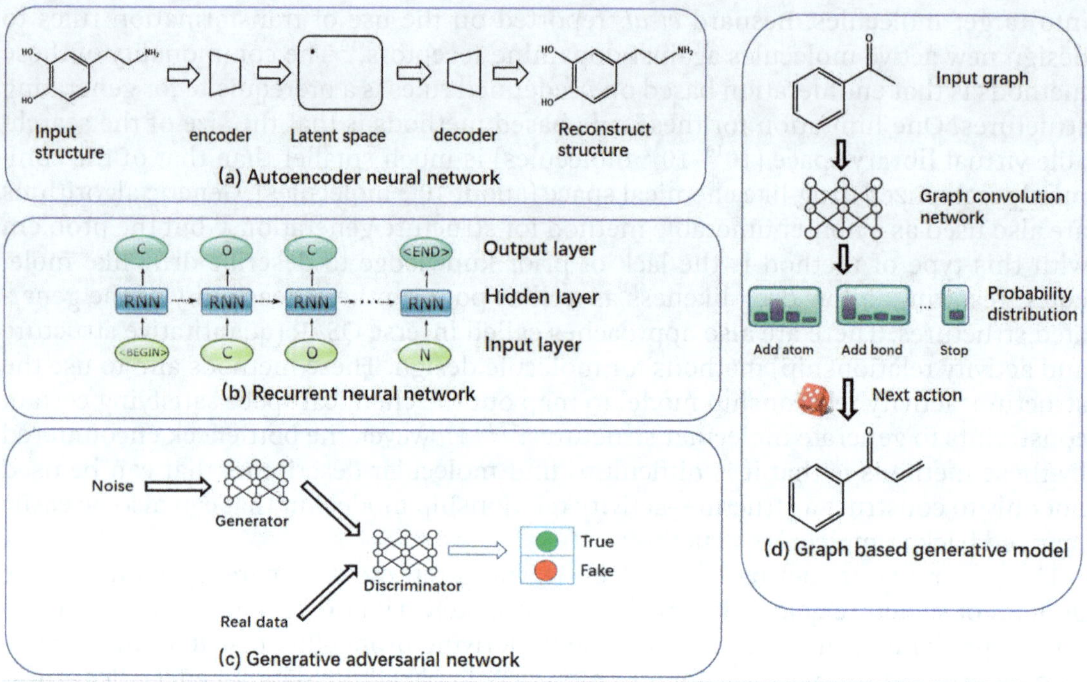


**Figure 6.1** Examples of common types of generative models for *de novo* molecular design.

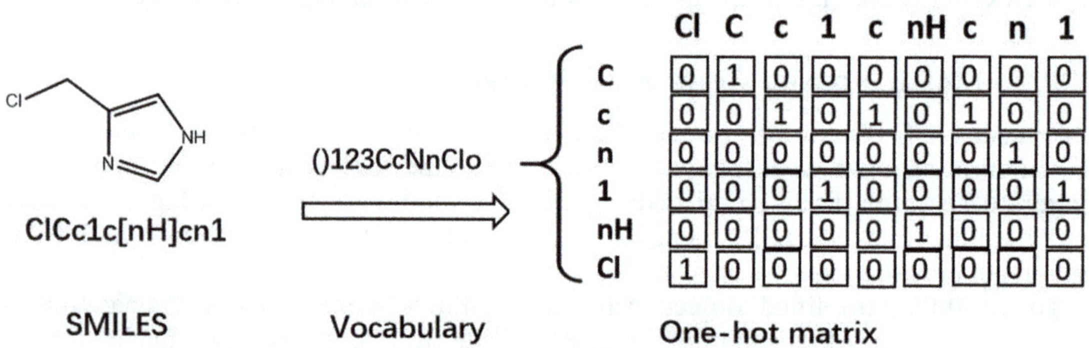


**Figure 6.2** Transformation of SMILES sequence.

one-hot matrix according to the vocabulary (as shown in Figure 6.2). One-hot is a group of bits among which the legal combinations of values are only those with a single high (1) bit with all the others low (0). Here the columns in the one-hot matrix correspond to the positions in the SMILES sequence and the rows refer to the all types of token defined in SMILES language, while the element in the matrix is a binary value, indicating if the token is used at certain position or not. Taking the one-hot matrix as input, different neural network architectures can be used for structural generation.

The architecture of a recurrent neural network (RNN) is shown in Figure 6.1b. Each layer of an RNN can be presented as a neural network unit which processes an input sequence recursively. For each iteration, the neural network receives two inputs: a vector of numbers and also a hidden state matrix (which contains information from the previous steps) and returns two outputs: an output vector and an updated hidden state matrix. For the next iteration the output and the hidden state from the previous iteration is input. This is repeated until all the input sequences are processed. Since SMILES itself can be regarded as a sequence of strings, RNN is very suitable to process SMILES. Segler[16] and Olivecrona[17] used Long Short Term Memory (LSTM) and Gated Recurrent Unit (GRU) RNN networks to generate molecular structures, respectively. Here LSTM and GRU are two types of neural network unit used in RNN and their architecture design enables them to keep the dependency from steps which are far ahead in the input sequence. By using a large number of SMILES as training sets, the trained RNN models can automatically generate highly drug-like random chemical structures, the accuracy of the generated SMILES can be as high as 90% (SMILES are valid according to the SMILES grammar and rules), and the diversity of molecular structures obtained is basically the same as the training set.

Due to the nature of SMILES representation, the same molecular structure can be represented by different SMILES sequences. Arús-Pous *et al.*[18] found that randomizing SMILES sequences can be used as a data augmentation technique to train the RNN model. Their study showed that the coverage of the chemical space for the GDB-13[19] database of RNN models trained by randomized SMILES is much better than that of the models trained with standard SMILES sequences. However, generating random molecular structures is not what we need. What we need is to be able to design drug-like molecule structures that can bind to specific targets. In order to gain a better control of the structures generated by neural networks, Segler *et al.*[16] employed transfer learning (TL) to generate molecules that are active to specific targets. Olivecrona *et al.*[17] proposed the REINVENT algorithm, combining RNN and an reinforcement learning algorithm (RL) to optimize the score of the generated molecules by fine-tuning the model parameters of RNN, which achieves the aim of controlling the molecular structure. Reinforcement learning penalises the RNN structure generation algorithm for generating structures we don't want and rewards generating structures we do want. It achieves this by using scoring functions, which might be ranges of calculated physical properties or predicted affinities *vs.* our target of interest.

Besides the RNN architecture, Gomez-Bombarelli[20] and Blaschke[21] explored a variational autoencoder (VAE) neural network architecture (as shown in Figure 6.1a) to generate structures. The autoencoder neural network contains two parts: the encoder and decoder networks. The encoder network converts the input structure into a multidimensional vector, aka latent vector, and the decoder network tries to convert the latent vector back to the input structure. A VAE neural network is an extension of autoencoder neural network, the main difference is that VAE restrains the latent vector under a certain distribution, *e.g.* a Gaussian distribution. In Gomez-Bombarelli's work, a special neural network, a convolutional neural network (CNN), is used as the encoder to map the molecular structure input information into latent variables, and RNN is used in the decoder part to restore the hidden variables to input information. After training, the variables sampled from the hidden space can be converted to structures by using the decoder. The common problems for these VAE methods is that macrocyclic compounds can often be generated and the validity of SMILES is only about 60%. Bjerrum[22] proposed a type of autoencoder model called a Heteroencoder, in which RNN is used as the encoder instead of CNN. The accuracy of SMILES can be increased to 80% and there are also fewer cases of macrocyclic compounds.

Another type of neural network architecture that can be used to generate molecular structures is the so-called generative adversarial network (GAN).[23] GAN contains two competing neural networks (as shown in Figure 6.1c), namely the generator and discriminator. The generator network generates random SMILES, while the discriminator attempts to distinguish random molecules from the target molecules in the training set. In each round of training, the generator is gradually improved so that the generated molecular structures become more and more similar to the target molecules. The training is terminated when the discriminator can no longer distinguish the molecules generated by the generator from the target molecules in the training set and the generator network can then be used to generate the required molecules. The ORGAN[24] and ORGANIC[25] algorithms proposed by Aspuru-Guzik are the earliest examples of using GAN to generate molecular structures. Researchers from Insilico Medicine proposed the algorithms RANC[26] and ATNC,[27] trying to combine GAN, reinforcement learning, and differential neural computing (Differential Neural Computer, DNC), a more sophisticated version of the GRU network for processing long-term memory for structure generation. Prykhodko *et al.*[28] proposed the LatentGAN algorithm, which combines an autoencoder and the GAN algorithm to perform molecular design work. Instead of directly using SMILES as the input to GAN, as in the ORGANIC model, the hidden variables generated by the autoencoder are used as the input to GAN. Their results show that a large number of new structures can be generated, and some molecules can even have new scaffolds.

### 6.2.3 Graph-based Generative Models

The above methods all use SMILES for structure generation. However, in the process of structure generation, unfinished SMILES sequences are not valid molecule structures and can not be attributed scores during reinforcement learning. Therefore, algorithms using molecular graphs for structure generation have also been explored. Researchers from Deepmind proposed a molecular-graph-based algorithm[29] for structure generation. This algorithm treats molecular structure generation as a sequence of actions for graph transformation. Each step is predicted by a graph convolution model to predict the next action, *i.e.* to add a new atom or to form a chemical bond with one of the existing atoms and so on. The molecules in the training set will first need to be converted into a series of graph transformation sequences and then used for training the graph convolution model. Li[30] also proposed a similar MolMP graph generation algorithm, using the molecular graph convolution model to predict the probability of the next action. You[31] proposed a graph convolution strategy model. This algorithm used a molecular graph convolution model to predict the chemical bond type at each step.

One disadvantage of the SMILES-based VAE model is that the validity of generated SMILES is lower than that of the RNN model. For addressing this problem, Jin[32] proposed the Junction Tree Neural Network (JTNN) algorithm to generate molecular structures based on a molecular graph instead. It first converts the molecular structure into a feature tree composed of pharmacophores, and then uses two different graph convolution models to encode the molecular graph and the feature tree into hidden vectors $Z_g$ and $Z_t$ respectively. Finally, the decoder network is used to restore the hidden vectors $Z_g$ and $Z_t$ into the original molecular structure. Since each node in the feature tree is composed of valid substructures, this ensures that the decoded molecular structure will be a 100% valid chemical structure. The molecular-graph-based algorithm is not very mature at present. Comparing with the SMILES-based generative model, the graph model mimicks the human way of drawing structures, *i.e.* drawing atom by atom, bond by bond. But this results in a much larger searching space at each step. Also in the graph model, each molecular structure needs to be decomposed into a series of substructures during training, therefore the amount of data in the training set is greatly increased. These two factors result in a slower training speed for the graph model.

Although the generative model method was only proposed three years ago, the field has developed very rapidly and generative models have been used for drug design. Zhavoronkov[33] recently published work using VAE and reinforcement learning to quickly design DDR1 inhibitors and obtained experimental verification. The use of generative models for drug design is essentially a matter of controlled molecular structure generation under parameter constraints. Using reinforcement learning can achieve optimization under multiparameter constraints to a certain extent, but there is still room for optimization efficiency and diversity of generated molecules. Currently most generative models are still based on two-dimensional information to design molecules; how to use 3D compound information and especially 3D information on the protein binding pocket as a constraint to generate molecular structures will be the next interesting research field. Thanks to the open source movement, the source codes for a many generative models are available on the internet.[34–36]

## 6.3 Advances in Deep Learning for ADMET Prediction

### 6.3.1 Prediction of ADMET Properties

In drug discovery, prediction of ADMET properties has played an important role in reducing the attrition rate of drugs.[37] It essentially originates from the concept of quantitative structure–activity relationships (QSAR), which was formally introduced to medicinal chemistry in the 1960s through the work of Corwin Hansch and Toshio Fujita,[38] who mathematically correlated the biological activities of molecules to a quantitative description of chemical structure features, although medicinal chemists have tried to relate physicochemical properties to the ADMET characteristics of chemicals for over a century. There is a large body of reviews summarizing the modeling methods and applications of ADMET prediction,[5,39] which shows that machine-learning-based artificial intelligence (AI) technologies lead the trend of *in silico* modeling of ADMET properties. Compared to early QSAR modeling with linear regression models, machine learning promotes ADMET prediction by fitting multiple variables to various endpoints using non-linear models. Up till now, multiple machine learning algorithms, such as random forest (RF), artificial neural network (ANN), support vector machine (SVM), decision tree (DT), *k*-nearest neighbours (*k*-NN) and so on, have been extensively applied for ADMET prediction.[39] However, overfitting is still a common problem in machine learning, where a model performs well on training data but does not generalize well to unseen data. Some of the recent ML technologies seem to avoid the overfitting problem through automatic feature engineering to reduce data redundancy and efficiently utilizing computer power to deal with a big "training set" for modeling.

In recent years, the next generation of AI represented by deep learning (DL) has begun to be applied for drug discovery.[6,40–42] It became popular in ADMET prediction, beginning with deep neural network (DNN) architecture-based DL modeling.[40] More recently, convolution neural networks (CNN), graph neural networks (GNN) and their combination have begun to be a new favorite for researchers (Figure 6.3).[43] DNN is also known as fully connected deep neural network. It contains multiple hidden layers, each layer comprises hundreds of non-linear process units (aka neurons) and neurons in neighboring layers are all inter-connected. CNN was originally used for image recognition. It usually contains several convolution layers and subsampling layers. The convolution layer consists of a set of small size matrices (aka filters or kernels) whose elements are learnable parameters. During the forward pass, each filter matrix is slid across the width and height of the input data matrix, calculating the dot product between the entries of the filter matrix and its receptive field in the input matrix and producing a 2D feature map of that filter. The subsampling layer is then used to reduce the size of the feature maps. CNN has the capability to do automatic feature selection, which makes the manual and specific feature selection procedure unnecessary. In essence, GNN is similar to CNN, but the input data is not in a matrix format but in the form of graph, and the sliding process is done on each node of the graph. Another important feature in DL is to carry out multitask learning for ADMET prediction,[44] which may be applied in the parallel multiparameter optimization of pharmacokinetic properties in drug discovery.

The purpose of this section is to summarize the recent applications of DL technology for ADMET prediction. Indeed, some of the latest reviews have paid attention to the DL approaches used in ADMET prediction.[45–47] Here, we focus on the recent progress in DL-based ADMET prediction, including discussion on the current challenge and future perspectives.

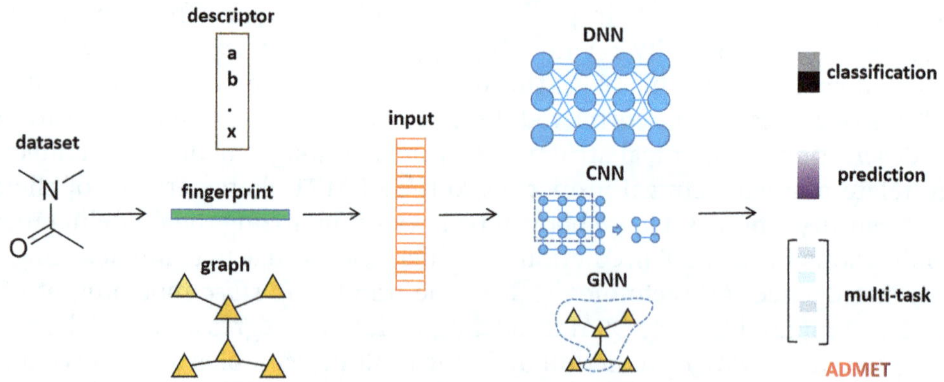


**Figure 6.3** Deep learning modeling for ADMET properties.

## 6.3.2 Applications of Deep Learning in ADMET Prediction

Comprehensive reviews on DL-based ADMET modeling are comparatively rare so far,[46] although continuous efforts have been made in this field. In this review, the focus is mainly on the applications of DL in ADMET prediction (Table 6.1).

### *6.3.2.1 Physicochemical Property Prediction*

Compound physicochemical properties have a long history of being used for compound quality evaluation. Early efforts had been focused on building rule-based models for evaluating compound quality. The most famous, called the "rule of five," was created as a compound druggability indicator.[48] Subsequently, *in silico* models especially built by machine learning methods were applied to predict the properties, such as solubility, $pK_a$, $\log P/D$, and so on, which are associated with ADMET behaviors. Many DL-based approaches have been developed on this topic, and some recent progress will be presented as follows.

**Table 6.1** Some examples of DL-based prediction of physicochemical and ADMET properties.

| Type | Models | Object | Accuracy | Ref. |
|---|---|---|---|---|
| Physico-chemical properties | DNN | $\log P$ | $R^2$: 0.66 | 49 |
| | DNN:TopP-S | $\log P$ and aqueous solubility | $R^2 > 0.90$ | 50 |
| | CNN:20-layer ResNet-like model | Aqueous solubility | $R^2$: 0.412 | 51 |
| | UG-RNN-CR-log P-Huusk-sub | Aqueous solubility | $R^2$: 0.67 | 52 |
| | GC-DNN | $pK_a$ | $R^2$: 0.437 | 53 |
| | CNN-Ab-oct-Deaq-representative | Aqueous solubility | MAE: 0.407 | 54 |
| | CNN-Br-tm-consensus | Melting point | MAE: 26.18 | 54 |
| | GCNN:Chemi-Net | Solubility | $R^2 > 0.5$ | 55 |
| | EAGCNconcat | Lipophilicity | $R^2$: 0.61 | 56 |
| ADMET properties | DNN | Human plasma protein binding | $R^2$: 0.598 | 63 |
| | DNN | Transport by P-glycoprotein | $R^2$: 0.616 | 63 |
| | DNN | Caco-2 permeability | Accuracy: 83.51% | 64 |
| | GCN | Mouse liver microsomal | Accuracy: 82.8% | 65 |
| | DNN | Metabolic lability | $R^2 > 0.5$ | 66 |
| | DNN-PBPK | Oral bioavailability in rats | Accuracy: 67% | 67 |
| | CNN | Human cytochrome P450 inhibition | Accuracy: 87.9% | 68 |
| | Autoencoder DNN | Human cytochrome P450 inhibition | Accuracy: 86.4% | 69 |
| | DNN:Deeppharm | Distribution at steady-state | Accuracy: 63.33% | 71 |
| | DNN:Deeppharm | Elimination half-life | Accuracy: 66.67% | 71 |
| | DNN:DeepTox | Tox21 challenge | AUC: 0.846 | 77 |
| | GCNN:IterRefLSTM | Tox21 challenge | AUC > 0.8 | 78 |
| | DNN | Chemically induced liver toxicity | $R^2$: 0.74 | 98 |
| | CNN | Tox21 challenge | AUC: 0.85 | 99 |
| | CNN | Clinic xerostomia | AUC > 0.65 | 100 |

Recently, Prasad *et al.* built a DNN model for the SAMPL6 challenge (Statistical Assessment of the Modeling of Proteins and Ligands – a community-wide blinded challenge focused on log$P$ prediction), which achieved an RMSE (root mean square error) of 0.41 log$P$ units.[49] Multitask DNN models built by Wu *et al.* made a similar achievement on the prediction of log$P$ and aqueous solubility.[50] Cui recently constructed a modified ResNet CNN model,[51] which shows excellent performance on aqueous solubility. Graph networks is another hot spot in physicochemical property prediction. Early in 2013, Lusci *et al.* constructed an undirected graph-based RNN model named UG-RNN specifically to predict aqueous solubility.[52] The molecular structure in this model was described as an undirected graph. This model demonstrated comparable performance to state-of-the-art machine learning despite using 60 compounds as the training set. Subsequently, a graph convolutional neural network (GCNN) was utilized by Hop *et al.* and Coley *et al.*[53,54] to predict properties such as p$K_a$, solubility, and melting point. As a result, solubility prediction showed better performance than traditional machine learning, while prediction of melting point did not reach a similar improvement. Recently, Liu *et al.* developed a GCNN model, called Chemi-Net,[55] which beat the commercial software Cubist used by Amgen in physicochemical property prediction. Other GNN variants were also recently reported.[56–61] The latest review gave a comprehensive summary of GNN models.[62] In short, DL is emerging as an all-round player in physicochemical properties prediction.

### 6.3.2.2 ADMET Property Prediction

In order to better describe the drug-like property of compounds, another strategy is to predict the parameters that directly indicate ADMET properties. Examples of these parameters are oral absorption, cellular permeability, bioavailability, volume of distribution, human plasma protein binding (hPPB), interaction profile of transport proteins, inhibition on metabolism enzymes, clearance, tumorigenicity, and so on.

For instance, Ma *et al.* developed DNN models superior to RF models for several ADMET endpoints,[63] such as transport by P-glycoprotein and human plasma protein binding. In addition, Shin *et al.* constructed a DNN model as a Caco-2 permeability classifier,[64] while Renn *et al.* built a model for mouse liver microsomal stability.[65] Recently, Wenzel *et al.* succeeded in the prediction of microsomal lability in different species and passive permeability in Caco-2/TC7 cells using multitask DNN models.[66] Schneckener *et al.* predicted oral bioavailability in rats with a DNN model,[67] which achieved an accuracy close to 70%. This study indicates that DL may provide an effective tool for the prediction of *in vivo* pharmacokinetic behaviors. Li *et al.* and Wu *et al.* successively constructed DL models to predict CYP450 inhibition using DNN,[68,69] but the later study showed that the ensemble modeling XGBoost derived a model with higher accuracy than the DL models. Similarly, the DL modeling did not show an obvious advantage over traditional machine learning,[70] although different datasets from Li's study were used. In fact, some efforts have been made to improve DL-based ADMET prediction. The most recent established a multitask GCNN model to predict a variety of ADMET properties using 31 assay datasets and exhibited significant improvement over both RF and single-task GCNN models.[60] Ye *et al.* integrated transfer learning and multitask learning, which significantly improved the prediction of oral bioavailability, plasma protein binding, volume of distribution at steady-state, and elimination half-life.[71] Peng *et al.* designed a hybrid framework using an RNN and a fully connected neural network to extract SMILES information and physicochemical properties, respectively, whose outputs were then combined as a input vector to train another fully connected neural network to predict chemical toxicity of drugs.[72] As a result, the hybrid model outperformed not only the traditional machine learning, but also available DL models, which indicates a possibility to improve the DL model through mixing different types of descriptors for learning.[73]

In recent years, drug toxicity prediction is an active area for DL modeling among ADMET prediction.[74–76] In 2016, a DL model called DeepTox won the Tox21 data challenge with excellent performance.[77] Altae-Tran *et al.* combined iterative refinement of long- and short-term memory and a GCNN model for toxicity prediction and achieved better performance than the traditional machine learning models.[78] So far, multiple DL models have been reported to predict various toxicities, such as drug-induced liver injury,[79] acute toxicity,[80] rectum toxicity,[81] hepatotoxicity,[82–86] hERG blocking,[87,88] receptor activity,[89,90] drug–drug interactions,[91–94] and so on. Most of the above-mentioned DL methods utilized 1-dimensional molecular descriptors or fingerprints as the input for the neural network, while several studies designed a 2-dimensional image-based neural network to predict ADMET properties such as CYP1A2 inhibitory potency, P-glycoprotein (P-gp) inhibitory activity, Blood–Brain Barrier (BBB) penetrating activity and toxicity.[95–97] Recently, Wang *et al.* constructed a DNN model based on transcriptomic data to predict chemically induced liver toxicity.[98] Last year, Yuan *et al.* reported a grid-based multichannel CNN with improved accuracy compared to traditional DL in toxicity prediction.[99] Another interesting field is predicting adverse effects from clinical data using DL technology. For example, Men *et al.* predicted xerostomia due to radiation therapy for head and neck squamous cell carcinoma from only 784 patients.[100]

### 6.3.3 Challenges and Opportunities in ADME Modeling

Since overfitting and gradient descent have been overcome for DL, the application of DL is continuously expanding. According to above reviews on DL-based ADMET modeling, most robust models available are derived to correlate the physicochemical and ADMET properties to molecular structures. Today there is still a lack of DL models specific for the modeling of *in vitro–in vivo* correlation that more intuitively reflects the pharmacokinetic risk in clinical setup.[74] Certainly, this field is more challenging, as small and local structural change of compounds may reverse the pharmacokinetic behaviors *in vivo*, for which local models would be more appropriate.

Many factors affect the success of DL modeling. Among them, data set size and quality of data play a critical role and seem more important than modeling methods.[101] In order to achieve better performance, DL models may require larger data sizes than the traditional machine learning methods. But, there was a report that multitask DL can achieve higher accuracy on small data sets.[102] When the data comes from different sources, it is usually hard to derive consistent models, although the DL technology allows more data heterogeneity. On the other hand, big pharmaceutical companies generally have massive proprietary experimental data with high quality and consistency. Therefore promoting open data to increase data accessibility could definitely boost the benchmark study of various DL technologies.[103]

Molecular representation also influences model quality.[104] Compared to traditional machine learning, DL can deal with various types of molecular representations, not only the traditional structural fingerprints and physicochemical descriptors, but also the contextual information that describes the molecule structure such as SMILES, molecular graphs, even 2D molecular sketch images. A molecular-graph-based DL model recently attracted a lot of attention, as it described the molecular structure in a higher level of detail compared to SMILES and fingerprints, where atom and bond information are mapped into nodes and edges in a graph. On the negative side, most DL modeling methods don't pay much attention directly to the contribution of molecular fragments, which was partially resolved by methods such as matched molecular pairs algorithms[105,106] and a "response map" algorithm reported by Wenzel *et al.*[66] Structure-based ADMET prediction strategy,[107] which employs protein–ligand interaction information to predict ADMET properties, is so far still not fully explored using DL methods and could be an interesting area to expand.

In 2012, the Merck Molecular Activity Challenge promoted the popularity of multitask DL,[108] which demonstrated that multitask learning is superior to traditional machine learning methods, but does not always outperform it.[109] More endeavors are required to improve this technology for ADMET prediction. Another challenge worthwhile mentioning is to predict ADMET properties toward new modalities such as peptides, PROTAC[110] *etc.*, which represent a totally new chemical space compared with conventional small molecules.

## 6.4 *In Silico* Protein Target Deconvolution

### 6.4.1 Structure- and Ligand-based Approaches Toward Protein–Ligand Prediction

Biochemical methods for target deconvolution are expensive and time-consuming and it is intractable to experimentally test small molecules for all possible on-target or off-target interactions.[111,112] *In silico* protein target deconvolution is a well-established computational technique offering an alternative avenue to infer protein–ligand interactions by combining computational techniques with known bioactivity data (ligand–target pairs) from biochemical experiments.[113,114]

Both structure- and ligand-based methods exist to annotate protein targets with predicted small molecule ligands.[114–119] The former describe approaches that exploit structural information of proteins of interest combined with scoring functions.[120–122] Ligand-based methods investigate preexisting structure–activity relationship (SAR) space, using methods that exploit chemical space similarity on large numbers of annotated protein–ligand pairs obtained from chemogenomic databases.[123–126] Both approaches are intended to help direct experimental resources for corroboration in biological confirmation afterward, given they are still only computational predictions and usually do not predict quantitative activity (*e.g.* affinity values).[127–129]

Alternative approaches to *quantitatively* model ligand–protein activity (*i.e.* more similar to multitarget QSAR methods) have recently been published, which, for a subset of proteins and chemical space, approach the reported reproducibility of assays. However, probabilities of activity and quantitative activity are two distinct aspects of compound bioactivity modeling and a trade-off between both axes exists (*i.e.* quantitative activity prediction, chemical coverage, and model performance cannot be optimized at the same time and independently of each other). Hence, both binary target prediction, which aims to annotate ligands with likelihoods of activity at a given threshold, and quantitative activity predictions have distinct strengths and weaknesses.

Similar to other approaches in this chapter, the emergence and progression of target prediction resulted from the continued advancement in three main areas; firstly are the developments of advanced machine learning algorithms, that are able to rationalize the non-linear target interactions between chemical and biological information from chemogenomic databases,[114,130,131] secondly are the growing access and reducing cost of increasingly powerful computational resources to apply these algorithms,[132] and, lastly, the developments in high-throughput techniques,[133–135] responsible for the expansion of freely available SAR data.[136–140]

## 6.4.2 Ligand-based Approaches

Ligand-based predictive models are founded upon the principle of chemical similarity and have existed for many years.[141] Such approaches rely on the relevant similarities of compound features annotated across different targets which are likely to be responsible for binding activity.[142,143] Similarity searching for ligand-based target prediction is considered the simplest form and is well established in literature.[114,119,124,144–147] Models base their predictions on the molecular similarity principle of identified bioactive compounds from chemogenomic databases.[143,147] The simplistic nature of these methods means they are only able to consider the molecule structure as a whole, significantly hindering their predictivity.

Building on the theme of similarity searching, data-mining algorithms are capable of considering multiple combinations of compound fragments by applying pattern recognition techniques. They gained traction for target prediction due to their demonstrated ability to more efficiently extrapolate predictions,[114] and are less time consuming when compared to other approaches.[117]

### *6.4.2.1 Publicly Available ML Tools*

One of the earliest and most widely used examples of data-mining target elucidation is the continuously curated and expanded Prediction of Activity Spectra for Substances (PASS) software,[118] trained on data assimilated from more than 270 000 compound–ligand pairs. The authors based the model on multilevel neighborhoods of atoms (MNA) descriptors, producing predictions based on Bayesian estimates of probabilities. The Multifingerprint Similarity Search Algorithm (MuSSeL) was also developed, exploiting a large collection of high quality experimental bioactivity data available from ChEMBL.[148] This algorithm combines, in a consensus-like approach, predictions resulting from a similarity search performed using 13 different fingerprint definitions. Another popular web-based target prediction protocol, SwissTargetPrediction, has been available since 2014 and the 2019 version of SwissTargetPrediction consisted of 2092 protein targets.[149] The approach applies a unique procedure calculating similarity between an input compound and those defined in experimental binding assays. The model was fitted using a multiple logistic regression on various size-related subsets of known actives in order to weight 2D and 3D similarity parameters in a so-called Combined-Score. The principle is that two similar molecules are represented by analogous vectors, which exhibit a quantified similarity close to 1. A Combined-Score higher than 0.5 predicts that molecules are likely to share a common protein target. More recently, the Perturbation Theory Machine Learning (PTML) method was used to search for QSAR models capable of simultaneous prediction of many target properties under several experimental conditions. Another publicly available tool is version 3 of the Prediction IncluDinG INactivity (PIDGIN) protocol, trained using Random Forests (RFs) on bioactivity data from PubChem and ChEMBL (https://zenodo.org/badge/latestdoi/142870938). The technique employs a modification of the Reliability-Density Neighbourhood (RDN) Applicability Domain (AD) analysis,[150] and offers NCBI pathway and DisGeNET disease enrichment annotations.

#### 6.4.2.2 Applications of Different Algorithms and Architectures

The Naïve Bayes (NB) classifiers have been a popular family of algorithms used for the prediction of bioactivity for compounds.[151–153,156] These methods offer quick training and prediction times and are relatively insensitive to noise.[154] Nidhi *et al.*[151] employed a multiclass Naïve Bayes classification algorithm trained on a data set comprised of over 960 target proteins extracted from the "World Of Molecular BioAcTivity" (WOMBAT) database.[155] Another target prediction algorithm developed by Koutsoukas *et al.*[113] was trained with a Laplacian-modified Naïve Bayes classifier and a Parzen–Rosenblatt Window (PRW) learner in a multiclass setting for 155 000 ligand–protein pairs from the ChEMBL database.[136] The algorithm encompassed 894 different human protein targets, and after benchmarking experiments it was found that the PRW learner outperformed the Naïve Bayes algorithm overall, achieving a recall and precision of 66.6% and 63.3%, respectively.[113]

Support Vector Machines (SVMs) have also been employed for the task of target prediction. These models have historically utilised smaller amounts of data in comparison to NB models, mostly due to the computational expense of the SVM algorithm. The Random Forest (RF) algorithm has also proved popular, as exemplified by the number of publicly available tools employing this algorithm in the section above. Examples in literature include kinase activity modeling,[157] iterative screening,[158] and a comprehensive study applied to 1121 targets indicated a recall rate of ~73.9% within the top 1% of predictions. Deep Neural Networks (DNN) have also been applied for the area of target prediction.[128,159–161] The aim of the networks is to discover multiple levels of distributed representations built from a hierarchy of related features, with higher levels representing more abstract concepts. Thus, a natural hierarchy of features arises, which translates as simple chemical features within the first layer of the network and the subsequent hidden layers forming larger substructures derived from combinations of fragments. Although this behavior gives deep learning superior performance over other prediction methods, DNN often rely on large amounts of training data in order to construct indicative features, and hence are more suited to targets with large number of bioactivity points.[162] Despite this, DNN were shown to be the top performing classifiers compared to NB, RF, SVM, and Logistic Regression when assessed using QSAR and proteochemometric (PCM) methods.[163] Moreover, the best method "DNN_PCM" performed significantly better at almost one standard deviation higher than the mean performance. The Polypharmacology Browser (PPB2) combines NB and DNN trained on ChEMBL with Nearest Neighbors (NN) metrics using molecular fingerprints encoding composition (MQN), molecular shape and pharmacophores (Xfp), and substructures (ECFP4).[164] Deep feed-forward neural networks (FNN) were also shown to generate the best results (while SEA showed the lowest predictivity) in another comparison study.[165]

A variety of modeling approaches or architectures have been evaluated for target prediction. For example, one study showed that a Bernoulli NB algorithm trained with both active (binding or functionally active) molecules from ChEMBL and large-scale inactive bioactivity data from PubChem outperformed a multilabel model trained on active bioactivity data alone.[166] Multitask learning (MTL) approaches (techniques for simultaneously co-modeling multiple properties within a single model) have also received recent attention.[44] Human cytochrome P450 inhibition for five kinases were predicted using a pre-trained autoencoder-based DNN,[69] where the authors proved that a multitarget DNN approach can significantly outperform single-target DNN. Other approaches can identify sparse features to be used directly with linear or kernel methods, or to provide features for training other methods. One such method is Macau,[167] based on Bayesian Probabilistic Matrix Factorisation (BPMF). BPMF allows inputting missing values in the matrix thus enabling the application of standard techniques, such as singular value decomposition and principal component analysis. In contrast to classical algorithms of matrix factorization, Macau is able to handle side relations and can work with multidimensional data and perform tensor decomposition. This technique was trained with inhibition activities of 15 073 compounds for 346 targets extracted from ChEMBL.[168] Results showed Macau was able to perform similar to DNN but did not require GPU-accelerated computing. Multitask bioactivity prediction for the ExCAPE database using Macau was also combined with side-information from cell morphology information (CellPaint) experiments.[169] Results showed that cell morphology information was able to improve the predictivity of multitask predictions for a variety of targets, such as β-catenin.

### 6.4.3 Extensions to *In Silico* Target Deconvolution Methods

Ligand-based predictions provide a basis for further analysis to rationalize compound Mechanism-of-Action (MOA). Liggi *et al.*[170] extended target output predictions from a PRW target prediction algorithm with annotated enriched targets implicated with a cytotoxic phenotype, using pathways from the GO[171,172] and KEGG[173,174] pathway databases. A similar approach was applied to understand cytotoxicity and cytostaticity in a High Throughput Screening (HTS) collection,[175] with pathway annotation of predicted targets to improve insight into both "toxic" and "static" MOAs. Other examples include the combination of target prediction and classification tree techniques for rationalizing phenotypic readouts from a rat model for hypnotics.[166,176] The authors derived interpretable decision trees for the observed phenotypes and inferred the combination of modulated targets that contribute towards good sleeping patterns. Other applications utilized the predicted target profiles as a descriptor (*i.e.* predicted bioactivity fingerprint) during model training.[177] Examples include using predicted bioactivity profiles to predict noval synergistic antimalarial compound combinations,[178] cytotoxicity prediction,[179] and acute toxicity prediction.[180]

### 6.4.4 Limitations and Future Concerns for Target Prediction Methods

#### *6.4.4.1 Neglecting Pharmacokinetic/Pharmacodynamic (PK/PD) Factors*

Target prediction methodologies assume that small molecules are ubiquitously capable of reaching and interacting with all proteins within the cell, and therefore do not consider the pharmacokinetic/pharmacodynamic (PK/PD) properties of compounds.[181] This is a problem for predictions as they reduce the biological responses, which are influenced by time and space, to a binary prediction about the modulation of a target.

#### *6.4.4.2 Applications to Functional Prediction*

One limitation for many target prediction approaches is that they usually do not predict compound functional effects, such as activation or inhibition (in the simplest case of allowing only for two types of functional effects), upon binding to their protein counterparts. This is important since protein activation or inhibition may positively or negatively modulate a pathway, which in turn may relate in different ways to an observed phenotype. Although SEA and PASS provide some functional predictions based on the MDL Drug Data Report (MDDR), these predictions are only for a small training set and many functional classes are not on the target level. Another approach classified agonist from antagonist but was limited to nuclear receptors only.[182] A more recent (proprietary) approach was trained using ~23 million compound–target annotations available at AstraZeneca, with 226 045 activating and 1 032 439 inhibiting compounds from functional assays across a range of G-protein-coupled receptors (GPCRs), nuclear hormone receptors (NHRs), ion channels, and transporter targets. Models cascaded predictions through "stage 1" target prediction and "stage 2" functional prediction, performing with overall precision and recall of 72% and 71%, highlighting that one limitation on this approach was the propagation of errors through both predictive stages of modeling. Hence, functional prediction remains a challenging aspect for the current approaches for target prediction.

#### *6.4.4.3 Data Quality (Training) Issues*

Predictive modeling approaches are data driven and hence the training data influences model performance and prediction outputs. One issue is hence data quality and assay variability (propagating error through to predictive results).[183] On this topic, many public repositories commissioned as training data have a range of inaccuracies, from errors in molecular structure and incorrect physicochemical properties, to incorrect accompanying bioactivity metadata.[184] Indeed, an analysis of commercial and public bioactivity databases highlighted various inconsistencies between vendors, with no absolute guarantee that compound records and accompanying protein interactions in activity information are observed in reality.[185] The ChEMBL[136] database identified this issue for many records of its bioactivity data, and has responded to the problem *via* the annotation of target confidence scores for its bioactivities.[186] Clearly, the reliability of a given bioactivity source needs evaluation in parallel with the extent of chemical and biological space encapsulated by the data.

#### 6.4.4.4 The Problem of Data Distribution

The chemogenomic data sets used for training can also not be considered identically, independently distributed (i.i.d).[187] This is because associations are based on highly different data distributions (*i.e.* different target family classes, number of annotated compound activities, and degree of diversity).[188] For example, training data was shown to comprise a greatly imbalanced number of compound annotations across the proteome in one study, with a median of 752 and (~6.5 times larger) standard deviation of 4954 compounds assayed per protein target.[189] Another study modelled 15 different protein families, with between 17 and 615 targets per family and a standard deviation of 174 individual targets per family.[190] Imbalance toward enzymes and kinase families (*e.g.* ~30% and ~34% of training data set size)[113] negatively influences multilabel probability estimates for minority protein families. Models are further influenced by the putative or experimental origin of negative (*i.e.* non-binding or functionally inactive) training instances,[191] the proportion of protein-target complexes (~6% of ChEMBL data),[192] and an imbalance towards the negative class[193] (*e.g.* "$pXC_{50} < 5{:}pXC_{50} > 5$" compound ratio of ~96, standard deviation of ~16).[194] The chemical space of the training data is also biased with often 10–30 compound exemplars per scaffold,[195] but also high numbers of singleton scaffolds present for some scaffold cases.[196] Biological data for ortholog proteins was also shown to comprise a distinct region of chemical space compared to human.[197] As a consequence, ortholog bioactivity data has been historically aggregated to improve bioactivity data completeness *via* incorporation of data from related species, helping to overcome biases in bioactivity space and increasing under-represented target data points.[197]

#### 6.4.4.5 Applicability Domain Estimation Remains an Issue

Since target prediction models are frequently deployed to a novel chemical space of interest, this routinely pushes the capabilities of the applicability domain (AD) to the limit, defined as the chemical space of the model. Hence the predictions may exceed the ranges or combinations of descriptor space, with increased risk they cannot be accurately relied upon. Different approaches are available and reviewed here.[198–200] Indeed, since *in silico* methods are also often incapable of maintaining predictive power far past compound training sets, precautions must be taken to ensure query datasets do not fall outside the

AD of models.[201] Hence, despite their advantages and proven successes in recent studies, such approaches are still faced with multiple limitations that should be evaluated.[170]

#### 6.4.4.6 Poor Calibration and Confidence Estimation

An important consideration for target prediction is providing an accurate likelihood of activity (not only their statistical quality). The accuracy of the algorithmic output to assign a probability estimate that reflects the ground (actual) probability for each individual prediction is important. For example, a raw probability score of 0.90 may represent a high estimate that a compound is active; however only 70% of the compounds with that corresponding score may be active in reality. Thus, the ground truth likelihood of a compound obtaining this score is lower than the relative output from the algorithm, and hence the model is poorly calibrated. In comparison, predictions from a perfectly calibrated (binary) single-label classifier would classify the samples such that, among the samples to which it gave a probability value of 0.90 (to belong to the active class), indeed 90% actually belong to the active class. A variety of calibration techniques have been applied to target prediction tasks to convert the output from models into more accurate (and interpretable) outputs.[202,203] The Venn ABERS method (based on isotonic regression) has been shown to produce the most reliable outputs across a wide variety of methods evaluated.[204]

## 6.5 Synthesis Prediction with Machine Learning

Synthetic route prediction has come a long way since the first rule-based programs appeared in the 1960s. The progress in the following decades was slow, but has accelerated significantly during the last few years. The reason for the faster development during recent years has been both access to more data and methodological development that have made synthesis prediction amenable to machine learning methods like deep learning. In this section we will focus on applying synthesis prediction to medicinal chemistry and on the corresponding machine learning methods used. There have also been several reviews covering this topic recently.[205–207] For readers interested in applying synthesis prediction to process chemistry and the use of quantum mechanical methods, there have also been several recent reviews.[208,209] The topics that will be covered in this section are chemical reaction data, forward synthesis prediction, and synthetic route prediction, which contains both retrosynthetic analysis as well as forward synthesis. The focus will be on key methodological progress and applications and not on commercially available tools for CASP (Computer Aided Synthesis Prediction). There are also several commercial products which have recently been discussed.[206]

### 6.5.1 Chemical Reaction Data

The availability of high-quality chemical reaction data is absolutely key for building a successful machine learning model to predict the synthetic route. Compared to other fields in drug discovery where ML has become popular, like affinity prediction, the amount of chemical reaction data present in the public domain is significantly smaller and of lower quality. Large reaction data sets for synthesis prediction have not become available until recent years and in the public domain only a reaction set based on text mining exists. The so far only open-access reaction data set of reasonable size was first published as part of a PhD student project and consists of chemical reactions extracted through text mining from USPTO patents.[210] The data set has later been updated.[211] Since the dataset is still the only reaction set available in the public domain, it has been part of numerous benchmark studies. While the set has been tremendously useful to develop and benchmark novel algorithms, it suffers from some inherent problems. Since the reactions are derived from patents, there are by definition only reactions that have worked and no negative examples. Also there might be a bias for reactions that are robust and therefore popular in an industrial setting. A recent study showed that the extracted reaction yields are not accurate enough to be used for building machine learning models.[212] There are several commercial sources for chemical reaction data. The Pistachio database[214] comprises 9.5 million reactions and not only contains reactions from the patent office of the United States, but also chemical reactions from the European Patent Office. A thorough analysis of the extracted chemical reaction data from patents with text mining has been published.[213] There exist several databases with manually curated chemical reaction data from the literature, SPRESI,[215] with 3.5 million reactions, Chemical Abstracts, with 127 million reactions,[216] and Reaxys, with 49 million reactions.[217] Of these databases, Reaxys is the database that has by far been the most important for developing novel algorithms for synthesis prediction. Many of the examples of methods discussed in this chapter have been developed and validated with the help of data from Reaxys. A lot of potentially useful data also resides in the ELNs (Electronic Laboratory Notebooks) of large pharmaceutical companies. A study describing extracting data from an ELN in a pharmaceutical company has been published.[218] The extracted reaction data was used to construct large virtual libraries. A large-scale comparison between internal pharmaceutical data, Reaxys, USPTO, and Pistachio has recently been published.[219] In the study, reaction templates were extracted for all of the databases. A reaction template consists of the atoms taking part in the reaction and their surroundings. As can be seen in Figure 6.4, the reaction templates from the different databases show little overlap, beside between the Pistachio and USPTO datasets, which both cover patents.

Large reaction datasets generated consistently through HTE (High Throughput Experimentation) is still under-represented in the public domain; however, recently two datasets have appeared.[220,221] Both datasets were generated in a pharmaceutical setting. There is a general appreciation that with large high-quality reaction data sets in the public domain, the development of novel algorithms will speed up. Recently a consortium has been set up to address the issue of lack of high-quality data.[222]

### 6.5.2 Forward Synthesis Prediction

Forward synthesis prediction covers, for a given set of building blocks, which reactions will occur (chemo-selectivity), how they will react (regio-selectivity), and which stereo isomers will be formed (chiral selectivity). In addition under which conditions

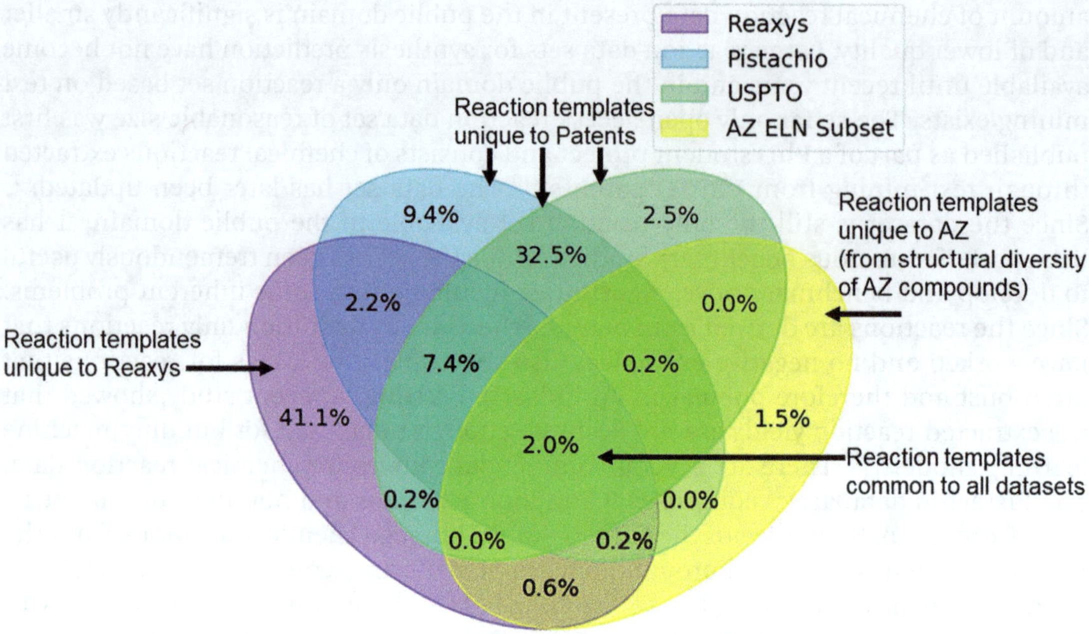


**Figure 6.4** Venn diagram showing the overlap of the patent datasets (USPTO, Pistachio), Reaxys and a subset of AstraZeneca ELN data. Percentages are expressed as being part of the combined dataset. Only 2% of the extracted templates are common between all datasets, and 11.6% between Reaxys and patent data. Reproduced from ref. 219 with permission from the Royal Society of Chemistry.

(*i.e.* solvent, catalyst, temperature base, *etc.*) will the reaction work and what will be the yield. There are two rather different ways to do forward synthesis prediction: either the method is based on a reaction template or it is template-free. The reaction template-based method has often been used in conjunction with synthetic route prediction. The reaction template is derived from the atoms participating in the reaction and its surrounding atoms. Programmatic template generation is a compromise. If too little of the surrounding atomic environment is taken into account, the template becomes very general and has difficulty distinguishing between working and non-working reactions. If too much of the surrounding atomic environment is included, the template becomes too specific and many reactions in a prospective test reaction set are not described by a template[219] and accordingly cannot be predicted. Several template-based methods for forward synthesis prediction have been published.[223,224] It has been observed that ring-forming reactions have been difficult to predict, therefore a more bespoke synthesis prediction tool has been developed to predict the synthesis of rings.[225] Reaction template-based methods for forward synthesis prediction have both pro and cons. An advantage is that the methods can associate a given reaction rule back to the original source, thus giving a synthetic chemist direct access to the relevant literature to understand which reaction conditions were used. A disadvantage is that the reaction template cannot generalize outside its definition, thus novel reactions that are not included in the training set cannot be proposed.

To solve the issue that reaction template-based methods cannot generalize outside their applicability domain, template-free methods have been proposed. These template-free methods are inspired by natural language translation, where the reactants can be seen as one language and the product another language. The first template-free method was based on the SMILES seq2seq approach.[226] However, almost at the same time, the first graph-based method was also published.[227] It was later followed by a graph convolutional method.[228] It has also been shown that the sequence-based molecular transformer architecture provided high accuracy.[229] The developed template-free methods performs very well on the public USPTO reaction data set, however, it is unclear how well they would generalize to a different reaction data set.

Other types of forward reaction prediction endpoints have been described in the literature, like reaction condition prediction,[230] based on a dataset from the Reaxys database. Forward reaction prediction is also key for high throughput experimentation (HTE). HTE has become popular in the last few years because of progress in automation and a couple of datasets have also been deposited in the public domain which can be used for modeling. In a recent study it was shown that active learning can be used to speed up modeling of HTE data.[231]

### 6.5.3 Synthetic Route Prediction

Accurate synthetic route prediction is the holy grail in synthesis prediction. Historically the methods used were rule-based going all the way back to Corey's pioneering work in the 1960s.[232] Manually curated rules were the norm in synthetic route prediction until the last few years. Deriving new reaction rules from literature is still an active research field.[233] However, in 2018 there was a breakthrough paper published on AI-based synthetic route prediction.[234] The paper combines several novel ideas into one system for predicting synthetic routes. Instead of manually extracting reaction rules, the reaction rules were extracted automatically from the Reaxys database and used as reaction templates for building machine learning models. Deep neural networks were trained both in the forward synthesis and backward synthesis (retro-synthesis) directions based on the extracted reaction templates. The trained networks were used together with a Monte Carlo Tree search algorithm to assess and score possible synthetic routes and proposed the highest ranked routes for synthesis, based on a set of building blocks used to halt the algorithm when the desired molecule can be synthesised from a set of building blocks. The authors showed in the article that their novel system outperformed rule-based systems. There also exists an open-source implementation in the public domain (https://github.com/MolecularAI/aizynthfinder) that can be freely used.[235] It should also be pointed out that the results will be highly dependent on which building blocks have been used to halt the algorithm, as the larger the building block set, the more likely it is that the program will find a solution to synthesize the desired molecule.

While significant progress have been made during the last years, it is inherently difficult to quantify the progress. Compared to affinity prediction it is a challenge to set up a fair competition to compare the different synthesis prediction tools that have been developed. Computer aided synthesis prediction tools can be more or less manual and have different purposes. Some are more dedicated for process chemists and require significant manual input, while others are more automatic and more suitable for discovery chemistry.

## 6.6 Conclusions

This chapter has tried to capture the recent fast developments in applying ML/AI to drug design that have occurred during the last few years. While ML/AI has been used in drug design since the 1990s, the current renaissance is remarkable and could hardly have been predicted five years ago. There are several reasons for the resurgence. The relentless pace of faster hardware and cheaper diskspace have definitely contributed to make algorithms like deep learning feasible and affordable. The flexibility of deep learning architectures makes it possible to tailor-make an architecture for a bespoke modeling challenge. Several different architectures have been developed that are suitable for *de novo* molecular design. However, while the innovations have been very fast, there are not many prospective success stories published in the literature so far applying ML/AI to drug design. This can, at least to some extent, be explained by the publication lag for commercially interesting projects until the relevant substance patents have been published, 18 months after the filing of the patent. It is noteworthy that the venture capital community have been investing heavily in start-up companies applying AI to drug design. Compared to historical molecular modeling in the pharmaceutical industry, ML/AI is much more open minded. The developed code is usually open source and in many cases the algorithm is validated with data in the public domain. Thus the barrier to entrance to developing novel algorithms is low. While the low barrier facilitates innovation, the shear number of novel algorithms makes benchmarking very difficult. For many tasks the developed algorithms perform very well for the retrospective benchmarks; however, performing well on known benchmarks doesn't always translate into superior performance in prospective studies. For instance, for affinity prediction the progress in the prospective SAMPL challenges has not been very impressive.[236] In other areas like synthesis prediction, it is a challenge to define a fair comparison between the developed tools, since many of them have different objectives.

While, as described in this chapter, the progress so far has been impressive, a key question is will the innovation continue at the current pace? The authors believe that progress will continue at a rapid pace, driven by automation and generation of large machine learning friendly datasets. An example is high throughput experimentation, that will produce chemical reaction data of high and consistent quality.[237] Also DNA-encoded library screening will generate large datasets.[238] Compound collections will in the future be profiled in information-rich assays like cell-painting[239] and transcriptomics[240] that can be used to create biological signatures for molecules. Precompetitive collaborations based on privacy preserving federated learning will also boost the data volumes used for model building.[241] In addition the progress in automation is fast and systems like the Chemputer for automatic synthesis of molecules will be much more common in the future.[242] The progress in automation also highlights the need to progress from building machine learning models to AI for making decisions under uncertainty.

## 6.7 Hints and Tips

Synthesis prediction:

1. Proper data curation is key for successful modeling of reactions.
2. Whether or not a retrosynthetic route can be identified will be dependent on the selected list of building blocks used.
3. Template-free methods are needed for extrapolation to novel reactions.

*De novo* design:

1. For SMILES-based generative models, randomized SMILES is a good way for data augmentation.
2. The diversity and novelty of the sampling set for generative model is a very important aspect. We want to generate novel and diverse structures.
3. Mode collapse is a common problem during reinforcement learning; diversity filters could be used to overcome the problem to some extent.

ADMET modeling:

1. The application of deep learning methods makes descriptor selection/engineering in ADMET modeling no longer needed.
2. For a lot of ADMET modeling work, choosing a proper dataset and improving data quality is more important than choosing the algorithm.
3. Predicting *in vivo* properties of drugs is still a challenging task.

*In silico* protein target deconvolution:

1. Publicly available target prediction tools are trained on chemogenomic repositories linking compound–target pairs.
2. A wide variety of algorithms have been applied and more complex approaches, such as multitask learning, are being applied.
3. The data-driven approach is influenced by training biases in chemical/biological space, so performance ranges widely between protein targets.

## Key References

P. Schneider, W. P. Walters, and A. T. Plowright, *et al.*, Rethinking drug design in the artificial intelligence era, *Nat. Rev. Drug Discovery*, 2020, **19**, 353–364.

M. Segler, M. Preuss, and M. Waller, Planning chemical syntheses with deep neural networks and symbolic AI, *Nature*, 2018, **555**, 604–610.

M. H. S. Segler, T. Kogej, C. Tyrchan, and M. P. Waller, *ACS Cent. Sci.*, 2018, **4**(1), 120–131.

## References


1. J. Howard, The business impact of deep learning, in *Proceedings of the 19th ACM SIGKDD International Conference on Knowledge Discovery and Data Mining, 2013*, 2013, pp. 1135–1135.
2. D. CeArley, B. Burke, S. Searle and M. J. Walker, Top 10 strategic technology trends for 2018, *The Top*, 2016, p. 10.
3. W. S. McCulloch and W. Pitts, A logical calculus of the ideas immanent in nervous activity, *Bull. Math. Biophys.*, 1943, **5**, 115–133.
4. H. Chen, O. Engkvist, Y. Wang, M. Olivecrona and T. Blaschke, The rise of deep learning in drug discovery, *Drug Discovery Today*, 2018, **23**, 1241–1250.
5. L. L. G. Ferreira and A. D. Andricopulo, ADMET modeling approaches in drug discovery, *Drug Discovery Today*, 2019, **24**, 1157–1165.
6. H. Chen, O. Engkvist, Y. Wang, M. Olivecrona and T. Blaschke, The rise of deep learning in drug discovery, *Drug Discovery Today*, 2018, **23**, 1241–1250.
7. H. J. Bohm, The computer program LUDI: a new method for the de novo design of enzyme inhibitors, *J. Comput.-Aided Mol. Des.*, 1992, **6**, 61–78.
8. V. J. Gillet, W. Newell, P. Mata, G. Myatt, S. Sike, Z. Zsoldos and A. P. Johnson, SPROUT: recent developments in the de novo design of molecules, *J. Chem. Inf. Comput. Sci.*, 1994, **34**, 207–217.
9. G. Schneider, T. Geppert, M. Hartenfeller, F. Reisen, A. Klenner, M. Reutlinger, V. Hahnke, J. A. Hiss, H. Zettl, S. Keppner, B. Spankuch and P. Schneider, Reaction-driven de novo design, synthesis and testing of potential type II kinase inhibitors, *Future Med. Chem.*, 2011, **3**, 415–424.
10. J. Besnard, G. F. Ruda, V. Setola, K. Abecassis, R. M. Rodriguiz, X. P. Huang, S. Norval, M. F. Sassano, A. I. Shin, L. A. Webster, F. R. Simeons, L. Stojanovski, A. Prat, N. G. Seidah, D. B. Constam, G. R. Bickerton, K. D. Read, W. C. Wetsel, I. H. Gilbert, B. L. Roth and A. L. Hopkins, Automated design of ligands to polypharmacological profiles, *Nature*, 2012, **492**, 215–220.
11. G. Schneider, M. L. Lee, M. Stahl and P. Schneider, De novo design of molecular architectures by evolutionary assembly of drug-derived building blocks, *J. Comput.-Aided Mol. Des.*, 2000, **14**, 487–494.
12. T. Miyao, H. Kaneko and K. Funatsu, Inverse QSPR/QSAR Analysis for Chemical Structure Generation (from y to x), *J. Chem. Inf. Model.*, 2016, **56**, 286–299.
13. C. J. Churchwell, M. D. Rintoul, S. Martin, D. P. Visco Jr., A. Kotu, R. S. Larson, L. O. Sillerud, D. C. Brown and J. L. Faulon, The signature molecular descriptor. 3. Inverse-quantitative structure-activity relationship of ICAM-1 inhibitory peptides, *J. Mol. Graph. Model.*, 2004, **22**, 263–273.
14. D. Weininger, SMILES, a chemical language and information system. 1. Introduction to methodology and encoding rules, *J. Chem. Inf. Comput. Sci.*, 1988, **28**, 31–36.
15. T. Engel, Representation of chemical compounds, *Chemoinformatics: A Textbook*, 2003, pp. 15–168.
16. M. H. S. Segler, T. Kogej, C. Tyrchan and M. P. Waller, Generating Focused Molecule Libraries for Drug Discovery with Recurrent Neural Networks, *ACS Cent. Sci.*, 2018, **4**, 120–131.
17. M. Olivecrona, T. Blaschke, O. Engkvist and H. Chen, Molecular de-novo design through deep reinforcement learning, *J. Cheminf.*, 2017, **9**, 48.
18. O. Arús-Pous, S. V. Johansson, O. Prykhodko, E. J. Bjerrum, C. Tyrchan, J.-L. Reymond, H. Chen and O. Engkvist, Randomized SMILES strings improve the quality of molecular generative models, *J. Cheminf.*, 2019, **11**, 71.
19. L. C. Blum and J. L. Reymond, 970 million druglike small molecules for virtual screening in the chemical universe database GDB-13, *J. Am. Chem. Soc.*, 2009, **131**, 8732–8733.
20. R. Gomez-Bombarelli, J. N. Wei, D. Duvenaud, J. M. Hernandez-Lobato, B. Sanchez-Lengeling, D. Sheberla, J. Aguilera-Iparraguirre, T. D. Hirzel, R. P. Adams and A. Aspuru-Guzik, Automatic Chemical Design Using a Data-Driven Continuous Representation of Molecules, *ACS Cent. Sci.*, 2018, **4**, 268–276.
21. T. Blaschke, M. Olivecrona, O. Engkvist, J. Bajorath and H. Chen, Application of Generative Autoencoder in De Novo Molecular Design, *Mol. Inf.*, 2018, **37**, 1700123.
22. E. J. Bjerrum and B. Sattarov, Improving Chemical Autoencoder Latent Space and Molecular De Novo Generation Diversity with Heteroencoders, *Biomolecules*, 2018, **8**, 1–17.
23. I. J. Goodfellow, J. Pouget-Abadie, M. Mirza, B. Xu, D. Warde-Farley, S. Ozair, A. Courville and Y. Bengio, Generative Adversarial Networks, *arXiv preprint* 2014, arXiv, 1406.2661.
24. G. L. Guimaraes, B. Sanchez-Lengeling, C. Outeiral, P. L. C. Farias and A. Aspuru-Guzik, Objective-Reinforced Generative Adversarial Networks (ORGAN) for Sequence Generation Models, *arXiv preprint* 2017, arXiv, 1705.10843.

25. B. Sanchez-Lengeling, C. Outeiral, G. L. Guimaraes and A. Aspuru-Guzik, Optimizing distributions over molecular space. An Objective-Reinforced Generative Adversarial Network for Inverse-design Chemistry (ORGANIC), *ChemRxiv preprint* 2017, ChemRxiv, 5309668.v3.
26. E. Putin, A. Asadulaev, Y. Ivanenkov, V. Aladinskiy, B. Sanchez-Lengeling, A. Aspuru-Guzik and A. Zhavoronkov, Reinforced Adversarial Neural Computer for de Novo Molecular Design, *J. Chem. Inf. Model.*, 2018, **58**, 1194–1204.
27. E. Putin, A. Asadulaev, Q. Vanhaelen, Y. Ivanenkov, A. V. Aladinskaya, A. Aliper and A. Zhavoronkov, Adversarial Threshold Neural Computer for Molecular de Novo Design, *Mol. Pharmaceutics*, 2018, **15**, 4386–4397.
28. O. Prykhodko, S. V. Johansson, P.-C. Kotsias, J. Arús-Pous, E. J. Bjerrum, O. Engkvist and H. Chen, A de novo molecular generation method using latent vector based generative adversarial network, *J. Cheminf.*, 2019, **11**, 74.
29. Y. Li, O. Vinyals, C. Dyer, R. Pascanu and P. Battaglia, Learning Deep Generative Models of Graphs, *arXiv preprint* 2018, arXiv, 1803.03324.
30. Y. Li, L. Zhang and Z. Liu, Multiobjective de novo drug design with conditional graph generative model, *J. Cheminf.*, 2018, **10**, 33.
31. J. You, B. Liu, R. Ying, V. Pande and J. Leskovec, Graph Convolutional Policy Network for Goal-Directed Molecular Graph Generation, *arXiv preprint* 2019, arXiv, 1806.02473.
32. W. Jin, R. Barzilay and T. Jaakkola, Junction Tree Variational Autoencoder for Molecular Graph Generation, *arXiv preprint* 2019, arXiv, 1802.04364.
33. A. Zhavoronkov, Y. A. Ivanenkov, A. Aliper, M. S. Veselov, V. A. Aladinskiy, A. V. Aladinskaya, V. A. Terentiev, D. A. Polykovskiy, M. D. Kuznetsov, A. Asadulaev, Y. Volkov, A. Zholus, R. R. Shayakhmetov, A. Zhebrak, L. I. Minaeva, B. A. Zagribelnyy, L. H. Lee, R. Soll, D. Madge, L. Xing, T. Guo and A. Aspuru-Guzik, Deep learning enables rapid identification of potent DDR1 kinase inhibitors, *Nat. Biotechnol.*, 2019, **37**, 1038–1040.
34. https://github.com/MolecularAI/Reinvent, 23 November 2020.
35. https://github.com/pcko1/Deep-Drug-Coder, 23 November 2020.
36. https://github.com/molecularsets/moses, 23 November 2020.
37. P. Barton and R. J. Riley, A new paradigm for navigating compound property related drug attrition, *Drug Discovery Today*, 2016, **21**, 72–81.
38. C. Hansch, P. P. Maloney, T. Fujita and R. M. Muir, Correlation of Biological Activity of Phenoxyacetic Acids with Hammett Substituent Constants and Partition Coefficients, *Nature*, 1962, **194**, 178–180.
39. V. G. Maltarollo, J. C. Gertrudes, P. R. Oliveira and K. M. Honorio, Applying machine learning techniques for ADME-Tox prediction: a review, *Expert Opin. Drug Metab. Toxicol.*, 2015, **11**, 259–271.
40. I. I. Baskin, D. Winkler and I. V. Tetko, A renaissance of neural networks in drug discovery, *Expert Opin. Drug Discovery*, 2016, **11**, 785–795.
41. N. Fleming, How artificial intelligence is changing drug discovery, *Nature*, 2018, **557**, S55–S57.
42. Y. C. Lo, S. E. Rensi, W. Torng and R. B. Altman, Machine learning in chemoinformatics and drug discovery, *Drug Discovery Today*, 2018, **23**, 1538–1546.
43. M. Sun, S. Zhao, C. Gilvary, O. Elemento, J. Zhou and F. Wang, Graph convolutional networks for computational drug development and discovery, *Briefings Bioinf.*, 2020, **21**, 919–935.
44. S. Sosnin, M. Vashurina, M. Withnall, P. Karpov, M. Fedorov and I. V. Tetko, A Survey of Multitask Learning Methods in Chemoinformatics, *Mol. Inf.*, 2019, **38**, e1800108.
45. J. Vamathevan, D. Clark, P. Czodrowski, I. Dunham, E. Ferran, G. Lee, B. Li, A. Madabhushi, P. Shah, M. Spitzer and S. Zhao, Applications of machine learning in drug discovery and development, *Nat. Rev. Drug Discovery*, 2019, **18**, 463–477.
46. B. Bhhatarai, W. P. Walters, C. Hop, G. Lanza and S. Ekins, Opportunities and challenges using artificial intelligence in ADME/Tox, *Nat. Mater.*, 2019, **18**, 418–422.
47. J. Panteleev, H. Gao and L. Jia, Recent applications of machine learning in medicinal chemistry, *Bioorg. Med. Chem. Lett.*, 2018, **28**, 2807–2815.
48. C. M. Chagas, S. Moss and L. Alisaraie, Drug metabolites and their effects on the development of adverse reactions: Revisiting Lipinski's Rule of Five, *Int. J. Pharm.*, 2018, **549**, 133–149.
49. S. Prasad and B. R. Brooks, A deep learning approach for the blind logP prediction in SAMPL6 challenge, *J. Comput.-Aided Mol. Des.*, 2020, **34**, 535–542.
50. K. Wu, Z. Zhao, R. Wang and G. W. Wei, TopP-S: Persistent homology-based multitask deep neural networks for simultaneous predictions of partition coefficient and aqueous solubility, *J. Comput. Chem.*, 2018, **39**, 1444–1454.

51. Q. Cui, S. Lu, B. Ni, X. Zeng, Y. Tan, Y. D. Chen and H. Zhao, Improved Prediction of Aqueous Solubility of Novel Compounds by Going Deeper With Deep Learning, *Front. Oncol.*, 2020, **10**, 121.
52. A. Lusci, G. Pollastri and P. Baldi, Deep architectures and deep learning in chemoinformatics: the prediction of aqueous solubility for drug-like molecules, *J. Chem. Inf. Model.*, 2013, **53**, 1563–1575.
53. P. Hop, B. Allgood and J. Yu, Geometric Deep Learning Autonomously Learns Chemical Features That Outperform Those Engineered by Domain Experts, *Mol. Pharm.*, 2018, **15**, 4371–4377.
54. C. W. Coley, R. Barzilay, W. H. Green, T. S. Jaakkola and K. F. Jensen, Convolutional Embedding of Attributed Molecular Graphs for Physical Property Prediction, *J. Chem. Inf. Model.*, 2017, **57**, 1757–1772.
55. K. Liu, X. Sun, L. Jia, J. Ma, H. Xing, J. Wu, H. Gao, Y. Sun, F. Boulnois and J. Fan, Chemi-Net: A Molecular Graph Convolutional Network for Accurate Drug Property Prediction, *Int. J. Mol. Sci.*, 2019, **20**, 3389.
56. C. Shang, Q. Liu, K.-S. Chen, J. Sun, J. Lu, J. Yi and J. Bi, Edge Attention-based MultiRelational Graph Convolutional Networks, *arXiv preprint* 2018, arXiv, 1802.04944.
57. X. Wang, Z. Li, M. Jiang, S. Wang, S. Zhang and Z. Wei, Molecule Property Prediction Based on Spatial Graph Embedding, *J. Chem. Inf. Model.*, 2019, **59**, 3817–3828.
58. X. Li, X. Yan, Q. Gu, H. Zhou, D. Wu and J. Xu, DeepChemStable: Chemical Stability Prediction with an Attention-Based Graph Convolution Network, *J. Chem. Inf. Model.*, 2019, **59**, 1044–1049.
59. S. Ryu, J. Lim, S. H. Hong and W. Y. Kim, Deeply learning molecular structure-property relationships using attention- and gate-augmented graph convolutional network, *arXiv preprint* 2018, arXiv, 1805.10988.
60. E. N. Feinberg, E. Joshi, V. S. Pande and A. C. Cheng, Improvement in ADMET Prediction with Multitask Deep Featurization, *J. Med. Chem.*, 2020, **63**, 8835–8848.
61. F. Montanari, L. Kuhnke, A. Ter Laak and D. A. Clevert, Modeling Physico-Chemical ADMET Endpoints with Multitask Graph Convolutional Networks, *Molecules*, 2019, **25**, 44.
62. Z. Wu, S. Pan, F. Chen, G. Long, C. Zhang and P. S. Yu, A Comprehensive Survey on Graph Neural Networks, *IEEE Trans. Neural Netw. Learn. Syst.*, 2020, **32**, 4–24.
63. J. Ma, R. P. Sheridan, A. Liaw, G. E. Dahl and V. Svetnik, Deep neural nets as a method for quantitative structure-activity relationships, *J. Chem. Inf. Model.*, 2015, **55**, 263–274.
64. M. Shin, D. Jang, H. Nam, K. H. Lee and D. Lee, Predicting the Absorption Potential of Chemical Compounds Through a Deep Learning Approach, *IEEE/ACM Trans. Comput. Biol. Bioinf.*, 2018, **15**, 432–440.
65. A. Renn, B.-H. Su, H. Liu, J. Sun and Y. J. Tseng, Advances in the prediction of mouse liver microsomal studies: From machine learning to deep learning, *Comput. Mol. Sci.*, 2020, e1479.
66. J. Wenzel, H. Matter and F. Schmidt, Predictive Multitask Deep Neural Network Models for ADME-Tox Properties: Learning from Large Data Sets, *J. Chem. Inf. Model.*, 2019, **59**, 1253–1268.
67. S. Schneckener, S. Grimbs, J. Hey, S. Menz, M. Osmers, S. Schaper, A. Hillisch and A. H. Goller, Prediction of Oral Bioavailability in Rats: Transferring Insights from in Vitro Correlations to (Deep) Machine Learning Models Using in Silico Model Outputs and Chemical Structure Parameters, *J. Chem. Inf. Model.*, 2019, **59**, 4893–4905.
68. Z. Wu, T. Lei, C. Shen, Z. Wang, D. Cao and T. Hou, ADMET Evaluation in Drug Discovery. 19. Reliable Prediction of Human Cytochrome P450 Inhibition Using Artificial Intelligence Approaches, *J. Chem. Inf. Model.*, 2019, **59**, 4587–4601.
69. X. Li, Y. Xu, L. Lai and J. Pei, Prediction of Human Cytochrome P450 Inhibition Using a Multitask Deep Autoencoder Neural Network, *Mol. Pharmaceutics*, 2018, **15**, 4336–4345.
70. R. Liu, M. Madore, K. P. Glover, M. G. Feasel and A. Wallqvist, Assessing Deep and Shallow Learning Methods for Quantitative Prediction of Acute Chemical Toxicity, *Toxicol. Sci.*, 2018, **164**, 512–526.
71. Z. Ye, Y. Yang, X. Li, D. Cao and D. Ouyang, An Integrated Transfer Learning and Multitask Learning Approach for Pharmacokinetic Parameter Prediction, *Mol. Pharmaceutics*, 2019, **16**, 533–541.
72. Y. Peng, Z. Zhang, Q. Jiang, J. Guan and S. Zhou, TOP: A Deep Mixture Representation Learning Method for Boosting Molecular Toxicity Prediction, *Methods*, 2020, **179**, 55–64.
73. D. Jimenez-Carretero, V. Abrishami, L. Fernandez-de-Manuel, I. Palacios, A. Quilez-Alvarez, A. Diez-Sanchez, M. A. Del Pozo and M. C. Montoya, Tox_(R)CNN: Deep learning-based nuclei profiling tool for drug toxicity screening, *PLoS Comput. Biol.*, 2018, **14**, e1006238.
74. A. O. Basile, A. Yahi and N. P. Tatonetti, Artificial Intelligence for Drug Toxicity and Safety, *Trends Pharmacol. Sci.*, 2019, **40**, 624–635.
75. W. Tang, J. Chen, Z. Wang, H. Xie and H. Hong, Deep learning for predicting toxicity of chemicals: a mini review, *J. Environ. Sci. Health, Part C: Environ. Carcinog. Ecotoxicol. Rev.*, 2018, **36**, 252–271.

76. A. H. Vo, T. R. Van Vleet, R. R. Gupta, M. J. Liguori and M. S. Rao, An Overview of Machine Learning and Big Data for Drug Toxicity Evaluation, *Chem. Res. Toxicol.*, 2020, **33**, 20–37.
77. A. Mayr, G. Klambauer, T. Unterthiner and S. Hochreite, DeepTox: Toxicity Prediction using Deep Learning, *Front. Environ. Sci.*, 2016, **3**, 1–15.
78. H. Altae-Tran, B. Ramsundar, A. S. Pappu and V. Pande, Low Data Drug Discovery with One-Shot Learning, *ACS Cent. Sci.*, 2017, **3**, 283–293.
79. Y. Matsuzaka and Y. Uesawa, Prediction Model with High-Performance Constitutive Androstane Receptor (CAR) Using DeepSnap-Deep Learning Approach from the Tox21 10K Compound Library, *Int. J. Mol. Sci.*, 2019, **20**, 4855.
80. Y. Xu, J. Pei and L. Lai, Deep Learning Based Regression and Multiclass Models for Acute Oral Toxicity Prediction with Automatic Chemical Feature Extraction, *J. Chem. Inf. Model.*, 2017, **57**, 2672–2685.
81. X. Zhen, J. Chen, Z. Zhong, B. Hrycushko, L. Zhou, S. Jiang, K. Albuquerque and X. Gu, Deep convolutional neural network with transfer learning for rectum toxicity prediction in cervical cancer radiotherapy: a feasibility study, *Phys. Med. Biol.*, 2017, **62**, 8246–8263.
82. K. Fraser, D. M. Bruckner and J. S. Dordick, Advancing Predictive Hepatotoxicity at the Intersection of Experimental, in Silico, and Artificial Intelligence Technologies, *Chem. Res. Toxicol.*, 2018, **31**, 412–430.
83. B. Ibragimov, D. Toesca, D. Chang, Y. Yuan, A. Koong and L. Xing, Development of deep neural network for individualized hepatobiliary toxicity prediction after liver SBRT, *Med. Phys.*, 2018, **45**, 4763–4774.
84. B. Ibragimov, D. A. S. Toesca, D. T. Chang, Y. Yuan, A. C. Koong, L. Xing and I. R. Vogelius, Deep learning for identification of critical regions associated with toxicities after liver stereotactic body radiation therapy, *Med. Phys.*, 2020, **47**, 3721–3731.
85. B. Ibragimov, D. A. S. Toesca, Y. Yuan, A. C. Koong, D. T. Chang and L. Xing, Neural Networks for Deep Radiotherapy Dose Analysis and Prediction of Liver SBRT Outcomes, *IEEE J. Biomed. Health Inf.*, 2019, **23**, 1821–1833.
86. Y. Matsuzaka, T. Hosaka, A. Ogaito, K. Yoshinari and Y. Uesawa, Prediction Model of Aryl Hydrocarbon Receptor Activation by a Novel QSAR Approach, DeepSnap-Deep Learning, *Molecules*, 2020, **25**, 1317.
87. Y. Wang, L. Huang, S. Jiang, Y. Wang, J. Zou, H. Fu and S. Yang, Capsule Networks Showed Excellent Performance in the Classification of hERG Blockers/Nonblockers, *Front. Pharmacol.*, 2019, **10**, 1631.
88. C. Cai, P. Guo, Y. Zhou, J. Zhou, Q. Wang, F. Zhang, J. Fang and F. Cheng, Deep Learning-Based Prediction of Drug-Induced Cardiotoxicity, *J. Chem. Inf. Model.*, 2019, **59**, 1073–1084.
89. G. Idakwo, S. Thangapandian, J. t. Luttrell, Z. Zhou, C. Zhang and P. Gong, Deep Learning-Based Structure-Activity Relationship Modeling for MultiCategory Toxicity Classification: A Case Study of 10K Tox21 Chemicals With High-Throughput Cell-Based Androgen Receptor Bioassay Data, *Front. Physiol.*, 2019, **10**, 1044.
90. Y. Matsuzaka and Y. Uesawa, DeepSnap-Deep Learning Approach Predicts Progesterone Receptor Antagonist Activity With High Performance, *Front. Bioeng. Biotechnol.*, 2019, **7**, 485.
91. G. Lee, C. Park and J. Ahn, Novel deep learning model for more accurate prediction of drug-drug interaction effects, *BMC Bioinf.*, 2019, **20**, 415.
92. Y. Deng, X. Xu, Y. Qiu, J. Xia, W. Zhang and S. Liu, A multimodal deep learning framework for predicting drug-drug interaction events, *Bioinformatics*, 2020, **36**, 4316–4322.
93. T. Zhang, J. Leng and Y. Liu, Deep learning for drug-drug interaction extraction from the literature: a review, *Briefings Bioinf.*, 2019, **21**, 1609–1627.
94. S. Kwon and S. Yoon, End-to-End Representation Learning for Chemical-Chemical Interaction Prediction, *IEEE/ACM Trans. Comput. Biol. Bioinf.*, 2019, **16**, 1436–1447.
95. Y. Matsuzaka and Y. Uesawa, Optimization of a Deep-Learning Method Based on the Classification of Images Generated by Parameterized Deep Snap a Novel Molecular-Image-Input Technique for Quantitative Structure-Activity Relationship (QSAR) Analysis, *Front. Bioeng. Biotechnol.*, 2019, **7**, 65.
96. M. Fernandez, F. Ban, G. Woo, M. Hsing, T. Yamazaki, E. LeBlanc, P. S. Rennie, W. J. Welch and A. Cherkasov, Toxic Colors: The Use of Deep Learning for Predicting Toxicity of Compounds Merely from Their Graphic Images, *J. Chem. Inf. Model.*, 2018, **58**, 1533–1543.
97. T. Shi, Y. Yang, S. Huang, L. Chen, Z. Kuang, Y. Heng and H. Mei, Molecular image-based convolutional neural network for the prediction of ADMET properties, *Chemom. Intell. Lab. Syst.*, 2019, **194**, 103853.
98. H. Wang, R. Liu, P. Schyman and A. Wallqvist, Deep Neural Network Models for Predicting Chemically Induced Liver Toxicity Endpoints From Transcriptomic Responses, *Front. Pharmacol.*, 2019, **10**, 42.

99. Q. Yuan, Z. Wei, X. Guan, M. Jiang, S. Wang, S. Zhang and Z. Li, Toxicity Prediction Method Based on MultiChannel Convolutional Neural Network, *Molecules*, 2019, **24**, 3383.
100. K. Men, H. Geng, H. Zhong, Y. Fan, A. Lin and Y. Xiao, A Deep Learning Model for Predicting Xerostomia Due to Radiation Therapy for Head and Neck Squamous Cell Carcinoma in the RTOG 0522 Clinical Trial, *Int. J. Radiat. Oncol., Biol., Phys.*, 2019, **105**, 440–447.
101. H. van de Waterbeemd, Improving compound quality through in vitro and in silico physicochemical profiling, *Chem. Biodiversity*, 2009, **6**, 1760–1766.
102. J. Jiang, R. Wang, M. Wang, K. Gao, D. D. Nguyen and G. W. Wei, Boosting Tree-Assisted Multitask Deep Learning for Small Scientific Datasets, *J. Chem. Inf. Model.*, 2020, **60**, 1235–1244.
103. Y. Zhou, S. Cahya, S. A. Combs, C. A. Nicolaou, J. Wang, P. V. Desai and J. Shen, Exploring Tunable Hyperparameters for Deep Neural Networks with Industrial ADME Data Sets, *J. Chem. Inf. Model.*, 2019, **59**, 1005–1016.
104. Y. Xu, H. Yao and K. Lin, An overview of neural networks for drug discovery and the inputs used, *Expert Opin. Drug Discovery*, 2018, **13**, 1091–1102.
105. S. Turk, B. Merget, F. Rippmann and S. Fulle, Coupling Matched Molecular Pairs with Machine Learning for Virtual Compound Optimization, *J. Chem. Inf. Model.*, 2017, **57**, 3079–3085.
106. L. Fu, L. Liu, Z. J. Yang, P. Li, J. J. Ding, Y. H. Yun, A. P. Lu, T. J. Hou and D. S. Cao, Systematic Modeling of logD7.4 Based on Ensemble Machine Learning, Group Contribution, and Matched Molecular Pair Analysis, *J. Chem. Inf. Model.*, 2020, **60**, 63–76.
107. G. Moroy, V. Y. Martiny, P. Vayer, B. O. Villoutreix and M. A. Miteva, Toward in silico structure-based ADMET prediction in drug discovery, *Drug Discovery Today*, 2012, **17**, 44–55.
108. G. E. Dahl, N. Jaitly and R. Salakhutdinov, Multitask Neural Networks for QSAR Predictions, *arXiv preprint* 2014, arXiv, 1406.1231.
109. B. Ramsundar, B. Liu, Z. Wu, A. Verras, M. Tudor, R. P. Sheridan and V. Pande, Is Multitask Deep Learning Practical for Pharma?, *J. Chem. Inf. Model.*, 2017, **57**, 2068–2076.
110. K. R. Chi, Drug developers delve into the cell's trash-disposal machinery, *Nat. Rev. Drug Discovery*, 2016, **15**, 295–297.
111. N. A. Meanwell, Improving drug candidates by design: a focus on physicochemical properties as a means of improving compound disposition and safety, *Chem. Res. Toxicol.*, 2011, **24**, 1420–1456.
112. F. Sams-Dodd, Is poor research the cause of the declining productivity of the pharmaceutical industry? An industry in need of a paradigm shift, *Drug Discovery Today*, 2013, **18**, 211–217.
113. A. Koutsoukas, R. Lowe, Y. Kalantarmotamedi, H. Y. Mussa, W. Klaffke, J. B. Mitchell, R. C. Glen and A. Bender, In silico target predictions: defining a benchmarking data set and comparison of performance of the multiclass Naïve Bayes and Parzen-Rosenblatt window, *J. Chem. Inf. Model.*, 2013, **53**, 1957–1966.
114. A. Koutsoukas, B. Simms, J. Kirchmair, P. J. Bond, A. V. Whitmore, S. Zimmer, M. P. Young, J. L. Jenkins, M. Glick, R. C. Glen and A. Bender, From in silico target prediction to multitarget drug design: current databases, methods and applications, *J. Proteomics*, 2011, **74**, 2554–2574.
115. E. Gregori-Puigjané and J. Mestres, A ligand-based approach to mining the chemogenomic space of drugs, *Comb. Chem. High Throughput Screening*, 2008, **11**, 669–676.
116. L. Jacob, B. Hoffmann, V. Stoven and J. P. Vert, Virtual screening of GPCRs: an in silico chemogenomics approach, *BMC Bioinf.*, 2008, **9**, 363.
117. J. L. Jenkins, A. Bender and J. W. Davies, In silico target fishing: Predicting biological targets from chemical structure, *Drug Discovery Today: Technol.*, 2007, **3**, 413–421.
118. A. Lagunin, A. Stepanchikova, D. Filimonov and V. Poroikov, PASS: prediction of activity spectra for biologically active substances, *Bioinformatics*, 2000, **16**, 747–748.
119. J. H. Nettles, J. L. Jenkins, A. Bender, Z. Deng, J. W. Davies and M. Glick, Bridging chemical and biological space: "target fishing" using 2D and 3D molecular descriptors, *J. Med. Chem.*, 2006, **49**, 6802–6810.
120. D. Rognan, Structure-based approaches to target fishing and ligand profiling, *Mol. Inf.*, 2010, **29**, 176–187.
121. X. Chen, C. Y. Ung and Y. Chen, Can an in silico drug-target search method be used to probe potential mechanisms of medicinal plant ingredients?, *Nat. Prod. Rep.*, 2003, **20**, 432–444.
122. Z. Gao, H. Li, H. Zhang, X. Liu, L. Kang, X. Luo, W. Zhu, K. Chen, X. Wang and H. Jiang, PDTD: a web-accessible protein database for drug target identification, *BMC Bioinf.*, 2008, **9**, 104.
123. A. Bender, D. Mikhailov, M. Glick, J. Scheiber, J. W. Davies, S. Cleaver, S. Marshall, J. A. Tallarico, E. Harrington, I. Cornella-Taracido and J. L. Jenkins, Use of ligand based models for protein domains to

predict novel molecular targets and applications to triage affinity chromatography data, *J. Proteome Res.*, 2009, **8**, 2575–2585.
124. A. E. Cleves and A. N. Jain, Robust ligand-based modeling of the biological targets of known drugs, *J. Med. Chem.*, 2006, **49**, 2921–2938.
125. F. Nigsch, A. Bender, J. L. Jenkins and J. B. Mitchell, Ligand-target prediction using Winnow and naive Bayesian algorithms and the implications of overall performance statistics, *J. Chem. Inf. Model.*, 2008, **48**, 2313–2325.
126. L. Wang, C. Ma, P. Wipf, H. Liu, W. Su and X. Q. Xie, TargetHunter: an in silico target identification tool for predicting therapeutic potential of small organic molecules based on chemogenomic database, *AAPS J.*, 2013, **15**, 395–406.
127. G. Drakakis, K. A. Wafford, S. C. Brewerton, M. J. Bodkin, D. A. Evans and A. Bender, Polypharmacological In Silico Bioactivity Profiling and Experimental Validation Uncovers Sedative-Hypnotic Effects of Approved and Experimental Drugs in Rat, *ACS Chem. Biol.*, 2017.
128. M. Wen, Z. Zhang, S. Niu, H. Sha, R. Yang, Y. Yun and H. Lu, Deep-Learning-Based Drug-Target Interaction Prediction, *J. Proteome Res.*, 2017, **16**, 1401–1409.
129. A. Lavecchia and C. Cerchia, In silico methods to address polypharmacology: current status, applications and future perspectives, *Drug Discovery Today*, 2016, **21**, 288–298.
130. A. Varnek and I. Baskin, Machine learning methods for property prediction in chemoinformatics: Quo Vadis?, *J. Chem. Inf. Model.*, 2012, **52**, 1413–1437.
131. A. Kümmel, D. Gabriel, C. N. Parker and A. Bender, Computational methods to support high-content screening: from compound selection and data analysis to postulating target hypotheses, *Expert Opin. Drug Discovery*, 2009, **4**, 5–13.
132. R. Guha, K. Gilbert, G. Fox, M. Pierce, D. Wild and H. Yuan, Advances in cheminformatics methodologies and infrastructure to support the data mining of large, heterogeneous chemical datasets, *Curr. Comput.-Aided Drug Des.*, 2010, **6**, 50–67.
133. S. Rees, P. Gribbon, K. Birmingham, W. P. Janzen and G. Pairaudeau, Towards a hit for every target, *Nat. Rev. Drug Discovery*, 2016, **15**, 1–2.
134. M. Schenone, V. Dančík, B. K. Wagner and P. A. Clemons, Target identification and mechanism of action in chemical biology and drug discovery, *Nat. Chem. Biol.*, 2013, **9**, 232–240.
135. R. Macarron, M. N. Banks, D. Bojanic, D. J. Burns, D. A. Cirovic, T. Garyantes, D. V. Green, R. P. Hertzberg, W. P. Janzen, J. W. Paslay, U. Schopfer and G. S. Sittampalam, Impact of high-throughput screening in biomedical research, *Nat. Rev. Drug Discovery*, 2011, **10**, 188–195.
136. A. Gaulton, L. J. Bellis, A. P. Bento, J. Chambers, M. Davies, A. Hersey, Y. Light, S. McGlinchey, D. Michalovich, B. Al-Lazikani and J. P. Overington, ChEMBL: a large-scale bioactivity database for drug discovery, *Nucleic Acids Res.*, 2012, **40**, D1100–D1107.
137. D. S. Wishart, C. Knox, A. C. Guo, S. Shrivastava, M. Hassanali, P. Stothard, Z. Chang and J. Woolsey, DrugBank: a comprehensive resource for in silico drug discovery and exploration, *Nucleic Acids Res.*, 2006, **34**, D668–D672.
138. Y. Wang, J. Xiao, T. O. Suzek, J. Zhang, J. Wang and S. H. Bryant, PubChem: a public information system for analyzing bioactivities of small molecules, *Nucleic Acids Res.*, 2009, **37**, W623–W633.
139. A. P. Bento, A. Gaulton, A. Hersey, L. J. Bellis, J. Chambers, M. Davies, F. A. Krüger, Y. Light, L. Mak, S. McGlinchey, M. Nowotka, G. Papadatos, R. Santos and J. P. Overington, The ChEMBL bioactivity database: an update, *Nucleic Acids Res.*, 2014, **42**, D1083–D1090.
140. N. R. Coordinators, Database resources of the National Center for Biotechnology Information, *Nucleic Acids Res.*, 2013, **41**, D8–D20.
141. E. N. Muratov, J. Bajorath, R. P. Sheridan, I. V. Tetko, D. Filimonov, V. Poroikov, T. I. Oprea, I. I. Baskin, A. Varnek, A. Roitberg, O. Isayev, S. Curtalolo, D. Fourches, Y. Cohen, A. Aspuru-Guzik, D. A. Winkler, D. Agrafiotis, A. Cherkasov and A. Tropsha, QSAR without borders, *Chem. Soc. Rev.*, 2020.
142. G. Maggiora, M. Vogt, D. Stumpfe and J. Bajorath, Molecular similarity in medicinal chemistry, *J. Med. Chem.*, 2014, **57**, 3186–3204.
143. A. Bender and R. C. Glen, Molecular similarity: a key technique in molecular informatics, *Org. Biomol. Chem.*, 2004, **2**, 3204–3218.
144. A. Schuffenhauer, P. Floersheim, P. Acklin and E. Jacoby, Similarity metrics for ligands reflecting the similarity of the target proteins, *J. Chem. Inf. Comput. Sci.*, 2003, **43**, 391–405.
145. A. Bender, J. L. Jenkins, J. Scheiber, S. C. Sukuru, M. Glick and J. W. Davies, How similar are similarity searching methods? A principal component analysis of molecular descriptor space, *J. Chem. Inf. Model.*, 2009, **49**, 108–119.

146. K. Birchall, V. J. Gillet, G. Harper and S. D. Pickett, Training similarity measures for specific activities: application to reduced graphs, *J. Chem. Inf. Model.*, 2006, **46**, 577–586.
147. P. Willett, J. M. Barnard and G. M. Downs, Chemical similarity searching, *J. Chem. Inf. Comput. Sci.*, 1998, **38**, 983–996.
148. D. Alberga, D. Trisciuzzi, M. Montaruli, F. Leonetti, G. F. Mangiatordi and O. Nicolotti, A New Approach for Drug Target and Bioactivity Prediction: The Multifingerprint Similarity Search Algorithm (MuSSeL), *J. Chem. Inf. Model.*, 2019, **59**, 586–596.
149. A. Daina, O. Michielin and V. Zoete, SwissTargetPrediction: updated data and new features for efficient prediction of protein targets of small molecules, *Nucleic Acids Res.*, 2019, **47**, W357–W364.
150. N. Aniceto, A. A. Freitas, A. Bender and T. Ghafourian, A novel applicability domain technique for mapping predictive reliability across the chemical space of a QSAR: reliability-density neighbourhood, *J. Cheminf.*, 2016, **8**, 69.
151. Nidhi, M. Glick, J. W. Davies and J. L. Jenkins, Prediction of biological targets for compounds using multiple-category Bayesian models trained on chemogenomics databases, *J. Chem. Inf. Model.*, 2006, **46**, 1124–1133.
152. A. Bender, H. Y. Mussa, R. C. Glen and S. Reiling, Molecular similarity searching using atom environments, information-based feature selection, and a naïve Bayesian classifier, *J. Chem. Inf. Comput. Sci.*, 2004, **44**, 170–178.
153. D. Plewczynski, M. von Grotthuss, S. A. Spieser, L. Rychlewski, L. S. Wyrwicz, K. Ginalski and U. Koch, Target specific compound identification using a support vector machine, *Comb. Chem. High Throughput Screening*, 2007, **10**, 189–196.
154. K. P. Murphy, *Naive Bayes Classifiers*. University of British Columbia, 2006.
155. M. Olah, M. Mracec, L. Ostopovici, R. Rad, A. Bora, N. Hadaruga, I. Olah, M. Banda, Z. Simon and M. Mracec, WOMBAT: world of molecular bioactivity, *Chemoinformatics in Drug Discovery*, 2004, p. 1.
156. H. Zhang, *The Optimality of Naive Bayes*. 2004.
157. B. Merget, S. Turk, S. Eid, F. Rippmann and S. Fulle, Profiling Prediction of Kinase Inhibitors: Toward the Virtual Assay, *J. Med. Chem.*, 2017, **60**, 474–485.
158. I. Cortes-Ciriano, N. C. Firth, A. Bender and O. Watson, Discovering Highly Potent Molecules from an Initial Set of Inactives Using Iterative Screening, *J. Chem. Inf. Model.*, 2018, **58**, 2000–2014.
159. J. B. Mitchell, Machine learning methods in chemoinformatics, *Wiley Interdiscip. Rev.: Comput. Mol. Sci.*, 2014, **4**, 468–481.
160. T. Unterthiner, A. Mayr, G. Klambauer, M. Steijaert, J. K. Wegner, H. Ceulemans and S. Hochreiter, Deep learning for drug target prediction, in Conference Neural Information Processing Systems Foundation (NIPS 2014), Workshop on Representation and Learning Methods for Complex Outputs, 2014, 2014.
161. T. Unterthiner, A. Mayr, G. Klambauer, M. Steijaert, J. K. Wegner, H. Ceulemans and S. Hochreiter, MultiTask Deep Networks for Drug Target Prediction, in *Neural Information Processing System, 2014*, 2014, pp. 1–4.
162. A. Mayr, G. Klambauer, T. Unterthiner and S. Hochreiter, DeepTox: Toxicity Prediction using Deep Learning, *Front. Environ. Sci.*, 2016, **3**.
163. E. B. Lenselink, N. Ten Dijke, B. Bongers, G. Papadatos, H. W. T. van Vlijmen, W. Kowalczyk, I. J. AP and G. J. P. van Westen, Beyond the hype: deep neural networks outperform established methods using a ChEMBL bioactivity benchmark set, *J. Cheminf.*, 2017, **9**, 45.
164. M. Awale and J. L. Reymond, Polypharmacology Browser PPB2: Target Prediction Combining Nearest Neighbors with Machine Learning, *J. Chem. Inf. Model.*, 2019, **59**, 10–17.
165. H. Luo, J. Chen, L. Shi, M. Mikailov, H. Zhu, K. Wang, L. He and L. Yang, DRAR-CPI: a server for identifying drug repositioning potential and adverse drug reactions via the chemical-protein interactome, *Nucleic Acids Res.*, 2011, **39**, W492–W498.
166. L. L. Parker, S. A. Walter, P. G. Young and H. Piwnica-Worms, Phosphorylation and inactivation of the mitotic inhibitor Wee1 by the nim1/cdr1 kinase, *Nature*, 1993, **363**, 736–738.
167. J. Simm, A. Arany, P. Zakeri, T. Haber, J. K. Wegner, V. Chupakhin, H. Ceulemans and Y. Moreau, Macau: scalable bayesian multirelational factorization with side information using MCMC, *arXiv preprint arXiv:1509.04610*, 2015.
168. A. de la Vega de Leon, B. Chen and V. J. Gillet, Effect of missing data on multitask prediction methods, *J. Cheminf.*, 2018, **10**, 26.
169. M.-A. Trapotsi, I. Barrett, L. Mervin, A. M. Afzal, N. Sturm, O. Engkvist and A. Bender, Multitask bioactivity predictions using structural chemical and cell morphology information, 2020, ChemRxiv, 12571241.v1.

170. S. Liggi, G. Drakakis, A. Koutsoukas, I. Cortes-Ciriano, P. Martínez-Alonso, T. E. Malliavin, A. Velazquez-Campoy, S. C. Brewerton, M. J. Bodkin, D. A. Evans, R. C. Glen, J. A. Carrodeguas and A. Bender, Extending in silico mechanism-of-action analysis by annotating targets with pathways: application to cellular cytotoxicity readouts, *Future Med. Chem.*, 2014, **6**, 2029–2056.
171. M. Ashburner, C. A. Ball, J. A. Blake, D. Botstein, H. Butler, J. M. Cherry, A. P. Davis, K. Dolinski, S. S. Dwight, J. T. Eppig, M. A. Harris, D. P. Hill, L. Issel-Tarver, A. Kasarskis, S. Lewis, J. C. Matese, J. E. Richardson, M. Ringwald, G. M. Rubin and G. Sherlock, Gene ontology: tool for the unification of biology. The Gene Ontology Consortium, *Nat. Genet.*, 2000, **25**, 25–29.
172. J. Lomax, Get ready to GO! A biologist's guide to the Gene Ontology, *Briefings Bioinf.*, 2005, **6**, 298–304.
173. M. Kanehisa, The KEGG database, *Novartis Found. Symp.*, 2002, **247**, 91–101; discussion 101-3, 119-28, 244-52.
174. M. Tanabe and M. Kanehisa, Using the KEGG database resource, *Curr Protoc Bioinformatics*, 2012, ch. 1, Unit1.12.
175. L. H. Mervin, Q. Cao, I. P. Barrett, M. A. Firth, D. Murray, L. McWilliams, M. Haddrick, M. Wigglesworth, O. Engkvist and A. Bender, Understanding Cytotoxicity and Cytostaticity in a High-Throughput Screening Collection, *ACS Chem. Biol.*, 2016, **11**, 3007–3023.
176. G. Drakakis, A. Koutsoukas, S. C. Brewerton, D. D. Evans and A. Bender, Using machine learning techniques for rationalising phenotypic readouts from a rat sleeping model, *J. Cheminf.*, 2013, **5**, 1.
177. A. Bender, D. W. Young, J. L. Jenkins, M. Serrano, D. Mikhailov, P. A. Clemons and J. W. Davies, Chemogenomic data analysis: prediction of small-molecule targets and the advent of biological fingerprint, *Comb. Chem. High Throughput Screening*, 2007, **10**, 719–731.
178. D. J. Mason, R. T. Eastman, R. P. I. Lewis, I. P. Stott, R. Guha and A. Bender, Using Machine Learning to Predict Synergistic Antimalarial Compound Combinations With Novel Structures, *Front. Pharmacol.*, 2018, **9**, 1096.
179. U. Norinder, O. Spjuth and F. Svensson, Using Predicted Bioactivity Profiles to Improve Predictive Modeling, *J. Chem. Inf. Model.*, 2020, **60**, 2830–2837.
180. C. H. G. Allen, L. H. Mervin, S. Y. Mahmoud and A. Bender, Leveraging heterogeneous data from GHS toxicity annotations, molecular and protein target descriptors and Tox21 assay readouts to predict and rationalise acute toxicity, *J. Cheminf.*, 2019, **11**, 36.
181. S. Liggi, G. Drakakis, A. E. Hendry, K. M. Hanson, S. C. Brewerton, G. N. Wheeler, M. J. Bodkin, D. A. Evans and A. Bender, Extensions to in silico bioactivity predictions using pathway annotations and differential pharmacology analysis: application to xenopus laevis phenotypic readouts, *Mol. Inf.*, 2013, **32**, 1009–1024.
182. N. Lagarde, S. Delahaye, A. Jérémie, N. Ben Nasr, H. Guillemain, C. Empereur-Mot, V. Laville, T. Labib, M. Réau, F. Langenfeld, J. F. Zagury and M. Montes, Discriminating Agonist from Antagonist Ligands of the Nuclear Receptors Using Different Chemoinformatics Approaches, *Mol. Inf.*, 2017, **36**.
183. K. Yang, K. Swanson, W. Jin, C. Coley, P. Eiden, H. Gao, A. Guzman-Perez, T. Hopper, B. Kelley, M. Mathea, A. Palmer, V. Settels, T. Jaakkola, K. Jensen and R. Barzilay, Analyzing Learned Molecular Representations for Property Prediction, *J. Chem. Inf. Model.*, 2019, **59**, 3370–3388.
184. A. Bauer-Mehren, L. I. Furlong and F. Sanz, Pathway databases and tools for their exploitation: benefits, current limitations and challenges, *Mol. Syst. Biol.*, 2009, **5**, 290.
185. A. J. Williams, S. Ekins and V. Tkachenko, Towards a gold standard: regarding quality in public domain chemistry databases and approaches to improving the situation, *Drug Discovery Today*, 2012, **17**, 685–701.
186. P. Tiikkainen and L. Franke, Analysis of commercial and public bioactivity databases, *J. Chem. Inf. Model.*, 2012, **52**, 319–326.
187. K. Jacobs, Independent identically distributed (iid) random variables, in *Discrete Stochastics*, Springer, 1992, pp. 65–101.
188. H. Zhu, Big Data and Artificial Intelligence Modeling for Drug Discovery, *Annu. Rev. Pharmacol. Toxicol.*, 2020, **60**, 573–589.
189. L. H. Mervin, A. M. Afzal, L. Brive, O. Engkvist and A. Bender, Extending in Silico Protein Target Prediction Models to Include Functional Effects, *Front. Pharmacol.*, 2018, **9**, 613.
190. L. H. Mervin, Q. Cao, I. P. Barrett, M. A. Firth, D. Murray, L. McWilliams, M. Haddrick, M. Wigglesworth, O. Engkvist and A. Bender, Understanding Cytotoxicity and Cytostaticity in a High-Throughput Screening Collection, *ACS Chem. Biol.*, 2016.

191. S. Smusz, R. Kurczab and A. J. Bojarski, The influence of the inactives subset generation on the performance of machine learning methods, *J. Cheminf.*, 2013, **5**, 17.
192. N. Bosc, F. Atkinson, E. Felix, A. Gaulton, A. Hersey and A. R. Leach, Large scale comparison of QSAR and conformal prediction methods and their applications in drug discovery, *J. Cheminf.*, 2019, **11**, 4.
193. R. Rodriguez-Perez, M. Vogt and J. Bajorath, Influence of Varying Training Set Composition and Size on Support Vector Machine-Based Prediction of Active Compounds, *J. Chem. Inf. Model.*, 2017, **57**, 710–716.
194. L. H. Mervin, A. M. Afzal, G. Drakakis, R. Lewis, O. Engkvist and A. Bender, Target prediction utilising negative bioactivity data covering large chemical space, *J. Cheminf.*, 2015, **7**, 51.
195. M. Krier, G. Bret and D. Rognan, Assessing the scaffold diversity of screening libraries, *J. Chem. Inf. Model.*, 2006, **46**, 512–524.
196. S. R. Langdon, N. Brown and J. Blagg, Scaffold diversity of exemplified medicinal chemistry space, *J. Chem. Inf. Model.*, 2011, **51**, 2174–2185.
197. L. H. Mervin, K. C. Bulusu, L. Kalash, A. Afzal, F. Svensson, M. A. Firth, I. Barrett, O. Engkvist and A. Bender, Orthologue chemical space and its influence on target prediction, *Bioinformatics*, 2017.
198. T. Hanser, C. Barber, S. Guesné, J. F. Marchaland and S. Werner, Applicability Domain: Towards a More Formal Framework to Express the Applicability of a Model and the Confidence in Individual Predictions, in *Advances in Computational Toxicology*, Springer, 2019, pp. 215–232.
199. W. Klingspohn, M. Mathea, A. Ter Laak, N. Heinrich and K. Baumann, Efficiency of different measures for defining the applicability domain of classification models, *J. Cheminf.*, 2017, **9**, 44.
200. D. Gadaleta, G. F. Mangiatordi, M. Catto, A. Carotti and O. Nicolotti, Applicability domain for QSAR models: where theory meets reality, *Int. J. Quant. Struct.-Prop. Relat.*, 2016, **1**, 45–63.
201. S. Weaver and M. P. Gleeson, The importance of the domain of applicability in QSAR modeling, *J. Mol. Graph. Model.*, 2008, **26**, 1315–1326.
202. B. Van Calster, D. J. McLernon, M. Van Smeden, L. Wynants and E. W. Steyerberg, Calibration: the Achilles heel of predictive analytics, *BMC Med.*, 2019, **17**, 1–7.
203. T. Pereira, S. Cardoso, M. Guerreiro, A. d. Mendonca and S. C. Madeira, Alzheimer's Disease Neuroimaging, I., Targeting the uncertainty of predictions at patient-level using an ensemble of classifiers coupled with calibration methods, Venn-ABERS, and Conformal Predictors: A case study in AD, *J. Biomed. Inf.*, 2020, **101**, 103350.
204. L. H. Mervin, A. M. Afzal, O. Engkvist and A. Bender, *J. Chem. Inf. Model.*, 2020, **60**, 4546–4559.
205. F. Strieth-Kalthoff, F. Sandfort, M. H. S. Segler and F. Glorius, Machine learning the ropes: principles, applications and directions in synthetic chemistry, *Chem. Soc. Rev.*, 2020.
206. S. Johansson, A. Thakkar, T. Kogej, E. Bjerrum, S. Genheden, T. Bastys, C. Kannas, A. Schliep, H. Chen and O. Engkvist, AI-assisted synthesis prediction, *Drug Discovery Today: Technol.*, 2020.
207. G. Ranjith, R. Parvathy, V. Vikas, K. Chandrasekharan and S. Nair, Machine learning methods for the classification of gliomas: Initial results using features extracted from MR spectroscopy, *Neuroradiol. J.*, 2015, **28**, 106–111.
208. O. Engkvist, P. O. Norrby, N. Selmi, Y. H. Lam, Z. Peng, E. C. Sherer, W. Amberg, T. Erhard and L. A. Smyth, Computational prediction of chemical reactions: current status and outlook, *Drug Discovery Today*, 2018, **23**, 1203–1218.
209. Y.-h. Lam, Y. A. Abramov, R. Ananthula, J. Elward, L. Hilden, S. Nilsson-Lill, P.-O. Norrby, A. Ramirez, E. C. Sherer and J. Mustakis, Applications of Quantum Chemistry in Pharmaceutical Process Development: Current State and Opportunities, *Org. Process Res. Dev.*, 2020.
210. D. M. Lowe *Extraction of Chemical Structures and Reactions from the Literature*. University of Cambridge, 2012.
211. D. Lowe, *Chemical Reactions from US Patents (1976-Sep2016)*, 2018.
212. P. Schwaller; A. C. Vaucher; T. Laino; J.-L. Reymond, *Prediction of Chemical Reaction Yields Using Deep Learning*. 2020.
213. N. Schneider, D. M. Lowe, R. A. Sayle, M. A. Tarselli and G. A. Landrum, Big Data from Pharmaceutical Patents: A Computational Analysis of Medicinal Chemists' Bread and Butter, *J. Med. Chem.*, 2016, **59**, 4385–4402.
214. J. Mayfield, D. Lowe and R. Sayle, Pistachio: Search and faceting of large reaction databases, in Abstracts of Papers of the American Chemical Society, 2017; AMER CHEMICAL SOC 1155 16TH ST, NW, WASHINGTON, DC 20036 USA: 2017; vol. 254.
215. A. Brethorst, *Core of the Spresi Reaction Network*, University of California, Irvine, 2012.
216. American Chemical Society, CAS, accessed 25 August 2020, https://www.cas.org/.

217. A. J. Lawson, J. Swienty-Busch, T. Géoui and D. Evans, The making of reaxys—towards unobstructed access to relevant chemistry information, in *The Future of the History of Chemical Information*, ACS Publications, 2014, pp. 127–148.
218. C. D. Christ, M. Zentgraf and J. M. Kriegl, Mining electronic laboratory notebooks: analysis, retrosynthesis, and reaction based enumeration, *J. Chem. Inf. Model.*, 2012, **52**, 1745–1756.
219. A. Thakkar, T. Kogej, J. L. Reymond, O. Engkvist and E. J. Bjerrum, Datasets and their influence on the development of computer assisted synthesis planning tools in the pharmaceutical domain, *Chem. Sci.*, 2020, **11**, 154–168.
220. D. T. Ahneman, J. G. Estrada, S. Lin, S. D. Dreher and A. G. Doyle, Predicting reaction performance in C-N cross-coupling using machine learning, *Science*, 2018, **360**, 186–190.
221. D. Perera, J. W. Tucker, S. Brahmbhatt, C. J. Helal, A. Chong, W. Farrell, P. Richardson and N. W. Sach, A platform for automated nanomole-scale reaction screening and micromole-scale synthesis in flow, *Science*, 2018, **359**, 429–434.
222. *Overview — Open Reaction Database Documentation* https://ordschema.readthedocs.io/en/latest/overview.html, accessed 25 August 2020.
223. M. H. S. Segler and M. P. Waller, Neural-Symbolic Machine Learning for Retrosynthesis and Reaction Prediction, *Chemistry*, 2017, **23**, 5966–5971.
224. C. W. Coley, R. Barzilay, T. S. Jaakkola, W. H. Green and K. F. Jensen, Prediction of Organic Reaction Outcomes Using Machine Learning, *ACS Cent. Sci.*, 2017, **3**, 434–443.
225. A. Thakkar, N. Selmi, J. L. Reymond, O. Engkvist and E. J. Bjerrum, "Ring Breaker": Neural Network Driven Synthesis Prediction of the Ring System Chemical Space, *J. Med. Chem.*, 2020.
226. B. Liu, B. Ramsundar, P. Kawthekar, J. Shi, J. Gomes, Q. Luu Nguyen, S. Ho, J. Sloane, P. Wender and V. Pande, Retrosynthetic Reaction Prediction Using Neural Sequence-to-Sequence Models, *ACS Cent. Sci.*, 2017, **3**, 1103–1113.
227. W. Jin, C. Coley, R. Barzilay and T. Jaakkola, Predicting organic reaction outcomes with weisfeiler-lehman network, in *Advances in Neural Information Processing Systems*, 2017, pp. 2607–2616.
228. C. W. Coley, W. Jin, L. Rogers, T. F. Jamison, T. S. Jaakkola, W. H. Green, R. Barzilay and K. F. Jensen, A graph-convolutional neural network model for the prediction of chemical reactivity, *Chem. Sci.*, 2019, **10**, 370–377.
229. P. Schwaller, T. Gaudin, D. Lanyi, C. Bekas and T. Laino, Found in Translation": predicting outcomes of complex organic chemistry reactions using neural sequence-to-sequence models, *Chem. Sci.*, 2018, **9**, 6091–6098.
230. H. Gao, T. J. Struble, C. W. Coley, Y. Wang, W. H. Green and K. F. Jensen, Using Machine Learning To Predict Suitable Conditions for Organic Reactions, *ACS Cent. Sci.*, 2018, **4**, 1465–1476.
231. N. Eyke, W. H. Green and K. F. Jensen, Iterative Experimental Design Based on Active Machine Learning Reduces the Experimental Burden Associated with Reaction Screening, *React. Chem. Eng.*, 2020, **5**, 1963–1972.
232. D. A. Pensak and E. Corey, *LHASA—logic and Heuristics Applied to Synthetic Analysis*, ACS Publications, 1977.
233. T. Klucznik, B. Mikulak-Klucznik, M. P. McCormack, H. Lima, S. Szymkuć, M. Bhowmick, K. Molga, Y. Zhou, L. Rickershauser and E. P. Gajewska, Efficient syntheses of diverse, medicinally relevant targets planned by computer and executed in the laboratory, *Chem*, 2018, **4**, 522–532.
234. M. H. S. Segler, M. Preuss and M. P. Waller, Planning chemical syntheses with deep neural networks and symbolic AI, *Nature*, 2018, **555**, 604–610.
235. S. Genheden, A. Thakkar, V. Chadimová, J.-L. Reymond, O. Engkvist and E. Bjerrum, AiZynthFinder: a fast, robust and flexible open-source software for retrosynthetic planning, *J. Cheminf.*, 2020, **12**, 70.
236. M. T. Geballe, A. G. Skillman, A. Nicholls, J. P. Guthrie and P. J. Taylor, The SAMPL2 blind prediction challenge: introduction and overview, *J. Comput.-Aided Mol. Des.*, 2010, **24**, 259–279.
237. S. M. Mennen, C. Alhambra, C. L. Allen, M. Barberis, S. Berritt, T. A. Brandt, A. D. Campbell, J. Castañón, A. H. Cherney and M. Christensen, The evolution of high-throughput experimentation in pharmaceutical development and perspectives on the future, *Org. Process Res. Dev.*, 2019, **23**, 1213–1242.
238. K. McCloskey, E. A. Sigel, S. Kearnes, L. Xue, X. Tian, D. Moccia, D. Gikunju, S. Bazzaz, B. Chan, M. A. Clark, J. W. Cuozzo, M. A. Guie, J. P. Guilinger, C. Huguet, C. D. Hupp, A. D. Keefe, C. J. Mulhern, Y. Zhang and P. Riley, Machine Learning on DNA-Encoded Libraries: A New Paradigm for Hit Finding, *J. Med. Chem.*, 2020.

239. M. A. Bray, S. Singh, H. Han, C. T. Davis, B. Borgeson, C. Hartland, M. Kost-Alimova, S. M. Gustafsdottir, C. C. Gibson and A. E. Carpenter, Cell Painting, a high-content image-based assay for morphological profiling using multiplexed fluorescent dyes, *Nat. Protoc.*, 2016, **11**, 1757–1774.
240. C. Ye, D. J. Ho, M. Neri, C. Yang, T. Kulkarni, R. Randhawa, M. Henault, N. Mostacci, P. Farmer, S. Renner, R. Ihry, L. Mansur, C. G. Keller, G. McAllister, M. Hild, J. Jenkins and A. Kaykas, DRUG-seq for miniaturized high-throughput transcriptome profiling in drug discovery, *Nat. Commun.*, 2018, **9**, 4307.
241. Machine Learning Ledger Orchestration for Drug Discovery (MELLODDY) https://www.melloddy.eu/, accessed 25 August 2020.
242. P. S. Gromski, J. M. Granda and L. Cronin, Universal Chemical Synthesis and Discovery with 'The Chemputer, *Trends Chem.*, 2020, **2**, 4–12.
243. P. Schneider, W. P. Walters and A. T. Plowright, *et al.*, Rethinking drug design in the artificial intelligence era, *Nat. Rev. Drug Discovery*, 2020, **19**, 353–364.

# 7 Drug Metabolism

R. Lock*[a], P. J. H. Webborn[b], C. W. Vose[c] and R. M. J. Ings[d]

[a]Aucuba Sciences Ltd, 67 Canterbury Innovation Centre, University Road, Canterbury, Kent CT27FG, UK; [b]PJHW Consultancy Ltd, Marton, Cheshire, SK11 9HD, UK; [c]Formerly of Centre for Integrated Drug Development, Quintiles Ltd, 500 Brook Drive, Green Park, Reading, Berkshire RG2 6UU, UK; [d]RMI-Pharmacokinetics, 1317, Bulrush Ct, Carlsbad, CA 92011, USA
*E-mail: ruth.lock@aucubasciences.com

## 7.1 Introduction

This chapter is intended as a general overview of drug metabolism for the medicinal chemist. Extensive references and a Recommended Reading section have been included to provide sources of more detailed information.

It is important for medicinal chemists to have a good understanding of drug metabolism for several reasons:

1. Metabolism is the predominant clearance mechanism of oral drugs[1]
2. Reducing the rate of metabolism is often a key design goal in the optimisation of hits and leads[2,3]
3. Metabolism to toxic or reactive species is a significant risk in discovery programmes
4. The formation of active metabolites may confound understanding of compound efficacy but may also offer opportunities
5. Metabolism can form the basis of prodrug strategies in medicinal chemistry, where metabolic activation of inactive prodrug leads to formation of the pharmacologically active drug. Approximately 10% of drugs used in therapy are administered as prodrugs[4]
6. Understanding the enzyme system that metabolises a compound enables assessment of the risk of drug–drug interactions through inhibition or induction by a comedication.

The Handbook of Medicinal Chemistry: Principles and Practice, 2nd Edition
Edited by Simon E. Ward and Andrew M. Davis

Published by the Royal Society of Chemistry, www.rsc.org

Living systems have evolved families of enzymes to aid elimination of the foreign substances to which they are exposed. A general principle is that these enzymes generate metabolites that are less lipophilic than the starting compound. Being less lipophilic, the metabolites bind less to tissues and to plasma proteins and are therefore more available to excretion in the kidney or bile.

## 7.2 Drug Metabolism Pathways

Classically, drug metabolism reactions have been classified into two types: Phase I and Phase II. Phase I reactions are those which produce or introduce a new chemical group into a molecule (Table 7.1). Most Phase I reactions are mediated by the cytochrome 450 (CYP) group of enzymes. There is a wide range of Phase I reactions which generally yield a product (metabolite) that is less lipophilic and thus more effectively excreted in urine than the drug and may also produce metabolites which are substrates for the Phase II reactions, leading to conjugated metabolites that may be more readily excreted in bile. There are exceptions to this basic rule: acetylation and methylation are biotransformation reactions that can yield metabolites that are more lipophilic. However, it is also important to note that some Phase I pathways may produce reactive, potentially toxic metabolites *e.g.* epoxides, quinone-imines, nitrosamines (see Section 7.7.3).

Oxidations, which are the most common Phase I reactions, include aromatic and aliphatic hydroxylation, *e.g.* propranolol and debrisoquine, oxidation at nitrogen or sulphur atoms, *e.g.* nicotine and sulindac, and *N*- or *O*-dealkylation, *e.g.* imipramine and misonidazole (Figure 7.1). Note: The dealkylation pathway is an oxidation, as the initial step is hydroxylation of the alkyl group adjacent to the heteroatom with subsequent cleavage of the C–heteroatom bond.

Reductions may also occur, *e.g.* of nitro or carbonyl groups leading to amines and alcohols, respectively (Figure 7.1), with consequent decreases in lipophilicity.

Hydrolysis of esters, amides or hydrazides yields the more water-soluble acids, alcohols, amines and hydrazines, respectively.

Phase II or conjugation reactions differ from Phase I pathways in that they link the drug and/or a Phase I metabolite of a drug with an endogenous molecule, *e.g.* glucuronic acid, sulphate, an amino acid (Table 7.2). The prerequisite for conjugation reactions is

**Table 7.1** Phase I metabolic pathways.

| Reaction type | Pathway |
|---|---|
| Oxidation | Aliphatic or aromatic hydroxylation<br>*N*- or *S*-Oxidation<br>*N*-, *O*- or *S*-Dealkylation |
| Reduction | Nitro reduction to hydroxylamine, amine<br>Carbonyl reduction to alcohol |
| Hydrolysis | Ester to acid and alcohol<br>Amide to acid and amine<br>Hydrazides to acid and substituted hydrazine |

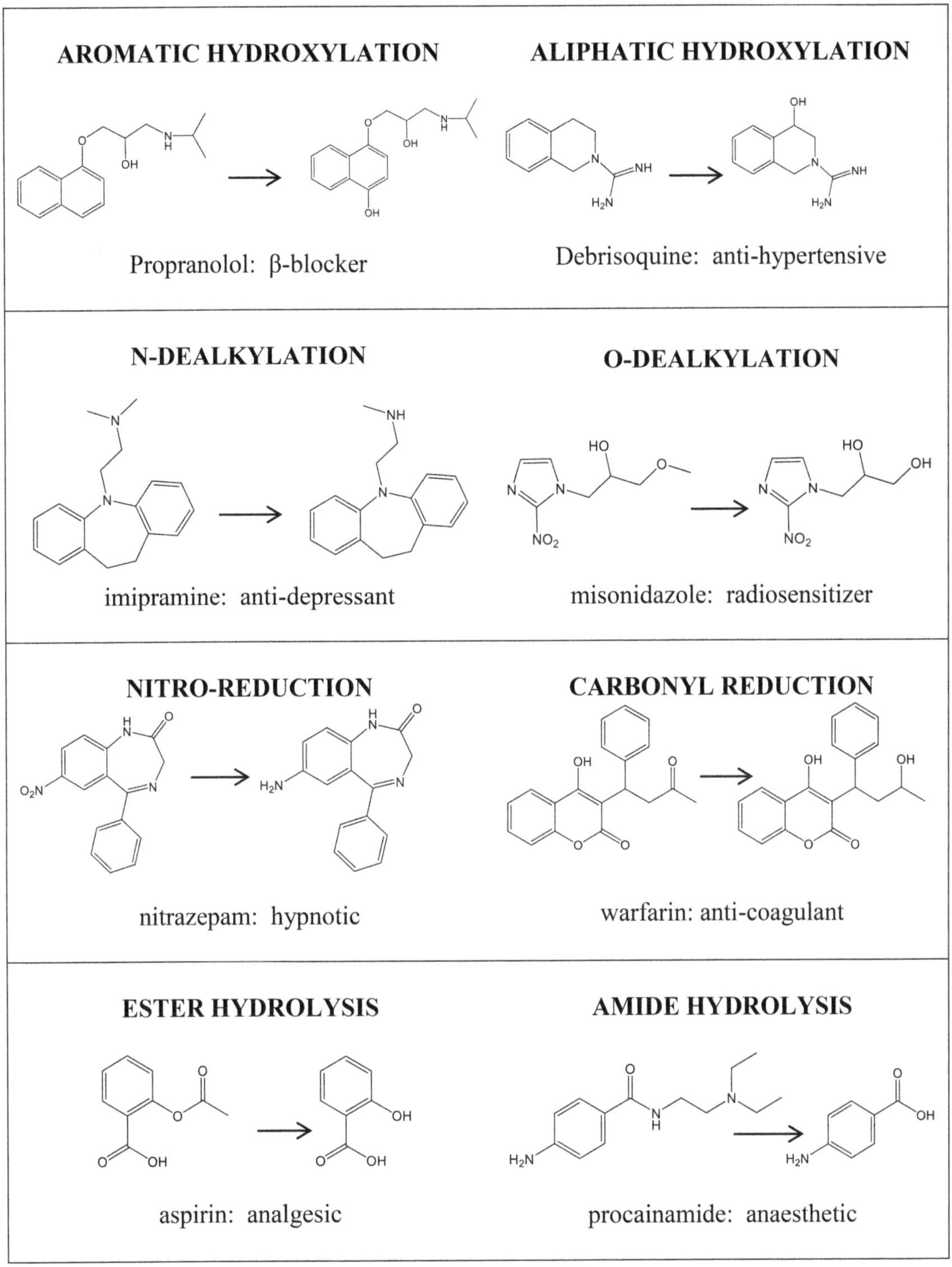


**Figure 7.1** Common Phase I metabolic pathways.

Table 7.2 Phase II conjugation pathways.

| Conjugation reaction | Endogenous reagent or substrate | Xenobiotic substrate |
|---|---|---|
| Glucuronidation | Uridine diphosphate glucuronic acid (UDPGA) | Carboxylic acid, alcohol, phenol, amine |
| Sulphation | 3′-Phosphoadenosine-5′-phosphosulphate (PAPS) | Alcohol, phenol, amine |
| Acetylation | Acetyl-CoA | Amine |
| Amino acid | Glycine, glutamine | Carboxylic acid |
| Glutathione conjugation | Glutathione | Epoxides, arene oxides, chloro compounds, quinone-imines |
| Methylation | *S*-Adenosyl methionine | Phenols, amines, thiols |

that the molecule (drug or Phase I metabolite) has a suitable chemical group, *e.g.* OH, $NH_2$, COOH with which the endogenous substrate can react. The conjugation of a drug or Phase I metabolite with glucuronic acid, sulphate, an amino-acid or glutathione (Figure 7.2) can add an ionic charge both reducing lipophilicity and making metabolites more suitable for secretion into bile. Additional conjugation pathways are *N*-acetylation of amines and *O*-, *N*-, and *S*-methylation. These, unlike other Phase II reactions, generally result in a more lipophilic product.

Some products of Phase II conjugation reactions may also contribute to drug toxicity, *e.g.* glucuronide or sulphate conjugates of certain substituted *N*-hydroxyamides have been implicated in the induction of bladder cancer[5] and acyl glucuronides of some carboxylic acids have been associated with hepatotoxicity.[6] The endogenous reagent and xenobiotic substrates are shown in Table 7.2 for the conjugation pathways.

## 7.3 The Key Role of Cytochrome P450 Enzymes

The cytochrome P450 (CYP) enzymes are a superfamily of haem-containing enzymes that act as monooxygenases in the metabolism of steroids and fatty acids, as well as drugs and other foreign compounds. These enzymes are by far the most important enzymes involved in the metabolism of drugs and chemical leads.

More than 60% of marketed drugs are metabolised by CYP enzymes.[7] Many marketed drugs are metabolised by more than one CYP enzyme, and these CYP enzymes or close analogues of them are also expressed in other mammalian species, *e.g.* rat, dog, monkey.[8,9] Human CYP3A4/5 accounts for about 40 to 50% of all CYP-dependent drug metabolism. By contrast, CYP2C9/19 and CYP2D6 (which are polymorphic) together account for approximately 40% of the metabolism of clinically used drugs. In addition, CYP1A2, CYP2A6 and CYP2B6 are polymorphic enzymes that contribute to xenobiotic metabolism.[10,11]

Table 7.3 shows the characteristics of several human CYP isozymes involved in the metabolism of xenobiotics, including drugs, and shows the overlaps in substrate specificity even between these major isozymes. Many of these enzymes are known to be

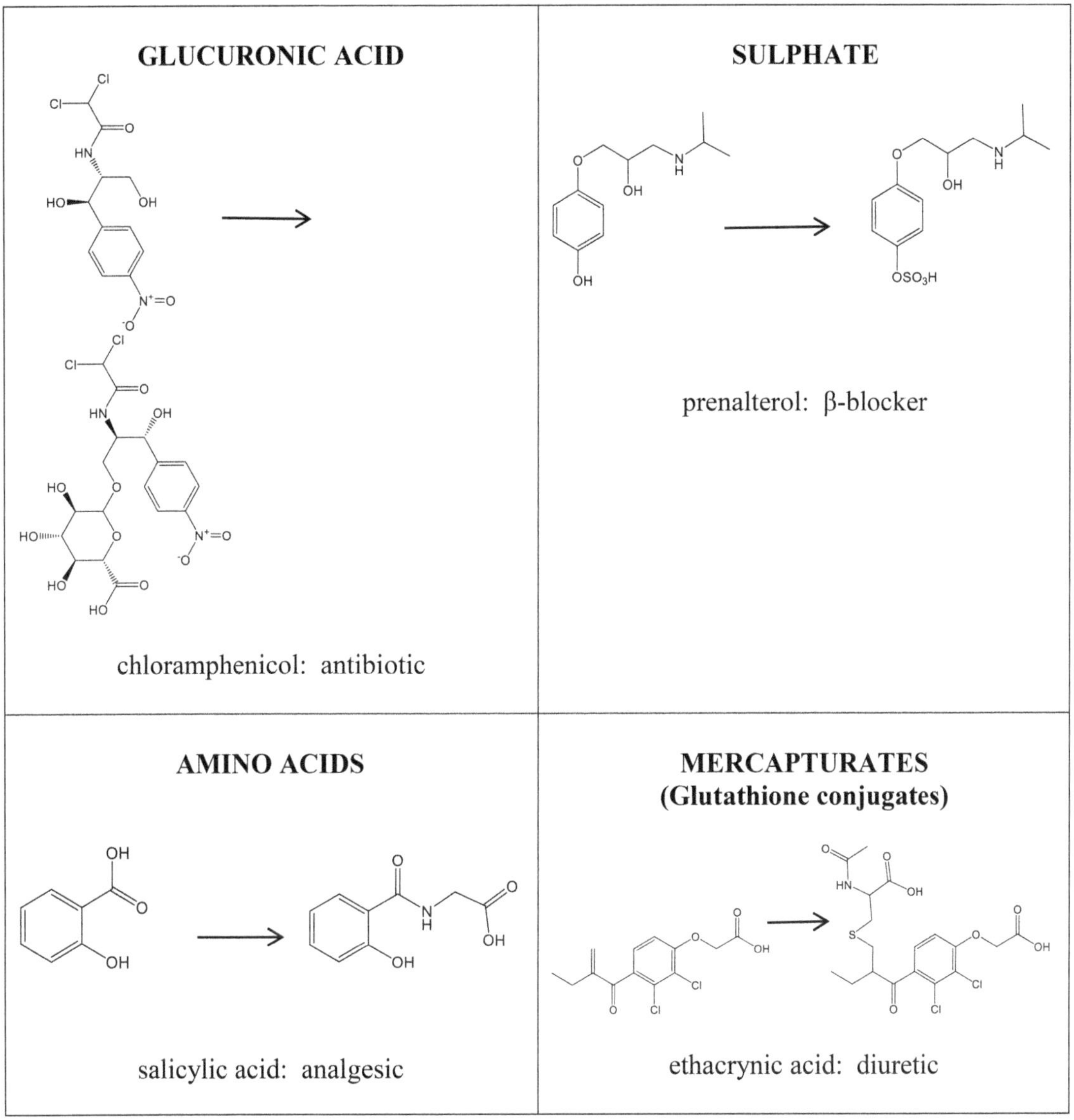


**Figure 7.2** Common Phase II conjugation pathways.

inhibited and/or induced by drugs and other xenobiotics, *e.g.* dietary components, and such effects can modulate the metabolism and thus the pharmacokinetics and pharmacodynamics of a drug that has metabolism by these enzymes as a major elimination route. A review in 2004 by Ingelman-Sundberg[12] provides comparative information on the CYP enzymes in animals and man.

The catalytic cycle of the CYP enzymes and the mechanisms of typical CYP-catalysed reactions is well covered in standard medicinal chemistry textbooks.[10,12]

**Table 7.3** Human cytochrome P-450 isozyme characteristics.

| Isozyme | Hepatic CYP450 (%) | Substrate examples | Reaction | Inhibition | Induction | Polymorphic |
|---|---|---|---|---|---|---|
| 1A1/2 | 13 | PAH | Epoxidation | ✓ | ✓ | ✓ |
| | | Caffeine | Hydroxylation | | | |
| | | Paracetamol | Hydroxylation | | | |
| | | Tacrine | Hydroxylation | | | |
| 2A6 | 4 | Basic, neutral | | ✓ | ✓ | ✓ |
| | | 7-Ethoxycoumarin | De-ethylation | | | |
| | | Nicotine | Oxidation; dealkylation | | | |
| | | Cyclophosphamide | Hydroxylation | | | |
| 2B6 | 0.2 | Efavirenz | Hydroxylation | ✓ | ✓ | ✓ |
| | | Bupropion | Hydroxylation | | | |
| 2C8 | 7 | Paclitaxel | Hydroxylation | ✓ | ✓ | ✓ |
| | | Repaglinide | Hydroxylation | | | |
| | | Rosiglitazone | Hydroxylation | | | |
| | | | Dealkylation | | | |
| 2C9 | 20 | Acidic | | ✓✓✓ | ✓ | ✓✓ Poor metabolisers |
| | | Phenytoin | Hydroxylation | | | 5–10% Caucasians |
| | | Tolbutamide | Hydroxylation | | | 23% Oriental |
| | | Retinol | Hydroxylation | | | |
| | | Ethylmorphine | Dealkylation | | | |
| | | Lidocaine | Dealkylation | | | |
| 2C19 | 2–5 | Basic | Hydroxylation | ✓✓✓ | ✓ | ✓✓ Poor metabolisers |
| | | *S*-Mephenytoin omeprazole | Hydroxylation | | | 5–10% Caucasians |
| | | Retinol | Hydroxylation | | | 5–10% Caucasians |
| | | Ethylmorphine | Dealkylation | | | |
| | | Lidocaine | Dealkylation | | | |
| 2D6 | 2–5 | β-Blockers | Hydroxylation | ✓✓✓ | — | ✓✓✓ Poor metabolisers |
| | | SSRIs | Dealkylation | | | 5–10% Caucasians |
| 2E1 | 7 | Paracetamol | Quinone-imine formation | ✓ | ✓ | ✓ |
| 3A4/5 | 30 | Basic, acidic, neutral | | ✓✓✓ | ✓✓ | N/A |
| | | Dihydropyridines | | | | High inter-individual variability |
| | | Cyclosporine | Aromatization | | | |
| | | Ethylmorphine | Dealkylation | | | |
| | | Benzodiazepines | Dealklation | | | |
| | | Steroids | Hydroxylation | | | |
| | | Macrolides | Hydroxylation | | | |

## 7.4 What Are the Key Organs that Metabolise Drugs?

Drug metabolism can occur in most tissues and organs of the body, *e.g.* liver, kidneys, intestine, lung, blood, plasma. The liver is by far the most important site of metabolism, having a high capacity for the most metabolic reactions and having a high flow of blood from both the heart and the intestine (particularly important for orally administered compounds). The kidneys and gut wall are important sites for Phase II or conjugation reactions and the mucosal cells of the small intestine express significant levels of CYP3A4 and CYP2C9 (accounting for 80 and 15%, respectively, of total immunoquantified CYPs),[13] and peptidases. It has been demonstrated that the mRNA levels of CYP isoforms diminish along the intestinal tract, with the highest CYP expression in the duodenum and the lowest in the colon.[14] The enzymes in the gut wall and liver contribute to the extensive metabolism that occurs with some drugs after absorption from the g.i. tract leading to low oral bioavailability. This is the source of the well-known "first-pass metabolism" of orally administered drugs. Metabolising enzymes are present in the lung (including CYPs, sulphotransferases, UDP-glucuronyltransferases and esterases) although at relatively low levels. The total lung CYP content is only approximately 1% of the liver. Hydrolysis of esters and amides may occur in most tissues, as well as in blood and plasma.

## 7.5 Relationship Between Chemical Structure and Rate of CYP Metabolism

At present it is not possible to accurately predict the rate of metabolism of a compound purely based on its chemical structure. Tools are available than can predict the likely sites of metabolism, and their relative likelihood (*e.g.* MetaSite, Molecular Discovery, UK and Stardrop, Optibrium, UK) but prediction of rates of metabolism is far more difficult. In broad terms the rate of metabolism is dependent upon lipophilicity, as a driver of binding to the active site, steric factors that restrict access of susceptible features to the haeme, and specific electronic features associated with the reaction in question, but which are common to chemical oxidations. Examples of such features are the electron density in aromatic systems, and the ease of α-hydrogen abstraction in *N*-dealkylation reactions and the stability of the transition states.

There can be confusion about the importance of the rate of metabolism and the extent of metabolism. From a drug design perspective, it is the rate that is critical. The extent of metabolism just reflects the relative rates of metabolic and non-metabolic clearance processes, *i.e.* for a compound that is 50% metabolised and excreted 50% unchanged in urine, the two clearance rates are equal; similarly if a compound is 90% metabolised and excreted 10% unchanged in urine, it just means that the rate of metabolism is ~10× that of the renal clearance.

Rates of metabolism are best understood in terms of "clearance", rather than half-life or % dose. Clearance concepts are well-described in the literature[1] and also in Chapter 8 of this publication.

The rate of metabolism within a chemical series is often positively correlated with lipophilicity *e.g.* β-blockers.[15] As a general rule, drugs with a $\log D > 0$ will undergo some metabolism. Thus, the antidepressant drug chlorpromazine (Figure 7.3) is very lipophilic ($\log P$ 5.14; $\log D_{7.4}$ 3.3), poorly water soluble, and has many potential sites of metabolism. It undergoes *N*-dealkylation, aromatic hydroxylation, sulphoxidation, *N*-oxidation and a combination of these Phase I processes. Some of the resulting Phase I metabolites are also substrates for Phase II conjugation reactions, *e.g.* glucuronidation, sulphation. This produces many metabolites which are excreted in urine and bile with limited excretion of unchanged drug. In contrast, the much less lipophilic atenolol ($\log P$ −0.11, $\log D_{7.4}$ −1.94) is excreted predominantly unchanged in urine. Only a small amount (≤5% dose) is metabolised to its monohydroxy metabolite.

A more targeted approach was used to design the $\beta_1$-adrenoceptor antagonist betaxolol, which had improved bioavailability (80%) and half-life in man (14–22 h) resulting from modifying the *p*-substituent in metoprolol (bioavailability about 50%; $t_{1/2}$ 3.5 h) (Figure 7.4). This work used *in vitro* metabolism studies in liver microsomes to select the most metabolically stable compounds.[16]

QSAR models have proven useful for understanding the relationships between chemical structure and rates of metabolism,[17,18] however, they tend to be more effective

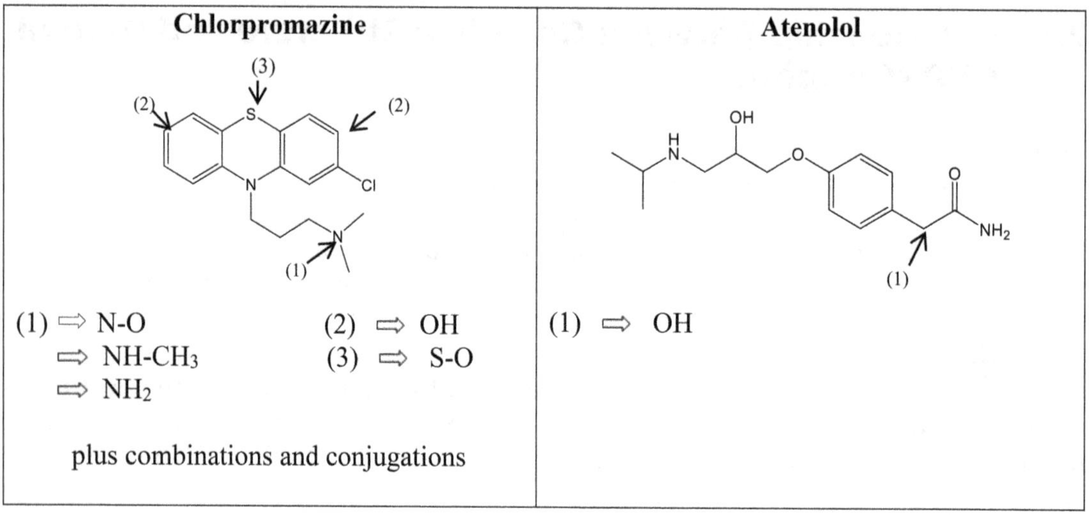


Figure 7.3 Comparison of metabolic pathways for chlorpromazine and atenolol.

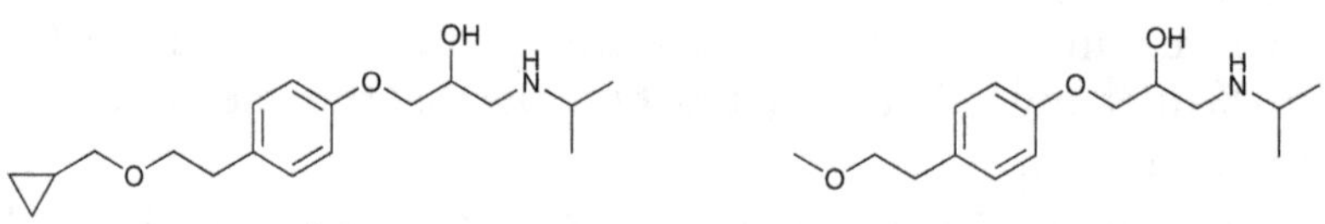


1 2

Figure 7.4 Structures of the β-blockers betaxolol (1) and metoprolol (2).

within a chemical series rather than globally. Matched molecular pair analysis (MMPA) is a tool capable of assessing the likely impact of specific changes in structure on rate of metabolism[19] (*e.g.* substitution of chlorine for methyl, fluorine for hydrogen).

## 7.6 How is Drug Metabolism Studied?

The metabolic fate of a compound is generally studied using HPLC linked to mass spectrometry. On occasions, when precise sites of oxidation need to be determined, proton NMR may also be used. An important part of the process is sample preparation, to make samples suitable for HPLC analysis (mainly a deproteination step). Mass spectrometry is carried out on triple quadrupole, ion-trap or increasingly on hybrid instruments. Most commonly the eluent from the chromatograph is delivered directly to the spectrometer, *e.g.* LC-MS, UHPLC-MS, LC-MS/MS, LC-NMR, enabling metabolite identification without the need for separate extraction, concentration and purification techniques. LC-MS or LC-MS/MS are also the most commonly used specific quantitative methods for a drug and its metabolite(s) in biological samples *e.g.* plasma, blood, urine.

In drug discovery, most learning comes from the analysis of metabolites formed *in vitro*, from microsome or hepatocyte incubations. Hepatocytes have the advantage that they contain a full range of drug metabolising enzymes. Study of the metabolites formed *in vivo* in pre-clinical species are assessed to understand the *in vitro in vivo* correlation (IVIVC) and confidence in the *in vitro* extrapolation to man. Analysis of metabolites circulating in plasma can, however, give a misleading view of the overall abundance of a metabolite or contribution of a particular metabolic pathway.[20,21] Metabolite concentrations that circulate will be conducted as part of the safety risk assessment and efficacy of a compound during development. The definitive study of the metabolism a compound is likely to be in human volunteers with a radiolabelled form of the drug.

The use of drugs radiolabelled with $^{14}C$, $^{3}H$ or in some cases $^{35}S$ provides a technique to detect and precisely quantify all drug-related material. Measurement of total radioactivity in blood, plasma, urine and faeces by liquid scintillation counting (LSC) gives information on the absorption and the routes, rates and extent (excretion balance) of excretion of drug related material. Total radioactivity is the sum of the concentrations of the drug (if present) and any radiolabelled metabolites, as shown for example in plasma (Figure 7.5).

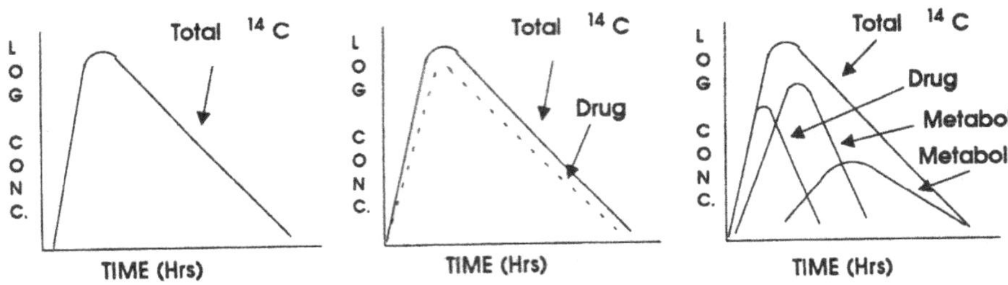


**Figure 7.5** Comparison of concentration–time profiles for total radioactivity, parent drug and metabolites.

Over the past 20 years accelerator mass spectrometry (AMS), which has been extensively used in radio-carbon dating of archaeological artefacts, has been applied to drug metabolism studies in man. AMS is approximately $10^6$ times more sensitive than liquid scintillation counting, thereby allowing the determination of pharmacokinetics, excretion balance, PK of parent drug and metabolite profile proportions of total radioactivity using microdoses (0.1–100 Bq) of radioactivity, whereas MBq doses are normally used for such studies in man.[22,23] Thus such investigations, if appropriate, can be incorporated into clinical studies in healthy volunteers and/or patients as part of single and multiple ascending doses in first-in-man studies and/or aligned to Phase II or III registration studies.

Thus, the appropriate combination of extraction procedures, LC-MS, LC-MS/MS and LC-NMR, with radiolabelled drug enables the characterisation of the absorption, metabolism and excretion of a drug. In particular, it provides information on the concentration of metabolites in biological samples. It may also be possible to carry out direct NMR analysis of biological samples (*e.g.* urine) with minimal sample preparation. This can provide very rapid metabolic information when relatively high doses have been administered and urinary excretion of drug and metabolites is rapid and extensive. Thus, it may be possible to identify metabolites and estimate their concentrations in small urine volumes by direct analysis of the samples or following freeze-drying and dissolution in $D_2O$ using proton NMR spectroscopy. Alternatively, solid-reverse-phase extraction and step gradient elution with water or aqueous buffer containing increasing proportions *e.g.* 0%, 20%, 40%, 80%, 100% of methanol or acetonitrile may provide sufficient purification and concentration of metabolite fractions from biological samples to enable identification by proton and/or $^{13}$C-NMR analysis.

The detection and identification of metabolites of drugs containing fluorine may be in some cases be obtained by direct $^{19}$F-NMR analysis of urine samples or deproteinated plasma samples, because, in contrast to proton NMR, there is essentially no background signal from endogenous components in biological samples, as shown by Wade *et al.* with trifluoromethylaniline[24] as a model compound. This approach was also used with imirestat to identify its metabolites in dog urine, including a metabolite resulting from an NIH fluorine shift (an NIH shift is a chemical migration of substituents in aromatic hydroxylation reactions).[25]

Drug metabolism may be studied *in vivo* or *in vitro*. Most commonly preparations from liver *e.g.* S-9 supernatants, microsomes (fragmented endoplasmic reticulum), hepatocytes or liver slices are used, to assess the *in vitro* metabolism of a drug and identify metabolites. S9 supernatants and microsomes can also be prepared from other tissues *e.g.* small intestine, lung. Centrifugation of the appropriate organ or tissue homogenate from the relevant species, *e.g.* rat, dog, monkey or man at 9000 to 12 000*g*, removes the nuclei and mitochondria to give the tissue S9 supernatant. Centrifuging the S9 fraction at about 136 000*g* produces microsomes from the relevant tissue.

S9 supernatants in phosphate buffer (pH7.4) incubated with the drug of interest and added NADPH (reduced nicotinamide-adenosine diphosphate), UDPGA (uridine diphosphate glucuronic acid) or PAPS (phosphoadenosine phosphosulphate) enables CYP Phase I metabolism, Phase II conjugation with glucuronic acid or with sulphate, respectively. Addition of all three factors allows all three pathways and their interactions to be investigated.

Microsomes in phosphate buffer (pH7.4) are most commonly used to investigate CYP metabolism when incubated with the drug of interest and added NADPH. However, the presence of added UDPGA and/or PAPS and a pore forming agent, *e.g.* alamethicin, allows investigation of Phase II conjugation with glucuronic acid and/or with sulphate, respectively.

Addition of glutathione in such systems also allows investigation of its conjugation with any reactive metabolites resulting from CYP oxidation.

Once a metabolite(s) has been identified, a specific quantitative analytical method can be developed where appropriate, to allow measurement of its concentrations in biological fluids and thus its pharmacokinetics.

## 7.7 Metabolites in Assessing Drug Safety and Efficacy

### 7.7.1 The Industry Perspective

Drug metabolism information provides a link between the animals used in pharmacology and toxicology studies and man. A comparison of the drug's fate in all species studied allows the interpretation of the relevance to man. A drug may be pharmacologically active, inert or toxic, as may a drug metabolite. A metabolite's pharmacological profile may be similar to that of its precursor drug or be completely different.

If the drug itself has low affinity for the target and one or more of its metabolites is the source of its activity, the drug is acting as a prodrug. In some cases, the prodrug is the result of a conscious drug design decision, *e.g.* the antibiotic pivampicillin, an ester prodrug which yields improved systemic exposure to ampicillin as the prodrug is more efficiently absorbed and then rapidly hydrolysed to ampicillin. For another drug, leflunomide (Figure 7.6), an immunomodulator used to treat rheumatoid arthritis (RA), its prodrug character was realised during early development when it was shown to be converted to teriflunomide. This major plasma metabolite is an inhibitor of dihydroorotate dehydrogenase and thus of *de novo* pyrimidine biosynthesis. This suppresses growth of rapidly dividing cells, including activated T cells and may explain the activity

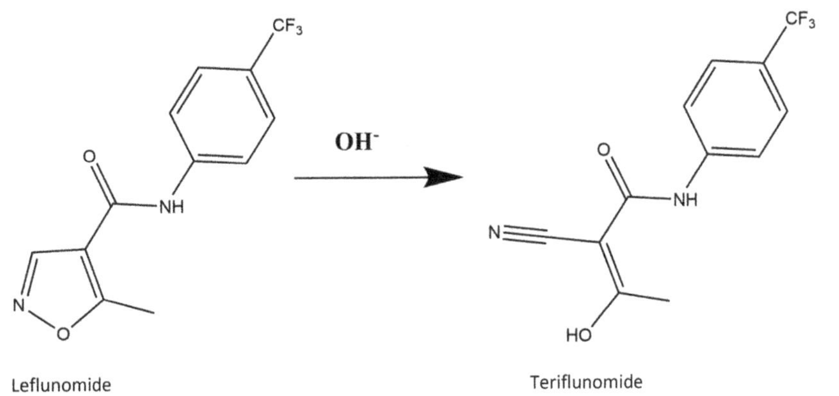


**Figure 7.6** Chemical structure of the prodrug leflunomide and it's active metabolite teriflunomide.

of leflunomide in RA and of teriflunomide which was approved by the FDA in 2012 as an oral treatment for multiple sclerosis.

Non-clinical evaluation of drug safety in animal toxicology studies usually includes assessment of parent drug plasma concentrations. These are used to aid selection of starting and maximum doses in first-in-man studies and to assess the relevance of potential risks suggested by non-clinical findings, and are used to guide monitoring in clinical trials. This is normally sufficient when the metabolic profile in humans is similar to that in at least one of the animal species used in non-clinical studies. However, metabolic profiles can vary across species both quantitatively and qualitatively, and in some cases clinically relevant metabolites may not have been identified or not been adequately evaluated during non-clinical safety studies. This situation can occur if the metabolite is formed only in humans and is absent in the animal test species or if the metabolite is present at higher levels in humans than in the animal species used in the standard non-clinical toxicity testing with the parent drug. Such a metabolite is called a disproportionate drug metabolite.[26] For zoniporide (Figure 7.7) both rat and dog resemble man in being exposed to parent drug and metabolites M1 and M3 with no evidence of disproportionate exposure to metabolites in man compared to rat and dog. A number of other metabolites were also detected in rat and dog. If a significant drug metabolite in man is not observed in the animal species used in pharmacology or toxicology studies, the potential pharmacologic or toxicologic effects of the metabolite in man may not be reflected in the non-clinical safety evaluation.

### 7.7.2 Guidance on Safety Testing of Metabolites

In 2008 the FDA issued guidance on the safety testing of metabolites, this has subsequently been revised in 2016 and 2020[26] to align with the ICH guidance for industry M3(R2) Nonclinical Safety Studies for the Conduct of Human Clinical Trials and Marketing Authorization for Pharmaceuticals (January 2010).[27] Both documents focus on the importance of metabolite profiling and metabolite quantification in supporting the safety evaluation in R and D, and ultimately marketing approval of a drug. The MIST (Metabolites in Safety Testing) guidelines focused on metabolites in human plasma that were either unique or were present at disproportionately higher concentrations compared to those of parent drug in man than in animals. In the original 2008 FDA guidance non-clinical characterisation would be required for a metabolite if at steady-state the metabolite plasma AUC was >10% of the parent drug in man and a similar or greater relative exposure was not observed in at least one toxicology species to provide coverage of its potential toxicity. The science behind the original MIST guidance has been widely discussed regarding commentary on the number of drug metabolites considered to be important for MIST being excessively high if a simple percentage-of-parent-drug criterion is used.[28–30] Experts in the field suggest that the need for further metabolite risk assessment should be considered with respect to (i) comparisons of absolute exposures (as circulating concentrations or total body burden), (ii) the nature of the toxicity mechanism, (iii) the biological matrix in which the metabolite was observed (circulatory *vs.* excretory) and (iv) consideration of the duration of exposure.

The ICH guidance (M3(R2)) broadened the criterion for non-clinical safety characterisation of a human metabolite so that it was only warranted when it was observed at

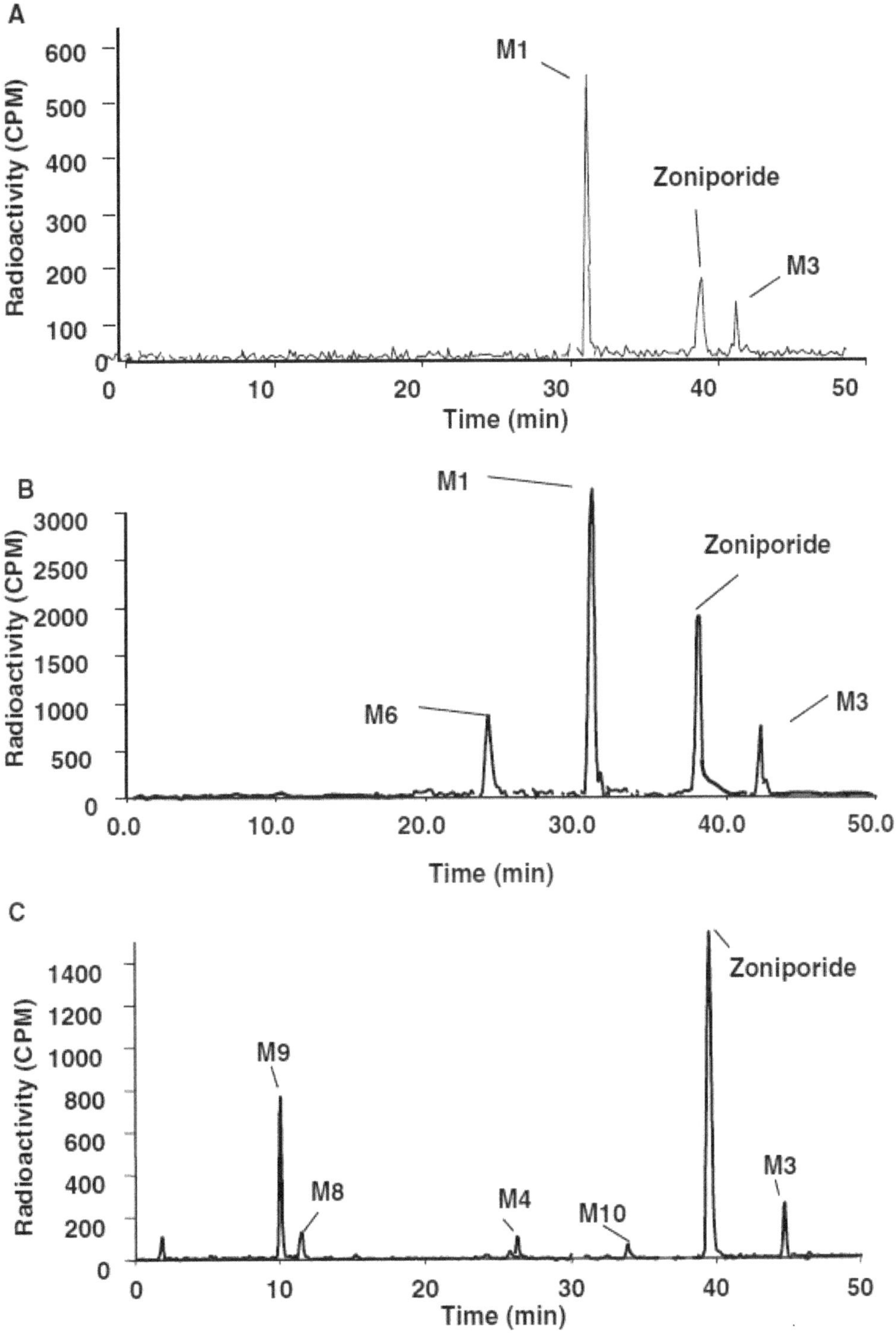


**Figure 7.7** Species comparison of [$^{14}$C]-zoniporide metabolism in plasma of healthy male volunteer (A), Sprague–Dawley rat (B) and beagle dog (C). Reproduced from ref. 71 with permission from American Society of Pharmacology and Experimental Therapeutics, Copyright 2010.

exposures >10% of *total* drug related exposure at steady state, and was at significantly greater levels in humans than the maximum exposure seen in the toxicity studies. The latest 2020 FDA guidance on the safety testing of metabolites reflects the change to >10% of drug-related material. Measurement of total drug related exposure may be based on comparison with total radioactivity or based on non-radioisotope methods to estimate total drug-related material and metabolite exposures.[31,32] This may also be expedited by using plasma sample pooling methods to reduce the number of samples that have to be analysed to provide the required exposure data.[33,34]

Clearly these guidelines have implications for drug R and D activities. If there are human metabolites not covered by the toxicology studies then specific toxicology studies on the metabolite(s), *e.g.* three-month toxicity, genotoxicity, reprotoxicity studies, may be required. An early understanding of the level of coverage for potential human metabolites during and following candidate selection will be important in assessing the need for a more extensive toxicology programme on metabolites to enable the clinical investigation and ultimately marketing of a drug candidate.

### 7.7.3 Reactive Metabolites

The metabolism of drugs to chemically reactive intermediates that bind covalently to endogenous proteins can, in certain cases, lead to organ damage or to immune-mediated adverse reactions. Thus, CYP mediated aromatic hydroxylation involves potentially reactive arene oxide intermediates. These can non-enzymatically convert to phenols, be metabolised to dihydrodiol metabolites by epoxide hydrolase and/or undergo glutathione-S-transferase catalysed conversion to mercapturic acid. Saturation of the enzyme catalysed pathways or glutathione depletion may in some circumstances result in covalent binding to cellular macromolecules. However, many drugs are metabolised *via* the arene oxide intermediate without significant associated toxicity.

Similarly, carboxylic acid drugs can undergo conjugation *via* the acid moiety with glucuronic acid to form 1β-D-acyl glucuronides or acyl-CoA thioesters. Such metabolites can in some circumstances react with cellular proteins. This can occur with acyl glucuronides by transacylation, transfer of the acyl group from the glucuronic acid to amino or hydroxyl groups in proteins. It is also possible for the acyl group of the acyl 1β-D-glucuronide to migrate to form the 2β, 3β or 4β isomers. These isomers have the ability to react with proteins *via* the 1β hemi-acetal group. Again, there are few examples where toxicity has been clearly linked to acyl glucuronide metabolite formation, and the importance is debated.[4] More recently, the safety assessment of acyl glucuronides, together with a proposal for how acyl glucuronides may best be considered in metabolites in safety testing (MIST) evaluations along with alternative (non-acyl glucuronide) mechanisms by which carboxylic acids may cause serious adverse reactions has been published.[35] A practical approach to compare systemic exposure to acyl glucuronide metabolites in humans to that in animal species used in pre-clinical safety assessment based on relative estimates of the total body burden of these circulating conjugates, is proposed.

The role of covalent protein binding in drug-induced toxicities is unclear and has been a controversial issue in drug discovery efforts. Various pharma companies have used *in vitro* microsomal metabolism screens, *e.g.* glutathione trapping or the extent of covalent binding of $^{14}C$-labelled drugs to protein, *e.g.* ≥50 pM drug equivalents per mg liver protein as the basis for rejecting candidates in early development due to concerns for their possible toxicity risks. These tests have overall been poorly predictive of the potential for toxicity, with ≥40% false positives or poor correlation with observed liver toxicity in non-clinical safety studies. Most companies appear to have abandoned such approaches because of these issues. However, there is still a desire within pharmaceutical companies to reduce reactive metabolite formation by chemical modification at early stages of drug discovery. Such practices minimise the potential for reactive metabolite formation of clinical candidates during preclinical drug optimisation. Such optimised candidates are expected to have a higher likelihood of succeeding throughout the development processes, resulting in safer drugs.

Reviews by Skonberg, Olsen *et al.*[36] (2008) and Park, Boobis *et al.*[37] (2011) provide significant insight into the challenges of interpreting the safety implications of such metabolites. This indicated that the risk of such toxicity appears to be greater, the higher the dose administered. R. A. Thompson *et al.*, at AstraZeneca, published an *in vitro* approach which explored both cellular effects and covalent binding (CVB) to assess idiosyncratic adverse drug reactions (IADR) risks for drug candidates using 36 drugs which caused different patterns and severities of IADRs in humans.[38] A comparison was made between *in vitro* CVB burden of the 36 $^{14}C$-labeled drugs and/or metabolites in human hepatocytes (determined as the fraction of metabolism leading to covalent binding, corrected for the maximum prescribed clinical dose) with the aggregated *in vitro* toxic effects of five cellular test systems. The five cellular systems comprised: (1) toxicity to THLE cells (SV40 T-antigen-immortalised human liver epithelial cells), which do not express P450s, (2) toxicity to a THLE cell line which selectively expresses P450 3A4, (3) cytotoxicity in HepG2 cells in glucose and galactose media, which is indicative of mitochondrial injury, (4) inhibition of the human bile salt export pump, BSEP, and (5) inhibition of the rat multidrug resistance associated protein 2, Mrp2. Combining the aggregated results from the *in vitro* cellular test systems, in the form of an aggregated *in vitro* panel score, with the CVB burden data (expressed as mg $day^{-1}$), discriminated, with high specificity and sensitivity, between 27 drug, which had severe or marked IADR concern, and 9 drugs which had low IADR concern. The authors propose that this detailed approach may offer the potential to select drug candidates with a lower risk of inducing such toxicity.[38]

More recently, hypotheses of how reactive metabolites induce an immune response that can lead to an IDR have been published.[39] The main hypotheses are the hapten and danger hypotheses. These are complementary hypotheses: a reactive metabolite can act as a hapten to produce neoantigens, and it can also cause cell damage leading to the release of danger-associated molecular pattern molecules that activate antigen presenting cells. Both are required for an immune response. In addition, drugs may induce an immune response through inflammasome activation. The ability to activate inflammasomes is believed to differentiate drugs that cause IADRs from similar drugs that do not. Advances are also being made in microphysiological systems (also known as organs-on-a-chip), with the potential to transform how the industry could risk assess reactive metabolites. Systems pharmacology approaches are also showing promising potential in reactive metabolite risk assessments.[40]

The successful registration of osimertinib and other epidermal growth factor receptor (EGFR)-tyrosine kinase inhibitors, has highlighted the difficulty of identifying "reactivity" as a simple defining property indicating hepatotoxicity. Osimertinib targets cysteine residues and covalently binds to albumin and to human hepatocytes at levels that would suggest significant risk.[7] With no validated, quantitative link between reactivity and drug toxicity, the strategy a project adopts to manage the toxicity risk from reactive metabolites tends to reflect the organisations overall attitude to pre-clinical safety risk management. For some organisations, even limited drug reactivity is seen as a fixable medicinal chemistry issue and therefore unacceptable. For others, *in vitro* based hazard data is a risk that can be carried through to more comprehensive safety assessment, taking into account the clinical context.

## 7.8 What Factors Influence the Metabolism of Drugs?

### 7.8.1 Dose Level

As the dose of drug is increased, the capacity of the metabolic enzyme systems may be saturated. This can lead to minor pathways becoming more significant and/or to a disproportionately high concentration of drug or of a toxic or active metabolite being present. This can result in exaggerated pharmacology and/or toxicity. Thus, paracetamol (Figure 7.8) is eliminated by conjugation with glucuronic acid and sulphate at therapeutic doses. At higher doses, sulphate and glucuronide conjugation become saturated and formation of a mercapturic acid by conjugation of reactive Phase I metabolites with glutathione is also observed. Overdose saturates glucuronidation and sulphation and depletes the glutathione. The reactive quinone-imine intermediates accumulate and cause damage to cell macromolecules with resultant liver and kidney toxicity. Thus, saturation of metabolic

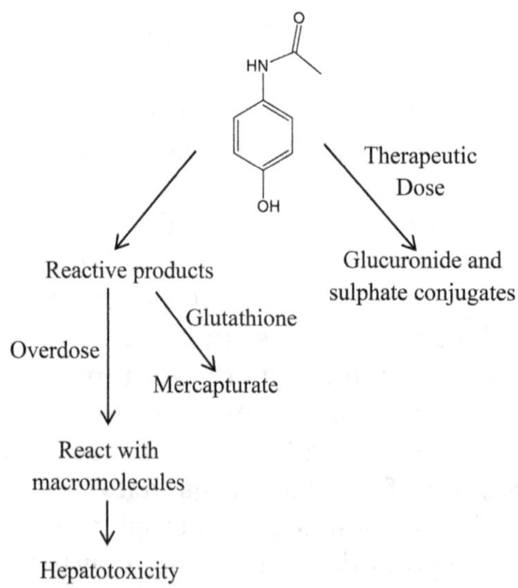


**Figure 7.8** Metabolic pathways for paracetamol.

elimination pathways at high doses can modify the exposure to parent drug and/or metabolites with consequent changes in pharmacology and toxicology. These effects should be considered when assessing the relevance of results from non-clinical toxicology studies to man. This is why the pharmacokinetics of drugs, and, where appropriate, metabolites, are studied in toxicology studies. This is often described as "toxicokinetics".

## 7.8.2 Route of Administration

Drugs given orally have to pass the digestive enzymes in the gut lumen, and drug metabolising enzymes of the intestinal wall and liver before reaching the systemic circulation. The gut microflora may also have a role in the absorption and metabolism of drugs that are absorbed from the large intestine.

Metabolism may occur at any or all of these sites and can reduce the drug concentration in the systemic circulation. If the drug itself is the active compound, this will affect the intensity of its pharmacodynamic effects. When this pre-systemic metabolism occurs in gut wall or liver, it is called "first-pass" metabolism or the "first-pass" effect.

Meptazinol (Figure 7.9) is an analgesic drug subject to a very high first-pass effect *via* conjugation with glucuronic acid or sulphate. This is markedly reduced if the drug is administered rectally since blood drainage from the rectum predominantly avoids the hepatic portal vein. Thus, much less drug is eliminated before reaching the systemic circulation, higher concentrations are obtained for a given dose and therefore it was a more effective analgesic when given rectally because of the decreased first-pass metabolism in gut wall and liver.[41] However, this was an extreme solution to avoid a problem inherent in the chemical structure of the drug. More typically, a discovery project would attempt to avoid such a problem using *in vitro* screening of intrinsic clearance to design more stable analogues. Drug administration by transdermal, sublingual, buccal or inhaled pulmonary routes has also been used to avoid "first pass" effects. Such strategies are generally considered if the non-oral route is a general feature of similar marketed drug classes and shouldn't be considered as a "quick fix" to avoid high "first pass" effects. A large "first-pass" effect does contribute to high inter-subject variability, which can be a major limiting factor in the clinical utility of a compound.

## 7.8.3 Species Difference in Metabolism

Species differences in drug metabolism may be attributed to (1) specific activity (product formed per unit time per unit enzyme) for a drug, (2) expression level of the metabolising enzyme(s), and in some cases, (3) differences between the inducible expression of the responsible enzyme(s).[42]

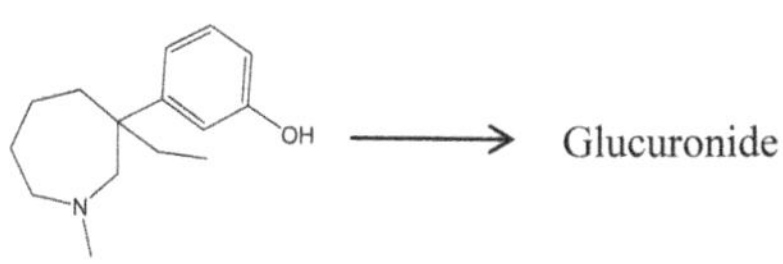


Peak plasma level after 50 mg dose:

| | |
|---|---|
| Orally | <0.01 μg/ml |
| Rectally | 0.05-0.2 μg/ml |

**Figure 7.9** Effects of route of administration on meptazinol metabolism and bioavailability.

There are frequently quantitative differences (same metabolic route but differing rates) in the Phase I pathways between species. These are at present in some cases difficult to predict and interpret. The general conclusion is that in man, oxidative metabolism is slower than in mouse, rat and dog, in part reflecting the changes in metabolic rate with changes in body weight and differences in hepatic blood flows, although this may vary for particular compounds owing to species differences in the abundance and activity of the specific enzymes involved. Different species may also have entirely different metabolic pathways for dealing with the same drug (*i.e.* qualitative differences). For example, in rat CYP2C is a major enzyme for nifedipine oxidation and lidocaine *N*-de-ethylation, whilst CYP3A is a major enzyme involved in (*S*)-mephenytoin hydroxylation. In contrast, CYP3A4/5 in man catalyses nifedipine oxidation and lidocaine *N*-de-ethylation, whilst CYP2C is the major enzyme involved in (*S*)-mephenytoin hydroxylation.[43] The CYP families 3A and 2D appear to show a remarkable conservation across species (human, dog, rat), with CYP2C being the least conserved. CYP2C is the largest and most complicated subfamily in several species. It shows sex dependent expression in rat and large differences in substrate specificities between human and animal. A study investigating mRNA and protein expression of dog liver CYPs in relation to the metabolism of human CYP2C substrates[44] showed marked differences in the metabolism of human CYP2C substrates in the beagle dog strain compared with humans with respect to rate of reaction, stereoselectivity and CYP enzyme selectivity. Dog livers expressed mRNA and CYP3A12, CYP2B11, CYP2C21 proteins, with no sex differences being found. Expression of CYP2C41 mRNA was undetectable in the livers of 6 of 11 dogs, consistent with other published data indicating a partial or complete deletion of the CYP2C41 gene in many dogs.[45] Correlation analysis suggested that CYP2B11 catalyses the 4′-hydroxylation of mephenytoin (mediated in humans by CYP2C19) in the dog, and that this enzyme and CYP3A12 contribute to S-warfarin 7-hydroxylation (mediated in humans by CYP2C9).

CYP1A2 is expressed almost exclusively in the liver of humans, rats and mice. In contrast, monkeys and dogs express CYP1A2 at low levels in the liver.[42] Furafylline and omeprazole are inhibitors and inducers of human CYP1A2, respectively, but they do not inhibit or induce CYP1A2 in rodents.[46]

The CYP2B family is expressed in all species in the liver; however, it is highly expressed in the intestine of mouse and rat but not in human.[47]

The species-specific isoforms of CYP1A, -2C, -2D and -3A show appreciable interspecies differences in terms of catalytic activity and a degree of caution should be applied when extrapolating metabolism data from animal models to humans. In contrast, CYP2E1 shows no large differences between species, and extrapolation between species appears to hold quite well.[47]

A number of qualitative differences are also seen for Phase II pathways. Dogs are unable to acetylate aromatic amines and are more sensitive to the pharmacologic and toxic effects of such compounds. Cats lack the ability to form glucuronide conjugates and only primates form amino-acid conjugates with glutamine.

UGT1A3 and UGT1A4 are expressed in the liver, intestine and colon and are the important enzymes in the glucuronidation of many tertiary amine or aromatic heterocycles to form quaternary ammonium glucuronides. The formation of quaternary ammonium glucuronides appears be highly species specific, with the highest activity being found in humans and monkeys. Rats and mice are generally incapable of forming quaternary ammonium glucuronides because the UGT1A3 and UGT1A4 isoforms are pseudogenes (non-functional segments of DNA that resemble functional genes) in these rodents.[42]

These differences can have implications for the screening of compounds in animal species other than man and also highlight the importance of selecting the appropriate rodent and non-rodent species for standard toxicity testing prior to first-in-human studies. Caution should be taken in extrapolation of animal data to humans; however, when *in vitro* metabolism studies with liver microsomes, hepatocytes and recombinant enzymes are available, the information can be incorporated into the decision-making process and can aid in the selection of the appropriate *in vivo* animal model.

It is important to remember that it is highly unlikely that any animal model can appropriately model all aspects of drug metabolism for a given compound, and in many cases, different species may be needed to answer specific questions.

### 7.8.4 Gender-related Differences

There can be significant differences in the rates of CYP mediated metabolism in male and female rodents, particularly rats. Thus, male rats required higher doses of hexobarbital to induce sleep than female rats because of their greater ability to inactivate the drug by aliphatic hydroxylation. Such differences tend to be much less common in non-rodent species. They are related to the effect of sex differences in the expression of CYP isozymes in the rat. However, such effects have been reported for several compounds in man, *e.g.* fluvoxamine, and should be investigated as part of the development of a new drug in man.

### 7.8.5 Age

Age is an important determinant of drug metabolism and is best studied in man. At either end of the age range, the liver (and other tissues) is (are) generally less capable of metabolic reactions, than in healthy volunteer subjects aged 18–45 typically used in early clinical studies. For example, neonates are essentially unable to conjugate chloramphenicol with glucuronic acid (Figure 7.2). This results in an accumulation of drug leading to toxic cardiovascular effects (grey baby syndrome). Similar problems occur in the aged liver (Table 7.4) with the reduced clearance of imipramine in the liver requiring changes in the administered dose, to avoid excessive drug accumulation and hence increased side-effects.

**Table 7.4** Age-dependent effects on imipramine pharmacokinetic parameters.[a]

| | Young | Old (>70) |
|---|---|---|
| Clearance (ml min$^{-1}$) | 950 | 570 |
| Half-life (h) | 17 | 30 |
| $C_{max}$ (ng ml$^{-1}$) | 10–20 | 40–45 |

[a]Volume of distribution and protein binding were unchanged: the decreased clearance is due to the reduced ability of the old liver to *N*-dealkylate.

The potential for age-related changes in pharmacokinetics and pharmacodynamics should be investigated for compounds ultimately intended to treat paediatric or elderly patients. The use of modelling and simulation in both industry and academia is becoming more widespread. Physiologically based pharmacokinetic (PBPK) modelling offers a unique opportunity to incorporate multiple levels of information to estimate age-specific pharmacokinetics.

### 7.8.6 Disease

Not surprisingly, drugs which are mainly eliminated by hepatic metabolism can show changes in their kinetics in patients with liver disease. Propranolol is more bioavailable in cirrhotic patients because of a much reduced first-pass effect in the damaged liver. Similarly, conversion of a prodrug to active compound may be decreased in cirrhotic patients. However, it is difficult to predict the effect of a particular liver disease on the fate of a specific drug, but based on the ADME characteristics of a drug such investigations in patients may be needed to support the safety evaluation of the drug and guide dosing in hepatically impaired patients. Regulatory guidance recommends a PK study in patients with impaired hepatic function if hepatic metabolism and/or excretion accounts for a substantial portion (>20% of the absorbed drug) of the elimination of a parent drug or active metabolite.[48,49] The timing of a stand-alone hepatic impairment study in development depends on a number of factors, but such studies are often run during Phase 2. Alternatively, if late-stage Phase 2/3 studies will be enriched for varying degrees of hepatic dysfunction then population PK analyses could be conducted.

Renal impairment (as a consequence of renal disease or ageing) can also influence hepatic metabolism of certain drugs by modifying CYP enzyme activity and transporter function.[50] Renal impairment has not only been associated with decreased renal excretion of drugs and metabolites, but also with changes in metabolism and active transport in the kidney, liver or gut. Effects of severe renal disease on non-renal elimination mechanisms have been suggested to be attributed to accumulation of uremic factors that inhibit or suppress metabolising enzymes and transport proteins. Thus, for most drugs that are likely to be administered to patients with renal impairment, including drugs that are not primarily excreted by the kidney, PK should be assessed in patients with renal impairment to provide appropriate dosing recommendations.[51,52]

### 7.8.7 Genetics

The majority of Phase I and Phase II drug-metabolising enzymes (DMEs) are polymorphic. Genetic polymorphism causes important interindividual differences in drug and metabolite exposure and can lead to wide population differences in the metabolic fate of a compound. For example, rapid and ultra-rapid metabolisers clear the drug very quickly, and the therapeutic concentration of the drug in the blood and tissues may not be reached. In patients termed poor metabolisers, the drug is metabolised so slowly that it accumulates in the blood stream. The higher concentration of the drug in the body creates a greater potential for adverse effects, particularly for drugs with a narrow therapeutic window. Clinically relevant examples of pharmacogenetic variation have been observed with CYP2C9 (for warfarin), CYP2C19 (for clopidogrel and omeprazole), CYP2D6 (for tamoxifen and codeine) and CYP3A5 (for tacrolimus).[53] In some instances, the resulting protein is still functional but exhibits reduced activity (*e.g.* CYP2C9); in other cases, the resulting variant protein may be completely devoid of activity or is not expressed (*e.g.* CYP2D6, CYP2C19 and CYP3A5).

Some 10% of the Caucasian population are unable to hydroxylate debrisoquine (Figure 7.1) and other basic drugs, *e.g.* β-blockers, SNRIs, metabolised by the same CYP isoenzyme (CYP2D6) with potential effects on their activity and side effects. The CYP2D6 polymorphism has influenced the adverse event profiles of CNS drugs such as venlafaxine[54] and haloperidol[55] with "poor metabolisers" showing increased incidences of adverse events compared to normal metabolisers. The population variability of CYP3A4 activity is extremely high (>100-fold), but genetic variants in the CYP3A4 gene have explained only a minor portion of this variability.[56] Significant variation in P450 activities has been found during development, from the prenatal period through birth, infancy, childhood, adolescence and adulthood.[57] CYP3A4 and CYP3A7 are differentially expressed at different developmental ages. CYP3A7 is the predominant CYP3A enzyme expressed in fetal and early postnatal liver tissues and then generally decreases over a few years to an undetectable level for the rest of life. Conversely, CYP3A4 is not detectable before birth but gradually increases postnatally and is the dominant P450 enzyme in the adult liver and intestine. These differences in catalytic activities and gene expression of CYP3A4 and CYP3A7 can lead to differences in drug metabolism and responses between paediatric and adult patients.

In addition to CYPs, polymorphisms exist in other DMEs. There are genetic differences in the ability to *N*-acetylate certain classes of drug, *e.g.* dapsone, isoniazid. Some 50% of Caucasians have a much lower capacity to carry out this reaction, which in turn influences the activity and side-effects of such compounds. Several UGT polymorphisms (UGT1A1, 1A7 and 1A9), are associated with an alteration in irinotecan metabolism and are receiving increasing attention in clinical settings.

## 7.9 Metabolism-based Drug–Drug Interactions

Hepatic metabolism occurs primarily through the CYP family of enzymes located in the hepatic endoplasmic reticulum, but can also occur through non-CYP enzymes, including Phase II glucuronosyl- and sulphotransferases. As many drugs are primarily eliminated by metabolism and the enzymes mediating these reactions can be subject to inhibition or induction by other compounds, the potential always exists for metabolism-mediated drug–drug interactions, with potential clinical safety and efficacy repercussions. This was highlighted by the discovery of a case of torsade de pointes, resulting from QT interval prolongation, in a patient receiving the antihistamine, terfenadine, with the antifungal agent, ketoconazole.[58] In normal circumstances, relatively lipophilic terfenadine is almost completely metabolised to the much more hydrophilic active species fexofenadine on its first pass through the liver *via* CYP3A4, so there are very low or no circulating plasma levels of the intact parent drug. However, in the presence of a potent CYP3A4 inhibitor, such as ketoconazole, this reaction is blocked, resulting in detectable plasma levels of terfenadine, which interacts with the cardiac hERG receptor causing a prolongation of the QT interval with the potential for torsade de pointes resulting in reported fatalities, ultimately leading to the withdrawal of terfenadine as a marketed product.

Clinical reports have indicated that ingestion of supplements or fruit juice can also alter systemic exposure of substrate drugs by modulating enzymes and transporters. Grapefruit juice has also been shown to inhibit CYP3A4, thereby decreasing the clearance and thus increasing steady-state plasma levels of drugs cleared extensively by 3A4 metabolism, *e.g.* terfenadine and statins, thus modifying their wanted and unwanted pharmacodynamic effects. Hence the detailed guidance or guidelines[59,60] now issued by most major regulatory authorities on testing for drug–drug interactions (covering both metabolising enzymes and transporters) and QT interval prolongation.

Although drug–drug interactions can cause an increase in the incidence of adverse events or a loss of therapeutic efficacy, not all drug–drug interactions are undesirable. For example, some HIV drugs, such as ritonavir, inhibit CYP3A4 and thereby improve the pharmacokinetic profile of other anti-HIV drugs, such as lopinavir and saquinavir. Tumours often overexpress transporters and GSTs, which can limit the effectiveness of some anticancer agents. Drugs that inhibit transporters and GST are being developed to enhance the efficacy of some anticancer drugs.[46]

The understanding of the number and type of metabolic drug–drug interactions has vastly improved since the introduction of *in vitro* technologies such as recombinant human cytochromes, as well as the use of microsomes and hepatocytes with specific and selective substrates and inhibitors. For many, a metabolic drug–drug interaction appears to be simply the inhibition of a CYP by a candidate compound, often identified in very early screening assays for CYP inhibition in the candidate drug selection process. However, it is much more complex than that and caution is advised on rejecting any compound based on the results of such tests alone, since potentially good compounds could be unnecessarily discarded and compounds with other types of metabolic drug–drug interaction liabilities missed as is discussed later when your drug is a target (victim) of a drug–drug interaction rather than being a causative (perpetrator) agent. Regarding perpetrator drug–drug interaction risk, to make a rational decision there needs to be data on the expected clinically relevant drug concentrations (systemic and, additionally, intestinal for orally administered drugs) and the extent of plasma protein binding. Also, it needs to be established that if an interaction occurs, it can it be successfully managed such as with the antiviral drugs where inhibitory interactions are even used to boost efficacy.[61]

The more common human CYPs involved with the metabolism of xenobiotics are listed in Table 7.5, together with examples of substrates, inhibitors and inducers. The FDA also provide a list of common CYP substrates, inhibitors and inducers: https://www.fda.gov/drugs/drug-interactions-labeling/drug-development-and-drug-interactions-table-substrates-inhibitors-and-inducers. A diverse range of chemical structures are seen in inhibitors and in inducers. Potent inhibitors tend to have a neutral nitrogen whose lone pair is able to strongly bind to the haem iron in the CYP active site, *e.g.* imidazole group as in ketoconazole, quinoline group as in quinidine, thiazole group as in ritonavir. Inducers vary from ethanol, phenobarbital, antiepileptic drugs,

**Table 7.5** Examples of substrates, inhibitors and inducers of different human CYP-450 isozymes.

| CYP-450 | Substrate | Inhibitor | Inducer |
|---|---|---|---|
| CYP1A2 | Alosetron/duloxetine/tizanidine | Ciprofloxacin/cimetidine/fluvoxamine | Omeprazole/montelukast/phenytoin |
| CYP2A6 | Coumarin/nicotine | Ritonavir/tranylcypromine | Phenobarbital/rifampicin |
| CYP2B6 | Bupropion/efavirenz | Clopidogrel/ticlopidine | Phenobarbital/efavirenz/rifampin |
| CYP2C8 | Paclitaxel/repaglinide | Anastrozole/gemfibrozil/trimethoprim | Phenobarbital/primidone/rifampin |
| CYP2C9 | Celecoxib/phenytoin/warfarin | Amiodarone/metronidazole/troglitazone | Rifampin/secobarbital/carbamazepine |
| CYP2C18 | *S*-Mephenytoin | Cimetidine | |
| CYP2C19 | Clobazam/omeprazole/*S*-Mephenytoin | Fluvoxamine/esomeprazole/ticlopidine | Carbamazepine/prednisone/rifampin |
| CYP2D6 | Desipramine/dextromethorphan/metoprolol | Buproprion/quinidine/terbinafine | |
| CYP2E1 | | Disulfiram/ritonavir | Ethanol/isoniazid |
| CYP3A4/5 | Cyclosporine/lovastatin/sildenafil | Clarithromycin/ketoconazole/saquinavir | Carbamazepine/rifampin/St. John's wort |

*e.g.* carbamazepine, to a complex cyclic antibiotic like rifampicin. A lot of emphasis has been placed on inhibitory metabolic drug–drug interactions since these tend to be the cause of safety concerns, but just as important can be metabolic drug–drug interactions resulting from enzyme induction. Induction of CYPs can impact the efficacy and safety of a drug upon multiple dosing with coadministered drugs. Also, there are two distinct directions in which the identification of metabolic drug–drug interaction must be approached. The first is as described above, where the drug or candidate compound is the causative agent or perpetrator of a metabolic drug–drug interaction. The second is when a drug or candidate compound is the target or a victim of a metabolic drug–drug interaction. Each of these aspects is equally important, but requires completely different strategies for their investigation.

*A perpetrator* of a metabolic drug–drug interaction can be by two routes, inhibition and induction. The mechanism of CYP inhibition can either be *via* a reversible or irreversible (time-dependent) interaction. If we first consider inhibition interactions, the most common studies, particularly in the early discovery screening phase are for direct inhibition of the five most relevant CYP isoforms, *i.e.* CYP1A2, CYP2C9, CYP2C19, CYP2D6 and CYP3A4, usually determining the percentage inhibition at a single concentration. By candidate nomination it is more common to estimate an $IC_{50}$ in an extended panel of human CYPs (CYP1A2, CYP2B6, CYP2C8, CYP2C9, CYP2C19, CYP2D6, CYP3A4/5), and $K_i$ for those CYPs where inhibition is observed. At this stage and for such studies it is advisable not only to examine for direct inhibition, but also for time-dependent inhibition (TDI). Direct inhibition involves the binding of the drug candidate to the CYP, and depending on the binding site, can be classified as competitive, non-competitive, uncompetitive or mixed inhibition. For this type of inhibition, usually human liver microsomes are used (although other options include pooled cryopreserved hepatocytes or individual microsomes expressing recombinant CYP enzymes) with specific model substrates, such as those recommended in the FDA Drug Interaction Guidance (2020)[59] to determine the $IC_{50}$ and $K_i$ (inhibition constant) of inhibitors, and different concentrations of the candidate compound, and, if the type of inhibition is being investigated, different substrate concentrations as well. If there is good evidence that the inhibition is competitive, the use of different substrate concentrations may be omitted since the $K_i$ is calculated by half the $IC_{50}$, but if not, the $K_i$ has to be calculated using the equations cited in the FDA and European guidances.[59,60] Based on the results of the *in vitro* studies ($K_i$) and the *in vivo* pharmacokinetics of the investigational drug, the risk of inhibition *in vivo* is evaluated. If it cannot be excluded that enzyme inhibition takes place *in vivo*, studies *in vivo* are recommended.

In addition to direct inhibition, some drugs display TDI. CYP mediated transformation of these drugs results in metabolites which can act as reversible inhibitors or chemically modify the CYP enzyme (*e.g. via* covalent bond formation). TDI can be divided into a number of mechanistic categories including irreversible (covalent) modification of the enzyme (mechanism-based inactivation), quasi-irreversible (metabolite–intermediate complex), reversible (metabolite is more potent inhibitor than parent), *etc.* TDI by a drug manifests as their inhibitory potency increasing with incubation time (a pre-incubation time of 30 minutes is standard practice). TDI is assessed by the difference in $IC_{50}$ values measured under two different conditions: pre-incubation of the drug with CYP enzyme and the cofactor NADPH and pre-incubation without NADPH. An $IC_{50}$ shift of greater than 1.5 is considered to be a significant shift and the compound is classed as a time dependent inhibitor. Further work should then be completed to evaluate the mechanism of time-dependent inhibition or determine $K_i$ and $k_{inact}$ values to predict the risk of drug–drug interactions *in vivo*. TDI inhibition is of particular importance because it may result in a long-lasting inhibition since usually *de novo* synthesis of the CYP enzyme is required to recover the CYP activity. The unwanted consequences of TDI can in some cases lead to termination of drug development, drug withdrawal or restrictions of use.

In addition to studying the inhibition of CYPs, regulatory guidance[60] recommended to study inhibition of UGTs known to be involved in drug interactions, including UGT1A1 and UGT2B7, if one of the major elimination pathways of the investigational drug is direct glucuronidation. Likewise, if the investigational drug is mainly metabolised by other enzymes (*e.g.* MAO), it is recommended to study the inhibitory effect on that specific enzyme if feasible. A metabolite with significant plasma exposure or pharmacological activities may need to be evaluated for its DDI potential as a substrate or as a perpetrator of metabolising enzymes.

Enzyme induction after multiple dosing is another possible means where a candidate drug could be a perpetrator of a metabolic drug–drug interaction and manifests in increased clearance of another drug (victim) or their own clearance (autoinduction). CYP induction is one of the major concerns in clinical practice and for the pharmaceutical industry. There are two major issues associated with CYP induction: a reduction in therapeutic efficacy of comedications and an induction in reactive metabolite-induced toxicity. Thus, it is highly desirable to develop new drug candidates that are not potent CYP inducers to avoid the potential of CYP induction-mediated drug interactions.

For this reason, today, many companies routinely include the assessment of CYP induction earlier in drug discovery as part of the selection processes of new drug candidates for further clinical development. Some xenobiotic compounds are able to interact with nuclear receptors such as aromatic hydrocarbon receptor (AhR), constitutive androstane receptor (CAR) and pregnane X receptor (PXR), each inducing sets of drug metabolising enzymes and transporters including the CYP1As, CYP2Bs, CYP2Cs, CYP3As, glucuronyl transferases and P-gp, depending on the receptor. Activation of these receptors, however, is species-specific so when investigating induction drug–drug interactions, it is recommended to always use human systems and not to be tempted to extrapolate animal induction data to the human situation.

During the early pre-clinical phase, an initial screening assay using human nuclear receptor binding assays (*e.g.* CAR, AhR, PXR) can be invaluable in understanding the SAR of potential induction issues and the risk of drug–drug interactions. Given that PXR is responsible for the transcriptional regulation of CYP3A, CYP2C and also P-gp, strategically, some companies focus on primarily assessing PXR, given most induction DDIs are related to CYP3A.[62] Towards candidate nomination, induction may be assessed in the hepatocyte-derived cell model (HepaRG); however, results from these studies are considered supportive rather than definitive in nature by the regulatory authorities. The more definitive study, accepted by regulators, uses a functional assay where different concentrations of the test compound are incubated with human hepatocytes for 2 to 3 days and the microsomal activities of the enzymes of interest compared before and after incubation using specific, model substrates. The $E_{max}$ and $EC_{50}$ for induction are determined and compared to those of positive controls run at the same time to assess the possible clinical impact of the induction. A major challenge of measuring only the enzyme's activity is that the induction may be masked in the presence of concomitant inhibition. Transcriptional analysis through the measurement of mRNA levels may address this challenge. Ultimately, regulatory guidance recommends *in vitro* evaluation of the potential of an investigational drug to induce CYP1A2, CYP2B6, CYP2C8, CYP2C9, CYP2C19 and CYP3A4.[59,60]

Although not approved as a biomarker by the regulatory agencies, urinary 6β-hydroxycortisol/cortisol and plasma 4β-hydroxycholesterol are selective CYP3A endogenous biomarkers and are increasingly used by companies in early clinical phase I studies as an indicator of drug candidate CYP induction liability. An early readout can be valuable, given that induction normally results in a reduction of efficacy, due to increased metabolism of drugs. Of particular concern is the induction of CYP3A4, since this can result in a reduction of plasma levels of oestrogens and progestins found in oral contraceptives, possibly resulting in unplanned pregnancy, and reduction in cyclosporine plasma levels resulting in transplant rejection due to increased cyclosporine clearance.

*A victim* of a metabolic drug–drug interaction is when the investigational drug is the target and requires a completely different strategy to that described above for perpetrators of a drug–drug interaction. When establishing if a test compound could be a victim of a drug–drug interaction, *i.e.* another coadministered compound alters its clearance, it is necessary to establish and quantify every route of elimination of the compound, including non-metabolic routes of elimination such as renal. The rationale is that the fewer the routes of elimination, the greater the potential for a compound to be a victim of a metabolic drug–drug interaction. The rule of thumb is that if any one route of elimination exceeds 25% of the total clearance of a compound, there may be a risk of a clinically meaningful drug–drug interaction. To evaluate this is not a simple process, since, for instance, if renal secretion or biliary/gut wall secretion separately is estimated to account for more than 25% of drug elimination, attempts should be made to identify the transporter(s) involved in the active secretion. To identify the metabolic component, often termed as reaction phenotyping, the extent of any non-CYP (*e.g.* aldehyde oxidase (AOX), flavin-containing mono-oxygenases (FMO), monoamine oxidases (MAO), UDP-glucuronosyl transferases (UGT), esterases, sulphotransferases (SULT), *N*-acetyltransferases (NAT) and glutathione S-transferases (GST)) and CYP metabolism will need to be established. Historically, one approach included pre-incubating human hepatocytes or human S9 fractions (these preparations contain the non-CYP enzymes, whereas microsomes may not) with 1-aminobenzotriazole (1-ABT) to inhibit all the CYP activity then determining how much of the test compound is still metabolised. If metabolism occurs in the presence of 1-ABT, the enzymes responsible would be identified, although the risk of a compound largely metabolised by non-CYP enzymes showing a clinically relevant drug–drug interaction tends to be lower than those primarily metabolised by CYPs. Other more common approaches now include the use of recombinant enzymes, expressing FMO, MAO, carboxylesterases (CE), AOX, UGT, SULT or NAT. Approaches using liver microsomes, S9, cytosol, or hepatocytes with enzyme-selective inhibitors are also sometimes used. There are two widely used methods for identifying the individual CYP enzymes responsible for a drug's metabolism: (1) the first method uses chemicals, drugs or antibodies as specific enzyme inhibitors in human liver microsomes or hepatocytes (*e.g.* a pool of more than 10 donors). Commonly used *in vitro* CYP enzyme inhibitors can be found on the FDA's website on Drug Development and Drug Interactions;[63] and (2) the second method uses individual human recombinant CYP enzymes. Regulators recommend the use of both methods to identify the specific enzymes responsible for a drug's metabolism. When using individual human recombinant CYP enzymes, it is recommended to consider the difference in the amount and enzyme activity of CYPs between the recombinant CYP enzyme systems and the human liver.

As can be seen from the above discussion, any understanding of the risk of a potential metabolic drug–drug interaction is much more than performing a quick CYP inhibition screen. It must be put into the context of whether it is viewed as a perpetrator or a victim of an interaction, as well as the final use of the drug. The therapeutic index of the drugs involved, together with the plasma concentrations of the candidate drug obtained at anticipated clinical doses, plasma protein binding, type of inhibition/induction, *etc.*, must all be brought into these considerations. It is now more commonplace to aim to design out any liabilities during lead optimisation so as to avoid the described complexities later in drug development. Furthermore, a metabolite with significant plasma exposure or pharmacological activities may need to be evaluated for its DDI potential as a substrate or as a perpetrator of metabolising enzymes. The European guidelines on drug–drug interactions provide a series of very useful decision trees to help in the interpretation of the *in vitro* inhibition and induction data.[60] Many of the interactions, once identified and quantified, can be manageable and sometimes may even be of benefit, such as ritonavir boosted protease inhibitors when treating HIV and probenecid with some β-lactam antibiotics.

Before embarking on expensive clinical studies, it is always possible to simulate the possible clinical consequences of any of these metabolic drug–drug interactions using physiological based pharmacokinetic (PBPK) models with programs such as GastroPlus® (https://www.simulations-plus.com/software/gastroplus/drug-interaction/) and Simcyp™ (www.simcyp.com). The DDI Module in GastroPlus® allows you to predict mechanistic and static drug–drug interactions (DDIs) among drugs and metabolites. You can also incorporate variability between subjects in your dynamic simulations and see the impact on victim, perpetrator and metabolite(s) concentrations and AUC ratios. Simcyp™ PBPK models allow investigation of metabolic DDIs due to competitive enzyme inhibition, mechanism-based inhibition, enzyme induction and polypharmacy. This program is population-based incorporating the variability of the distribution of different human cytochromes, so it is possible to simulate not just the average effect but also the extremes where often the real clinical problems lie. Also, if there are multiple major elimination pathways (≥25% of total clearance), it is possible to simulate the effect of different drug–drug interaction scenarios.

## 7.10 How Transporter Proteins Affect Drug Metabolism

Uptake and efflux transporter proteins can have an important role in the distribution and elimination of some drugs. Efflux proteins are ATP dependent and primarily function to reduce the amount of compound either entering the body (*e.g.* in the G.I. tract) or specific organs (*e.g.* the brain), or to facilitate the excretion of compounds (*e.g.* bile canaliculus and kidney proximal tubule). Uptake proteins are driven by an ion gradient and facilitate the entry of compounds into cells and organs.

Endogenous and exogenous compounds with even moderate lipophilicity can enter cells primarily by simple diffusion through the lipid bilayer that forms the cell membrane. For more polar compounds, such diffusion is limited, and uptake transporters facilitate their entry (*e.g.* glucose, amino acids). Uptake transporters in the liver influence the metabolism of drugs by raising the free drug concentrations at the site of the metabolising enzymes (*e.g.* atorvastatin), in the intestine the effect is to aid absorption (*e.g.* acyclovir), and in the kidney the primary effect is to increase renal secretion (*e.g.* metformin). Conversely, efflux transporters reduce the free drug concentrations to which the metabolising enzymes are exposed, reducing the rate of metabolism.

The impact of drug transporters on metabolism is best understood in terms of competing elimination pathways and in terms of the impact on the ratio of the free concentration inside the cell, relative to that in plasma.[64,65]

The understanding of transporters and their role in the overall ADME of drugs has gathered momentum over recent years with the identification of many different proteins, both for transporting xenobiotics and endogenous compounds. This, combined with the development of experimental systems to identify xenobiotic substrates, inhibitors and inducers of the specific transporters has provided a much better awareness of their impact on drug pharmacokinetics. The subject has now grown to an extent that it would be impossible to provide a detailed and comprehensive overview in this chapter and the interested reader should refer to the many excellent reviews that are available including those by Russel (2010),[66]; Giacomini *et al.* (2018)[67]; Zamek-Gliszczynski *et al.* (2018)[68] and associated literature of The International Transporter Consortium (https://www.itc-transporter.org/).

The transporters of particular interest can be divided into four broad super-families. There are two categories of solute carrier transporters (SLC), one of which acts mainly on transporting anionic compounds such as benzylpenicillin, furosemide, ibuprofen and the statins (OATs and OATPs) and the other transports mainly cations such as cimetidine, ranitidine and metformin (OCTs, OCNTs and MATEs). Then there are the ATP binding cassette (ABC) efflux transporters that transport a wide range of anionic, cationic and neutral compounds (*e.g.* digoxin and doxorubicin) and, as the name suggests, rely on ATP hydrolysis to actively move substrates across membranes. The SLC transporters can undertake both drug uptake and efflux, whereas the ABC type of transporter only undertakes efflux. Finally, there are the peptide transporters, which can be especially important for the absorption and elimination of certain peptide-like compounds such as the β-lactam antibiotics, lisinopril and oseltamivir (Tamiflu). The major human transporters are listed in Table 7.6, together with some known substrates.

The main tissues where these transporters are found include the intestine, liver, kidney and brain, as summarised in Table 7.6 and Figure 7.10. The brain has been

**Table 7.6** Summary of the major human drug transporters and their substrates (data collated from Russel (2010);[66] International Transporter Consortium (https://www.itc-transporter.org/); FDA guidance on drug–drug Interactions, 2020[59]).[a]

| Transporter | Typical tissue distribution | Membrane distribution | Substrate examples |
|---|---|---|---|
| PEPT1 | Intestine/kidney | BBM | Ampicillin/amoxicillin/cefaclor/cefadroxil/enalapril |
| PEPT2 | Kidney | BBM | Amoxacillin/bestatin/cefaclor/valganciclovir |
| OCT1 | Intestine/liver | BLM/SM | Acyclovir/ganciclovir/metformin/cimetidine/quinine |
| OCT2 | Kidney/brain | BLM | Cimetidine/ranitidine/metformin/propanolol/zidovudine |
| OCT3 | Liver | BLM | Cimetidine |
| OCTN1 | Intestine/kidney | BBM | Mepyramine/quinidine/verapamil/gabapentin |
| OCTN2 | Intestine/kidney | BBM | Mepyramine/quinidine/valproate/cephaloridine/ematine |
| OAT1 | Kidney | BLM | Adefovir/methotrexate/furosemide/ibuprofen/cimetidine |
| OAT2 | Liver | SM | Erythromycin/cimetidine/taxol/butetanide/salicylate |
| OAT3 | Kidney/liver/muscle/heart | BLM | Benzylpenicillin/tetracycline/ranitidine/ketoprofen/pravastatin |
| OAT4 | Kidney | BBM | Tetratcycline/zidovudine/bumetanide/ketoprofen/salicylate |
| MATE1 | Liver/kidney | CM/BBM | Cimetidine/procainamide/metformin/cephalexin/fexofenadine |
| MATE2 | Kidney | BBM | Cimetidine/procainamide/metformin/fexofenadine/oxaliplatin |
| OATP1A2 | Intestine/kidney | BBM | Fexofenadine/enalapril/rosuvastatin/imatinib/saquinavir |

**Table 7.6** *(continued)*

| Transporter | Typical tissue distribution | Membrane distribution | Substrate examples |
|---|---|---|---|
| OATP1B1 | Liver | BBM | Benzylpenicillin/rifampicin/pravastatin/valsartan/troglitazone |
| OATP1B3 | Liver | BLM | Digoxin/rifampicin/enalapril/fluvastatin/valsartan/paclitaxel |
| OATP2B1 | Liver/intestine | SM/BBM | Benzylpenicillin/bosentan/pravastatin/glibenclamide |
| OATP4C1 | Kidney | BLM | Digoxin/ouabain/methotrexate |
| MDR1 (P-gp) | Intestine/liver/kidney/brain | BBM/CM/BBM | Vincristine/doxorubicin/paclitaxel/digoxin/ritonavir/cyclosporin |
| MDR3 | Liver | CM | Digoxin/paclitaxel/vinblastine |
| MRP2 | Intestine/liver/kidney/brain | BBM/CM/BBM | Vinblastine/doxorubicin/ritonavir/glutathione conjugates |
| MRP3 | Intestine/liver/kidney | BLM/SM/BLM | Glucuronide conjugates/methotrexate |
| MRP4 | Intestine/liver/kidney | BBM/SM/BBM | Topotecan/6-thioguanine/tenovir/cefazolin/furosemide |
| BCRP | Intestine/liver/kidney | BLM/CM/BBM | Topotecan/SN38/imatinib/nelfinavir/rosuvastatin/ofloxacin |

[a]BLM – basal lateral membrane; BBM – brush border membrane; SM – sinusoidal membrane; CM – canalicular membrane.

highlighted, in addition to the excretory organs, because it can be especially important when developing CNS acting drugs, with the efflux transporters forming an integral component of the blood–brain barrier.

Drug transporters are another potential source of drug–drug interactions. This issue has been reviewed in detail by the International Transporter Consortium (2018) and was subsequently followed up by regulatory guidance from the FDA (2020)[59] and a discussion document from the EMEA (2017).[69]

## 7.11 Summary

Optimisation of a chemical series to yield bioavailable, long half-life compounds suitable for use as oral drugs often includes reducing the rate of metabolism (intrinsic clearance) of hit and lead compounds. Due to the high dependence upon lipophilicity, modulation of log$D$ is likely to form an important part of the optimisation strategy. However, because of the common inverse correlation between lipophilicity and potency, there is often limited scope for substantial reductions. Insights into the sites of metabolic vulnerability and the associated mechanisms of metabolism, aligned with determination of the key metabolites formed *in vitro*, gives great scope for more targeted improvements. Attention also needs to be paid to the nature of the metabolites formed, as metabolites can have significant impact on drug toxicity and efficacy.

One of the principles upon which our understanding of the pharmacokinetics of drugs is based, is that at equilibrium (*i.e.* not at early time points, and not in very poorly perfused regions, *e.g.* tumours), the free concentration in tissues is the same as that in plasma.[70] This allows a quantitative understanding of metabolism ($CL_{int}$, $K_m$ and $V_{max}$) and drug–drug interaction potential in terms of the free plasma concentrations.

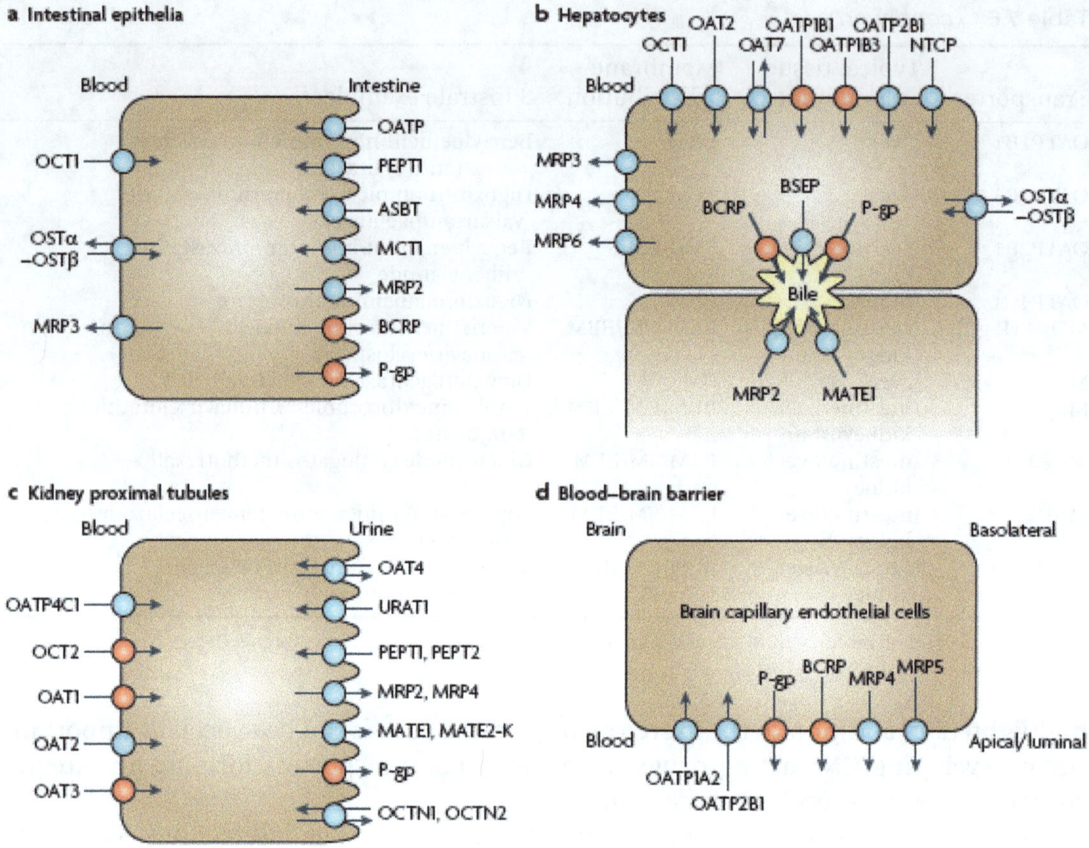


**Figure 7.10** A summary of the human transporter proteins involved with xenobiotic and endogenous compound transport across cell walls. Reproduced from ref. 72 with permission from Springer Nature, Copyright 1969. Transporters not identified in Table 7.6 are ASBT (ileal apical sodium/bile acid co-transporter), MRCT1 (monocarboxylic acid transporter), NTCP (sodium/taurocholate co-transporter), $OST_\alpha$ and $OST_\beta$ (heteromic organic solute transporter) and URAT1 (urate transporter 1).

It should be noted that drug transporter proteins alter this equilibrium and make extrapolation from plasma concentration data more complex. This effect is the source of the term "transporter interplay" that is common in the literature.

## 7.12 Drug Metabolism Hints and Tips

- The rate of metabolism and how it impacts drug kinetics (half-life and bioavailability) is best understood in terms of drug clearance, rather than half-life, or percentage of compound metabolised.
- Within a series of compounds, the rate of metabolism generally increases with increasing lipophilicity of the drug.[4]
- Understanding how a compound is metabolised can aid targeted medicinal chemistry strategies to reduce the rate of metabolic clearance. Classic steps include:

  - o Deactivate aromatic rings, introduce electron-withdrawing groups, $CF_3$, $SO_2$, heterocycles, F
  - o Block aromatic oxidation sites with halogens
  - o Remove potential for *N*-, and *O*-dealkylation,
  - o Replace labile groups (bioisosteres), change ester to amide or heterocycle, look at ester bioisosteres
  - o Block/replace possible sites for conjugation, avoid phenols, unhindered alcohols, carboxylic acids.
- As the rate of metabolic clearance is reduced within a chemical series, other clearance mechanisms may well become of increased importance.
- The levels of metabolites formed from low clearance compounds tend to be lower than those from high clearance compounds, purely because the metabolites are formed at a much slower rate.
- Studying rates of metabolism in hepatocytes covers the full range of liver enzymes. You need to be mindful that if microsomes are used, additional enzyme systems may play a role.
- Metabolism can form the basis of prodrug strategies in medicinal chemistry, where metabolic activation of inactive prodrug leads to formation of the pharmacologically active drug.
- It is recommended that by candidate selection, an *in vitro* profile of the metabolites formed in the key animal species and in humans is obtained.
- Understanding the activity and safety implications of key metabolites early in development can be critical to the overall evaluation of the drug product, since metabolites can confer pharmacological activity and possible toxicity beyond that of the parent drug.
- If a significant drug metabolite in man is not observed in the animal species used in safety pharmacology or toxicology studies or is only seen at much lower levels than those in man, the potential pharmacologic or toxicologic effects of the metabolite in man may not be reflected in the non-clinical safety evaluation.
- Drug administration by transdermal, sublingual, subcutaneous, intramuscular, buccal, inhaled pulmonary or rectal routes have been used for some drugs to avoid "first pass" effects. However, such strategies shouldn't be considered as a "quick fix" if the non-oral route is not a general feature of similar marketed drug classes.
- The FDA and European guidelines on drug–drug interactions provide a series of very useful equations and decision trees to help in the interpretation of the *in vitro* inhibition and induction data and the potential necessity to investigate potential DDIs by conducting a clinical DDI study.

## Recommended Reading

FDA guidance to Industry M3(R2) nonclinical safety studies for the conduct of human clinical trials & marketing authorization for pharmaceuticals, 2010.

D. A. Smith, Discovery and ADMET: Where are we now, *Curr. Top. Med. Chem.*, 2011, **11**, 467–481.

B. Williamson, N. Colclough, A. J. Fretland, B. C. Jones, R. D. O. Jones, and D. F. McGinnity, Further Considerations Towards an Effective and Efficient Oncology Drug Discovery DMPK Strategy, *Curr. Drug Metab.*, 2020, **21**, 145–162.
B. Testa, A. Pedretti, and G. Vistoli, Foundation review: Reactions and enzymes in the Metabolism of drugs and other Xenobiotics, *Drug Discovery Today*, 2012, **17**(11–12), p549–p560, 12p.
D.A. Smith, K. Beaumont, T. S. Maurer, and L. Di, Clearance in Drug Design, *J. Med. Chem.*, 2019, **62**, 2245–2255.

## References


1. D. A. Smith, K. Beaumont, T. S. Maurer and L. Di, *J. Med. Chem.*, 2019, **62**, 2245–2255.
2. P. Ballard, P. Brassil, K. H. Bui, H. Dolgos, C. Petersson, A. Tunek and P. J. H. Webborn, *Drug Metab. Rev.*, 2012, **44**, 224–252.
3. B. Williamson, N. Colclough, A. J. Fretland, B. C. Jones, R. D. O. Jones and D. F. McGinnity, *Curr. Drug Metab.*, 2020, **21**, 145–162.
4. K. Hajnal, H. Gabriel, R. Aura, V. Erzsébet and S. S. Blanka, *Acta Med. Marisiensis*, 2016, **62**, 356–362.
5. G. Grimmer, G. Dettbarn, A. Seidel and J. . Jacob, *Sci. Total Environ.*, 2000, **247**(1), 81–90.
6. S. L. Regan, J. L. Maggs, T. G. Hammond, C. Lambert, D. P. Williams and B. Kevin Park, *Biopharm. Drug Dispos.*, 2010, **31**(7), 367–395.
7. R. J. Bertz and G. R. Granneman, *Clin. Pharmacokinet.*, 1997, **32**(3), 210–258.
8. D. Smith, *Drug Metab. Rev.*, 1991, **23**, 255.
9. M. Murray, *Clin. Pharmacol.*, 1992, **23**, 132.
10. T. Shimada, *et al.*, *J. Pharmacol. Exp. Ther.*, 1994, **270**, 414–423.
11. S. Sim and M. Ingelman-Sundberg, *Hum. Genomics*, 2020, **4**, 278–281.
12. M. Ingelman-Sundberg, *Naunyn-Schmiedeberg's Arch. Pharmacol.*, 2004, **369**, 89–104.
13. M. Paine, H. Hart, S. Ludington, R. Haining, A. Rettie and D. Zeldin, *Drug Metab. Dispos.*, 2006, **34**(5), 880–886.
14. R. Iswandana, M. Ika Irianti, D. Oosterhuis, H. Hofker, M. Merema, M. de Jager, H. Mutsaers and P. Olinga, *Drug Metab. Dispos.*, 2018, **46**(12), 1879–1885.
15. G. R. Bourne, in *Progress in Drug Metabolism*, ed. J. W. Bridges and L. F. Chasseaud, Wiley, London, 1981, vol. 6, pp. 77–110.
16. P. M. Manoury, *et al.*, *J. Med. Chem.*, 1987, **30**(6), 1003–1011.
17. J. G. Cumming, A. M. Davis, S. Muresan, M. Haeberlein and H. Chen, *Nat. Rev. Drug Discovery*, 2013, **12**, 948–962.
18. L. George, T. Fotios, G. Costas and T.-K. Anna, Journal, 2017, 339.
19. E. J. Griffen, A. G. Dossetter and A. G. Leach, *J. Med. Chem.*, 2020, **63**, 8695–8704.
20. D. A. Smith and D. Dalvie, *Xenobiotica*, 2012, **42**, 107–126.
21. C.-M. Loi, D. A. Smith and D. Dalvie, *Drug Metab. Dispos.*, 2013, **41**, 933–951.
22. G. Lappin and L. Stevens, *Expert Opin. Drug Metab. Toxicol.*, 2008, **4**, 1021–1033.
23. G. Lappin, M. Rowland and R. C. Garner, *Expert Opin. Drug Metab. Toxicol.*, 2006, **2**, 419–427.
24. K. R. Wade, J. Troke, C. M. Macdonald, I. D. Wilson and J. K. Nicholson, in *Methodological Surveys in Biochemistry and Analysis, Bioanalysis of Drugs and Metabolites Especially Anti-inflammatory and Cardiovascular*, ed. E. Reid, J. D. Robinson and I. D. Wilson, Plenum Press, New York and London, 1987, vol. 18, F-5, pp. 383–88.
25. P. J. Gilbert, *et al.*, *Xenobiotica*, 1992, **22**, 775–787.
26. Safety Testing of Drug Metabolites Guidance for Industry, FDA, March 2020, Revision 2.
27. ICH M3 (R2) Non-clinical safety studies for conduct of human clinical trials and marketing authorisation for pharmaceuticals, 2010.
28. D. A. Smith, R. S. Obach, D. P. Williams and B. K. Park, *Chem.-Biol. Interact.*, 2009, **179**, 60–67.
29. D. A. Smith and R. S. Obach, *Chem. Res. Toxicol.*, 2009, **22**, 267–279.
30. D. A. Smith and R. S. Obach, *Bioanalysis*, 2010, **2**, 1223–1233.
31. I. C. Yu, *et al.*, *Rapid Commun. Mass Spectrom.*, 2007, **21**, 497.
32. L. Leclercq, *et al.*, *Chem. Res. Toxicol.*, 2009, **22**, 280–293.

33. R. A. Hamilton, *et al.*, *Clin. Pharmacol. Ther.*, 1981, **29**, 408–413.
34. C. E. C. A. Hop, *et al.*, *J. Pharm. Sci.*, 1998, **87**, 901–903.
35. D. A. Smith, T. Hammond and T. A. Baillie, *Drug Metab. Dispos.*, 2018, **46**(6), 908–912.
36. C. Skonberg and J. Olsen, *et al.*, *Expert Opin. Drug Metab. Toxicol.*, 2008, **4**, 425–438.
37. B. K. Park and A. Boobis, *et al.*, *Nat. Rev. Drug Discovery*, 2011, **10**, 292–306.
38. R. A. Thompson and E. M. Isin, *et al.*, *Chem. Res. Toxicol.*, 2012, **25**, 1616–1623.
39. T. Cho and J. Uetrecht, *Chem. Res. Toxicol.*, 2017, **30**(1), 295–314.
40. R. A. Thompson, E. M. Isin, M. O. Ogese, J. T. Mettetal and D. P. Williams, *Chem. Res. Toxicol.*, 2016, **29**(4), 505–533.
41. R. A. Franklin, *Xenobiotica*, 1988, **18**(1), 105–112.
42. J. G. Dekeyser and M. Shou, *Encyclopedia of Drug Metabolism and Interactions*, 2012.
43. D. A. Smith, *Drug Metab. Rev.*, 1991, **23**, 353–373.
44. M. J. Graham, A. R. Bell, H. K. Crewe, C. L. Moorcraft, L. Walker, E. F. Whittaker and M. S. Lennard, *Xenobiotica*, 2003, **33**(3), 225–237.
45. M. H. Court, *Vet. Clin. North Am.: Small Anim. Pract.*, 2013, **43**(5), 1027–1038.
46. A. Parkinson, B. Ogilvie, D. Buckely, F. Kazmi, M. Czerwinski and O. Parkinson, Biotransformation of Xenobiotics, *Casarett & Doull's Toxicology, the Basic Science of Poisons*, 8th edn, 2013, ch. 6.
47. M. Martignoni, G. M. M. Groothuis and R. de Kanter, *Expert Opin. Drug Metab. Toxicol.*, 2006, **2**(6), 875–894.
48. FDA Guidance for Industry, Pharmacokinetics in Patients with Impaired Hepatic Function: Study Design, Data Analysis, and Impact on Dosing and Labeling, 2003.
49. EMA Guideline on the evaluation of the pharmacokinetics of medicinal products in patients with impaired hepatic function, August 2005.
50. C. K. Yeung, D. D. Shen, K. E. Thummel and J. Himmelfarb, *Kidney Int.*, 2014, **85**(3), 522–528.
51. FDA Guidance for Industry, Pharmacokinetics in Patients with Impaired Renal Function –Study Design, Data Analysis, and Impact on Dosing, Draft, Sept 2020.
52. EMA Guideline on the evaluation of the pharmacokinetics of medicinal products in patients with decreased renal function, August 2014.
53. T. S. Tracy, A. S. Chaudhry, B. Prasad, K. E. Thummel, E. G. Schuetz, X.-b. Zhong, Y.-C. Tien, H. Jeong, X. Pan, L. M. Shireman, J. Tay-Sontheimer and Y. S. Lin, *Drug Metab. Dispos.*, 2016, **44**(3), 343–351.
54. M. E. Shams, *et al.*, *J. Clin. Pharmacol. Ther.*, 2006, **31**(5), 493–502.
55. J. G. Brockmoller, *et al.*, *Clin. Pharmacol. Ther.*, 2002, **72**, 438–452.
56. A. N. Werk and I. Cascorbi, *Clin. Pharmacol. Ther.*, 2014, **96**(3), 340–348.
57. R. N. Hines, *J. Biochem. Mol. Toxicol.*, 2007, **21**, 169–175.
58. B. P. Monahan and C. L. Fergason, *et al.*, *J. Am. Med. Assoc.*, 1990, **254**, 2788–2790.
59. FDA Guidance for Industry: *In vitro* Drug Interaction Studies — Cytochrome P450 Enzyme and Transporter-Mediated Drug Interactions, January 2020.
60. EMA Guideline on the Investigation of Drug Interactions, CPMP/EWP/560/95/Rev1 Corr2**, 2012.
61. J. G. Gerber, *Clin. Infect. Dis.*, 2000, **30**(Suppl 2), S123–S129.
62. B. C. Jones, H. Rollison, S. Johansson, K. P. Kanebratt, C. Lambert, K. Vishwanathan and T. B. Andersson, *Drug Metab. Dispos.*, 2017, **45**(1), 35–41.
63. www.fda.gov/Drugs/DevelopmentApprovalProcess/DevelopmentResources/DrugInteractionsLabeling/ucm0 93664.htm#table1-2.
64. P. J. H. Webborn, A. J. Parker, R. L. Denton and R. J. Riley, *Xenobiotica*, 2007, **37**, 1090–1109.
65. S. W. Paine, A. J. Parker, P. Gardiner, P. J. H. Webborn and R. J. Riley, *Drug Metab. Dispos.*, 2008, **36**, 1365–1374.
66. F. G. M. Russel, Transporters: Importance in drug absorption, distribution, and removal, in *Enzyme- and Transporter-based Drug–Drug Interactions Progress and Future Challenges*, ed. K. S. Pang, A. D. Rodrigues and R. M. Peter, *Am. Ass. Pharm. Sci.*, 2010, pp. 27–40.
67. K. M. Giacomini, A. Galetin and S. M. Huang, *Clin. Pharmacol. Ther.*, 2018, **104**, 766–771.
68. M. J. Zamek-Gliszczynski, M. E. Taub, P. P. Chothe, X. Chu, K. M. Giacomini, R. B. Kim, A. S. Ray, S. L. Stocker, J. D. Unadkat, M. B. Wittwer, C. Xia, S.-W. Yee, L. Zhang and Y. Zhang, *Clin. Pharmacol. Ther.*, 2018, **104**, 890–899.
69. Concept paper on a revision of the Guideline on the investigation of drug interactions, EMEA/CHMP/694687/2016, 23 March 2017.
70. D. A. Smith and M. Rowland, *Drug Metab. Dispos.*, 2019, **47**, 665–672.
71. D. Dalvie, *et al.*, *Drug Metab. Dispos.*, 2010, **38**, 641–654.
72. The International Transporter Consortium, Membrane transporters in drug development, *Nat. Rev. Drug Discovery*, 2010, **9**, 215–236.

# 8 ADME Optimization in Drug Discovery

Dermot F. McGinnity*[a] and Ken Grime[b]

[a]DMPK, Oncology R&D, AstraZeneca, Cambridge, UK; [b]DMPK, Respiratory & Immunology, Biopharma R&D, AstraZeneca, Gothenburg, Sweden
*E-mail: Dermot.F.McGinnity@astrazeneca.com

## 8.1 Introduction

The application of pharmacokinetic principles in drug discovery and development is now widespread due to the recognition of the role of drug concentrations as a surrogate for measuring pharmacological effects. A basic tenet of pharmacology is that the magnitude of a pharmacological response is a function of the drug concentration at the site of action. Thus, the objective of therapy may be achieved by maintaining sufficient concentration of drug at the site of action for the necessary duration, yet not so high as to elicit a deleterious effect. The concentration of drug is typically measured in blood or plasma, as direct measurement at the site of action is challenging.

Pharmacokinetics (PK) is defined as the study of change of drug concentration over time and describes a systematic approach to relating dose to amount of drug in the body and is typically separated into the distinct physiological processes of Absorption, Distribution, Metabolism and Excretion (ADME). The pharmaceutical industry is currently increasing the diversity of approaches to therapeutic intervention, including evaluation of many different new modality concepts in part in order to expand the druggable proteome. Small molecule chemistry is being diversified beyond previously established physicochemical guidelines for oral therapies such as the "Rule-of-5". For example PROteolysis Targeting Chimeras (PROTACs) are bifunctional high molecular weight (typically >650 Da) new chemical entities designed to target proteins for degradation by engaging the ubiquitin proteasome system and further considerations on the ADME properties for this exciting new therapeutic modality are considered later in the chapter.

The Handbook of Medicinal Chemistry: Principles and Practice, 2nd Edition
Edited by Simon E. Ward and Andrew M. Davis

Published by the Royal Society of Chemistry, www.rsc.org

The route of administration for potential therapies is an important consideration in drug discovery and design. The oral route is most common and favoured because of convenience and patient preference and ADME concepts for new chemical entities *via* the oral route of administration is the primary focus of this chapter. Parenteral (avoiding the gastrointestinal tract) routes will be covered with a section covering inhaled, topical and intravenous therapies.

It is now recognised in the pharmaceutical industry that acceptable human PK parameters and minimised drug–drug interaction potential increases the probability of a promising candidate becoming a successful therapy. Moreover, the role of DMPK scientists in drug discovery is not to merely provide project teams with measurements and data from the plethora of DMPK related assays and models that have been developed and implemented in screening cascades over the last 10–20 years, but to develop a mechanistic understanding of the disposition of the candidate drugs towards the optimisation and confident prediction of key properties associated with *human* drug absorption, clearance, distribution and elimination.[1] This is achievable from a consideration of physicochemical properties and data from *in vitro* assays with human-derived material and from *in vivo* animal studies. This chapter is targeted at medicinal chemists and drug design teams and provides general definitions of the fundamental PK parameters, together with such characterisation, prediction and optimisation strategies employed at AstraZeneca.

### 8.1.1 Absorption

Oral absorption can be defined as the irreversible transfer of a drug from the gut lumen across the mucosal membranes of the gastrointestinal tract. This is just one step in a multi-faceted process which transfers a drug from the site of administration (*i.e.* mouth) to the systemic circulation. The active pharmaceutical ingredient (API) typically taken using tablets or capsules in the mouth needs to dissolve in the fluids of the gastrointestinal tract where, prior to the absorptive step, it may be degraded by the acidic pH of the gastric fluid and gut flora enzymatic activity. The small intestine is the primary site of absorption due to its high surface area, drug permeability properties and high blood flow. Additionally drug movement through the gastrointestinal membranes is dependent on the physicochemical properties of the drug molecule. Drugs may be transported passively, *via* the transcellular route, that is, through the cell, passing through both apical and basolateral membranes, or the paracellular route, that is, between the cells. The majority of drugs are absorbed transcellularly, since paracellular permeability through water-filled tight junctions between cells decreases significantly with increasing molecular size (>250 Mwt) and lipophilicity ($\log P > 0$).[2] Absorption may also be facilitated or hindered by uptake and efflux transporter proteins.

It is important for the medicinal chemist to be able to differentiate the definitions of absorption *versus* oral bioavailability ($F$) which is the fraction of the dose of administered drug that reaches, in an unchanged form, the systemic circulation and is a measure of a compound's ability to avoid all the processes that protect the body from exposure to xenobiotics. These processes include the physical barrier of the gut wall, active transport into the gut lumen, metabolism in the gut, metabolism in the liver and biliary elimination. Thus *F* is a product of the fraction of dose that is absorbed through the gut and the fraction of drug that escapes elimination by the intestinal tract and liver, so called "first-pass" elimination. High extraction drugs that are rapidly metabolised will have low systemic exposure following an oral dose and low *F*, whereas low extraction drugs that are relatively stable to metabolism, assuming they are absorbed across the gut wall will have high systemic exposure following an oral dose and high *F*. Bioavailability is estimated from $F = \text{AUC}_{\text{oral}}/\text{AUC}_{\text{IV}}$, for an equivalent dose. Thus there exists an interplay between the physiology of gastrointestinal tract and compounds' biopharmaceutical, physicochemical and structure–activity properties with drug metabolising enzymes and transporters that are required to be understood to facilitate optimisation of new chemical entities to enable acceptable oral absorption and bioavailability.

## 8.1.2 Distribution

Drug distribution describes the reversible transfer of drug from one location to another. For an orally administered drug, distribution occurs from the bloodstream into the interstitial and intercellular fluids. Volume of distribution ($V_d$) is the theoretical volume that would have been available for the drug to disperse everywhere in the body were it at the same concentration as in the blood and can be derived following intravenous (IV) administration (Figure 8.1). A measured dose is administered and drug levels in plasma are determined over time. Early concentrations are back-extrapolated to estimate the concentration at $t = 0$, and simple mass balance considerations allow estimation of the volume that the dose would have to be distributed in to yield that concentration. This is the initial volume of distribution with units of L or L kg$^{-1}$ (Figure 8.1). If there is a mono exponential decline in plasma concentrations, this is the $V_d$. $V_d$ is most usefully thought of as a measure of the relative affinity of the compound for tissues over the sampled blood or plasma, and hence the ratio of the total amount of drug in the body to the concentration in the blood. The volume term that most accurately describes this measure, for multi-exponential profiles is the volume of distribution at steady-state ($V_{ss}$), since this is an estimate of drug distribution independent of elimination processes (steady state referring to the pseudo-equilibrium achieved between drug entering the tissues from the systemic blood and drug being eliminated from the body).

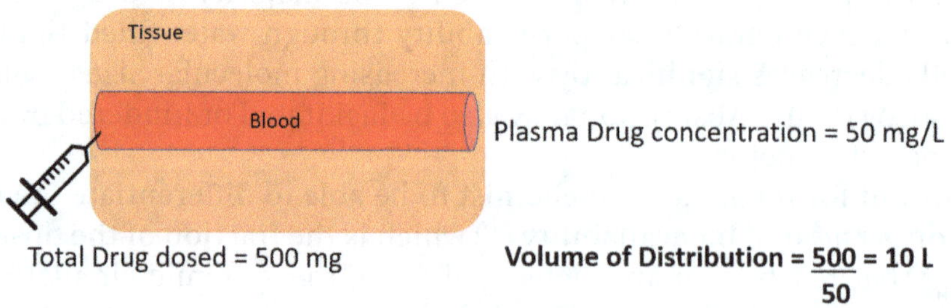


**Figure 8.1** Volume of distribution.

### 8.1.3 Metabolism

Xenobiotic metabolism can be defined as chemical transformation by a biological system, usually *via* drug metabolising enzymes, which typically converts relatively lipophilic compounds into more readily excreted hydrophilic metabolites. Drug metabolites may be pharmacologically active, weakly active, inactive or indeed reactive with endogenous macromolecules. The liver is the principal site of drug metabolism, moreover hepatic metabolic clearance is the predominant elimination route for oral marketed drugs.[3] The most important drug metabolism enzyme family are the cytochrome P-450s, a superfamily of membrane-bound isoenzymes that catalyses the oxidation of many drugs. In addition to oxidation, reduction and hydrolysis are common xenobiotic metabolism pathways and conjugation with endogenous polar substrates such as glucuronic acid and glutathione may occur directly to the parent molecule or after an initial transformation.

Clearance (CL) is the parameter that best describes the efficiency of the eliminating process. The area under the plasma concentration–time profile (AUC) for a given dose is a measure of how efficiently a compound is removed from the body. Compounds yielding low AUCs are eliminated by efficient processes. This ratio (dose/AUC) is used to derive the CL of a compound and has units of flow (mL $min^{-1}$ $kg^{-1}$). CL relates the rate of elimination (ng $min^{-1}$) to the substrate concentration (ng $mL^{-1}$) *i.e.* CL = rate of elimination/[substrate]. CL has units of flow and can be related to physiological parameters such as organ blood flows. A CL to hepatic blood flow ratio of 1 : 2 means 50% of the drug is extracted in a passage through the liver.

### 8.1.4 Excretion

Metabolism together with renal and biliary excretion are the major drug elimination routes in humans and preclinical species. Clearances are additive, if the processes are parallel. As human glomerular filtration rate (GFR) is only ~1.7 mL $min^{-1}$ $kg^{-1}$ and as the majority of drugs are to various extents bound to plasma proteins, CL *via* renal elimination is typically low, whereas biliary excretion can be an important route of elimination and remains challenging to predict to human.

An important PK parameter obtained from a simple fit of IV data is the half-life ($T_{1/2}$). Of course multi-exponential plasma drug concentration–time profiles have half-lives associated with each exponential phase of the decline (where the $T_{1/2}$ is ln(2)/exponential rate constant). The simplest case is often a profile that has an initial drug distribution phase (where the drug is subject to elimination, but the major process is distribution from the central systemic circulation into the tissues) and an elimination phase (in which the majority of the drug in the body is eliminated). It is this latter phase that accounts for the largest proportion of the AUC (since the drug is being eliminated) and approximates to $\ln(2) \times V_{ss}/\mathrm{CL}$. This is only the terminal $T_{1/2}$ if there is no later phase observed in the dose interval. Further phases of the plasma profile can occur beyond the elimination phase when, for example, the drug distributes into tissues or body compartments that release the drug with a rate lower than the elimination rate. This is typically true for lipophilic or basic drugs that have good distribution properties, but not for acidic drugs that do not distribute extensively beyond the plasma. The most important $T_{1/2}$ depends on the key phase of the profile for maintaining the drug concentration above the level required for efficacy. Generally the elimination $T_{1/2}$ is the most important, as it describes the decrease in plasma concentration associated with the largest proportion of the AUC and therefore largest drop in plasma (or blood) concentration of drug. This $T_{1/2}$ is consequently often the most influential in maintaining the drug concentration above the required minimum effective concentration. $T_{1/2}$ does not describe the efficiency of eliminating processes (this is CL) but is related to CL by the equation $T_{1/2} = \ln(2) \times V_d/CL$. Since there is only one value for CL, each $T_{1/2}$ is associated with a different distribution volume (*e.g.* initial, $V_0$, steady state, $V_{ss}$, terminal, $V_z$) and can be modulated accordingly by changing the $V_d$ or CL.

After identification of a relevant druggable target, maximising the likelihood of a chemical series yielding a candidate drug which subsequently becomes a marketed therapy can be achieved by optimising potency and selectivity for the target protein together with a strategy that achieves an adequate pharmacokinetic profile in patients with minimal drug–drug interaction potential. A drug discovery approach of optimising *key* properties in parallel undoubtedly maximises the probability of success. What can assist in this difficult, and at times seemingly insurmountable challenge, is that the key PK parameters of drugs are often strongly associated with their inherent physicochemical properties. Understanding these relationships is a key element of drug design. The most important physicochemical properties, in this context, are molecular size, hydrophobicity, aqueous solubility and ionisation state at physiological pH. These properties, to a greater or lesser extent, effect dissolution in the gastrointestinal tract and membrane permeability (and therefore oral absorption), susceptibility to drug metabolising enzymes and other elimination processes.

The sections below outline the authors' view of current best practice for optimising and predicting the key ADME parameters in human. It is intended to be a practical guide directing both optimisation strategies and mechanistic understanding for ADME properties in drug discovery and development. There are many literature sources that provide more fundamental information. The authors can strongly advocate *Metabolism, Pharmacokinetics and Toxicity of Functional* groups edited by Dennis Smith.[4] For a comprehensive analysis of pharmacokinetics and full derivation of equations the authoritative reference, *Clinical Pharmacokinetics* by Rowland and Tozer[5] is recommended.

## 8.2 Optimization and Prediction of Key Human Pharmacokinetic Parameters in Drug Discovery

Both human PK and clinically efficacious dose may be estimated from *in vitro* experiments utilising human-derived material and by *in vivo* animal studies. Prediction of clinical dose is a useful parameter in the optimisation of compounds as a holistic measure of "quality" that relies on both human PK estimates and on the anticipated therapeutic concentration.[6] The prediction and refinement of therapeutic concentrations in relevant patient populations is vital. It is built on the foundation of a quantitative understanding between target engagement and relevant biomarkers, from an integrated assessment, in which the pharmacology and the role of the biological target in the pathophysiology of the disease are considered to establish an exposure and target engagement profile most likely to deliver clinical efficacy. Thus pharmacokinetic–pharmacodynamic (PKPD) relationships should be derived from clinical precedents, preclinical PD or disease models and mechanistic studies of the drug–target interaction, and refined throughout the life of a project. The optimization and prediction of human PK and the clinical dose that delivers the required extent and duration of target engagement are essential elements of drug discovery projects.[1,6]

In addition to potency and selectivity against the target, the focus for oral drug design teams with respect to optimization strategies, should be on the influential PK parameters, $F_{abs,}$ CL and $V_{ss}$. Establishing a set of quantitative criteria for these parameters upfront in programs facilitates optimization towards, and discovery of, a promising candidate drug as rapidly and efficiently as possible. A PK property that remains challenging to determine is the free concentration of drug at the site of pharmacological action, which is dependent on the involvement of drug transporters, a rapidly developing yet still immature area of ADME science. The next sections outline the authors' experience and view of current best practice for predicting the key PK parameters for patients.

## 8.2.1 Oral Absorption

Inter-patient variability in drug exposure is inversely related to bioavailability,[7] and therefore absolute bioavailability in humans of greater than 30% is an appropriate target for acceptable inter-subject variability, and effect on dose size. As $F$ is a product of the fraction of absorbed drug, the fraction escaping intestinal metabolism and liver extraction as it passes from the portal vein to the systemic circulation ($F = F_{abs} \times F_g \times F_h$) targeting a human absorption of ≥50% is appropriate.

It is important to understand the relevance of the contribution of first pass hepatic and intestinal metabolism, and of intestinal permeability, and not just determine $F$ in preclinical species. As animal *in vivo* PK may poorly predict human kinetics, good PK properties in animals *per se* are not necessarily a sign of quality in molecules; likewise a low animal bioavailability value and/or suboptimal PK profile is not necessarily an indicator of poor human PK. The real value of animal PK data is to validate, or otherwise, the approaches that are used to predict PK in the clinic. Fundamentally, low bioavailability in animals may impact in limiting exposure in preclinical PD, efficacy and safety testing.

An assessment of the role of intestinal drug extraction is a component of the human $F$ prediction. Intestinal drug metabolizing enzymes are well characterized with CYP3A, CYP2C9 and uridine 5′-diphospho-glucuronosyltransferase (UGT) predominating.[8–13] Mathematical modeling can enable *in vitro* data to be used in the prediction of $F_g$ and extraction by the intestine can be similar to or exceed hepatic extraction, despite much less intestinal compared to hepatic cytochrome P450 (CYP).[14–18] Intestinal extraction is typically associated with metabolically unstable drugs. Efficient location of drug metabolizing enzymes including CYP3A4 and p-glycoprotein efflux transporter (which also share substrate specificity), in the villus tip of enterocytes, facilitates cycling of drugs, thereby prolonging exposure and therefore, intestinal metabolism.[14,15,19,20] Compounds of limited permeability, that are also good substrates for efflux transporters and drug metabolizing enzymes are likely to be efficiently extracted by the intestine. If optimization strategies early in the drug discovery process are effective at mitigating these properties, intestinal metabolism should rarely be a significant issue for candidate drugs.

Optimizing towards compounds with appropriate physicochemical properties that ensure sufficient solubility of crystalline API, and transmembrane permeability should maximize oral absorptive potential of candidate drugs. The apparent permeability measure ($P_{app}$) is typically obtained from assessment of drug flux across a monolayer of cells intended to mimic the intestinal barrier, most commonly determined using Madin–Darby canine kidney (MDCK) or Caco-2 cell lines.[14,21] $P_{app}$ values are transformed into effective permeability ($P_{eff}$) values, describing intestinal permeability per unit surface area, as a prerequisite to develop relationships between *in vitro* permeability and human absorption.[14,22]

It is now widely accepted that efflux by p-glycoprotein or other intestinal drug transporters is unlikely in most cases to limit absorption of drugs with good permeability and solubility.[23,24] However, *in vivo* p-glycoprotein dependent efflux can be clinically relevant if the $K_m$ between substrate-p-glycoprotein is high (>10s of μM) and/or the dose is low (<1 mg kg$^{-1}$).[25] The intestinal drug concentration range sufficient for interacting with p-glycoprotein may be estimated from the maximum dose taken per 250 mL (intestinal fluid volume) or alternatively, *via* an estimation of the maximum concentration in the enterocyte ($F_{abs} \times k_a \times$ dose/$Q_{ent}$, where $Q_{ent}$ is enterocyte blood flow).[14,20]

In our laboratory, a solubility–permeability heat map has been generated (Figure 8.2), and is used as a visual and simple tool which demonstrates for a 1 mg kg$^{-1}$ dose a fraction absorbed in human of ≥50% (green circles) requires a crystalline solubility of 100 μM and a Caco-2 $P_{app}$ of 5 × 10$^{-6}$ cm s$^{-1}$.[26] Especially for compounds that have borderline physicochemical properties, supplementary dynamic simulations incorporating measured *in vitro* permeability and dissolution rate measures, such as commercial software Gastroplus® or SimCYP®, validated with known clinical data, are valuable at providing additional information for decision making.[25,27,28] Indeed more generally,

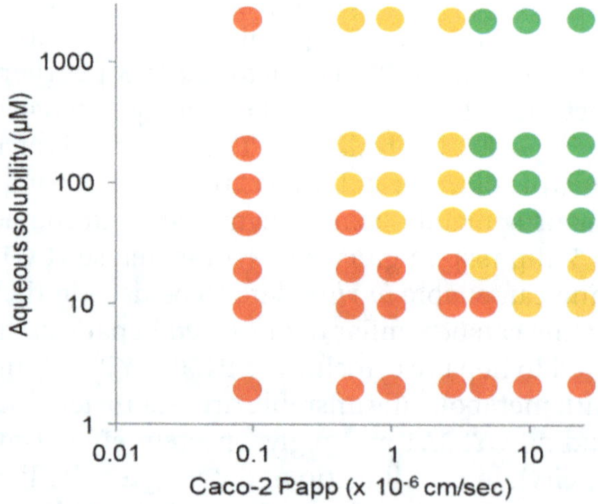


**Figure 8.2** Absorption heat map.

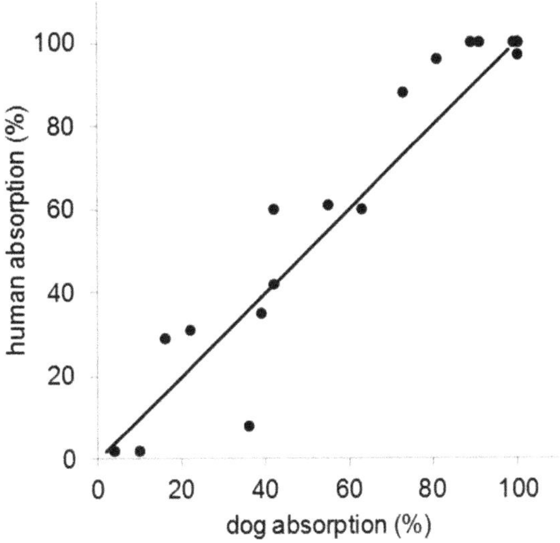


**Figure 8.3** Relationship showing correlation between human absorption and dog absorption for compounds with Mwt >325. The line of unity is shown. Reproduced from ref. 6 with permission from Bentham Science, Copyright 2007.

physiologically based pharmacokinetic (PBPK) modeling approaches have great utility in the prediction and simulation of PK profiles, including the potential for assessing likely variability in patients.

In oral drug discovery programs, an estimate of rat oral bioavailability is likely important for determining if safety or PD/efficacy studies can be adequately performed, yet poor oral absorption in the rat should not *per se* preclude progression of compounds. In our experience rat oral absorption is, generally, not a good predictor of human absorption.[6] This is most likely explained, at least in part, by the fact that once normalized for body surface area, the rat small intestine has a four times lower surface area compared to human.[29] Predicting human absorption from preclinical *in vivo* data is more successful using dog as a model, since the dog to human absorption correlation appears strong for high molecular weight (>325) compounds, when absorption is not by the paracellular route oral (Figure 8.3, adapted from McGinnity *et al.*[6]). In our experience, for drugs absorbed by the transcellular route, not only does dog PK data indicate a systematically greater absorption than in rat, but also that dog absorption, using crystalline API and an appropriate formulation, is more akin to human. Good oral drug-like physicochemical properties providing sufficient aqueous solubility of the crystalline form and passive transcellular permeability can support a confident and acceptable human absorption prediction of ≥50%, which can be further strengthened by good *in vivo* absorption in the dog.

## 8.2.2 Volume of Distribution

$V_d$ is a measure of the relative affinity of a drug for tissues and plasma, thus correlating with the relative affinity of compound for tissues. This is expressed by the equation: $V_d = [fu_p/fu_T] \times V_T + V_P$, with units of L $kg^{-1}$, where $fu_p$ is the unbound drug fraction in the plasma; $fu_T$ is the unbound drug fraction in the tissue; $V_T$ is the volume of the tissue (~1 L kg$^{-1}$) and $V_P$ is the volume of the plasma (0.03 L kg$^{-1}$). As $V_T \gg V_P$, changes in $fu_p$ will directly affect $V_d$.[5] Moreover, Øie and Tozer's approach defines the key driver of inter-species differences in $V_d$ to be differences in ppb on the assumption that inter-species differences in tissue binding are minimal.[30] Using preclinical *in vivo* PK data and correcting for species ppb differences, $V_d$ or $V_{ss}$ as the most predictable of PK parameters: if unbound volumes are consistent across species, human volume can be predicted from animal data, by estimating $V_u$ (Figure 8.4). Based on our experience, unbound $V_{ss}$ is usually conserved within 2-fold across species.

In general, bulk physicochemical properties rather than specific pharmacophores determine $V_d$ values, albeit transporters can modulate distribution into and out of tissues. Typically, for drug-like molecules, acids have low (<1 L kg$^{-1}$), neutrals and zwitterions moderate (1–3 L kg$^{-1}$), monobases high (>3 L kg$^{-1}$) and dibases very high (>10 L kg$^{-1}$) steady-state $V_d$ values (Figure 8.5). Basic drugs tend to have similar ppb to neutral drugs, in contrast to acids, which show higher binding, even for a given $\log D_{7.4}$.[31] The overriding influence on the distribution of acidic drugs is that of extensive binding to albumin in plasma. Apparent distribution volumes thus approach that of albumin, approximately 0.1 L kg$^{-1}$ and do not typically exceed 0.3 L kg$^{-1}$ unless active hepatic uptake or entero-hepatic re-circulation is a factor. Re-circulation of parent drug after elimination in bile (of parent or glucuronide that can be hydrolyzed to parent in the gastrointestinal tract) can lead to an extended

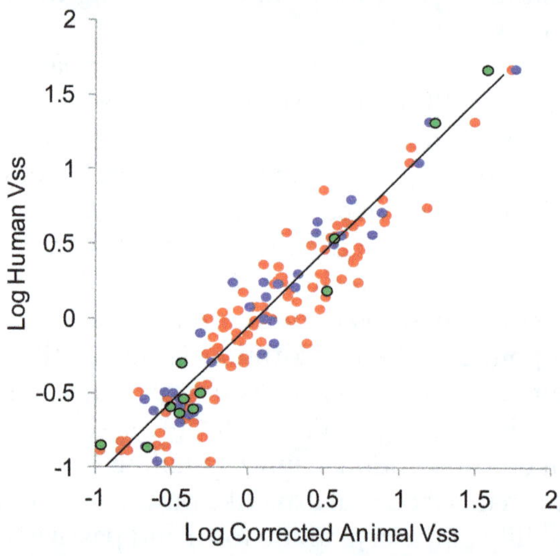


**Figure 8.4** Using preclinical species to predict human $V_{ss}$. Reproduced from ref. 6 with permission from Bentham Science, Copyright 2007. Relationship between human $V_{ss}$ values and preclinical animal $V_{ss}$ values corrected for human/animal differences in ppb as detailed in McGinnity *et al.*, 2007.[6] Red circles are data from rats, green from mice and blue from dogs. The dataset includes both data generated in this laboratory and literature data from rat, dog and mouse, and compared to clinical $V_{ss}$. Line of regression shown with the equation $\log y = 1.\log x + 0.06$, $r^2 = 0.93$, $p = 4.6 \times 10^{-101}$, afe = 1.36. Thus human $V_{ss}$ can be predicted from preclinical animals using eqn (8.1).

PK profile and a larger apparent $V_{ss}$. Moreover, this can yield incorrect predictions if extrapolating to a species where re-circulation does not occur to same extent. The $V_d$ for neutral drugs is governed by hydrophobic interactions with plasma proteins and tissue membranes. Increasing lipophilicity raises tissue affinity, but also has the counter effect of restricting tissue distribution due to an increase in ppb. Being positively charged at physiological pH, bases have favorable interactions with anionic phospholipid head groups leading to higher tissue affinity and therefore for the same ppb as a neutral compound, a base will tend to have a higher tissue distribution.[32] Ion trapping in lysosomes, sub-cellular acidic organelles abundant in liver and lung, also contribute.[33] $V_d$ is not by itself a parameter that should typically be optimized in drug discovery, rather, estimates of the boundaries of $V_d$ for a given chemical series can be transformed into a strategy for obtaining the necessary human elimination $T_{1/2}$ *via* optimizing the elimination processes towards a target CL value. Modification of a neutral molecule by adding a basic group can be successfully employed, for example in the discovery of the dihydropyridine calcium channel blocker, amlodipine, which, compared to the neutral analogue nifedipine, has a long plasma half-life (35 h) due, in large part, to the resultant high volume of distribution.[34] However in the authors' experience this apparently straightforward strategy to increase $T_{1/2}$ is not often successful due to the basic centre introducing other deleterious properties, including increasing $CL_{int}$.

$V_{ss}$ is reasonably predictable from physicochemical properties, *in silico* approaches,[35,36] and *in vitro* data.[37–39] However, the Oie and Tozer method from preclinical species PK appears superior for making human predictions, as demonstrated by several

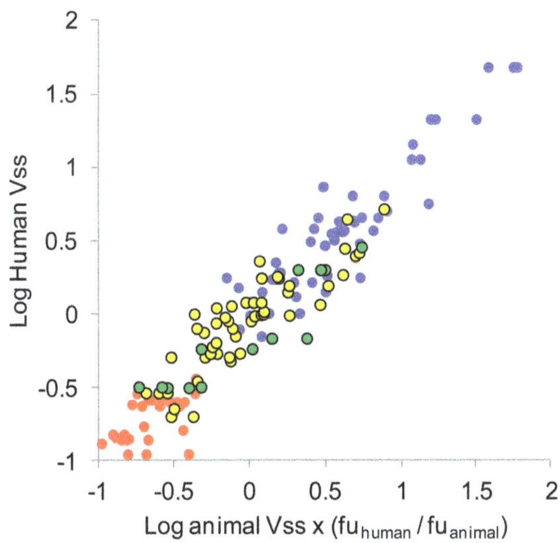


**Figure 8.5** Using preclinical species to predict human $V_{ss}$ for compounds with a range of physicochemical properties. Relationship between human $V_{ss}$ values and preclinical animal $V_{ss}$ values corrected for human/animal differences in ppb. Red circles are acids, green – zwitterions, yellow – neutrals and blue – bases. Same data as included in Figure 8.4 and McGinnity *et al.*, 2007.[6]

laboratories.[1,6,40–42] Also, as determination of PK profiles are required for several reasons in at least two species before clinical candidate selection this is the preferred predictive methodology (*via* eqn (8.1)) in our laboratory for candidate drugs.

$$\log(V_{\text{SS}_{\text{human}}}) = \log\left(V_{\text{SS}_{\text{animal}}}\frac{\text{fu}_{\text{human}}}{\text{fu}_{\text{animal}}} + 0.1\left(1 - \frac{\text{fu}_{\text{human}}}{\text{fu}_{\text{animal}}}\right)\right) - 0.06 \quad (8.1)$$

## 8.2.3 Distribution into Central Nervous System

The blood–brain barrier (BBB) consists of endothelial cells with tight junctions and drug movement into the brain occurs *via* passive transcellular diffusion or active uptake. The endothelial cells of the BBB contain efflux transporters, including p-glycoprotein (P-gp) and breast cancer resistance protein (BCRP), which actively pump drugs from the brain into the blood, thus restricting exposure of drugs to the brain and limiting efficacy for CNS therapies.

At AstraZeneca, good brain penetrance properties is an important design criteria for oncology drugs that are aimed at treating primary brain tumours and secondary metastases. We have developed a set of preclinical assays and models, incorporating assessment of human transporter substrate activity, unbound brain/plasma ratios ($K_{\text{puu}}$) and positron emission tomography (PET) imaging studies in rodents and cynomolgus monkeys.[43] This strategy has recently been validated with the discovery of brain penetrant ATM inhibitors,[44] being investigated for the treatment of glioblastoma, building on the success of brain penetrant osimertinib, a third generation irreversible tyrosine kinase inhibitor approved for first line treatment of patients with EGFRm and T790M positive non-small cell lung cancer, and demonstrated to be effective in treating CNS malignancies.[45]

Compounds that demonstrate good BBB penetrance (*i.e.* $K_{\text{puu}}$ approaching unity) are both passively permeable and not substrates of the major human BBB efflux transporters. Consequently, *in vitro* assays that determine intrinsic passive permeability and human P-gp and BCRP transporter activity are important to have as first line assays to direct compound design. *In vitro* cell culture monolayers from Madin–Darby canine kidney (MDCK) cells overexpressing human efflux transporters P-gp and BCRP, both individually and as dual transfected cell lines provide useful models. The efflux ratio of compounds in these assays can be determined by the apparent permeability ($P_{\text{app}}$) in the B to A direction across the monolayer divided by the A to B $P_{\text{app}}$. Progression criteria in drug discovery programs drive compound design to reduce efflux ratios as low as possible towards 1. In our experience, rat brain $K_{\text{puu}}$ represents a useful *in vivo* model for human $K_{\text{puu}}$, therefore $K_{\text{puu}}$ rodent determinations and imaging techniques ensure a complementary range of BBB models can be exploited to design and identify brain penetrant drugs. In practical terms, in drug discovery a $K_{\text{puu}}$ target of >0.3 is often used, whilst poorly BBB penetrant compounds have $K_{\text{puu}}$ values <0.05. PET microdosing allows the distribution of compounds in the healthy brain of primates to be studied. This can be employed for candidate drugs, as primates represent the closest brain model to human with *in vivo* studies to date supporting good concordance between the species.

### 8.2.4 Human Clearance

Identification of the elimination route and rate in preclinical species and optimization of human CL are major challenges and goals of most drug discovery projects. The major drug CL routes in humans and preclinical species are metabolic, biliary and renal, and as there is currently no reliable way to predict human elimination from purely *in silico* or *in vitro* methods, a combination of determining CL routes in preclinical species and use of *in vitro* human tools is required to predict human CL.

Liver is the major xenobiotic metabolizing organ and it is now widely accepted that *in vitro–in vivo* extrapolation (IVIVE) can be used to estimate hepatic metabolic CL in human and animals, *via in vitro* determination of rates of turnover and a mathematical liver model.[46–52] The model describes hepatic metabolic CL ($CL_H$), *via* terms for liver blood flow ($Q_h$), hepatic intrinsic clearance ($CL_{int}$) and blood binding ($fu_b$). Hepatocytes are the optimal *in vitro* system for predicting *in vivo* metabolic hepatic CL, as they contain the full complement of drug metabolizing enzymes and transporters. However, data from subcellular liver fractions such as microsomes, which define the oxidative metabolic component, and which have a larger dynamic range than hepatocytes, can add value by increasing the mechanistic understanding of the primary metabolic pathways for chemical series and key compounds. Both hepatic microsomes and hepatocytes are used routinely for this purpose in our laboratory. A panel of recombinant heterologously expressed CYPs can also be used to predict metabolic CL and to determine the individual CYPs responsible for the metabolism of key compounds. This information is important to understand likely variability of CL in the population associated with metabolism *via* polymorphic CYPs, potential intestinal CL contributions (*e.g.* if *via* CYP3A and 2C9) and to determine the risk of drug–drug interactions as victims of coadministered inhibitors of the CYPs involved. There is less drug–drug interaction risk associated with compounds that are cleared *via* multiple CYPs and other elimination routes. For this reason alone it is important to attempt to quantify all elimination pathways as far as possible.

Predicting *in vivo* hepatic metabolic CL involves initially building *in vivo–in vitro* $CL_{int}$ models for each species using a training set of compounds with estimated *in vivo* hepatic metabolic CL values, *via* subtracting non-hepatic metabolic CL from total CL values. Hepatocyte $CL_{int}$ is measured and the fraction unbound in the incubation ($fu_{inc}$) incorporated to calculate unbound *in vitro* $CL_{int}$, which is scaled up to a whole liver unbound $CL_{int}$.[46] To establish prediction accuracy, the unbound *in vivo* $CL_{int}$ of the test compound is calculated from *in vivo* hepatic metabolic CL adjusted for *in vivo* blood binding. The derived unbound *in vitro* and *in vivo* $CL_{int}$ values form a line of correlation from which estimations of unbound *in vivo* $CL_{int}$ values for test compounds can be made after determination of *in vitro* $CL_{int}$.[46,47,49,52] Evaluation of the predictive accuracy for the test compound is made against the *linear* relationship of unbound *in vitro vs. in vivo* $CL_{int}$, not CL. Figure 8.6 is a schematic that demonstrates the approach, using all the *in vitro* measured terms on the *X*-axis and predicting *in vivo* $CL_{int}$ from the *Y*-axis. Intrinsic clearance estimates from human liver microsome or hepatocyte incubations ($CL_{int}$) are scaled to a liver $CL_{int}$ according to:

$$\text{Scaled liver } CL_{int} = CL_{int} \times \text{Scaling Factor} \times fu_b/fu_{inc}$$

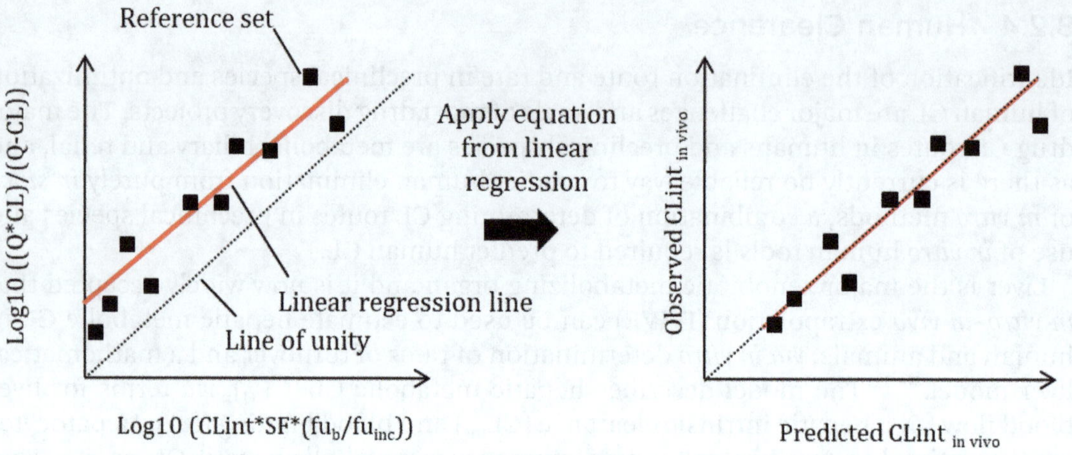


**Figure 8.6** Schematic showing how the regression offset is applied to empirically correct the scaled *in vitro* data.

where the "Scaling Factor" (SF) for microsomes represents the product of microsomal product yield ($mg_{protein}\ g_{liver}^{-1}$) and liver weight ($g_{liver}\ kg_{body\ weight}^{-1}$) and for hepatocytes represents the product of hepatocellularity ($10^6$ cells per $g_{liver}$) and liver weight ($g_{liver}\ kg_{body\ weight}^{-1}$).

The resultant scaled liver $CL_{int}$ is converted to a "Predicted $CL_{int\ in\ vivo}$" using a regression line established for a reference set of drugs ($n = 57$). As can be observed from Figure 8.6, this approach yields a systematic underprediction of *in vivo* $CL_{int}$ for reasons not yet mechanistically understood, although several explanations have been proposed. However, it is important to appreciate that this underprediction factor, corrected *via* use of the regression line, is associated with the assay, not the compounds and is observed across laboratories, microsomes or hepatocytes and species. Predicted hepatic metabolic (blood) clearance is then calculated from "Predicted $CL_{int\ in\ vivo}$" by application of the well-stirred model:

$$\text{Hepatic Metabolic CL} = \text{LBF} \times \text{Predicted } CL_{int\ in\ vivo}/(\text{LBF} + \text{Predicted } CL_{int\ in\ vivo})$$

In general this "regression offset correction"-based IVIVE method has been found to predict hepatic metabolic $CL_{int\ in\ vivo}$ within 3-fold for ~60% of compounds and within 5-fold for ~80% of compounds. Absolute average fold-error is generally ~2.5-fold.

More recently in our laboratory and others, compounds demonstrating significantly higher human liver microsomal $CL_{int}$ relative to human hepatocyte $CL_{int}$ have been encountered, the majority being CYP3A substrates.[53] A mechanistic explanation for this phenomenon is subject to ongoing research. Using hepatocyte $CL_{int}$ for CYP3A substrates, the current IVIVE regression offset approach remains an appropriate strategy to predict $CL_{met}$. However, using the same approach for HLM significantly overpredicts $CL_{met}$ for CYP3A substrates, highlighting that a different IVIVE regression offset is required for CYP3A substrates using microsomes.[53]

If the unbound *in vivo* $CL_{int}$ has been accurately predicted in animals, typically rat and dog, the approach can be used in humans with some confidence that a similar relationship may apply. Moreover, if rat and dog hepatic metabolic *in vivo* $CL_{int}$ *cannot* be predicted from *in vitro* data there should be little confidence that a similar approach will predict human $CL_{int}$. Importantly for candidate drugs, a quantitative mechanistic understanding of rates and routes of elimination pathways in human-derived *in vitro* milieu and preclinical species is critical to increase the likelihood of successful prediction of rates and routes in humans.

In our laboratory the instances of "lack of scaling" of *in vitro* to *in vivo* $CL_{int}$ in chemical series or key compounds are relatively frequent and require a systematic approach to investigate the possible causes of such disconnects. It is advisable that the first step should always be a close examination of existing *in vitro* $CL_{int}$ and *in vivo* PK data, as several experimental and/or biological phenomena may have led to an under- or overestimation of *in vitro* or *in vivo* $CL_{int}$. An understanding of the known rates, and metabolic and excretion routes, from structurally related compounds may provide more understanding and an experimental investigation of the key *in vitro* measured terms, $CL_{int}$, B:P, ppb and $fu_{inc}$, can follow. Often discovering the cause of poor CL predictions adds to the mechanistic understanding of the compound's disposition, which may increase, or indeed decrease, the confidence in an accurate human CL prediction.

Consideration of significant extra-hepatic metabolic CL may include experimental identification of the enzymes responsible for metabolism. These may include amidases, esterases, amine oxidases and transferases, for example, and experiments using hepatic and non-hepatic subcellular fractions and blood or plasma can be useful. Plasma hydrolysis of drugs can be scaled to whole body CL from *in vitro* data by multiplying the measured *in vitro* elimination rate constant ($\ln(2)/T_{1/2}$) by the volume of plasma. Unless the rate is rapid, hydrolysis solely in plasma is unlikely to be a major CL pathway, but hydrolysis can occur at a number of sites throughout the body and the cumulative CL can thus be both high and challenging to estimate. Indeed, for compounds cleared *via* drug metabolizing enzymes other than the CYPs or UGTs on which the IVIVE approaches have been predominantly validated may require additional experimentation and refined methodologies can be applied as appropriate.

A common misconception is that high ppb is to be avoided or designed away from and decreasing ppb will result in a lower efficacious dose through the generation of higher circulating free drug concentrations available to the pharmacological target. However, this neglects the fact that decreasing ppb also results in higher CL. Thus for most drugs, decreasing ppb has no effect on the *in vivo* unbound drug concentration. The $T_{1/2}$ is, in most cases, also largely unaffected, since CL and $V_d$ are impacted similarly by ppb changes. The only notable exception to this is when ppb is so high that drug distribution volume is restricted to that of plasma proteins. At this lower limiting value for $V_d$, increasing ppb further does indeed lower CL but with $V_d$ unaffected, $T_{1/2}$ increases. These concepts are elegantly and comprehensively outlined by DA Smith *et al.*, 2010,[32] which provides guidance on the use of ppb in drug discovery. Therefore the focus should be on physiochemical parameters such as $\log P$, $pK_a$ and PSA or structural modifications based on knowledge of the metabolically liable functional groups to affect a change in unbound CL, in order to optimize free drug concentration. Lowering lipophilicity in isolation may prove unproductive due to concomitant effects on unbound CL and unbound $V_d$, thus leaving $T_{1/2}$ unchanged.

Renal excretion of untransformed compounds can be complex and may involve both passive and active components. The high pressure and relatively large pores in the glomerulus result in free drug in blood entering the proximal tubule. The filtration rate, as a CL, is the product of the compound's fraction unbound in blood and GFR (approximately 1.7 mL $min^{-1}$ $kg^{-1}$ in humans), and thus can be readily estimated. As the majority of drugs are highly bound to blood proteins, passive renal CL is low in particular, relative to hepatic CL. Furthermore only compounds with negative $\log D_{7.4}$ values are passively renally cleared to any extent as the kidney tubules passively reabsorbs molecules of sufficient lipophilicity back into the blood.[54] Uptake transporter proteins may recover compounds if sufficient structural similarities exist to their physiological endogenous substrates. Active renal secretion consists of uptake across the basolateral membrane of the proximal tubule then egress across the apical membrane *via* combinations of different transporters polarized to the apical or basolateral membrane. In humans the principal transporters in the basolateral membrane are organic anion transporters OAT1 and OAT3 and organic cation transporter OCT2, whilst the apical transporters include P-gp, BCRP, multidrug resistance protein (MRP2, MRP4), organic anion transporters OAT4 and URAT1, and organic cation transporters OCTN1, OCTN2 and MATE-1.[55] Intuitively, transporter dependent renal CL is likely to be less predictable across species than when flow dependent passive processes predominate. However, in our laboratory, a reasonable prediction using dog renal CL corrected for ppb and kidney blood flow species differences emerged for a diverse set of 36 actively secreted drugs, forming the basis of our approach to predicting renal CL in human for candidate drugs (Figure 8.7).[56] Male rat renal CL correlated less well with human possibly due to poor species cross-over for OAT substrates or sex differences for rat OATP substrates.[57,58] The continued development of human-derived *in vitro* models for the prediction of active human renal CL and kidney transporter mediated drug–drug interactions is an area of ongoing research.

Biliary excretion is an important elimination route, but in part due to the lack of high-quality definitive clinical data there remains no consensus on the best practice strategy to predict human biliary CL and human-derived *in vitro* models are still in active development.[59,60] As for renal elimination, biliary excretion of drugs can be a two-step process involving the hepatic uptake transporters organic anion transporting polypeptide (OATP), OAT and OCT, and bile canalicular efflux transporters P-gp, BCRP, MRP1 and MRP2.[60–63] High biliary CL is most often observed with acids, likely due to synergy between OATP and MRP transporters. Indeed in our experience it is acids where biliary CL and renal CL typically contribute most to total CL and therefore for acids, these determinations should be made routinely.[64] In the authors' laboratory, rat, dog and human biliary CL data from drugs of different chemotypes and therapeutic classes were compared (Figure 8.8).[65] For the majority of the compounds studied, rat unbound biliary CL values, when corrected for body weight and ppb differences, were >10-fold higher than the human value with some >100-fold. Interestingly, these compounds appeared to be substrates for hepatic uptake OATP transporters. This is in line with the observation that rat uptake transporters are typically more efficient than the human and dog counterparts.[65,66] Albeit based on relatively few compounds, dog biliary CL, when corrected for body weight and ppb differences appears to be more

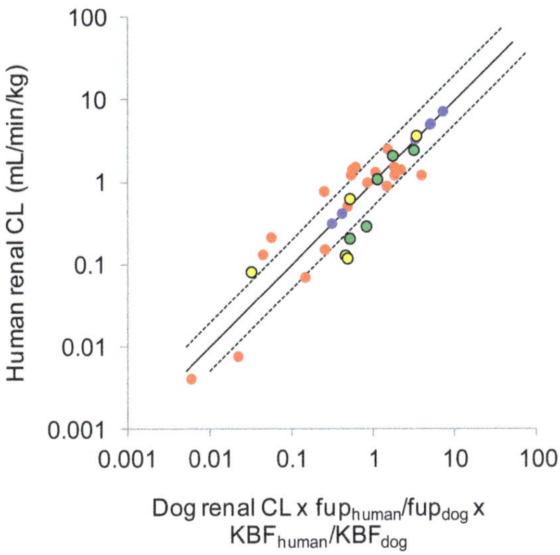


**Figure 8.7** Relationship between human renal clearance and dog renal clearance corrected for human/dog differences in ppb and kidney blood flow. Red circles are acids, blue - bases, yellow - neutrals and green - zwitterions. Reproduced from ref. 56 with permission from The American Society for Pharmacology and Experimental Therapeutics, Copyright 2011.

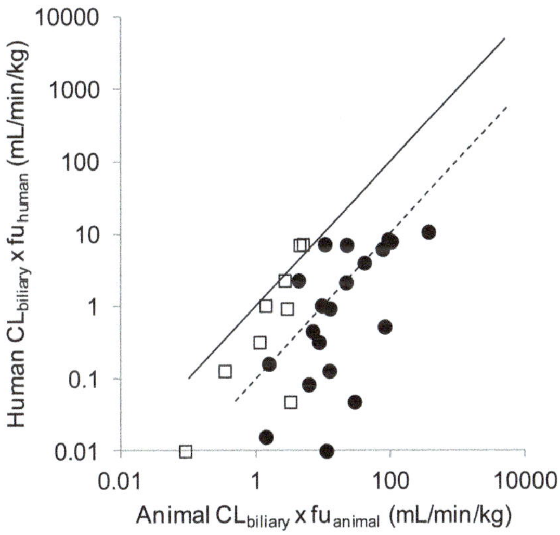


**Figure 8.8** Relationship between unbound human biliary clearance and unbound rat (solid circles) and unbound dog (open squares) biliary clearance. Reproduced from ref. 65 with permission from American Chemical Society, Copyright 2013.

comparable to human than rat. However, for drugs that seemingly have no significant active hepatic uptake component, rat, dog and human biliary CL were similar.

In the literature, several inter-species allometric scaling methodologies for biliary CL have been evaluated,[67–69] but a consensus is not apparent, likely due to the relatively few compounds analyzed, the fact that some used total drug-related material rather than parent and that allometry underpredicts human biliary CL for some compounds but not others.[70,71] Simple allometry using unbound CL and an exponent of 0.66 gave the best predictions of 18 drugs between rat and human.[72] Human predictions were within 3-fold of observed values for 12 of the compounds, yet for others human CL was overestimated by one to two orders of magnitude. Compared to rat alone, multiple species allometry using biliary CL data corrected for ppb yielded improved predictions.[72]

Intuitively, because CL predictions require several input parameters (hepatocyte $CL_{int}$, extra hepatic $CL_{int}$, renal and biliary CL, ppb, *in vitro* incubational binding, B:P) human estimates are more uncertain than for oral absorption or $V_{ss}$. In summary, human CL can be predicted as follows: human hepatic metabolic CL from human hepatocyte $CL_{int}$, human renal CL from dog renal CL and human biliary CL tentatively estimated from the dog or rat biliary CL for non-OATP substrates. Both prediction of renal and biliary CL remain important challenges from human-derived *in vitro* tools. Publications from GSK, J&J and Novartis.[73–75] confirm the authors' view that allometric scaling approaches offer fairly poor predictivity of human clearance, in particular for metabolic clearance where there may be clear species differences in metabolic rates and routes. However, for a key candidate drug an allometric prediction in agreement with the more mechanistic and validated approaches presented here may increase the confidence in that human CL prediction, thus adding value to decision making.

## 8.3 ADME Considerations for PROTACs

PROteolysis Targeting Chimeras (PROTACs) are bifunctional molecules that target both the protein of interest and an ubiquitin E3 ligase, thus marking the protein for proteasomal degradation *via* the ubiquitin proteasome system. As such, PROTACs are an exciting new therapeutic modality that should expand the druggable proteome. The first PROTAC therapeutics have now reached the clinic, yet drug discovery optimisation strategies regarding ADME properties are only beginning to be published. Indeed our laboratory has recently shared some of our initial experiences and lessons learned to date regarding ADME properties of PROTACs and the reader is directed to this publication and references therein for a broader discussion of this exciting emerging topic.[76]

In short, the common structural features of two separate pharmacophores connected by a linker chain mandate a relatively high (>500 Da) molecular weight for PROTACs, thus forcing divergence from accepted small molecule oral drug-like property space with respect to lipophilicity, hydrogen bond donors/acceptors, rotatable bonds and polar surface area *etc.* Unexpectedly, using cereblon E3 ligands, acceptable rodent (mouse and rat) pharmacokinetics, including relatively high oral bioavailability (>30%) has been relatively routinely achieved with multiple protein-of-interest ligands and preferred linkers. However, profiling compounds from this much higher lipophilicity range ($\log D_{pH7.4}$ values >4) than usual for traditional small molecules, has resulted in multiple challenges to standard ADME *in vitro* screening cascades. Issues include poor aqueous solubility, very high levels of non-specific binding to labware and protein, as well as chemical instability. These have resulted in challenges in accurate determinations of values such as Caco-2 $P_{apps}$, plasma protein and tissue binding, and aqueous solubility values, amongst other experimental measurements.

High metabolic stability in liver fractions have been achievable, even for highly lipophilic PROTACs (unbound $CL_{int}$ may be high) and compounds were selected for mouse and rat PK largely on this property rather than from the plethora of *in vitro* values, including solubility and permeability, that typically precede *in vivo* evaluation of conventional small molecules. Due to the bifunctional nature of PROTACs, understanding metabolic fate can be particularly complex. Of particular note is the potential to generate metabolites that retain affinity to the POI and/or E3 ligase, which may compete with the parent PROTAC to block the mode of action. Therefore evaluation of circulating metabolites should be incorporated into *in vivo* PK/PD and efficacy studies. Overall hepatic metabolic clearance appears to predominate as the major disposition route for PROTACs, as for the few examples we have tested, biliary and renal clearance are not major clearance pathways and overall *in vivo* clearance is well estimated from hepatocyte $CL_{int}$.

In comparison to the depth of understanding of the physicochemical and ADME properties of conventional small molecules, derived from a large diverse data set over many years, our understanding of PROTAC ADME properties is nascent. Nevertheless our emerging experience with PROTACs suggests it is possible to regularly achieve robust oral bioavailability, often despite apparently unfavorable physicochemical properties.

## 8.4 Inhaled, Topical and Intravenous Routes of Administration

Direct delivery of drugs to the lung can facilitate high local concentrations driving therapeutic effect at lower doses than required following oral drug administration, where systemic exposure drives effect.[77] However, inhaled drugs for the treatment of pulmonary disease require optimization of molecular structure and/or formulation in order to have sufficient unbound drug exposure and pharmacokinetic duration in the lung. The two main strategies for such optimization involve maintaining a reservoir of drug in the airways, through low solubility and slow dissolution rate, or in the lung tissue through the distribution properties of the drug.[78] The former case is exemplified by the inhaled corticosteroids (ICS) and the latter by bronchodilators, where longer half-life in the lung has been achieved by increasing the overall basicity of the molecules, giving higher tissue affinity through mechanisms such as lysosomal trapping.[78,79] Prior to pulmonary absorption and/or pharmacological target interaction, inhaled particles dissolve in the epithelial lining fluid (ELF), whilst undissolved particles may be transported towards the pharynx by mucociliary clearance (MCC) and eventually swallowed. The MCC transport rate varies across the lung with a maximum velocity in the trachea, but typical half-lives for the overall clearance are in the range 0.5–2 hours.[80] Absorption rates from conducting airways to central (bronchial) blood and from small airways/alveoli to peripheral (pulmonary) blood vary due to epithelial depth differences (60 µm in the central airways to less than 3 µm in the small airways/alveoli) and differences in the flow of the two blood supply routes.[81] A large percentage of the dose is likely to be absorbed in the first hour or two after dose. For soluble mono-basic small molecule drugs, this can be approximately 90% of the dose, but may be as low as 50% for di-basic molecules that distribute extensively into the lung tissue and considerably less than this for low solubility molecules that reside in the airways until dissolved.[80,82] Much of this absorption occurs in the peripheral airways and alveolar region, where the epithelial barrier is thin and the pulmonary blood supply (100% of cardiac output) provides a sink and steep concentration gradient.[83,84] Whilst permeability influences the speed and extent of this initial (alpha phase, 0–2 h) absorption, our data indicates that it has little impact on the beta phase that essentially drives the duration of pharmacodynamic effect. Nevertheless, the physico-chemical properties of the drug that influence this initial absorption rate through altering permeability, clearly do influence the amount of drug (and therefore overall exposure) in the pharmacokinetic beta phase. Thus, low permeability influences inhaled dose. All these aspects have a role to play in defining the lung pharmacokinetic profile and therefore can influence the overall therapeutic effectiveness of the inhaled medicine. Physiologically based pharmacokinetic (PBPK) models have been developed to address these complexities. These models have been shown to effectively predict not only preclinical lung and systemic PK, but also clinical PK and target engagement biomarkers demonstrating the ability to predict unbound drug concentration at different target locations in the lung.[82–84]

By understanding what properties drive the lung pharmacokinetics generally and/or within in a particular chemical series, it is possible to optimize the design of an inhaled drug using preclinical data. A clear advantage of low permeability is the likelihood of low oral bioavailability which greatly reduces the risk of unwanted systemic side effects. It should also be noted that the anti-muscarinic agents ipratropium and tiotropium have extremely low permeability due to the fact that they both have the same structural feature of a permanently charged nitrogen. This clearly does not impede their usefulness as inhaled drugs. However, the fact that both are substrates of organic cation transporter proteins (OCTs) may facilitate their transport through the lungs, since this family of drug transporters is expressed in the lung.[85,86] High lung deposition of material with poor aqueous solubility (typically <1 μM) can lead to duration of many hours as inhaled particles dissolve slowly within the lung tissue as a prelude to absorption into the systemic circulation. Whilst this approach can yield high lung concentrations and long half-lives, the approach is highly dependent on the physical characteristics of the crystal form of the compound and in early discovery programs material properties are generally poorly characterized and not optimized.

Pulmonary drug metabolism is another consideration, since first pass metabolism of an inhaled therapeutic could have implications for drug safety or pharmacologically relevant local drug exposure. Many drug metabolizing enzymes have been shown to be present, including CYP1A1, CYP1B1, CYP2A6, CYP2A13, CYP2B6, CYP2C8/18, CYP2D6, CYP2E1, CYP2F1, CYP2J2, CYP2S1, CYP3A4/5, CYP3A43, CYP4B1, EHs and FMOs.[87] However, expression levels and functional activity are generally low compared to hepatic.[87]

The skin is the largest organ in humans and functions as a protective, homeostasis and sensing barrier. Drugs, such as antifungal or steroid creams for dermatological conditions can be delivered topically to deliver a local pharmacodynamic effect in the skin, whereas transdermal drug delivery is used to drive a systemic pharmacodynamic effect, such as for birth control and hormone replacement therapy. Likewise, treatment of ocular diseases may use topical formulations and drug disposition in the eye has been summarized.[88]

Many techniques, including *in vitro* assays, *ex vivo* models of animal and human skin, as well as animal and human *in vivo* studies have been developed to evaluate the permeation of topical and transdermal drugs.[89,90] As for oral therapies, skin permeation is associated with the physicochemical properties of the drug molecule, including lipophilicity. Drug formulation is also critical to enhancing skin permeation. Studies on the xenobiotic metabolic properties of the skin have been compared and contrasted to the major hepatic drug metabolizing enzyme families, more often at the level of mRNA and protein more so than enzyme activity,[91] which limits the translational understanding. Overall the activity of drug metabolizing enzymes is significantly lower in the skin compared to the liver, but considering the relative organ sizes, skin metabolism may still be therapeutically relevant and worthy of continued study.

Drugs administered by the intravenous (IV) route, avoid a first pass through the liver and may be given as a bolus or more typically by an infusion over a defined time at a constant rate to allows precise control of plasma drug concentrations, important for anesthetics and drugs with a very narrow therapeutic index. Upon infusion, once the drug has reached the plateau or steady-state, the rate of drug eliminated is equal to the rate of drug infusion. For oncology indications, narrow therapeutic index drugs that need relatively short target engagement to drive tumor cell kill can utilize the IV route to maintain target plasma concentrations up until the end of infusion. In drug design, considerations include targeting high CL and low $V_{ss}$ resulting in short $T_{1/2}$ drugs to minimize systemic drug concentrations after the end of infusion and limit systemic toxicity. Likewise, establishing the lack of active major metabolites and victim drug interaction potential as well as clearance *via* a non-polymorphic drug metabolizing enzyme pathway are additional important considerations to minimize excessive variability of active species within a patient population. However, the invasiveness and inconvenience caused to patients using the IV administration route restricts its utility to specific indications and drug targets.

## 8.5 Hints and Tips

In this section are a list of hints and tips for applying some of the principles outlined in this chapter in drug discovery programs:

- $F$ = AUCpo/AUCiv (if equivalent doses given). Target $F > 30\%$ (and $F_{abs} > 50\%$) in humans to avoid excessive inter-individual variation. A crystalline solubility of 100 µM and a Caco-2 $P_{app}$ of $5 \times 10^{-6}$ cm s$^{-1}$ will likely result in an acceptable $F_{abs}$ in humans of >50%; specific values will depend on assays in any given laboratory. Intestinal P-gp efflux is unlikely to be clinically relevant for compounds with high permeability and solubility. Rat oral absorption is not a good predictor of human, but vital for determining if toxicological studies can be adequately performed. Frequently dog is a better model for human absorption.

- $V_d$ correlates with the relative affinity of compound for tissues. $V_{ss}$ values for acids are low (0.1–0.3 L $kg^{-1}$), neutrals moderate (1–3 L $kg^{-1}$) and bases are high (>3 L $kg^{-1}$). Using animal PK data corrected for species ppb, $V_{ss}$ is the most predictable of PK parameters: unbound $V_{ss}$ should be conserved within 2-fold across species.
- Compounds that demonstrate good BBB penetrance are passively permeable, are not substrates of the major human BBB efflux transporters and have $K_{puu}$ values determined in preclinical species approaching unity.
- CL is the parameter that best describes the efficiency of an eliminating process CL = dose/AUC. CL is influenced by ppb. Relating the rate of removal to the concentration of unbound drug in plasma, gives $CL_{int}$ or "intrinsic clearance". Confidence in predicting human hepatic metabolic *in vivo* $CL_{int}$ is increased if *in vivo*/*in vitro* $CL_{int}$ is <2 for rat and dog. For poor preclinical predictions of metabolic CL from *in vitro* data, investigate *in vitro* and *in vivo* variables to gain a better mechanistic understanding. Human hepatic metabolic CL can be predicted from human hepatocyte $CL_{int}$, human renal CL predicted from dog renal CL and human biliary CL from rat biliary CL, when drugs do not require active hepatic uptake to access the liver. Comparing human microsomal and hepatocyte $CL_{int}$ values is valuable in increasing mechanistic understanding. Allometric scaling approaches offer fairly poor predictivity of human CL. However, they do offer a "sense-check" on human predictions made from more mechanistic approaches, *e.g.* human elimination $T_{1/2}$ frequently approximates to 4× rat $T_{1/2}$ and 2× dog $T_{1/2}$. This may be applicable when cross-species *in vitro* hepatic stability/CL routes are comparable.
- *In vivo* efficacy is determined by unbound drug concentration at the target, which is modulated primarily by $CL_{int}$, not ppb. Thus, decreasing ppb has no effect on the *in vivo* unbound drug concentration, $AUC_u$ or $T_{1/2}$ for most compounds, and so is typically not a suitable parameter for optimization in drug discovery. Focus on physiochemical parameters such as log*P*, p$K_a$ and PSA, as well as specific structural insights to lower CL and raise absorption, to optimize free drug concentration.
- Emerging experience with PROTACs suggests it is possible to achieve robust oral bioavailability and good PK, despite apparently unfavorable physicochemical properties.
- For QD dosing, a human $T_{1/2}$ target of approximately 16 h is appropriate, since being 2-fold out (*e.g.* 16 to 8 or 32 h) changes the dose and $C_{max}$ only by 2-fold.

## 8.6 Summary

AstraZeneca drug project teams use a five-dimensional framework to maximize the probability of project success and pipeline quality, described as the five "Rs": the right target, right patient, right tissue and exposure, right safety and right commercial potential.[92] Under this overarching framework the focus of AstraZeneca drug design teams, with respect to clinical PK optimization, are on the key parameters that support PK profiles CL, $V_{ss}$ and $F_{abs}$, underpinned by an understanding of the candidate drug's exposure–effect relationship.[1,93] Other parameters, such as those related to mitigating against drug–drug interactions are incorporated as necessary.

As outlined above, PK parameters have strong interdependencies with the physicochemical properties of compounds, and thus optimizing these fundamental properties may be a focus for project teams. However, a recent and extensive analysis of the relationship between physicochemical properties and drug attrition concluded further refinement of physicochemical properties within the oral drug-like space is unlikely to have a significant effect on attrition rates for small molecule drug candidates.[94] Indeed PROTACs often breach "rule-of-5" limits, but oral bioavailability and acceptable PK remains achievable, yet the wide range of physicochemical properties can challenge ADME assays.[76] It is critical, in the authors' view, to develop as full a mechanistic understanding of the ADME disposition properties of key candidate drug(s) during drug discovery *via* detailed experimentation and thorough investigations to optimize towards a candidate drug with acceptable human PK profile and attain a sufficient degree of confidence in the predicted clinical PK parameters to make informed investment decisions. Pharmacokinetics is complex and all predictions are fraught with uncertainty, and, somewhat paradoxically, the establishment, in the last two decades, of a plethora of *in silico* methods, *in vitro* screens and *in vivo* models could lead to a box-ticking checklist approach to drug discovery, generating in our opinion only a superficial understanding of a compound's disposition properties. Excellent ADME science contribution to drug design teams requires additional intellectual and experimental input by experienced and expert scientists. Furthermore the limitation of predictive accuracy should be appreciated. It is commonly and subjectively accepted within the DMPK community that a prediction within 2-fold of the measured value is a success. However, a successful prediction of individual parameters may not equate to a successful prediction of clinical dose and exposure due to the cumulative impact of 2-fold errors in CL and $V_{ss}$ predictions on $T_{1/2}$, exposure and dose.[1,6] This understanding of uncertainty and risk explains, for example, why for once-daily dosing of a candidate drug, a human $T_{1/2}$ prediction of approximately 16 h is desirable, if drug effect is related to trough concentration, since being 2-fold out in either direction elevates the dose and $C_{max}$ by only 2-fold for a 8 h $T_{1/2}$ or results in only a 4-fold accumulation from single dose to steady-state for a 32 h $T_{1/2}$.

Based on a robust understanding of the interdependencies between physicochemical properties and key PK parameters and with targeted experimentation using well-validated assays and models as a foundation, together with bespoke experiments designed to test specific hypotheses, an ADME optimization strategy towards clinical candidates with an acceptable clinical PK profile is achievable. DMPK scientists working in partnership with medicinal chemists and drug design teams can maximize the probability of success *via* building predictions, knowledge and developing a thorough mechanistic understanding of the ADME disposition properties of the relevant chemical series and candidate drug.

## References


1. M. Davies, R. D. O. Jones, K. Grime, R. Jansson-Löfmark, A. J. Fretland, S. Winiwarter, P. Morgan and D. F. McGinnity, Improving the Accuracy of Predicted Human Pharmacokinetics: Lessons Learned from the AstraZeneca Drug Pipeline Over Two Decades, *Trends Pharmacol. Sci.*, 2020, **41**(6), 390–408.
2. H. Lennernäs, Does fluid flow across the intestinal mucosa affect quantitative oral drug absorption? Is it time for a reevaluation?, *Pharm. Res.*, 1995, **12**(11), 1573–1582.

3. R. J. Bertz and G. R. Granneman, Use of in vitro and in vivo data to estimate the likelihood of metabolic pharmacokinetic interactions, *Clin. Pharmacokinet.*, 1997, 32(3), 210–258.
4. D. A. Smith, *Metabolism, Pharmacokinetics and Toxicity of Functional Groups*, ed. D. A. Smith, RSC Drug Discovery Series No. 1, 2010.
5. M. Rowland and T. N. Tozer, *Clinical Pharmacokinetics – Concepts and Applications*, Williams and Wilkins, 3rd edn, 1989.
6. D. F. McGinnity, J. Collington, R. Austin and R. Riley, Evaluation of human pharmacokinetics, therapeutic dose and exposure predictions using marketed oral drugs, *Curr. Drug Metab.*, 2007, **8**, 463.
7. E. T. Hellriegel, T. D. Bjornsson and W. W. Hauck, Interpatient variability in bioavailability is related to the extent of absorption: implications for bioavailability and bioequivalence studies, *Clin. Pharmacol. Ther.*, 1996, **60**, 601.
8. H. Komura and M. Iwaki, In vitro and in vivo small intestinal metabolism of CYP3A and UGT substrates in preclinical animal species and humans: species differences, *Drug Metab. Rev.*, 2011, **43**, 476.
9. A. Galetin, M. Gertz and J. B. Houston, Contribution of intestinal cytochrome p450-mediated metabolism to drug–drug inhibition and induction interactions, *Drug Metab. Pharmacokinet.*, 2010, **25**, 28.
10. K. Thelen and J. B. Dressman, Cytochrome P450-mediated metabolism in the human gut wall, *J. Pharm. Pharmacol.*, 2009, **61**, 541.
11. M. F. Paine, H. L. Hart, S. S. Ludington, R. L. Haining, A. E. Rettie and D. C. Zeldin, The human intestinal cytochrome P450 "pie", *Drug Metab. Dispos.*, 2006, **34**, 880.
12. Q. Y. Zhang, D. Dunbar, A. Ostrowska, S. Zeisloft, J. Yang and L. S. Kaminsky, Characterization of human small intestinal cytochromes P-450, *Drug Metab. Dispos.*, 1999, **27**, 804.
13. T. Prueksaritanont, L. M. Gorham, J. H. Hochman, L. O. Tran and K. P. Vyas, Comparative studies of drug-metabolizing enzymes in dog, monkey, and human small intestines, and in Caco-2 cells, *Drug Metab. Dispos.*, 1996, **24**, 634.
14. J. Yang, M. Jamei, K. R. Yeo, G. T. Tucker and A. Rostami-Hodjegan, Prediction of intestinal first-pass drug metabolism, *Curr. Drug Metab.*, 2007, **8**, 676.
15. M. M. Doherty and W. N. Charman, The mucosa of the small intestine: how clinically relevant as an organ of drug metabolism?, *Clin. Pharmacokinet.*, 2002, **41**, 235.
16. M. F. Paine, M. Khalighi, J. M. Fisher, D. D. Shen, K. L. Kunze, C. L. Marsh, J. D. Perkins and K. E. Thummel, Characterization of interintestinal and intraintestinal variations in human CYP3A-dependent metabolism, *J. Pharmacol. Exp. Ther.*, 1997, **283**, 1552.
17. A. Galetin and J. B. Houston, Intestinal and hepatic metabolic activity of five cytochrome P450 enzymes: impact on prediction of first-pass metabolism, *J. Pharmacol. Exp. Ther.*, 2006, **318**, 1220.
18. A. Galetin, Intestinal first-pass metabolism: bridging the gap between in vitro and in vivo, *Curr. Drug Metab.*, 2007, **8**, 643.
19. Y. Zhang and L. Z. Benet, The gut as a barrier to drug absorption: combined role of cytochrome P450 3A and P-glycoprotein, *Clin. Pharmacokinet.*, 2001, **40**, 159.
20. *Guidance for Industry Drug Interaction Studies - Study Design, Data Analysis, Implications for Dosing and Labeling Recommendations*, U.S. Department of Health and Human Services Food and Drug Administration Center for Drug Evaluation and Research (CDER). 2012.
21. I. J. Hidalgo, T. J. Raub and R. T. Borchardt, Characterization of the human colon carcinoma cell line (Caco-2) as a model system for intestinal epithelial permeability, *Gastroenterology*, 1989, **96**, 736.
22. D. Sun, H. Lennernas, L. S. Welage, J. L. Barnett, C. P. Landowski, D. Foster, D. Fleisher, K. D. Lee and G. L. Amidon, Comparison of human duodenum and Caco-2 gene expression profiles for 12,000 gene sequences tags and correlation with permeability of 26 drugs, *Pharmacol. Res.*, 2002, **19**, 1400.
23. X. Lin, S. Skolnik, X. Chen and J. Wang, Attenuation of intestinal absorption by major efflux transporters: quantitative tools and strategies using a Caco-2 model, *Drug Metab. Dispos.*, 2011, **39**, 265.
24. T. Murakami and M. Takano, Intestinal efflux transporters and drug absorption, *Expert Opin. Drug Metab. Toxicol.*, 2008, **4**, 923.
25. M. B. Bolger, V. Lukacova and W. S. Woltosz, Simulations of the nonlinear dose dependence for substrates of influx and efflux transporters in the human intestine, *AAPS J.*, 2009, **11**, 353.
26. K. H. Grime, P. Barton and D. F. McGinnity, Application of in silico, in vitro and preclinical pharmacokinetic data for the effective and efficient prediction of human pharmacokinetics, *Mol. Pharm.*, 2013, **10**, 1191.
27. M. Jamei, S. Marciniak, K. Feng, A. Barnett, G. Tucker and A. Rostami-Hodjegan, The Simcyp population-based ADME simulator, *Expert Opin. Drug Metab. Toxicol.*, 2009, **5**, 211.

28. V. K. Sinha, J. Snoeys, N. V. Osselaer, A. V. Peer, C. Mackie and D. Heald, From preclinical to human-prediction of oral absorption and drug–drug interaction potential using physiologically based pharmacokinetic (PBPK) modeling approach in an industrial setting: a workflow by using case example, *Biopharm. Drug Dispos.*, 2012, **33**, 111.
29. J. M. DeSesso and C. F. Jacobson, Anatomical and physiological parameters affecting gastrointestinal absorption in humans and rats, *Food Chem. Toxicol.*, 2001, **39**, 209.
30. S. Øie and T. N. Tozer, Effect of altered plasma protein binding on apparent volume of distribution, *J. Pharm. Sci.*, 1979, **68**, 1203.
31. R. J. Riley, I. J. Martin and A. E. Cooper, The influence of DMPK as an integrated partner in modern drug discovery, *Curr. Drug Metab.*, 2002, **3**, 527.
32. D. A. Smith, L. Di and E. H. Kerns, The effect of plasma protein binding on in vivo efficacy: misconceptions in drug discovery, *Nat. Rev. Drug Discovery*, 2010, **9**, 929.
33. A. C. MacIntyre and D. J. Cutler, The potential role of lysosomes in tissue distribution of weak bases, *Biopharm. Drug Dispos.*, 1988, **9**, 513.
34. D. A. Smith, B. C. Jones and D. K. Walker, Design of drugs involving the concepts and theories of drug metabolism and pharmacokinetics, *Med. Res. Rev.*, 1996, **16**, 243.
35. G. Berellini, C. Springer, N. J. Waters and F. Lombardo, In silico prediction of volume of distribution in human using linear and nonlinear models on a 669 compound data set, *Med. Chem.*, 2009, **52**, 4488.
36. M. P. Gleeson, N. J. Waters and S. W. Paine, Davis AM, In silico human and rat Vss quantitative structure-activity relationship models, *J. Med. Chem.*, 2006, **49**, 1953.
37. R. S. Obach, Prediction of human volume of distribution using in vivo, in vitro, and in silico approaches, *Annu. Rep. Med. Chem.*, 2007, **42**, 469–488.
38. L. M. Berry, C. Li and Z. Zhao, Species differences in distribution and prediction of human V(ss) from preclinical data, *Drug Metab. Dispos.*, 2011, **39**, 2103–2116.
39. L. M. Berezhkovskiy, On the accuracy of determination of unbound drug fraction in tissue using diluted tissue homogenate, *J. Pharm. Sci.*, 2012, **101**, 1909–1916.
40. P. Zou, N. Zheng, Y. Yang, L. X. Yu and D. Sun, Prediction of volume of distribution at steady state in humans: comparison of different approaches, *Expert Opin. Drug Metab. Toxicol.*, 2012, **8**, 855.
41. R. D. Jones, H. M. Jones, M. Rowland, C. R. Gibson, J. W. Yates, J. Y. Chien, B. J. Ring, K. K. Adkison, M. S. Ku, H. He, R. Vuppugalla, P. Marathe, V. Fischer, S. Dutta, V. K. Sinha, T. Björnsson, T. Lavé and P. Poulin, PhRMA CPCDC initiative on predictive models of human pharmacokinetics, part 2: comparative assessment of prediction methods of human volume of distribution, *J. Pharm. Sci.*, 2011, **100**, 4074.
42. F. Lombardo, N. J. Waters, U. A. Argikar, M. K. Dennehy, J. Zhan, M. Gunduz, S. P. Harriman, G. Berellini, I. Liric Rajlic and R. S. Obach, Comprehensive assessment of human pharmacokinetic prediction based on in vivo animal pharmacokinetic data, part 1: volume of distribution at steady state, *J. Clin. Pharmacol.*, 2013, **53**, 178.
43. N. Colclough, K. Chen, P. Johnström, M. Fridén and D. F. McGinnity, Building on the success of osimertinib: achieving CNS exposure in oncology drug discovery, *Drug Discovery Today*, 2019, 1067.
44. A. Jucaite, P. Stenkrona, Z. Cselényi, S. De Vita, N. Buil-Bruna, K. Varnäs, A. Savage, A. Varrone, P. Johnström, M. Schou, C. Davison, A. Sykes, V. P. Reddy, M. Hoch, A. Vazquez-Romero, M. M. Moein, C. Halldin, M. S. Merchant, M. Pass and L. Farde, Brain exposure of the ATM inhibitor AZD1390 in humans - a positron emission tomography (PET) study, *Neuro Oncol.*, 2021, **23**(4), 687–696.
45. N. Colclough, K. Chen, P. Johnström, N. Strittmatter, Y. Yan, G. L. Wrigley, M. Schou, R. Goodwin, K. Varnäs, S. J. Adua, M. Zhao, D. X. Nguyen, G. Maglennon, P. Barton, J. Atkinson, L. Zhang, A. Janefeldt, J. Wilson, A. Smith, A. Takano, R. Arakawa, M. Kondrashov, J. Malmquist, E. Revunov, A. Vazquez-Romero, M. Mahdi Moein, A. D. Windhorst, N. D. Karp, R. V. Finlay, R. A. Ward, J. W. T. Yates, P. D. Smith, L. Farde, Z. Cheng and D. A. E. Cross, Preclinical Comparison of the Blood–brain barrier Permeability of Osimertinib with Other EGFR TKI, *Clin. Cancer Res.*, 2021, **27**(1), 189–201.
46. K. Grime and R. J. Riley, The impact of in vitro binding on in vitro-in vivo extrapolations, projections of metabolic clearance and clinical drug–drug interactions, *Curr. Drug Metab.*, 2006, 7, 251.
47. A.-K. Sohlenius-Sternbeck, C. Jones, D. Ferguson, B. J. Middleton, D. Projean, E. Floby, J. Bylund and L. Afzelius, Practical use of the regression offset approach for the prediction of in vivo intrinsic clearance from hepatocytes, *Xenobiotica*, 2012, **42**, 841.
48. T. Lavé, K. Chapman, P. Goldsmith and M. Rowland, Human clearance prediction: shifting the paradigm, *Expert Opin. Drug Metab. Toxicol.*, 2009, **9**, 1039.
49. K. Ito and J. B. Houston, Prediction of human drug clearance from in vitro and preclinical data using physiologically based and empirical approaches, *Pharm. Res.*, 2005, **22**, 103.

50. R. S. Obach, Predicting clearance in humans from in vitro data, *Curr. Top. Med. Chem.*, 2011, **11**, 334.
51. J. B. Houston, Utility of in vitro drug metabolism data in predicting in vivo metabolic clearance, *Biochem. Pharmacol.*, 1994, **47**, 1469.
52. R. J. Riley, D. F. McGinnity and R. P. Austin, A unified model for predicting human hepatic, metabolic clearance from in vitro intrinsic clearance data in hepatocytes and microsomes, *Drug Metab. Dispos.*, 2005, **33**, 1304.
53. B. Williamson, S. Harlfinger and D. F. McGinnity, Evaluation of the disconnect between hepatocyte and microsome intrinsic clearance and in vitro in vivo extrapolation performance, *Drug Metab. Dispos.*, 2020, 1137.
54. *Pharmacokinetics and Metabolism in Drug Design*, ed. D. A. Smith, C. Allerton and A. S. Kalgutkar, Wiley-VCH, 3rd edn, Methods and Principles in Medicinal Chemistry, 2012, vol. 51.
55. C. D. A. Brown, R. Sayer, A. S. Windass, I. S. Haslam, M. E. De Broe, P. C. D'Haese and A. Verhulst, Characterisation of human tubular cell monolayers as a model of proximal tubular xenobiotic handling, *Toxicol. Appl. Pharmacol.*, 2008, **233**, 428.
56. S. W. Paine, K. Menochet, R. Denton, D. F. McGinnity and R. J. Riley, Prediction of human renal clearance from preclinical species for a diverse set of drugs that exhibit both active secretion and net reabsorption, *Drug Metab. Dispos.*, 2011, **39**, 1008.
57. H. Tahara, M. Shono, H. Kusuhara, H. Kinoshita, E. Fuse, A. Takadate, M. Otagiri and Y. Sugiyama, Molecular cloning and functional analyses of OAT1 and OAT3 from cynomolgus monkey kidney, *Pharm. Res.*, 2005, **22**, 647.
58. Y. Kato, K. Kuge, H. Kusuhara, P. J. Meier and Y. Sugiyama, Gender difference in the urinary excretion of organic anions in rats, *J. Pharmacol. Exp. Ther.*, 2002, **302**, 483.
59. Y. Shitara, T. Horie and Y. Sugiyama, Transporters as a determinant of drug clearance and tissue distribution, *Eur. J. Pharm. Sci.*, 2006, **27**, 425.
60. T. Ishikawa, K. Akimaru, M. T. Kuo, W. Priebe and M. Suzuki, How does the MRP/GS-X pump export doxorubicin?, *J. Natl. Cancer Inst.*, 1995, **87**, 1639–1640.
61. D. Keppler, I. Leier and G. Jedlitschky, Transport of glutathione conjugates and glucuronides by the multidrug resistance proteins MRP1 and MRP2, *Biol. Chem.*, 1997, **378**, 787–791.
62. M. Müller and P. L. Jansen, Molecular aspects of hepatobiliary transport, *Am. J. Physiol.*, 1997, **272**, G1285–G1303.
63. P. Chandra and K. L. Brouwer, The complexities of hepatic drug transport: current knowledge and emerging concepts, *Pharm. Res.*, 2004, **21**, 719–735.
64. B. Williamson, N. Colclough, A. J. Fretland, B. C. Jones, R. D. O. Jones and D. F. McGinnity, Further Considerations Towards an Effective and Efficient Oncology Drug Discovery DMPK Strategy, *Curr. Drug Metab.*, 2020, **21**, 145.
65. K. H. Grime and S. W. Paine, Species differences in biliary clearance and possible relevance of hepatic uptake and efflux transporters involvement, *Drug Metab. Dispos.*, 2013, **41**, 372.
66. M. G. Soars, D. F. McGinnity, K. Grime and R. J. Riley, The pivotal role of hepatocytes in drug discovery, *Chem.-Biol. Interact.*, 2007, **168**, 2.
67. P. Gardiner and S. W. Paine, The impact of hepatic uptake on the pharmacokinetics of organic anions, *Drug Metab. Dispos.*, 2011, **39**, 1930.
68. I. Mahmood, Interspecies scaling of biliary excreted drugs: a comparison of several methods, *J. Pharm. Sci.*, 2005, **94**, 883.
69. I. Mahmood and C. Sahajwalla, Interspecies scaling of biliary excreted drugs, *J. Pharm. Sci.*, 2002, **91**, 1908.
70. J. A. Scatina, D. R. Hicks, M. Kraml and M. N. Cayen, Disposition of a new tetrahydrocarbazole analgesic drug in laboratory animals and human, *Xenobiotica*, 1989, **19**, 991.
71. I. Påhlman, M. Edholm, S. Kankaanranta and M.-L. Odell, Pharmacokinetics of susalimod, a highly biliary-excreted sulphasalazine analogue, in various species. Nonpredictable human clearance by allometric scaling, *Pharm. Pharmacol. Commun.*, 1998, **4**, 493–498.
72. M. Morris, Y. Yang, Y. A. Gandhi, S. G. Bhansalia and L. J. Benincosa, Interspecies scaling: prediction of human biliary clearance and comparison with QSPKR, *Biopharm. Drug Dispos.*, 2012, **33**, 1.
73. K. W. Ward and B. R. I. Smith, A comprehensive quantitative and qualitative evaluation of extrapolation of intravenous pharmacokinetic parameters from rat, dog, and monkey to humans. I. Clearance, *Drug Metab. Dispos.*, 2004, **32**, 603.
74. G. W. Caldwell, J. A. Masucci, Z. Yan and W. Hageman, Allometric scaling of pharmacokinetic parameters in drug discovery: can human CL, Vss and t1/2 be predicted from in-vivo rat data? *Eur. J. Drug Metab. Pharmacokinet.*, 2004, **29**, 133.

75. F. Lombardo, N. J. Waters, U. A. Argikar, M. K. Dennehy, J. Zhan, M. Gunduz, S. P. Harriman, G. Berellini, I. Liric Rajlic and R. S. Obach, Comprehensive assessment of human pharmacokinetic prediction based on in vivo animal pharmacokinetic data, part 2: clearance, *J. Clin. Pharmacol.*, 2013, **53**, 178.
76. A. Pike, B. Williamson, S. Harlfinger, S. Martin and D. F. McGinnity, Optimising proteolysis-targeting chimeras (PROTACs) for oral drug delivery: a drug metabolism and pharmacokinetics perspective, *Drug Discovery Today*, 2020, **25**(10), 1793–1800.
77. P. Backman, H. Adelmann, G. Petersson and C. B. Jones, Advances in inhaled technologies: understanding the therapeutic challenge, predicting clinical performance, and designing the optimal inhaled product, *Clin. Pharmacol. Ther.*, 2014, **95**, 509–520.
78. A. E. Cooper, D. Ferguson and K. Grime, Optimisation of DMPK by the inhaled route: challenges and approaches, *Curr. Drug Metab.*, 2012, **13**, 457–473.
79. E. Bäckström, E. Boger, A. Lundqvist, M. Hammarlund-Udenaes and M. Fridén, Lung Retention by Lysosomal Trapping of Inhaled Drugs Can Be Predicted In Vitro With Lung Slices, *J. Pharm. Sci.*, 2016, **105**, 3432–3439.
80. M. Sakagami and P. R. Byron, Respirable microspheres for inhalation: the potential of manipulating pulmonary disposition for improved therapeutic efficacy, *Clin. Pharmacokinet.*, 2005, **44**, 263–277.
81. N. R. Labiris and M. B. Dolovich, *Br. J. Clin. Pharmacol.*, 2003, **56**, 588–599.
82. R. Hendrickx, E. Lamm Bergström, D. L. I. Janzén, M. Fridén, U. Eriksson, K. Grime and D. Ferguson, Translational model to predict pulmonary pharmacokinetics and efficacy in human for inhaled bronchodilators, *CPT: Pharmacometrics Syst. Pharmacol.*, 2018, **7**, 147–157.
83. E. Boger, N. Evans, M. Chappell, A. Lundqvist, P. Ewing, A. Wigenborg and M. Fridén, Systems Pharmacology Approach for Prediction of Pulmonary and Systemic Pharmacokinetics and Receptor Occupancy of Inhaled Drugs, *CPT: Pharmacometrics Syst. Pharmacol.*, 2016, **5**, 201–210.
84. E. Boger and M. Fridén, Physiologically Based Pharmacokinetic/Pharmacodynamic Modelling Accurately Predicts the Better Broncho-dilatory Effect of Inhaled Versus Oral Salbutamol Dosage Forms, *J. Aerosol Med. Pulm. Drug Delivery*, 2019, **32**, s1–s12.
85. T. Nakanishi, T. Haruta, Y. Shirasaka and I. Tamai, Organic cation transporter-mediated renal secretion of ipratropium and tiotropium in rats and humans, *Drug Metab. Dispos.*, 2011, **39**, 117–122.
86. H. Koepsell, Polyspecific organic cation transporters: their functions and interactions with drugs, *Trends Pharmacol. Sci.*, 2004, **25**, 375–381.
87. K. Rubin, P. Ewing, E. Bäckström, A. Abrahamsson, B. Bonn, S. Kamata and K. Grime, Pulmonary Metabolism of Substrates for Key Drug-Metabolizing Enzymes by Human Alveolar Type II Cells, Human and Rat Lung Microsomes, and the Isolated Perfused Rat Lung Model, *Pharmaceutics*, 2020, **12**, 117–129.
88. U. A. Argikar, J. L. Dumouchel, V. M. Kramlinger, A. L. Cirello, M. Gunduz, C. E. Dunne and B. Sohal, Do We Need to Study Metabolism and Distribution in the Eye: Why, When, and Are We There Yet?, *J. Pharm. Sci.*, 2017, 2276.
89. S. Supe and P. Takudage, Methods for evaluating penetration of drug into the skin: A review, *Skin Res. Technol.*, 2021, **27**(3), 299–308.
90. N. Couto, J. R. A. Newton, C. Russo, E. Karunakaran, B. Achour, Z. M. Al-Majdoub, J. Sidaway, A. Rostami-Hodjegan, M. R. Clench and J. Barber, Label-Free Quantitative Proteomics and Substrate-Based Mass Spectrometry Imaging of Xenobiotic Metabolizing Enzymes in Ex Vivo Human Skin and a Human Living Skin Equivalent Model, *Drug Metab. Dispos.*, 2021, 39.
91. S. Kazem, E. C. Linssen and S. Gibbs, Skin metabolism phase I and phase II enzymes in native and reconstructed human skin: a short review, *Drug Discovery Today*, 2019, 1899.
92. D. Cook, D. Brown, R. Alexander, R. March, P. Morgan, G. Satterthwaite and M. N. Pangalos, Lessons learned from the fate of AstraZeneca's drug pipeline: a five-dimensional framework, *Nat. Rev. Drug Discovery*, 2014, **13**, 419–431.
93. S. A. Visser, M. Aurell, R. D. Jones, V. J. Schuck, A. C. Egnell, S. A. Peters, L. Brynne, J. W. Yates, R. Jansson-Löfmark, B. Tan, M. Cooke, S. T. Barry, A. Hughes and U. Bredberg, Model-based drug discovery: implementation and impact, *Drug Discovery Today*, 2013, **18**, 764–775.
94. M. J. Waring, J. Arrowsmith, A. R. Leach, P. D. Leeson, S. Mandrell, R. M. Owen, G. Pairaudeau, W. D. Pennie, S. D. Pickett, J. Wang, O. Wallace and A. Weir, An analysis of the attrition of drug candidates from four major pharmaceutical companies, *Nat. Rev. Drug Discovery*, 2015, **14**, 475–486.

# 9 Molecular Biology for Medicinal Chemists

N. M. Ahmad[a], E. Bush[b], B. Nancolas[b], N. Macabuag[b] and P. I. Racz*[c]

[a]Charles River Laboratories, 8-9 Spire Green Centre, Harlow, Essex, CM19 5TR, UK; [b]Charles River Laboratories, Chesterford Research Park, CB10 1XL, UK; [c]Darwinweg 24, 2333 CR, Leiden, Netherlands
*E-mail: peter.racz@crl.com

## 9.1 A Brief History of Molecular Biology

As the name suggests, molecular biology pertains to a branch of biology that is concerned with understanding life on a molecular level. It is difficult to accurately ascertain when molecular biology was born as an independent scientific approach, but the consensus is the early part of the 20th century, when attempts to isolate and characterise molecules prevalent in organisms became tractable with the advent of novel technologies. Technologies such as X-ray crystallography and electron microscopy acted as tremendous catalysts in the progression of molecular biology and allowed scientists, for the first time, to visualise and gain a mechanistic understanding of the organisation of the molecular world that had remained in obscurity until then.

Molecular biology has placed what was once deemed to be the realm of science fiction firmly in the realm of science reality; Dolly the first cloned sheep is a prominent example.[1] Apart from such sensational examples, molecular biology has had a profound effect on various aspects of drug discovery; this is the main topic of this chapter. In this section we will highlight the basics of molecular biology described through a historical perspective and go on to outline how the discipline is helping to shape drug discovery pipelines.

Investigations as early as 1928 had indicated the basis of the mechanisms of heredity,[2] with deoxyribonucleic acid (DNA) increasingly suspected as the molecule responsible for transmission of genetic information;[3] a landmark publication in 1952 by Alfred Hershey and Martha Chase definitively confirmed this.[4] The work showed specific uptake of

The Handbook of Medicinal Chemistry: Principles and Practice, 2nd Edition
Edited by Simon E. Ward and Andrew M. Davis

Published by the Royal Society of Chemistry, www.rsc.org

$^{32}P$-labelled bacteriophage DNA into bacteria, with $^{35}S$-labelled protein remaining in the culture medium. They concluded that whilst the protein portion of the bacteriophage likely had no role in infection, DNA probably had some function: "This protein probably has no function in the growth of intracellular phage. The DNA has some function. Further chemical inferences should not be drawn from the experiments presented." Hershey and others went on to win a Nobel Prize for this and related findings; however, it was the ground-breaking discovery published in 1953 that is widely acknowledged as the beginning of modern genetics.

In 1953, James Watson and Francis Crick presented the three-dimensional structure of DNA that, despite its apparent simplicity of two intertwined helical chains, showed novel features that hinted at "considerable biological importance".[5] The key feature was the manner in which the purine and pyrimidine bases were paired, and which held the two chains together. Based on the assumption that these nitrogen bases were found in their most common keto rather than enol configuration, then adenine (purine) could only pair with thymine (pyrimidine) and guanine (purine) could only pair with cytosine (pyrimidine). This direct observation from the model of the X-ray diffraction was supported by the experimental observation that in natural DNA, of multiple organisms, the ratios of guanine to cytosine and adenine to thymine were always close to unity. The implication of this specific base pairing rule was not lost on Watson and Crick; they correctly suggested that it was a copying mechanism for the genetic material. A few years later Matthew Meselson and Franklin Stahl very elegantly showed that DNA was indeed replicated in a semiconservative fashion, whereby each helix acts as the template for the synthesis of the next new strand.[6]

Further discoveries in the 1950s and 1960s included the proposal of the central dogma model of molecular biology, with RNA acting as the intermediate between DNA and protein.[7] Semiconservative replication, hinted at by Watson and Crick, was demonstrated by Meselson and Stahl in 1958[6] and the key enzyme in the process, DNA polymerase, was also discovered.[8] After the discovery that the language of DNA is coded in triplets,[9] several scientists "cracked" the genetic code, with Nirenberg, Holley and Khorana winning the 1968 Nobel Prize.

Har Gorbind Khorana led the efforts in deciphering the language of DNA by taking a chemical approach to crack the code. Taking advantage of recently developed cell-free protein expression systems, and his method of generating synthetic polynucleotides of defined sequences, Khorana managed to decode the entire genetic code. He started off by synthesising a long DNA polymer consisting of two repeating guanine and thymine nucleotides (GT)n, which would constitute two triplets of GTG and TGT. Such a polymer was predicted to direct the synthesis of two amino acids in strictly alternating sequence. The subsequent cell-free protein synthesis reaction showed that the sequence led to the generation of a polypeptide with repeating valine and cysteine sequences. Expanding this strategy to generate triplet and quadruplet repeats allowed Khorana to determine the entire combination of the genetic code in a systematic way.[10] The final version revealed that the genetic code exhibited degeneracy, which meant that most of the amino acids were coded for by more than one codon. Codon degeneracy became apparent as there were more codon combinations than the number of amino acids; the total possible number of triplet combinations for coding 20 common amino acids using the four bases was 64. In reality, the 20 common amino acids were coded for by 61 codons out of the possible 64, with the remaining three encoding for stop codons that signal the termination point of protein synthesis. It was thought that the genetic redundancy was a mechanism to increase the potential of the genomes to absorb errors by increasing the chances of silent mutations.

By 1970, the big pieces of the molecular biology puzzle were in place and there was good mechanistic understanding of how cells use the genetic information as a recipe for synthesising proteins. These insights allowed the field of molecular biology to enter a new phase of technological development that resulted in the creation of a set of tools that have collectively ushered in the era of recombinant technology. One of the earliest examples of these is the discovery and characterisation of restriction enzymes – groups of enzymes that recognise a specific sequence of DNA and create a double-stranded cut in the DNA. These reagents are an indispensable part of the cloning kit, allowing for rapid and facile cloning of DNA fragments.

The full potential of restriction enzymes as tools in molecular biology was only fully realised by the invention of the Polymerase Chain Reaction (PCR) in 1986. This technique allows exponential amplification of a specific region of DNA utilising DNA polymerase to copy a single-stranded DNA template. The key feature of the polymerases employed in PCRs is that they are heat-stable, such as the *Taq* polymerase, an enzyme originally isolated from the thermophilic bacterium *Thermus aquaticus*. Kary Mullis was awarded the Nobel Prize in Chemistry for his invention;[11] he shared the prize with Michael Smith who invented an equally powerful technology called site-directed mutagenesis.[12] This technology allows for the introduction of a specific mutation in a specific location in the DNA, thereby enabling investigators to study the effect of a single mutation in a single gene. The final piece of technological advancement developed in the late 1970s was the DNA sequencing technology developed by Fredrick Sanger and colleagues that allowed for the determination of the nucleotide order in DNA using *in vitro* DNA synthesis reactions terminated by incorporation of dideoxynucleotides.[13] Together this slew of technological developments placed the field of molecular biology in a position to effectively and accurately manipulate genetic material and provide detailed mechanistic answers to specific questions. This eventually led to several large initiatives designed to provide large-scale datasets, most famously the Human Genome Project.[14]

Being able to map every gene in the genome has been a fundamental breakthrough in identifying and validating novel drug targets. The Human Genome Project (1990–2003)[14] was an international scientific research project with the initial aims of determining the complete sequence of the human genome, to physically and functionally map all the estimated 20 000–25 000 human genes, and to make them accessible for further study. It followed on from, and utilised, many technological developments made *via* the sequencing of the genomes of several species of bacteria and other model organisms. The massive amount of data generated from the sequencing of the human genome is a source of potentially thousands of novel drug targets.

In response to the large quantities of sequencing data being produced, and along with the rapid development of computing power and software sophistication, bioinformatics developed as a new field of research. This enabled key insights such as prediction of gene function from sequence, discovery of noncoding DNA structures such as promoters and enhancers, and the involvement of specific genes in metabolic and signalling pathways, which differ in varying disease states. Many bioinformatic tools have also been developed to identify sequence homology, which is used to identify members of proteins with similar functions (*e.g.*, the G-protein coupled receptor superfamily, tumour necrosis factor (TNF)-related apoptosis-inducing ligand (TRAIL) isoforms as members of the TNF family), BLAST (Basic Local Alignment Search Tool), HMMER (Hidden Markov Model profiler), and SAM (Sequence Alignment Modeller). These are publicly available tools that are curated by the National Centre for Biotechnology Information.[15]

In the 21st century, following the completion of the Human Genome Project and its technical legacy, additional mass data-driven molecular biology projects to further expand our understanding and knowledge of genetic variation, and subsequent influences on humans, have been initiated. The variations in DNA sequence where individuals differ at a single DNA base are called single nucleotide polymorphisms (SNPs). A pattern of SNPs on the same chromosome, which are inherited as a block, is called a haplotype. The International HapMap Project, led by National Human Genome Research Institute, was a global initiative to develop a haplotype map ("HapMap") of the human genome, a tool that allows researchers to find genes and genetic variations that affect health and disease. The effort was not only to associate the genetic factors with diseases, but to also study variations in response to environmental factors, in susceptibility to infection, and in the effectiveness of, and adverse responses to, drugs and vaccines. The final data set was published in 2010.[16]

Genomes contain vast regions of non-coding DNA sequences which are instructions for the cellular proteins and RNAs to execute their actions in a timely manner and with appropriate magnitudes. The aim of the Encyclopaedia of DNA Elements (ENCODE) project, which began in 2003, is to delineate these functional elements of the human and mouse genomes based on experimental data sets, and link changes in the expression of certain genes to the development of various diseases. All data to date are available through the ENCODE data portal (https://www.encodeproject.org).[17] Functional elements of the mouse and human genomes are defined as discrete, linearly ordered sequence features that specify molecular products (*e.g.*, protein-coding genes, non-coding RNAs) or regulatory roles (*e.g.*, transcriptional promotors or enhancers). Since the biological functions of these elements differ between different cell types and their sources, the ENCODE data now contains 503 biological cell or tissue types from 1369 biological sample sources to better represent their annotations. It is anticipated that emerging technologies, involving genome or epigenome editing, will provide more precise and accurate functional annotations to develop this into a more powerful tool for diagnosis and identification of new targets to treat diverse diseases.

In this century, there have been significant advances in molecular biology technologies which will continue to enable new discoveries in the understanding of diseases and development of new treatments. Following the discovery of PCR in the 1980s, the adaptation of this technique has enabled absolute quantification of mRNA using real-time reverse transcription PCR (also known as RT-qPCR) which is now a widely used technique in molecular biology research and disease diagnosis.[18] Its most prominent role in recent time is in the diagnosis of COVID-19 (SARS-CoV-2) and it is currently the only reliable test for the presence of acute infection with adequate turnaround time.[19] Massive parallel or deep sequencing technology (also known as next-generation sequencing (NGS)), that first emerged in the 1990s, has developed significantly in the last 20 years, and cost per genome has now declined to $1000 from $3 billion (estimated for the Human Genome Project), making it more accessible for wide-scale research and diagnosis of diseases.

Another prominent aspect of molecular biology in this century was the discovery of induced pluripotent stem cells (iPSCs). In 1962 John B. Gurdon originally challenged the hypothesis that mature cells had specialised characteristics that were irreversible. Forty years later, Shinya Yamanaka and his group demonstrated induction of pluripotent stem cells from adult fibroblasts by introducing just four transcription factors: Oct3/4, Sox2, c-Myc and Klf4[20] that enabled the cells to develop into all the different tissues of the body. The Nobel Prize in Physiology or Medicine was later awarded for this work in 2012. The use of pluripotent stem cells (iPSCs) circumvented ethical issues arising from the use of embryonic stem cells. iPSCs can now be generated from human skin cells, including patients' cells, and live cells derived from iPSCs now allow scientists to study disease mechanisms in new ways. Clinical trials involving iPSCs are still on a small scale; however, there are several such trials ongoing to treat conditions such as macular degeneration and Parkinson's disease.[21]

The CRISPR/Cas9 system of genome editing is arguably one of the most important developments of the 21st century in molecular biology thus far, providing great promise for gene therapy. DNA sequences which were repeated and separated by different spacer sequences were first identified in archaea and in other microbes by Ishino and his colleagues in 1987, and later named by Jansen in 2002 as CRISPR (Clustered Regularly Interspaced Short Palindromic Repeats).[22] In 2011, microbiologist Emmanuelle Charpentier discovered trans-activating CRISPR RNA (tracrRNA) as part of bacteria's ancient immune system. Bacteria protect themselves by cleaving viral DNA from viruses that are infecting them.[23] Together with Jennifer Doudna, an experienced biochemist, they succeeded in turning this mechanism into genetic scissors for genome editing in 2012.[24] This work was awarded a Nobel Prize in Chemistry in 2020. CRISPR/Cas9 has made genome editing simpler and accessible, and it has revolutionised science. Molecular biology will continue to shape the drug discovery landscape, and, in this chapter, we will describe the various techniques used in molecular biology to enable successful drug discovery.

## 9.2 Sequencing

### 9.2.1 History of Sequencing

Determining the sequence of DNA or RNA in biological samples is an integral component of molecular biology research. Over the last fifty years, techniques and technologies for sequencing DNA and RNA molecules have evolved rapidly, from sequencing short oligonucleotides in bacteria and yeast to a whole human genome. In 1977, the first DNA genome was resolved by Frederick Sanger and his colleagues for bacteriophage ϕX174 or "PhiX", which is still used in many sequencing labs today as a positive control genome.[25] The "plus and minus technique" used to sequence this genome utilises DNA polymerase to synthesise from a primer, incorporating $^{32}$P radiolabelled nucleotides. By running the products on a polyacrylamide gel and comparing between the eight lanes (*i.e.* +A. +T, +C, +G, −A, −T, −C, −G), the nucleotides at each position can be inferred in the covered sequence.

## 9.2.2 Sanger Sequencing

Shortly after, "chain-termination" or the dideoxy technique was developed by Sanger, widely known as Sanger sequencing (Figure 9.1), which is still widely used in small-scale sequencing today.[13] The chain-termination technique makes use of dideoxynucleotides (ddNTPs), which are chemical analogues of the monomers of DNA strands. When ddNTPs get incorporated into a newly synthesised DNA, they halt extension of the DNA strand as ddNTP does not contain a reactive group required for incorporation of the next nucleotide. Mixing labelled ddNTPs into a DNA extension reaction, at a fraction of the concentration of standard nucleotides, results in the production of DNA strands of each possible length as the ddNTPs get randomly incorporated. By performing four

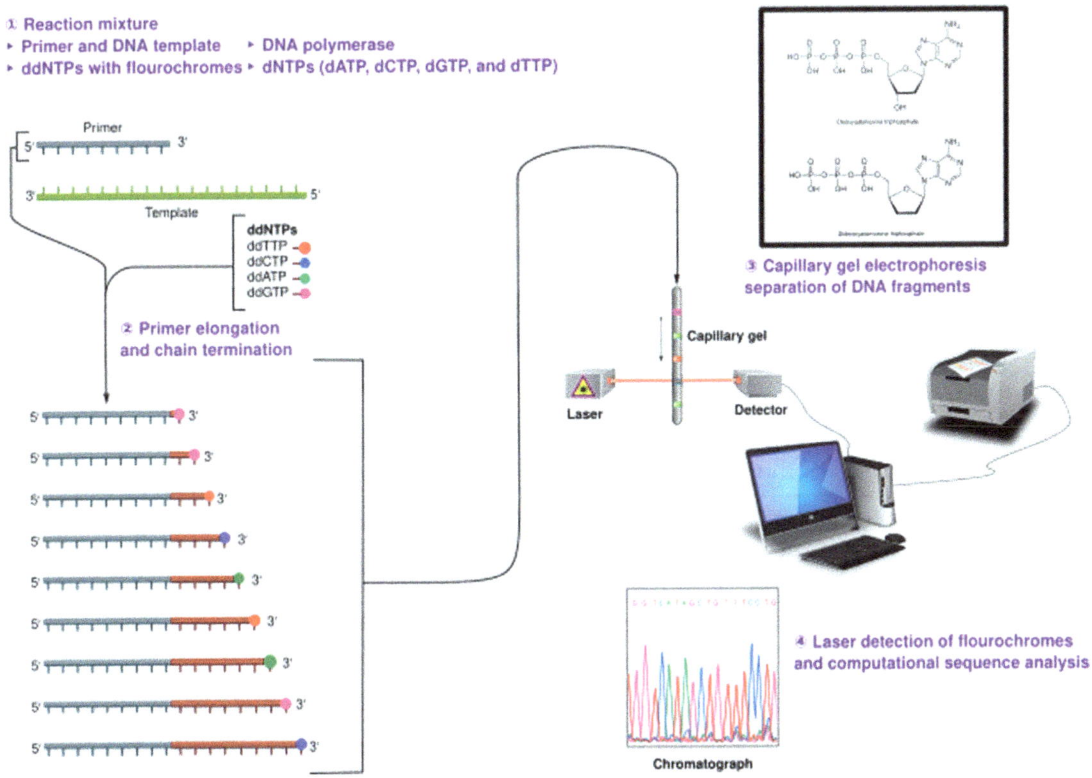


**Figure 9.1** Sanger sequencing. Reproduced from https://commons.wikimedia.org/wiki/File:Sanger-sequencing.svg, under the terms of the CC BY 3.0 license, https://creativecommons.org/licenses/by-sa/3.0/deed.en. Image credit: Estevezj.

parallel reactions containing each individual ddNTP base, and running the reactions on four lanes of a polyacrylamide gel, a DNA sequence of interest can be inferred by the distances at which each fragment with labelled ddNTP migrates under electrophoresis. Automated Sanger sequencing platforms utilise capillary electrophoresis for resolving DNA fragments containing fluorescently labelled ddNTPs. These can produce reads slightly less than 1000 bases in length. To analyse longer sequences, overlapping DNA fragments were cloned and sequenced separately, and then assembled into one contiguous sequence *in silico*. This is known as shotgun sequencing, and this is still applied today with next-generation sequencing, which is faster than Sanger sequencing. Sanger sequencing is still, however, a more cost-effective sequencing technique with faster turnaround for shorter oligonucleotides, ideal for small-scale experiments such as confirming sequences of target genes for cloning.

### 9.2.3 Next-generation Sequencing

Next-generation sequencing (NGS) is massive parallel or deep DNA sequencing that revolutionised genomic research. The previous Sanger sequencing technology that was used to decipher the human genome took more than a decade during the Human Genome Project,[14] whereas using NGS an entire human genome can be sequenced in a day.

There are currently several different NGS platforms using different sequencing technologies; these are summarised in Table 9.1. All NGS technologies utilise DNA polymerase amplification from template sequences by PCR first, which are called the sequencing libraries. In most NGS platforms, these amplified DNA templates are specially segregated and are sequenced simultaneously in a massive parallel manner to achieve much increased throughputs.[26,27] These three major NGS technologies are illustrated in Figure 9.2. The most widely used NGS technology today is the bridge amplification sequencing by Illumina, adapted from a patent published by Roger Y. Tsien *et al.* (WO1991006678A1). Adaptors are added to the ends of DNA molecules for sequencing. These are passed over a lawn of complementary oligonucleotides bound to a flow-cell. These sequences are amplified by solid-phase PCR, producing clusters of

**Table 9.1** Comparison of the three most widely use NGS technologies.

| NGS technologies | Bead-based pyrosequencing (Roche 454) | Bridge amplification sequencing (Illumina) | Ion semiconductor sequencing (Ion Torrent) |
|---|---|---|---|
| Amplification method | Bead-based emulsion PCR | Bridge amplification in flow-cell | Amplification on semi-conductor chip |
| Detection signal | Luminescent | Fluorescence | Hydrogen ion |
| Advantages over other NGS technologies | No modifications required to nucleotides, longer read length | Large data output capability, able to decipher homopolymers (*e.g.*, TTTTTTT...) better | Fast sequencing, high throughput, more cost effective for small-scale applications |
| Disadvantage over other NGS technologies | Unable to decipher homopolymers well, discontinued in 2016 | High cost, short read length | Unable to decipher homopolymers well, short read length |

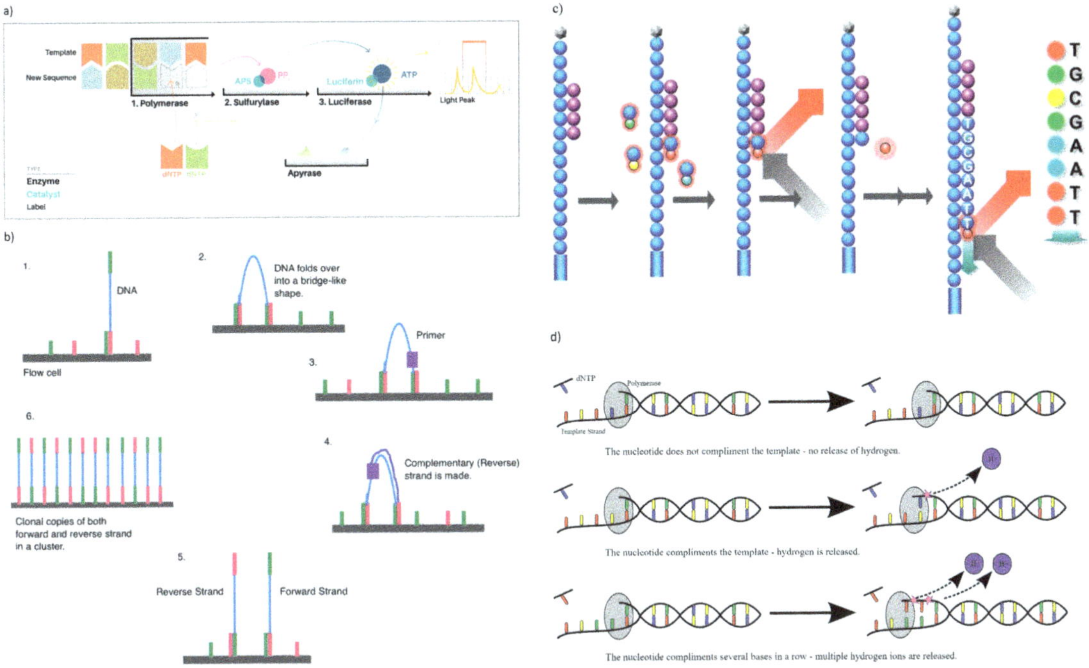


**Figure 9.2** Next-generation sequencing. (a) Pyrosequencing. Reproduced from https://commons.wikimedia.org/wiki/File:How_Pyrosequencing_Works.svg, under the terms of the CC BY-SA 4.0 license, https://creativecommons.org/licenses/by-sa/4.0/deed.en. Image Credit: Jacopo Pompilii, DensityDesign Research Lab. (b) Bridge amplification in Illumina sequencers. Reproduced from https://commons.wikimedia.org/wiki/File:Cluster_Generation.png, under the terms of the CC BY-SA 4.0 license, https://creativecommons.org/licenses/by-sa/4.0/deed.en. Image Credit: DMLapato. (c) Reversible terminator chemistry of Illumina's sequencer, incorporating fluorescently labelled nucleotides for detection. Reproduced from https://en.wikipedia.org/wiki/File:Sequencing_by_synthesis_Reversible_terminators.png, under the terms of the CC BY-SA 3.0 license, https://creativecommons.org/licenses/by-sa/3.0/. Image Credit: Abizar Lakdawalla. (d) Ion semiconductor sequencing by Ion Torrent. Reproduced from https://commons.wikimedia.org/wiki/File:DNTP_nucletide_incorporation_events.svg, under the terms of the CC BY-SA 3.0 license, https://creativecommons.org/licenses/by-sa/3.0/deed.en. Image Credit: David Tack.

clonal populations from each of the individual original flow-cells. The process is known as bridge amplification as the DNA strand bridges over during the amplification process (Figure 9.2b). Sequencing itself is performed in the presence of DNA polymerase and fluorescent "reversible-terminator" dNTPs, which cannot immediately bind the next nucleotide as the fluorophore occupies the position for the next nucleotide. This is cleaved away before the next nucleotide is added thus allowing the sequencing to occur in a synchronous manner. The fluorophore of the newly incorporated nucleotide is excited by appropriate lasers and its fluorescent is captured by CCD camera, before the fluorophores blocking the next nucleotide extension are removed by enzymatic rection (Figure 9.2c).

### 9.2.4 RNA Sequencing

RNA sequencing (RNA-Seq) is a powerful method which uses next-generation sequencing (NGS) of cDNA to perform transcriptome analysis in a biological sample at a certain moment. Over the past decade, this technique has become a ubiquitous tool of transcriptomics both for qualitative (*i.e.* discovering new transcripts) and quantitative (*i.e.* measuring relative quantities for transcripts) analyses to better understand the genomic function.[28–32]

Before RNA-Seq was developed, transcriptome annotations were carried out using cDNA libraries, then by high-throughput techniques such as hybridisation-based microarrays and sequencing-based methods. However, due to several issues with microarrays, sequencing gained more ground in the field of transcriptomics.[33,34] These progressed from Sanger sequencing, and chemical tag-based methods to the now widely used Illumina short-read sequencing technology.[35,36]

Short-read RNA-seq is most often used for analysing differential gene expression (DGE).[32] However, to date, almost 100 distinct methods have been derived from the standard RNA-seq protocol to study many different aspects of RNA biology, such as revealing the extent of mRNA splicing, the regulation of gene expression by non-coding RNAs and enhancer RNAs, single-cell gene expression, translation (the translatome), RNA structure (the structurome) and spatial transcriptomics (spatialomics).[32,37–40]

### 9.2.5 Third-generation DNA Sequencing

The latest generation DNA sequencing, which is often referred to as third-generation DNA sequencing, is capable of sequencing single DNA or RNA molecules, negating the requirement for DNA amplification shared by all predecessor technologies.

The most widely used third-generation technology is the single molecule real time (SMRT) platform from Pacific Biosciences.[41] The SMRT platform consists of arrays of microfabricated nanostructures called zero-mode waveguides (ZMWs) which are essentially tiny holes in a metallic film covering a chip (Figure 9.3). Inside a ZMW, a DNA polymerase is affixed at the bottom of the hole. As the diameter of these holes is smaller than the wavelength of the light passing through, which causes it to decay exponentially, it allows visualisation of a single nucleotide. During SMRT sequencing, the DNA library of interest and fluorescent dNTPs are added to the DNA polymerase and the extension of DNA chains by a single nucleotide can be monitored in real-time as a fluorescent nucleotide being incorporated. Only the newly incorporated nucleotide will give a fluorescent signal as the dye is cleaved away immediately afterwards. This process is much faster than next-generation sequencing platforms and is capable of producing exceptionally long reads (>10 kb in length), which are useful for *de novo* genome assembly. The disadvantage in this platform is that it can result in a greater error rate than some other next-generation sequencing platforms.

Nanopore is another third-generation sequencing technique that can produce incredibly long reads but does not rely on DNA amplification, which makes sequencing data far cheaper and faster than was previously possible, and avoids PCR bias in

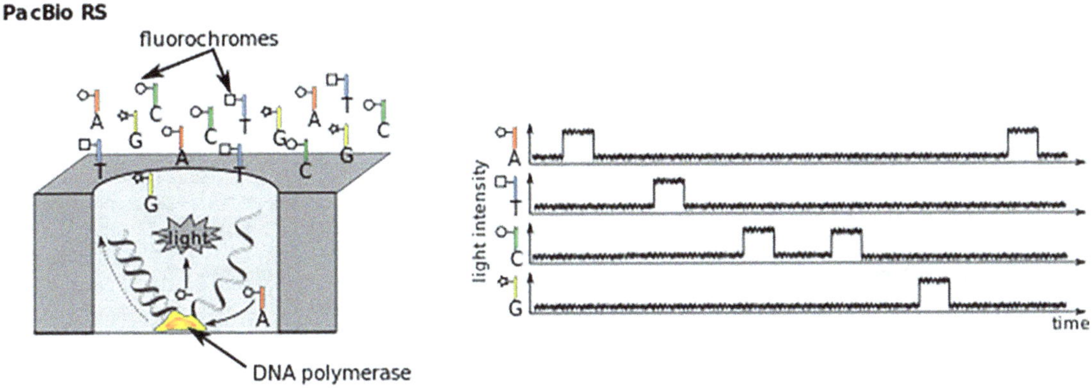


**Figure 9.3** Nucleotide detection in a zero-mode waveguide (ZMW), as featured in PacBio's SMRT sequencers. Reproduced from https://commons.wikimedia.org/wiki/File:-From_second_to_fourth-generation_sequencing,_illustration_on_TAGGCT_template.svg, under the terms of the CC BY-SA 3.0 license, https://creativecommons.org/licenses/by-sa/3.0/deed.en. Image Credit: Philippe Hupé.

sequencing data.[41] The first-generation nanopore consists of α-haemolysin protein which creates tiny holes (1 nm) that are large enough for a single DNA nucleotide to pass through.[42] These nanopores are embedded in an electro-resistant membrane, and each nanopore is connected to an electrode connected to a channel and sensor chip. Double-stranded DNA gets denatured by a processive enzyme or motor protein which ratchets one of the strands through a nanopore. When single-stranded DNA or RNA for sequencing passes through the nanopore, the current is disrupted and produces a unique pattern which is detected by the sensor chip. This pattern is then decoded using base-calling algorithms to determine the DNA or RNA sequence in real-time (Figure 9.4). MinION sequencer marketed by Oxford Nanopore Technologies (ONT) can generate up to 50 Gb of real-time sequencing data on a bench-top scale, which presents the opportunity to decentralise sequencing and make it more available in ordinary laboratories or even in the field setting where samples are collected, rather than being carried out at sequencing core facilities that are common today (https://nanoporetech.com/).

Comparison of Illumina's next-generation sequencing and PacBio/ONT's third-generation sequencing is shown in Table 9.2. Illumina's sequencers provide the highest throughput and the lowest cost per sequencing data, coupled with the highest accuracy. Nevertheless, this is limited by the short maximum read lengths, and interpretation of output is challenging if the sequence contains long nucleotide repeats. PacBio and ONT provide considerable advantages on long read lengths without a requirement for PCR-based amplification in the DNA library preparation. However, the sequence accuracy tends be lower and is more expensive than Illumina at this moment in time. Nevertheless, OTN's pocket-sized sequencers are paradigm-shifting, and with further research and development on its nanopores, these may bring in a new era for molecular biology research and hence revolutionize drug discovery.

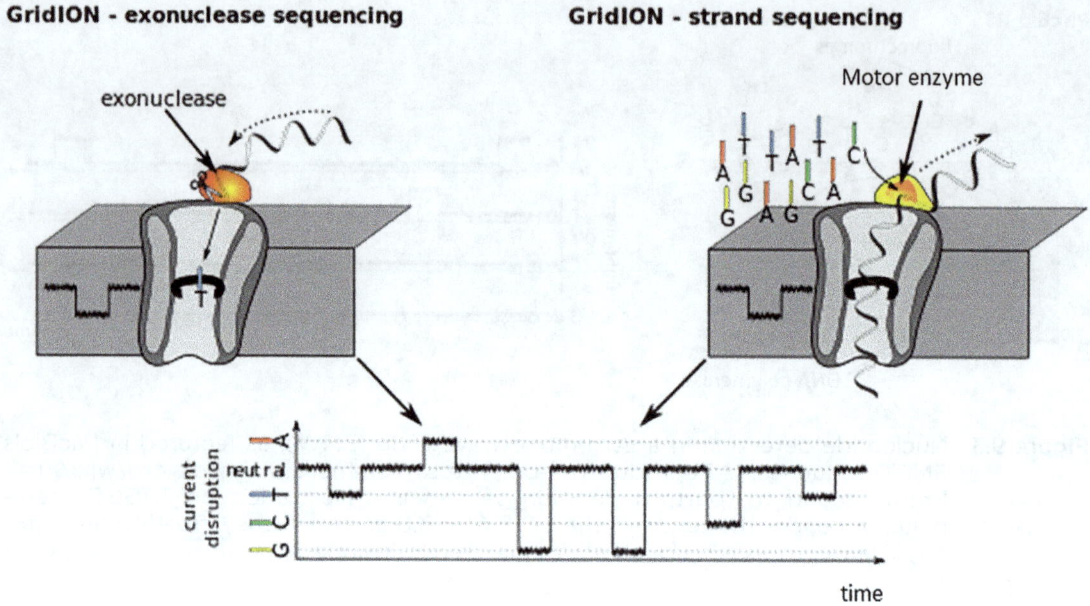


**Figure 9.4** Nanopore DNA sequencing as employed in Oxford Nanopore Technologies' MinION sequencer. Reproduced from https://commons.wikimedia.org/wiki/File:From_second_to_fourth-generation_sequencing,_illustration_on_TAGGCT_template.svg, under the terms of the CC BY-SA 3.0 license, https://creativecommons.org/licenses/by-sa/3.0/deed.en. Image Credit: Philippe Hupé.

**Table 9.2** Comparison of various platforms of PacBio, ONT and Illumina sequencing read lengths, accuracy throughput and cost. (Adapted from Logsdon *et al. Nature Reviews Genetics*. 2020.).

| Sequencing technology/ platform | Read length (kb) | Read accuracy (%) | Maximum throughput per flow cell (Gb) | Estimated cost per Gb (US$) |
|---|---|---|---|---|
| Pacific Biosciences (PacBio)/RS II | >60 | 87–92 | 2 | 333–933 |
| Oxford Nanopore Technologies (ONT)/MinION/GridION | >1000 | 87–98 | 30 | 50–500 |
| Illumina/NextSeq550 | 0.15 | >99.9 | >30 | 50–63 |

## 9.3 Gene-editing Methods

Targeted genome editing can be used to modify any sequence of interest in cells or organisms. Knock-in and knock-out of specific genes or sequences use engineered nucleases: artificial enzymes composed of a sequence-specific DNA-binding domain, fused to a nuclease that cleaves DNA non-specifically. The nucleases usually induce double-stranded breaks at specific DNA sites, which are then repaired by endogenous cellular mechanisms. These mechanisms are exploited *via* these techniques, creating sequence alterations by their innate inaccuracies which lead to gene expression alterations.

Three key genome-editing tools, zinc finger nucleases, transcription activator-like effector nucleases (TALENs) and CRISPR/Cas9, have evolved and transformed molecular biology and drug discovery research over the last 20 years. In this section we describe different gene editing techniques in molecular biology.

### 9.3.1 Zinc Finger Nucleases (ZFNs)

Zinc finger nucleases (ZFNs), discovered in 1996,[43] can be thought of as highly specific genomic scissors before the arrival of CRISPR/Cas genome editing, capable of creating double-stranded DNA breaks at user-specified locations. The ZFN is comprised of two components: a zinc finger domain and a FokI endonuclease domain. Zinc finger domains are naturally occurring transcription factors, typically recognising a 9 base-pair target specific for the DNA sequence to be edited. The FokI endonuclease must dimerise for activity, meaning the double-strand DNA cleavage will only occur at sites where two ZFNs are bound on opposite DNA strands, limiting off-target cleavage. The double-stranded break created by the ZFN will activate the native DNA damage response pathway, leading to repair by one of two cellular processes: homologous recombination or non-homologous end joining. If a repair template is co-transfected into the cell, homologous recombination will result in gene integration or modification (knock-in). If a repair template is not available, non-homologous end joining will take place, resulting in mis-repair and ultimately gene deletion (knock-out).[44]

The first use of ZFNs relied on viral vector delivery to the cell, but studies generally now use mRNA delivery *via* electroporation. High levels of expression can be obtained in this way, but expression is only transient, with the mRNA half-life shorter than that of DNA.[45]

### 9.3.2 Transcription Activator-like Effector Nucleases (TALENs)

Like ZFNs, TALENs also comprise a DNA-binding domain fused to the FokI endonuclease; however, in place of the zinc finger motif, here the Fokl nuclease is fused to a bacterial transcription activator-like effector protein (TALE).[46] TALENs contain DNA-binding domains composed of 33–35 amino acid repeats, with specificity determined by just two variable amino acids. Since a single TALEN motif recognises just one nucleotide, sequence specificity is determined by arrays of individual TALENs. This single-base recognition allows greater design flexibility than the triplet configuration of ZFNs; however, cloning of the TALEN arrays presents a technical challenge due to large identical repeat sequences. Like ZFNs, mRNA delivery *via* electroporation is used as the vector for TALENs. Although the TALEN system was named as one of the methods of the year for precise genome editing in 2011 by *Nature Methods*,[47] due to its complexity in molecular cloning methods and difficulty in delivery of large functional components, this technique has been overshadowed by the CRISPR/Cas system since its emergence shortly after. Both ZFNs and TALENs are in early clinical trials to demonstrate their therapeutic applications.[45]

### 9.3.3 CRISPR

CRISPR (Clustered Regularly Interspaced Short Palindromic Repeat) gene-editing technology is composed of an endonuclease protein and a short guide RNA giving DNA targeting specificity. The repeat elements, separated by non-repeating DNA sequences called spacers, were first noted in the bacteria *E. coli* in 1987.[48] It then took over a decade for researchers to recognise the importance of CRISPR in the adaptive immunity of bacteria and archaea.[24,49] In bacteria, resistance to certain viruses can be ascertained by incorporation of a small fragment of the virus genome into the CRISPR sequence after infection, allowing subsequent infection to be targeted for destruction *via* DNA cleavage. The endonucleases responsible for DNA cleavage are Cas proteins; the most well-known and relevant for gene editing is Cas9.

The Cas9 nuclease is coupled to two types of RNA: trans-activating crRNA (tracrRNA) and a CRISPR RNA (crRNA) that recognises the target DNA sequence by Watson–Crick base pairing, guiding Cas9 to the target site where it stimulates DNA strand-break (Figure 9.5). In research using single guide RNA (sgRNA) which contains tracrRNA fused with crRNA, which is synthetically generated, is now more prevalent. This DNA cleavage can be a double-stranded break in the case of the wild-type Cas9, or a single-stranded break if mutant Cas9 variants known as nickases are employed. Multiple double-stranded breaks can also be exploited to mediate larger deletions in the genome. For more precise gene editing, repair templates in the form of double-stranded DNAs, or single-stranded oligonucleotides, are utilised, leading to homology-directed repair pathways that are mediated by endogenous DNA repair enzymes. This repair method is effective for making small changes in the genome, such as introducing single-nucleotide mutations. However, its efficiency is dependent on cell types, states, and genomic sites and repair templates.

The CRISPR/Cas9 system has many advantages over ZFNs and TALENs due to its ability to be guided by RNA–DNA interactions, easy design, cost-effectiveness, facile prediction of off-target effects, and the possibility of multiplexing to modify several genomic sites simultaneously.[50] These features also make the CRISPR/Cas9 system well-suited for high-throughput gene-editing screening. Key features of the three genome editing tools are compared in Table 9.3.

One of the major concerns for CRISPR/Cas9 gene editing is off-target effects, which refers to non-specific and unintended genomic site modifications. The Cas9 nickase variant that induces single-stranded breaks has been shown to minimise the off-target effects, along with various other Cas9 that are engineered with the intention to reduce the off-target effects. Improved guide-RNA design can also help to reduce the off-target effects of CRISPR. Several tools have been developed to generate optimised guide-RNA sequences for specific genes, for example, E-Crisp (http://www.e-crisp.org/E-CRISP/) and CasOFFinder (http://www.rgenome.net/cas-offinder/). Limitations for this type of platform are that they are based on computational algorithms that rely on experimental data and may lack generalisability across different experimental setups. Recently, a more robust and widely applicable design tool called sgDesigner (http://crispr.wustl.edu) was developed to address these limitations by a group at Washington University and is freely available as a web application.

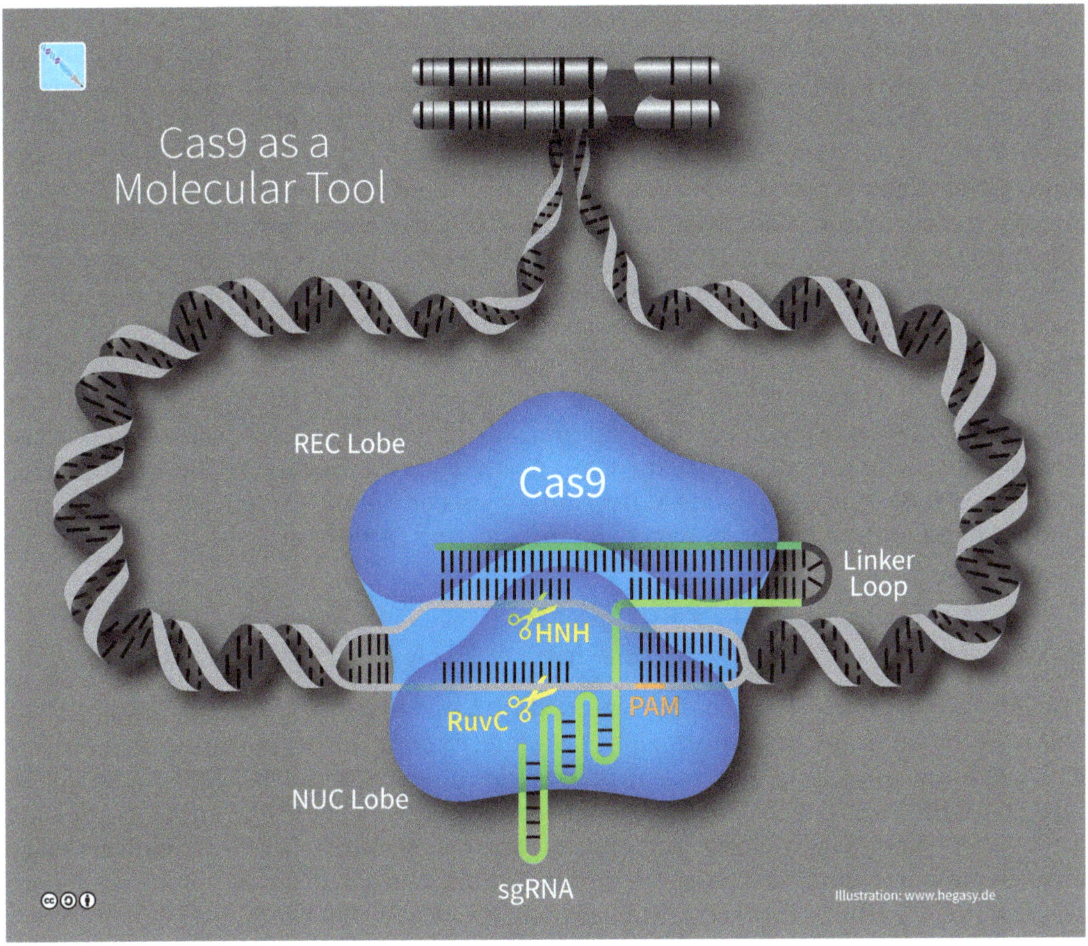


**Figure 9.5** CRISPR/Cas9, sgRNA, PAM. Reproduced from https://commons.wikimedia.org/wiki/File:15_Hegasy_Cas9_DNA_Tool_Wiki_E_CCBYSA.png, under the terms of the CC BY-SA 4.0 license, https://creativecommons.org/licenses/by-sa/4.0/deed.en. Image Credit: Guido4.

**Table 9.3** Technology differences between genome editing techniques (adapted from S. H. Khan, Genome-Editing Technologies: Concept, Pros, and Cons of Various Genome-Editing Techniques and Bioethical Concerns for Clinical Application, *Mol. Ther. Nucleic Acids*, 2019).

| Parameter | ZFN | TALEN | CRISPR/Cas9 |
|---|---|---|---|
| Mechanism of target DNA recognition | DNA–protein interaction | DNA–protein interaction | DNA–RNA interaction |
| Mechanism of DNA cleavage | Double-strand break by *FokI* | Double-strand break by *FokI* | Single- or double-strand break by Cas9 |
| Design simplicity | Moderate | Easy–moderate | Easy |
| Assembly | Difficult | Moderate | Easy |
| Cost | Low | High | Low |
| Specificity | Low | Higher | Highest |

While some factors influence which sequences can be selected as targets of CRIPSR/Cas (*e.g.*, presence of similar off-target sequences, GC content, internal secondary structure of sgRNA), almost any DNA sequences can be targeted for editing. Nevertheless, one limitation of flexibility in DNA targeting by the CRISPR/Cas system is that it requires a short sequence (usually 2–6 base pairs long) called a protospacer adjacent motif (PAM) flanking each target sequence.[51] In bacteria, for example, the well-known *Streptococcus pyogenes* Cas9 (SpCas9) requires target recognition of the NGG motif, where N can be A, C, G, or T. PAMs are used to discriminate self and non-self to protect their genome from being targeted by their own CRISPR/Cas system. PAMs also allow a more efficient search for the target sequences in viruses. This is because the Cas nucleases scan available DNA for a PAM before looking for the specific target sequence by sgRNA binding. Consequently, a sequence with a perfect match between sgRNA in Cas and target genome sequence will be ignored without the presence of a PAM. To date, over 900 distinct naturally occurring Cas9 homologues with varying PAM recognition profiles have been identified.[52] Altering and/or relaxing PAM recognition by mutating a homologue of Cas9 has been beneficial for allowing CRISPR enzymes to access more of the genome.

### 9.3.4 Gene Expression Modulation by RNA Interference (RNAi)

The gene silencing effect of double-stranded RNA was discovered in *C. elegans* in 1998, and later in plants and other animals.[53] RNA interference (RNAi) is a conserved process which is initiated with the processing of long, double-stranded RNA (dsRNA) molecules into small interfering RNA (siRNA) by the endonuclease Dicer. The siRNA complexes are 21–25 nucleotides (nt) long, and have distinctive termini, with the 3′ end carrying a dinucleotide overhand, while the 5′ end has a monophosphate group. Both the length and termini are critical for recognition of the siRNA by the RNA-induced silencing complex, or RISC. Once generated, the siRNA duplex is loaded onto the Argonaute (AGO2) component of RISC, by Dicer and the RNA binding protein TRBP. AGO2 then cleaves the mRNA target and the cleaved product is released, leaving behind the single-stranded guide RNA within the RISC. The RISC is subsequently recycled, using the same guide strand for several other rounds of target mRNA cleavage.

Use of RNAi to screen for the effects of the knockdown of target gene expression is now a widely used tool in the pharmaceutical industry for pharmacological target identification and validation. It can be undertaken at a high-throughput level with an adaptation of modern screening platforms, developed for small molecules. The most powerful RNAi screens cover the whole genome of model organisms or cell lines, which are commercially available. Such screens have been carried out to investigate signal transduction pathways, differentiation and pathogen interactions.[54] Although CRISPR whole-genome screens have become a popular choice in recent years, RNAi still has a couple of advantages in certain areas: (1) RNAi can still be designed if an organism's transcriptome is sequenced but not the whole genome, (2) RNAi targets mRNA in the cytoplasm and not genomic DNA in the nucleus. Hence, accessibility does not appear to be impaired by chromatin states, as observed for CRISPR-based approaches.[55]

For screening purposes, various RNAi reagents are used to exploit the endogenous processing mechanisms, including synthetic siRNAs, small hairpin RNAs (shRNAs) and dsRNAs. dsRNAs are not used in mammalian systems as they trigger the interferon responses, however, they are used frequently as *in vivo* RNAi screening tools in model organisms such as *C. elegans* and *Drosophila* to study the effect of gene silencing in a complex, multicellular system. Long dsRNAs are usually 200–500 nt in length, and can be injected directly, delivered *via* bacteria, in which they are expressed as transgenes, or simply by incubating with cultured cells.

The use of synthetic siRNAs was first described by Elbashir *et al.* in 2001.[56] They are transfected into cells chemically by electroporation, viral delivery or directly injected in model organisms. More recently, there are chemically modified siRNAs with self-delivering capability which enable RNAi in difficult-to-transfect cells such as immunological and neuronal cells by conventional methods. The effects of the siRNAs are transient, especially in actively dividing cells, as they are not stable outside of the RISC and the silencing effect is only at mRNA level and not a change in the genome.

This contrasts with shRNA vectors, which are DNA sequences that allow for controlled or continuous expression of small single-stranded RNA (50–70 nt) transcripts, complementary to the selected mRNA target. shRNA vectors are either transfected into cells as plasmid DNA or delivered using viral particles, particularly into cells that are difficult to transfect. Long RNA transcripts fold back to form stem-loop structures (hence the name hairpin). The shRNAs are then processed in the cytoplasm by Dicer to generate siRNAs, as described above. shRNA vectors can be placed under the control of inducible promoters, restricting expression temporally or spatially.[54,57]

Cell-based RNAi screening can be combined with small molecule screening to provide additional information or a more focused screen. For example, cells can be sensitised with a drug prior to a whole-genome RNAi screen for synergistic phenotypes. This was undertaken with neratinib (Nerlynx®), a small molecule tyrosine kinase inhibitor of the ErbB receptor family used as treatment for breast cancer.[58] A genome-wide functional RNAi screen was combined with a lethal dose of neratinib in the SKBR-3 breast cancer cell line to discover chemo-resistant interactions with the drug. This screen identified novel mediators of cellular resistance to the kinase inhibitor that could lead to the identification of new drug targets. These can be used in conjunction with neratinib and help prevent drug resistance.[58,59]

Genome-wide RNAi screening has been carried out extensively in *C. elegans in vivo*, as it is particularly amenable to this mechanism.[58] Ashrafi *et al.* carried out an RNAi screen to identify novel components involved in lipid metabolism.[58] The use of Nile Red, a fluorescent dye that can be fed to the worms and is taken up into fat, allowed for a relatively simple screen of the visualisation and quantification of fluorescent lipid droplets. Knock-down of 305 of the genes tested increased the accumulation of fat, whilst 112 genes decreased fat levels when inactivated. Many of these genes have human homologues, some of which are known to be involved in lipid metabolism. Other represented genes not previously implicated in fat regulation were identified and may eventually become targets for the treatment of obesity. Genome-wide RNAi screens have also been carried out *in vivo* in *Drosophila* on systems such as pain perception, obesity, heart function, bacterial infections of the gut, neural stem cell self-renewal and neurological disease. RNAi approaches have also been used *in vivo* in mice. RNAi can be introduced into embryonic stem cells from which transgenic mice can then be generated. Lentiviral-based RNAi constructs can also be applied to tissues such as skin. An *ex vivo* approach has proved to be useful in the study of cancer development, whereby RNAi can be added to tumour cells in culture; these cells can then be introduced into mice to assess the effect of the gene knockdown on tumourigenesis.[53]

RNAi-based gene silencing has revolutionised functional genomics due to its relative ease and ability to provide a powerful reverse genetic approach, particularly in organisms in which classical genetic approaches are otherwise difficult or have not been developed.[60] Its ease of use has made RNAi the method of choice for deciphering gene function. However, RNAi does not knock down its target gene expression, which does not always mirror the complete loss of function that often occurs with genetic mutation.[55] Too much RNAi can displace microRNAs from RISC. This can impair the functions of endogenous microRNAs, leading to alterations in gene transcript levels and consequently to off-target phenotypes.[126] Furthermore, the reproducibility of RNAi screen hits is approximately 32–49% overlap, dependent on the types of analysis between two separate screens for 21 853 genes comparing the top 200 and 500 targets.[59]

RNAi is still a popular choice for molecular biology experiments due to its accessibility to commercially available pre-validated tools, ease of application and the speed at which the effect can be observed relative to CRISPR/Cas9 in cellular assays. Furthermore, RNAi leads to a reversible, hypomorphic knockdown of the gene of interest, which could be advantageous if a complete, permanent knockdown is lethal or presents unfavourable phenotypes.

## 9.4 Model Systems

Model systems are used by researchers to study biological systems in a physiologically relevant setting, with the practice being based upon the fundamental idea that biological systems and processes are evolutionarily conserved. During the late 20th and early 21st centuries, research has been focused upon a handful of model organisms. This section will outline some of the most used model systems, detailing the advantages and disadvantages to utilising these for research purposes, with a summary provided in Table 9.4.

### 9.4.1 Cellular Systems

Bacteria have long been hailed as powerful model systems for studying the fundamentals of molecular biology.[61] One major advantage of bacterial systems is their rapid growth rate, with some strains dividing every 45 minutes. This means that a single bacterial cell can produce enough DNA or protein for purification and further study within as little as 16 hours. Comparing this to the doubling time of mammalian cells, approximately 18 hours, several days of growth are required to obtain the same level of cell numbers. The most frequently used bacterial species in molecular

**Table 9.4** Comparison of common model systems, their advantages and comments as to their usage and relevance.

| System | Advantages | Comments |
|---|---|---|
| Bacteria | Rapid growth rate | Over 400 prokaryote genome sequences published |
| | Ease of genetic manipulation and genetic replication | Mapping mutations allows for identification of resistance mechanisms |
| | Low cost | |
| *S.cerevisiae/S. pombe* | Ease of genetic manipulation *e.g.*, introduction of exogenous DNA, gene deletion, gene replacement | High degree of sequence conservation with humans |
| | Genome-wide screening | Characterisation of metabolic pathways and signal transduction *e.g.*, cyclin-dependent kinases, cholesterol synthesis, GPCRs and MAPKs |
| | Low cost | Investigation of protein–protein interactions using yeast two-hybrid systems |
| *C. elegans* | Ease of genetic manipulation, in particular RNAi gene silencing | First multicellular organism to have its genome sequenced (1998) |
| | High conservation of biochemical pathways between worms and humans | 75% human genes have homologues in *C. elegans* |
| | Low cost | Pathways such as RAS-MAPK, insulin signalling and apoptotic pathways highly conserved in *C. elegans* |
| | Forms complex structures such as nervous system and digestive tract | |
| *D. melanogaster* | Short life-cycle | 77% human disease-linked genes have homologues in *Drosophila* |
| | Low cost | A single *Drosophila* gene often has multiple human counterparts *e.g.*, p53 has three isoforms in humans, p53, p63 and p73 beneficial in target identification as redundancy is removed |
| | Distinct developmental stages | |
| | Simple genetics | |
| | Disease causing mutations present in humans also relevant in *Drosophila* | |
| *D. rerio* | Can be assessed in multiwell formats | Traditionally used for the study of embryogenesis |
| | Rapid development | 70% protein coding human genes related to zebrafish genes |
| | Low cost | Mutations gave been identified that cause disease phenotypes similar to those seen in humans *e.g.*, polycystic kidney disease, heart disease, leukaemia and nervous system disorders |
| | | Can be used for ADME, PK, safety and toxicology studies |
| Mammalian cells | Closest in physiological response to human disease state | 3D cell cultures can closely mimic physiology, making them more disease-relevant models *e.g.*, tumours |
| | Various models can be adopted *e.g.*, immortalised cell lines, primary cells and stem cells | Primary cells from donor tissue do not require any genetic manipulation in order to exhibit disease phenotype |
| *M. musculus* | Higher proteomic and functional genetic conservation with humans | 95% genes conserved between humans and mice |
| | Allows for transplantation, gene knock-out or knock-in | Various mouse models exist to mimic human diseases *e.g.*, NOD (non-obese diabetic) mice develop type I diabetes |
| | | SCID (severe combined immune deficiency) mice lack an immune system |

biology is *Escherichia coli* (*E. coli*). Commonly used laboratory *E. coli* strains do not carry toxins and are considered non-pathogenic. There are many uses of *E. coli* in molecular biology, such as cloning of genes and growing plasmid DNA from many different organisms. DNA from any source can be inserted into a plasmid and replicated in *E. coli*.

Despite the advantages of bacterial systems, arguably mammalian cells are the most important model system in biology and medicine. The culture of cells and tissues has been documented since the late 1800s; however, routine culturing of mammalian cells was not possible until the 1950s. There are three types of mammalian cells cultured *in vitro* that are commonly used in molecular biology and drug discovery research: immortalised cells, primary cells and stem cells.

### 9.4.2 Immortalised Cells

These cells are "immortal" because they undergo cell division and proliferate almost infinitely. There are various immortalised cell lines which have been derived from numerous sources. Some of them are derived from stem cells and are naturally proliferative, while others contain mutations that deregulate the normal cell cycles leading to uncontrolled proliferation. The most well-known example of these are the cervical cancer biopsy cells of Mrs Henrietta Lacks. The cells, now known as HeLa cells, have enabled several biological and medical breakthroughs, including the discovery of the first effective polio vaccine.[62]

One of the advantages of use of immortalised cell lines is consistency; with consistent cell culture conditions these cells reliably multiply for scaling up purposes, and the variability between the different batches of cells tends to be minimal. Another advantage of these cell lines is their potential for being in culture for a relatively long period. These two attributes are particularly important for high throughput screening, where a consistent baseline response is expected across assay multiwell plates, and over days or even weeks of screening, to compare the therapeutic responses accurately.

### 9.4.3 Primary Cells

Primary cells are directly taken from tissues by dissociation using enzymatic or mechanical methods and re-established under optimised culture conditions. These could be taken from healthy human tissues, patient's diseased tissues or tissues from animal models (*e.g.*, transgenic rodents). As they are directly derived from tissues and cultured as unmodified, they may represent a more *in vivo* state and exhibit normal physiology. The disadvantages of using primary cells are that they have limited growth potential and there is a limit on their life span, even under optimal growth conditions. However, use of primary cells may avoid many ethical objections raised towards animal experiments and can reduce cost. Primary cells can also enable experiments on human tissues which otherwise could not have been carried out *in vivo*, and this is the only tool to allow studies of donor-to-donor variability preclinically.

### 9.4.4 Stem Cells

Despite the effectiveness of animal and immortal cell line models, the inherent disadvantage is that their physiology is different to that of patient cells, which lends an explanation as to why many drug candidates are not efficacious once they reach clinical trials. The use of patient-specific stem cells for the generation of human disease models is one way in which this issue can be addressed. Stem cells possess limitless self-renewal and differentiation properties, which allow them to produce large quantities of specific cell types for research models. An advantage of patient-specific disease models lies in the fact that the cells carry the same genotype as the donor patient, who displays an observable phenotype. In theory, these cells can generate a translational disease model. Three types of commonly utilised stem cells include adult stem cells, human embryonic stem cells (hESCs), and induced pluripotent stem cells (iPSCs).

- *Adult stem cells*
  Neural stem cells (NSCs) can be successfully derived from human adult tissue and cultured as self-renewing cell lines.[63,64] Human neural cultures that are derived from biopsy specimens or post-mortem tissue terminally differentiate following prolonged passaging and are cultured as neurospheres that contain a mixture of neural progenitor cells (NPCs), neurons and glial cells. Two examples of successful patient-derived NPC disease models have been from patients with fragile X syndrome (FXS)[65] and amyotrophic lateral sclerosis (ALS).[66] The ability to isolate cells from patients with end-stage disease means that NPCs do not require any genetic or epigenetic manipulation in order to be relevant for disease modelling.
  Despite their advantages and examples of success, NPCs are not ideally suited to modelling human disease. Adult NSCs are extremely difficult to expand in culture for long periods of time due to the complicated culture conditions required to recapitulate the *in vivo* environment. Furthermore, adult NSCs possess limited ability to differentiate to specific neuronal subtypes and eventually become exclusively glionic when in culture.

- *Human embryonic stem cells*
  Human embryonic stem cells (hESCs) were the first pluripotent stem cells (PSCs) to be isolated and are derived from pre-implanted embryos. They require genetic manipulation to manifest adult disease phenotypes. Despite initial derivation in 1998 by Thomson and colleagues,[67] the development of hESC models and their widespread adoption has been slow due to ethical considerations around the derivation process. There are two main approaches to the derivation of hESCs, the first involves manipulation of the hESC genome. This approach is exemplified by the generation of a model of Lesh–Nyhan Syndrome. Gene targeting was used to generate the model, introducing a mutated form of the HPRT1 gene, with the generated hESC lines exhibiting disease phenotypes such as lack of HPRT1 activity and elevated levels of uric acid.[68] The second approach is known as pre-implantation genetic diagnosis (PGD).[69] In this approach, an embryo is screened when one or both parents are known to carry a known disease-linked mutation or chromosomal

disorder. There have been several studies that utilise PGD-derived disease models, including those for Huntington's,[70] fragile X syndrome,[68] and cystic fibrosis.[71] There are disadvantages to this approach of model generation, for example, it is dependent upon access to PGD embryos carrying the desired disease state and, in general, there is a lack of widely available patient information.

- *Induced pluripotent stem cells*
  Owing to the disadvantages and ethical considerations surrounding the use of hESCs, researchers often choose to utilise induced pluripotent stem cells (iPSCs) in their place. iPSCs were first described in 2006 and were generated from mouse embryonic fibroblasts (MEFs) following the induction of four key transcription factors; Oct3/4, Sox2, Klf4 and c-Myc.[20] The generation of human iPSCs quickly followed in 2007,[72,73] with the promise of providing new opportunities for disease modelling and screening for new drugs.[74] iPSC models have proven to be a powerful and reliable tool in disease modelling. For example, the first iPSC-based disease model generated was for the neurodegenerative disorder spinal muscular atrophy (SMA), which results from a loss of function in the SMN1 gene. The model successfully showed that motor neurons which were differentiated from diseased iPSCs degenerated significantly faster than a wild-type control. This was the first study to show patient-specific iPSC-derived cells with disease-associated phenotypes.[75]

The most used model organisms are the yeast species *Saccharomyces cerevisiae* (*S. cerevisiae*), the nematode worm *Caenorhabditis elegans* (*C. elegans*), the humble fruit fly *Drosophila melanogaster* (*D. melanogaster*), zebrafish (*D. rerio*) and the mouse (*M. musculus*). These systems were chosen due to being robust and fast-growing while producing many offspring and being cost effective to propagate within a laboratory. The genomes of these commonly used model systems have been published and widely available, a key advantage to utilising these systems, allowing for an integrated systems biology approach to research. For example the genome sequence of *S. cerevisiae* was made publicly available in 1996 and was the first eukaryotic genome to be sequenced.[76] The genome of *C. elegans* followed in 1998 and was the first multicellular organism to be sequenced,[77] with an annotated version of the genome being widely available on the open-source software WormBase (www.wormbase.org).

These commonly used model systems share a large amount of homology with humans, 60–80% of genes in *C. elegans* have human orthologues with approximately 42% of human disease genes having orthologues in *C. elegans*.[78–80] Similarly the *Drosophila* genome shares 60% homology with humans, with approximately 65% of human disease genes having homologues in flies.[81,82] A significant proportion of these human homologues perform an equivalent function in the model system as they do in humans.

The mouse is the most well-characterised *in vivo* mammalian model system with the murine genome first published in 2002.[83] There is a high similarity between the mouse and the human genome, with 95% of genes being conserved between the two species. There are several disease models that have been successfully generated in mice *via* natural breeding techniques. These include NOD (non-obese diabetic) mice, which develop type I diabetes, and SCID (severe combined immune deficiency) mice, which almost completely lack an immune system.

In addition to disease models generated through natural breeding, mouse knock-out models are extremely powerful in identifying gene function in mammalian systems. This was demonstrated in an analysis of the 100-best selling drugs in 2003. These 100 drugs targeted 43 host proteins (14 of the drugs were anti-infectives and did not target human proteins) with 34 of the 43 targets having been knocked out in mice. Many of these mouse knock-out models provided invaluable information regarding gene function and pharmaceutical relevance, leading to a direct correlation between the knock-out phenotype and the therapeutic effect of the drug.[84]

## 9.5 Gene Expression Studies and Their Application

For each cell to function and adapt to their environment, numerous proteins with diverse roles are produced. Genes encode proteins, and the process by which their information is used for protein production is called gene expression. The flow of genetic information starts with transcription from DNA to RNA, which is followed by translation from RNA to protein. These two main steps are separated by time and by space; DNA is transcribed in the nucleus, before being transported to the cytoplasm as messenger RNA (mRNA) where it engages with ribosomes and other regulatory proteins to direct the translation process. This process results in a sequence of amino acids, building blocks for protein synthesis. The amino acid chain then self-folds to form a mature, functional protein. The regulation of transcription and translation is critical for the proper function of a cell. Only a fraction of all genes is expressed at any one time, with the amount and type of mRNA molecules present reflecting the function of the cell.

The application of gene expression studies in a drug discovery campaign are of extreme importance, playing critical roles from target identification and validation, through to determination of mechanism of action and off-target toxicity studies. Molecular biologists rely upon the understanding of gene function, the dysregulation of this function in a disease state, and the impact of this upon a cellular phenotype to inform drug development projects. There are several expression-profiling methodologies that have emerged in order to investigate and monitor changes in the expression of genes in response to therapeutic modulation; these are described below.

### 9.5.1 Application of PCR

The invention of PCR (Polymerase Chain Reaction) has revolutionised the field of research.[11,85,86] Today, it is one of the most used techniques due to its simplicity, high accuracy, sensitivity and low cost. The process of the PCR consists of heating and cooling cycles (Figure 9.6), allowing for denaturation and annealing of DNA strands. The initial denaturation cycle is set at a high temperature for a long period of time to linearize and melt the double-stranded structure of the DNA. After this, the reaction is cooled to the annealing temperature. In the annealing step (30 seconds to 1 minute) the primers bind in a complementary manner to the target sequence. The final step in the reaction is the extension, or elongation step (~1 minute), during which the DNA polymerase extends the primers from the 3′ end. The DNA polymerase usually extends

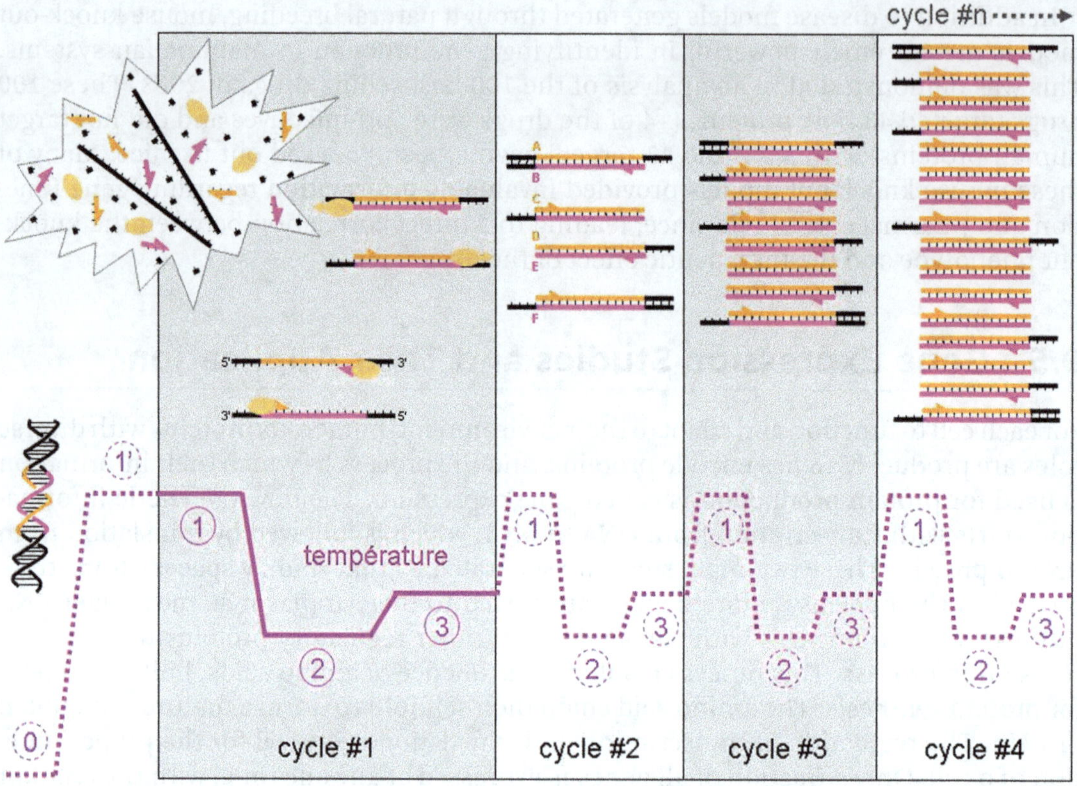


**Figure 9.6** Polymerase chain reaction (PCR). Polymerase chain reaction can be divided three (3) main steps. During the first step the DNA template will be denatured into single strands at high temperature; in the second step, the temperature will drop, the primers will anneal to each of DNA strands and polymerase will bind to the primers. The last step of the temperature will increase again slightly where the polymerase can synthetize the new DNA strands. Reproduced from https://commons.wikimedia.org/wiki/File:PCR_basic_principle1.jpg, under the terms of the CC BY-SA 3.0 license, https://creativecommons.org/licenses/by-sa/3.0/deed.en. Image Credit: Ygonaar.

with a rate of 1 kilobase per minute. This step can be extended if longer amplicons are needed. The amount of template DNA doubles during each cycle of the reaction and the cycling step is repeated 30–40 times, depending on the starting material, as more cycles are required for a smaller input or a rare sequence. At the end of the PCR reaction, the amplicons are visualised by gel electrophoresis. Currently, endpoint PCR is mostly used to amplify specific sections of DNA for sequencing and cloning.

### 9.5.2 Studying Gene Expression by Quantitative Reverse Transcription PCR (qRT-PCR)

For PCR assays that have RNA as a starting material, a reverse transcription reaction must take place prior to the PCR reaction. When the PCR reaction is quantified, this is called a quantitative reverse transcription PCR or qRT-PCR (or qPCR for short). It is most often used for the quantification of gene expression in a sample of interest.[87–89]

The first step of a qRT-PCR involves the synthesis of the RNA molecule into a complementary DNA (cDNA) molecule. This is carried out by incubating the RNA molecule, at a specific temperature and for a defined period, with primers and a reverse transcriptase enzyme. The second step is performing a qPCR reaction. As the cDNA is single-stranded after the synthesis, it is also called first-strand cDNA synthesis, with the second strand of the DNA molecule being primed and elongated during the first PCR cycle.

There are two different ways in which sample fluorescence can be measured during qRT-PCR: the use of an intercalating dye provides non-specific fluorescent signal or the use of a fluorescent probe, which provides specific fluorescent signal.

Dye-based detection is performed by the incorporation of a binding or intercalating dye in the PCR. These dyes are non-specific and bind tightly, but reversibly, to any double-stranded DNA (dsDNA) generated during amplification, resulting in the emission of fluorescence at each cycle as the template yield increases. The most used dyes are SYBR green and the newer, more stable, EvaGreen. The main advantage of this method is that the dyes are cheap and easy to use; however, the main disadvantage comes with their non-specificity, which could lead to false positive signals.

Probe-based quantitation uses sequence-specific DNA-based fluorescent reporter probes, which result in the quantification of the sequence of interest only, not all dsDNA, as is the case with intercalating dyes. These probes contain a fluorescent reporter at the 5′ end and a non-fluorescent quencher (NFQ) at the 3′ end to prevent fluorescence. Common fluorescence reporters include derivatives of fluorescein, rhodamine and cyanine.

The most used linear probe is the TaqMan or hydrolysis probe. The TaqMan method relies on the 5′-3′ exonuclease activity of *Thermus aquaticus* (Taq) DNA polymerase to cleave a labelled probe when it is annealed to its complementary sequence.[90,91]

The TaqMan method can be described in three steps:

**Step 1:** The temperature of the reaction is raised to denature the dsDNA. During this step the fluorescent dye on the 5′ end of the TaqMan probe is quenched by the NFQ at the 3′ end.

**Step 2:** The reaction temperature is lowered, allowing for the probes to bind to their specific complementary sequence if available.

**Step 3:** During this step, Taq DNA polymerase synthesises new strands of DNA. When it encounters the TaqMan probe the double-strand-specific 5′-3′ nuclease activity of the enzyme displaces the 5′ end of the probe and then degrades it. This releases the fluorophore and quencher into solution, separating them, leading to an irreversible increase in fluorescence.

The fluorescence of a sample is measured during the PCR run, and an amplification plot is created. The amplification plot is divided into three phases: the baseline fluorescence phase, the exponential amplification phase and the plateau phase. The cycle at which the fluorescence is detected above the baseline, called the cycle threshold (Ct), is one of qPCR's most important factors. During the first phase of amplification, the sample fluorescence is too low to be detected by the instrument. This is the baseline or background fluorescence and is usually due to the low input of starting material. The lower the input, the longer it will take for the fluorescence to be detected above the threshold, and *vice versa*. Once enough fluorescence has accumulated to enable detection, the exponential phase of the amplification can be visualised and is usually a steep slope. As soon as the reaction components are depleted, the reaction reaches the plateau phase and there is no further increase in the fluorescent signal.

qPCR can be employed at many stages during a drug discovery campaign and provides meaningful information throughout. For example, in the target validation stage the method is a reliable tool to provide information on the effects of target knock-out/-down upon gene expression further down the biological pathway. Similarly, the method can be employed much later in the drug discovery lifecycle to play a vital role in the measurement of clinical biomarkers.

### 9.5.3 Digital PCR

Digital PCR (dPCR) is the third generation of PCR and allows for absolute quantification of DNA, where the product is measured at the end of the amplification cycle.[92–94] During dPCR, each sample is diluted and partitioned into individual wells, to ensure that each well contains one or no copies of the intended target. Each well is then amplified independently using a fluorescent label, and the fluorescence is measured at the end of the amplification. In theory, each well that contained a copy of the target generates a signal, and the wells with no target generate no signal. The number of positive and negative wells is then used to measure the initial concentration of the sample tested. As more than one copy can be partitioned into each well, the sample's dispersal is considered to follow a Poisson distribution.

dPCR is a relatively new technology, but there are many instruments available on the market. dPCR is more advantageous than qPCR as it is highly sensitive, reaching up to 0.01% or in some cases 0.001% sensitivity. When compared to the PCR, which only reaches 1%, dPCR has been found to be much more applicable for detection of trace DNA, rare mutations and circulating tumour DNA.[95]

Another advantage of dPCR is that it does not rely on amplification efficiency, and it has a more comprehensive dynamic range than qPCR. The dynamic range is instrument-dependent and dictated by the number of total partitions an instrument can create.

Despite these key advantages, dPCR is extremely costly, both in the initial high cost of the instruments as well as the cost of the consumables. Other disadvantages include greater complexity and lower throughput as well as the fact that is not as widely used and understood by scientists as qPCR. It is these limitations that have so far slowed its incorporation into clinical laboratories.[96]

### 9.5.4 Reporter Cell Lines

Reporter cell lines are modified immortalised cells, containing an extra "reporter" gene in the genome, allowing various biological processes to be visualised. The central concept of a reporter gene is simple; it is a defined nucleotide sequence, which, when introduced into a biological system, yields a readily measurable phenotype upon expression.[97] Reporter molecules can be fluorescent, like Green Fluorescent Protein (GFP), luminescent, such as firefly's luciferase protein, or biochemical tags (β-galactosidase).[98–100] Reporter genes, and the associated detection methodologies, have contributed to many discoveries in molecular biology and revealed underlying cellular processes of diseases. During stable reporter cell line generation, the reporter gene sequence, with or without the gene of interest, must integrate into the genome. There are three main steps of reporter cell line generation: (1) generation of reporter construct, (2) transfer of the reporter construct to the nucleus of the cells to be modified, (3) validation of the integration and function of the reporter gene. Generation of the reporter constructs involves designing a vector that contains the sequence-of-interest cloned upstream of a reporter gene. It has an origin of replication (ORI), a selection marker, and a cloning site. The special sequence of the Open Reading Frame (ORI) allows replication initiation through recruiting replication machinery proteins within the cells. For example, the selection marker could be an antibiotic-resistant gene that enables selecting the positively transfected cells upon antibiotic treatments. The cloning site is a short segment of DNA which contains several restriction sites, allowing for the easy insertion of DNA.[101–103]

The cells' delivery method can be virus-mediated (transduction) or non-virus mediated delivery (transfection). Transduction occurs when foreign DNA or RNA is introduced into bacterial (bacteriophage) or eukaryotic cells *via* a virus or viral vector. The most used viral vectors for gene transfer are retrovirus, lentivirus, adenovirus, adeno-associated virus, and Herpes simplex virus. Transfection is a non-viral gene transfer methodology to deliver the negatively charged molecules (*e.g.*, DNA and RNA) into the cells through the negatively charged cell membrane. Chemicals such as calcium phosphate and diethyl aminoethyl (DEAE)-dextran, or cationic lipid-based reagents, coat the DNA, then neutralise, or even impart an overall positive charge on the molecule, thus making it easier for the DNA-transfection reagent complex to cross the cell membrane.[35,104,105] Physical methods like microinjection or electroporation can also be employed; such methods simply punch through the membrane and introduce DNA directly into the cytoplasm.[106,107]

Confirmation of successful reporter line generation involves the determination of the integration sites by sequencing, and validation of the function using suitable detection methods like Flow Cytometry Cell Sorting (FACS) or High Content Analyses (HCA).

Early applications of reporter genes focused primarily on the analysis of *cis*-acting genetic elements (gene regulatory elements), usually promoters and enhancers.[108–110] Today's reporter assays have expanded to provide information about gene expression, cellular response, protein–protein interaction, protein trafficking, drug screening, toxicology research and many more. For example, in one study Cox *et al.*[111] constructed a panel of fifteen different reporter cell lines to monitor the morphologies of multiple subcellular organelles and the activation status of various intracellular signalling pathways in the presence of 1008 small molecules for phenotypic profiling. They selected three cell types – each from a different lineage – for gene-editing, to express a diverse set of fluorescent markers: the A549 lung adenocarcinoma, the HepG2 hepatocellular carcinoma and the WPMY1 prostatic stromal myofibroblast lines. Each reporter cell line carried a BFP segmentation cassette that enabled detection of the nuclear and cell boundaries. Each reporter cell line expressed a GFP- and a RFP/FusionRed-tagged organelle, or pathway marker, from its endogenous chromosomal locus. These markers were selected to cover a broad array of organelles, cellular structures and regulatory pathways.

## 9.6 Proteomics in Drug Discovery

Mass spectrometry-based proteomics research techniques have been adopted by drug discovery scientists since the early 2000s to identify protein targets from phenotypic assays and to understand on- and off-target engagement of novel therapeutic compounds. Fundamentally, proteomic analysis by mass spectrometry uses the mass to charge ($m/z$) ratio of ionised fragments to identify targets in a sample matrix. Tandem mass spectrometry or peptide fingerprinting techniques are adopted to gain information about the amino acid sequence and relative abundance of the ionised fragments within the samples. As the proteome is inherently dynamic, unlike the genome, proteomic analysis provides a functional snapshot of the cell at a given time point. There are many challenges in drug discovery that proteomics has helped to address in recent years, for example target deconvolution in phenotypic screens and off-target toxicity studies, biomarker identification and protein interactions. Below, a brief introduction to some of the recent developments in proteomic techniques is outlined, with examples of relevance and success in the drug discovery setting.

### 9.6.1 Protein Microarrays

Traditional proteome profiling techniques originally combined mass-spectrometry with separation tools such as 2D-electrophoresis or multidimensional liquid chromatography and allowed for the simultaneous analysis of dozens of proteins. However, these techniques were labour intensive and required large amounts of biological material. These major disadvantages have led to the development of protein microarrays (PMAs), a miniaturised tool for the investigation of proteomes.

There are three types of PMA: functional protein arrays, analytical/capture protein arrays, and reverse-phase protein arrays (Figure 9.7). Functional protein arrays are used to assay functional properties of protein, for example, identify targets for post-translational modification, investigating enzymatic activity and screening for molecular interactions. These arrays display folded and active protein immobilised on a solid surface in a high-density dot matrix configuration.[112] Analytical, or capture arrays, consist of affinity reagents such as antibodies that are arrayed on the solid surface and enable the expression of proteins to be profiled, or for the quantification of antibodies in complex samples such as serum. Such arrays are used for purposes such as biomarker discovery and deconvoluting protein activity within signalling cascades.[113] Reverse-phase protein arrays allow for the measurement of protein levels across many biological samples at the same time. This technique is quantitative when coupled with the use of highly specific antibodies. In this type of array, it is the biological sample (*e.g.*, cell lysate, serum, urine) that is immobilised on the solid surface and analysis is achieved by probing the array with antibodies, which can be multiplexed to detect multiple proteins simultaneously.[114,115]

PMAs have been successfully adopted to profile various molecular interactions that have then led to the discovery of potential drug targets at the molecular level. These include protein–protein, protein–DNA/RNA, protein–lipid and protein–small-molecule interactions. The first example of the application of a protein array to

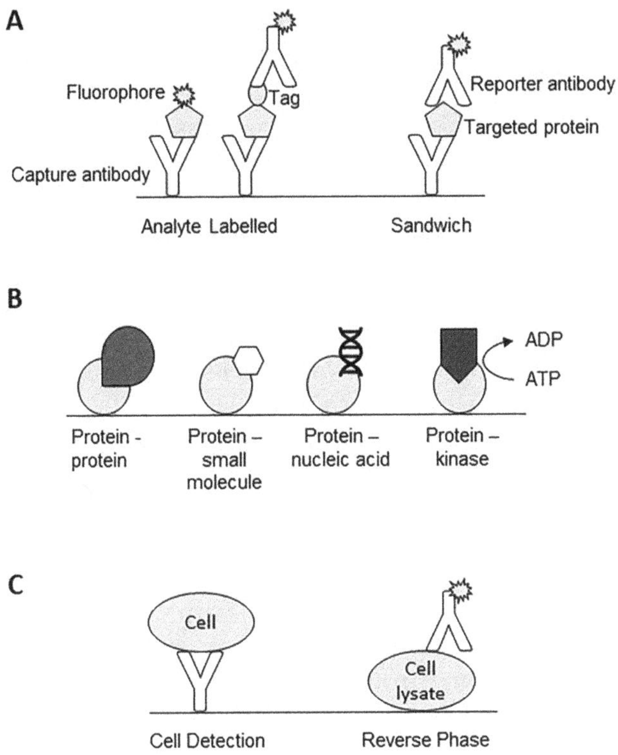


**Figure 9.7** Diagram representing the three categories of protein microarrays. (A) Analytical protein microarrays are usually antibody arrays and focus mainly on protein detection. Targeted proteins can be detected by direct labelling or using a reporter antibody in a sandwich assay format. (B) Functional microarrays have a wide range of applications investigating molecular interactions. (C) Reverse-phase protein microarrays allow for the measurement of protein levels across biological samples by immobilising different lysate samples on the same chip. Adapted from ref. 125 with permission from John Wiley & Sons, Copyright © 2013 John Wiley & Sons, Inc.

investigate protein–small-molecule interactions was in 2000 by MacBeath and Schreiber, where interactions between FKBP12 and three small molecules labelled with fluorophores were identified. The differences in the binding affinities were demonstrated.[116] Another early example of the utilisation of PMAs for the identification of protein–small-molecule interactions was by Schreiber *et al.*, whereby six small molecule inhibitors of rapamycin (SMIR), that had previously been identified through a phenotypic assay, were screened against immobilised His- and GST-tagged proteins. This screen was successful in identifying a previously unknown member of the target of rapamycin (TOR) signalling pathway.[117]

## 9.6.2 Kinase Profiling

A major hurdle in the development of kinase inhibitors comes from the conservation of the ATP binding site amongst family members, therefore target selectivity *via* competitive binding to the ATP binding site is difficult to achieve. To date, ATP-competitive kinase inhibitors have been approved for cancer treatment and often demonstrate otherwise unacceptable toxicities due to off-target effects. To address this issue in the development of kinase inhibitors, Patricelli and colleagues have developed a chemoproteomic technique for the profiling of kinases in native systems; this system is known as KiNativ®.[118]

Using the Kinativ® approach, soluble probes consisting of ATP or ADP linked to biotin through an acyl-phosphate bond are utilised. Upon interacting with a kinase, the probes covalently modify conserved lysine residues that are present in the active sites of kinases, hence labelling the kinase active site. The sample is then subject to tryptic digestion and streptavidin enrichment, allowing for probe-labelled peptides to be characterised and quantified using mass spectrometry. When coupled with powerful mass spectrometry-based analysis platforms, KiNativ® probes can be used to detect >300 endogenous kinases from a biological sample.[118]

KiNativ® technology is now the industry-leading kinase profiling platform and has been successfully applied to aid the drug discovery process. For example, a highly selective Mitogen-activated protein kinase 7 (also known as ERK5) inhibitor, AX15836 was developed in 2016 by optimising a first-generation ERK5 inhibitor, XMD8-92.[119] The group were able to identify off-target activity of compounds exemplified by XMD8-92 against Bromo- and Extra-Terminal domain (BET) family proteins, which was previously unidentified, and demonstrated that the efficacy of said compounds was due to this off-target interaction, rather than through ERK5. Within this study the ERK5 inhibitors were also incubated with live cells prior to washing, lysis and analysis. This application of the KiNativ® platform allows for the investigation of cellular permeability of compounds and intracellular target engagement and any potential intracellular off-target engagement, which may not be detected from cellular lysate.[119]

### 9.6.3 Label-free Proteome Profiling

Significant advances in the target identification of small molecules *via* label-free proteome profiling techniques have been made in recent years. These recent advances are due in part to the improvement of high-resolution mass-spectrometry techniques and a more in-depth understanding of protein stability, with most label-free target deconvolution techniques depending upon inherent changes in protein stability upon compound binding. Thermal proteome profiling (TPP) involves the thermal perturbation of a protein matrix and the measurement of the intact protein state. Proteins unfold when subjected to thermal stress and expose their hydrophobic regions, which leads to aggregation. Protein aggregates can then be removed from the matrix through precipitation, thus allowing for unfolded proteins to be recovered and identified.

In a recent publication Saei and colleagues utilised TPP in conjunction with other proteomic techniques to deconvolute the targets of auranofin (Ridaura®).[120] Auranofin was first approved in 1985 for the treatment of rheumatoid arthritis, however, there had been many recent clinical trials in which the drug is being repurposed for cancer therapy. This repurposing led to the need for a comprehensive characterisation of the protein targets and downstream effects in cancer cells. Using an unbiased approach to target deconvolution, the group were successful in identifying thioredoxin reductase 1 (TXNRD1), nuclear factor NF-κB (NFKB2) and Cysteine and Histidine Rich Domain

Containing 1 protein (CHORDC1) as cognate targets of auranofin in cancer cells. This publication is a demonstration of the powerful influence and complementarity of proteomic techniques in the deconvolution of small molecule targets and the overall impact upon drug discovery in general.[120]

Another example of label-free proteomic analysis is that of drug affinity responsive target stability (DARTS). Binding of ligands to proteins can induce stabilisation through resistance to proteolysis, and this change in stabilisation can be detected through the DARTS methodology. Following ligand exposure, samples are exposed to a protease such as thermolysin or pronase, which cleaves exposed regions of proteins, while protein regions that are bound to the ligand will remain protected from proteolytic cleavage. The cleaved samples are then subject to separation by SDS-PAGE and the identification of protein bands that have been protected from proteolytic cleavage. These bands are then extracted and subjected to analysis by mass spectrometry, allowing for the identification of the protein(s). The main advantages of the DARTS technique are that it utilises the native small molecule, without any prior immobilisation or chemical modification, and that it is an unbiased approach to target deconvolution.[121]

An illustration of the application of the DARTS technique in drug discovery was the identification of disulfiram (DSF) as a therapeutic for triple-negative breast cancer by Robinson *et al.* in 2013.[122] In this study Robinson and colleagues carried out a high-throughput screen of 3185 drugs against various triple-negative breast cancer cell lines with the view to identify novel therapeutics using DARTS. This screen identified that DSF, an FDA-approved anti-alcoholism drug, bound to IQ motif-containing factors IQ Motif Containing GTPase Activating Protein 1 (IQGAP1). Some years later, the use of DFS together with copper was shown to have an anti-cancer effect in tumour-initiating cells, which are thought to be the mechanism for driving chemoresistance and tumour recurrence[123] and in many other preclinical studies. Since then, open-label Phase II clinical trials have been initiated with this 60-year-old drug as a re-purposed anti-cancer drug which is currently being tested in metastatic breast cancer patients.[124]

## 9.7 Hints and Tips

The field of molecular biology has transformed modern drug discovery, having a huge impact from target identification and validation, through to detection of clinical biomarkers and off-target toxicity. The aim of this chapter has been to outline the key principles of molecular biology and how these can be applied to support and progress a successful medicinal chemistry campaign. Below are outlined some key take home messages from this chapter:

- Next-generation sequencing (NGS) has allowed for the rise of genetics-informed drug development; however, third-generation sequencing techniques are beginning to have an impact in the field.
- CRISPR/Cas9 has made genome editing in cells and animal models relatively easy to achieve and has become an important tool for generating genetically modified organisms and target validation.

- Selecting the right model system for your drug discovery campaign is critical. Areas of consideration include target conservation across species, drug metabolism in the chosen system and physiological relevance. By selecting the most appropriate model systems early in the process, chances of clinical success are heightened.
- Gene expression studies are highly informative; however, levels of expressed mRNA within a cell are not always indicative of protein levels that are observed.
- The field of proteomics is evolving and can provide key information regarding disease mechanisms, off-target interactions and mode of action of lead compounds; however, sensitivity can be an issue when investigating low abundance proteins and data complexity can provide challenges.

## References


1. I. Wilmut, A. E. Schnieke, J. McWhir, A. J. Kind and K. H. S. Campbell, Viable offspring derived from fetal and adult mammalian cells, *Nature*, 1997, **385**(6619), 810–813.
2. F. Griffith, The Significance of Pneumococcal Types, *J. Hyg.*, 1928, **27**(2), 113–159.
3. O. T. Avery, C. M. Macleod and M. McCarty, Studies on the chemical nature of the substance inducing transformation of pneumococcal types: Induction of transformation by a desoxyribonucleic acid fraction isolated from pneumococcus type iii, *J. Exp. Med.*, 1944, **79**(2), 137–158.
4. A. D. Hershey and M. Chase, Independent functions of viral protein and nucleic acid in growth of bacteriophage, *J. Gen. Physiol.*, 1952, **36**(1), 39–56.
5. J. D. Watson and F. H. C. Crick, Molecular structure of nucleic acids: A structure for deoxyribose nucleic acid, *Nature*, 1953, **171**(4356), 737–738.
6. M. Meselson and F. W. Stahl, The replication of DNA in Escherichia coli, *Proc. Natl. Acad. Sci. U. S. A.*, 1958, **44**(7), 671–682.
7. V. Singh, F. H. C. Crick, F. R. S. Leslie Barnett, S. Brenner and R. J. Watts-Tobin, General Nature of the Genetic Code for Proteins, *Resonance*, 2019, **24**(10), 1171–1178.
8. I. R. Lehman, M. J. Bessman, E. S. Simms and A. Kornberg, Enzymatic synthesis of deoxyribonucleic acid. I. Preparation of substrates and partial purification of an enzyme from Escherichia coli, *J. Biol. Chem.*, 1958, **233**(1), 163–170.
9. M. W. Nirenberg and J. H. Matthaei, The dependence of cell-free protein synthesis in E. coli upon naturally occurring or synthetic polyribonucleotides, *Proc. Natl. Acad. Sci. U. S. A.*, 1961, **47**, 1588–1602.
10. D. Söll, E. Ohtsuka, D. S. Jones, R. Lohrmann, H. Hayatsu and S. Nishimura, *et al.*, Studies on polynucleotides, XLIX. Stimulation of the binding of aminoacyl-sRNA's to ribosomes by ribotrinucleotides and a survey of codon assignments for 20 amino acids, *Proc. Natl. Acad. Sci. U. S. A.*, 1965, **54**(5), 1378–1385.
11. K. Mullis, F. Faloona, S. Scharf, R. Saiki, G. Horn and H. Erlich, Specific enzymatic amplification of DNA in vitro: The polymerase chain reaction, *Cold Spring Harbor Symp. Quant. Biol.*, 1986, **51**(1), 263–273.
12. C. A. Hutchison, S. Phillips, M. H. Edgell, S. Gillam, P. Jahnke and M. Smith, Mutagenesis at a specific position in a DNA sequence, *J. Biol. Chem.*, 1978, **253**(18), 6551–6560.
13. F. Sanger, S. Nicklen and A. R. Coulson, DNA sequencing with chain-terminating inhibitors, *Proc. Natl. Acad. Sci. U. S. A.*, 1977, **74**(12), 5463–5467.
14. E. S. Lander, L. M. Linton, B. Birren, C. Nusbaum, M. C. Zody and J. Baldwin, *et al.*, Initial sequencing and analysis of the human genome, *Nature*, 2001, **409**(6822), 860–921.
15. H. Walczak, R. E. Miller, K. Ariail, B. Gliniak, T. S. Griffith and M. Kubin, *et al.*, Tumoricidal activity of tumor necrosis factor-related apoptosis-inducing ligand in vivo, *Nat. Med.*, 1999, **5**(2), 157–163.
16. D. M. Altshuler, R. A. Gibbs, L. Peltonen, S. F. Schaffner, F. Yu and E. Dermitzakis, *et al.*, Integrating common and rare genetic variation in diverse human populations, *Nature*, 2010, **467**(7311), 52–58.
17. F. Abascal, R. Acosta, N. J. Addleman, J. Adrian, V. Afzal and B. Aken, *et al.*, Expanded encyclopaedias of DNA elements in the human and mouse genomes, *Nature*, 2020, **583**(7818), 699–710.
18. S. A. Bustin, Absolute quantification of mrna using real-time reverse transcription polymerase chain reaction assays, *J. Mol. Endocrinol.*, 2000, **25**, 169–193.

19. S. A. Bustin and T. Nolan, RT-QPCR testing of SARS-COV-2: A primer, *Int. J. Mol. Sci.*, 2020, **21**(8), E3004.
20. K. Takahashi and S. Yamanaka, Induction of Pluripotent Stem Cells from Mouse Embryonic and Adult Fibroblast Cultures by Defined Factors, *Cell*, 2006, **126**(4), 663–676.
21. J. Deinsberger, D. Reisinger and B. Weber, Global trends in clinical trials involving pluripotent stem cells: a systematic multidatabase analysis, *npj Regener. Med.*, 2020, **5**(1), 15.
22. R. Jansen, J. D. A. van Embden, W. Gaastra and L. M. Schouls, Identification of genes that are associated with DNA repeats in prokaryotes, *Mol. Microbiol.*, 2002, **43**(6), 1565–1575.
23. E. Deltcheva, K. Chylinski, C. M. Sharma, K. Gonzales, Y. Chao and Z. A. Pirzada, *et al.*, CRISPR RNA maturation by trans-encoded small RNA and host factor RNase III, *Nature*, 2011, **471**(7340), 602–607.
24. M. Jinek, K. Chylinski, I. Fonfara, M. Hauer, J. A. Doudna and E. Charpentier, A programmable dual-RNA-guided DNA endonuclease in adaptive bacterial immunity, *Science*, 2012, **337**(6096), 816–821.
25. F. Sanger, G. M. Air, B. G. Barrell, N. L. Brown, A. R. Coulson and J. C. Fiddes, *et al.*, Nucleotide sequence of bacteriophage φx174 DNA, *Nature*, 1977, **265**(5596), 687–695.
26. J. M. Heather and B. Chain, The sequence of sequencers: The history of sequencing DNA, *Genomics*, 2016, **107**, 1–8.
27. M. W. Anderson and I. Schrijver, Next generation DNA sequencing and the future of genomic medicine, *Genes*, 2010, **1**, 38–69.
28. F. Ozsolak and P. M. Milos, RNA sequencing: Advances, challenges and opportunities, *Nat. Rev. Genet.*, 2011, **12**, 87–98.
29. S. Maekawa, A. Suzuki, S. Sugano and Y. Suzuki, RNA sequencing: From sample preparation to analysis, *Methods Mol. Biol.*, 2014, **1164**, 51–65.
30. K. R. Kukurba and S. B. Montgomery, RNA sequencing and analysis, *Cold Spring Harbor Protoc.*, 2015, **2015**(11), 951–969.
31. H. Zhang, L. He and L. Cai, Transcriptome sequencing: RNA-seq, *Methods Mol. Biol.*, 2018, **1754**, 15–27.
32. R. Stark, M. Grzelak and J. Hadfield, RNA sequencing: the teenage years, *Nat. Rev. Genet.*, 2019, **20**, 631–656.
33. G. P. Page, S. O. Zakharkin, K. Kim, T. Mehta, L. Chen and K. Zhang, Microarray analysis, *Methods Mol. Biol.*, 2007, **404**, 409–430.
34. V. Bolón-Canedo, A. Alonso-Betanzos, I. López-de-Ullibarri and R. Cao, Challenges and Future Trends for Microarray Analysis, *Methods Mol. Biol.*, 2019, 283–293.
35. K. Kumar, M. Cowley and R. Davis, *Semin. Thromb. Hemostasis*, 2019, **45**(7), 661–673.
36. W. R. McCombie, J. D. McPherson and E. R. Mardis, Next-generation sequencing technologies, *Cold Spring Harbor Perspect. Med.*, 2019, **9**(11), a036798.
37. E. Papalexi and R. Satija, Single-cell RNA sequencing to explore immune cell heterogeneity, *Nat. Rev. Immunol.*, 2018, **18**, 35–45.
38. S. Vickovic, G. Eraslan, F. Salmén, J. Klughammer, L. Stenbeck and D. Schapiro, *et al.*, High-definition spatial transcriptomics for in situ tissue profiling, *Nat. Methods*, 2019, **16**(10), 987–990.
39. S. Oikonomopoulos, A. Bayega, S. Fahiminiya, H. Djambazian, P. Berube and J. Ragoussis, Methodologies for Transcript Profiling Using Long-Read Technologies, *Front. Genet.*, 2020, **11**, 606.
40. P. Uapinyoying, J. Goecks, S. M. Knoblac, K. Panchapakesan, C. G. Bonneman and T. A. Partridg, *et al.*, A long-read RNA-seq approach to identify novel transcripts of very large genes, *Genome Res.*, 2020, **30**(6), 885–897.
41. E. L. van Dijk, Y. Jaszczyszyn, D. Naquin and C. Thermes, The Third Revolution in Sequencing Technology, *Trends Genet.*, 2018, **34**, 666–681.
42. R. M. A. Manara, S. Tomasio and S. Khalid, The nucleotide capture region of alpha hemolysin: Insights into nanopore design for DNA sequencing from molecular dynamics simulations, *Nanomaterials*, 2015, **5**(1), 144–153.
43. Y. G. Kim, J. Cha and S. Chandrasegaran, Hybrid restriction enzymes: Zinc finger fusions to Fok I cleavage domain, *Proc. Natl. Acad. Sci. U. S. A.*, 1996, **93**(3), 1156–1160.
44. D. Carroll, Genome engineering with zinc-finger nucleases, *Genetics*, 2011, **188**(4), 773–782.
45. C. Ashmore-Harris and G. O. Fruhwirth, The clinical potential of gene editing as a tool to engineer cell-based therapeutics, *Clin. Transl. Med.*, 2020, **9**(1), 15.
46. M. Christian, T. Cermak, E. L. Doyle, C. Schmidt, F. Zhang and A. Hummel, *et al.*, Targeting DNA double-strand breaks with TAL effector nucleases, *Genetics*, 2010, **186**(2), 757–761.
47. Method of the Year 2011, *Nat. Methods*, 2012, **9**, 1.

48. Y. Ishino, H. Shinagawa, K. Makino, M. Amemura and A. Nakatura, Nucleotide sequence of the iap gene, responsible for alkaline phosphatase isoenzyme conversion in Escherichia coli, and identification of the gene product, *J. Bacteriol.*, 1987, **169**(12), 5429–5433.
49. Y. Ishino, M. Krupovic and P. Forterre, History of CRISPR-Cas from encounter with a mysterious repeated sequence to genome editing technology, *J. Bacteriol.*, 2018, **200**(7), e00580-17.
50. L. Cong, F. A. Ran, D. Cox, S. Lin, R. Barretto and N. Habib, *et al.*, Multiplex genome engineering using CRISPR/Cas systems, *Science*, 2013, **339**(6121), 819–823.
51. D. Collias and C. L. Beisel, CRISPR technologies and the search for the PAM-free nuclease, *Nat. Commun.*, 2021, **12**, 555.
52. K. S. Makarova, Y. I. Wolf, J. Iranzo, S. A. Shmakov, O. S. Alkhnbashi and S. J. J. Brouns, *et al.*, Evolutionary classification of CRISPR–Cas systems: a burst of class 2 and derived variants, *Nat. Rev. Microbiol.*, 2020, **18**, 67–83.
53. A. Fire, S. Xu, M. K. Montgomery, S. A. Kostas, S. E. Driver and C. C. Mello, Potent and specific genetic interference by double-stranded RNA in caenorhabditis elegans, *Nature*, 1998, **391**(6669), 806–811.
54. S. E. Mohr and N. Perrimon, RNAi screening: New approaches, understandings, and organisms, *Wiley Interdiscip. Rev.: RNA*, 2012, **3**, 145–158.
55. M. Boettcher and M. T. McManus, Choosing the Right Tool for the Job: RNAi, TALEN, or CRISPR, *Mol. Cell*, 2015, **58**, 575–585.
56. S. M. Elbashir, J. Harborth, W. Lendeckel, A. Yalcin, K. Weber and T. Tuschl, Duplexes of 21-nucleotide RNAs mediate RNA interference in cultured mammalian cells, *Nature*, 2001, **411**(6836), 494–498.
57. A. A. Seyhan, U. Varadarajan, S. Choe, W. Liu and T. E. Ryan, A genome-wide RNAi screen identifies novel targets of neratinib resistance leading to identification of potential drug resistant genetic markers, *Mol. BioSyst.*, 2012, **8**(5), 1553–1570.
58. K. Ashrafi, F. Y. Chang, J. L. Watts, A. G. Fraser, R. S. Kamath and J. Ahringer, *et al.*, Genome-wide RNAi analysis of Caenorhabditis elegans fat regulatory genes, *Nature*, 2003, **421**(6920), 268–272.
59. N. J. Barrows, C. le Sommer, M. A. Garcia-Blanco and J. L. Pearson, Factors affecting reproducibility between genome-scale siRNA-based screens, *J. Biomol. Screening*, 2010, **15**(7), 735–747.
60. K. Gavrilov and W. M. Saltzman, Therapeutic siRNA: Principles, challenges, and strategies, *Yale J. Biol. Med.*, 2012, **85**, 187–200.
61. Z. D. Blount, *Elife*, 2015, **25**(4), e05826.
62. British Poliomyelitis Vaccines, *Lancet*, 1956, **267**(6915), 319.
63. T. D. Palmer, P. H. Schwartz, P. Taupin, B. Kaspar, S. A. Stein and F. H. Gage, Progenitor cells from human brain after death, *Nature*, 2001, **411**(6833), 42–43.
64. P. H. Schwartz, P. J. Bryant, T. J. Fuja, H. Su, D. K. O'Dowd and H. Klassen, Isolation and Characterization of Neural Progenitor Cells from Post-Mortem Human Cortex, *J. Neurosci. Res.*, 2003, **74**(6), 838–851.
65. P. H. Schwartz, F. Tassone, C. M. Greco, H. E. Nethercott, B. Ziaeian and R. J. Hagerman, *et al.*, Neural progenitor cells from an adult patient with fragile X syndrome, *BMC Med. Genet.*, 2005, **6**, 2.
66. A. M. Haidet-Phillips, M. E. Hester, C. J. Miranda, K. Meyer, L. Braun and A. Frakes, *et al.*, Astrocytes from familial and sporadic ALS patients are toxic to motor neurons, *Nat. Biotechnol.*, 2011, **29**(9), 824–828.
67. J. A. Thomson, Embryonic stem cell lines derived from human blastocysts, *Science*, 1998, **282**(5391), 1145–1147.
68. A. Urbach, O. Bar-Nur, G. Q. Daley and N. Benvenisty, Differential modeling of fragile X syndrome by human embryonic stem cells and induced pluripotent stem cells, *Cell Stem Cell*, 2010, **6**, 407–411.
69. D. Ben-Yosef, M. Malcov and R. Eiges, PGD-derived human embryonic stem cell lines as a powerful tool for the study of human genetic disorders, *Mol. Cell. Endocrinol.*, 2008, **282**, 153–158.
70. C. K. Bradley, H. A. Scott, O. Chami, T. T. Peura, B. Dumevska and U. Schmidt, *et al.*, Derivation of Huntington's disease-affected human embryonic stem cell lines, *Stem Cells Dev.*, 2011, **20**(3), 495–502.
71. S. J. Pickering, S. L. Minger, M. Patel, H. Taylor, C. Black and C. J. Burns, *et al.*, Generation of a human embryonic stem cell line encoding the cystic fibrosis mutation ΔF508, using preimplantation genetic diagnosis, *Reprod. BioMed. Online*, 2005, **10**(3), 390–397.
72. J. Yu, M. A. Vodyanik, K. Smuga-Otto, J. Antosiewicz-Bourget, J. L. Frane and S. Tian, *et al.*, Induced pluripotent stem cell lines derived from human somatic cells, *Science*, 2007, **318**(5858), 1917–1920.
73. K. Takahashi, K. Okita, M. Nakagawa and S. Yamanaka, Induction of pluripotent stem cells from fibroblast cultures, *Nat. Protoc.*, 2007, **2**(12), 3081–3089.
74. Y. Mochiduki and K. Okita, Methods for iPS cell generation for basic research and clinical applications, *Biotechnol. J.*, 2012, **7**, 789–797.

75. A. D. Ebert, J. Yu, F. F. Rose, V. B. Mattis, C. L. Lorson and J. A. Thomson, *et al.*, Induced pluripotent stem cells from a spinal muscular atrophy patient, *Nature*, 2009, **457**(7227), 277–280.
76. A. Goffeau, G. Barrell, H. Bussey, R. W. Davis, B. Dujon and H. Feldmann, *et al.*, Life with 6000 genes, *Science*, 1996, **274**(5287), 546, 563–567.
77. The C. elegans Sequencing Consortium, Genome sequence of the nematode C. elegans: A platform for investigating biology, *Science*, 1998, **282**, 2012–2018.
78. T. W. Harris, N. Chen, F. Cunningham, M. Tello-Ruiz, I. Antoshechkin and C. Bastiani, *et al.*, WormBase: A multispecies resource for nematode biology and genomics, *Nucleic Acids Res.*, 2004, **32**, (DATABASE ISS.), D411–D417.
79. R. Baumeister and L. Ge, The worm in us - Caenorhabditis elegans as a model of human disease, *Trends Biotechnol.*, 2002, **20**, 147–148.
80. G. Poulin, R. Nandakumar and J. Ahringer, Genome-wide RNAi screens in Caenorhabditis elegans: Impact on cancer research, *Oncogene*, 2004, **23**, 8340–8345.
81. S. Chien, L. T. Reiter, E. Bier and M. Gribskov, Homophila: Human disease gene cognates in Drosophila, *Nucleic Acids Res.*, 2002, **30**(1), 149–151.
82. S. Yamamoto, M. Jaiswal, W. L. Charng, T. Gambin, E. Karaca and G. Mirzaa, *et al.*, A drosophila genetic resource of mutants to study mechanisms underlying human genetic diseases, *Cell*, 2014, **159**(1), 200–214.
83. R. H. Waterston, K. Lindblad-Toh, E. Birney, J. Rogers, J. F. Abril and P. Agarwal, *et al.*, Initial sequencing and comparative analysis of the mouse genome, *Nature*, 2002, **420**(6915), 520–562.
84. B. P. Zambrowicz and A. T. Sands, Knockouts model the 100 best-selling drugs - Will they model the next 100?, *Nat. Rev. Drug Discovery*, 2003, **2**, 38–51.
85. K. A. Eckert and T. A. Kunkel, DNA polymerase fidelity and the polymerase chain reaction, *Genome Res.*, 1991, **1**(1), 17–24.
86. M. R. Green and J. Sambrook, Polymerase Chain Reaction, *Cold Spring Harbor Protoc.*, 2019, DOI: 10.1101/pdb.top095109.
87. S. N. Peirson and J. N. Butler, Quantitative Polymerase Chain Reaction, *Methods Mol. Biol.*, 2007, **362**, 349–362.
88. S. C. Taylor and E. M. Mrkusich, The state of RT-quantitative PCR: Firsthand observations of implementation of minimum information for the publication of quantitative real-time PCR experiments (MIQE), *J. Mol. Microbiol. Biotechnol.*, 2014, **24**(1), 46–52.
89. M. Dooms, A. Chango and A. Abdel-Nour, La PCR quantitative (qPCR) et le guide de bonnes pratiques MIQE: adaptation et pertinence dans le contexte de la biologie clinique, *Ann. Biol. Clin.*, 2014, **72**(3), 265–269.
90. C. A. Heid, J. Stevens, K. J. Livak and P. M. Williams, Real time quantitative PCR, *Genome Res.*, 1996, **6**(10), 986–994.
91. E. Navarro, G. Serrano-Heras, M. J. Castaño and J. Solera, Real-time PCR detection chemistry, *Clin. Chim. Acta*, 2015, **439**, 231–250.
92. A. A. Morley, Digital PCR: A brief history, *Biomol. Detect. Quantif.*, 2014, **1**, 1–2.
93. R. Kanagal-Shamanna, Digital PCR: Principles and applications, *Methods Mol. Biol.*, 2016, 43–50.
94. A. S. Whale, W. de Spiegelaere, W. Trypsteen, A. A. Nour, Y.-K. Bae and V. Benes, *et al.*, The Digital MIQE Guidelines Update: Minimum Information for Publication of Quantitative Digital PCR Experiments for 2020, *Clin. Chem.*, 2020, **66**(8), 1012–1029.
95. X. Mao, C. Liu, H. Tong, Y. Chen and K. Liu, Principles of digital PCR and its applications in current obstetrical and gynecological diseases, *Am. J. Transl. Res.*, 2019, **11**, 7209–7222.
96. J. Kuypers and K. R. Jerome, Applications of digital PCR for clinical microbiology, *J. Clin. Microbiol.*, 2017, **55**, 1621–1628.
97. K. v. Wood, Marker proteins for gene expression, *Curr. Opin. Biotechnol.*, 1995, **6**(1), 50–58.
98. O. Shimomura, F. H. Johnson and Y. Saiga, Extraction, purification and properties of aequorin, a bioluminescent, *J. Cell. Comp. Physiol.*, 1962, **59**, 223–239.
99. G. R. MacGregor, A. E. Mogg, J. F. Burke and C. T. Caskey, Histochemical staining of clonal mammalian cell lines expressing E.coli β galactosidase indicates heterogeneous expression of the bacterial gene, *Somatic Cell Mol. Genet.*, 1987, **13**(3), 253–265.
100. H. Tanahashi, T. Ito, S. Inouye, F. I. Tsuji and Y. Sakaki, Photoprotein aequorin: use as a reporter enzyme in studying gene expression in mammalian cells, *Gene*, 1990, **96**(2), 249–255.
101. E. Schenborn and D. Groskreutz, Reporter gene vectors and assays, *Appl. Biochem. Biotechnol., Part B*, 1999, **13**, 29–44.
102. A. M. F. Liu, D. C. New, R. K. H. Lo and Y. H. Wong, Reporter gene assays, *Methods Mol. Biol.*, 2009, **486**, 109–123.

103. B. Ekundayo and F. Bleichert, Origins of DNA replication, *PLoS Genet.*, 2019, **15**, e1008320.
104. P. Kumar, A. Nagarajan and P. D. Uchil, *Cold Spring Harbor Protoc.*, 2018, DOI: 10.1101/pdb.top096263.
105. T. K. Kim and J. H. Eberwine, Mammalian cell transfection: The present and the future, *Anal. Bioanal. Chem.*, 2010, **397**(8), 3173–3178.
106. J. Shi, Y. Ma, J. Zhu, Y. Chen, Y. Sun and Y. Yao, *et al.*, A review on electroporation-based intracellular delivery, *Molecules*, 2018, **23**, E3044.
107. P. Kumar, A. Nagarajan and P. D. Uchil, Electroporation, *Cold Spring Harbor Protoc.*, 2019, DOI: 10.1101/pdb.top096271.
108. S. A. Godambe, D. D. Chaplin, T. Takova, L. M. Read and C. J. Bellone, A novel cis-acting element required for lipopolysaccharide-induced transcription of the murine interleukin-1 beta gene, *Mol. Cell. Biol.*, 1995, **15**(1), 112–119.
109. S. J. Kim, T. Park and K. K. Lee, Identification of a novel cis-acting positive element responsible for the cell-specific expression of the NK-1 homeobox gene, *Biochem. Biophys. Res. Commun.*, 1999, **257**(2), 538–544.
110. B. D. Wyse, S. L. Linas and T. J. Thekkurnkara, Functional role of a novel cis-acting element (GAGA box) in human type-1 angiotensin II receptor gene transcription, *J. Mol. Endocrinol.*, 2000, **25**(1), 97–108.
111. M. J. Cox, S. Jaensch, J. van de Waeter, L. Cougnaud, D. Seynaeve and S. Benalla, *et al.*, Tales of 1,008 small molecules: phenomic profiling through live-cell imaging in a panel of reporter cell lines, *Sci. Rep.*, 2020, **10**(1), 13262.
112. S. Hu, Z. Xie, J. Qian, S. Blackshaw and H. Zhu, Functional protein microarray technology, *Wiley Interdiscip. Rev.: Syst. Biol. Med.*, 2011, 3(3), 255–268.
113. D. Hamelinck, H. Zhou, L. Li, C. Verweij, D. Dillon and Z. Feng, *et al.*, Optimized normalization for antibody microarrays and application to serum-protein profiling, *Mol. Cell. Proteomics*, 2005, **4**(6), 773–784.
114. M. Hartmann, M. Schrenk, A. Döttinger, S. Nagel, J. Roeraade and T. O. Joos, *et al.*, Expanding assay dynamics: A combined competitive and direct assay system for the quantification of proteins in multiplexed immunoassays, *Clin. Chem.*, 2008, **54**(6), 956–963.
115. C. P. Pjaweletz, L. Charboneau, V. E. Bichsel, N. L. Simone, T. Chen and J. W. Gillespie, *et al.*, Reverse phase protein microarrays which capture disease progression show activation of pro-survival pathways at the cancer invasion front, *Oncogene*, 2001, **20**(16), 1981–1989.
116. G. MacBeath and S. L. Schreiber, Printing proteins as microarrays for high-throughput function determination, *Science*, 2000, **289**(5485), 1760–1763.
117. J. Huang, H. Zhu, S. J. Haggarty, D. R. Spring, H. Hwang and F. Jin, *et al.*, Finding new components of the target of rapamycin (TOR) signaling network through chemical genetics and proteome chips, *Proc. Natl. Acad. Sci. U. S. A.*, 2004, **101**(47), 16594–16599.
118. M. P. Patricelli, T. K. Nomanbhoy, J. Wu, H. Brown, D. Zhou and J. Zhang, *et al.*, In situ kinase profiling reveals functionally relevant properties of native kinases, *Chem. Biol.*, 2011, **18**(6), 699–710.
119. E. C. K. Lin, C. M. Amantea, T. K. Nomanbhoy, H. Weissig, J. Ishiyama and Y. Hu, *et al.*, ERK5 kinase activity is dispensable for cellular immune response and proliferation, *Proc. Natl. Acad. Sci. U. S. A.*, 2016, **113**(42), 11865–11870.
120. A. A. Saei, H. Gullberg, P. Sabatier, C. M. Beusch, K. Johansson and B. Lundgren, *et al.*, Comprehensive chemical proteomics for target deconvolution of the redox active drug auranofin, *Redox Biol.*, 2020, **32**, 101491.
121. M. Y. Pai, B. Lomenick, H. Hwang, R. Schiestl, W. McBride and J. A. Loo, *et al.*, Drug affinity responsive target stability (DARTS) for small-molecule target identification, *Methods Mol. Biol.*, 2015, **1263**, 287–298.
122. T. J. Robinson, M. Pai, J. C. Liu, F. Vizeacoumar, T. Sun and S. E. Egan, *et al.*, High-throughput screen identifies disulfiram as a potential therapeutic for triple-negative breast cancer cells: Interaction with IQ motif-containing factors, *Cell Cycle*, 2013, **12**(18), 3013–3024.
123. L. Wu, F. Meng, L. Dong, C. J. Block, A. v. Mitchell and J. Wu, *et al.*, Disulfiram and BKM120 in Combination with Chemotherapy Impede Tumor Progression and Delay Tumor Recurrence in Tumor Initiating Cell-Rich TNBC, *Sci. Rep.*, 2019, **9**(1), 236.
124. C. Lu, X. Li, Y. Ren and X. Zhang, Disulfiram: a novel repurposed drug for cancer therapy, *Cancer Chemother. Pharmacol.*, 2021, **87**, 159–172.
125. F. X. R. Sutandy, J. Qian, C.-S. Chen and H. Zhu, Overview of Protein Microarrays, *Curr. Protoc. Protein Sci.*, 2013, **72**, 27.1.1–27.1.16.
126. A. A. Khan, D. Betel, M. L. Miller, C. Sander, C. S. Leslie and D. S. Marks, *Nat. Biotechnol.*, 2009, **27**(6), 549–555.

# 10 Assays[†]

Barbara Saxty*[a], Peter J. Coombs*[a]

[a]LifeArc, Accelerator Building, Open Innovation Campus, Stevenage, SG1 2FX, UK
*E-mail: barbarasaxty@btinternet.com, peter.coombs@lifearc.org

## 10.1 Assay Detection Technologies

There are a large number of assay techniques available to the drug discovery bioscientist; each is designed to generate information from measurements such as optical spectroscopy, mass spectroscopy, radiometric techniques, nuclear magnetic resonance and surface plasmon resonance. Whilst there is utility in all of these methods, the design of assays for routine prosecution in drug discovery ultimately utilises three optical signal measurements: absorbance, fluorescence and luminescence. Within these three categories there are subcategories defined by the nature of photon generation, and each technology has advantages and disadvantages.

### 10.1.1 Absorbance

Absorbance is the oldest spectrophotometric method used to measure the concentration of a substance in solution. Absorbance-based assays are extremely useful for measuring the activity of enzymes and countless methods have been described utilising the absorbance of natural metabolites (*e.g.* NADH absorbs at 340 nm) or surrogate enzyme substrates such as paranitrophenol phosphate (pNPP) for phosphatase enzymes.[1] For drug discovery purposes, absorbance assays have the attraction of being relatively simple (*i.e.* few components) and cheap, but caution needs to be practised with respect to wavelengths used in homogeneous assays where compound interference in the 330–450 nm range will be common.

[†]Updated from Tim Hammonds and Peter B. Simpson, 2015.

The Handbook of Medicinal Chemistry: Principles and Practice, 2nd Edition
Edited by Simon E. Ward and Andrew M. Davis

Published by the Royal Society of Chemistry, www.rsc.org

## 10.1.2 Fluorescence

Fluorescence assays have revolutionised the HTS process since they began to be introduced in the late 1980s. Fluorescent molecules with excitation and emission wavelengths above 450 nm have been available for many years, and many have been used as labelling moieties (tags) for other, non-fluorescent molecules (for a good insight into what is available see *Molecular Probes® Handbook* from ThermoFisher.com). With time, reagent suppliers have marketed fluorescent tags with higher wavelengths and increased emission ratios to avoid compound interference and increase assay sensitivity. The parallel development of more sensitive plate readers with the ability to pick up weaker fluorescence signals led to the development of high throughput assays not only for fluorescence intensity (FI), but also for fluorescence resonance energy transfer (FRET), time resolved fluorescence (TRF and TR-FRET) and fluorescence polarisation (FP). The principles involved in these assays are illustrated in Figure 10.1. These techniques allow the assay scientist not only to measure the intrinsic fluorescence intensity

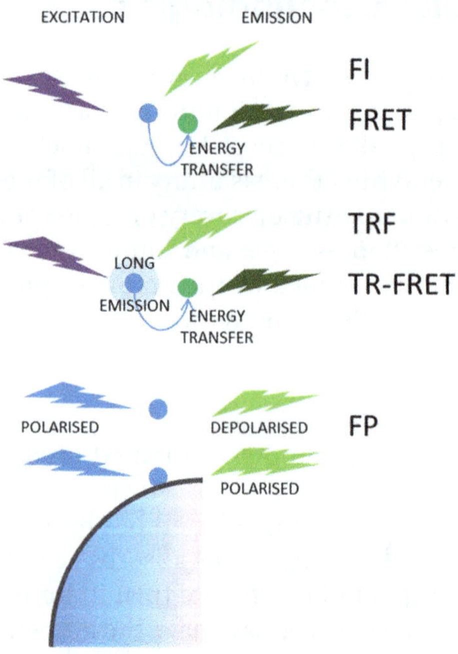


**Figure 10.1** Fluorescence techniques for drug discovery assays. Five mechanisms of measurement are shown, each emission (green flash) is the direct or indirect product of excitation (blue flash). Fluorescent molecules (fluors) are shown as spheres and resonant energy transfer by arrows. FI = Fluorescence intensity is directly measured from a single fluor. FRET = Fluorescence energy resonance transfer, where energy is transferred between fluors before emission. TR = Time resolved, the lifetime of decay and fluorescence of the primary (fluor) is relatively long, allowing for measures of FI or FRET to be made after background or interfering signals have decayed. FP = Fluorescent polarisation, a polarised mixture of excitation is used and the ratio of polarised emitted light is proportional to the apparent size of a fluor in solution, binding to a large protein or affinity bead can be detected by a change in the FP measure.

of a molecule, but also its proximity to another molecule *via* FRET or its apparent size in solution by FP. This ability to measure proximity by fluorescence ultimately has all but replaced radioactive proximity assays such as scintillation proximity assays (SPA). Time resolved fluorescence assays bring an extra dimension in that the emission fluorescence of one assay component is relatively long lived, *i.e.* in the order of milliseconds compared to nanoseconds. By adjusting the time at which the fluorescence is read, potentially interfering auto-fluorescent molecules are ignored by the assay system, decreasing the rate of false data. A combination of both TR fluorescence and FRET is known as TR-FRET.

### 10.1.3 Luminescence

Luminescence assays rely on a chemiluminescent reaction to generate an excited intermediate molecule, which decays to a ground state and emits a photon of defined wavelength. There are many enzymes that create chemiluminescence, but for drug discovery assays the most commonly used are firefly luciferase, Renilla luciferase and aequorin.[2] The reaction for firefly and Renilla luciferase is described in Figure 10.2. Like Renilla luciferase, aequorin also binds coelenterezine, but only activates it to emit luminescence upon calcium binding. All reagents for these luminescence reactions are commercially available, therefore if an assay can be developed that generates any component of a luminescence reaction then that assay can be supplemented with the remaining reagents and the resulting luminescence is a measure of the initial reaction. Luminescent assays have the major advantage that they do not rely upon any other source of light. As such, very low

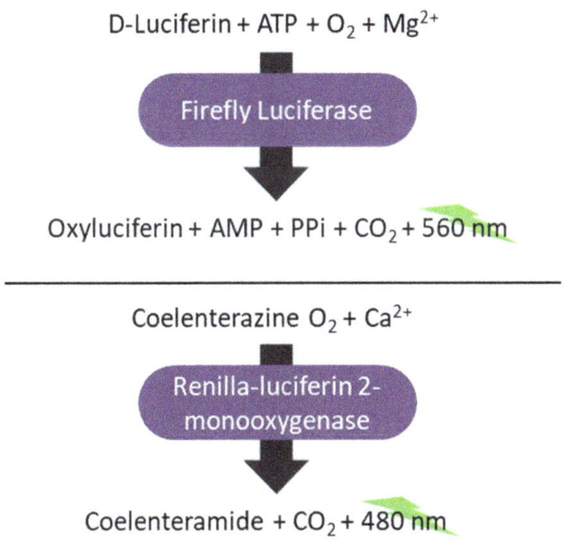


**Figure 10.2** Common luminescence reactions for drug discovery assays. The two most common reactions used to detect luminescence; each enzyme utilises a number of cofactors to give an emitted photon (green flash). Measurement of any of the cofactors or the concentration of the enzyme itself can be achieved using these systems. Emitted light is in the blue/green region of the spectrum.

levels of luminescence can be detected and these assays have an excellent limit of sensitivity. Luciferase assays are very robust and amenable to HTS and so they have a key role in biochemical and cell-based assays. Luciferases and aequorin can also be genetically engineered into cellular assays to allow the measurement of intracellular processes such as gene expression (Molecular Biology, Chapter 9 and Section 10.2.5).

As they perform a reaction in their own right, luminescence assay systems will attract a number of false positives *via* direct inhibition of the luciferase enzyme.[3] These can easily be detected by running test compounds against the reconstituted assay, but care should be taken to ensure identical conditions are created. Alphascreen™/AlphaLISA™ (PerkinElmer) are bead-based technologies that can be configured to measure biomolecular binding events in a biochemical or cell-based assay. The term Alpha is an acronym for amplified luminescent proximity homogeneous assay. Two bead types are required in the assay; donor beads and acceptor beads. Donor beads contain phthalocyanine, which converts ambient oxygen to an excited form, singlet oxygen, when illuminated at 680 nm. Within its 4 μs half-life, singlet oxygen can diffuse approximately 200 nm in solution. This is a much greater distance than can be achieved with fluorescent energy transfer. If an acceptor bead is within that proximity, energy is transferred from the singlet oxygen to thioxene derivatives within the acceptor bead, producing light emission. Acceptor beads for the two technologies differ. Both contain thioxene, but Alphascreen beads contain two other dyes, anthracene and rubrene, which result in a broad emission of light 520–620 nm, whereas AlphaLISA is coupled to an europium chelate which has an intense narrow emission wavelength 605–625 nM (see Figure 10.3). The proximity of acceptor to donor beads depends on the interaction between the biomolecules that are bound to them. For example, if a receptor is attached to donor beads and the relevant ligand to acceptor beads, then when the ligand binds its receptor, energy is transferred from donor to acceptor beads and a signal is produced. So, addition of compounds which displace the ligand will reduce the light signal and allow measurement of the affinity of that compound. AlphaScreen has limitations in assay sensitivity, which restricts its use to fairly abundant proteins. It also suffers practical issues with assay plates needing protection from long exposure to ambient light, compounds in screening libraries can scavenge the singlet oxygen thereby interfering with the detection and donor beads photo-bleaching limits the assay format to a single read.[4] AlphaLISA used in conjunction with selective antibody detection reagents (see Section 10.1.4, Figure 10.3) and have been widely employed in cell-based assays for proximal biomarkers. AlphaLISA™ assays require small sample volumes yet they have over a 100-fold greater analytical range than ELISAs. Uptake of this technology has been mixed so far, perhaps reflecting the multitude of options now available to the screener (Fluorescence Polarisation, Time Resolved Fluorescence, Meso Scale Detection) that all can be satisfactory for many drug target assays – though they may well detect overlapping but certainly non-identical sets of active compounds.[5]

### 10.1.4 Antibody-based Assays

An enzyme-linked immunosorbent assay (ELISA) uses an enzyme coupled to an antibody, or antigen, to detect a specific protein. This can be either a biochemical *in vitro* assay, or a cellular assay typically measuring protein abundance in a cell lysate.

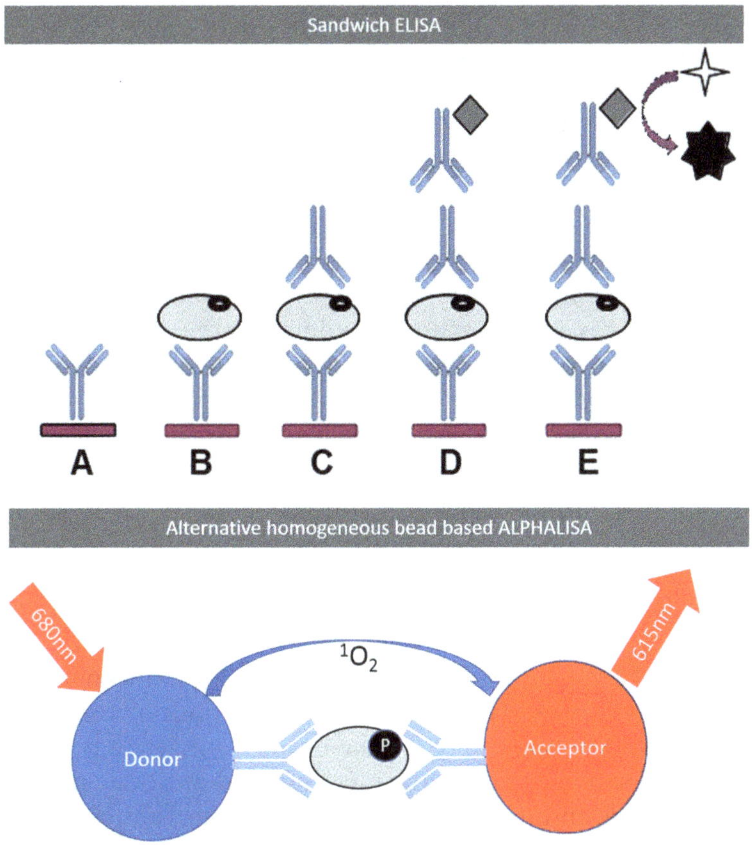


**Figure 10.3** Adaptation of the sandwich ELISA to a homogeneous assay format for high throughput assays. Upper panel: Sandwich ELISA protocol. (A) The microplate well is coated with capture antibody. (B) The assay sample is added and antigen binds to the capture antibody. Non-binding components are washed away. (C) The detection antibody, which binds captured antigen, is added. Unbound antibody is washed off. (D) An enzyme-conjugated secondary antibody is added. This binds to the secondary antibody. Unbound antibody is washed off. (E) Enzyme substrate is added, converted to a detectable product and the signal is produced. Lower panel: AlphaLisa bead-based detection in solution. No wash steps are involved; the specific antibodies are attached to the beads *via* affinity (*e.g.* biotin streptavidin binding) or conjugation. The specificity of the signal relies on the close proximity of the beads when bound to the analyte. Similar configurations using FRET and TR-FRET are possible.

There are multiple versions of the basic ELISA principle shown in Figure 10.3.[6] Performing an ELISA assay therefore involves having at least one antibody with high specificity for the particular antigen in the target protein, as a very high level of specificity is important for building a reliable assay. However, as a preferred technology they are relatively laborious in nature. There are multiple addition steps, and washes, required over the course of an extended period of time.[7] For screeners, the more steps there are in an assay, the more things there are to go wrong or to increase data variability between testing occasions, such as automation failures, reagents degrading, batch-to-batch differences, or screener error. The major drawback with ELISA assays is that they require repeat wash steps – which even using current high-quality automated equipment can increase assay noise, length of time required for plate processing and assay failure rates. ELISA-type assays have a role to play in confirming target engagement for the analysis of cellular protein abundance and post-translational modification. Where possible, substitution of a homogeneous fluorescence-based detection format is preferred for throughput. For established target classes a broad range of validated kits are commercially available. A variant of the basic ELISA, for use in fluorescence microscopy, utilises fluorophore-conjugated antibodies. This version enables multiple assays within each well, as different detection antibodies can be coupled to fluorophores which emit at different wavelengths.[8] This is discussed in more detail in the cell imaging Section 10.1.8.

Alternative technologies permit multiplexing multiple read-outs using antibodies.[9] Meso Scale Discovery have developed an instrument which uses specialised microtiter plates containing electrodes and antibodies labelled with an electrochemiluminescent tag for detection following conventional ELISA-like protocols. When electricity is passed across the plate, antibody bound to antigen in close proximity to the surface emits light. This detection technology has ultra-low sensitivity and broad dynamic range such that dilution to accommodate high and low expression levels are not needed. The signal generated is localised within the plate and it is possible to multiplex the detection of 4–10 antigens in one well by spotting capture antibodies in a grid pattern in the well. Luminex® bead-based technologies and advances in automated flow cytometry instrumentation have given rise to advanced multiplex options to interrogate complex biology in 96, 384 and 1536 formats. Here the beads themselves contain dye to distinguish different analytes, and phycoerythrin-conjugated antibody detected to quantify the amount of analyte bound. Panels of secreted proteins, adhesion molecules, cytokines, enzymes, receptors and growth factors can be quantified from one sample using cell lines, cocultures, primary cells or plasma, thus providing a broader picture of the impact of compounds on multiple pathways and saving time and sample reagents to process multiple ELISAs.

### 10.1.5 Mass Spectrometry

For many years, liquid chromatography-mass spectrometry (LC-MS) has been an important, but late, component of drug testing cascades, commonly applied in *in vitro* ADME assays.[10] From a target assay perspective, mass spectrometry can be highly desirable as it offers highly specific detection and is suitable for target molecules that are not amenable to most other conventional assays.[11] For example, minor changes in a metabolite can be detected *via* mass spectrometry where it would be impossible to generate a specific, selective antibody-based assay. In many cases, labelling of proteins is not required, and sensitivity is sufficiently high for assays to be performed in native or primary cells. With advances in pre-processing, automation and analysis platforms, mass spec now has a place at all stages of the discovery process.

Primary biochemical assays have been automated using commercial LC-MS systems such as the RapidFire 360 High-throughput MS System[12] (Agilent). With processing speeds of under 10 seconds per sample this technology has been widely adopted for profiling compounds as an orthogonal read-out from conventional fluorescence-based

HTS assays. However recent technological advances in development are coupling acoustic dispensing to mass spec, acoustic mist ionisation (AMI-MS), to achieve increased sample processing to sub-second time frames, enabling HTS throughputs of 100 000 samples per day.[13]

Methods to approach target engagement have also been developed using mass spec. The first of these is affinity selection mass spec to detect label-free small molecule target binding.[14] This has the advantage over conventional approaches which require the attachment of a probe to the small molecule, which itself may interfere with binding. Target compound–protein complexes are separated from unbound compounds using size exclusion separation. Known ligands, cofactors or substrates can be included in the assay to gain insight into competition of binding sites. Cellular target engagement can be explored using thermal proteome profiling (TPP) or thermal-stability profiling allowing the simultaneous measurement of the entire melting proteome, typically ~4000 proteins.[15] Compounds are added to cell lysates or intact cells over a dose–response range consistent with biological effect. Cells are lysed and thermally treated. Soluble proteins are fractionated and digested and peptides tagged prior to detection on the mass spec. Proteomic data analysis is applied to identify proteins showing significant stabilisation following temperature-dependent thermal aggregation (see CETSA, Section 10.1.8). In intact cells, more proteins may be identified than in cell lysates; these represent both direct binders (in common with cell lysate) and indirect consequences of changes to stability of near neighbours in the pathway. This is a powerful data-rich technology upon which project teams can prioritise progression of the best leads based on cellular selectivity.

An exciting ongoing challenge is to broaden the applicability of higher throughput MALDI-TOF metabolomic and proteomic profiling in cellular assays for drug discovery. Separation and quantitation of multiple parallel readouts from interfering cellular components in a timely way is becoming highly enabling for detailed mechanism-of-action studies and identification of disease biomarkers. Cell LC/MS screening assays are an attractive option, *e.g.* for metabolism assays in which multiple pathway components may be affected by a compound, and inhibition at one point can be counteracted by compensation elsewhere in the pathway or network. Whilst bespoke biochemical assays can measure a change in the ratios of individual, or pairs of, key cellular cofactors, *e.g.* ATP : ADP, glutamine : glutamate, or NAD : NADH, to indicate a phenotypic metabolic switch or stress response, metabolomics assays by mass spec can rapidly measure many tens or hundreds of individual metabolites and generate phenotypic responses associated with disease states and responses to chemical agents.[16]

Using MALDI-TOF, unique molecular mass signatures are first identified, which characterise a response to a stimulus or disease state. Then phenotypic assays quantifying the changes in these markers in response to compounds are developed.[17] The low sample volumes and sensitivity of mass spec allow the same markers identified in cell assays to be detected in tissue. For low abundance biomarkers ($<10$ ng ml$^{-1}$) affinity selection can be applied to enrich samples either by depletion of high abundance proteins (*e.g.* sera) or selection using antibodies, ligands, dyes or metal-coated affinity resins.[18] The development of MALDI imaging mass spec provides a powerful tool to multiplex detection of hundreds of proteins, peptides, lipids and metabolites in discrete tissue regions with 1–10 μM resolution.[19] From these studies we can confirm our lead compound (or metabolites thereof) arrived at the site of action *in vivo* and gain insight to the pharmacological and toxicological impact of the treatment.

### 10.1.6 Surface Plasmon Resonance

SPR is a label-free technique that allows the sensitive detection of the addition of mass to a sensor chip surface in real time. In practical terms, this typically means by immobilising a target protein on a surface and exposing it to a potential small molecule binding partner, it is possible to observe their interaction directly. The real time measurements, plotted as a sensorgram, are a real strength of SPR, allowing the determination of kinetic rates of association and dissociation.[20] SPR can also give an indication of stoichiometry of binding partners, although ITC is often the preferred biophysical technique for stoichiometry determination if it is available or practical, due to very high protein requirements. Non-specific binding observed in SPR experiments can be an indicator of non-desirable mechanism of action by hit compounds, for example hits identified by a biochemical inhibition assay screen may be working by aggregation, though on occasion the SPR setup or immobilisation may be an issue and an alternative assay format, for example an in-solution method such as NMR or MST, may be needed.

SPR can have particular impact on challenging targets such as non-enzymatic targets or PPIs, where biochemical assays are complicated or low-throughput, or enzyme targets that reach the tight-binding limit. The latest high-throughput instruments, such as the Biacore 8K+, are capable of measuring thousands of interactions against targets in less than a day. Typically instruments are also highly sensitive, making them ideal for fragment screening and to support fragment-based drug discovery projects (see Chapter 5).[21] SPR, alongside other biophysical techniques, is commonly used to validate hits from biochemical assays and to confirm target engagement (see Section 10.3.2).

Other comparable technologies that can deliver similar real-time, biosensor-based data include the Fortebio Octet, which uses BLI (Bio Layer Interferometry) and Creoptix instruments which use GCI (Grating-Coupled Interferometry). While perhaps less established than SPR, they may have advantages in terms of reduced problems with buffer effects, though it should be noted that current BLI instruments are less sensitive, and therefore often not as suitable with regards to small molecule work.

### 10.1.7 Microscale Thermophoresis (MST)

Microscale thermophoresis has become an established alternative biophysical technique for looking at target–ligand interactions over the last 10 years with the Monolith series of instruments from NanoTemper.[22] The technique monitors changes in thermophoretic movement, *i.e.* motion of molecules in a temperature gradient, and differences in this upon ligand binding. Detection is *via* fluorescence, which can either be intrinsic to the protein target or ligand, or extrinsic, such as a conjugated fluorescent label or GFP. The MST signal is sensitive to temperature-related intensity changes of the fluorescent probe, movement in the temperature gradient, as well as changes in the chemical microenvironment and hydration shell. By comparing the MST signal in the presence and absence of a potential binding partner, and ultimately in a dose–response experiment, it is possible to determine the affinity of the interaction. Experiments are set up in a series of glass capillaries, each typically containing a fixed concentration of labelled target and a specific concentration of ligand to be tested. MST is an in-solution method, so immobilisation is not necessary, which may have advantages in some situations. Compared to alternative in-solution biophysical methods, ITC and NMR, the protein requirements are very low, and it is particularly well suited for studying protein complexes, which may not be sufficiently stable to study in a flow-based SPR system.

### 10.1.8 Protein Thermal Shift and CETSA

Changes in protein stability can be measured in thermal stability assays. This relies on protein stabilisation as a result of ligand binding. When unbound proteins are exposed to a heat gradient, they begin to unfold or "melt" at a certain temperature, exposing hydrophobic patches onto which a dye binds (typically Sypro Orange) and becomes fluorescent, emitting a signal – usually detected on a real-time PCR thermal cycler instrument. The mid-point of these transitions, *i.e.* where the concentrations of native and denatured proteins are the same, is generally referred to as the melting temperature ($T_m$). Ligand-bound proteins, however, are stabilised by their interacting partner and will therefore melt at a higher temperature when exposed to the same heat gradient, resulting in a so-called $T_m$ shift. An adaptation of $T_m$ shift assays for use in whole cells is CETSA (cellular thermal shift assay).[23] The assay is based on quantification of the remaining levels of stabilised protein following irreversible aggregation of thermally unfolded proteins. Proteins are detected using antibodies or mass spec technologies. To reflect the non-equilibrium nature of these experiments, the ligand-induced stabilisation is more appropriately referred to as thermal aggregation temperature ($T_{agg}$) shifts. The magnitude of thermal shifts vary broadly among proteins and ligands. The technique is limited to soluble proteins and altered by changes to protein complex binding and is therefore not applicable for all targets. It is not reliant on recombinant protein and can be applied across the cascade, from live cell assays to *ex vivo* tissue biopsies to confirm cellular target engagement.[24] Coupled with mass spec detection it offers powerful target deconvolution and target specificity profiling for mechanism of action studies (see thermal proteome profiling mass spec, Section 10.1.5).[25]

### 10.1.9 Cell Imaging

High content screening (HCS) methods for drug discovery employ fluorescent labelling of cellular components, and microscopy-based cell image acquisition, combined with quantitation of the resultant fluorescent image by specific analytical algorithms. There are several automated platforms available suitable for adherent cells (InCell Analyser (GE Healthcare), Opera Phenix (PerkinElmer) and Image Xpress (Molecular Devices)) which combine automation and data analysis software to achieve the throughput required for drug discovery. Stains for cell nuclei and membranes are used as markers for individual cells, and each cell is automatically counted and scored individually for a response in the assay. This enables visualisation and measurement of specific protein changes, post translational modification, translocation between compartments or altered abundance, within individual cells.

There are currently two predominant types of high content assay: fixed cell antibody and stain-based detection systems, and live imaging systems based on fluorescent protein expression and non-toxic cell stains. In the fixed cell format the assay is similar to the ELISAs detailed above and is illustrated in Figure 10.4. After treatment of cells with compounds, the antigens within cells are fixed *in situ* by an agent such as paraformaldehyde. An agent to permeabilise cells may also be used. An antibody against the antigen of interest is added to the well, incubated, then excess unbound antibody is washed off. A second antibody that is coupled to a fluorophore is then added that binds to the first antibody.[26] By varying the fluorophore used, it is possible to differentially fluorescently label multiple cellular components to build up a more sophisticated view of the cell and therefore of the impact of compound treatment on the cell or even subpopulation of cells within a complex 3D network or coculture of cells. HCS can be used to determine the mode of action, potency, and selectivity of potential drug molecules within a biologically relevant cellular context, and also provides information on off-target liabilities and cytotoxicity.[27]

Imaging of complex 3D structures requires instrument and analytical adaptations to allow for imaging through the vertical layers of the 3D structure, so called Z-stack. This inevitably increases the volume of data and time to capture images; for example, a 384-well plate of 3D spheroids imaged at 4× magnification will generate 50–100 GB of data. This is sufficient to view shape and size of spheroids or microtissues embedded in a gel matrix. For single-cell resolution to monitor impact on different subpopulations, higher magnification, 10×, can be used, but this brings additional data analysis challenges to

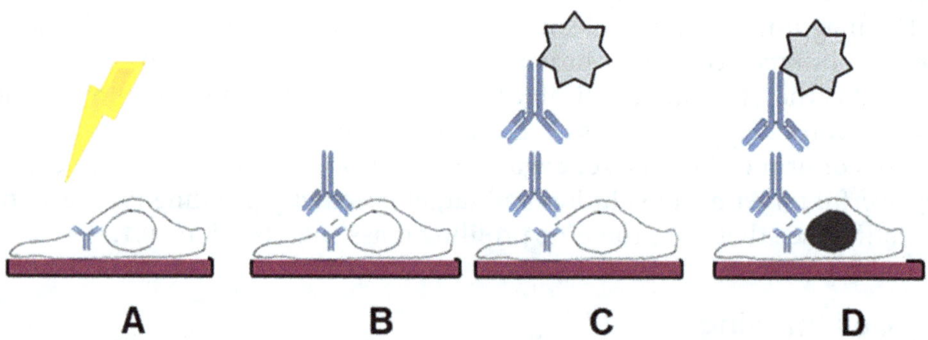


**Figure 10.4** Outline of a typical fixed cell HCS protocol. (A) Adherent cells are fixed and permeabilised to ensure antigens are in position. Cells are washed. (B) The antigen detection antibody is added and binds to antigen. Cells are washed to remove unbound antibody. (C) The secondary antibody, labelled with a fluorophore is added and binds to the antigen detection antibody. Cells are washed to remove unbound antibody. (D) DNA is visualised using a fluorescent DNA intercalating dye. The cells are visualised at both the antibody and DNA fluor wavelengths. The images are combined to show the amount of antigen present and its localisation relative to the cell nucleus. By the addition of additional fluor-labelled antibodies and stains for subcellular structures, multiparametric assays of increasing complexity can be configured.

retain cellular architecture and colocalisation of fluorescent objects through the stack. Higher resolution and live cell imaging, which can be achieved in 2D, requires further software development for "on-the-fly" object recognition in 3D. Using such approaches the mechanism of action of compounds in complex disease-relevant models can be differentiated, desirable and undesirable compound features identified and the best series selected for progression.[28]

In an advancement from conventional analysis of a small number of defined read-outs, automated data analysis is enabling high content morphological cell profiling. Here, hundreds of biological features with single cell resolution are measured by multiplexing several fluorescent dyes to stain various subcellular structures and then quantifying a large amount of morphological data from the microscopy images to generate an unbiased cellular profile or phenotype in a technique called cell painting.[29] There is also potential for combining profiles from multiple methodologies (*e.g.* imaging + gene expression) in the same experiment to capture a broader range of cell activities. These types of assays give rise to very large data sets and the size, complexity and multiparametric nature of such data sets make automated analysis strategies necessary to identify cellular phenotypes that differ from the wild type. As a consequence, many profiling studies are turning to supervised or unsupervised machine learning strategies to capture and evaluate phenotypic changes of single cells or cell populations.[30] This unbiased approach allows comparison of compounds to identify those with a similar activity or differentiated mode of action relative to a reference compound to avoid unwanted effects or to identify unexpected target associations for drug repurposing.[31] Another useful application is in complex disease biology to screen small molecules to highlight candidates that reverse a disease-associated phenotype back to the wild-type phenotype.

Bright-field imaging systems, such as IncuCyte (Essen Instruments), facilitate a range of experimental studies on long-term live cellular behaviour, as they can be left in the cell incubator for extended time periods, and are now available with fluorescent options enabling combined use of cell shape changes with fluorescent detection of biological events within the cell. This is useful for understanding mode of action in long-term growth assays and tracking movement of cells (see Section 10.2.6).

## 10.2 Assay Design

From a drug discovery perspective, an assay is an estimate of the ability of a project compound to inhibit, activate or modulate a biological process, and the development of appropriate robust (*i.e.* accurate and reproducible) assays is essential to project progression. The word "estimate" is used very deliberately here – it is important to understand from the outset that all assays performed in drug discovery are estimates, be they single point estimates of percentage activity or multipoint estimates of compound potency. The error in assays is brought about by their multiparametric nature, and the more variables an assay has, then, in principle, the less exact it may become.

Assays come in various "shapes and sizes" and assay developers often describe assays by parameters concerning their build and output. The technologies described above are combined with bespoke reagents to generate assays fit for different purposes. In order to understand better the design, function and potential issues of an assay it is useful to describe the assay parameters governing the build and output; these are summarised in Table 10.1. The simplest and theoretically easiest assays to work with are homogenous, direct product accumulation assays, *i.e.* the substrate is directly transformed to product

**Table 10.1** Common assay nomenclature. Combinations of these parameters and descriptors will be used to describe the format and readout of assays.

| Operational descriptor | Definition | Pros | Cons |
|---|---|---|---|
| Homogenous | All components can be added sequentially | Easy for HTS | Compounds may interfere |
| Washed | Components must be removed and replaced during the assay operation | Low compound interference<br>Allows technically difficult assays | Cumbersome for HTS |
| Stopped | The assay is designed to have a fixed signal endpoint | Easy for HTS<br>Ideal for potency | Must be well timed<br>Not ideal for kinetics |
| Kinetic | The reaction/signal continues unabated during the testing process | Gold standard for kinetics | Difficult for HTS |
| **Readout value** | | | |
| Accumulation (bottom up) | Measures product generated from zero | Best for kinetic analysis | |
| Depletion (top down) | Measures the loss of one reagent | Poor for kinetics if enzyme activity is weak | Often more noisy<br>May require high % conversion |
| Ratiometric | Measures the balance between two species | Dispensing errors are adjusted for in ratio<br>Often very robust | Poor linearity<br>May be limited for kinetics |
| Binding/displacement | Detects two molecules interacting | Direct measures of drug affinity possible | Binding may not be a direct measure of inhibition |
| **Readout type** | | | |
| Number | Cell number, number of mitochondria, cell protrusion *etc.* | Robust measure allows for easy statistics | Cell assays are biology and as such more error prone |
| Direct | The reaction of interest generates the signal | Ideal reaction to measure | |
| Coupled | A series of other reactions generate assay output from the initial reaction | May increase the rate of product-inhibited enzymes<br>Allows measurement of any common cell metabolite | Prone to interference from compounds and contaminating enzymes<br>May be complex and expensive reagents involved |
| Proximity | The signal relies upon two objects being close to each other in space | Robust<br>Allows for many non-enzymatic measurements | Poor for kinetics |
| **Measure** | | | |
| Product | The reaction product that one is interested in the cell | Ideal measure | |
| Cofactor | Any other reaction component that goes to make product | Many assays exist for cellular cofactors | More prone to contaminant protein interferences |
| Probe | Labelled versions of any assay component | Ideal for binding reactions | Not a direct measure of enzyme activity |

by the target in question and the reaction can be read once all of the reagents are added to the sample well. For HTS, this assay would also be stopped to ensure an even signal across plates tested at various times in the automation process. In reality, assays have to be developed to various designs utilising either entire commercial kits, or by combining in-house and purchased reagents. Signal generation is the one area where recent advances have expanded the number of assays that can be developed. Aside from the ongoing development of novel direct substrates and coupling systems, proximity assays are of particular importance as they have allowed a far more flexible approach to assay development. In theory, the development of an antibody or affinity media that specifically binds a substrate or product of a reaction allows for that component to be measured *via* associated off-the-shelf FP, FRET or TR-FRET reagents from a variety of manufactures.

Once a stable signal has been established, then assay development proper can begin, and each parameter could significantly affect the assay performance and thus project progression. The assay scientist may spend many experiments adjusting the buffer conditions to obtain optimal robustness of signal performance, spend time miniaturising an existing assay to be more cost effective or increase capacity, or adjust conditions in an assay to give reproducible $IC_{50}$ data on a regular basis.

Regardless of the origin and nature of the expression system, it is increasingly clear that poor attention to reagent design, and/or using criteria based solely on signal, accuracy and precision, will most likely lead to poorly predictive data. Most worryingly, such data may not at first appear to be misleading and otherwise meet pass/fail criteria, greatly wasting precious time, energy and cost. Key to long-term success is functional validation of reagents using known pharmacological standards, ideally those tested in the clinic. Sadly, when leading from the front on novel targets, for which there may be few or no available standards, drug discovery assays are progressed at risk. In the absence of well validated tools against your target-of-interest substrate analogues, products of the reaction or known modulatory protein binding partners will serve for assay validation. If these are not practical, then pilot screening of a small pharmacologically active sets (*circa* 1000 compounds) can reveal useful tools. They may not be selective for your target or may be non-drug-like, but will suffice for the purpose of benchmarking an assay. Imperative is also early testing in non-clonal or "native" expression systems which tend to be more physiologically predictive.

## 10.2.1 Biophysical Assays

Biophysical techniques are a key component of many drug discovery cascades, fulfilling an important role alongside biochemical and cell-based assays. The techniques that fall under biophysics are many and varied,[32] measuring various physical phenomena to examine direct interactions between protein target and ligand. These include surface plasmon resonance spectroscopy (SPR), microscale thermophoresis (MST), protein thermal shift assays (TSA) and some applications of mass spectrometry (see Section 10.1.5), as described above, as well as isothermal titration calorimetry (ITC), nuclear magnetic resonance (NMR), X-ray crystallography, cryo-electron microscopy (cryo-EM), and some less commonly used techniques such as kinetic exclusion assay (KinExa), second harmonic generation (SHG) and DNA nanolevers (SwitchSense), which have more niche roles. Although all of these techniques address the central question of whether the ligand binds the target, each technique can provide different information, and may be useful at different stages of the drug discovery process. Table 10.2 presents a summary of biophysical techniques that can be used for affinity determination. In practice, specific techniques may lend themselves to the affinity determination or target engagement confirmation for a particular target, whilst others may not be viable for a variety of reasons; it is important to be pragmatic about which biophysical technique may be most appropriate and practical, and it is good to keep options open if one does not work out well. The concept of a toolbox of biophysical approaches to be drawn upon as needed can be a useful way to think about it. Improvements in speed and sensitivity of the instrumentation associated with many, though not all, of these techniques has meant that the throughput, quality and resolution of the data collected has improved dramatically over time. As such, some biophysical instruments, particularly when combined with robotic automation, are capable of measuring 100s, if not 1000s, of protein–ligand interactions in a day. High-quality protein is key, and biophysical techniques can also help with checking this as part of a quality control process.

In SPR, immobilisation of the target on the sensor chip can be both beneficial and problematic, where some proteins will be stabilised and behave well when immobilised and others will not. There are many options for how to immobilise the target of interest on the sensor chip, and often it may be necessary to try more than one to hit upon a productive setup. The factors affecting the choice of immobilisation may be availability of reagents, availability of tags or antibodies, the stability of the protein target over time and the strength of the interaction being studied. For very tight interactions (*e.g.* typically associated with low to sub-nM affinities), dissociation back to baseline could take hours for each concentration tested, so to avoid extremely long experiments, regeneration of the sensor chip may be required. Immobilisation strategies for SPR can be *via* covalent coupling, *e.g. via* amine or thiol coupling to protein surface lysine/cysteine side chains, though this can have deleterious effects on the protein due to the location of the coupled residues on the protein or the exposure to low pH required. Capture techniques are also an option, where an anti-target or anti-tag antibody can be used to capture the target. A highly specific, high affinity antibody with low non-specific binding is needed for this approach to be successful for small molecule work, though it does have the advantage of potential regeneration, where the target can be stripped off the antibody and fresh target recoated. The generally preferred options for target immobilisation for small molecule work are biotin–streptavidin or His-tag-Nickel-NTA. Biotinylation of the protein target can be achieved chemically, *e.g.* NHS-PEG4-Biotin from Thermo Scientific, attaching to surface lysines and the N-terminus, where generally the preference is to label at a stoichiometric level so as to not saturate the surface of the protein with biotin. The alternative is the use of the Avi-tag system, where a ~14–15 amino acid sequence is incorporated into the protein construct that is recognised by the enzyme biotin ligase, which can be used to add a single biotin molecule onto a lysine within the sequence, giving a specifically biotinylated protein.[33] The biotinylated protein is then immobilised on a streptavidin chip, which given the affinity of streptavidin for biotin, is effectively irreversible, and gives a surface with a very stable baseline. Histidine-tagged

**Table 10.2** Selected biophysical techniques for small molecule affinity determination work pros and cons.

| Technology | Pros | Cons |
|---|---|---|
| Surface plasmon resonance (SPR) | High-throughput (plate-based)<br>High sensitivity (suitable for fragment work)<br>Low protein requirement<br>Real time measurement of kinetics<br>Stoichiometry & thermodynamic measurements possible | Required immobilisation on sensor surface may affect target structure, stability or accessibility<br>Sensitive to changes in high refractive index components in buffers and samples (*e.g.* DMSO)<br>Microfluidic system requires regular maintenance |
| Grating-coupled interferometry (GCI) | Real-time measurement of kinetics<br>High sensitivity (suitable for fragment work)<br>Less buffer composition sensitivity than SPR | Required immobilisation on sensor surface may affect target structure or accessibility<br>Throughput not yet as high as for leading SPR instruments |
| Bio layer interferometry (BLI) | Real time measurement of kinetics<br>Broad buffer tolerance<br>Long interaction measurements don't require more reagents<br>Plate-based with no fluidics<br>Small molecule competition experiment setup can be viable | Required immobilisation on sensor surface may affect target structure or accessibility<br>Low sensitivity severely limits direct binding measurements of low molecular weight molecules |
| Microscale thermophoresis (MST) | Very low protein requirement.<br>In solution<br>Protein complexes and solubilised membrane proteins can be studied<br>High sensitivity (suitable for fragment work) | Requires fluorescent labelling or strong intrinsic fluorescence<br>Susceptible to fluorescence interference<br>Medium throughput |
| Differential scanning fluorimetry/protein Thermal shift assay (DSF/TSA) | High-throughput (plate-based)<br>Low protein requirement<br>Ease of setup and access to equipment (qPCR)<br>Useful for buffer screening to optimise target stability | Low sensitivity<br>Potential for false negatives & positives – degree of stabilisation target- & binding site-dependent, fluorescent quenching possible<br>Requires fluorescent dye<br>Susceptible to fluorescence interference<br>Not suitable for accurate KD determination – comparative data allows compound ranking<br>Not suitable for hydrophobic proteins |
| nanoDSF | Intrinsic fluorescence detection means no labelling required<br>Easy setup<br>Low protein requirement | Low sensitivity<br>Potential for false negatives & positives – degree of stabilisation target- & binding site-dependent-Target must have suitable intrinsic fluorescence (*i.e.* well-located tryptophan residues) to obtain good dataSusceptible to fluorescence interference<br>Not suitable for accurate KD determination – comparative data allows compound ranking<br>Not suitable for hydrophobic proteins |

(*continued*)

**Table 10.2** *(continued)*

| Technology | Pros | Cons |
|---|---|---|
| Isothermal titration calorimetry (ITC) | In solution<br>Direct determination of thermodynamic properties (enthalpy ($\Delta H$) and entropy ($\Delta S$))<br>Accurate determination of stoichiometry | Very high protein requirement<br>Requires high compound solubility<br>Low throughput |
| Ligand-observed NMR (STD, Water-LOGSY, CPMG, $^{19}$F) | In solution<br>Sensitive and suitable for fragment screening<br>No labelling or immobilisation of protein target<br>Protein and ligand integrity information<br>Suitable for competitor ligand experiments | High protein requirement<br>Medium throughput (high if using compound cocktails)<br>Not suitable for accurate KD determination – comparative data allows compound ranking |
| Protein-observed NMR | Determination of $K_D$ by titration experiments<br>Binding epitope determinable if NMR spectrum is assigned<br>Protein integrity information | High isotopically-labelled (e.g. 15N) protein requirement<br>Low throughput<br>Not suitable for large proteins (>40 kDa) |

proteins, commonly used for purification, can be immobilised on Nickel-NTA coated sensor chips, which can be very convenient. The major problem with this is that for a monomeric protein with a single hexahistidine (His-6) tag, the affinity of the His-tag for the Ni-NTA on the chip is not sufficient for a stable baseline, and the baseline will drift down over time as the protein dissociates from the chip surface. However, incorporation of a longer or double-His-tag allows a higher avidity interaction with the chip and should provide a sufficiently stable baseline for conducting small molecule binding measurements.[34]

The other factors that may require thought and optimisation are the SPR buffer and temperature, with key parameters being keeping the protein target happy and, buffer-wise, including detergent (typically 0.05% Tween-20). One complication of using SPR for small molecule work that should be noted is the effect of DMSO on Biacore signals. Due to the high refractive index of DMSO, SPR signals are highly sensitive to its presence and efforts must be made to match the amount of DMSO in the running buffer with the samples as closely as possible and to include a solvent correction as part of each experiment. However, in a well-setup experiment with concentrated compound stocks with low/no water absorption, DMSO issues should be minimal.

Positive control compounds, when available, will facilitate the SPR assay optimisation – this may be existing literature inhibitors (or activators), other ligands, cofactors or enzyme substrates. In the ideal situation, controls are in the low μM $K_D$ range with relatively fast dissociation to enable quicker experiments without having to wait for lengthy dissociation between cycles.

As for any assay, following assay development and any potential single point screening, it is important to see good dose–response data to have confidence in the assay and

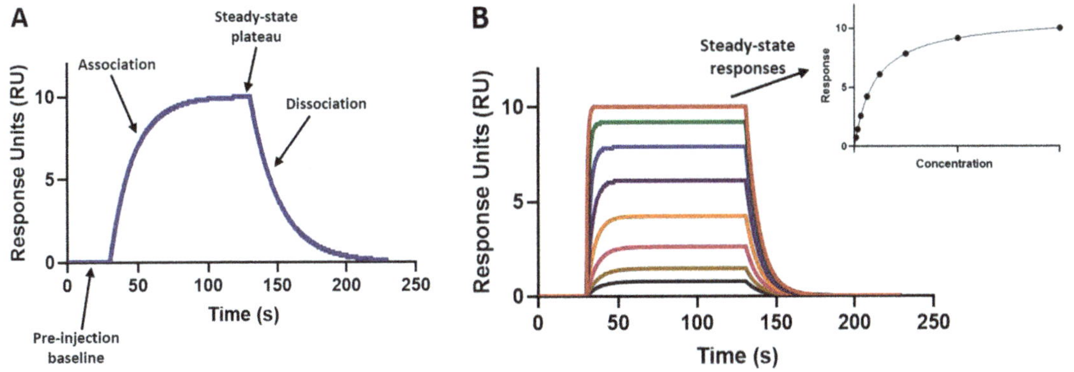


**Figure 10.5** (A) Example annotated SPR sensorgram of small molecule binding to a protein target showing a typical 1:1 kinetic binding interaction at a single compound concentration. (B) Overlay of dose–response sensorgrams for steady state analysis from which $R_{max}$ (maximum binding response at saturation) and $K_D$ can be estimated from the secondary plot shown in the inset. The amplitude of the response signal from ligand binding should be proportional to the amount of target protein immobilised on the sensor chip at a ratio of their respective molecular weights, such that $R_{max}$ = small molecule molecular weight/target molecular weight × immobilised target response units (*e.g.* 250 Da compound/50 000 Da protein × 2000 RU immobilised protein = 10 RU $R_{max}$). This estimated $R_{max}$ is somewhat approximate and can depend on the amount of active target on the sensor chip (which itself can be estimated by additional SPR experiments); a good rule-of-thumb is that anything within ~2-fold of calculated $R_{max}$ is likely fine.

ligand binding. The SPR experimental setup should always strive to measure a simple 1:1 binding event. For weak interactions, equilibrium or steady state measurements are the preferred option, ideally measured at concentrations ~1/10 $K_D$ to 10× $K_D$, and a plot of response *vs.* concentration should provide a binding curve to allow a 1:1 fit and $K_D$ estimation (Figure 10.5). For slow or tighter interactions, for example as projects progress through Hit-to-Lead, experiments should be designed for kinetic analysis where the rate of association ($k_{on}$) and rate of dissociation ($k_{off}$) can be measured, and $K_D$ calculated ($k_{off}/k_{on}$). The amplitude of the response signal from ligand binding should be proportional to the amount of target protein immobilised on the sensor chip at a ratio of their respective molecular weights. A comparison between the measured $R_{max}$ (maximum binding response at saturation) of several binding compounds, and in particular a positive control, can give an indication of the approximate "real" $R_{max}$ for the setup. A consequence of the proportionality of response to binding and molecular weight allows the determination, or at least a good indication, of the stoichiometry of binding by looking at the response amplitude, for example a response twice as high as expected $R_{max}$ suggests a 2:1 binding interaction.

## 10.2.2 Enzyme Assays

A simple enzyme inhibition reaction scheme is shown in Figure 10.6. Any component of an enzyme reaction can theoretically be assayed as a measure of enzyme activity utilising fluorescent tags, enzyme coupling, antibodies or mass spec technologies described

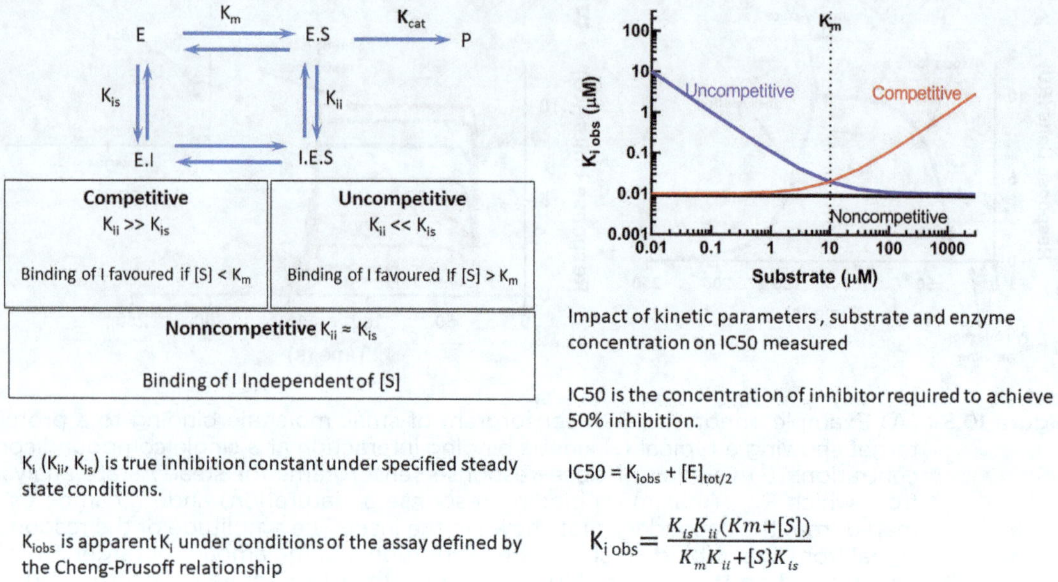


**Figure 10.6** Enzyme mode of inhibition and impact of kinetic parameters on the apparent inhibition observed. A schematic of a classical reversible enzyme inhibition reaction and classification of the different modes of inhibition, where E = Enzyme, I = Inhibitor, S = Substrate, and inhibition constant $K_i$. A theoretical plot is shown to exemplify how the observed $K_i$ changes with respect to substrate concentration, depending on the mode of inhibition for an inhibitor (true $K_i$ = 10 nM). For unbiased screening of all enzyme forms or comparison across multiple targets, selection of $K_m$ conditions in the assay is optimal for selectivity ranking. Here $IC_{50}$ approximates to 1–2 × $K_i$ for all mechanisms of action. This is true until enzyme limiting conditions are met, where $K_i$ for a tight binder is a lot lower than the enzyme concentration used in the assay. These conditions impact a dose-response curve in two ways, the $IC_{50}$ becomes a constant and the Hill slope becomes steeper. The minimum observed $IC_{50}$ is equivalent to half the total active enzyme concentration in the assay and once this is reached the assay can no longer drive SAR decisions.

above. The ability of the enzyme to tolerate fluorescently labelled substrates or the availability of validated affinity reagents to detect products of the reaction will determine the choice of assay. In addition to kinetic factors such as concentration of substrate, protein construct used or sensitivity to product conversion the $IC_{50}$ value can (and does) vary in response to a vast array of parameters. Buffer composition, *e.g.* metal ion, or a change in ionic strength, pH, temperature can affect protein stability and enzyme activity/aggregation. Physical or mechanical variables too can have an impact; for example, automation, mode of serial compound dilution and plate plastics used, resulting in variable reagent concentrations. Finally one must not forget compound-related variables such as compound batch, compound reweighing from the same batch, solubility or free concentration in the assay, which can be reduced by the presence of carrier proteins, *e.g.* serum/BSA due to non-specific binding. As a consequence, each and every one of these variables must be accounted for and/or measured in order to maximise the long-term accuracy of $IC_{50}$ values throughout the lifetime of a project. Most important is the quality of the enzyme used, which must be pure, functional and stable.

The first steps in designing an enzyme assay is to assess the dose dependency and linearity of the enzyme reaction. In general, it is better to measure the accumulation of low levels of product rather than depletion of substrate over time. For some enzymes, product inhibition can be an issue and complete turnover of the substrate cannot be achieved. Ideally, assays should be sensitive enough to detect less than 10% turnover. This is essential for kinetic mode of action studies but is often not the case for high throughput assays using fluorescent tagged substrates, where more than 50% turnover is required to generate a robust signal. Optimisation of all the components of an assay follows to find the best activity for the lowest amount of enzyme. Having established a linear reaction over a fixed time frame, it is important to confirm that the activity measured is dependent on the target enzyme. No enzyme controls will show any background conversion of substrate and can be accounted for easily in appropriate controls in the HTS. The half maximal concentration of substrate, $K_m$, required for maximal activity should be determined and compared to literature values to confirm that they are within the expected range. Ideally this concentration is then used for profiling compounds, such that, independent of mode of inhibition, the $IC_{50}$ measured approximates to $K_i$ (see Figure 10.6). However, the substrate concentration selected may be influenced by the desired mode of inhibition or driven by more pragmatic decisions, such as signal detection and cost. If known inhibitors exist, these should be tested and $IC_{50}$ values and ranking compared. The use of labelled non-specific substrates or detection of common agents such as ATP should be used with caution, as low levels of highly active enzymes can be copurified with your protein of interest. In the absence of known inhibitors, an important control as part of assay development is to check that an enzyme-dead version of your protein is inactive in the assay. Here a single amino-acid modification at the active site of the enzyme is made and expressed and purified in the same way as the wild-type enzyme.

For HTS, stopped reactions are used for ease of automation. Stop reagents are designed to rapidly inactivate the enzyme reaction without effecting the signal generated. Acid to drop the pH or EDTA to chelate essential metal ions are commonly used. Kinetic assays capable of measuring activity under saturating substrate conditions are required to conduct reliable mechanism of inhibition assays. The effects of measured $IC_{50}$ over a range of substrate concentrations ($K_m/10$ to $10K_m$) should be measured, and multivariate non-linear regression used to predict mechanism and determine $K_i$. These are detailed studies, not amenable to high throughput, but can be applied to leads. For larger numbers of compounds to prioritise clusters for progression during lead identification, a simpler profiling study can be performed to measure the ratio of $IC_{50}$ measured at high and low substrate concentrations (ideally, $10K_m$ and $K_m/10$). Based on the Cheng–Prussoff relationship,[35] the $IC_{50}$ for competitive inhibitors targeting the substrate pocket will have a ratio >3, uncompetitive inhibitors which bind only in the presence of substrate will have a ratio <0.3 and non-competitive inhibitors targeting an allosteric pocket will not change, ratio ~1.

Enzyme assays, irrespective of the detection technology used, are prone to non-specific inhibition by pan assay interfering compounds – PAINS[36] in compound collections, particularly aggregators. It is therefore important post-HTS to confirm mode of binding before wasting chemistry effort trying to optimise a non-specific mechanism.

Chemical software tools and identification of steep binding curves provide good flags, but there are a number of assays that can be employed to confirm that compounds have the desired mechanism of action. Technology hitters can be ruled out by confirming activity in an orthogonal assay. This could be an alternative enzyme assay using a different readout or a binding assay. Non-stoichiometric binding can be identified by measuring the ratio of $IC_{50}$ measured at high and low enzyme concentrations; this should equal 1 for stoichiometric binders. Irreversible mechanisms can be identified using a rapid dilution method. Enzyme and compound are pre-incubated and then rapidly diluted 10-fold into the reaction mix and the activity followed. Reversible inhibitors immediately recover activity, tight binders may show a slow recovery, while irreversible binders remain inactive.

There is one important limitation of enzyme assays to be aware of during Hit-to-Lead: enzyme concentration. The relationship between $IC_{50}$ and enzyme concentration is shown in Figure 10.6. As potency increases, the value of $K_{iobs}$ decreases and under tight binding conditions may be significantly less than the total amount of enzyme in the assay. In practise the minimum $IC_{50}$ that can be measured is equal to half the total enzyme concentration used in the assay, so-called enzyme limiting conditions. This is a common problem as more potent compounds are generated, and manifests as increasing Hill slopes indicative of tight binding and measured $IC_{50}$s plateau, hindering SAR decision making. If the assay cannot be reconfigured, then alternative methods such as biophysical or cell-based assays should be employed to drive the SAR.

### 10.2.3 Ion Channel Assays

Ion channels are a drug target class of importance to a range of therapeutic areas, notably within pain, psychiatry and cognitive diseases, and within cardiovascular conditions.[37] It is often desirable to avoid activity against certain ion channels (*e.g.* hERG block, which was linked to QTc syndrome), while being highly desirable to inhibit, potentiate, activate or modulate activity at other, yet closely related, ion channels. Broadly there are two main classes of ion channels – voltage gated, and ligand gated. These are differentiated by their activation mechanism and require different assay approaches. Originally, the main methods for assessing ion channels were either radioligand binding assays and patch clamp electrophysiology. "Manual" patch clamp (MPC) electrophysiology remains a gold standard assay, giving high temporal resolution on channel kinetics, and informs the scientists on a wide range of functional channel properties. It is, however, highly specialised, requires extensive user training and experience, and is labour intensive and low throughput. Although MPC offers deep understanding of channel function, these *operational* factors largely limit utility in iterative compound optimisation and developing SAR. Recent technical advances have greatly improved the throughput of these types of assays and "automated" patch clamp (APC) electrophysiology has enabled the use of this label-free, phenotypic, physiologically predictive assessment, earlier in drug discovery campaigns. Combined, APC and MPC allow study of the biophysical properties and kinetics of an ion channels, *e.g.* current–voltage relationships, active- or passive-channel properties and state dependence. These are pivotal in predicting compound effects in disease-relevant pathophysiology, but are not easily understood using assays relying on a surrogate of channel activity, *e.g.* fluorescence or radioligand binding. Despite the advent of APC, modern medicinal chemistry programmes, and particularly primary HTS, still demand throughputs beyond that achievable with patch clamp. Historically, this led to the emergence of kinetic fluorescence-based methods[37–40] and these remain central to ion channel drug discovery programmes, albeit, typically in a capacity of hit ID and triage prior to APC. For ligand-gated channels, it became relatively straightforward to pre-incubate cells with molecules, add the ligand, then measure changes in intracellular ions ($Ca^{2+}$, or pH changes linked to $Cl^-$) or membrane potential, using kinetic plate readers such as a Fluorometric Imaging Plate Reader FLIPR™. Second-generation voltage dyes have improved fluorescence screening approaches as well as the use of fluorescent indicators tailored to monitor specific ion channel function and ion flux. Examples include fluorescent thallium labels,[41] whereby thallium influx is used to monitor potassium channel function. Interestingly, when biological systems are thoughtfully designed (see GPCR Section 10.2.4), data obtained using thallium flux assays can align well with that of APC/MPC. Sophion, Nanion, Axion, Molecular Devices and others have released increasingly sophisticated APC platforms, each offering subtly different functionality and throughput.[42–44] In addition to optimising activity at the primary therapeutic target, patch clamp and particularly APC, have improved early understanding of off-target ion channel activity that might otherwise lead to poor side effect profiles. This is particularly pertinent to ion channel drug discovery programmes because many cardiac liabilities are imparted by the same, or homologous, ion channels to the primary target. Again, APC has enabled safety assessment assays to be incorporated earlier into medical chemistry initiatives. Moreover, increases in throughput and technical ease have driven down assay costs to a point where external contract screening providers offer standard or bespoke profiling "panels" encompassing targets most likely to cause undesirable side effect(s). Such assays are also employed in drug discovery programmes beyond ion channels.

In addition to technical advances in hardware, much attention has recently been given to design of the biological assay system itself, with the aim of improving pharmacological and physiological predictability. It has become increasingly clear that the 'underpinning' reagent(s), typically cell lines overexpressing the desired target, are highly impactful on alignment of data with that of downstream (more holistic) assays, *e.g.* animal studies. Aside from relatively obvious considerations such as achievable signal : noise, accuracy and precision, it is particularly difficult to "clonally" express ion channels at high levels due to cellular toxicity imparted by the channels themselves. Largely because ion channels control central cellular functions essential for life, *e.g.* homeostasis, resting membrane potential (of excitable cells) and flow into/out of the cell, high or "unbalanced" ion channel expression tends to be toxic. It is therefore imperative to try to obtain expression levels suitable for both screening purposes, yet which also allow cells to grow at a scale and speed suitable to support robust high throughput assays. Moreover, this is further complicated by the fact that ion channels are often made up of multiple protein subunits which naturally reconstitute as active "pore-forming" channels. Achieving appropriate stoichiometry of these subunits, not least considering the above challenges, is highly complex and necessitates testing of potential useful reagents in functional assays. Despite this, many regents have now been developed which recapitulate pharmacologically predictive ion channel function. In a somewhat reciprocating fashion, ion channel reagent development has itself led to innovation in genetic manipulation and expression systems. For example, toxicity can sometimes be avoided by use of transient rather than stable channel expression. Viral gene delivery has also been increasingly used including both BacMam and lentivirus systems, the former being particularly useful in *titrating* a desired expression level.[45] Toxicity can be also avoided, during cell growth phases, by use of inducible expression systems.

### 10.2.4 GPCR Assays

G protein-coupled receptors (GPCRs) are a large superfamily of seven transmembrane domain proteins which sense changes in *concentration* of a myriad of "ligands" outside of cells and transduce this into a variety of intracellular signals. GPCR activators, often in common with ion channels and indeed classified in the same pharmacophoric family, include photons, protons, low $M_w$ compounds, peptides, hormones, proteins and antibodies, as well as ligand-free mechanical activation, *e.g.* pressure and stretch. Stimulation of a GPCR results in conformational changes, which in turn leads to the activation of an associated G protein heterotrimer. The activated G protein modulates intracellular enzymes, which control the production of key intracellular second messengers. These second messengers then act on many downstream targets that regulate gene transcription and a plethora of cell functions. In addition, activated G proteins also recruit other cellular proteins, including β-arrestin, which itself acts as a physiologically relevant signalling molecule, but also drives receptor internalisation, desensitisation and recycling. Both directly, and indirectly *via* second messengers/β-arrestin, GPCR activation reciprocally modulates ion channel and other membrane bound protein functions. In this way, different targets classes integrate to sense, monitor and modulate the cellular milieu.

There are four subclasses of G protein to which different GPCRs may couple; most GPCRs can couple to more than one type although may show a preference. Coupling to the different types of G protein ($G\alpha_s$, $G\alpha_i$, $G\alpha_{q/11}$, $G\alpha_{12/13}$) can lead to multiple, often parallel and interacting, signal pathways being activated,[46] as shown in Figure 10.7. While this can make the biological consequences of GPCR inhibition/activation challenging to predict, it opens up a wide variety of types of assays which screeners can build for this drug target family. Similarly, more recent developments have opened numerous ways in which to monitor β-aArrestin-mediated function, including BRET/FRET and enzyme fragment complementation.

Some assay classes discussed elsewhere, such as AlphaScreen™ (PerkinElmer), and FLIPR™ (Molecular Devices), are suitable for detecting major signalling pathways activated by GPCRs. In the last decade, test systems of this kind have proliferated and include LANCE™ (PerkinElmer), HTRF™ (Cisbio), and both HitHunter™ and PathHunter™ from DiscoverX, which utilise a common detection technology for both second messenger and β-arrestin functions.

For example, GPCRs can couple *via* $G\alpha_{q/11}$ proteins to convert lipid phosphates to inositol trisphosphate (IP3), which releases cytosolic $Ca^{2+}$ from the endoplasmic reticulum. $Ca^{2+}$-sensitive dyes lead to an increasing fluorescence signal, detected by high

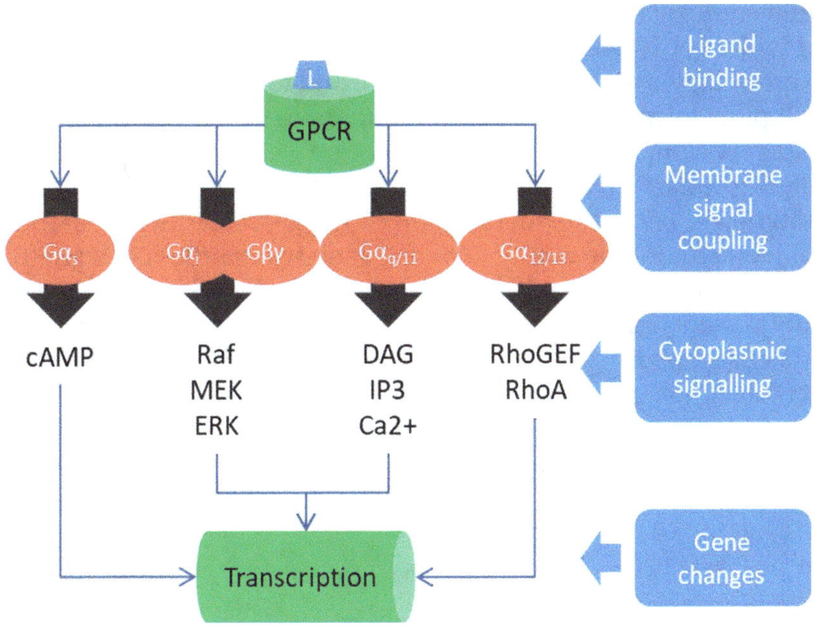


**Figure 10.7** Common points of intervention for GPCR assay design and development. As assays move further from the GPCR itself and into downstream signalling events, so they become more prone to off-target false positives.

throughput kinetic plate readers such as FLIPR.[47] Higher cellular and subcellular resolution may also be obtained, using the wide variety of available high-content readers, albeit typically measuring single cell events rather than a population response. IP3 signalling is relatively transient, so for screeners with a lower budget or a preference for less time-dependent readouts, *e.g.* an accumulation-based endpoint, alternative detection can rely on the breakdown of IP3 back to inositol monophosphate (IP1). Lithium can prevent recycling of IP1, allowing accumulation of IP1 and endpoint detection by immunoassay. One popular kit for IP1 detection is IPOne™ (CisBio), a time-resolved fluorescence-based immunoassay detection kit that involves competition between the cell lysate and labelled IP1 for an anti-IP1 monoclonal antibody.[48] Coupling to $G\alpha_s$ leads to activation of adenylate cyclase, which catalyses conversion of adenosine trisphosphate to the signalling molecule cyclic adenosine monophosphate (cAMP). Conversely, coupling to $G\alpha_i$ proteins leads to inhibition of adenylate cyclase. Both immunoassay detection kits and enzyme complementation assays are commonly used for detection of cAMP levels. Alternatively, multiple G proteins lead to downstream signalling consequences on a widespread protein called ERK. A change in the phosphorylation level of ERK is a relatively generic indicator of GPCR activity that can be measured in various assay kits, from AlphaScreen™ to HTRF and beyond. Based largely on the ease/low cost with which systems such as the FLIPR can be used, as well as the desire to fully utilise expensive hardware, systems have been designed to monitor $G\alpha_s$-and/or $G\alpha_i$-activation using calcium as a readout. Non-native coupling of this type typically employs chimeric or promiscuous G-proteins *e.g.* $G\alpha_{qi5}$ and $G\alpha_{16}$, respectively. In the case of $G\alpha_{qi5}$, the five C-terminal amino acids of $G\alpha_q$ have been replaced with those of $G\alpha_I$, thus, enabling activation of typically $G\alpha_i$-coupled GPCR to signal *via* calcium. Almost regardless of the underlying technology, systems are now reliable and robust enough to support 96-, 384- and 1536-well plate formats, depending on the required (and changeable) throughput of a drug discovery campaign.

For so-called "orphan" GPCRs where the ligand and intracellular coupling mechanisms are unknown, efforts to "deorphanize" these receptors (*i.e.* identify native or synthetic ligands) require the ability to detect activity regardless of signalling pathway. Some assays are now available which do not specifically rely upon the type of G protein or signal transduction pathway activated. For example, Corning's Epic™ platform detects shape changes, or mass redistribution within cells, using resonant waveguide grating (RWG) technology. Changes in cell confluence, adhesion, cytoskeletal rearrangement and activation status in response to addition of a compound are detected in a generic readout. This approach, or conceptually similar impedance-based detection, can be used for screening for ligands of the GPCR, or for detection of modulators or inhibitors.[49]

## 10.2.5 Cell Reporter Gene

Cell reporter genes (CRG) assays measure the production of an intercellular enzyme known as a reporter enzyme. The basic principle of reporter gene assays is outlined in Figure 10.8. Cellular production of the reporter enzyme is coupled to the intracellular activity of a target protein or target cellular pathway. After pathway stimulation, by for example a receptor ligand, the resulting reporter enzyme is quantitated by adding back the components of the reporter enzyme reaction either to whole cells or after a cell lysis step. Positive data from CRG assays will often result in a compound being described as exhibiting "on pathway" activity, *i.e.* capable of blocking or activating the target signalling pathway of interest in a cellular setting. Typical intracellular reporter enzymes used

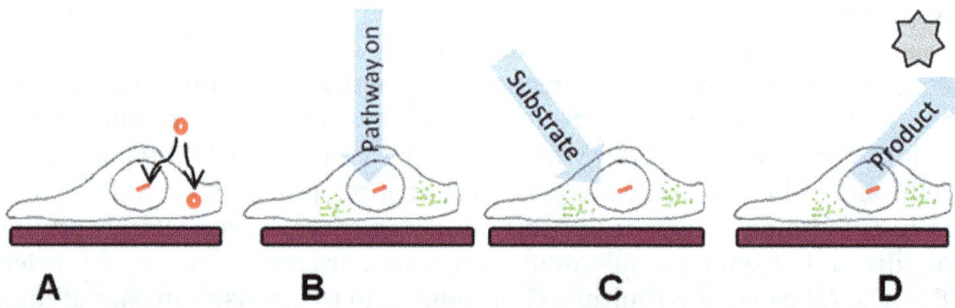


**Figure 10.8** Cell reporter gene assay principle. (A) The gene encoding the reporter enzyme is genetically engineered into the host cell, either as a transient plasmid, or *via* incorporation into the genome. (B) Upon pathway stimulation, reporter enzyme (green dots) is produced, the strength of pathway signal being proportional to the amount of enzyme produced. (C) The enzyme is exposed to a substrate and (D) converts this substrate to a product that can be quantitated by standard technologies (*e.g.* luminescence). Stages (C) and (D) may be performed after a cell lysis step, depending on the type of reporter enzyme produced.

for compound analysis are firefly luciferase, Renilla luciferase and β-galactosidase. The luciferases give rise to luminescence signals, as previously described, whilst β-galactosidase can be used to give an absorbance- or fluorescence-based signal *via* modified substrates.[50] An adaptation of these reporters exploits the ability to express subdomains of luciferase (Nanobit, Promega) or β-galactosidase (HitHunter, DiscoverX) on different proteins within the cell. Active enzyme is reconstituted when the two domains are in close proximity, enzyme fragment complementation, as a result of protein binding. In this way protein complexes or translocation events can be measured in the cell, *e.g.* β-arrestin recruitment to activated receptor.[51,52] Reporter genes can also be secreted into the media, *e.g.* placental alkaline phosphatase (Phospha-Light™), or be fluorescent proteins in their own right such as green fluorescent protein (GFP). The signal from enzyme-based CRG assays is very high compared to the number of molecules produced as the product of the assay is an enzyme, which in turn allows for a degree of signal amplification during the detection reaction. With major suppliers offering ready to use kits and contract services for the creation of bespoke cell reporter assays these assays have become common in discovery cascades. There are two main types of CRG assays: transient transfection, where a plasmid is introduced directly into the cell during the assay process, and stable transfection, where the reporter gene is permanently incorporated into the host genome of a cell. Transient transfection assays may be difficult to make robust as the transfection process is prone to variation, whereas stable transfection assays can be extremely robust and as such can be used for compound profiling and for "target agnostic" or "pathway" HTS.[53] The main drawbacks of CRG assays are the potential for off-target activity of test compounds. Inhibition of any component of the transcriptional or translational complexes in the cell, cell toxicity or inhibition of the reporter enzyme will all give false positives. All of these false positives are easily removed *via* a parallel, non-target-based CRG assay of similar readout and a counterscreen assay of this type is therefore a prerequisite of any CRG cascade assay.

### 10.2.6 Cell Phenotypic Assays

A cellular phenotype is based on an observation of something that a cell does as a whole entity, rather than an estimate of protein or pathway modulation. In these assays we are only concerned with counting whole cell phenomena that are part of or recapitulate the disease state to be targeted. Since 2010, drug discovery has seen a trend towards phenotypic screening for the identification of first-in-class drugs.[54,55] In target-based assay cascades the incorporation of disease-relevant phenotypic assays typically represent the final *in vitro* assay before an animal model of disease is utilised and compounds that show activity are said to have cellular phenotypic efficacy. Phenotypic assays give rise to a measure of cell number, cell morphology, cellular chemistry or cell movement. These generic categories can be further subdivided to more specific phenotypes such as cell cycle status, apoptosis induction, cell differentiation, neurite outgrowth, pseudopodia formation, cell invasion, cell migration, cellular metabolic status *etc.* Each of these subtypes are suitable for more detailed analysis that will also show an associated number, shape chemistry (including biochemistry) or movement phenotype.

### 10.2.6.1 Cell Proliferation, Cell Death

The simplest cell phenotype is a measure of cell number, this can give rise to a measure of direct toxicity, *i.e.* how many of the original cells died? Or cell growth, *i.e.* how many more cells do I have than when I started? Early assays relied on manual microscopy cell counting, *e.g.* by trypan blue exclusion, but these were not amenable to HTS. HTS assays began with assays such as the sulforhodamine blue (SRB) assay which stains an adhered monolayer and uses the amount of adsorbed stain as a measure of biomass (cells) remaining after compound treatment.[56] As these involve a washing step to remove unbound stain, advances were made when specific reagents were developed that reacted with intracellular dehydrogenases to give an absorbance or fluorescence signal (*e.g.* MTT, MTS) allowing for homogenous assays for viability.[57] Assays based on cellular enzyme levels give a good estimate of cell number with adherent or non-adherent cells but suffer from the drawback that dead cells may still release active dehydrogenases into the media and thus give a slightly false reading. The CellTitre-Glo assay (Promega) is similar in that it measures the amount of ATP in each well as a surrogate for cell number *via* the luciferin–luciferase system. This assay is also a homogenous mix and read system, has been reported to accurately measure as few as 100 cells per well and is one of the most accurate and robust high throughput measures of cell number available. Along with simple estimates of cell number, biochemical reagents are now available for cellular assays that can estimate the number of live and dead cells and the induction of specific cellular pathways. Assays are often multiplexed *via* kits, *e.g.* the ApoTox-Glo™ caspase-live-dead from Promega which utilises three different fluorescent substrates to gives a simultaneous measure of all three listed outputs.

The advent of high content plate readers that take images of multiple cells in each well has brought the cell survival assay full circle, automating the staining and counting of cells stained as live or dead. This method can be the most accurate estimate of live cell number, also allowing for cocultures and specific labelling of cell types to be targeted or spared. Another recent innovation in cell growth assays is the ability to measure cells growing in real time. Bright-field imaging systems, such as the IncuCyte can give growth curves over many days. This is particularly useful when looking at compounds which have more subtle growth inhibitory effects or which may have a delay in cell toxicity, dependent upon their mechanism of action. It is worth noting here that in all assays to measure cell number and compound toxicity, the number of cells that one starts with and the duration of incubation can have marked effects on the apparent potency of compounds. Cells in culture will rarely survive happily in microplates for more than 4 or 5 days without showing some signs of nutrient deprivation or edge effects due to evaporation in outer plate wells. As a consequence the number of cells seeded and the duration of incubation should always be tightly controlled. The most sensitive assays for cell survival are clonogenic assays, where cells are treated as individual cell suspensions and plated for colony formation. These slow, long-term assays can often reveal subtle long-term toxicities missed in monolayer experiments, but they are tedious to prepare in a reasonable throughput.

### 10.2.6.2 Cell Movement

Assays for cell movement are exemplified by chemotaxis assays, cell migration assays and cell invasion assays. Cell migration monitors the random movement of cells in 2D and often model wound healing. These assays have been adapted from low throughput experiments to higher throughput modalities with the availability of real-time imaging systems such as the Incucyte mentioned above. Assay formats take the form of Scratch Wound approaches, which removes an area of cells from a confluent monolayer, or technologies such as The Platypus Technologies Oris system, which is designed to leave spaces for migrating cells using a preformed template. Quantitation of these assays ranges from simply measuring the size of area "closed" or the distance migrated, to in-depth analysis of the movement of individual cells.[58] In comparison, chemotaxis assays measure the directed movement of cells in response to a chemical stimulus. These assays use plates containing a membrane of specific pore size, which creates two chambers in the well or, with more advanced systems such as the Bellbrook Iuvo assay plate system, utilises a capillary to allow distance travelled to be measured as well as number of migrating cells. However, there is a large degree of noise associated with these assays due to the essentially random movement of the cells and the overlapping effects of toxicity, cell growth and true (anti-)migratory effects on the measured signal. Whilst experimentally they are becoming easier to run, this inherent variability often leads to issues in gaining robustness for day to day use. Both cell migration and chemotaxis assays can be converted into invasion assays with the incorporation of an extracellular matrix. Although it should be noted that invasion assays present all the issues of migration assays multiplied by the issues of working in and assaying cells in 3D cultures. There are companies that sell kits and specialist plates for invasion assays but even with these, design and robust prosecution of invasion assays on a regular basis is not for the faint-hearted and should be given due time and consideration.

### 10.2.6.3 Complex Cell Models

Co-coculture experiments are a step towards mimicking the interplay between cells seen *in vivo* and which may drive pathology. The effects of one population on another can be visualised using high content screening assays and cellular signalling multiparametric end point assays. The use of primary cells, for example human immune cells isolated from blood and primary embryonic endothelial or epithelial cells have been combined to generate models of vascular, immune, hepatic, cardiac and cancer stromal environments against which lead compounds can be profiled and responses compared to known drugs to predict efficacy or unwanted toxic side effects.[59]

3D assays offer a more physiologically relevant system. They can vary in complexity from spheroids derived from single cell lines to microtissues composed of multiple cell types grown in an extra-cellular matrix to organoids derived from primary tissue or stem cells. The generation of spheroids is easy to automate and combined with a simple end point readout for growth have been widely adopted in the cancer field for profiling inhibitors.[60] Here cells are grown in an anchorage-independent context using the hanging drop or ultra-low attachment plates. As the cells divide, the cells adhere to each other to form spheroids. The less flattened cell architecture, cellular matrix and nutrient gradients which exist across the spheroid structure formed impacts cellular signalling, cellular differentiation, survival and drug responses.

Given the limited availability of patient-derived tissue, human induced pluripotent stem cells (hiPSC) provide an alternative for developing disease-relevant models for profiling lead compounds. hiPSCs can be cultured and therefore are scalable to provide sufficient quantities for screening. Under selective conditions they can be differentiated into specific cell types – hepatic, cardiac, neuronal, immune cells *etc.* and have the ability to self-organise into multicellular organoids. This technology in combination with automated-imaging high content analysis platforms has been adopted for drug toxicity profiling (beyond the scope of this chapter) where it could replace conventional hERG and other cardiac ion channel profiling in time. From a disease biology perspective, aberrant tissue organisation/cell communication is a feature of many disease pathologies, *e.g.* neurodegeneration, fibrosis and cancer, which cannot be captured effectively in 2D assays.

## 10.3 Building the Cascade

Assay development for drug discovery is the process of defining each assay in the cascade and making it fit for purpose. The primary goal is to analyse the reaction at hand and decide upon a format that will detect one of the assay components. Using a mixture of purchased and bespoke reagents, the assays scientist will then attempt to establish an assay signal. Achieving an assay signal is only the first stage of assay development, and much effort is then spent developing the basic assay. When an assay is fully developed and producing robust and useful data it is described as "fit for purpose". One should always start with the end goal in mind and remember that an assay will only be considered developed when it is routinely delivering data to the project team that can be used to make decisions on project progress.

### 10.3.1 Primary Assay

Many target-based discovery projects begin in high throughput screening and whilst assays for HTS must retain a functional link to the cellular process to be targeted, the requirements for these assays are largely dictated by the ability of the assay to withstand the automated HTS process. The HTS assay, or a variant thereof, is typically used for routine potency assessment ($IC_{50}$) as these also require a high throughput and becomes the primary driver of compound structure–activity relationships. By way of example consider a generic protein kinase reaction in a cellular context illustrated in Figure 10.9 alongside the typical kinase assay developed for HTS. Herein is a good example of how HTS arrives at a much simpler assay based on pragmatic considerations, with the assumption that an inhibitor of the phosphorylation of a short substrate peptide by the isolated kinase domain of a protein will also inhibit the full length kinase protein in a cellular context. Whilst this may seem unrealistic, the development of many kinase inhibitors from outputs of HTS prosecuted *via* these assays has to some extent borne out this model of drug discovery.[61]

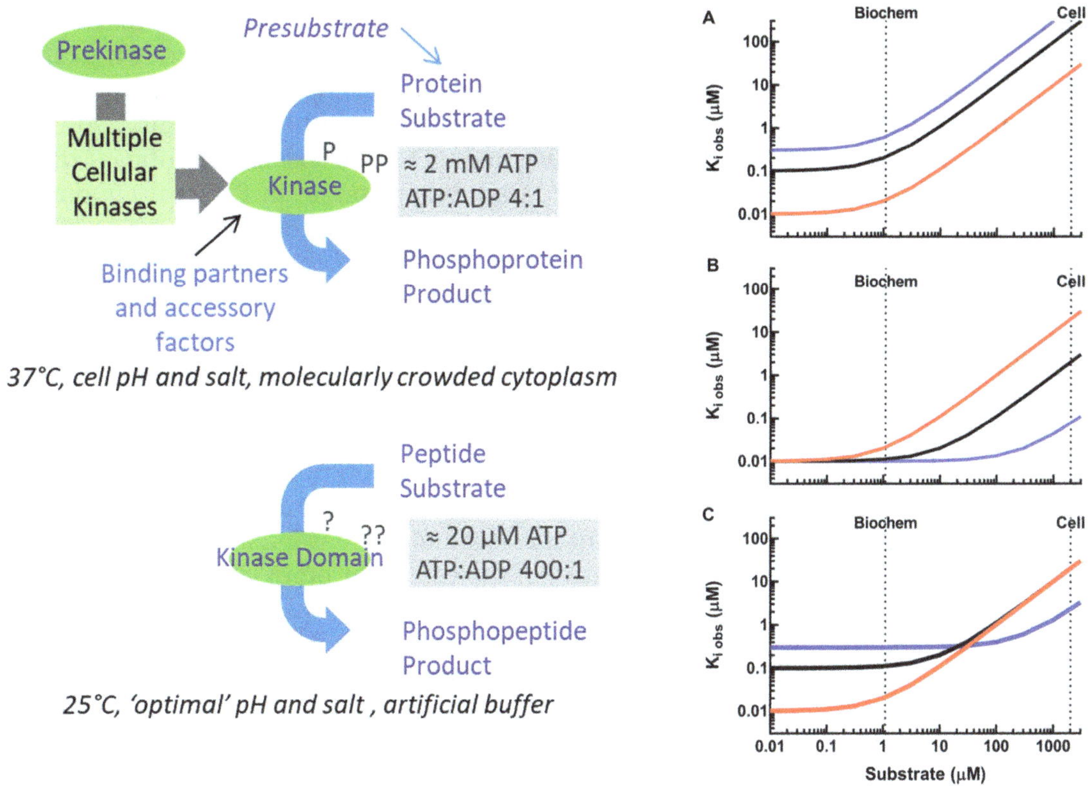


**Figure 10.9** Schematic of cellular and HTS kinase reactions. Whilst both produce a phospho product and ADP, cellular kinases and their substrates are often the products of pre-reactions and take place in a high viscosity cytoplasmic environment surrounded by many other proteins and cofactors. For the purposes of HTS this reaction is often simplified to a single domain of the protein and a peptide from the substrate in buffer conditions optimised for HTS and not for comparison to the cellular environment. Phosphorylation status and absence of binding partners may alter the conformation and affinity for ligands. The theoretical impact on inhibition observed between the two formats is illustrated in the plots A–C. These describe how $K_{\mathrm{iobs}}$ measured for a competitive inhibitor changes with substrate concentration for three related targets: 1 $K_i$ = 10 nM (red), 2 $K_i$ = 100 nM (blue), 3 $K_i$ = 300 nM (black) and how apparent selectivity changes in the three scenarios shown. This is dependent on $K_m$ of the three targets. (A) First scenario, all targets share same affinity for substrate, $K_m$ = 10 µM for all – $IC_{50}$s are shifted in the cell but ranking is conserved across assays. (B) Second scenario, inhibitors are equipotent $K_i$ = 10 nM, $K_m$ differs, target 1 $K_m$ 1 µM, target 2 $K_m$ 10 µM, target 3 $K_m$ 300 µM – apparent cellular selectivity observed. (C) Final scenario to show impact of changes in $K_m$, target 1 $K_m$ 1 µM, target 2 $K_m$ 10 µM, target 3 $K_m$ 300 µM – apparent selectivity reversed across assays.

For established target classes a plethora of validated commercial reagents may exist, and the choice of detection reagents may be selected on the basis of past experience. This has two advantages. First, established automation protocols will already exist, thus shortening the assay development time. Second, compounds interfering with the assay technology used will already be known, which will aid hit selection. For novel targets, reagents will have to be designed from scratch, adding significantly to the assay development time for a project and will carry the added the risk of unknown druggability. This can be mitigated using fragment-based approaches to assess ligandability by probing for pockets prior to any large-scale high-throughput campaigns.[62] Alternatively, target-focussed cell assays can be designed – the options and significant differences between assay formats are illustrated for a kinase target in Figure 10.9, but are equally true for any intracellular target. Simple, two-fluorophore cell imaging assays have proved to be robust for this purpose and often report a relatively high success rate[63] There are pros and cons to both approaches. Biochemical/biophysical assays offer simple systems with which compounds can be profiled against a defined target. To generate a robust assay using recombinantly expressed protein, assay developers often need to make compromises. For example, for ease of expression, a single domain may be used rather than full length protein, cellular binding partners are not present, post translational modification absent or buffer conditions non-physiological. All of these factors could cause changes in the folding or behaviour of the protein and consequently the shape or accessibility of the pocket of interest and there is a risk that the predominant form in the assay is not representative of the cellular protein. Such assays are also prone to aggregators, leading to false positive hits. These issues are alleviated using cell assays targeting the endogenous protein. Careful assay design to include toxicity and unwanted off-target activity can be used to triage hits. Interpretation of structure–activity relationships however, can be more challenging for intracellular targets, as protein binding, cellular penetrance, cellular efflux and potency are all factored into the measured response.

Generation of pharmacologically predictive data is imperative. Although not always the case, development of reagents with high expression, largely driven by the need to continually improve S : N, such as when using increasingly low assay volumes and high well density formats, data tend to become less well aligned with more intact and physiologically relevant readouts. Examples of this include perfectly predictable but gross overestimation of GPCR agonist potencies ($pEC_{50}$) at very high expression level, due to receptor-driven signal amplification. On the face of it this would appear to be problematic but increasingly researchers are able to exploit such phenomenon. For example, during early phase hit ID it is typically desirable to overamplify detection to pick up weak binders. Systems can thus be designed and sensitised, "on a hair trigger", given that researchers appreciate that potencies are likely to drop dramatically later in the screening cascade. Conversely, systems designed to be more physiologically predictive require lower expression. The development and thoughtful use of "controllable" expression systems, *e.g.* BacMam, has afforded researchers the ability to build distinct systems, with different expression levels, tailored specifically, with different goals in mind.[64] Given that detection technologies are nonetheless common, screening cascades can accommodate both hit ID and physiology profiling. Of clear importance is also the modality of the targeted molecule. The above amplification is generally only relevant for agonist and partial agonists, or activators in the case of some ion channels. If a drug discovery programme target is an inhibitor, researchers might be less concerned about expression level and opt for the highest expression available. In this sense reagents need to be specifically tailored to the aim of the assay and are not generally interchangeable, even when the target itself and assay readout are identical. This is never more so than when targeting allosteric modalities for GPCRs, whereby expression levels and system design are even more impactful. Unknowing or thoughtless interchange of "historical" reagents between projects has undoubtedly led to failed or ineffective drug discovery campaigns in the past.

### 10.3.2 Target Engagement

As discussed above, many compromises may have been made to deliver a robust primary assay. It is important to ensure that there is not a disconnect between the biochemical/biophysical or cellular target early in the process. A key reason for this is to ensure that compounds identified from a primary screen are acting in the expected and desired way, rather than interfering with the assay detection process before the investment of extensive time and effort is spent in optimising that compound into a lead series. Biophysical methods such as SPR or MST are useful to establish target binding and ruling out non-stoichiometric binding or undesirable mechanisms of HTS hits. Such methods are not always feasible or can be extremely challenging to develop, depending on the target, and a negative result cannot always be interpreted as evidence of non-binding to the target if assay conditions (buffers, salts or presence of cofactors) are very different between the biochemical and a biophysical assay. Confirmation of binding of a biochemical assay hit in a biophysical assay that is dose-dependent and stoichiometric can give real confidence in being on target and the worth of progressing the hit series.

Cellular target engagement is an important step in the path to translation. On-target activity may be inferred from changes to target-specific substrates/products, pathway or protein stability. Proximal biomarker assays and cellular reporter-based assays can be configured to generate robust cellular assays for endogenously expressed protein with the necessary capacity to support Hit-to Lead campaigns and are widely used for this purpose.

For proximal biomarkers the selectivity of the antibodies used and specificity of the target are crucial. For example, in kinase signalling there are thousands of proteins, including hundreds of kinases and substrates, and consequently there are many thousands of different phosphorylation sites.[65] If the assay format does not have antibody tools that detect only the target of interest, the project team can be readily misled as to the activity of their lead compounds in cells. To deliver a cellular ELISA whose data can be correctly interpreted by the project team therefore requires highly specific assay tools, and well-validated cell assays, to prevent such misinterpretation of profiling data.[66] Most screeners have learnt the painful lesson that not all commercially available antibodies are anything like as target-specific as the vendor claims.[67] Western blots, combined with cell imaging assays, can build confidence that the antibody is binding only (or predominantly) to a protein of the expected molecular weight, located in the expected cellular component. The remaining issue to be addressed is an understanding that the reaction is unique to the target of interest. The use of overexpression systems, which can be turned on or off can control for this.

Ligand binding often leads to changes in protein stability within the cell. Protein abundance can be measured using antibody detection or the target itself may be conjugated to a reporter to monitor expression. Cellular target engagement thermal shift assays in live cells rely solely on ligand-induced thermodynamic stabilisation of proteins, thus eliminating the requirements for protein engineering and is applicable to primary cells, tissues, animal models and patient-derived material.[68] Recombinant cellular assays carry the risk that the protein construct used is not representative of the native protein and could lead to lack of translation when more disease-relevant cells and assays are used later in the cascade. The application of MS detection removes the dependency on antibodies and opens up the possibility to track drug target engagement throughout the discovery process, in principle from primary screening to the treated patient. This information will help to ensure resources are invested on the best candidate compounds in target-based drug discovery programmes.

### 10.3.3 Mode of Action

Demonstration of biochemical, biophysical and cellular potency tracking and expected mode of action are important milestones for the drug discovery project on route to effective translation. It is important here to move away from recombinant overexpression systems and test effects on native targets in a disease-relevant cellular context, ideally using primary cells. Cell lines offer well-characterised systems in which to test compounds, but relevance to disease can be a limitation, given their immortalised phenotype, altered cell cycle and metabolism. Cellular mode-of-action studies encompass a range of cellular assays to relate changes in biomarkers, pathways and phenotype relevant to the disease biology or predictive toxicology to generate data-rich profiles of a few lead compounds.

Structural, binding and mechanistic studies are complementary methods used to understand the mode of binding of hits. Application of some or all the biophysical and mode of inhibition studies described in Section 10.2 will help to understand structure–activity relationships (SAR) and cluster series for progression. For enzymes determining the mode of inhibition – competitive, uncompetitive or non-competitive – provides indirect information on the binding site and the inhibition constant $K_i$ can be determined for definitive ranking of inhibitors with different modes of inhibition. Biophysical methods on the other hand, which can measure binding $K_D$ in the presence or absence of ligand, does not predict effect on activity. $k_{on}/k_{off}$ rates offer insight which may be important for occupancy and duration of action. For a full picture both measurements are required. It cannot be assumed that because an inhibitor is competitive for a ligand binding pocket in a biophysical assay, it is also competitive in the enzyme assay. An example of this is mycophenolic acid which binds at the NAD+ site of IMP dehydrogenase requiring binding of both inositol monophosphate and NAD+ and exhibits uncompetitive inhibition in activity assays.[69] The converse is also true, competitive inhibition does not mean that the substrate pocket is the target. Examples of this include kinase inhibitors which target a selectivity pocket close to the ATP-site, *e.g.* pyrazolourea inhibition of P38α, which has important implications for selectivity and cellular activity.[70]

Divergent mechanisms result from binding to different complexes, pockets or conformation of the target, which will in turn influence cellular potency and subsequent *in vivo* efficacy. The desired mode of inhibition selected should be driven by the known disease biology. When dealing with a novel target, where little is known about the active species or ligand concentrations present in the disease setting, progressing multiple series with different modes of binding will maintain diversity and reduce risk of failure to translate to later phenotypic cellular assays or *in vivo*. This can be exemplified for GPCR targets in CNS disorders where it may be known that the ligand secretion is reduced in the disease setting and an agonist activity is needed to compensate. However, overstimulation of the GPCR may result in undesirable pharmacology. A better mode of action therefore may be an allosteric activator, which can boost the signal from the small amount of ligand present.[71]

As part of lead optimisation, selectivity of your compound *vs.* closely related targets will become an issue. For predicted closely related enzymes sharing the same substrates and with high homology at the active site, it is usual to generate recombinant biochemical assays for each of the targets, most likely using modifications of the existing assay used for the primary target. For established drug targets, *e.g.* kinases, ion channels and GPCRS, panels for selectivity profiling exist commercially and are useful to quantify unpredicted off-target activity. Early assessment of hit series against selectivity panels can help prioritise the best cores as starting points based on relative selectivity. How selective a compound needs to be to have impact in the cell environment will depend on the kinetic parameters and mode of action of your inhibitor. If careful thought is not considered in the assay design, the apparent selectivity at different assay concentrations can be misleading. Figure 10.9 illustrates how the $IC_{50}$ ranking for a competitive inhibitor can theoretically reverse across three targets between biochemical and cell conditions, dependent on $K_m$. An example of apparent selectivity switching at different ATP concentrations has been reported for dual PIM1/PIM2 inhibitors.[72] Figure 10.9 also serves to illustrate the magnitude of drop-off one can expect between biochemical and cell-based assays. Lack of activity in cell-based assays in the early stages of the project before optimisation of potency has taken place may be mechanism related. Unexpected cell potency, on the other hand, may indicate off-target mechanisms at play.

Cellular selectivity can be addressed using thermal proteome profiling (TPP) to detect both direct ligand and pathway interactions in the cell. Proteomic analysis confirms on the one hand expected target engagement and proximal pathway modulation and on the other reveals off-target activities, or unexpected target-driven pathways. These unwanted mechanisms of action can be followed up in conventional biochemical or cell-based assays to optimise compound selectivity. For novel targets, deconvolution of on- and off-target pathway activity can be challenging.

Cells grown as monolayers on tissue-culture plastic in nutrient-rich media may lack the complexity to recapitulate the disease phenotype or sensitivity to detect a particular mode of action. Consider one of the easiest phenotypes to measure – cell number. The "blunt" nature and potential for off-target false positives in a simple direct toxicity measurement based on cell number often means that they are replaced by project-specific surrogates such as measures of cell replication (*e.g.* bromovinyldeoxyuridine (BrdU incorporation) or apoptosis (caspase induction)) with the assumption that this is the desired mode of cell death or arrest and that a positive in a shorter duration, possibly more robust assay will give rise to the desired gross phenotype in a longer term clinical setting. However, grown as mono-layers the cells have a deregulated cell cycle, such that they double in number approximately every 24 hours. This is in contrast to the *in vivo* setting, where typically there are only a few percent of actively dividing cells in the tumour and only a marginal increase in the rate of proliferation relative to healthy tissue. 3D spheroid assays recapitulate the nutrient gradients and hypoxic environment found within tumours and are now used in preference. Ideally, patient-derived cells would be used to faithfully mimic the genetic and epigenetic features of the disease state, however access to these is limited. In the cancer field, an alternative offered by several commercial organisations is to use patient-derived xenograft (PDX) material.[73] Pre-profiling of leads *in vitro* prior to *in vivo* testing in the autologous tumour model offers a higher level of confidence for translation.

Advancements in high content imaging, mass spec and human induced pluripotent stem cell (hIPSC) platforms are enabling the development of more disease-relevant 2D and 3D assays. Mixed cell populations can be distinguished using fluorescent markers of each cell type of interest and all analysis can be related back to only those cells expressing that marker, thereby avoiding interference from other cells within the well, *e.g.* differentiated stem cell subpopulations. Using multiplex antibody detection or high content screening assays it is possible to track, in parallel, the primary target–drug interaction event within cells, *e.g.* autophosphorylation of a kinase, and in the same well, track off-target effects, *e.g.* phosphorylation of substrates mediated by other related kinases, or downstream events within the pathway of interest, *e.g.* cytokine release. This combination of both proof of principle and proof of mechanism in a single experiment can provide evidence that a compound enters the cell and inhibits the target, and that the appropriate downstream consequences are delivered.

## 10.4 The Cascade in Practise

Once assays are in place and are part of the project it is essential to correctly analyse data that they produce and to continually monitor assay robustness. Data analysis is the estimate of a value assignable to a compound activity; this is done objectively *via* statistical analysis and curve fitting. Robustness is estimated from the analysed data *via* a series of quality control measurements designed to constantly monitor the "fit for purpose" nature of the assay. This is therefore an objective collection of statistics followed by a subjective analysis of their importance for data accuracy. Where these two come together is in the interpretation of individual datasets against large collections of assay data collated over the lifetime of a project, robustness indicators will often explain data anomalies and allow useable data from otherwise unusual values.

### 10.4.1 Data Analysis

Most assays will arrive at a number indicating the percentage activity or inhibition of an assay compared to the maximum assay signal, or the concentration of compound at which that assay gives half maximum output. Depending on the assay type and the preferences of discovery teams, there are differences in the way these data are calculated. Common measures of compound effects are summarised in Table 10.3.

**Table 10.3** Common reported parameters.[a]

| Measure | Definition |
|---|---|
| % Of control | The percentage of IR remaining |
| % Inhibition | Percentage of IR that is inhibited |
| % Or fold stimulation | Increase in signal above the positive control as a function of IR |
| $IC_{50}$ | Concentration required to give 50% of the IR |
| $EC_{50}$ | Concentration at which an agonist gives 50% of the maximum possible induced response for that agonist |
| $GI_{50}$ | Concentration at which organisms grow to 50% of the control value |
| $LD_{50}$ | Concentration at which 50% of organisms are dead |
| $K_D$ | Equilibrium dissociation constant at which 50% binding sites are occupied |
| $T_m$ | Mid-point of a melting curve halfway between fully folded and fully unfolded target |

[a]IR = inhibitable response, *i.e.* the difference between the maximum and minimum assay signals.

Because assay data can be presented in various formats, misreading, mislabelling and subsequent misunderstanding of the data is possible unless a standard data format is agreed upon for each assay. Though it seems obvious, if a team is used to seeing percentage inhibition data, when confronted with a table of percentage of control data (*i.e.* 100% inhibition) confusion often ensues. There are also many other measurements that are presented as indicators of compound potency, particularly in GPCR inhibitor discovery[38] and it is worth asking your assay scientist exactly what is being measured and presented.

To generate any of these types of data, the assay must have a series of internal controls and reference compounds that the assay scientist uses to set estimates of full reaction signal and no reaction signal. For maximum accuracy of compound testing, the design of controls and blanks should be such that the positive control (100% signal) recapitulates the activity of the assay in the absence of only the test compound, and the negative control (0% signal) recapitulates a fully compound-inhibited system. Commonly used positive and negative controls are solvent only and commonly used negative controls are reactions lacking enzyme, or reaction with a saturating amount of a known inhibitor. The number of control well replicates is kept high per assay so as to accurately estimate the 100% and 0% values. With accurate estimates of each of these, all of the associated, often high throughput, test compounds can be more robustly analysed for significant effects on the assay. A standard measure of robustness for an assay is the $Z'$ factor[74] (eqn (10.1)):

$$1-\frac{3(\mathrm{STDEV}_{\mathrm{control}})+3(\mathrm{STDEV}_{\mathrm{blank}})}{(\mathrm{VALUE}_{\mathrm{control}}-\mathrm{VALUE}_{\mathrm{blank}})} \tag{10.1}$$

where STDEV = standard deviation of the control or blank and VALUE = the measured mean value of each parameter. The $Z'$ factor takes into account the variation in the controls and blanks and it is set against a basic hypothesis that if you cannot accurately and repeatedly distinguish between control and blank wells, then you cannot designate intermediate test readings as significantly different from either. The $Z'$ factor has added to or supplanted measures such as signal-to-background and signal-to-noise as measures of assay robustness. Indeed, assays with traditionally "poor" signal-to-background values <1.5 are now commonplace for HTS as the very low errors associated with readouts give very robust $Z'$ scores and negate the need for a large signal window. $Z'$ factors of 0.5 or above are typically classed as acceptable but it should be remembered that the $Z'$ factor is a guide and is ultimately used subjectively; assays with $Z'$ scores of 0.4 are commonly passed if inspection of the data suggests that potency estimates are most likely robust. Once an assay $Z'$ is calculated and the assay is declared as having run robustly, then values can be assigned to compounds. Outside of HTS where percentage inhibition is the commonest value calculated, the most common measure reported is compound potency as the $IC_{50}$. Dose–response curves are plotted in a log-linear fashion and the $IC_{50}$ is typically estimated from a fit of the curve to 7–12 datapoints corresponding to different compound concentrations, usually at 3-fold dilutions or thereabouts. The most common equation used to estimate the $IC_{50}$ is the four parameter logistic model, or Hill slope model.[38] This generates an $IC_{50}$ and a fitting error associated with this value (based not on multiple $IC_{50}$ values, but on the variance of individual values from the fitted curve). It also generates a Hill slope; in an ideal system (*i.e.* "ideal" in the sense of the gas equation, a kinetically perfect assay with a perfectly competitive inhibitor) the Hill slope should have a value of 1. However, not all reactions are "ideal" and whilst shallower or steeper Hill slope gradients can be an indicator of inappropriate compound mechanism,[75] this value has an acceptable range of 0.5–2.0. Assay scientists will look at each individual $IC_{50}$ curve and employ standard curve-fitting rules and regulations before passing each curve as adequately fitted. For example, there will be a minimum number of points on the curve that may be designated as outlier errors and ignored, the Hill slope and maximum and minimum values will be investigated and $IC_{50}$ values should not be extrapolated and at least one (preferably more than two) datapoints should lie on either side of the calculated $IC_{50}$ value. It is important to realise that $IC_{50}$ values generated are not absolute measures of how potent a compound is, as previously discussed, they are estimated values highly dependent upon the reaction conditions under which they are gathered. As such, no two $IC_{50}$ experiments will ever give truly identical data and the role of the $IC_{50}$ is to provide a relative ranking of compound potency against other compounds tested in a particular assay.

### 10.4.2 Biophysical Assay Data Analysis

In the majority of biophysical assays, the key parameter to be determined is the equilibrium dissociation constant $K_D$, which measures the affinity of binding of ligand to target. Each biophysical technique has its own parameters and factors to consider in terms of data analysis, but universally positive and negative control data should be used for comparison, dose-dependency should be evaluated and overinterpretation of data avoided. The use of complex fitting models should be avoided unless completely justified and strongly supported by other data.

Specifically for SPR data, as discussed in the previous sections, it can be challenging to spot and deal with all the potential misleading or non-ideal data issues when analysing the data, such as presence of non-specific binding, binding to control surfaces, non 1:1 behaviour, bulk shift (signal jumps due to differences in refractive index of the sample and running buffer), overfitting, stoichiometric discrepancies and mass transport limitations (issues in transfer of analyte from bulk solution to the sensor chip surface under flow).[76] Caution and expert consultation should be taken and, as for all assays, reproducibility is key.

The advances in instrumentation and throughput for several biophysical assay formats means that large amounts of data can be generated readily once assays have been developed. Fragment screens can run to 1000s of compounds against many targets.[62] Processing all the data generated can then become the bottleneck for progression, where to cast an expert eye over every sensorgram curve can take many days or weeks. Fortunately, automated procedures to help with this are being developed by multiple companies, which, combined with further robotic automation and computation, should allow even higher throughput and speed of data generation and analysis in the future.

### 10.4.3 Robustness Analysis and Data Comparison

Potency data are generated on a regular basis and as such generate large datasets that require constant monitoring for drift and error. To ensure a reliable $IC_{50}$ ranking system, standard compounds are included in each assay run and compared with historic data to ensure data robustness with time. The hypothesis here is that if the standard compounds are grossly inaccurate, so are the novel compounds tested in that run. To guard against false alarms, more than one standard compound per plate is advised and both have to shift significantly to warrant wholesale data rejection. Once a batch of assays is passed and a compound has a validated $IC_{50}$, it can be compared to the historic dataset and ranked accordingly. In comparing compound $IC_{50}$ data, it is essential to look at the ratio of $IC_{50}$ values and not the absolute difference.[38] Equations based on the variance of fit error and controls can give degrees of confidence that data are different or similar, but as rule of thumb, with average assay robustness, if two values of $IC_{50}$ are within 3-fold of each other they cannot be definitively classed as different. So a compound with an $IC_{50}$ at 60 nM is not more potent than to one at 100 nM, whereas an $IC_{50}$ of 1 nM is more potent than 6 nM despite only being "5 nM different"; it is in fact six times lower. For an in-depth mathematical analysis of $IC_{50}$ measurement and comparison the *Assay Guidance Manual*[38] is recommended.

### 10.4.4 When Assays Fail

So, this will happen to you: an assay whose data you are depending on for the next round of chemistry decisions, doesn't deliver. Sometimes assays "fall over" for lengthy periods and the assay scientist will have to re-optimise conditions to restore the assay to a robust state. Sometimes, the assay scientist will know why it failed – the robot dropped the plate, their student didn't put the detection reagent into the wells, the cells are infected. Often, though, an immediate answer and resolution is less satisfactory than those examples. Perhaps the assay has reached its limit of sensitivity or poorly correlates with other assays in the cascade and alternative assays need to be deployed to drive SAR. In these cases, time out from the design–make–test cycle may be beneficial for the team, giving the assay scientists time to troubleshoot any assay issues or if the original hypothesis is in question to establish the best assays to drive SAR against the most disease-relevant forms of the target.

As well as tracking compound potency, all assay performance parameters are tracked with time. Analysis of all historical assay data gives an indication of "assay drift" towards a lack of robustness and rather than have whole runs failed on the basis of gross variance of the assay, the assay developers can intercept and fix the assay to ensure continuous performance.

### 10.4.5 The SAR Doesn't Track Across Assays in the Cascade

As a senior project chemist who has read this chapter you should by now expect assays to give somewhat variable data, but there will be times when things start to make less and less sense *vs.* the hypotheses being tested. Forearmed is forewarned in these circumstances. Get to know the inherent variability of each of the assays in the project cascade and keep an eye on the robustness as the project progresses. Simply asking how the assay went each time is a reasonably good way to keep on top of any changes in assay with time. Flagging poorly soluble, potentially reactive or unstable series in advance and presenting the assay history at each project meeting is also good practise. This is by no way a chemistry-only problem, two-way communications are critical, the assay scientist may observe that a compound was yellow/green in solution in the morning and colourless two hours later, leading to swift conclusions on compound stability and deprioritisation. It is also worth noting here that whilst it is rare that an assay goes wrong for a specific compound amongst other compounds, it can happen (misfiring liquid dispensers, empty compound wells, *etc*). Once you have established that there is an issue with data, then retesting is always the first port of call, explain your concerns and ask for retests and see if the data was indeed just a blip.

If every compound in the assay "shifts" in potency then the assay or automation conditions will most likely need to be redeveloped somewhat to bring the numbers back on track, similar to the situation in Section 10.4.4. If an isolated compound or series repeatedly gives no-robust or unexpected data, then it is most likely a compound issue and this can include compound handling as well physical and chemical properties of the compound at hand. Solubility is by far the most common reason that compounds do not give reproducibly accurate data in assays, couple this to a variable assay and the situation can quickly become unreadable. It is therefore also helpful to learn to read and understand $IC_{50}$ data and hill slopes and to look for signs of shift (all data points move) or poor solubility (top concentration data points are poor quality) as you go along.

As projects progress, issues with ranking potent compounds can arise. A tell-tale sign that enzyme-limiting conditions have been reached is the observation of loss of linearity of measured $IC_{50}$ tracking at high potencies, with an asymptote having been reached, common to multiple series, approximately equal to half the active enzyme concentration. In addition, examination of the enzyme activity dose response curves of some compounds at the asymptote may show an increase in Hill slope. For enzyme activity assays, caution should always be exercised when interpreting ranking when the $IC_{50}$s measured are close to the total amount of enzyme added to the reaction. However, note that the actual amount of active enzyme in a prep may not be accurately known. The proportion of active enzyme to total enzyme added may be small, especially true when active complexes are involved.

## 10.5 Hints and Tips

When assay data are robust and reliable, there are few issues surrounding the relationship between the project chemist and the assay scientist, and mutual trust prevails. But there will be times when data are not making sense and at this time it is critical for the project chemist and assay scientist to use their acquired knowledge of each other's roles to help to determine whether a problem exists and, where it does, to assist each other in resolving it such that the project can once again function effectively.

### 10.5.1 Assay Design Fundamental Questions

It seems obvious but at the outset of a project there should be a clear hypothesis that target X is involved in disease Y. Depending on the level of knowledge around a target, the level of confidence in the hypothesis may be high or low. Drug discovery is, after all, not without risk. Taking a top down approach to designing and incorporating appropriate assays into your cascade will improve translatability. However, be prepared for hypotheses to change during the course of a project in the light of new data, and adapt accordingly. Consider the following questions for assay design.

1. What disease? The phenotypic change associated with the disease is the driver for disease-relevant models. Are there patient-derived cells or tissues available for testing compounds or surrogate cell models that can be used?
2. Where in the body? This leads to selection of appropriate cell lines to use for cellular target engagement and mechanistic studies. Ask why are we using an embryonic kidney cell for a neuronal target? Are there environmental conditions to be factored into the assays, *e.g.* nutrient stress, hypoxia, DNA damaging agents.
3. How? The pathways and signalling molecules dysregulated in the disease state define the outputs of cell assays to confirm mechanism of action. Consider the tools available to measure these changes and possibilities for multiplex cellular assays.
4. When to modulate? The desired mode of action needed – allosteric modulator, competitive inhibitor or protein stabiliser? Long- or short-acting? Is the pathway permanently activated or in response to a stimulus?
5. Which target? Identify the driver of a pathway. Construct design and assay conditions should factor in the desired mode of action to favour that the correct form of target is present in the assay. Related targets and assays should be considered for selectivity screening.

### 10.5.2 Assay Troubleshooting

When an assay fails there will follow a period of time whereby the root cause is established and fixed. This may be lengthy because, as discussed in Section 10.4.3, there may be many parameters to re-optimise. Typical troubleshooting ideas that assay scientists go through to fix broken assays will include:

(1) Check whether the SOP (standard operating protocol) for the assay was followed correctly?
(2) Check whether the dispensers and reader were functional and correctly calibrated. Or if they have just been serviced, if the old data were generated on pre-calibrated equipment and data can (rarely) shift slightly after an annual service, or (more commonly) upon using a new piece of hardware for the same task.
(3) What is the recent historical pattern of the assay in terms of signal window and assay robustness. Assay parameters and control compounds should be routinely tracked with each submission so that any loss of performance can be mitigated before the assay reaches 'failure' point, *e.g.* by scheduling a new batch of active protein to be made if activity loss is observed.
(4) How old were the reagents being used? Cell lines, for example, do change behaviour/assay performance after a certain number of passages in culture; also proteins "go off" over time and become no longer useable in a biochemical assay or as detection reagents; check kit reagent shelf life.
(5) Has any component of the assay involved a recent new batch (protein, detection reagent, *etc*). Has this batch been properly demonstrated to perform as well as the previous batch? Failing an easy answer to this and the previous question, it is not uncommon for assay scientists to start afresh with new batches of every reagent. If the assay behaves again, this is quicker than a laborious examination of each component and data can again be generated. In the long term it is good to know which reagent is most likely to be the cause and this can be followed up separately.

### 10.5.3 What Can You Do When Your Data Looks Odd?

If an assay apparently works but the data are confusing, here are some thoughts on good questions to ask and things to think of when data do not match hypotheses.

(1) Did the control compound values match previous values? *Sometimes assays will misbehave for certain compounds or compound series. A major variable here is compound solubility, but it may be that compounds stray into reactive or protein aggregating space. If the assay and standards are accurate but the test compounds are not, look to the sample management and MOA and then to the assay.*
(2) Is the synthesis batch of the test compounds the same as that evaluated in the assay previously? *The commonest reason for changes in potency is batch-to-batch variation or variance due to reweighing from the same batch.*
(3) What is the inherent occasion-to-occasion variability on this assay? *It may be that the differences you see in potency between test occasions for the compounds are within the expectations of a "noisy" assay – and the bioassay scientist should know how variable their assay is.*

(4) How good was the curve fit? *It is possible the raw data is fine, but the $IC_{50}$ value is inaccurate due to a poor curve fit. Hopefully the bioscientist has noticed this, but in a large screening run it may have been missed. For large datasets, it is good practice to flag poor fits in the database to facilitate exclusion from decision making.*
(5) Have enzyme limiting conditions been reached? *During the latter stages of Hit to Lead, despondency within teams can set in as favourable modifications to compounds are combined and predictive gains in potency do not follow. Suspicion of enzyme limiting conditions should be raised if $IC_{50}$ values reported are close to the enzyme concentration used in the assay and there is evidence of increasing Hill slopes. Reconfiguration of the assay will be required to increase the sensitivity to tight binders or use biophysical or cell-based assays for ranking potent compounds.*
(6) Compound activity does not track across assays – is the hypothesis correct? *Theory is by definition malleable, but data are what they are. If you understand what the assay was designed to do and you know that it performed appropriately, then use the data it tells you to change the theory, rather than try to change or repeat the data to fit the theory.*

## Key References

*Assay Guidance Manual*, ed. S. Markossian, A. Grossman and K. Brimacombe, Bethesda (MD): Eli Lilly & Company and the National Center for Advancing Translational Sciences, 2004. Online. http://www.ncbi.nlm.nih.gov/books/NBK53196/ This assay guidance manual is a web-based resource that is produced by Eli Lilly and is a comprehensive overview of assay development and data analysis. It is a more detailed one stop shop for further information on all of the areas covered in this chapter. We would particularly recommend Chapter 13: "Basics of Enzymatic Assays for HTS".
J. H. Zhang, T. D. Chung and K. R. Oldenburg, *J. Biomol. Screening*, 1999, **4**, 67. The original paper to describe the *Z*-factor, essential reading to understand what assay scientists mean when they talk about assay robustness and how they measure it.
R. Zhang and X. Xie, *Acta Pharmacol. Sin.*, 2012, **33**, 372. An excellent overview on the workings of and assays available for GPCRs, a major class of cell surface proteins recognised as one of the most successful therapeutic targets for a broad spectrum of diseases.

J. P. Renaud, C. W. Chung, U. H. Danielson, U. Hennig, R. E. Hubbard and H. Nar, *Nat. Rev. Drug Discovery*, 2016, **15**, 679–698. The array of biophysical techniques available continues to expand, for a recent review covering the vast majority and their application the article 'Biophysics in drug discovery: impact, challenges and opportunities' is an excellent reference.

## References


1. C. MacKintosh, in *Protein Phosphorylation: A Practical Approach*, ed. D. G. Hardie, IRL Press, New York, 1993, p. 221.
2. L. Rowe, E. Dikici and S. Daunert, *Anal. Chem.*, 2009, **81**, 8662.

3. D. S. Auld, N. T. Southall, A. Jadhav, R. L. Johnson, D. J. Diller, A. Simeonov, A. Austin and J. M. Inglese, *J. Med. Chem.*, 2008, **51**, 2372.
4. R. M. Eglen, T. Reisine, P. Roby, N. Rouleau, C. Illy, R. Bosse and M. Bielefeld, *Curr. Chem. Genomics*, 2008, **1**, 2.
5. M. A. Sills, D. Weiss, Q. Pham, R. Schweitzer, X. Wu and J. J. Wu, *J. Biomol. Screening*, 2002, **7**, 191.
6. R. M. Lequin, *Clin. Chem.*, 2005, **51**, 2415.
7. M. A. Macmillan, J. P. Orme and K. Roberts, *J. Biomol. Screening*, 2011, **16**, 967.
8. G. R. Richards, J. E. Kerby, G. K. Y. Chan and P. B. Simpson, *Methods Mol. Biol.*, 2006, **356**, 109.
9. A. Günther, M. Becker, J. Göpfert, T. Joos and N. Schneiderhan-Marra, *Front. Immunol.*, 2020, **11**, 572634.
10. M. S. Lee, *LC/MS Applications in Drug Development*, Wiley, New York, 2002.
11. E. F. Langsdorf, A. Malikzay, W. A. Lamarr, D. Daubaras, C. Kravec, R. Zhang, R. Hart, F. Monsma, T. Black, C. C. Ozbal, L. Miesel and C. A. Lunn, *J. Biomol. Screening*, 2010, **15**, 52.
12. X. Wu, J. Wang, L. Tan, J. Bui, E. Gjerstad, K. McMillan and W. Zhang, *J. Biomol. Screening*, 2012, **17**, 761.
13. I. Sinclair, G. Davies and H. Semple, *Expert Opin. Drug Discovery*, 2019, **14**, 609.
14. T. Motoyaji, *Chem. Pharm. Bull.*, 2020, **68**, 191.
15. H. Franken, T. Mathieson, D. Childs, G. M. A. Sweetman, T. Werner, I. Tögel, C. Doce, S. Gade, M. Bantscheff, G. Drewes, F. B. Reinhard, W. Huber and M. Savitski, *Nat. Protoc.*, 2015, **10**, 1567.
16. G. J. Patti, O. Yanes and G. Siuzdak, *Nat. Rev. Mol. Biol.*, 2012, **13**, 263.
17. R. E. Heap, A. G. Hope, L.-A. Pearson, K. M. S. E. Reyskens, S. P. McElroy, C. J. Hastie, D. W. Porter, J. S. C. Arthur, D. W. Gray and M. Trost, *SLAS Discovery*, 2017, **22**, 1193.
18. B. Kim, R. Araujo, M. Howard, R. Magni, L. A. Liotta and A. Luchini, *Expert Rev. Proteomics*, 2018, **15**, 353.
19. O. Karlsson and T. Hanreider, *Arch. Toxicol.*, 2017, **91**, 2283.
20. T. A. Morton and D. G. Myszka, *Methods Enzymol.*, 1998, **295**, 268.
21. A. M. Giannetti, *Methods Enzymol.*, 2011, **493**, 169.
22. M. Jerabek-Willemsen, C. J. Wienken, D. Braun, P. Baaske and S. Duhr, *Assay Drug Dev. Technol.*, 2011, **9**, 342.
23. R. Jafari, H. Almqvist, H. Axelsson, M. Ignatushchenko, T. Lundback, P. Nordlund and D. M. Molina, *Nat. Protoc.*, 2014, **9**, 2100.
24. D. M. Molina, R. Jafari, M. Ignatushchenko, T. Seki, E. A. Larsson, C. Dan, L. Sreekumar, Y. Cao and P. Nordlund, *Science*, 2013, **341**, 84.
25. T. Friman, *Bioorg. Med. Chem.*, 2020, **28**, 115174.
26. G. R. Richards, J. E. Kerby, G. K. Y. Chan and P. B. Simpson, *Methods Mol. Biol.*, 2006, **356**, 109.
27. J. Comley, *Drug Discovery World*, 2015, **17**, 25.
28. T. H. Booij, L. S. Price and E. H. J. Danen, *SLAS Discovery*, 2018, **24**, 615.
29. M. A. Bray, *Nat. Protoc.*, 2016, **9**, 1757.
30. C. Scheeder, F. Herigwer and M. Bouros, *Curr. Opin. Syst. Biol.*, 2018, **10**, 43–52.
31. J. C. Caicedo, S. Singh and A. E. Carpenter, *Curr. Opin. Biotechnol.*, 2016, **39**, 134.
32. J. P. Renaud, C. W. Chung, U. H. Danielson, U. Hennig, R. E. Hubbard and H. Nar, *Nat. Rev. Drug Discovery*, 2016, **15**, 679.
33. M. Fairhead and M. Howarth, *Methods Mol. Biol.*, 2015, **1266**, 171.
34. F. Khan, M. He and M. J. Taussi, *Anal. Chem.*, 2006, **78**, 3072.
35. Y.-C. Cheng and W. H. Prusoff, *Biochem. Pharmacol.*, 1973, **222**, 3099.
36. J. Baell and M. A. Walters, *Nature*, 2014, **513**, 481.
37. G. J. Kaczorowski, O. B. McManus, B. T. Priest and M. L. Garcia, *J. Gen. Physiol.*, 2008, **131**, 399.
38. *Assay Guidance Manual*, ed. S. Markossian, A. Grossman and K. Brimacombe, Bethesda (MD): Eli Lilly & Company and the National Center for Advancing Translational Sciences, 2004.
39. A. J. Smith and P. B. Simpson, *Anal. Bioanal. Chem.*, 2003, **377**, 843.
40. J. E. González and M. P. Maher, *Recept. Channels*, 2002, **24**(8), 283.
41. C. D. Weaver, D. Harden, S. I. Dworetsky, B. Robertson and R. J. Knox, *J. Biomol. Screening*, 2004, **8**, 671.
42. S. Friis, M. H. Holmqvist, L. D. Løjkner, M. K. Jensen and M. Sunesen, *Biophys. J.*, 2011, **100**, 270.
43. M. H. Bridgland-Taylor, A. C. Hargreaves, A. Easter, A. Orme, D. C. Henthorn, M. Ding, A. M. David, B. G. Small, C. G. Heapy, N. Abi-Gerges, F. Persson, I. Jacobson, M. Sullivan, N. Albertson, T. G. Hammond, E. Sullivan, J. P. Valentin and C. E. Pollard, *J. Pharmacol. Toxicol. Methods*, 2006, **54**, 189.
44. C. Farre, A. Haythornthwaite, C. Haarmann, S. Stoelzle, M. Kreir, M. George, A. Brüggemann and N. Fertig, *Comb. Chem. High Throughput Screening*, 2009, **12**, 24.
45. D. McCoull, E. Ococks, J. M. Large, D. C. Tickle, A. Mathie, J. Jerman and P. D. Wright, *SLAS Discovery*, 2021, **26**, 428.
46. R. Zhang and X. Xie, *Acta Pharmacol. Sin.*, 2012, **33**, 372.

47. P. B. Simpson, A. Woollacott, R. Hill and G. Seabrook, *Eur. J. Pharmacol.*, 2000, **392**, 1.
48. E. Trinquet, M. Fink, H. Bazin, F. Grillet, F. Maurin, E. Bourrier, H. Ansanay, C. Leroy, A. Michau, T. Durroux, D. Maurel, F. Malhaire, C. Goudet, J. P. Pin, M. Navale, O. Hernoute, F. Chrétiene, Y. Chapleure and G. Mathis, *Anal. Biochem.*, 2006, **358**, 126.
49. K. Dodgson, L. Gedge, D. C. Murray and M. J. Coldwell, *Recept. Signal Transduction*, 2009, **29**, 163.
50. K. R. Gee, W. C. Sun, M. K. Bhalgat, R. H. Upson, D. H. Klaubert, K. A. Latham and R. P. Haugland, *Anal. Biochem.*, 1999, **273**, 41.
51. Y.-X. Yan, D. M. Boldt-Houle, B. P. Tillotson, M. A. Gee, B. J. D'Eon, X.-J. Chang, C. E. M. Oleson and M. A. Palmer, *J. Biomol. Screening*, 2002, **7**, 451.
52. A. S. Dixon, M. K. Schwinn, M. P. Hall, K. Zimmerman, P. Otto, T. H. Lubben, B. L. Butler, B. F. Binkowski, T. Machleidt, T. A. Kirkland, M. G. Wood, C. T. Eggers, L. P. Encell and K. V. Wood, *ACS Chem. Biol.*, 2016, **11**, 400.
53. E. Siebring-van Olst, C. Vermeulen, R. X. de Menezes, M. Howell, E. F. Smit and V. W. van Beusechem, *J. Biomol. Screening*, 2013, **18**, 453.
54. P. Morgan, D. G. Brown, S. Lennard, M. J. Anderton, J. C. Barrett, U. Eriksson, M. Fidock, B. Hamrén, A. Johnson, R. E. March, J. Matcham, J. Metteral, D. J. Nicholls, S. Rees, M. A. Snowden and M. N. Pangalos, *Nat. Rev. Drug Discovery*, 2018, **17**, 167.
55. D. Haasen, U. Schopfer, C. Antczak, C. Guy, F. Fuchs and P. Selzer, *Assay Drug Dev. Technol.*, 2017, **15**, 239.
56. E. Vega-Avila and M. K. Pugsley, *Proc. West. Pharmacol. Soc.*, 2011, **54**, 10.
57. M. V. Berridge, P. M. Herst and A. S. Tan, *Biotechnol. Annu. Rev.*, 2005, **11**, 127.
58. J. Huth, M. Buchholz, J. M Kraus, M. Schmucker, G. von Wichert, D. Krndija, T. Seufferlein, T. M. Gress and H. A. Kestler, *BMC Cell Biol.*, 2010, **11**, 24.
59. E. L. Berg, *Drug Discovery Today: Technol.*, 2017, **23**, 53.
60. R. E. Eglen and T. Reisine, *SLAS Technol.*, 2019, **24**, 18.
61. H. Ma, S. Deacon and K. Horiuch, *Expert Opin. Drug Discovery*, 2008, **3**, 607.
62. P. Canning, K. Birchall, C. A. Kettleborough, A. M. Merritt and P. J. Coombs, *Drug Discovery Today*, 2020, **25**, 2030.
63. P. Alcock, C. Bath, C. Blackett and P. B. Simpson, *Eur. Pharm. Rev.*, 2010, **15**, 13.
64. E. A. Davenport, P. Nuthulaganti and R. S. Ames, Methods in Molecular Biology (Methods and Protocols), in *G Protein-Coupled Receptors in Drug Discovery*, ed. W. Leifert, Humana Press, Totowa, NJ, 2009, vol. 552, doi:10.1007/978-1-60327-317-6_14.
65. S. Pearlman, Z. Serber and J. Ferrell, *Cell*, 2011, **117**, 934.
66. G. Høyer-Hansen, M. Hamers, A. N. Pedersen, H. J. Nielsen, N. Brünner, K. Danø and R. W. Stephens, *J. Immunol. Methods*, 2001, **235**, 91.
67. J. Benicky, R. Hafko, E. Sanchez-Lemus, G. Aguilera and J. M. Saavedra, *Cell. Mol. Neurobiol.*, 2012, **32**, 1353.
68. D. Martinez Molina, R. Jafari, M. Ignatushchenko, T. Seki, E. A. Larsson, C. Dan, L. Sreekumar, Y. Cao and P. Norlund, *Science*, 2013, **341**, 84.
69. T. J. Franklin, W. P. Morris, V. N. Jacobs, E. J. Culbert, C. A. Heys, W. H. Ward, P. N. Cook, F. Jung and P. Pié, *Biochem. Pharmacol.*, 1999, **58**, 867.
70. J. E. Sullivan, G. A. Holdgate, D. Campbell, D. Timms, S. Gerhardt, J. Breed, A. L. Breeze, A. Bermingham, R. A. Pauptit, R. A. Norman, K. J. Embrey, J. Read, W. S. VanScyoc and W. H. Ward, *Biochemistry*, 2005, **44**, 16475.
71. D. J. Foster and P. J. Conn, *Neuron*, 2017, **94**, 431.
72. K. Quian, L. Wang, C. L. Cywin, B. T. Farmer 2nd, E. Hickey, C. Homon, S. Jakes, M. A. Kashem, G. L. Lee, S. Leonard, J. Li, R. Magboo, W. Mao, E. Pack, C. Peng, A. Prokopowicz 3rd, M. Welzel, J. Wolak and T. Morwick, *J. Med. Chem.*, 2009, **52**, 1814.
73. M. Hidalgo, F. Amant, A. V. Biankin, E. Budinská, A. T. Byme, C. Caldas, R. B. Clarke, S. de Jong, J. Jonkers, G. M. Maelandsmo, S. Roman-Roman, J. Seoane, L. Trusolino and A. Villanueva, *Cancer Discovery*, 2014, **4**, 998.
74. J. H. Zhang, T. D. Chung and K. R. Oldenburg, *J. Biomol. Screening*, 1999, **4**, 67.
75. B. K. Shoichet, *J. Med. Chem.*, 2006, **49**, 7274.
76. L. Rich and D. G. Myszka, *J. Mol. Recognit.*, 2010, **23**, 389.

# 11 *In Vitro* Biology: Measuring Pharmacological Activity that Will Translate to Clinical Efficacy

Iain G. Dougall[a], Rachel L. Grimley[b] and Per Erik Strömstedt[c]

[a]IGD Consultancy Ltd, UK; [b]Cancer Research, UK; [c]AstraZeneca, Gothenburg, Sweden
*E-mail: igdconsultancy@btinternet.com, Rachel.Grimley@cancer.org.uk, Per-Erik.Stromstedt@astrazeneca.com

## 11.1 Introduction: Importance of Detailed Mechanistic Understanding

Target identification and validation methods have evolved rapidly over the past decade, affording drug-hunters the ability to focus on previously untouched targets. We are now in an era where technology such as genomics, transcriptomics, metabolomics, proteomics and gene-editing methods such as CRISPR, have revolutionised our ability to identify targets linked to specific diseases more comprehensively, and to undertake rapid genetic validation of their function.[1] Increasingly, more novel (less well-precedented) targets are being identified, some of which are poorly characterised at the molecular level in terms of their mechanism: indeed, a higher proportion of targets of "unknown" function are being implicated in disease through genetic association.[2] Classical mechanistic studies on enzyme and receptor targets are now returning to the forefront of drug discovery efforts, with the ambition of using more physiologically relevant, *in vitro* pharmacology and mechanistic enzymology studies during the lead identification and optimization phases to understand as fully as possible the target, and consequences of drug intervention. There is increased appreciation that classical enzymology and pharmacology is essential to the creation of relevant hit-identification campaigns and downstream project assay cascades.[3,4] Importantly, the latter also need to be capable of characterising inhibitors more fully

The Handbook of Medicinal Chemistry: Principles and Practice, 2nd Edition
Edited by Simon E. Ward and Andrew M. Davis

Published by the Royal Society of Chemistry, www.rsc.org

than solely by traditional $IC_{50}$ values. While useful for cross-comparing the effects of small molecule/other modulation within a standard set of assay conditions (such as time, substrate concentration), the information characteristic of $IC_{50}$ values cannot indicate a change in inhibitory mechanism (for example, a shift from uncompetitive to mixed-type inhibition) in a series of lead compounds. Such understanding is critical to drive SAR and enable more accurate dose predictions, both for *in vivo* efficacy and toxicity studies, and also for translation through to the patient. Furthermore, $IC_{50}$ values on their own are poorly correlative with the potential drugs' pharmacodynamic action, as they give no insight into the *time-dependency* of target modulation, such as potential slow onset of inhibition, and no quantitation of the period of time the compound "resides" on its target and hence can effect the activity (residence time).[5]

Detailed mechanism of action (MoA) studies are critical to understanding the interaction of a compound with its target, and defining how natural ligands at physiological concentrations (*i.e.*, in the disease-relevant cellular context) will modulate this activity. In order to enable the selection and optimisation of those series most likely to translate into efficacious drugs, hit compounds should be characterised in terms of potency, selectivity *vs.* homologous targets and mode of inhibition or activation, as well as the standard early safety profiling and physico-chemical assessment.[4] As "best-practice", a fully comprehensive data package should be provided for all Lead and Candidate molecules: this should incorporate characterisation of the target–ligand interactions from the molecular to the cellular level, using increasingly complex and disease relevant assays (from "reductionist" isolated enzyme or receptor assays through to human tissues). Such packages should also incorporate structural biology insights, knowledge of metabolic pathways, and more comprehensive systems pharmacology knowledge. Together, these facilitate the progressive journey of lead compounds through to clinical candidates with defined mechanism of action, cellular efficacy and the appropriate safety and pharmacokinetic properties. Such best-practice also enables the identification and prioritisation of a range of diverse mechanisms (not just diverse chemotypes), and hence a number of truly differentiated options to achieve the desired biological effect *in vivo*. Having such alternatives can be the key factor to achieving the final combination of a safe, well-tolerated, efficacious drug, that can be dosed to the minimum level and period of time possible.

## 11.2 A Desire to Work With More Physiologically Relevant Systems

Classical drug discovery campaigns generally include a combination of biochemical, biophysical, and cell biology assays and methodologies to identify and characterise modulators of key targets and pathways of interest. Of course, translation through to the clinical disease setting is of paramount importance, and so several key points need to be considered when characterising the *in vitro* biological effects of drug–target interactions.

### 11.2.1 Target Integrity

In order to enable the design and employment of more physiologically relevant assays, a comprehensive understanding of the molecular environment of the target of interest is crucial. This is particularly pertinent when targeting less well-characterised proteins. Recent years have seen the pharmaceutical industry move away from the use of isolated, usually recombinant domains, and model or generic substrates, re-focussing on systems more likely to be of higher relevance and "translatability". These systems include assays employing full-length proteins, complex partners and native substrates/ligands.[4] It is important to remember that in the highly complex physiological environment, full-length, multidomain targets comprise multiple functional domains; for example, catalytic domains are frequently regulated by non-catalytic domains in a manner which controls activity, and often, substrate (or ligand) specificity. This is of particular note in the epigenetic modulator target space. Moreover, post-translational modification status, activation state and artificial modifications, such as affinity tags, can all affect the kinetic integrity of the target of interest. Therefore a thorough understanding of the relevant form(s) of the target is crucial.[6]

The Akt Ser/Thr protein kinases (protein kinase B; Akts 1–3) provide a salutary tale to remind us about careful decision-making during early drug discovery. Recombinant expression of the kinase domain of the Akt kinases could be considered to shorten timelines, as well as being more amenable to structural characterization, in a world where there is an ever-pressing need to move drugs through to patients as rapidly as possible. However, profiling the native, full-length protein, as opposed to a recombinant fragment encompassing only the catalytic domain of this membrane-associated protein kinase, enabled the identification of the novel allosteric site on the amino-terminal pleckstrin-homology domain that ultimately provided an exploitable site for inhibitor discovery by Merck, amongst others.[7,8] Merck identified two Akt inhibitors from a HTS campaign that exhibited isoenzyme specificity. The first (Akt-I-1) inhibits only Akt1 ($IC_{50}$ 4.6 μM), while the second (Akt-I-1,2) inhibits both Akt1 ($IC_{50}$ 2.7 μM) and Akt2 ($IC_{50}$ 21 μM). Neither compound inhibits Akt3 nor mutants lacking the pleckstrin homology domain at concentrations up to 250 μM. These compounds are reversible, cell-active inhibitors, and show mixed inhibition with respect to ATP. In addition to inhibiting kinase activity of individual Akt isoforms, the phosphorylation and concomitant activation of the corresponding Akt isoforms by PDK1 (phosphoinositide-dependent kinase 1) is also blocked by these inhibitors. A model supports these inhibitors binding to a site formed only in the presence of the pleckstrin homology domain, where inhibitor-binding is postulated to promote the formation of an inactive conformation.

Another high impact example is where the addition of a 19 amino-acid juxta membrane domain to the catalytic domain of Vascular Endothelial Growth Factor Receptor (VEGFR) increases the affinity of a small molecule inhibitor by approximately 40-fold from 1100 pM to 28 pM;[9] again an important reminder of the need for detailed understanding of the target, and ensuring that any "reductionist" systems used are still able to provide translation through to more disease-relevant systems.

### 11.2.2 Complex Binding Partners and Cofactors

Complex binding partners can also exert significant influence on the catalytic activity of the associated protein, and, as a consequence, affect inhibitor binding. A classic example is the cyclin partners of the CDK enzymes, where activation of the cyclin-dependent kinases involves a two-step process comprising cyclin binding followed by phosphorylation at a conserved threonine residue within the kinase activation loop.[10] Knowledge of such events enables the potential to modulate different forms of the target. For example, Targeting Protein for XLPA2 (TPX2) is a physiological binding partner that positively regulates Aurora A kinase. TPX2 has no effect *per se* on the enzyme turnover or reaction mechanism; however, it does affect the binding affinity of Aurora A kinase's substrates; moreover, the binding of TPX2 also affects the SAR of inhibitors binding to a hydrophobic pocket adjacent to the ATP binding site.[11]

There are also numerous similar examples for receptors, *e.g.* G-protein coupled receptors (GPCRs)[12] and nuclear hormone receptors (NHRs).[13]

Profiling in the presence of the native binding partner (at appropriate levels and stoichiometry to assure complex formation) can clearly enhance the probability of identifying molecules more likely to translate through into the native cellular environment. This is particularly important where several complex partners affect the overall competence of the target. The protein methyltransferase EZH2 is a well-known example where the enzyme is only fully catalytically competent to methylate histone H3 lysine 27 in the presence of its associated partners comprising its full pentameric PRC2 complex.[14] Historical drug discovery initiatives for this target which utilised "simple" screening cascades (*e.g.* isolated EZH2 and a histone peptide substrate) failed to yield suitable equity.

Clearly, an understanding of the physiologically relevant protein complex, and its native substrate and cofactors/coregulators is key to ensuring that the correct form of the target is represented in the assay biology system of choice. Importantly, there may be specific complexes associated with healthy- and disease-relevant states of the target, knowledge of which might help to drive selectivity; as part of the early target characterisation, immuno-precipitation from disease-relevant cells coupled with mass-spectrometry analysis can help to identify complex partners and their associated stoichiometry.[15]

### 11.2.3 Binding Interactions and Catalytic Mechanisms

Binding interactions between macromolecular substrates and enzymes can occur at sites distal to the active site, and indeed can contribute to the overall binding energy for the formation of the initial enzyme–substrate encounter complex. Therefore the identity of enzyme substrates is also another important consideration, particularly if specific conformational changes accompany the binding of the native substrate.[16] Substitution of the native substrate with a shorter peptide, for example in the case of a protease or kinase, could affect both the enzyme's kinetic mechanism, and also the ability to identify inhibitors which might prevent formation of the ES complex by binding to distal sites. For example, specific inhibitor pockets are revealed upon $tRNA^{Gln}$ binding in some bacterial Glu-amidotransferases.[17] The enzyme 3-Phosphoinositide-dependent Protein Kinase 1 (PDK1) is a classic example where the catalytic mechanism, and hence the potential for identifying differentiated drug molecules, is influenced by the choice of substrate. Phosphorylation of the endogenous substrate S6K1 protein kinase, occurs through a steady-state ordered mechanism where binding of S6K1 precludes association of MgATP.[18] However, phosphorylation of an extended peptide substrate containing a single distal recognition element proceeds through a rapid equilibrium random mechanism.[19] In an even more compelling example, differential substrate selectivity in the cellular context for MAPKp38α (ATF2 *versus* MK2a) is able to define the particular pathways perturbed by small molecules. This offers the opportunity for careful control of drugs targeting those specific, disease-relevant p38α catalytic events and, potentially, fewer unwanted side-effects.[20,21]

In the diverse and important field of epigenetics, the importance of using native nucleosome substrates in preference to short, histone N-terminal tail peptides as surrogates, has been increasingly recognised in order to identify small molecule inhibitors that translate through to the cellular context and target the desired activity of the enzyme. For the histone methyltransferase NSD2, the choice of a nucleosome substrate *versus* a histone octamer substrate in the presence of short ss- or ds-DNA directs the specificity of lysine methylation.[22,23] Histone acetyl transferases are but one of numerous examples in which the kinetic mechanism, and small molecule affinity is directly influenced by the choice of substrate.[24]

Since many enzymes can catalyse low-level activity with suboptimal substrates, it is of critical importance that the physiological relevance of any catalytic activity is ascertained to be a true reflection of the endogenous activity.[25] It is especially important to convert assay signal (such as fluorescence units per second) into the amount of product formed over the specified period of time; by doing so, it is possible to quantify this activity and relate back to the core kinetic properties of the enzyme to ensure that any "assay window" or signal is relevant. Furthermore, it may not always be feasible to perform high throughput hit-finding campaigns with full-length protein and native substrates, due to parameters such as challenge in protein reagent scale-up, or cost. It is therefore crucial to understand the level of compromise introduced by the use of simpler systems by careful characterisation and comparison with the more native system, and to define a compelling strategy to relate any activities back to the cellular context, particularly in the lead optimisation stage.

## 11.3 Pharmacological Profiling

A thorough knowledge of the target's molecular environment in the disease-relevant setting enables the informed targeting of specific mechanisms of interest. For example, it can be of benefit to identify inhibitors that are not competitive with the native substrate where the cellular concentration of the latter is high, and hence minimise the amount of dose that needs to be applied. Kinase drug discovery is an example where drug-hunting is evolving to focus on the identification of inhibitors which are either non-competitive or uncompetitive with respect to ATP in order to mitigate the challenge of high cellular concentrations of the latter.[26,27] Specific examples include MK-2206 (an allosteric Akt inhibitor which binds at the interface of the pleckstrin homology domain and the catalytic domain, and locks the kinase in an inactive state[28]), and all four of the clinically approved MEK inhibitors;[29] these bind in the MEK allosteric site in BRAF/MEK complexes, stabilising the MEK activation loop in a conformation that is resistant to BRAF-mediated dual phosphorylation required for full activation of MEK.

An understanding of the rate-limiting step(s) of a target enzyme or series of receptor binding events affords the ability to target specifically the different steps of the overall reaction. Furthermore, consideration of the rates of binding and dissociation, $k_{on}$ and $k_{off}$, can also inform the design of inhibitors that exhibit "kinetic selectivity", where the drug–target complex has a longer half-life than off-target–drug complexes. A significant number of marketed drugs have slow-binding inhibition kinetics;[30] for example, all of the FDA-approved COX2 inhibitors that have been taken to the clinic work by a similar slow-binding, induced-fit mechanism of isozyme selective inhibition.[31] The slow off-rate of lapatinib (GW572016) from EGFR (Erb-1) and Erb-2 correlates with a prolonged down-regulation of receptor tyrosine phosphorylation in tumour cells.[32] The translation of such kinetics into cellular and *in vivo* contexts is underpinned in part by the concept of residence time.[5,33] An extreme example is the recent resurgence in irreversible covalent inhibition as a desired mechanism.

## 11.3.1 The Challenge with $IC_{50}$

Conventional drug discovery of enzyme inhibitors or receptor antagonists tends to focus on $IC_{50}$ assessments, *i.e.* the inhibitor concentration giving a 50% decrease in rate or maximum phenotypic response *under the specific assay conditions employed*:

$$\frac{v_i}{v_o} = \frac{1}{1 + \left(\frac{[I]}{IC_{50}}\right)^h} \tag{11.1}$$

where $\frac{v_i}{v_o}$ is the fractional velocity, [I] is the concentration of inhibitor, and $h$ is the Hill Coefficient, related to the stoichiometry of the enzyme–inhibitor interaction.[34]

It is important to remember that the $IC_{50}$ value itself is often not a true reflection of inhibitor affinity; it is a thermodynamic estimate measured under equilibrium conditions. The measured value can be significantly affected by the experimental conditions, particularly the concentration of the substrate to which the inhibitor could be competitive and the specific timing of the assay readout. Furthermore, potential differences associated with buffer components, pH and ionic strength effects can also compromise true understanding of the overall inhibition. Binding often involves protein flexibility[35] and changes in conformation during induced-fit processes, and the value of $IC_{50}$ may be modified by changes in substrate identity and concentration as well as enzyme concentration. Crucially, for slow-binding inhibitors, the "$IC_{50}$" simply represents a snapshot in time under the specific assay conditions. Therefore, undertaking more detailed experimentation to define the true $K_i^{(\prime)}$, (equilibrium dissociation constant for the E(S)I complex), coupled together with the rates of drug–target association and dissociation, is a far more correct and explicit strategy to determine how to optimise the potential drug ("structural kinetic relationship" as opposed to "structural activity relationship").

This is exemplified when assessing selectivity; whereas the $IC_{50}$ values ("thermodynamic selectivity") may be equivalent for related targets, determination of the "kinetic selectivity"[36,37] can open up a significant therapeutic window between the desired, and off-target effects (as described further in Section 11.3.3.2 on "residence time").

## 11.3.2 Mechanism of Enzyme Inhibition

Understanding the mechanism of inhibition is key to drug design. Coupled with structural analysis it can help to define key molecular interactions and binding poses. Importantly, it can also predict how *in vitro* analysis at the molecular level will translate through to the cellular level. For example, depending on the mechanism of inhibition, there may be a predictable "drop-off" between biochemical and cellular potency data, or there may be a specific mechanism that better translates to a particular disease state. A number of classical enzymology texts describe the mechanisms of inhibition in exquisite detail and so only a brief description is afforded here.[37,38]

Competitive inhibition is common, where the inhibitor binds to the target before the substrate, *i.e.* they bind preferentially to the free form of the enzyme (E). Often inhibitors are either designed to mimic the substrates of an enzyme reaction or to bind at the substrate binding site. Rational drug design in such cases can be more predictable, however there is often the challenge of a significant drop in potency when testing in a cellular context if the substrate with which the molecule is competitive is present in the cell at higher concentrations than the enzyme's $K_m$: for example, many kinases have $K_{m(ATP)}$ values in the range of 1–50 μM, whereas the cellular [ATP] is in the range of ~1–5 mM. In such cases, the apparent potency can shift between biochemical and cellular contexts by up to 1000-fold, according to equation (11.2).

- Competitive inhibition: Inhibitor binds only before substrate binding ($K_i$). This does not prove it binds at the same site as the varied substrate
- Uncompetitive inhibition: Inhibitor binds only after substrate has bound ($\alpha K_i$). This does not prove it binds at a different site to the varied substrate
- Mixed inhibition: Inhibitor binds both before and after substrate has bound. If $K_i = \alpha K_i$ (*i.e.* $\alpha = 1$, the inhibitor binds before and after substrate with the same affinity) this is known as pure non-competitive inhibition.

Equations that describe competitive, uncompetitive and mixed inhibition can be derived assuming that the scheme above is in rapid equilibrium and that [E] is $\ll$ than $K_i/\alpha K_i$. Schemes can also be derived for mechanisms where the ESI complex is catalytically active (partial inhibition) or substrate inhibition (ESS complex) occurs.

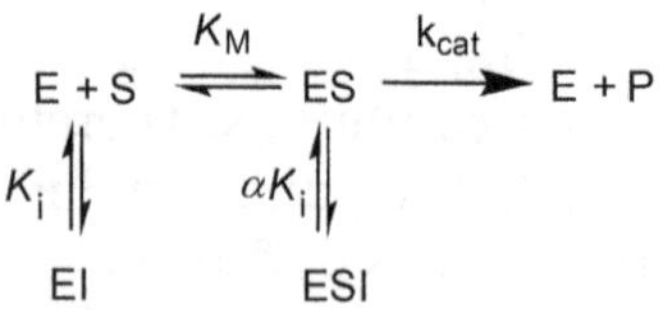


**Figure 11.1** Mechanisms of reversible inhibition.

Equations

$$\text{Competitive inhibition } v = \frac{v_{\max}[S]}{[S] + K_m\left(1 + \left(\frac{[I]}{K_i}\right)\right)} \tag{11.2}$$

Competitive inhibitors increase the apparent $K_m$, but have no effect on the apparent $V_{max}$.

Other mechanisms include non-competitive kinetics, where test compound may bind both before and after substrate binding with equivalent affinity, *i.e.* to both the free form of the enzyme (E) or the enzyme–substrate complex (ES); mixed inhibition is a case of non-competitive inhibition where the affinities for the free enzyme and enzyme substrate complex are not equivalent. Uncompetitive inhibition occurs when the inhibitor binds only after the substrate has bound to the enzyme (ES complex), and often is rarer.[39] However, one can imagine scenarios (*e.g.* in the kinase field) whereby uncompetitive inhibition (with respect to ATP) could be favourable, to avoid the challenge of competing with high intracellular concentrations of the substrate.

$$\text{Uncompetitive inhibition } v = \frac{v_{\max}[S]}{[S]\left(1 + \left(\frac{[I]}{\alpha K_i}\right)\right) + K_m} \tag{11.3}$$

Uncompetitive inhibitors decrease both the apparent $K_m$ and $V_{max}$.

$$\text{Mixed inhibition } v = \frac{v_{\max}[S]}{[S]\left(1 + \left(\frac{[I]}{\alpha K_i}\right)\right) + K_m\left(1 + \left(\frac{[I]}{K_i}\right)\right)} \tag{11.4}$$

Mixed inhibitors have varying effects, depending on whether the inhibitor has higher affinity for the free (E) or bound form (ES) of the enzyme. Pure non-competitive inhibitors have no effect on the apparent $K_m$ and decrease the apparent $V_{max}$ ($\alpha = 1$).

An additional important rationale for understanding the inhibitor mechanism-of-inhibition is to ensure appropriate assessment of selectivity, such that the individual $K_m$ values and relevant substrate concentrations can be taken into account when cross-comparing different datasets.

The mechanism, and true $(\alpha)K_i$ (equilibrium dissociation constant for the E(S)I complex) should be ascertained through full matrix experiments where [S] and [I] are varied: such experiments are more compelling and definitive than simplified substrate-shift experiments, for example where the inhibition is assessed at $K_m$ and $10 \times K_m$ substrate concentrations. It should be remembered that once the data are fit to global models of inhibition, the model suitability should be assessed using statistical analyses such as Akaike Information Criterion[40] or F-test.[41]

If the inhibition modality is confirmed to be either competitive, non-competitive or uncompetitive, the Cheng–Prusoff relationship can be utilised to convert $IC_{50}$ values into dissociation constants.[42]

$$IC_{50} = K_i\left(1 + \frac{[S]}{K_m}\right) \quad \text{Competitive}$$

$$IC_{50} = \alpha K_i \left(1 + \frac{K_m}{[S]}\right) \quad \text{Uncompetitive}$$

$$IC_{50} = \frac{[S] + K_m}{\frac{K_m}{K_i} + \frac{[S]}{\alpha K_i}} \quad \text{Non-competitive(note when } \alpha = 1, IC_{50} = K_i)$$

However, this "correction" does not address the issue of potential time-dependency of inhibition. To this end, there is a drive to move from SAR to SKR ("structural kinetic relationship") profiling to enable more impactful data to drive drug design. This involves running assays in a kinetic, rather than end-point, mode in order to deliver key parameters relating to the mechanism, and time-dependency, of inhibition. Indeed, the assessment of drug–target kinetics is critical to enable the deployment of drugs with optimised kinetic properties and duration of action.[43,44]

## 11.3.3 Slow-binding and Tight-binding Enzyme Inhibition

Enzyme inhibitors may act either reversibly or irreversibly. It should be noted that whilst irreversible inhibitors form covalent bonds, there may also be covalent bond formation between a reversible inhibitor and the enzyme. Compounds which fall in the continuum of reversible and irreversible inhibition are described as "slow-binding inhibitors".[45]

### *11.3.3.1 Slow-binding Inhibition*

Inhibitors can bind to, or dissociate from, their targets slowly, thus leading to a time-dependence for the onset of inhibition.[45,46] As a consequence, the degree of inhibition for a slow-binding inhibitor increases with time, therefore the $IC_{50}$ also changes with time; the $IC_{50}$ value obtained at a single time point is unlikely to be a reliable measure of inhibitory potency. It is therefore critical to analyse time courses for inhibitors suspected to be slow-binding (for example, the majority of inhibitors of sub-nM affinity), or irreversible, rather than using single time points for dose–response analysis, and to characterise the individual rate constants for the steps involved in forming the enzyme–inhibitor complexes. This enables the optimisation through SKR, where specific forms of the EI complex may be targeted. An elegant example is the study of slow-binding inhibition of *Mycobacterium tuberculosis* shikimate kinase by manzamine alkaloids,[47] where the various rate and inhibition constants have been characterised for the two-step binding interactions of a range of inhibitors in order to select the most efficacious.

There are two primary mechanisms that account for the majority of slow-binding interactions,[48] simple reversible slow-binding, and a two-step reaction where there is a rapid formation of an initial collision complex (EI) which subsequently undergoes a slow isomerisation to a higher affinity complex (EI*). There are numerous texts that describe these mechanisms in detail beyond the scope of this chapter, and the reader is referred to Chapter 6 in the seminal book by Robert Copeland.[37]

Simple reversible slow-binding can occur because reactions at low concentrations will proceed more slowly, according to the law of mass action. When an inhibitor has a low $K_i$ value and [I] is varied in the region of this, the value for the pseudo-first order rate constant for the formation of the non-covalent EI complex ($k_3 \cdot [I]_t$) would be low, irrespective of whether $k_3$ is of the order expected for a diffusion-controlled reaction ($10^8$ $M^{-1}$ $s^{-1}$) or lower; the dissociation rate constant ($k_4$) could also be low. Such a mechanism is represented in Figure 11.2. It can be also be seen that if [E] is very low, for example if the majority of $[E]_t$ is actually in the form ES, due to very high competing substrate, then slow binding may result.

Slow-binding inhibition can also arise if there is a rapid equilibrium formation of an initial encounter complex (EI) which subsequently undergoes a slow isomerisation to a higher affinity complex (EI*), as represented in Scheme B in Figure 11.2. This can also be referred to as the "induced fit mechanism". Here, the initial affinity of the encounter complex EI = $K_i = k_3/k_4$. The isomerisation step, $k_5$, is much slower than the reversible steps associated with the formation of EI; dissociation of the inhibitor from the EI* complex is rate-limited by the reverse isomerisation step, governed by $k_6$. The overall "true" affinity of the inhibitor $K_i^*$ cannot be assessed until the formation of the EI* complex:

$$K_i^* = \frac{K_i}{1 + \frac{k_5}{k_6}} \tag{11.5}$$

As a consequence, values for $K_i$, $k_5$ and $k_6$ can also be tuned as part of the SKR profiling.

Literature suggests that the majority of slow-binding and slow, tight-binding inhibitions occur according to mechanism B.[45] For inhibition to conform to mechanism B above, $K_i^*$ must be lower than $K_i$, therefore $k_6$ must be lower than $k_5$. Also, the values of

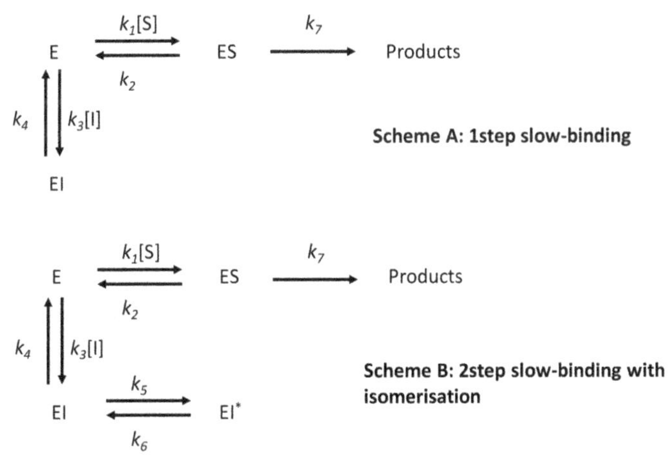


**Figure 11.2** Exemplar mechanisms of slow-binding inhibition. Scheme A describes the 1step slow-binding mechanism, where the formation of the non-covalent enzyme–inhibitor (EI) complex is slow. Scheme B describes the 2step slow-binding mechanism, in which encounter complex EI is formed rapidly but is then slowly converted to the higher affinity EI* complex through enzyme isomerisation. ES, non-covalent enzyme–substrate complex; [I], inhibitor concentration; [S], substrate concentration; $k_{1-7}$ rate constant of the specific step.

$k_5$ and $k_6$ must be of a magnitude which allows observation of the attainment of equilibrium between EI and EI*.

It is possible to distinguish between these two different mechanisms of slow-binding inhibition by following the progress curves for inhibition in reactions initiated with enzyme. The progress curves display a characteristic "bending" from an initial rate ($v_i$) to a steady-state inhibited rate ($v_s$). Data are fit to the classic Morrison–Walsh slow-binding equation:[46]

$$[\mathrm{P}] = v_s t + \frac{v_i - v_s}{k_{obs}}\left[1 - e^{(-k_{obs} t)}\right] \tag{11.6}$$

The initial ($v_i$) and steady state ($v_s$) velocities are defined by the slope values in the early and late stages of the progress curve, [P] defines the concentration of product, and $t$ = time.

Secondary plots of $k_{obs}$ *versus* [I] are linear for the one-step mechanism and hyperbolic for the two-step mechanism, and the individual rate constants can be estimated.[37] Assessment of these individual steps and constants facilitates the dissection of the mechanism of inhibition, and optimisation through SKR profiling. A complementary approach to the characterisation of the progress curves defining the slow onset of inhibition is to carry out jump-dilution experiments, where the pre-equilibrated EI complex is diluted rapidly into the assay and recovery of enzyme activity is measured over time as the inhibitor dissociates from the complex (rapidly, slowly or not at all in the case of irreversible inhibitors).[49] This method can be easily translated into the cellular context in the form of washout experiments. Traditional graphical fitting packages (such as Grafit, GraphPad Prism) can be augmented with more specialised modelling and simulation packages (such as KinTek Explorer[50]), enabling the experimenter to define and test specific hypotheses *in silico* and design experiments to support or refute these.

### *11.3.3.2 Drug–Target Residence Time*

The drug–target residence time model was first introduced in 2006.[5] Here, the concept of including the residence time ($T$) of the binary drug–target complex in drug optimisation was first captured.

$$T = 1/k_{off}$$

Taken together in context with an understanding of the protein–target's kinetics of degradation and re-synthesis, and the terminal pharmacokinetic half-life of the drug in systemic circulation,[33] the residence time can be used to predict the pharmacological durability of the drug *in vivo*. Assuming differential residence times for the drug on any potential off-targets, a true quantitation of the safety and/or selectivity window can also be ascertained. Here, whilst an "$IC_{50}$ snapshot" may show similar thermodynamic binding properties, the additional kinetic profiling can reveal therapeutic differentiation which may otherwise have been missed, as in the case of roniciclib (BAY1000394 [51]) for CDK2/9. Here, the prolonged residence times of roniciclib on CDK2 and CDK9 (as opposed to the transient residence times on other CDK enzymes) are reflected in a sustained inhibitory effect on retinoblastoma protein (RB) phosphorylation in tumour cells, indicating that the target residence time on CDK2 may contribute to sustained target engagement and antitumour efficacy. Over the past 15 years, the residence time concept has increasingly been used to drive molecules to the clinic.[52–54]

Taken together, these detailed interrogations of the target–ligand interactions enable the medicinal chemist to derive SKR based on informed intervention at the mechanistic step(s) of most relevance, and to drive more accurate dose prediction, both *in vivo* and in the clinic.

#### *11.3.3.3 Tight-binding Inhibition and Ligand Depletion*

Whilst generally desirable, high affinity compounds are challenging to characterise correctly. In order to rank compounds correctly it is important to realise that true $K_i$ values must be compared: $IC_{50}$ values will not give an accurate representation of affinity where ligand depletion occurs. This situation is often termed "tight-binding", the classical definition of which is a situation where the active enzyme concentration is approximately equal to, or even higher than, the apparent inhibition constant. Goldstein described this phenomenon in 1944[55,55] with the relationship between $IC_{50}$, $K_i'$ (the apparent $K_i$) and $[E]_t$ being described by:

$$IC_{50} = K_i' + [E]_t/2 \tag{11.7}$$

where $K_i' = K_i/(1 + [S]/K_m)$ for a competitive inhibitor.

It is clear that the measured $IC_{50}$ is limited to half of the functional enzyme concentration as the $K_i'$ value becomes very small; essentially, at this point, the enzyme concentration is literally being titrated by the inhibitor, and any measurement of $IC_{50}$ could be highly misleading in terms of significantly underestimating the true affinity. In such cases, alternative approaches must be taken to fully understand the true affinity.

The quadratic equation described below by Morrison[46] is a data-fitting approach that does not assume that the free concentration of inhibitor equals the total concentration. However, even these methods become unreliable as the affinity increases beyond around 10-fold below the functional enzyme concentration.

$$v_i = v_0 \cdot \frac{-([I]_t - [E]_t + K_i') + \sqrt{([I]_t - [E]_t + K_i')^2 - 4K_i'[E]_t}}{2[E]_t} \tag{11.8}$$

where $v_i$ is the inhibited rate, $v_0$ is the uninhibited rate, $K_i'$ is the apparent $K_i$ (uncorrected for mechanism) and $[I]_t$ is the total inhibitor concentration. When $[I]_t = IC_{50}$, $v_i = 0.5v_0$ and eqn (11.8) may be re-arranged to provide eqn (11.7).

In order to circumvent this issue, experimental approaches to decrease the functional enzyme concentration or raise the apparent $K_i$ by the use of increased concentrations of competing substrate may increase the scope of the measurement. Ideally biophysical methods (*e.g.* surface plasmon resonance) should be employed to quantify $K_d$, and relate it to $K_i$, $K_i'$, assuming that the mechanism of inhibition is known. In addition, a number of sophisticated simulation packages are available to help to build more comprehensive models to enable estimation of key parameters with more confidence, once the key components have been carefully ascertained.[56]

### 11.3.3.4 Irreversible Covalent Compounds

Irreversible covalent inhibition is enjoying a resurgence, where there is now increased confidence that tuning the balance between the initial molecular recognition event and the chemical reactivity can lead to the desired target selectivity without compromising safety and concern for off-target toxicity.[57–59] It is important to note that irreversible, covalent compounds are, by definition, unable to be ranked in terms of effectiveness using an equilibrium dissociation constant, $K_d$ or $K_i$. $IC_{50}$ values are also not useful or meaningful in ranking these types of compounds given the time-dependent nature of the inhibition; any irreversible inhibitor, added at half the enzyme concentration, will, allowing sufficient time for all of the added inhibitor to covalently modify the enzyme, lead to a 50% decrease in control rate. This can be deduced as the extreme case in eqn (11.7), where $K_i^*$ = zero and so $IC_{50}$ = $[E]_t/2$. Irreversible inhibitors should be assessed using the kinetic parameter $k_{inact}/K_I$ which is ascertained from time-course experiments with varying inhibitor concentrations to assess $k_{obs}$ (rate of conversion from initial EI encounter complex to the irreversible covalent complex). Here, the $K_I$ term describes the concentration of inhibitor required for one-half of the maximum rate of covalent bond formation and should not be confused with $K_i$ describing the dissociation of the initial EI encounter complex, which is not affected by covalent bond formation. Attempts have also been made to derive these parameters from time-dependent $IC_{50}$ values;[60,61] however, the advantage of using a kinetic approach to measure $k_{inact}/K_I$ is clear. Firstly, it uses valid parameters to describe the inhibition. It also allows the effectiveness of the irreversible inhibition to be dissected into initial molecular recognition and chemical reaction steps, in an analogous way to understanding the steps in the slow two-step binding mechanism described earlier. This information can then be used for further SKR optimisation, and also PKPD modelling and dose prediction. Further dissection to characterise $K_I$ and $K_i$ can be employed through the use of stopped-flow spectrophotometry, as recently very elegantly described for the detailed characterisation of osimertinibb.[62,62] Osimertinib is an irreversible covalent, third-generation epidermal growth factor receptor (EGFR) tyrosine kinase inhibitor (TKI) approved for treating non-small-cell lung cancer patients with activating EGFR mutations (Exon19del or L858R) or with the T790M resistance mutation following disease progression on first- or second-generation EGFR TKIs. Zhai *et al.* combined steady-state and pre-steady-state kinetics in a set of very elegant studies to determine the covalent inactivation rates ($k_{inact}$) and reversible binding affinities ($K_i$) for osimertinib against WT, L858R and L858R/T790M EGFR. They compared these data to the inhibition kinetics of earlier generations of EGFR TKIs to rationalize and understand how osimertinib achieves mutant EGFR selectivity over the wild-type (WT). The work shows that osimertinib overcomes the T790M mutation through improved affinities from stronger hydrophobic interactions with Met790 *versus* Thr790 and an improved rate of covalent bond formation *via* better positioning of the acrylamide warhead; conversely, osimertinib targets the L858R mutation through better affinities and reactivities with the mutant in the context of differential binding affinities of the competing substrate ATP. Such detailed characterisation of irreversible inhibitors is essential in order to modulate the interplay between initial non-covalent interactions that help to improve recognition for the target protein, and intrinsic compound reactivity, which may lead to a lack of selectivity and the potential for off-target toxicity.

A key consideration in all of the above for the cellular context is the rate of protein turnover and re-synthesis.[63] In particular, the efficacy of irreversible inhibitors is dependent on the lifetime of the protein; proteins with a short half-life are not afforded the benefit of drugs with a long residence time, due to their rapid turnover. It is also precedented for engagement of the target with small molecules to affect significantly the rate of protein turnover; indeed such a concept is becoming of wider interest in the protein degradation field.[64]

A further consideration needs to be the quantitation of the intracellular compound concentration, ideally at the site of action,[65] which is still regarding as an experimental "Holy Grail". This is not trivial; however, mass-spectrometry methods are becoming ever more sensitive and sophisticated, enabling this important parameter to be more accessible[66] and to feed forward into more accurate modelling for dose prediction.

## 11.4 Translating Through to Dosing: Target Occupancy

It is therefore appreciated that a detailed understanding of the target, and its interaction with its ligand(s), is key to ensuring optimal, rational design of inhibitors/modulators. The overarching aim is to design a safe and efficacious drug that will translate from *in vitro* experiments through to the clinical setting. A combination of classical enzymology and pharmacology, characterising from the molecular to the cellular level, is critical to enabling confidence in translation, and also in dose prediction. Importantly, such a combination can help to predict the amount of target that should be occupied by the drug at any particular time and any particular dose. These data can be combined into a mechanistic PKPD model to improve clinical prediction. A recent example from Walkup *et al.* describes the impact of such modelling to define a prospective mechanistic pharmacodynamic model to predict dose–response curves for inhibitors of the LpxC enzyme from *Pseudomonas aeruginosa* in an animal model of infection.[67] Here, drug–target kinetic parameters, including the on- and off-rates for the formation and breakdown of the drug–target complex, are incorporated together with protein turnover data and compound PK to generate more confidence in specific dose prediction. Moving forward, this sets the precedence for incorporating drug–target kinetic data into PD models to enable selection of those molecules most likely to generate the best candidate drugs.

## 11.5 Introduction: Receptors

Receptors are a class of cellular macromolecules that can be divided into four main classes: ion channels, G-protein coupled receptors (GPCRs), enzyme-linked receptors and nuclear receptors.[68]

*Ion channel* targets are channels with a receptor site localized on the cell membrane coupled directly to the ion channel. They are made up of multiple subunit proteins which form cation or anion channels. The channel properties are determined by the composition of the subunit isoforms. Hence, their activity can be regulated by varying composition of different subunits, *e.g.* GABAA[69] agonistic ligands open the channel resulting in "activation", while antagonists prevent agonists from opening the channel. Inverse agonists close open channels.

*G-protein coupled receptors* are composed of seven transmembrane helices which have an extracellular domain, the ligand binding site and an intracellular domain that couples to a specific G-protein. The GPCRs do not act directly as effectors, they act as integrators of multiple stimuli and the G-proteins can regulate multiple intracellular messengers/effectors. G-protein coupled receptors amplify signalling through several effector systems such as ion channels, the adenylate cyclase-cAMP system and the phospholipase-C-inositol phosphate system.[70]

The *enzyme-linked receptors* are directly linked to tyrosine kinase (*e.g.* VEGF, GH) or guanylate cyclase (*e.g.* atrial natriuretic peptide).

The *nuclear receptor* family (*e.g.* PPARs, GR, ER) bind to lipophilic ligands (*e.g.* retinoids, steroids) to affect transcriptional regulations of specific target genes.[71]

Receptors interact specifically and directly with ligand-dependent signalling within a cell and between cells. The binding of a ligand to a receptor is governed by the laws of thermodynamics and is typically saturable and reversible. Binding of an endogenous ligand will trigger a signalling event leading to a functional response. Hence, a receptor displays at least two major functional domains, a ligand binding domain and an effector domain. The conformational state of the ligand binding site is not necessarily complementary to the preferred conformation of the ligand. Adaptation of both the ligand and the ligand binding site is a dynamic process referred to as binding plasticity.[72] Conformational changes as a result of mutually induced fit in a receptor are translated into biological effect. However, the response can also be influenced by the number of receptors available/present (referred to as receptor density), differences in signal transduction mechanisms, alternative second messengers and/or other factors affecting gene regulation, protein synthesis and/or other aspects of cellular homeostasis. Binding of a ligand to the active site on a receptor regulates the activity of a receptor directly. For instance, agonists are ligands that display affinity as well as intrinsic activity, while antagonists are ligands which display affinity but no intrinsic activity.[73,74] Receptors usually exist in two principal conformations, the active state ($R_a$) and the inactive state ($R_i$), and the reader is referred to excellent texts as cited here.[75,76]

An agonist has higher affinity for the active conformation ($R_a$) than for the inactive ($R_i$), while an antagonist binds either of these conformations with equal affinity without shifting the equilibrium in any direction. Partial agonists display a slightly higher affinity for the active form than the inactive form and thereby shift the equilibrium towards the active form, but to a lesser extent compared to a full agonist.

An inverse agonist reverses constitutive receptor activity causing repression of basal activity. Hence, an inverse agonist can cause an opposite effect to that of an agonist even in the absence of an agonist. More recently, the concept of multistate models with intermediate conformational states has been brought forward. Ligand-induced receptor conformations may cause receptors to interact with different second messenger systems and thus only activate some of the downstream functions of the receptor.[77]

### 11.5.1 Agonist Concentration-effect Curves

The agonist concentration-effect (E/[A] or dose–response) curve has become one of the hallmarks of modern pharmacology. The generation of such data requires an assay system which can deliver robust and reproducible functional responses elicited solely *via* activation of the target under investigation. Under these conditions, E/[A] curves are typically sigmoidal when plotted in semi-logarithmic form (E/$\log_{10}$[A]) and are described by four parameters: (1) a lower asymptote ($\beta$) which represents the basal state of the system, (2) an upper asymptote ($\alpha$) which represents the maximum effect that the agonist produces in the system, (3) a location or potency ([$A_{50}$] or $EC_{50}$), which represents the concentration of agonist that produces an effect equal to 50% of $\alpha - \beta$ and (4) a slope parameter ($n$), which is a measure of the gradient of the curve at the [$A_{50}$] level. Estimates of these parameters are typically made by fitting experimental E/[A] curve data to the following form of the Hill equation (a saturable function that adequately describes curves of varying gradients):

$$E = \beta + \frac{(\alpha - \beta)[\mathrm{A}]^n}{[\mathrm{A}]^n + [\mathrm{A}_{50}]^n} \tag{11.9}$$

In practice, in the majority of cases $\beta = 0$, that is, the basal effect level is ascribed a value of zero, and therefore most E/[A] curve data can be adequately described by a three-parameter Hill equation as illustrated in Figure 11.3. It is the analysis of how these three curve parameters ($\alpha$, [$A_{50}$] and $n$) are affected by the efforts of the medicinal chemist that drives the optimisation of the pharmacological properties of new compounds. As antagonists do not elicit functional responses, their activity is derived from analysis of how they affect agonist responses.

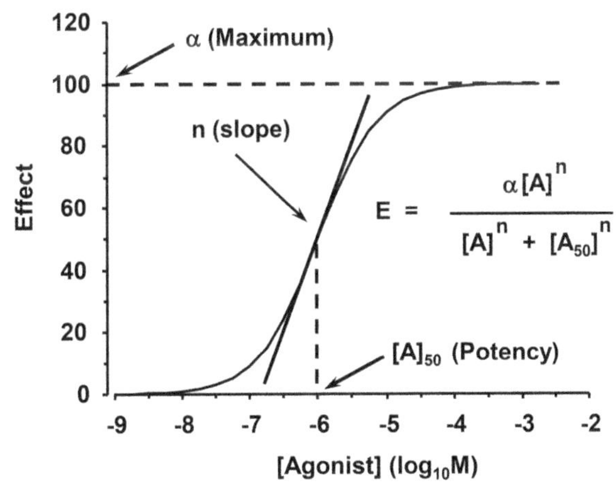


**Figure 11.3** Agonist concentration-effect curves. A simulated curve highlighting the parameters that define it, $\alpha$ (the maximum effect), [$A_{50}$] (potency) the concentration of agonist that produces 50% of $\alpha$ and $n$, a measure of the slope. [$A_{50}$] values are often quoted as $pA_{50}$ ($-\log_{10}[A_{50}]$). In this example the [$A_{50}$] is $10^{-6}$ M and the $pA_{50}$ is 6.0. Real examples of agonist E/[A] curves are shown in many of the following figures.

### 11.5.2 Full Agonists, Partial Agonists and Inverse Agonists

The first step in agonist action is the formation of a reversible agonist–receptor (AR) complex, a process that is generally assumed to be governed by the Law of Mass Action. Accordingly, the equilibrium concentration of agonist-occupied receptors is a rectangular hyperbolic (a special case of the Hill function where $n = 1$) function of the agonist concentration. This curve is defined by a maximal value of $[R_{tot}]$, the total receptor concentration, and a midpoint value of $K_A$, the agonist dissociation constant. In theory, $K_A$ is a purely drug-dependent parameter, and it determines how well the agonist binds; that is, it is a measure of the affinity (the reciprocal of the dissociation constant) of the agonist for its receptors. Agonist occupancy is subsequently converted into functional effect by the biochemical/biophysical machinery of the cell/tissue, and this is what is measured experimentally in the form of an E/[A] curve. The efficiency of this transduction process can vary between agonists and across systems, that is, it is both drug and tissue dependent. Agonist efficacy is a measure of the efficiency of the transduction process. Full agonists have high efficacies and therefore can elicit the maximum effect ($E_{max}$) that the test system can generate. Partial agonists, by contrast, have low efficacy and cannot elicit a maximum response (Figure 11.4).

Measuring the efficacy (and affinity) of full agonists is not straightforward. This is because it requires an experimental manipulation that decreases the efficacy of the agonist to a level where it behaves as a partial agonist. Irreversible antagonists have been used for this purpose as they covalently modify receptors, thereby decreasing $[R_{tot}]$.

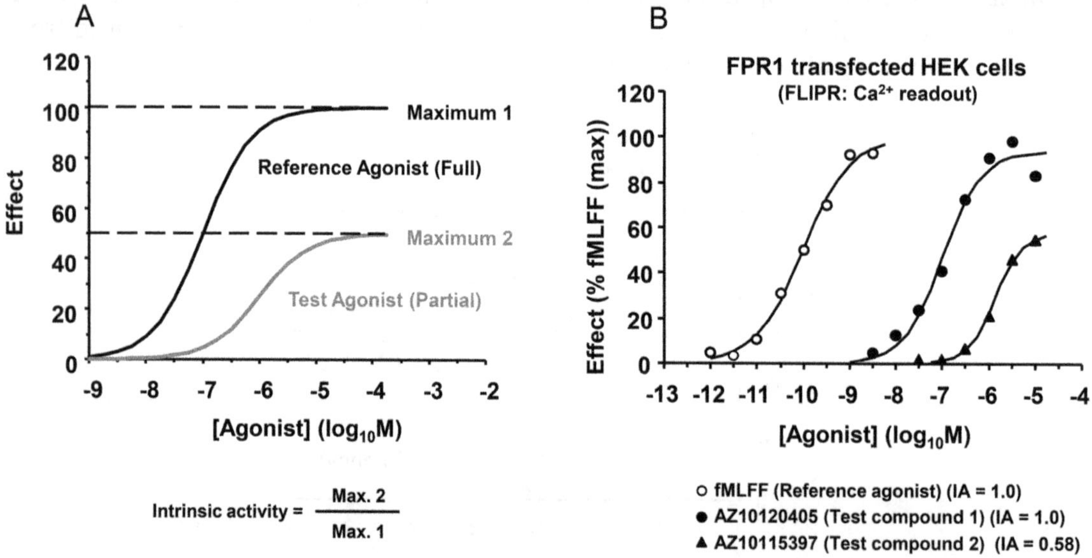


**Figure 11.4** Full agonists, partial agonists, and intrinsic activity. Panel A shows simulated curves for a reference full agonist and a test partial agonist and how intrinsic activity is calculated. In this example IA of the partial agonist is 0.5. Panel B shows experimental data (increases in intracellular $Ca^{2+}$ levels) for a reference full agonist, fMLFF and two test agonists in HEK cells stably expressing the human FPR1 receptor. AZ10120405 is a full agonist (IA = 1.0) but AZ10115397 exhibits partial agonism (IA = 0.58). Unpublished data.

Their utility in estimating agonist efficacy and affinity is described below. An important consequence of efficacy being both a drug and a system-dependent parameter is that an agonist can demonstrate different behaviours in different systems. Thus, a drug that exhibits partial agonism in one system may be a full agonist in another (with higher $[R_{tot}]$ or more efficient transduction machinery) or effectively an antagonist in yet another (with lower $[R_{tot}]$ or less efficient transduction machinery) (Figure 11.5). As alluded to above, it can be difficult to measure the affinity and efficacy of agonists, and typically the information reported to the chemist is the potency ($[A_{50}]$ or more often, $pA_{50}$ ($-\log_{10}[A_{50}]$)) and the intrinsic activity (IA) of the compound. The latter is a measure of the maximal activity of the test compound relative to a reference full agonist. If the test agonist produces a maximum response less than the reference agonist then the IA will be <1.0; for example, if it produces a maximum effect that is 50% of the reference, it will have an IA of 0.5 and exhibit partial agonism (Figure 11.4A). Such compounds are useful to the medicinal chemist as they help direct efforts to optimise the efficacy of compounds for therapeutic benefit, for example, identification of partial agonists were important staging posts in the development of the antagonists propranolol[78] and cimetidine.[79] Finally, it is important to emphasise that the IA scale does not discriminate between full agonists, that is, all full agonists will have an IA of 1.0 (Figure 11.4B), but they may have different efficacies.

Until relatively recently agonist efficacy was considered only as a positive vector associated with increased receptor activity. This dogma was challenged by the discovery of the phenomenon of constitutive receptor activation and compounds that showed inverse

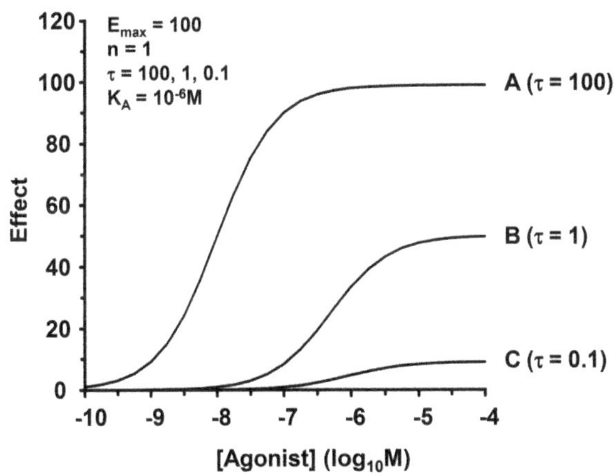


**Figure 11.5** System dependence of drug effects. Simulated curves showing how the curve parameters of an agonist change in systems with varying receptor expression. The receptor expression range is 1000-fold from curve A to curve C. In system A, the drug exhibits full agonism (IA = 1.0 and high efficacy ($\tau$ = 100)); in system B, it shows partial agonism (IA = 0.5 and low efficacy ($\tau$ = 1)) and in system C, it shows very weak partial agonism (IA = 0.09 and very low efficacy ($\tau$ = 0.1)). In system C the drug effectively behaves as an antagonist as this level of IA is difficult to detect in most assay systems. The Operational Model of Agonism[106] was used to simulate the data. In this model, $\tau$ is a measure of the efficacy of the agonist and incorporates both drug (intrinsic efficacy) and system (receptor number ($[R_{tot}]$) and coupling efficiency) parameters.

agonism,[80] that is, they decreased the level of constitutive activation, demonstrating negative efficacy (Figure 11.6). The most likely mechanism for inverse agonism is that such compounds have a selectively higher affinity for the inactive state of the receptor and thereby uncouple spontaneously coupled (active) receptor species.[81] The identification of receptor conformations that display clear preference for different ligands supports this hypothesis and may allow the functional characterisation of ligands by measuring their affinity for a pair (or more) of G protein-coupled receptor conformations.[82] To date, inverse agonism has largely been a property detected in genetically engineered systems where receptors (or modified receptors) can be expressed at very high levels. Many of the compounds that exhibit inverse agonism in such systems behave as competitive (neutral) antagonists with zero efficacy in more physiologically relevant assays. As such, the therapeutic relevance of inverse agonism remains largely unknown, but this now well-documented phenomenon has changed the way pharmacologists view drug–receptor interactions, as well as resulting in the re-classification of drugs that were formerly thought to be competitive antagonists (*e.g.* ranitidine and propranolol). Moreover, as more diseases are identified that are linked to constitutive receptor activation it seems likely that inverse agonists will become increasingly important tools in addressing unmet clinical needs.

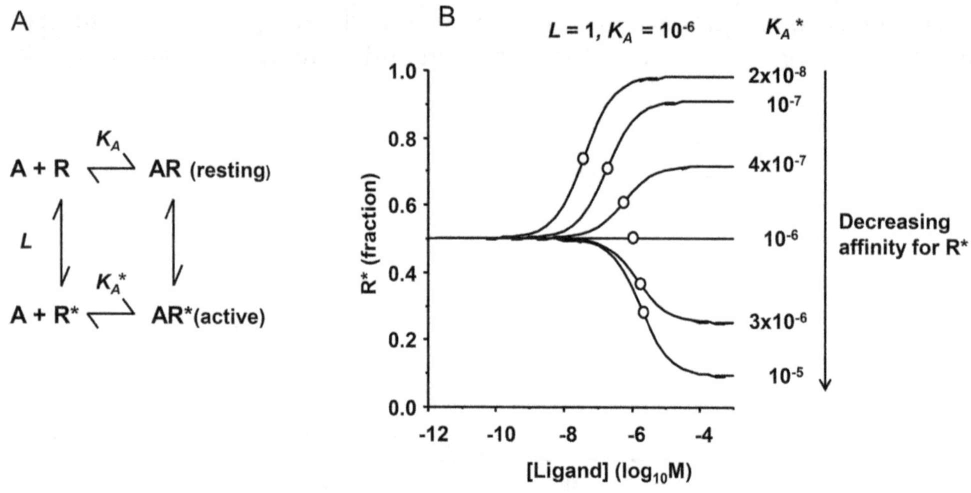


**Figure 11.6** Inverse agonism. Panel A shows a simple two-state model in which the receptor exists in R (resting) or R* (active) states. In the absence of agonist (A) the distribution of the two states is governed by the equilibrium constant $L$. The agonist has affinities for the two states governed by the dissociation equilibrium constants, $K_A$ and $K_A^*$. Panel B shows a simulation that represents the effects of six ligands with different $K_A:K_A^*$ values. Effect is determined by the fraction of receptors in the R* form. $L$ is set to 1 in this example so under basal conditions the receptors are equally distributed between the two states. In such a system inverse agonism is easily detectable. For agonists with higher affinity for R*, positive agonism is observed; for agonists with higher affinity for R, inverse agonism is observed. Ligands with equal affinity for the two states are neutral and behave as antagonists of positive and inverse agonists. Reproduced from ref. 81 with permission from Elsevier, Copyright 1995.

#### *11.5.2.1 Biased Agonists*

A single receptor can activate multiple signalling pathways. For example, it is now commonly recognised that GPCRs can interact with multiple G-proteins and other signalling molecules such as arrestins, and that recruitment of β-arrestin, that occurs following activation of the majority of GPCRs, results in receptor desensitisation and subsequent internalisation. Biased agonists are proposed to stabilize receptor conformations, preferentially stimulating one of these pathways, and therefore allow a more targeted modulation of cell function and treatment of disease. Biased antagonists have also been reported that can inhibit one signalling pathway and not another.

A highly cited application of the concept of biased agonism is the discovery of opioid receptor agonists that exhibit analgesic effects but with little constipation and/or respiratory suppression.[83] It was demonstrated that β-arrestin 2 knock-out mice exhibited enhanced analgesia in response to opioid receptor agonists but less tolerance development and little constipation or respiratory suppression. This suggested that μ-opioid receptor agonists, biased for G-protein activation, with little arrestin-mediated effects, may exhibit a beneficial profile in the treatment of pain. Inspired by these findings, oliceridine was developed,[84] a μ-opioid receptor agonist which exhibited robust G-protein activation with a potency and efficacy similar to that of morphine, but which caused far less arrestin recruitment and receptor internalization. A clinical Phase 2 study confirmed that oliceridine acted as a potent analgesic drug in patients, producing similar analgesia compared with morphine but with fewer adverse events. The FDA approved oliceridine in August 2020 based on the results of three Phase 3 trials. However, not everything is clear cut, and the biased agonism "arrestin hypothesis" has been challenged by the persistence of morphine- and fentanyl-induced side effects, including respiratory depression and constipation, in a knock-in mouse expressing a phospho-deficient μ-opioid receptor mutant that is unable to recruit β-arrestin, and by the persistence of morphine-induced respiratory depression in the β-arrestin 2 knock-out mouse. In addition, robust physiological evidence demonstrates that classical G-protein signalling from the μ-opioid receptor contributes substantially to respiratory depression, as well as to other side effects, such as constipation. Recent evidence suggests oliceridine's beneficial profile may be more related to its low intrinsic activity, rather than biased agonism.[85]

Biased ligands offer exciting new therapeutic opportunities, but many challenges remain to be addressed to capitalise on the unique properties of such ligands. Amongst these are the need to establish robust assays to capture functional selectivity (not assay artifacts), and clear definition of compound profiles that are likely to be clinically relevant.

### 11.5.3 Optimising Agonists

As discussed above, agonists both bind and activate receptors. The optimisation of agonist properties relies on designing compounds with both good affinity and appropriate efficacy. These needs dictate the assays used in agonist-focussed drug discovery programmes. Affinity can be measured in ligand binding assays, similar to those illustrated in Figure 11.9. Such assays have the benefit of confirming that the compounds do indeed bind to the target of interest, but in most instances give no information on efficacy. Functional assays are required to provide estimates of IA or efficacy. These often take the form of simple second messenger readouts such as changes in intracellular calcium or cyclic adenosine monophosphate (cAMP) levels, and are nowadays routinely conducted in cell lines expressing the human version of the target receptor. Such systems have the advantage of high throughput and are generally very robust. A disadvantage is that the agonist responses observed may poorly reflect those observed in the biologically relevant cells/tissues due to differences in receptor number and/or coupling and the readout. Testing of compounds in more relevant cellular and tissue systems is therefore essential before progressing to *in vivo* testing. An example of the assays employed, and the data generated in a typical agonist programme is shown in Figure 11.7. Here, both binding and functional assays were used to assess activity of $\beta_2$-receptor agonists and, as expected, compounds with higher intrinsic activity (and therefore efficacy) showed a greater discrepancy between their binding activity and their functional potency ($pA_{50}$). (As highlighted earlier, the binding affinity of full agonists is a poor measure of their functional potency, as $pA_{50}$ is dependent on both agonist affinity and efficacy.)

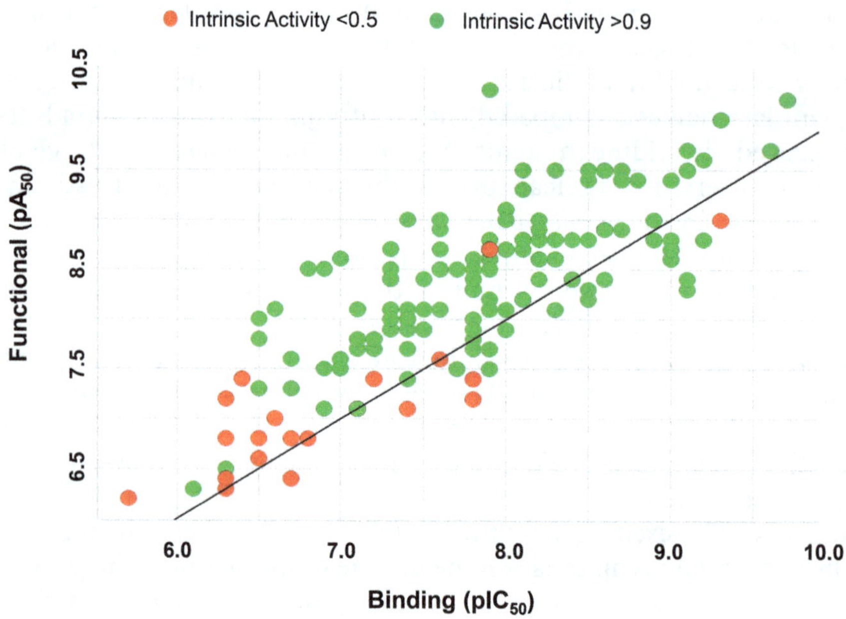


**Figure 11.7** Optimising agonists. The binding activities ($pIC_{50}$) and functional potencies ($pA_{50}$) of a range of $\beta_2$-agonists are shown. The binding activities were measured by displacement of $^{125}$I-labelled cyanopindolol in HEK293 cells stably transfected with the human $\beta_2$-adrenoceptor, and the functional potencies were assessed by measuring increases in cAMP levels in H292 cells, a human lung epithelial cell line that endogenously expresses the $\beta_2$-adrenoceptor. In the latter assay, the intrinsic activity of compounds was assessed relative to the full agonist, formoterol. Compounds are grouped into those with an intrinsic activity <0.5 (red) and those with an intrinsic activity >0.9 (green). As expected, compounds largely lie above the "equi-activity" lines, that is, the functional activities are greater than the binding activities and this discrepancy is generally larger for compounds with higher intrinsic activity.

In most cases, the aim of agonist-based projects is to identify high potency, high efficacy agonists so that the drug dose ultimately administered will be small and the effect large. In some instances, however, partial agonists can have therapeutic advantages. Thus, if the desirable therapeutic effect is observed in a tissue with high receptor number/coupling but an undesirable side-effect is mediated in a tissue with low receptor number/coupling, a partial agonist of appropriate efficacy could produce agonism in the former but be "silent" in the latter (compare curves A and C in Figure 11.5).

## 11.5.4 Antagonists

Several different classes of antagonists with distinct mechanisms of action including irreversible competitive, reversible competitive, non-competitive and allosteric have been identified. Their blockade of agonist-induced effects can be surmountable (rightward displacement of the E/[A] curve with no depression of the maximum ($\alpha$)) or insurmountable (depression of the maximal agonist response ($\alpha$)). It is important to realise that the profile of antagonism observed can show system dependence, that is, an antagonist can exhibit surmountable activity in one assay system and insurmountable activity in another, despite having the same mechanism of action (see Figure 11.12A and B). A common example of this phenomenon is the behaviour of high affinity competitive antagonists in FLIPR® assays, in which the changes in intracellular calcium levels measured are typically transient in nature. In these circumstances, true equilibrium is not reached, and the agonist cannot access antagonist bound receptors, resulting in non-surmountable antagonism.[86] This contrasts with the behaviour of such antagonists in systems where the agonists responses are sustained (for example isolated tissues), true equilibrium is reached, and the antagonism is surmountable.

The interaction of an antagonist with its receptors is described by a single parameter, affinity which equates to potency (unlike agonists where potency is dependent on both affinity and efficacy). By definition, antagonists have an IA = 0 in functional assays, in which their affinity is measured by studying their interaction with an agonist. The affinity of antagonists can also be measured in binding assays, although if such systems are used it is essential to confirm lack of efficacy by subsequent testing in functional assays. The following sections discuss the properties and analysis of the various classes of antagonists.

### *11.5.4.1 Irreversible Competitive Antagonists*

Irreversible competitive antagonists are relatively rare, but they are worthy of discussion as they form the basis of the receptor inactivation method developed by Furchgott[87] that allows the estimation of the efficacy and affinity of full agonists. These agents (for example phenoxybenzamine) bind covalently to receptors and thereby decrease $[R_{tot}]$ by making a portion of the receptor pool unavailable for agonist binding. As outlined above, agonist efficacy is partly dependent on $[R_{tot}]$, so this chemical inactivation of receptors decreases agonist efficacy and converts full agonists into partial agonists. Under these conditions the $[A_{50}]$ (or $pA_{50}$) of the partial agonist curve yields a good estimate of the affinity ($K_A$ or $pK_A$) of the agonist; the lower the maximum effect ($\alpha$) the

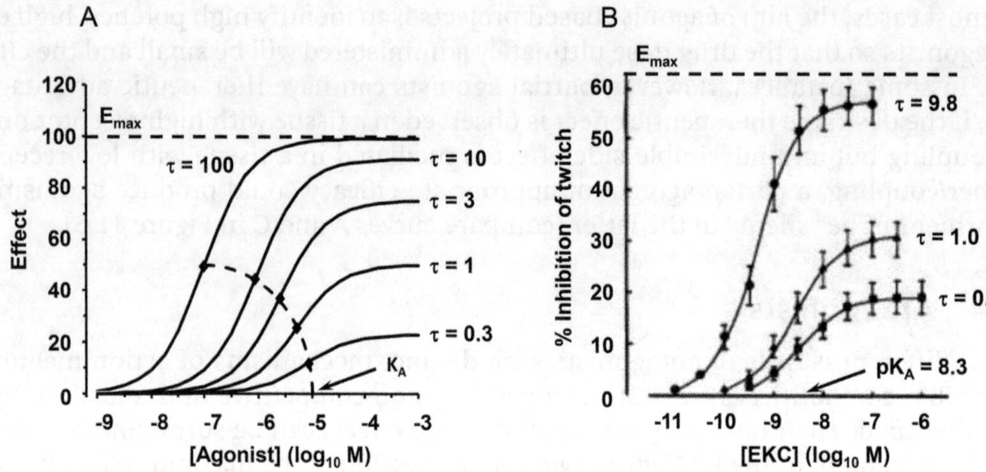


**Figure 11.8** Irreversible antagonism. Panel A shows a simulation of the effects of an irreversible antagonist on the response of a full agonist. Increasing concentrations of the irreversible antagonist cause rightward displacement of the control agonist E/[A] curve ($\tau$ = 100) with depression of the maximum response ($\alpha$). As the curves become increasingly depressed, the $[A]_{50}$ approaches the $K_A$ affording an estimate of the agonist affinity. The data was generated using the Operational Model of Agonism[106] by varying $[R_{tot}]$, which has the effect of reducing agonist efficacy ($\tau$). Panel B shows an example of irreversible antagonism of the effects of the κ-opioid agonist ethylketocyclazocine by the alkylating agent β-chlornaltrexamine (β-CNA) in isolated, coaxially stimulated guinea-pig ileum. E/[A] curves are shown in the absence of (•) or following 30 minutes exposure to 10 nM (▲) or 30 nM (■) β-CNA. The lines drawn through the data are the results of fitting the data to the Operational Model of Agonism. The estimates of p$K_A$ (affinity) and $\tau$ (efficacy) for EKC were 8.3 and 9.8 respectively. Panel B: Reproduced from ref. 107 with permission from John Wiley & Sons, Copyright 1989 British Pharmacological Society.

better the $[A_{50}]$ of the E/[A] curve serves as an estimate of agonist affinity. The $[A_{50}]$ estimate obtained under the "low efficacy" condition divided by the $[A_{50}]$ of the control curve (no irreversible antagonist) serves as an approximate measure of the agonist efficacy. In practice, such data can be fitted to mathematical models[88] that give accurate estimates of the parameters of affinity and efficacy (Figure 11.8). Unfortunately, the lack of appropriate irreversible antagonists for many receptors precludes this sort of analysis in most cases. The "potency" of the antagonists themselves in such experiments is somewhat meaningless as occupancy does not reach a steady state but rather increases with exposure time, and unbound antagonist is removed before assessment of the agonist effects.

#### 11.5.4.2 Reversible Competitive Antagonists

Reversible competitive antagonists are probably the most important class of antagonists and many clinically used drugs fall into this class. As outlined above for agonists, the first step in the action of these drugs is the formation of a reversible, relatively short-lasting, drug–receptor complex governed by the Law of Mass Action. This can be measured directly in binding studies used labelled (for example, radioactively or fluorescently) compounds with the binding describing a saturable rectangular hyperbolic function. The concentration of antagonist that binds 50% [$R_{tot}$] defines the antagonist dissociation constant ($K_D$ or $K_B$ in functional studies) (Figure 11.9A). Binding of a competitive antagonist precludes the binding of other drugs to the same sites on the receptor. This mutually exclusive binding allows test compounds to be assessed for their ability to displace a labelled compound (L), a practice that is routinely used in drug screening to derive an estimate of potency. Such indirect analysis is important as it is impractical to label all test compounds. These displacement experiments typically yield a sigmoidal curve (which can be fitted to a Hill equation similar to eqn (11.9)) from which the $IC_{50}$ (concentration of the test compound that produces 50% displacement of the specific binding of the labelled compound) can be measured (Figure 11.9B). Assuming that the interaction between the labelled compound and the test compound is competitive then the dissociation constant ($K_I$) of the test compound can be calculated using a modified Cheng–Prusoff equation:[89]

$$K_I = \frac{IC_{50}}{1 + [L]/K_D} \tag{11.10}$$

Proof of the assumption that the interaction is competitive requires further experimentation, such as studying the displacement by the test compound, of different concentrations of the labelled ligand. As is evident from the Cheng–Prusoff equation, at concentrations of L in excess of $K_D$, the $IC_{50}$ estimate will increase proportionately, that is, higher concentrations of L will require higher concentrations of test compound to displace it. It is therefore imperative that the activities of different test compounds are

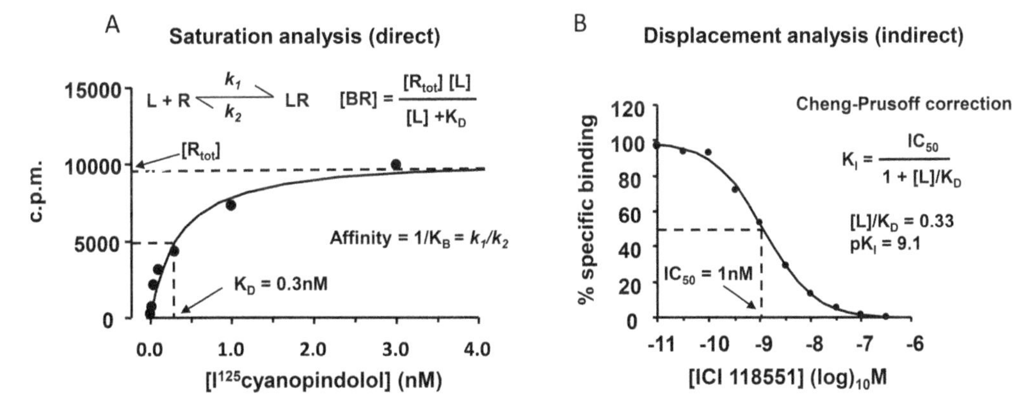


**Figure 11.9** Competitive antagonism: binding assays. Panel A shows a direct binding assay using $^{125}$I-labelled cyanopindolol as a $\beta_2$-adrenoceptor ligand. The curve describes a rectangular hyperbola which saturates at high ligand concentration. The ligand dissociation constant ($K_D$) was estimated as 0.3 nM and is a measure of the ligand affinity ($1/K_D$). Panel B shows a typical displacement analysis in the same system using 0.1 nM labelled cyanopindolol. The displacing ligand, the selective $\beta_2$-adrenoceptor antagonist ICI 118551, produces complete displacement of the specific binding yielding an $IC_{50}$ of 1 nM. In this instance $[L]/K_D$ is <1.0 so the $IC_{50}$ is a good estimate of the $K_I$, as calculated by the Cheng–Prusoff equation. Unpublished data.

compared under identical conditions, that is, $[L]/K_D$ should be constant. Since $IC_{50}$ values do not infer a particular mechanism of action, they are routinely used to compare the activities of compounds in binding assays rather than calculated $K_I$ values.

The affinity of competitive antagonists can also be measured in functional assays. In this case, the presence of the antagonist (B) decreases the probability that an agonist–receptor interaction will occur. To achieve the same degree of agonist occupancy and therefore the same effect, in the presence of the antagonist as in its absence, the agonist concentration must be increased. The factor ($r$) by which it must be increased depends on both the concentration of antagonist ([B]) used and on how well it binds ($K_B$). This relationship, which was first described by Schild,[90] is shown in eqn (11.11):

$$r - 1 = [B]^n/K_B \tag{11.11}$$

where $r = [A_{50}]/[A_{50}]^c$ (location parameter of the E/[A] curve in the presence of the antagonist/location parameter of the E/[A] curve in the absence of the antagonist), $K_B$ is the antagonist equilibrium dissociation constant and $n$ represents the order of reaction between the antagonist and the receptors (for a first order reaction $n = 1$, that is, one molecule of antagonist binds to one receptor molecule).

Experimentally, a $K_B$ is estimated by studying the interaction of an agonist and antagonist over a wide range of antagonist concentrations (the wider, the better). This is necessary because drugs which are not reversible competitive antagonists may appear to be so within a narrow range of concentrations (see Figures 11.12A and 11.13A). If the antagonist is truly competitive then it should produce parallel rightward displacement (that is, no change in midpoint slope ($n$) occurs) of the E/[A] curves with no change in the maximal response ($\alpha$) (Figure 11.10A), that is, surmountable antagonism is observed. This is intuitively obvious, since the antagonist is merely decreasing the probability that an agonist–receptor interaction will occur, an effect that can always be overcome by increasing the agonist concentration. The analysis involves fitting experimentally derived values of $r$ at different concentrations of antagonist to the following form of eqn (11.11)[91] (Figure 11.10B).

$$\log_{10}(r - 1) = n\log_{10}[B] - \log_{10}K_B \tag{11.12}$$

Adherence of the data to this equation is judged by the finding of a linear plot with unit slope. Under these conditions the intercept on the $x$-axis ($\log_{10}[B]$) gives an estimate of $K_B$. When $n$ is significantly different from 1 then the intercept gives an estimate of $pA_2$ ($-\log_{10}K_B/n$) The $pA_2$ is an empirical estimate of antagonist affinity and equates to the negative logarithm of the concentration of antagonist that produces a two-fold rightward shift ($r = 2$) of the control E/[A] curve. Non-linearity and slopes other than unity can result from many causes. For example, a slope of greater than 1 may indicate incomplete equilibration with the antagonist or removal of the antagonist from the biophase (receptor compartment). A slope that is significantly less than 1 may indicate removal of the agonist by a saturable uptake process, or it may result from the interaction of the agonist with more than one receptor. In the latter case the Schild plot may be non-linear, with a clear inflexion.[92] All these potential complicating factors have been described in detail previously by Kenakin.[93]

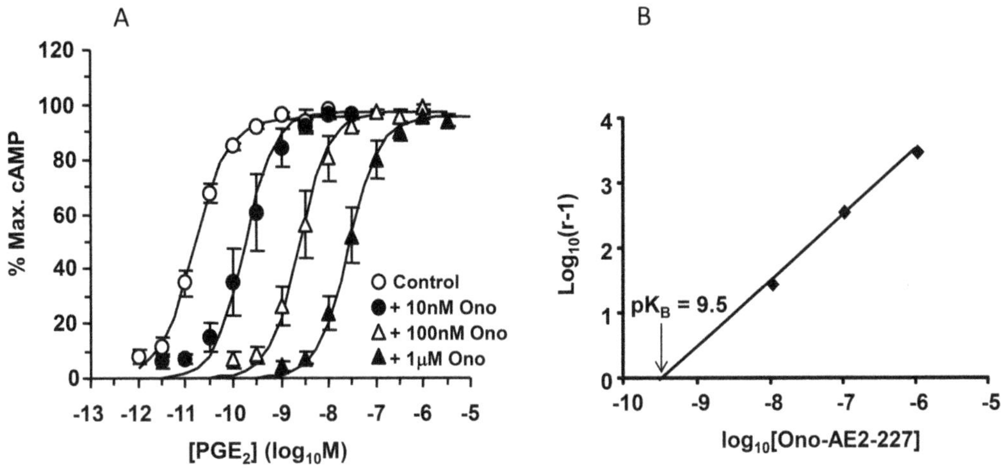


**Figure 11.10** Competitive antagonism: functional assays. Antagonism of the $PGE_2$-mediated induction of cAMP by the competitive antagonist Ono-AE2-227, in CHO cells stably transfected with the human $EP_4$ receptor (Panel A). Note the concentration-dependent parallel rightward displacement of the control curves. Panel B illustrates the displacements (*r* values) in Schild plot form derived for one of the five experiments that make up the data shown in panel A. The plot has a slope of unity and the intercept on the *x*-axis yields an estimate of 9.5 for the $pK_B$ ($-\log_{10}K_B$). Adapted from ref. 108 with permission from European Respiratory Society, Copyright 2007.

Although Schild-type analysis is the most robust method of assessing antagonist behaviour in functional assays, the needs of modern high throughput drug discovery programmes dictate that it is used sparingly to assess the mechanism of action for priority compounds. Routine screening of antagonist properties will more likely be assessed by doing a functional Cheng–Prusoff type experiment (Figure 11.11) in which the effects of several concentrations of the test compound on the response to a single concentration of agonist are studied. The experimental data can then be fitted to eqn (11.13):[94]

$$K_B = \frac{IC_{50}}{(2 + ([A]/[A_{50}])^n)^{1/n} - 1} \tag{11.13}$$

As was outlined above for binding studies, the estimated $IC_{50}$ is dependent on the concentration of ligand employed. In this case the concentration of agonist (A) relative to its $[A_{50}]$ dictates the $IC_{50}$ (and hence the estimated $K_B$). Practically, the experimenter usually employs a concentration of agonist that is as close to the $[A_{50}]$ as possible so that the $IC_{50}$ is a good estimate of the $K_B$. The shape of the agonist E/[A] curve is also important, as evidenced by the inclusion of the slope parameter ($n$) in this form of the Cheng–Prusoff equation. When $n = 1$ the equation simplifies to a form equivalent to eqn (11.10). Such analysis, although higher throughput, does not discriminate different modes of action of test compounds, for example it will not differentiate competitive from non-competitive compounds. Without additional proof that the interaction of agonist and antagonist is competitive it is more appropriate to use the measured $IC_{50}$ as a measurement of antagonist potency rather than calculating a $K_B$.

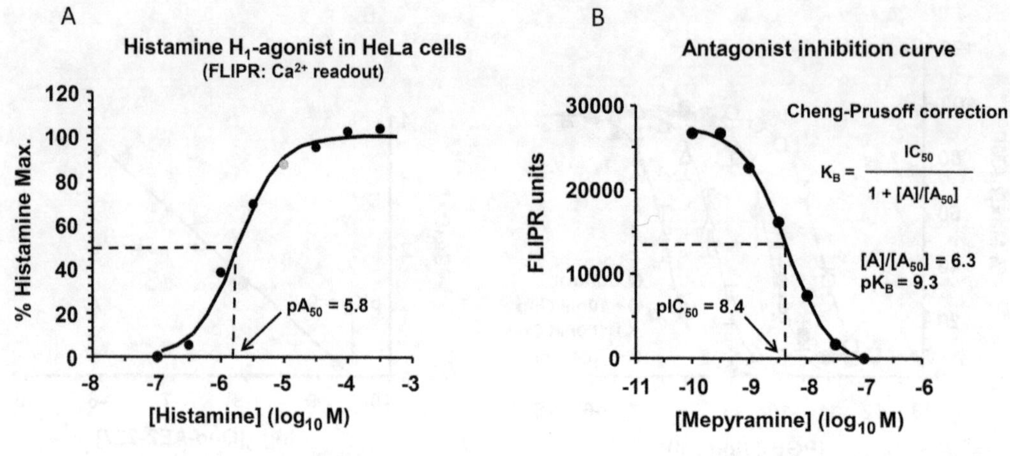


**Figure 11.11** Cheng-Prusoff analysis of antagonism in functional assays. Panel A shows a histamine concentration effect curve generated in HeLa cells which endogenously express the human $H_1$-receptor. 10 μM histamine (grey symbol) was chosen as the concentration of agonist to be used to assess the inhibitory effects of the $H_1$-receptor antagonist mepyramine (Panel B). Mepyramine completely inhibited the $Ca^{2+}$-induced histamine response and yielded a $pIC_{50}$ value of 8.4. As $[A]/[A_{50}]$ was significantly greater than 1, the affinity ($pK_B$) estimate (9.1) is considerably greater than the $pIC_{50}$. In this case the slope of the histamine E/[A] curve was 1 so eqn (11.13) simplifies to the equation shown in panel B. Unpublished data.

### *11.5.4.3 Non-competitive Antagonists*

Non-competitive antagonists bind to receptors and make them functionally inoperative either by preclusion of agonist binding or through some other biochemical mechanism that obviates agonist effect. Under these circumstances, increasing the agonist concentration cannot overcome the effect of the antagonist and therefore a distinctive feature of non-competitive antagonists is the depressive effect they have on the maximal agonist response, that is, they exhibit insurmountable antagonism (Figure 11.12). This mechanism has the potential therapeutic advantage that high concentrations of endogenous agonists, (for example those associated with tumours such as prolactinomas) are less likely to overcome the antagonist effects. The magnitude of the depression will, however, depend on the agonist under study and the system used. This relates to the concept of receptor reserve whereby maximum agonist effects can be achieved at low levels of receptor occupancy (binding). For example, if an agonist can elicit a maximum response by activation of 10% of the receptor population, then there will be a 90% receptor reserve. Receptor reserve depends on both the receptor number ($[R_{tot}]$) and the efficiency of stimulus-response coupling, as well as the intrinsic efficacy of the agonist, hence non-competitive antagonists will have differing capabilities to depress the maximal response to the same agonist in different systems (compare Figures 11.12A and 11.12B). The same will be true for different agonists in the same system. In terms of measuring the potency of insurmountable antagonists the data can be fitted to several models to yield estimates of $K_B$.[95]

Slowly dissociating reversible competitive antagonists exhibit non-competitive behaviour when their rate of offset prevents correct re-equilibration of agonist,

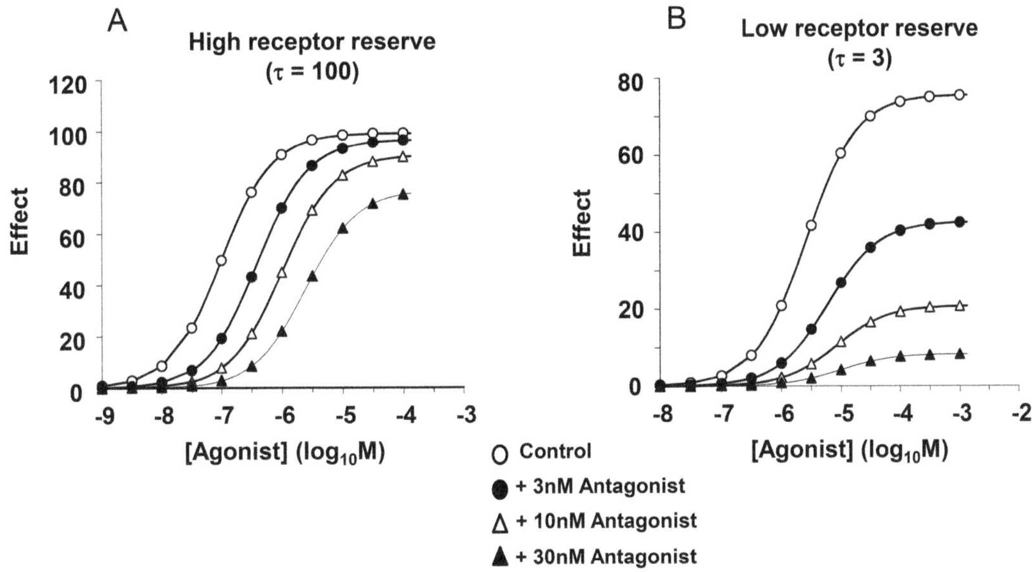


**Figure 11.12** Non-competitive antagonism. Simulations showing the effect of a non-competitive antagonist on responses to the same agonist in a system with high receptor reserve (A) or low receptor reserve (B). Increasing concentrations of the antagonist (3, 10, 30 nM) cause more marked depression of the agonist maximum effect in the low reserve system. Data was simulated using a form of the Operational Model of Agonism that assumes that antagonist binding precludes binding of the agonist.[109] The model parameters used were $E_m$ = 100, $n$ = 1, $\tau$ = 100 (high reserve) or $\tau$ = 3 (low reserve), p$K_A$ = 5.0, p$K_B$ = 9.0.

antagonist and receptors during the period of agonist response measurement. Under these conditions, a pseudo-irreversible blockade of the receptors occurs whereby the agonist cannot access antagonist-bound receptors. Antagonists with very slow off-rates offer a means of extending the duration of action (pharmacodynamic effect) of therapeutic agents distinct from (or complementary to) optimising their pharmacokinetic profiles.[96]

In practice this requires the identification of very high potency (nanomolar–picomolar range) compounds, although factors such as the rate of free diffusion away from the receptor compartment are also important in determining duration of action.

#### *11.5.4.4 Allosteric Antagonists*

The modes of antagonism described above are orthosteric, that is, the antagonist blocks access of the agonist to its binding site through steric hindrance. Allosteric antagonists in contrast bind to their own site on the receptor to induce a change in conformation of the receptor, which in turns alters the affinity or efficacy of the receptor for the agonist. It is now clear that allosteric ligands can both increase (for example benzodiazepines at $GABA_A$ receptors) and decrease the affinity and efficacy of other ligands, so allosteric modulators is a more appropriate term. One of the key properties of allosteric modulators is their saturability of effect, which can be evidenced in functional experiments

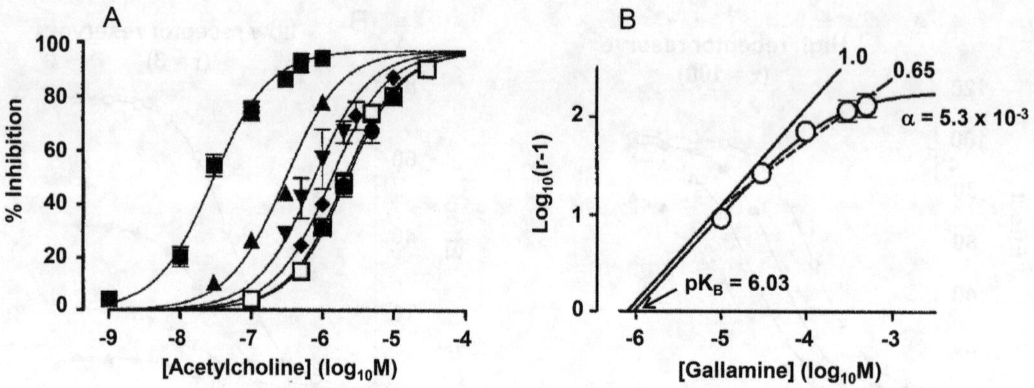


**Figure 11.13** Allosteric antagonism. Panel A shows the effects of acetylcholine (Ach) on the electrically evoked contractions of the guinea pig left atrium in the absence (■) or presence of the allosteric modulator gallamine at the following concentrations: 10 μM (▲), 30 μM (▼), 100 μM (◆), 300 μM (□) and 500 μM (•). Panel B shows the Schild plot of the data shown in A. The solid line (slope = 1) denotes the behaviour expected for a competitive antagonist, whereas the dashed line shows the best fit linear regression (and associated slope factor) through the points. The curve through the points, and associated parameter estimates, represent the fit to an allosteric model. The estimated $pK_B$ was 6.03 and the $\alpha$ values of $5.3 \times 10^{-3}$ equates to a gallamine-induced decrease in the affinity of ACh of 189-fold. Reproduced from ref. 97 with permission from American Society for Pharmacology and Experimental Therapeutics, Copyright 2002.

such as Schild analysis where a curvilinear plot is observed (Figure 11.13; contrast this with the competitive antagonist in Figure 11.10).[97] This results from the fact that while the allosterically modified receptor may have diminished affinity (and/or efficacy) for the agonist, the agonist can still produce receptor activation in the presence of the modulator. A detailed discussion of the complex behaviour of allosteric modulators is beyond the scope of this chapter but the interested reader is referred to some recent reviews.[98–101]

Allosteric modulation offers several potential advantages over orthosteric antagonists. Firstly, they can modify (that is, reduce or increase by a small amount) endogenous agonist signals without completely blocking them, thus allowing fine-tuning of responses. Secondly, there is the potential to increase the duration of allosteric effect by loading the receptor compartment with high concentrations of modulator. Such large concentrations will have no further effect than to prolong the saturated allosteric effect, that is, the saturability of the allosteric ligand can be used to limit effect but increase duration. Another potential advantage of allosterism is increased selectivity. Orthosteric antagonists often have limited selectivity across receptor subtypes, for example, most muscarinic receptor antagonists exhibit poor selectivity between the five known subtypes ($M_1$–$M_5$), presumably because they are competing with acetylcholine for very similar recognition sites. However, the surrounding protein structure of the receptors are sufficiently different to offer the potential for selective stabilization of receptor conformations by allosteric modulators. The identification of several allosteric antagonists with selectivity for the $M_2$-receptor supports this hypothesis.[102] Allosteric ligands also exert effects that are probe dependent, meaning that their effects are not the same towards all agonists (in contrast to orthosteric antagonists which typically show the same degree of blockade of all agonists). This may offer further advantages if different agonists induce different responses (or degrees of response) following receptor activation, that is, allosteric antagonists in theory could block the adverse effect of one agonist without affecting the beneficial effect of another. An example of where this approach may bear fruit is the HIV co-receptor CXCR4, as there is evidence of dissociation of virus binding and chemokine peptide activity.[103] This raises the possibility that allosteric molecules that block HIV entry but do not interfere with SDF-1α-mediated chemokine function could be found, thus avoiding the undesirable side-effects of blocking the important physiological roles of CXCR4. A corollary of the above is that it is important to use the physiological/pathophysiological agonist(s) in experiments where possible rather than synthetic agonists. All of the above-mentioned potential therapeutic advantages of allosteric modulators remain largely theoretical as very few such agents have reached the market. Nevertheless, the approval of the CCR5 antagonist maraviroc for the treatment of HIV demonstrates the feasibility of the approach. This compound inhibits the entry of the virus into cells by binding to a receptor site distinct from where the viral gp120 envelope protein binds.[104,105]

## 11.6 Conclusions

The applications of the principles and various analyses described in this chapter are the cornerstone of structure–activity relationships. They have also significantly advanced our understanding of enzyme inhibitors, receptor agonists and antagonists, and ultimately facilitated the discovery of new drugs. While the measurement of biological activity of compounds emanating directly from the medicinal chemists' bench is just the start of the drug discovery process, design of appropriate assays and understanding compound mode of action influences all subsequent steps of the drug discovery process, including clinical testing. Accordingly, the initial interface between the disciplines of medicinal chemistry and biology remains one of the most important rewarding and exciting areas of drug discovery and development.

## 11.7 Hints and Tips

- Detailed mechanistic understanding of protein targets, and their interaction with ligands, from the molecular to the cellular level is essential to enable discovery of the best molecules, with the right mechanism of action and the highest chance of patient benefit.
- It is important to be aware of the limitations of $IC_{50}$ measurements, and to add further context to inhibition data with respect to time-dependence and substrate concentration effects (amongst others).
- Moving from Structural Activity Relationship (SAR) profiling to Structural Kinetic Relationship (SKR) profiling enables better-informed decision-making, using

kinetic paraments such as $k_{off}$ and $k_{on}$ for optimization, assessment of selectivity and prediction of pharmacological duration of action.

- For agonists, ligand binding assays have the benefit of confirming that compounds bind to the target of interest but give no information on efficacy. Functional assays are required to provide estimates of intrinsic activity or efficacy.
- As drug efficacy is both a drug- and system-dependent parameter, an agonist can demonstrate different behaviours in different systems. Testing agonists in cell systems overexpressing the target of interest offers the advantage of high throughput and robustness, but agonist responses may poorly reflect those in biologically relevant systems due to differences in receptor number and/or coupling and readout. Testing in more relevant (translational) cell or tissue systems is therefore important before progressing to *in vivo* testing.
- Partial agonists are good staging posts towards the design of antagonists.
- Allosteric modulators offer the potential of increased selectivity over orthosteric modulators. As allosteric modulators can block the effects of one agonist and not another it is important to use physiologically relevant agonists in experiments rather than synthetic agonists.

## Key References


- R. A. Copeland, *Evaluation of Enzyme Inhibitors in Drug Discovery: A Guide for Medicinal Chemists and Pharmacologists*, John Wiley & Sons, 2013. This seminal enzymology book is an invaluable resource for all drug-hunters
- T. Kenakin, *Pharmacology in Drug Discovery and Development: Understanding Drug Response*, Academic Press, 2016. This seminal pharmacology book is an invaluable resource for all drug-hunters
- G. K. Walkup, Z. You, P. L. Ross, E. K. Allen, F. Daryaee, M. R. Hale, J. O'Donnell, D. E. Ehmann, V. J. Schuck, E. T. Buurman, A. L. Choy, L. Hajec, K. Murphy-Benenato, V. Marone, S. A. Patey, L. A. Grosser, M. Johnstone, S. G. Walker, P. J. Tonge and S. L. Fisher, *Nat. Chem. Biol.*, 2015, **11**, 416–423 This paper describes a mechanistic pharmacodynamic model that includes drug–target kinetic parameters. It has been applied to predict dose–response curves for inhibitors in an animal model of infection.


## Glossary

**Competitive inhibition** Type of inhibition where inhibitor binds only before the varied substrate is bound.

**Constitutively active receptor** A receptor that displays a biological response in the absence of a bound ligand.

**$IC_{50}$** The inhibitor concentration giving a 50% decrease in rate or maximum phenotypic response *under the specific assay conditions employed.*

**Intrinsic activity** A scale of agonist activity referring to the fractional maximum response to an agonist relative to a standard "full agonist" in the same system (where a full agonist produces the full system maximum response).

**Inverse agonist** A ligand that reverses constitutive receptor activity.

**Irreversible inhibition** Inhibition that cannot be reversed on the timescale of the assay. Truly irreversible inhibitors never dissociate from the target: they are characterised by an inactivation rate constant, not a dissociation constant. It should be noted that irreversible inhibitors do not necessarily have to be covalently bound.

**Mechanism** Comprehensive process by which a reaction takes place. This is determined when all the intermediates, complexes and conformational states of an enzyme or receptor target are characterised, with the rate constants associated with the conversion between them quantified. Term often used in inhibition studies to distinguish between different modes of inhibition.

**Mixed inhibition** Inhibition in which inhibitor binds both before and after the varied substrate, with different affinity.

**Neutral antagonist** A ligand with no activity in the absence of an agonist or inverse agonist but can block the activity of either.

**Non-competitive inhibition** Inhibition in which inhibitor binds with equal affinity both before and after the varied substrate.

**Ordered mechanism (enzyme)** Reaction mechanism in which one of the two substrates preferentially binds to the enzyme first to form a binary complex, followed by the other to form a ternary complex.

**Potency** The concentration (usually molar) of a drug that produces a defined effect. Often, potencies of agonists are defined in terms of $EC_{50}$ ($A_{50}$) or $pEC_{50}$ ($pA_{50}$) values. In the case of agonists, potency is the product of compound binding (affinity) and compound efficacy. For antagonists and inhibitors, it is defined by compound binding (affinity).

**Random mechanism (enzyme)** Reaction mechanism in which either of the two substrates may bind to the enzyme first to form a binary complex, followed by the other to form a ternary complex.

**Reversible inhibition** Inhibition that can be reversed on the timescale of the assay, by competition or dilution. It should be noted that reversible inhibitors are not precluded from forming covalent bonds with the target.

**Slow-binding inhibition** Inhibition which occurs slowly on the timescale of the assay, as the target–inhibitor complex concentration increases to its steady state level.

**Tight-binding inhibition** Type of inhibition occurring under conditions when the concentration of inhibitor required to cause inhibition is similar to the enzyme concentration, leading to depletion of the free inhibitor concentration. This leads to breakdown of the usual assumptions leading to simple inhibition kinetics and requires a more complex rate equation. In receptor pharmacology, this is often defined as receptor (or ligand) depletion.

**Uncompetitive inhibition** Inhibition in which the inhibitor binds only after the varied substrate is bound.

## References


1. T. I. Oprea, C. G. Bologa, S. Brunak, A. Campbell, G. N. Gan, A. Gaulton, S. M. Gomez, R. Guha, A. Hersey, J. Holmes, A. Jadhav, L. J. Jensen, G. L. Johnson, A. Karlson, A. R. Leach, A. Ma'ayan, A. Malovannaya, S. Mani, S. L. Mathias, M. T. McManus, T. F. Meehan, C. von Mering, D. Muthas, D. T. Nguyen, J. P. Overington, G. Papadatos, J. Qin, C. Reich, B. L. Roth, S. C. Schurer, A. Simeonov, L. A. Sklar, N. Southall, S. Tomita, I. Tudose, O. Ursu, D. Vidovic, A. Waller, D. Westergaard, J. J. Yang and G. Zahoranszky-Kohalmi, *Nat. Rev. Drug Discovery*, 2018, **17**, 377.
2. J. P. Overington, B. Al-Lazikani and A. L. Hopkins, *Nat. Rev. Drug Discovery*, 2006, **5**, 993–996.
3. R. A. Copeland, *Anal. Biochem.*, 2003, **320**, 1–12.
4. G. A. Holdgate, T. D. Meek and R. L. Grimley, *Nat. Rev. Drug Discovery*, 2018, **17**, 115–132.
5. R. A. Copeland, D. L. Pompliano and T. D. Meek, *Nat. Rev. Drug Discovery*, 2006, **5**, 730–739.
6. M. E. Bunnage, A. M. Gilbert, L. H. Jones and E. C. Hett, *Nat. Chem. Biol.*, 2015, **11**, 368–372.
7. C. W. Lindsley, Z. Zhao, W. H. Leister, R. G. Robinson, S. F. Barnett, D. Defeo-Jones, R. E. Jones, G. D. Hartman, J. R. Huff and H. E. Huber, *Bioorg. Med. Chem. Lett.*, 2005, **15**, 761–764.
8. S. F. Barnett, D. Defeo-Jones, S. Fu, P. J. Hancock, K. M. Haskell, R. E. Jones, J. A. Kahana, A. M. Kral, K. Leander, L. L. Lee, J. Malinowski, E. M. McAvoy, D. D. Nahas, R. G. Robinson and H. E. Huber, *Biochem. J.*, 2005, **385**, 399–408.
9. J. Solowiej, S. Bergqvist, M. A. McTigue, T. Marrone, T. Quenzer, M. Cobbs, K. Ryan, R. S. Kania, W. Diehl and B. W. Murray, *Biochemistry*, 2009, **48**, 7019–7031.
10. L. M. Stevenson, M. S. Deal, J. C. Hagopian and J. Lew, *Biochemistry*, 2002, **41**, 8528–8534.
11. K. Anderson, J. Yang, K. Koretke, K. Nurse, A. Calamari, R. B. Kirkpatrick, D. Patrick, D. Silva, P. J. Tummino, R. A. Copeland and Z. Lai, *Biochemistry*, 2007, **46**, 10287–10295.
12. H. Gronemeyer, J.-Å. Gustafsson and V. Laudet, *Nat. Rev. Drug Discovery*, 2004, **3**, 950–964.
13. D. Wacker, R. C. Stevens and B. L. Roth, *Cell*, 2017, **170**, 414–427.
14. A. Kuzmichev, K. Nishioka, H. Erdjument-Bromage, P. Tempst and D. Reinberg, *Genes Dev.*, 2002, **16**, 2893–2905.
15. K. Drew, C. Lee, R. L. Huizar, F. Tu, B. Borgeson, C. D. McWhite, Y. Ma, J. B. Wallingford and E. M. Marcotte, *Mol. Syst. Biol.*, 2017, **13**, 932.
16. S. Krishnaswamy and A. Betz, *Biochemistry*, 1997, **36**, 12080–12086.
17. M. R. Harpel, K. Y. Horiuchi, Y. Luo, L. Shen, W. Jiang, D. J. Nelson, K. C. Rogers, C. P. Decicco and R. A. Copeland, *Biochemistry*, 2002, **41**, 6398–6407.
18. M. M. Keshwani, X. Gao and T. K. Harris, *J. Biol. Chem.*, 2009, **284**, 22611–22624.
19. X. Gao and T. K. Harris, *J. Biol. Chem.*, 2006, **281**, 21670–21681.
20. C. Pargellis, T. Liang, L. Churchill, P. F. Cirillo, T. Gilmore, A. G. Graham, P. M. Grob, E. R. Hickey, N. Moss and S. Pav, *Nat. Struct. Mol. Biol.*, 2002, **9**, 268.
21. W. Davidson, L. Frego, G. W. Peet, R. R. Kroe, M. E. Labadia, S. M. Lukas, R. J. Snow, S. Jakes, C. A. Grygon and C. Pargellis, *Biochemistry*, 2004, **43**, 11658–11671.
22. Y. Li, P. Trojer, C. F. Xu, P. Cheung, A. Kuo, W. J. Drury 3rd, Q. Qiao, T. A. Neubert, R. M. Xu, O. Gozani and D. Reinberg, *J. Biol. Chem.*, 2009, **284**, 34283–34295.
23. M. B. Poulin, J. L. Schneck, R. E. Matico, P. J. McDevitt, M. J. Huddleston, W. Hou, N. W. Johnson, S. H. Thrall, T. D. Meek and V. L. Schramm, *Proc. Natl. Acad. Sci. U. S. A.*, 2016, **113**, 1197–1201.
24. H. Wapenaar and F. J. Dekker, *Clin. Epigenet.*, 2016, **8**, 59.
25. A. Bar-Even, E. Noor, Y. Savir, W. Liebermeister, D. Davidi, D. S. Tawfik and R. Milo, *Biochemistry*, 2011, **50**, 4402–4410.
26. X. Lu, J. B. Smaill and K. Ding, *Angew. Chem.*, 2020, **59**, 13764–13776.
27. M. M. Attwood, D. Fabbro, A. V. Sokolov, S. Knapp and H. B. Schiöth, *Nat. Rev. Drug Discovery*, 2021, **20**, 839–861.
28. H. Hirai, H. Sootome, Y. Nakatsuru, K. Miyama, S. Taguchi, K. Tsujioka, Y. Ueno, H. Hatch, P. K. Majumder and B.-S. Pan, *Mol. Cancer Ther.*, 2010, **9**, 1956–1967.
29. G. L. Gonzalez-Del Pino, K. Li, E. Park, A. M. Schmoker, B. H. Ha and M. J. Eck, *Proc. Natl. Acad. Sci. U. S. A.*, 2021, **118**, e2107207118.
30. D. C. Swinney, *Nat. Rev. Drug Discovery*, 2004, **3**, 801–808.
31. A. S. Nies and M. J. Gresser, *Adv. Protein Chem.*, 2001, **56**, 115–141.
32. E. R. Wood, A. T. Truesdale, O. B. McDonald, D. Yuan, A. Hassell, S. H. Dickerson, B. Ellis, C. Pennisi, E. Horne and K. Lackey, *Cancer Res.*, 2004, **64**, 6652–6659.
33. G. Dahl and T. Akerud, *Drug Discovery Today*, 2013, **18**, 697–707.

34. H. C. Cheng, *J. Pharmacol. Toxicol. Methods*, 2001, **46**, 61–71.
35. S. J. Teague, *Nat. Rev. Drug Discovery*, 2003, **2**, 527–541.
36. W. E. de Witte, M. Danhof, P. H. van der Graaf and E. C. de Lange, *Trends Pharmacol. Sci.*, 2016, **37**, 831–842.
37. R. A. Copeland, *Evaluation of Enzyme Inhibitors in Drug Discovery: A Guide for Medicinal Chemists and Pharmacologists*, John Wiley & Sons, 2013.
38. A. Cornish-Bowden, *Perspect. Sci.*, 2014, **1**, 121–125.
39. A. Cornish-Bowden, *FEBS Lett.*, 1986, **203**, 3–6.
40. K. P. Burnham and D. R. Anderson, *Model Selection and Multimodel Inference: A Practical Information-Theoretic Approach*, Springer New York, 2007.
41. R. G. Lomax, *Statistical Concepts: A Second Course*, Lawrence Erlbaum Associates Publishers, Mahwah, NJ, US, 3rd edn, 2007.
42. C. Yung-Chi and W. H. Prusoff, *Biochem. Pharmacol.*, 1973, **22**, 3099–3108.
43. P. J. Tonge, *ACS Chem. Neurosci.*, 2018, **9**, 29–39.
44. H. Lu, J. N. Iuliano and P. J. Tonge, *Curr. Opin. Chem. Biol.*, 2018, **44**, 101–109.
45. J. F. Morrison and C. T. Walsh, *Adv. Enzymol. Relat. Areas Mol. Biol.*, 1988, **61**, 201–301.
46. J. F. Morrison, *Biochim. Biophys. Acta*, 1969, **185**, 269–286.
47. J. Simithy, N. R. Fuanta, M. Alturki, J. V. Hobrath, A. E. Wahba, I. Pina, J. Rath, M. T. Hamann, J. DeRuiter, D. C. Goodwin and A. I. Calderón, *Biochemistry*, 2018, **57**, 4923–4933.
48. M. J. Sculley, J. F. Morrison and W. W. Cleland, *Biochim. Biophys. Acta, Protein Struct. Mol. Enzymol.*, 1996, **1298**, 78–86.
49. R. A. Copeland, A. Basavapathruni, M. Moyer and M. P. Scott, *Anal. Biochem.*, 2011, **416**, 206–210.
50. K. A. Johnson, *Methods Enzymol.*, 2009, **467**, 601–626.
51. P. Ayaz, D. Andres, D. A. Kwiatkowski, C.-C. Kolbe, P. Lienau, G. Siemeister, U. Lücking and C. M. Stegmann, *ACS Chem. Biol.*, 2016, **11**, 1710–1719.
52. R. A. Copeland, *Nat. Rev. Drug Discovery*, 2016, **15**, 87–95.
53. G. S. Van Aller, M. B. Pappalardi, H. M. Ott, E. Diaz, M. Brandt, B. J. Schwartz, W. H. Miller, D. Dhanak, M. T. McCabe and S. K. Verma, *ACS Chem. Biol.*, 2014, **9**, 622–629.
54. K. P. Cusack, Y. Wang, M. Z. Hoemann, J. Marjanovic, R. G. Heym and A. Vasudevan, *Bioorg. Med. Chem. Lett.*, 2015, **25**, 2019–2027.
55. A. Goldstein, *J. Gen. Physiol.*, 1944, **27**, 529–580.
56. D. J. Murphy, *Anal. Biochem.*, 2004, **327**, 61–67.
57. D. S. Johnson, E. Weerapana and B. F. Cravatt, *Future Med. Chem.*, 2010, **2**, 949–964.
58. S. De Cesco, J. Kurian, C. Dufresne, A. Mittermaier and N. Moitessier, *Eur. J. Med. Chem.*, 2017, **58**, 138, 96–114.
59. J. M. Strelow, *SLAS Discovery*, 2017, **22**, 3–20.
60. B. F. Krippendorff, R. Neuhaus, P. Lienau, A. Reichel and W. Huisinga, *J. Biomol. Screening*, 2009, **14**, 913–923.
61. A. Thorarensen, P. Balbo, M. E. Banker, R. M. Czerwinski, M. Kuhn, T. S. Maurer, J.-B. Telliez, F. Vincent and A. J. Wittwer, *Bioorg. Med. Chem.*, 2021, **29**, 115865.
62. X. Zhai, R. A. Ward, P. Doig and A. Argyrou, *Biochemistry*, 2020, **59**, 1428–1441.
63. T. Mathieson, H. Franken, J. Kosinski, N. Kurzawa, N. Zinn, G. Sweetman, D. Poeckel, V. S. Ratnu, M. Schramm, I. Becher, M. Steidel, K.-M. Noh, G. Bergamini, M. Beck, M. Bantscheff and M. M. Savitski, *Nat. Commun.*, 2018, **9**, 689.
64. M. Kostic and L. H. Jones, *Trends Pharmacol. Sci.*, 2020, **41**, 305–317.
65. M. E. Bunnage, E. L. P. Chekler and L. H. Jones, *Nat. Chem. Biol.*, 2013, **9**, 195–199.
66. L. J. Gordon, M. Allen, P. Artursson, M. M. Hann, B. J. Leavens, A. Mateus, S. Readshaw, K. Valko, G. J. Wayne and A. West, *J. Biomol. Screening*, 2016, **21**, 156–164.
67. G. K. Walkup, Z. You, P. L. Ross, E. K. Allen, F. Daryaee, M. R. Hale, J. O'Donnell, D. E. Ehmann, V. J. Schuck, E. T. Buurman, A. L. Choy, L. Hajec, K. Murphy-Benenato, V. Marone, S. A. Patey, L. A. Grosser, M. Johnstone, S. G. Walker, P. J. Tonge and S. L. Fisher, *Nat. Chem. Biol.*, 2015, **11**, 416–423.
68. S. P. Alexander, E. Kelly, N. V. Marrion, J. A. Peters, E. Faccenda, S. D. Harding, A. J. Pawson, J. L. Sharman, C. Southan, O. P. Buneman, J. A. Cidlowski, A. Christopoulos, A. P. Davenport, D. Fabbro, M. Spedding, J. Striessnig and J. A. Davies, *Br. J. Pharmacol.*, 2017, **174**(Suppl 1), S1–S16.
69. E. A. Everington, A. G. Gibbard, J. D. Swinny and M. Seifi, *Front. Mol. Neurosci.*, 2018, **11**, 18.
70. D. M. Rosenbaum, S. G. F. Rasmussen and B. K. Kobilka, *Nature*, 2009, **459**, 356–363.
71. E. R. Weikum, X. Liu and E. A. Ortlund, *Protein Sci.*, 2018, **27**, 1876–1892.
72. X. Du, Y. Li, Y. L. Xia, S. M. Ai, J. Liang, P. Sang, X. L. Ji and S. Q. Liu, *Int. J. Mol. Sci.*, 2016, **17**, 144.

73. P. G. Strange, *Br. J. Pharmacol.*, 2008, **153**, 1353–1363.
74. D. Jack, *Br. J. Clin. Pharmacol.*, 1991, **31**, 501–514.
75. P. Buchwald, *Front. Pharmacol.*, 2019, **10**, 605.
76. T. Kenakin, *Pharmacology in Drug Discovery and Development: Understanding Drug Response*, Academic Press, 2016.
77. T. Kenakin, *Pharmacol. Rev.*, 2019, **71**, 267–315.
78. M. P. Stapleton, *Texas Heart Inst. J.*, 1997, **24**, 336.
79. M. E. Parsons, *Receptor Based Drug Design*, ed. P. Leff, Marcel Dekker, Inc, New York, 1998, vol. 89, pp. 195–206.
80. T. Costa and A. Herz, *Proc. Natl. Acad. Sci. U. S. A.*, 1989, **86**, 7321; P. Chidiac, T. E. Hebert, M. Valiquette, M. Dennis and M. Bouvier, *Mol. Pharmacol.*, 1994, **45**, 490.
81. P. Leff, *Trends Pharmacol. Sci.*, 1995, **16**, 89.
82. K. A. Bennett, B. Tehan, G. Lebon, C. G. Tate, M. Weir, F. H. Marshall and C. J. Langmead, *Mol. Pharmacol.*, 2013, **83**, 949.
83. M. C. Michel and S. J. Charlton, *Mol. Pharmacol.*, 2018, **93**(4), 259–265.
84. S. M. DeWire, D. S. Yamashita, D. H. Rominger, G. Liu, C. L. Cowan, T. M. Graczyk, X. T. Chen, P. M. Pitis, D. Gotchev and C. Yuan, *et al.*, A G protein-biased ligand at the $\mu$-opioid receptor is potently analgesic with reduced gastrointestinal and respiratory dysfunction compared with morphine, *J. Pharmacol. Exp. Ther.*, 2013, **344**, 708–717.
85. A. Gillis, A. B. Gondin, A. Kliewer, J. Sanchez, H. D. Lim, C. Alamein, P. Manandhar, M. Santiago, S. Fritzwanker, F. Schmiedel, T. A. Katte, T. Reekie, N. L. Grimsey, M. Kassiou, B. Kellam, C. Krasel, M. L. Halls, M. Connor, J. R. Lane, S. Schulz, M. J. Christie and M. Canals, Low intrinsic efficacy for G protein activation can explain the improved side effect profiles of new opioid agonists, *Sci. Signaling*, 2020, **13**(625), eaaz3140.
86. T. R. Miller, D. G. Witte, L. M. Ireland, C. H. Kang, J. M. Roch, J. N. Masters, T. A. Esbenshade and A. A. Hancock, *J. Biomol. Screening*, 1999, **4**, 249.
87. R. F. Furchgott, *Adv Drug Res*, ed. N. J. Harper and A. B. Simmonds, Academic Press, New York, 1966, vol. 3, pp. 21–55.
88. M. K. James, P. H. Morgan and H. F. Leighton, *J. Pharmacol. Exp. Ther.*, 1989, **249**, 61.
89. Y. C. Cheng and W. H. Prusoff, *Biochem. Pharmacol.*, 1973, **22**, 3099.
90. H. O. Schild, *Br. J. Pharmacol.*, 1949, **4**, 277.
91. O. Arunlakshana and H. O. Schild, *Br. J. Pharmacol.*, 1959, **14**, 48.
92. S. J. Lydford, K. C. W. McKechnie and P. Leff, *Prostaglandins*, 1996, **52**, 125b.
93. T. P. Kenakin, *Can. J. Physiol. Pharmacol.*, 1982, **60**, 249.
94. P. Leff and I. G. Dougall, *Trends Pharmacol. Sci.*, 1993, **14**, 110.
95. T. P. Kenakin, *A Pharmacology Primer: Theory, Applications and Methods*, ed. T. Kenakin, Elsevier Academic Press, Burlington MA USA, 3rd edn, 2009, ch. 6, pp. 116–119.
96. D. C. Swinney, *Curr. Opin. Drug Discovery Dev.*, 2009, **12**, 31; G. Vauquelin and S. J. Charlton, *Br. J. Pharmacol.*, 2010, **161**, 488.
97. A. Christopoulos and T. Kenakin, *Pharmacol. Rev.*, 2002, **54**, 323.
98. M. De Amici, C. Dallanoce, U. Holzgrabe, C. Tränkle and K. Mohr, *Med. Res. Rev.*, 2010, **30**, 463; J. P. Changeux, *Annu. Rev. Biophys.*, 2012, **41**, 103.
99. P. Keov, P. M. Sexton and A. Christopoulos, *Neuropharmacology*, 2011, **60**, 24.
100. C. E. Müller, A. C. Schiedel and Y. Baqi, *Pharmacol. Ther.*, 2012, **135**, 292; S. Urwyler, *Pharmacol. Rev.*, 2011, **63**, 59.
101. D. J. Scholten, M. Canals, D. Maussang, L. Roumen, M. J. Smit, M. Wijtmans, C. de Graaf, H. F. Vischer and R. Leurs, *Br. J. Pharmacol.*, 2012, **165**, 1617.
102. C. E. Müller, A. C. Schiedel and Y. Baqi, *Pharmacol. Ther.*, 2012, **135**, 292.
103. N. Heveker, M. Montes, L. Germeroth, A. Amara, A. Trautmann, M. Alizon and J. Schneider-Mergener, *Curr. Biol.*, 1998, **8**, 369.
104. C. Watson, S. Jenkinson, W. Kazmierski and T. Kenakin, *Mol. Pharmacol.*, 2005, **67**, 1268.
105. V. M. Muniz-Medina, S. Jones, J. M. Maglich, C. Galardi, R. E. Hollingsworth, W. M. Kazmierski, R. G. Ferris, M. P. Edelstein, K. E. Chiswell and T. P. Kenakin, *Mol. Pharmacol.*, 2009, **75**, 490.
106. J. W. Black and P. Leff, *Proc. R. Soc. London, Ser. B*, 1983, **220**, 141.
107. P. Leff and I. G. Dougall, *Br. J. Pharmacol.*, 1989, **96**, 702.
108. M. J. Ratcliffe, A. Walding, P. A. Shelton, A. Flaherty and I. G. Dougall, *Eur. Respir. J.*, 2007, **29**, 986.
109. J. A. Schmidt, F. M. Bell, E. Akam, C. Marshall, I. A. Dainty, A. Heinemann, I. G. Dougall, R. V. Bonnert and C. A. Sargent, *Br. J. Pharmacol.*, 2013, **168**, 1626.

# 12 Animal Models: Practical Use and Considerations

L. A. Lione*[a], M. Lanigan[a,b] and A. Fisher[b,c]

[a]University of Hertfordshire de Havilland Campus, Hatfield, AL10 9EU, UK; [b]Transpharmation Ltd., The London Bioscience Innovation Centre, 2 Royal College Street, London, NW1 0NH, UK; [c]Pharmaceuticals, Sovereign House, Histon, Cambridge, CB24 9BZ
*E-mail: l.lione@herts.ac.uk

## 12.1 Introduction

It is commonly accepted that, in general, animals, particularly mammalian species, share many common aspects that engender and sustain life. For example, mammals have a complex and dynamic central and autonomic nervous system that regulates multifaceted physiological processes such as digestion, body temperature regulation, respiration, circulation and so on. Thus, the advancement of biomedical sciences is and has been substantially predicated on the thesis that animal physiology can be exploited to learn human biology. Over the past century a wide variety of animal models used in research (including, but not limited to *Drosophila*, *C. elegans*, mice, rats, rabbits, dogs, cats and non-human primates) have been integral to advancing our knowledge of disease, to test new drugs, and to assure their safety before moving them into the clinical phase with human subjects. The use of these animal models in research has resulted in the advancement of knowledge for how diseases affect animals and humans and has also led to the effective and safe treatment of disease symptoms or in many cases disease cures. Unfortunately, the translatability of animal model data into the clinical arena continues to be subject to seemingly everlasting debate of the utility, validity and limitations of animal models[1] (Table 12.1). Nonetheless, due to significant pipeline attrition of new drugs in patient trials, the pharmaceutical industry is utilizing several strategies, including improved pharmacokinetic-pharmacodynamic (PKPD) and mechanistic approaches, to enhance the probability of successfully advancing novel compounds from the bench to human patients.

The Handbook of Medicinal Chemistry: Principles and Practice, 2nd Edition
Edited by Simon E. Ward and Andrew M. Davis

Published by the Royal Society of Chemistry, www.rsc.org

**Table 12.1** Balancing the rationale use of animal models in drug discovery. Reproduced from ref. 1 with permission from the Royal Society of Chemistry.

| Limitations | Advantages |
|---|---|
| Inconsistent clinical pharmacological translatability *e.g.* stroke, chronic pain, Alzheimer's disease | Animal models are the most relevant available for modelling *in vivo* disease processes (*e.g.* hypertension) |
| Acute uniform models of acute responses in adult animals (*e.g.* amyloid deposition models) | Historically used to inform physiology/pathology |
| Major anatomical differences (*e.g.* prefrontal cortical processing in schizophrenia) | Useful for PKPD modelling (*e.g.* allometric scaling for human dosing) |
| Comparable human endpoint measurements are often difficult in animals (*e.g.* reported level of pain intensity, delusions) | Integrates "efficacy" with safety and disease biology |
| Animal models do not capture the chronicity or the heterogeneity of human diseases (*e.g.* neuropathic pain, Alzheimer's disease) | |
| Lack of a PD target engagement biomarker in animals (*e.g.* CNS targets often require fPET, phMRI) | |
| PK/PD and TI to model efficacious dosing is unknown for novel "first in class" unprecedented (novel) targets | |

In this chapter we make a distinction between pathway biology pharmacodynamic (PD), disease mechanism and toxicology animal models (Figure 12.1). PKPD modelling is applied to all types of animal model. We define a pathway biology PD model as being a model with a relatively high throughput/quick turnaround and a relatively simple measurable output, or endpoint, that informs on drug action (efficacy/potency) and target engagement along a specific biological process or pathway (Figure 12.1). While this type of model can be used in any phase of drug discovery (*i.e.* target validation, lead identification or lead optimization), it is more often used in lead optimization, where there are efforts by a scientific team to screen and advance the "best" *in vivo* compound from an inventory of related drugs/drug series that may share similar physiochemical and pharmacological properties. The next step is to screen/profile the lead molecule(s) in a disease-related mechanism model (Figure 12.1). No animal model encapsulates all the complexities (*i.e.* chronicity, heterogeneity, *etc.*) of human disease (see Section 12.4 on validity). Indeed, these models typically only share some limited feature(s) of human diseases, hence they are "models of" human disease/mechanism. Consequently, we refer to this second type of model as being a disease mechanism model (Figure 12.1) which ideally (as reviewed by McGonigle and Ruggeri[2]) should possess: (a) similar genetic basis, (b) similar anatomy and physiology, (c) similar pathological response(s) and underlying mechanism(s), (d) similar phenotypic endpoints as clinical studies, and be (e) responsive to known drugs with clinical efficacy and (f) predictive of clinical efficacy (Figure 12.2). For many human diseases, both (e) responsive to known drugs with clinical efficacy and (f) predictive of clinical efficacy are still unknown (*e.g.* disease-modifying therapies for Alzheimer's disease (AD)). Disease mechanism model screening will identify the "best" *in vivo* compound based upon its PKPD, its exposure and efficacy on its target mechanism (minimum anticipated biological effect level

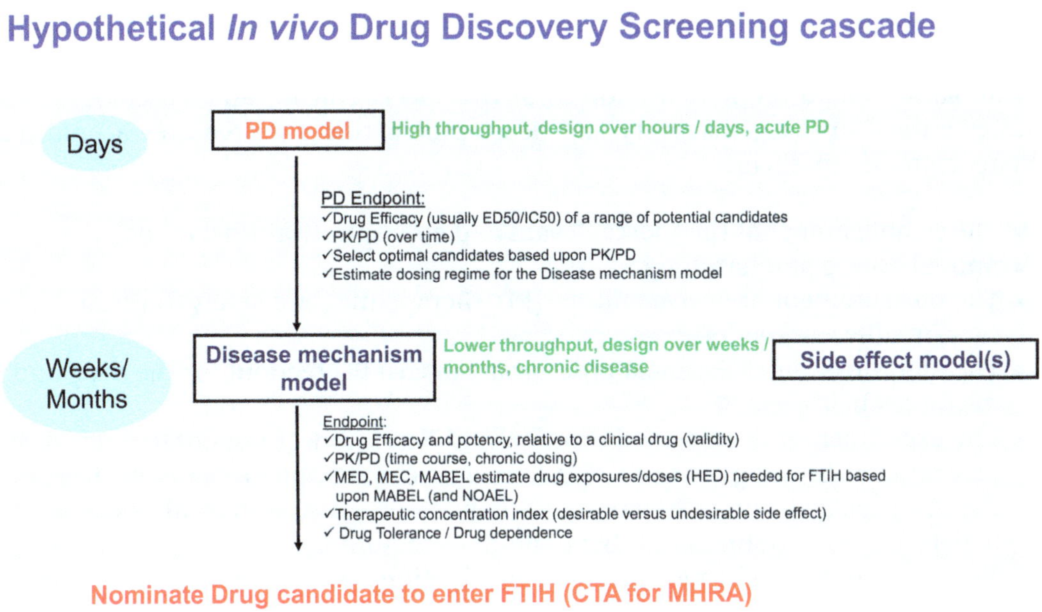


**Figure 12.1** Hypothetical *in vivo* drug discovery screening cascade. PD (pharmacodynamic), FTIH (first time in human); CTA (clinical trial authorization); HED (human equivalent dose); MED (minimum effective dose); MEC (minimum effective concentration); MABEL (minimum anticipated biological effect level); NOAEL (no observed adverse effect level), MHRA (Medicines & Healthcare products Regulatory Agency).

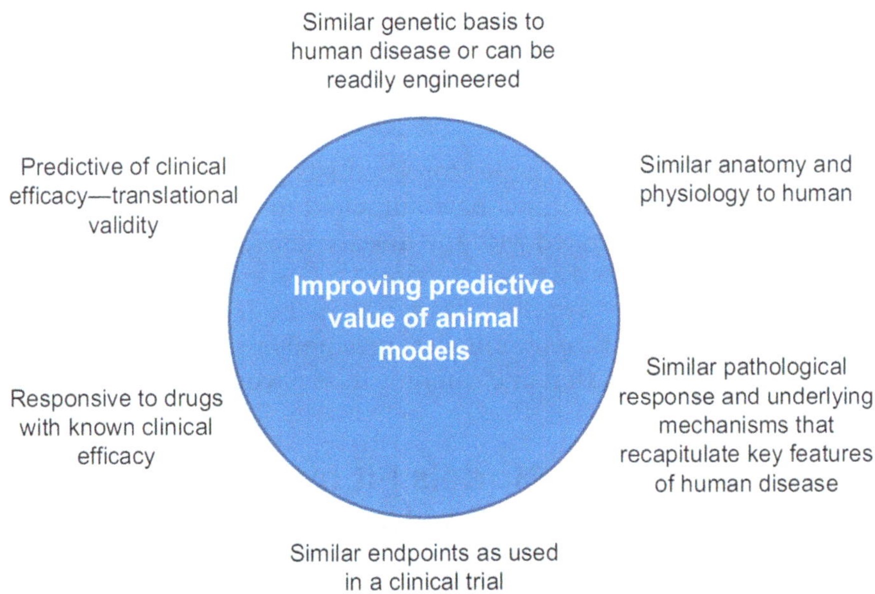


**Figure 12.2** The ideal disease mechanism animal model. Validity characteristics if aligned may improve the translatability of disease mechanism animal models. Reproduced from ref. 1 with permission from the Royal Society of Chemistry.

(MABEL)) and its safety (no adverse effect level (NOAEL), toxicology model screening) and will then be nominated to enter first time in humans (FTIH) clinical trials.

The planning and implementation of *in vivo* PKPD efficacy and toxicology animal studies critical for drug discovery and development therefore requires a multidisciplinary team of experts in:

- The establishment of the most relevant and appropriate animal model(s).
- Animal dosing and handling.
- The measurement of *in vivo* efficacy (PD, therapeutic) and safety (undesirable efficacy) in different models.
- The identification of the most appropriate *in vivo* PD readout for the drug and for the model being tested.
- The experimental design, optimization and execution of quantitative PD/disease mechanism/toxicology models and/or measurements, including consideration of the 3Rs (Replacement, Reduction and Refinement) and statistical power analysis to determine the optimal number of animals required.
- The measurement of drug concentrations in different tissue matrices.
- The evaluation and analysis of *in vivo* PK data.
- The analysis of relationships between PK, PD and efficacy (therapeutic and undesirable).

The aim of this chapter is to provide information on the basic principles of the effective use of pathway biology PD models, disease mechanism models and toxicology models for drug discovery. We discuss practical aspects of experimental design for *in vivo* studies and offer useful considerations for the medicinal chemist and other biomedical scientists. Ethics, relevant species and strain choice, group size, statistics, PD end point and PKPD relationship are addressed. Additionally, examples of pathway biology PD, disease mechanism animal models and toxicology models are provided in relation to their validity.

It is worth remembering that in order for scientists to successfully model relevant aspects of a human disease, they must have sufficient understanding of the pathological mechanism changes associated with the disease itself, the clinical phenotype and its underlying causality (Figure 12.2, see Section 12.4 on validity). The clinical phenotype and underlying causality are not always understood. As a consequence, *in vivo* researchers can only model pathophysiological mechanisms that are currently available to them, the implication being that one can only model what one knows at that time.

## 12.2 Where Do Animal Models Fit into the Process of Drug Discovery and Development?

Animal models are essential in the pharmaceutical drug discovery and development process to: (a) characterize disease pathophysiology and target pathway mechanisms (target validation), (b) discover new drug-target molecules and PD biomarkers (target identification/engagement), (c) evaluate evidence of downstream pharmacology, *i.e.* PD response (lead optimization, proof of mechanism) and (d) determine safety margins, *i.e.* PD *versus* toxicity responses to estimate clinical dosing regimens (Figure 12.3).

A major use of animal models is to explore the relationship between the drug's PK profile (absorption, distribution, metabolism, clearance and exposure (ADME)), the timing and magnitude of a PD biomarker (*e.g.* inhibition of a cellular response, inhibition of mediator production, cell proliferation or migration) and/or a clinically meaningful PD phenotypic response (*e.g.* anti-inflammatory, analgesic, anxiolytic, anti-cancer) (Figure 12.4). Animal models are essential to demonstrate whether the new drug is orally bioavailable and to gain a first insight into *in vivo* PK parameters that can subsequently be used to predict human values (Figures 12.4 and 12.5). Ideally, the data from the animal models should support an integrative platform of evidence, building with a line of sight to a clinical proof of concept (Figure 12.5). Mathematical modelling and *in silico* simulation experiments are critical parts in formulating the PKPD hypothesis, which can then inform the design of later preclinical (Figures 12.3 and 12.5) and subsequently clinical studies (Figure 12.4). Understanding the PKPD profile builds confidence that modulation of the chosen biological target mechanism is indeed driving the pharmacology, rather than some as yet undefined off-target effect.

There is a key difference between a PD biomarker readout and a pharmacology efficacy readout. The former is typically a molecular event taking place in the close proximity of the target of a therapeutic intervention, whereas the latter is a later event, in most cases relying on clinical phenotypic measures (see also Section 12.3). A PD biomarker is defined as "a characteristic that is objectively measured and assessed as an indicator of normal biological or pathogenic processes or pharmacological responses to a therapeutic intervention". PD biomarkers are a critical tool in preclinical decision-making

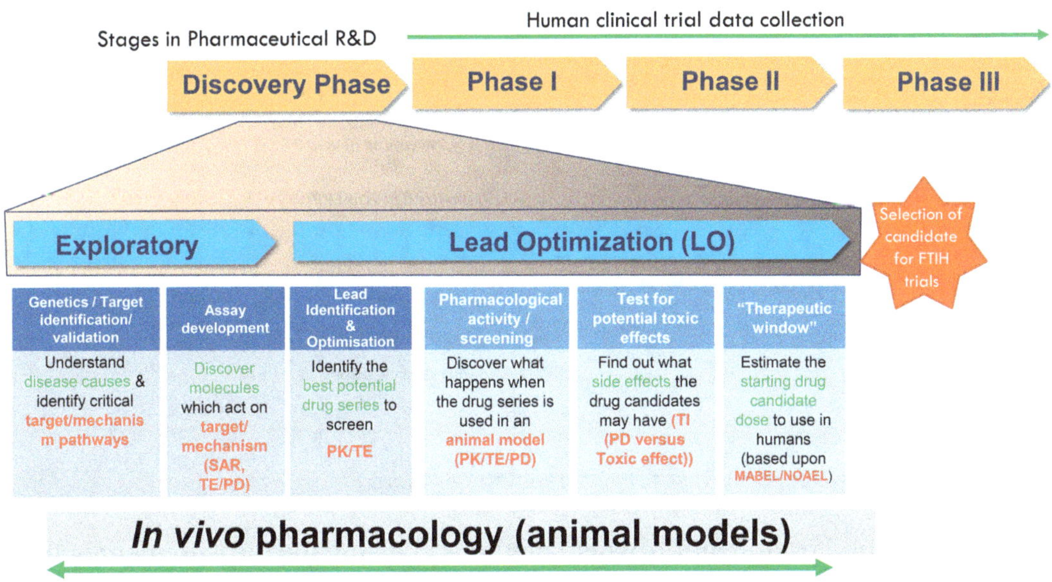


**Figure 12.3** Where animals fit into the drug discovery and development process. Image Credit: Dr Sorif Uddin.

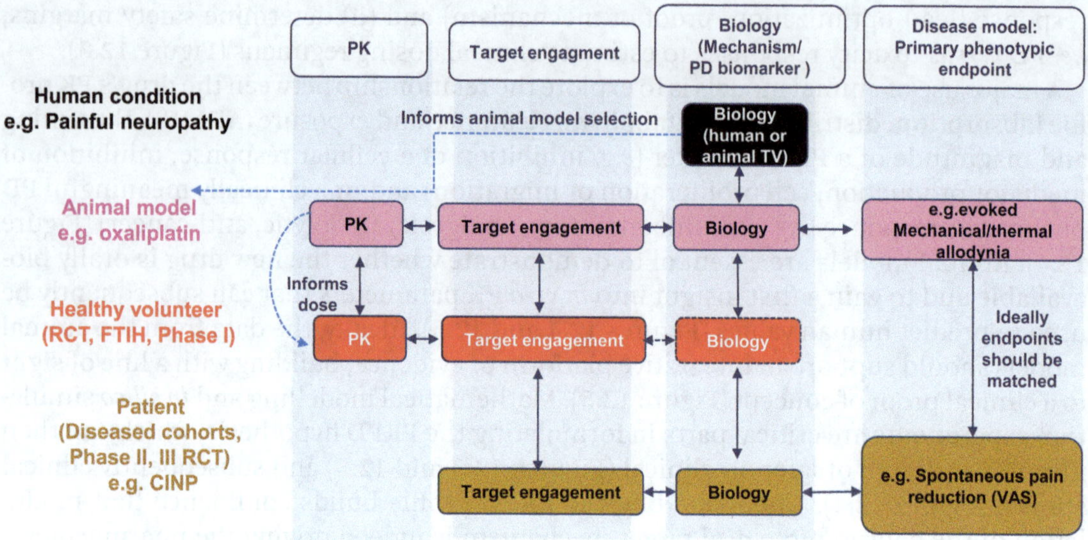


**Figure 12.4** Integrated bidirectional research approach linking animal and human PK, target engagement, PD biomarker, PKPD and pharmacology phenotypic data. RCT (randomised clinical trial), FTIH (first time in human), TV (target validation), CINP (chemotherapy-induced neuropathic pain), VAS (visual analogue scale). Reproduced from ref. 4, https://doi.org/10.3389/fphar.2020.614990, under the terms of the CC BY 4.0 license, https://creativecommons.org/licenses/by/4.0/.

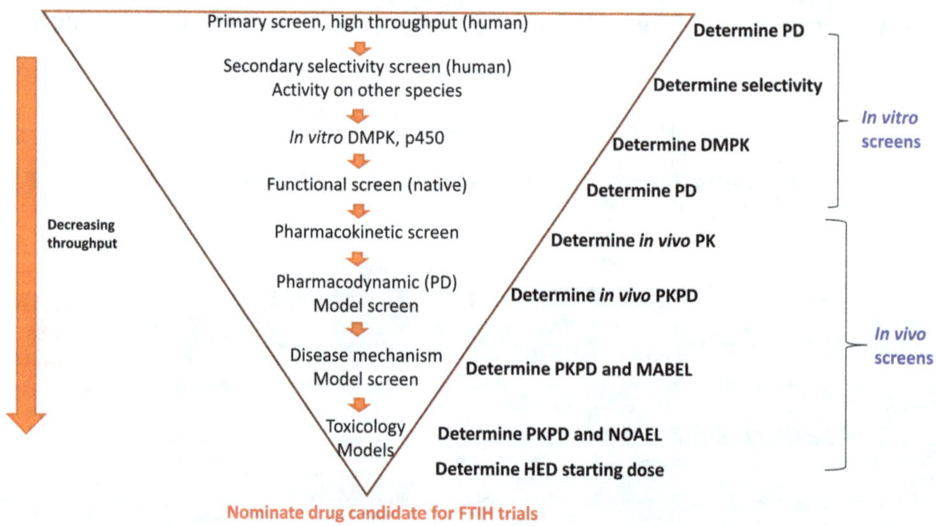


**Figure 12.5** Hypothetical drug discovery screening cascade.

and lead compound prioritization, where methods allowing the measurement of drug–target interactions in cells and tissues can be used *in vivo* to better understand the PKPD relationship and assess whether engagement of the target has any impact on a disease phenotype. PD biomarkers are also critical components of the translational process, allowing a direct link between what can objectively be measured in the animal model and the human model (volunteers and patients) (Figure 12.4). However, developing and validating a PD biomarker for a drug target can be a major undertaking in both time and complexity, especially in the context of developing first in class novel chemical entities (NCEs) and targets with a central nervous system (CNS) site of action where often pharmacological magnetic resonance imaging (MRI) or functional positron emission tomography (PET) ligands are required.

Important questions that can be answered with PKPD animal models include:

- What degree of "occupancy" of the biological target mechanism is required to generate a meaningful PD response? The PD effect is often produced by the drug binding to its target receptor to either activate or antagonise the receptor. For example, if the measured PD effect is maximum and the fractional occupancy of the biological target is known, the effect for any given concentration of a ligand could be determined, *e.g.* the neurokinin-1(NK-1) receptor antagonist, antiemetic aprepitant at clinically safe and tolerable doses, occupies and engages >90% of its central target.[3]
- What degree of "occupancy" of the biological target mechanism is required in the CNS (*e.g.* CNS tissue, cerebrospinal fluid (CSF)) and plasma to generate a meaningful PD response?
- Does the drug have to be present at high enough concentrations to engage the biological mechanism throughout the dosing period, or can the drug use a hit-and-run mechanism (*i.e.* maximum attainable plasma concentration ($C_{max}$)-driven PKPD relationship)?
- How long does the target need to be engaged before a meaningful PD effect can be measured?
- How do the PK and PD profiles relate to any adverse events that can also be measured (maybe at higher doses)?
- Understanding and modelling PKPD in one animal species can then allow predictions to be made for other species. Comparing PKPD relationships across multiple species allows one to estimate the PKPD relationship in humans prior to clinical trials.

It is good practice to consider the following guiding principles before embarking on designing PKPD *in vivo* models. Although some practical aspects of animal modelling may vary across different research areas, there is unanimous agreement on how to build the animal model or a tool, in order to study and understand the PKPD relationship and achieve the end product.

*Specificity Models*: Should be induced with specific stimulus that is relevant to the target/pathway of interest. In order to understand PKPD, researchers must understand their model and select a biomarker that links to the clinical end point (*i.e.* which cells or tissue produce biomarkers/readouts of interest). It is worth remembering some basic principles: (a) identify the tissue of interest, (b) understand the target expression of the tissue and (c) understand compound exposure at the site of action. The combination of all these parameters can enable assessment of both target engagement and the PKPD relationship.

*Robustness*: The induction of the model needs to be sufficient in magnitude (assay window) in order to allow differentiation between the compound doses (*i.e.* treatment groups). Although this is often assay dependent, any assay windows less than three-fold are generally considered insufficient for detailed pharmacological evaluation and PKPD assessment, particularly if there is a high degree of experimental variance around the treatment means.

*Reproducibility*: It is essential to have a reproducible response in the model, enabling direct comparison across different experiments. Monitoring baseline and induction responses longitudinally is essential.

*Simplicity*: Whenever possible, models should be simplified. Complex model design with multiple or cocktail drug induction challenges tends to result in a large number of variables, which in turn often leads to a reduction in reproducibility.

*Tools and Reagents*: It is important to have adequate tools in order to generate a robust PKPD model. For example, the use of supra-maximal doses of human-specific reagents (*i.e.* cytokines), in order to overcome non-specificity of the reagents. The implications of using non-specific tools can often lead to an off-target effect or response within the model.

In addition to the aforementioned, it is also very important that *in vivo* pharmacology and PK data are captured within a designated data base, in order to be available for further analysis, monitoring reproducibility and legal/regulatory purposes.

Target understanding and the relationship between exposure and PD response in a translatable animal model is critical in enhancing the human dose prediction. Prediction of human ADME properties, likely therapeutic dose and exposure of NCEs is an integral component of compound optimization in drug discovery and preclinical animal models are a key to understanding the ADME characteristics of the NCE, thereby enabling prediction of human PK.

## 12.3 Type of Animal Studies Required in Drug Discovery and Development (see Figure 12.5)

### 12.3.1 *In Vivo* PK Screening

Key drug series beginning to meet the *in vitro* human and animal target potency and selectivity, as well as most of the physicochemical and *in vitro* ADME targets, should next be assessed for *in vivo* PK (Figures 12.4 and 12.5) *i.e.* in the whole animal to determine the impact the whole body has on the compound/drug series.

*In vivo* PK (ADME) screening is critical to ensure drug candidate series have appropriate PK properties (bioavailability, total exposure (area under curve (AUC)), clearance, half-life, volume of distribution, $C_{max}$, and minimum attainable plasma concentration ($C_{min}$)) in the appropriate animal species being used to model PD, disease mechanism pharmacology and toxicology. Absorption critically determines the bioavailability, *i.e.* the percentage of drug that is absorbed by the body as defined by quantity in plasma. Bioavailability studies are generally conducted *in vivo* on drug candidates intended to be administered by a non-intravenous route, *e.g.* orally and intended to cross the blood–brain barrier whose target lies within the CNS. One would normally be aiming for a half-life of greater than 60 minutes when the drug series is administered intravenously and a fraction in excess of 20% absorbed following oral dosing although sometimes, different targets require very different PK profiles. *In vivo* PK screening provides required information on the $C_{max}$, the time after dose administration to $C_{max}$ ($T_{max}$) and the mean residence time in the plasma, to determine the dosing regimen (amount and dose frequency) of the drug candidates for *in vivo* evaluation in PD and disease mechanism screening. An *in vivo* PK profile needs to be in line with the dosing regimen required in humans, for example, if a once a day tablet is required then the drug series needs to have a half-life *in vivo* suitable to achieve this.

### 12.3.2 *In Vivo* PD Screening

The next step is to determine *in vivo* PD (Figures 12.4 and 12.5), *i.e.* in whole animals, to determine the net biological impact (efficacy) of a compound on all the macromolecules, tissues and organs that it distributes to. To prove efficacious, a drug delivered into the patient must reach the necessary concentration in plasma and in relevant tissues (as measured by *in vivo* PK studies, see Section 12.3). This is necessary to effectively engage and modulate the activity of the target protein (as measured by *in vivo* PD studies) in the body. PD biomarkers are used to identify whether biological processes and/or pathways regulated by the targeted protein are modulated by the drug. The ideal PD biomarker should be quantifiable, should be modulated in a dose-dependent manner, and should correlate with phenotypic therapeutic efficacy (see Section 12.3.3).

PD screening assays (see Figures 12.1 and 12.5) we define as a pathway biology PD model with a relatively high throughput/quick turnaround and a relatively simple measurable output, or endpoint, that informs on *in vivo* drug action (efficacy/potency) and target engagement along a specific biological process or pathway. The *in vivo* PD screen provides:

- A measure of the degree the target tissue is reached by active molecules is obtained.
- A determination of the minimal efficacious modulation of the target can be estimated.
- The ranking of compounds with different pharmacokinetics is improved.

The ultimate goal in lead optimization is to screen and advance the "best" *in vivo* drug series/candidates establishing a PKPD correlation, where the right dosage required to generate a meaningful biological event at the target tissue is determined with the aim of producing a therapeutic effect in the next screening stage (disease mechanism model).

Examples of PD screening simple measurable outputs of drug-target engagement include:

- *Measures of cell migration*. For example, measurement of peripheral blood mononuclear cells (PBMCs) or other blood cells in animal and human. The PD biomarker lymphopenia was successfully used to guide clinical dose selection and forward translation of natalizumab (immune selective inhibitor of T cell migration) and fingolimod (immune selective sequester of T cells in lymph nodes) for relapsing remitting multiple sclerosis.[5]

- *Signalling pathway measures.* For example *ex vivo via* immunoassays such as cyclo-oxygenase-2 (COX-2) lipopolysaccharide (LPS)-stimulated prostaglandin-E2 (PGE2) production from animal and human whole blood.[6] A more recent example of plasma dipeptidyl-peptidase-4 (DPP4) activity in animal and human provided a PD marker to successfully guide clinical dose selection of sitagliptin.[7]
- *Target protein levels in relevant biofluids* (*e.g.* detection of CNS gene therapy target proteins in animal and human CSF).
- *Physiological pathway measures.* For example, measuring change in body temperature using telemetry or non-invasive thermal imaging is a suitable PD marker of transient receptor potential vanilloid subtype 1 (TRPV1) antagonism reversal of capsaicin-induced hypothermia.[8] Another example is measuring increased water intake (drinking) to determine central activation of histamine $H_3$ receptors in rodents. A high throughput α-methylhistamine induced dipsogenia PD drinking screening assay was adopted to predict brain penetration, potency and duration of action of $H_3$ antagonist drug candidates in less than 18 months for progression into disease mechanism screening models of AD.[9] GSK189254 was ultimately selected as the optimal selective $H_3$ antagonist drug candidate that improved cognitive performance in aged animals and entered clinical development in patients with mild to moderate AD.
- *Behavioural pathway measures.* High throughput simple behavioural measures predictive of target mechanism/drug class modulation. Reproducibility of any behavioural PD output measure is dependent on several methodological challenges, including the complex interaction between genotype (strain, species) and environment (inter-laboratory and inter-group variability) and generalizability of rodent models to human disease and disorders.[10] Importantly, a predictive behavioural PD screening model does not need to look like the human disease, *e.g.* forced swim test (FST) of rodent mobile (swimming) behaviour does not need to measure depression, which it doesn't, but simply needs to predict that drug candidates that reverse immobility, *e.g.* recently United States Food and Drug Administration (FDA) approved S(+)-ketamine[11] then produce a therapeutic antidepressant effect in the next screening stage (disease mechanism model).

### 12.3.3 Disease/Mechanism Models

The next step is to screen the lead compound(s) in a disease mechanism model (Figures 12.1, 12.3 and 12.5) that models what we understand of the human disease mechanisms (pathway biology) to determine if the lead compound(s) are *likely* to have a therapeutic effect in patients. Screening drug candidates in the optimal disease mechanism model will identify the "best" compound based upon its PKPD, its exposure and efficacy (MABEL) on its target mechanism-driven phenotypic response (*e.g.* anti-inflammatory, analgesic, anxiolytic, anti-cancer) and if its safety allows (see Section 12.3.4 on Toxicology Models and NOAEL) it will be nominated to enter FTIH clinical trials, subject to regulatory approval. The Medicines and Healthcare products Regulatory Agency (MHRA) and other regulators require proof of efficacy and safety (see also Section 12.3.4) in animal disease mechanism models to be convinced that the nominated drug candidate is *likely* to be safe and effective in human trials before they will allow a new compound to be tested in human trials.

The ideal disease mechanism animal model should replicate a human disease phenotype, disease mechanism(s) (often heterogenous) and its underlying causality (see Section 12.4 on validity). In many instances, causality is not clearly understood, and many clinically diagnosed diseases are umbrella terms for heterogeneous groups of disorders representing different phenotypes/mechanisms which share common symptoms (*e.g.* neuropathic pain, asthma) making the gap between the patient and the animal model of their disease state challenging. For example, in patients with neuropathic pain, one mechanism can underlie many different symptoms, the same symptom in two patients may be caused by different mechanisms, more than one mechanism can operate in a single patient, and these mechanisms may change with time.[12] Many mechanisms are also still to be elucidated. Another important consideration in attempting to translate preclinical drug candidate efficacy to clinical efficacy is ensuring that the goal of treatment in the animal model corresponds to the goal of treatment in the patient. This is often not a reality (Figure 12.4). Verbal self-reporting is the clinical gold standard of pain and analgesia assessment, which is impossible to measure in animals who cannot verbally rate how they feel. Standardised primary assessment of pain and analgesia in animals is stimulus-evoked sensory endpoints (*e.g.* heat, cold or mechanical) delivered and inferred by humans[13] (Figure 12.6). In Figure 12.6 we illustrate the gold standard licenced treatment of peripheral and central neuropathic pain conditions. Pregabalin dose-dependently reduces evoked mechanical and thermal allodynia in rodent models of chemotherapy (oxaliplatin[14,15])-induced peripheral neuropathy (CIPN) providing decision-making efficacy and potency analgesia data to support clinical trials for CIPN.[16] Preclinical scientists and clinicians have become acutely aware of these methodological phenotypic mismatch issues and consequently it is becoming more conventional to consider markers in patients that can help design more clinically relevant pain assessment tests in animals (see Section 12.11 and recent review on bidirectional research).[4] *In vivo* scientists can only model pathophysiological mechanisms that are currently available to them; the implication being that one can only model what one knows at the time.

In contrast, some human diseases have clear target mechanisms elucidated with *matched* objective phenotypic preclinical and clinical endpoints and hence disease mechanism animal models are far more straightforward and translatable, such as endocrine disorders and hypertension. For example, natalizumab and fingolimod, successfully developed and licenced for relapsing remitting multiple sclerosis, block the migration of leukocytes into the brain or sequester leukocytes in the lymph nodes, respectively, and both suppress neuroinflammation in animals and in volunteers and patients.[5,17] Licensed statins (*e.g.* atorvastatin) reduce plasma cholesterol in animals fed a high cholesterol diet and similarly in humans with hypercholesterolemia.[18]

Disease mechanism model screening assays (see Figures 12.1 and 12.5) have a relatively low throughput and turnaround (weeks/months; especially if modelling a chronic human disease) and ideally an objective measurable output, or endpoint, that informs on *in vivo* drug action (efficacy/potency) and target engagement of therapeutic response (*e.g.* analgesic, Figure 12.6).

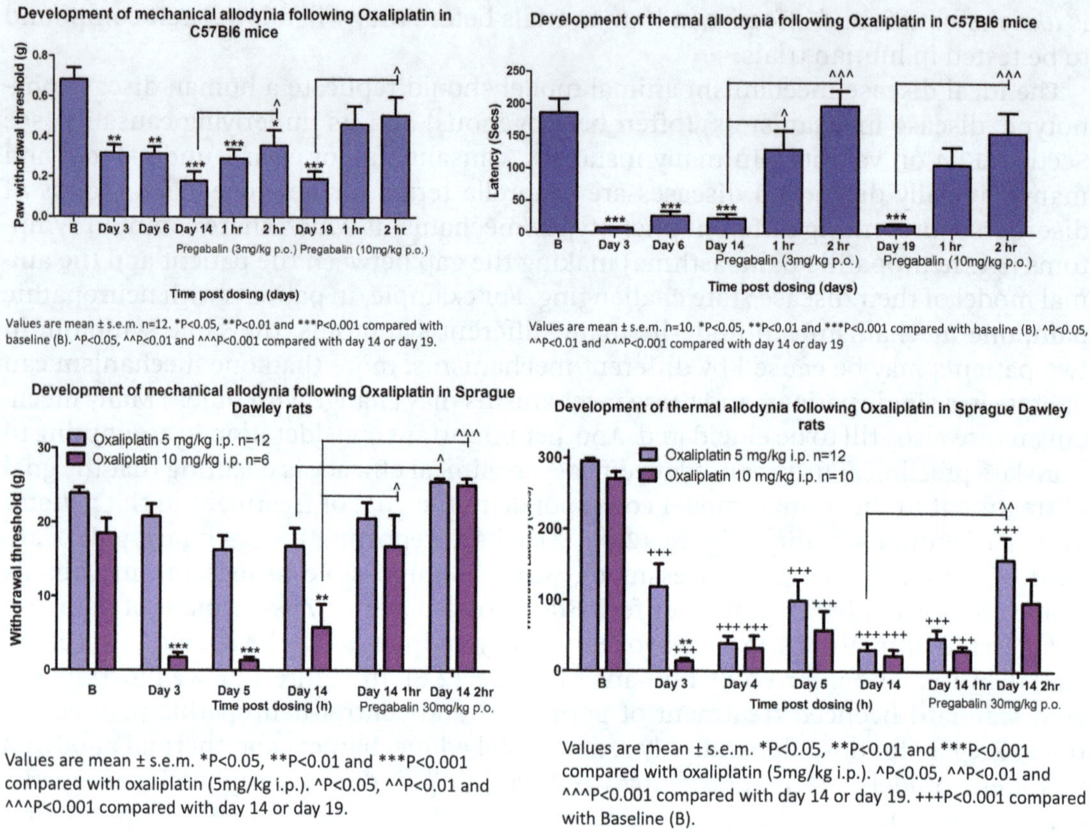


**Figure 12.6** Disease mechanism model. Pregabalin dose-dependently reverses allodynia in rodent models of oxaliplatin-induced peripheral neuropathy. Reproduced from ref. 14 with permission from the authors.

*In vivo* PKPD-efficacy relationship studies in disease mechanism models are designed to:

- Provide a quantitative analysis of dose–response relationships (PKPD) to determine ranking of compounds.
- Describe and predict the time-course effects resulting from one or multiple drug doses to determine steady state and any propensity for tolerance or dependence.
- Understand for how long and how much the target must be modulated to observe statistically significant therapeutic efficacy (steady state).
- Identify any unexpected/expected toxicity and/or off-target effects *in vivo*.
- Identify efficacious dosing regimens with an acceptable therapeutic index (TI).
- Determine MABEL and estimate human equivalent starting dose (HED) based on body surface area.[19]

Whole animal studies determine the net biological impact of a compound on all macromolecules, tissues and organs that it distributes to, and will include all biological targets that it interacts and engages with at specific doses. It is therefore important to monitor more than one physiological response (desirable and undesirable, Figure 12.1 and 12.3) as the effective dose for 50% of the population (ED50) and half maximal effective concentration (EC50) for each physiological response may be different. Knowledge of the compound dose dependency of both the desired and undesired biological responses allow the determination of the therapeutic window and TI, which considers the ratio of the highest non-toxic drug exposure to the exposure producing the desired efficacy (Figure 12.3). For example, if a compound reduces pain at a dose of 1 mg $kg^{-1}$ (therapeutic), but causes hyperthermia at 10 mg $kg^{-1}$ (side effect) then the TI of that compound is 10. Therefore, the "best" compound with optimal therapeutic efficacy in the disease mechanism model requires sufficient and acceptable TI, usually of >3.[20] Determining the therapeutic window based upon concentration over time is generally more challenging in practice.

The inclusion of *in vivo* PKPD-efficacy studies in the chosen disease mechanism model at early stages during the lead identification and optimization stages of a drug development programme can significantly accelerate the selection of the most promising and safe compound series.

Despite modelling challenges and limitations, animal disease mechanism models of human disease continue to be decision-making in evaluating NCEs as potential drug candidates, despite numerous unsuccessful attempts to demonstrate efficacy in humans *e.g.* stroke, migraine, neuropathic pain, AD, chronic obstructive pulmonary disease (COPD), severe asthma (see Section 12.4 on validity). Advancing an NCE into experimental human trials that has a measurable therapeutic effect and acceptable TI in an animal model of human disease is often a better use of resources than additional animal testing (see also Section 12.10 on The Future).

### 12.3.4 Toxicology Models

Paracelsus (1493–1541) is widely credited as the founding "Father of Toxicology" and stated back in 1538 that "all substances are poisonous, there is none which is not a poison. The *right dose* differentiates a poison and a remedy". Moreover, the final step required before regulatory submission for FTIH trials is preclinical *in vivo* toxicity and safety screening of your nominated candidate NCE to determine the *safe dose* (Figures 12.5 and 12.7). The MHRA and other regulators require proof of efficacy *and* safety in animal models (and/or occupancy/target engagement in other cell systems) to be convinced that the nominated drug candidate is *likely* to be safe and effective in human trials. Hence, the nominated drug candidate must produce a benefit (therapeutic effect) that substantially outweighs the risk of leaving the human condition untreated *and* any risk (toxicity) associated with the drug candidate itself.

*In vivo* toxicology studies must be performed under good laboratory practice (GLP) conditions as part of the overall preclinical safety assessment included in an Investigational Medicinal Product Dossier (IMPD) and Investigational Brochure (IB) application to the regulatory body. Safety data from at least two laboratory animal species, one rodent (rat or mouse) and one non-rodent (typically dog, but non-human primates can be used if justified) are always required to meet the IMPD application requirements (Figure 12.7).

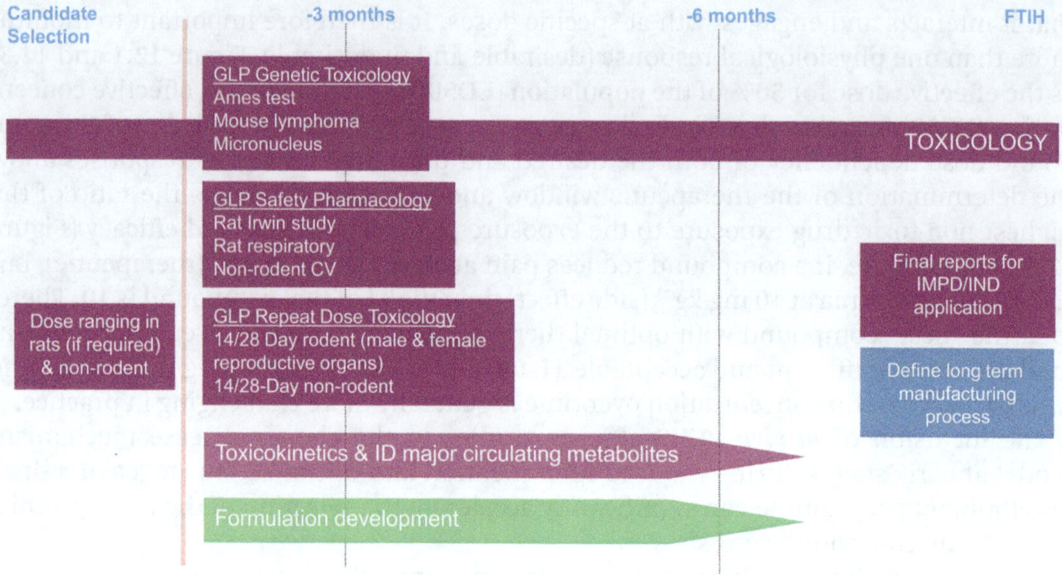


**Figure 12.7** *In vivo* toxicology models required for a drug candidate before FTIH. Image Credit: Dr Mike Kelly. GLP (good laboratory practice, ID (identification)), IMPD (Investigational Medicinal Product Dossier), IND (Investigational New Drug), FTIH (First Time in Human).

The primary goals of *in vivo* preclinical toxicology animal studies are:

- To determine whether the drug candidate has the potential to cause unexpected and undesirable effects.
- To detect unexpected and undesirable effects of the drug candidate in organ systems that cannot be evaluated in clinical trials.
- To identify target organ, toxicity and safety markers of the drug candidate for clinical monitoring of potential unexpected and undesirable effects.
- To determine the highest dose/exposure of the drug candidate at which no toxicity is observed, the NOAEL or maximum tolerable dose (MTD).[21]
- To estimate initial HED based on body surface area.[19]

Guidelines for *in vivo* toxicology assessment are defined by the International Conference on Harmonisation of Technical Requirements for Registrations of Pharmaceuticals for Human Use (ICH).[22] Toxicology assessment includes: (a) GLP safety pharmacology (*e.g.* Functional Observational Battery), (b) genetic toxicology (*e.g.* bacterial/mammalian genetic mutation/chromosomal damage) and (c) GLP acute and (d) sub-chronic toxicology, ADME studies, toxicokinetic, reproductive toxicity (Figure 12.7).

A low dose, intermediate dose and high dose of the drug candidate and a comparative control group is used in *in vivo* animal toxicity tests to provide the no observed effect level (NOEL), dose–response relationship, PKPD, dose linearity and target organ toxicity in animals, respectively. Doses are usually determined from dose range studies up to maximum 1000 mg $kg^{-1}$ $day^{-1}$, or maximum feasible, or 50× clinical

AUC study, and the maximum selected dose should be sufficient to identify the target organ toxicity. Initial dose range-finding and toxicity studies include single- and multiple-dose administration protocols with varied observation times in only a few animals, and one sex (one animal per dose level) and usually the rodent species as they require less candidate compound. These earliest initial studies are intended to determine the MTD, identify observable signs of toxicity and any ADME problems of a new chemical series leading to undesirable PK. Once a suitable dose range is identified, group sizes are increased to at least three per sex per dose level to allow for statistical comparisons.

The initial *in vivo* animal toxicology studies are often single dose assessments (single ascending dose study (SAD)) to determine the MTD and define both the NOEL and NOAEL in the acute setting. If the drug candidate has an acceptable TI, repeat dosing studies are performed to identify the MTD, NOEL, NOAEL and TI for extended administration. The duration of repeat dose toxicity studies in two species (rodent and non-rodent) is dependent on the proposed exposure in clinical trials, but is typically 7–28 days (Figure 12.7) in line with ICHM3 guidance.[22] Endpoints will include clinical signs, bodyweight, food consumption, ophthalmology, electrocardiography (ECG) (non-rodents), clinical chemistry and haematology, urinary examination and toxicokinetics. Toxicokinetic studies are critical to determining the TI of the drug candidate as a function of systemic concentration (PKPD). If the TI is too low in either the acute or repeat dosing studies or if the toxicology is deemed too severe, the progression of the drug candidate will be terminated and it will not submitted for regulatory approval. If the drug candidate has an acceptable TI in both acute and repeat dose toxicology models, an empirical PKPD modelling guided approach uses the NOAEL and estimates HED based upon body surface area (Rockville, 2005). Estimating the initial HED safe starting dose using the minimum risk of toxicity (NOAEL) rather than the minimum pharmacologic activity (MABEL) applies an arbitrary safety factor making the approach very conservative with a good safety record.[23]

Importantly, all animal models (PD, disease, toxicology) build a platform of drug discovery evidence, in the context of *in vitro* and PK data, to bridge preclinical pharmacology to clinical success.

## 12.4 Validity of Animal Models

As discussed previously, discovery and development of novel chemical or biological entities for a variety of therapeutic indications requires extensive research in both academic and industrial environments and preclinical animal models (*in vitro*, *ex vivo* and *in vivo*) are used at all stages of research for identification of novel targets, mechanisms as well as estimation of efficacy and therapeutic window.

Animal models form an essential part of translation of drug findings from bench to bedside as well as back translation from the clinic to the bench. Therefore, before commencement of any *in vivo* preclinical study the choice of animal model must be validated against three main criteria, first proposed by Willner in 1984;[24] face, construct and predictive validity in order to assess translational relevance.

### 12.4.1 Face Validity

Face validity is how well the model replicates the disease phenotype in humans, that is, similar clinical signs (*e.g.* hyperglycaemia), similar pathology (*e.g.* amyloid), similar mechanism (*e.g.* dopamine-induced stereotypy), similar biological markers (*e.g.* insulin), similar neural structure and function, similar behaviour (*e.g.* spontaneous seizure) and metabolites. Many early animal models of disease (1970–80s) were developed to model particular aspects of the human disease, such as individual clinical signs and symptoms (*e.g.* spontaneous seizure, hypertension) or individual pathway/mechanism (*e.g.* dopamine or glutamate-induced stereotypy, Table 12.2), as this was how human disease was understood at this time. These early models with good face validity for aspects of human diseases were critical and acknowledged in extrapolating new symptomatic therapeutic drugs into patient populations (Table 12.2, see also Section 12.4.3). However, good face validity for clinical signs and symptoms is a challenge for fundamentally *human* diseases, *e.g.* schizophrenia, autism, Tourette's syndrome, aphasia, pain. How do you model human subjective emotion or endpoints that require verbal communication in an animal model?

There are actually very few models of human disease in animals that have perfect face validity, that is, can reproduce *all* aspects of the human pathophysiology *and* symptomatology (Figure 12.2). This is not surprising, as most human diseases are highly heterogenous and have unknown causality (as discussed in Section 12.3.3).

### 12.4.2 Construct Validity

Construct validity is the extent to which the *cause* of human disease is reproduced in animal models, such as human infections, cancer and genetic diseases. With the advent of the completed human genome sequence and genetically engineered models in the latter part of the 20th century, mice and other species were modified to better reflect human disease pathways, *e.g.* transgenic, knock-out, knock-in and severe combined immunodeficient (SCID) mice susceptible to human infectious diseases and transplanted tumours. These predominantly rodent models have good construct validity (human causality) even if face validity is limited. An example is the APP/PSEN1/PSEN2 transgenic mouse models of AD, which uses human mutations responsible for a small percentage of AD patients (early onset). Although the models are relatively rapid and mimic some aspects of symptomatology and pathology, none of them exhibit the neurofibrillary tangles and neurodegeneration that are characteristic of AD pathology[25,26] (Table 12.1) and none of the therapeutics developed using these models have been successful in slowing down the disease in patients.[27] One of the biggest limitations of genetic construct models is that they often model rare causative forms of the human disease (with some exceptions, *e.g.* genetic models of autosomal dominant human diseases such as Huntington's disease[28]).

### 12.4.3 Predictive Validity

Predictive validity of animal models is the *most important* validity for drug discovery as it encompasses how well an animal model can predict the new treatment response (efficacy and toxicity) or human disease mechanisms/pathway (Figure 12.2). It is the

**Table 12.2** Validity of animal models.

| Animal model/Procedure | Human disease | Face validity (symptom, pathology, mechanism, biomarker) | Construct validity | Predictive validity |
|---|---|---|---|---|
| Post seizure models: various procedures, *e.g.* injection of kainate, stimulation of amygdala evoke ongoing spontaneous seizures | Recurring epileptic seizures | Good for spontaneous seizures, latent period after initial trigger.<br>Replicates histological including neurodegeneration | Probably good for some clinical forms of epilepsy | Good for anti-seizure drugs against partial and generalised tonic-clonic seizures (symptomatic)<br>Poor for epileptogenesis (no proven clinical examples) |
| Hypertension models: various procedures: *e.g.* spontaneous hypertension, Dahl salt-resistant rats, infusion of Ang II or DOCA (with and without high-salt diet), surgical (vessel constriction) | Primary/chronic hypertension | Good. Increase in blood pressure, some models develop secondary hypertension-related disturbances, *e.g.* ventricular hypertrophy, metabolic abnormalities, heart failure, renal damage | Moderate: differences between humans and animals with respect to causative factors that influence BP, *e.g.* genetics, physiology, anatomy, behaviour, environment | Good for anti-hypertensive drugs *e.g.* beta blockers, diuretics, ACE enzyme inhibitors, calcium channel blockers |
| Mouse experimental autoimmune encephalomyelitis (EAE) model | Human inflammatory demyelinating disease, relapsing remitting multiple sclerosis (MS) | Good for key early pathological features of MS: inflammation, demyelination, remyelination, axonal loss and gliosis<br>Poor for progressive neurodegeneration | Poor (unknown causality): artificially induced immunization required in animals; in humans sensitization to autoantigens (auto-immune) | Good for immunomodulatory disease-modifying drugs against rrMS (pathway specific)<br>Poor for progressive MS (no proven clinical examples) |
| MK-801 or apomorphine-induced locomotor activity and stereotyped sniffing | A mechanistic PD model in the treatment of schizophrenia | Good for dopamine antagonism mechanism<br>Poor for symptoms (human expression) | Poor: modulates mechanistic pathway in animals; in humans it is heterogenous and often neurodevelopmental | Good for typical and atypical antipsychotic (neuroleptic) drugs |
| Drug self-administration, conditioned place preference, and drug discrimination paradigms | Substance abuse and addiction and dependency | Good, exposure to drugs is sufficient to motivate and reinforce drug-taking behaviour<br>Drugs act as universal reinforcers | Good: drugs cause abuse and addiction in animals and humans<br>Moderate: model does not reflect pre-existing conditions | Good for predicting abuse and addictive potential of new drugs |

(*continued*)

**Table 12.2** *(continued)*

| Animal model/Procedure | Human disease | Face validity (symptom, pathology, mechanism, biomarker) | Construct validity | Predictive validity |
|---|---|---|---|---|
| APP/PSEN1/PSEN2 transgenic mouse or various protocols *e.g.* injection of scopolamine, surgical lesion of hippocampus, aged rodents | Alzheimer's disease | Good for cognitive deficits symptoms | Good for genetic models as uses early onset causative human genetic mutations (rare form) | Poor for neuroprotection/disease progression modification (300 different drugs effective APP mouse and rodent AD models; none effective in human trials). |
| | | Moderate for pathology: amyloid deposition but not tau, LTP deficits, no neurodegeneration | Poor for sporadic late onset human disease (unknown cause) | Moderate for symptomatic: five clinical drugs approved, many mechanisms have failed Replication in at least two independent laboratories is required |
| Ischaemic stroke models: various protocols, intraluminal filament MCAO (transient or permanent), photothrombotic, thromboembolic | Ischemic strokes *e.g.* caused by thromboembolism | Good for pathology (ischaemic penumbra) and some (*e.g.* MCAO) are good for duration (*e.g.* reperfusion injury) and mechanisms excitotoxicity, apoptosis), oxidative stress, vascular damage, injury to the BBB, neuroinflammation | Moderate: artificially induced thromboembolic clot/occlusion of MCA, similar to that observed in majority of human cases | Poor for neuroprotective interventions: |
| | | Moderate for symptoms (spatial neglect only in primates) and temporal mechanisms | | Two proven clinical drugs (tPA and aspirin, not neuroprotective) out of 100s of different drugs effective in ischaemic animal models |

| | | | | |
|---|---|---|---|---|
| Chronic pain: various protocols: injection of *e.g.* Freunds adjuvant or sodium iodoacetate induced joint inflammation, surgical sciatic nerve injury *e.g.* CCI, SNL | Arthritic or neuropathic chronic pain | Good for peripheral sensitization mechanisms, hypersensory symptoms<br>Poor for central sensitization mechanisms, hyposensory and reported pain intensity and Daily living (QoL) (mismatch primary assessment measures) | Moderate: artificially induced nerve injury, artificially induced joint inflammation, heterogenous human diseases with different causes *e.g.* metabolic, viral, auto-immune | Moderate for symptomatic interventions for inflammatory pain: opioid and non opioid approaches<br>Poor for symptomatic and disease-modifying interventions for neuropathic pain, one proven clinical drug (pregabalin) forward translated from 100s different drugs effective in animal models |
| HIV injection into non-human primates/mice | Human immune-deficiency Virus injection | Good: reproduce the complex biology of HIV transmission | Good, injection of causative human HIV virus | Poor for preventative vaccination 30–40 HIV vaccines in approx. 90 clinical trials failed; all vaccine candidates immunogenic in non-human primates and mice |

extent to which drug efficacy and safety in the animal model is predictive of efficacy and safety in the human patient (forward translation). As discussed in Section 12.4.1, animal models with good face validity for *aspects* of human disease (clinical signs, symptoms, known precedented mechanism) tend to have good predictive validity for these same aspects, Table 12.2).

Without a doubt, animal models have contributed to our understanding mechanisms/pathways of human disease and normal animal physiology and biochemistry, leading to many medicines that we have today. For example, drugs/drug classes (*e.g.* benzodiazepines) that modulate the gamma aminobutyric acid (GABA) mechanism are critical in animal disease mechanism models and human anxiety and epilepsy, and drugs that modulate dopamine and glutamate mechanism (*e.g.* haloperidol, clozapine) are critical in animals (stereotypy) and human psychosis (Table 12.2). Similarly, compounds that block the influx of leukocytes into the CNS and hence suppress neuroinflammation, in animals, healthy volunteers and in patients, slow down progression of relapsing remitting multiple sclerosis (Table 12.2). Understanding the central mechanisms/pathways important in animals and human disease is therefore key (see also Section 12.10) for improving the likelihood of forward/back translation.

Focusing on animal models of mechanism, rather than animal models of disease seems a sensible strategy; however, the ability of the predictive animal model to discriminate between different mechanisms/pathways is an important consideration to ensure no false negatives. A case in point, the Geller–Seifter conflict animal model of anxiety predicted benzodiazepine drug class efficacy (first predictive class) into the clinic, but the novel partial 5HT1a agonist, buspirone failed in this decision-making disease/mechanism screening model (no efficacy), so was disregarded from further development (false negative). The anxiolytic clinical efficacy of buspirone was only later recognised when it was investigated as a possible antipsychotic drug in patients with schizophrenia.[29] It is therefore important not to place too much reliance on precedented mechanistic predictivity of an animal model, as it is only clinical efficacy that will truly validate the mechanism. At the same time, translatability between preclinical and clinical models are improved by having some historical precedence. For example, if you are interested in developing a novel analgesic anti-inflammatory for rheumatoid arthritis, given the successful development of drugs like celecoxib and ibuprofen, it may be reasonable to use analogous tactics, including animal experiments, to advance your new drug entity. Indeed, we would be likely to use several of these drugs as positive comparators in our pathway biology PD and disease mechanism models.

The predictive validity of animal models carries inherent positive bias, as drugs that are nominated and proceed into clinical trials will have proved effective in the respective animal disease/mechanism model(s). In contrast, the drugs that are ineffective in the model (*e.g.* buspirone) are unlikely to have been developed or for that matter, reported (see Section 12.8.2 on Scientific Reporting). As a result, screening for efficacy in disease/mechanism models will lead to far more false positives than false negatives (*e.g.* buspirone). The record for animal models predicting *novel mechanistic* treatment effectiveness and toxicity, or preventive/disease-modifying strategies in human trials is particularly bleak. In reality, if predictive validity relies solely on existing precedented therapeutic knowledge, this is not conducive to innovative drug discovery, where the scientific research team are often aiming to screen and produce a mechanistically novel drug for aspects of human disease that currently have no existing treatment (*e.g.* disease modification of stroke, neurodegenerative disease, chronic pain). In these cases, in particular, the predictive validity of the animal models remains poor, despite many years and in some cases 100s of failed clinical trials (Table 12.2).

The failure of data in animal models of disease to forward translate into meaningful data in the clinic has critically hampered drug development and has led researchers and others to question the validity (face, construct *and* predictive) of these particular disease/mechanism models. Based upon a longitudinal review of small-molecule drug projects from 2005 to 2010, AstraZeneca have established a 5Rs framework of determining project success and pipeline quality: the right target, the right patient, the right tissue, the right safety and the right commercial potential.[30] The major reasons for compound failure in the clinic are lack of efficacy in patients and unexpected or dose-limiting toxicity. In some examples, target exposure, target engagement and/or pharmacological activity at the target was not established in patients, particularly if there was no easily translatable direct PD marker (*e.g.* CNS) so the target efficacy was not validated or invalidated.

Success rates of Phase II clinical projects with available efficacy PD markers are significantly higher than Phase II projects without such biomarkers.[30] Further, it is sometimes difficult to estimate the required novel compound exposure (*e.g.* anti-amyloid) at the target for activity in the human disease based upon the animal disease models, with their limitations, *e.g.* difficulty replicating the temporal nature and gradual neurodegeneration of the human disease. In contrast, animal models of ischaemia-induced acute neurodegeneration have good face (pathology, duration, mechanisms) and construct validities, and consistently demonstrated convincing neuroprotection with several novel drug mechanisms, over several hours after the ischaemic event; however, all failed in patients (Table 12.2). It is clear that these animal and human models need to be comparable for the timing of drug intervention, efficacy endpoints (histological and functional outcomes, *e.g.* spatial neglect), replication in at least two independent laboratories and perfusion/diffusion collateral blood flow in the compromised infarcted area for the drug to be able to reach the cells/target and halt/protect against delayed cell death.

A contributing factor for the lack of predictive validity of diverse novel analgesic mechanisms in chronic inflammatory and neuropathic pain animal models is the mismatch of *primary* neuropathic pain and analgesia assessment in animals *versus* humans. The predominant clinical feature of chronic neuropathic pain conditions is spontaneous pain, as opposed to evoked pain, hence randomised clinical trials primarily assess the verbal self-reporting of spontaneous pain intensity reduction, *e.g.* visual analogue or numerical pain scales, typically influenced by comorbidities.[31] In contrast, the industry standard primary measure of pain in animals is evoking (heat, cold or mechanical) stimuli delivered by an experimenter to assess loss and gain of function of different afferent fibre classes.[13] Hence, preclinical analgesic efficacy assessment is based upon the significant reduction of hyper-sensory phenomena (*e.g.* allodynia, hyperalgesia), an endpoint infrequently reported and measured in patients.[32]

Restricting evaluation of pain and analgesia in animals to exclusively subjective, reflexive outcomes is both oversimplified and can be argued not clinically relevant, given the continuous lack of forward translation across diverse mechanisms (Table 12.2). Assessment of spontaneous pain and other comorbidities, such as anxiety, depression, sleep issues and cognitive deficits so often associated with chronic pain patients, present developments in the animal model field for measuring matched objective signatures of chronic pain[4] (Figure 12.8). An ideal marker for chronic pain and analgesia is likely one that is objective in both humans and animals, and can be directly translated between the two, such as data from electroencephalography (EEG) recordings, which can be conducted in both species with no human subjectivity involved (see Section 12.10, Figure 12.8).

It is clear that no one animal model can accurately reflect the patient population entirely and therefore the challenge is to understand which mechanisms a particular disease model can address and how it correlates to signs and symptoms in a defined patient population.[33] There is much focus on improving construct, face and ultimately predictive validity of animal models (see Section 12.10), measuring the same or equivalent mechanisms, endpoints or biomarkers in both animal and human experiments and showing comparable pharmacological responses between animal models and proof of concept studies in humans.

| Preclinical endpoints | Human RCT endpoints |
|---|---|
| * Stimulus evoked sensory endpoints | Reflex QST |
| Spontaneous pain and Daily living (QoL)<br>Companion animal pain scale (*pets)<br>Pain stimulated and supressed behaviours<br>e.g. Grimace scales, ultrasonic vocalisation<br>burrowing, hoarding, nesting, gait | *Reported pain intensity and Daily living (QoL)<br>(e.g. VAS numerical rating pain scale) |
| Affective/Cognitive state<br>depression, anxiety,<br>sucrose preference, sleep<br>Operant place preference/avoidance, self administration | Affective/Cognitive state<br>depression, anxiety, motivation, sleep<br>anticipation of pain (preference/avoidance) |
| Objective markers<br>EEG, microneurography | Objective markers<br>EEG, microneurography, neuroimaging |

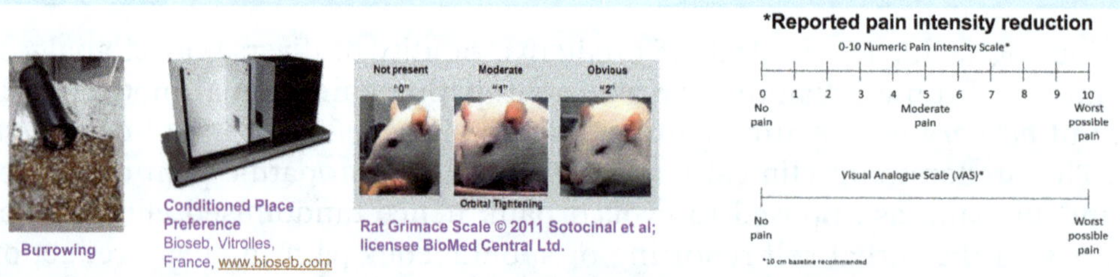


**Figure 12.8** Multiple preclinical pain assessment endpoints are under validation to improve face validity and translatability of preclinical to clinical research. *Primary endpoint, RCT (randomised clinical trial), EEG (electroencephalogram), QoL (quality of life). Reproduced from ref. 4, https://doi.org/10.3389/fphar.2020.614990, under the terms of the CC BY 4.0 license, https://creativecommons.org/licenses/by/4.0/.

## 12.5 Before the Study

Before the conduct of any *in vivo* animal experiments, it is important to address the following basic regulatory requirements and milestones for successful animal model experimentation.

### 12.5.1 Ethics

The UK, European Union and the USA legally require researchers planning any experiment using protected animals (vertebrates) to justify whether the objective of that experiment can be achieved using an alternative approach. A protected animal is defined as any living vertebrate except man (including some immature forms) and cephalopods (excluding embryonic forms). Animals used in research in the UK are protected by law (Animals Scientific Procedures Act (ASPA), 1986[34]) and in Europe by the European directive 2010/63/EU. These laws cover the people carrying out the research, the research project itself and the location of the research. Primates, cats, dogs and horses are given special status under the ASPA. They can only be used if no alternative research model would suffice and if their use can be justified by the scientist. Breeding facilities are also regulated by law and are formally licensed by the Home Office. Russell and Burch in 1959 developed an effective tool to assist the researcher in planning the use of animal models called the "3Rs" Replacement, Reduction and Refinement[35] (Table 12.3). Further details of these principles can be found on the National Centre for the Replacement, Refinement and Reduction of Animals in Research (NC3Rs) website,[36] including self-assessment tools that research groups and institutions can use to collate, track and benchmark their 3Rs activities.[37]

Conducting research in animals is a great responsibility and as such requires strict governance to ensure appropriate implementation. Any procedure done for a scientific (including experimental) or educational purpose which may cause a protected animal pain, suffering, distress or lasting harm, equivalent to or greater than the introduction of a hypodermic needle, is a regulated procedure under the ASPA and therefore is subject to strict licencing and regulations (see Section 1.4.2). The ASPA also regulates the breeding of animals for use of their organs or tissues in procedures.

**Table 12.3** Definitions of the 3Rs. Reproduced from nc3rs.org.uk/3rs-advice-project-licence-applicants with permission from the National Centre for the Replacement Refinement & Reduction of Animals in Research.

| | Standard | Contemporary |
|---|---|---|
| Replacement | Methods which avoid or replace the use of animals | Accelerating the development and use of models and tools, based on the latest science and technologies, to address important scientific questions without the use of animals |
| Reduction | Methods which minimise the number of animals used per experiment | Appropriately designed and analysed animal experiments that are robust and reproducible, and truly add to the knowledge base |
| Refinement | Methods which minimise animal suffering and improve welfare | Advancing animal welfare by exploiting the latest *in vivo* technologies and by improving understanding of the impact of welfare on scientific outcomes |

The UK has two tiers of regulation: local and national. Projects must be approved by an institution's Animal Welfare and Ethical Review Body (AWERB), who will also advise the principal investigator on matters relating to animal welfare and the 3Rs (Table 12.3). The project must then be approved by the Home Office, who will carry out a harm/benefit analysis to assess whether the expected benefits outweigh any possible adverse effects to the animal. The work of the Home Office in processing applications and inspecting animal facilities is scrutinised by the Animals in Science Committee, which is made up of a diverse membership including scientists, animal advocates, lay persons and a vet.

### 12.5.2 Licence Types

ASPA involves three levels of legal regulation (law) which covers the person carrying out the research, the research project and the location of the research itself. The person conducting the studies must be covered by a personal licence (PIL). The PIL is granted after a period of training and assessment. The programme of work is governed by the granting of a project licence (PPL) and the location at which the research is conducted is controlled by the granting of an establishment licence (PEL). Licences are granted for veterinary, scientific and environmental research.

## 12.6 Study Design

When considering the design of the study there are a number of essential steps that should be considered; these include formulation of the hypothesis/objective along with clearly defined aims. Simultaneously, the study should also be designed with a clear idea of how the results will be analysed. There should be clear identification of the "experimental unit" (the unit of replication, *e.g.* the individual animal) which should be as uniform as possible in order to control the variation, since the control of variability is crucial to the successful outcome of any study. What is becoming increasingly important in the drug discovery process is that preclinical animal studies should follow as closely as possible the established practices and end-points applied in the human clinical trials (see Section 12.4), where standardized requirements have been enforced for reporting statistical power, randomization procedures and patient stratification factors.

### 12.6.1 Selecting the Species

Preclinical applied research is primarily conducted within a relevant disease mechanism model and consequently the species of choice will be dictated by the availability of the model in that species (Table 12.3).

The most frequently used species are rats, mice, fish and birds that account for over 96% of all procedures (Table 12.5). Other mammals such as hamsters, guinea pigs, gerbils, rabbits and dogs are sometimes used, whilst larger species such as dogs, pigs and primates account for 0.2% of all procedures, particularly regulatory studies.

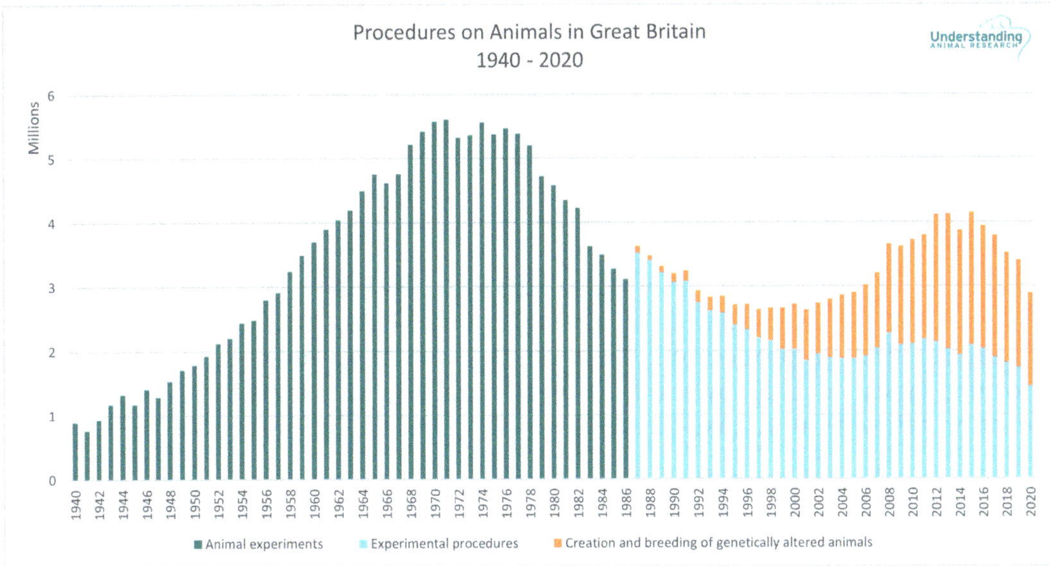


**Figure 12.9** Procedures on animals in Great Britain 1940–2020. Reproduced from ref. 38 with permission from Understanding Animal Research, Copyright 2020.

Mouse models carry a large amount of favour within the preclinical research space since they are small, economical and there is an array of transgenic phenotypes/varieties available (see Section 12.4.2). Dogs, cats, primates and horses have special protections, in that they can only be used if no other animals, *e.g.* a rodent or fish, will suffice.

Figure 12.9 illustrates the total numbers of regulated procedures on animals and trends over 80 years from 1940 to 2020, illustrating how the number of animals used in research grew steadily from 1940 to the mid-1970s, where it peaked at approximately 5.5 million experiments, reflecting the early years of drug discovery where animal phenotypic screening were a high-up (or first) assay in the cascade, until the end of the last century. The numbers then declined steadily until around 2000, to 2.6 million procedures (a slight change to the counting methodology took place from 1987). Since then, the numbers have risen to around 4 million, before levelling off in 2015. This reflects an increase in the production and use of animals with genetic modification or defects (mainly "breeding" category) and the steady decline in the numbers of genetically normal animals. In 2019, 49% (1 671 871) of procedures were for the creation of genetically altered animals, whilst 51% (1 729 646) reflected experimental procedures for basic research (56.9%, 984 316 procedures), regulatory toxicology/safety research (25.3%, 437 124 procedures) and applied R&D (16%, 277 303 procedures).

### 12.6.1.1 Choice of Animals

Given that diseased animals are usually more variable than healthy animals, it is desirable to use, "Specific Pathogen Free" (SPF) animals. These animals are regularly tested by the breeder to ensure they are free from a specific list of common and harmful pathogens that could otherwise interfere with preclinical testing. This approach reduces the number of animals required and allows greater statistical precision. SPF animals are widely available from commercial breeders. Care needs to be taken to avoid infection within the animal unit as infections can potentially have a detrimental effect on animal models or readouts.

#### 12.6.1.2 Species Choice

In general, species choice is mainly governed by: (a) physiology, (b) relevant translatability to humans, (c) availability of the model across different species, (d) model robustness and (e) model reproducibility (Tables 12.4 and 12.5). For example, if research is performed for cancer therapy and the objective is to investigate the role of a particular gene or protein within disease-like settings, the most likely strategy would be to use a

**Table 12.4** Typical species used in research setting. Reproduced from ref. 1 with permission from the Royal Society of Chemistry.

| Species average longevity (years) | Adult weight (g) | Weight at birth (g) |
|---|---|---|
| Mice 1–3 | 25–30 | 1–2 |
| Rats 2–3 | 50–600 | 5–6 |
| Hamster 2.5–3 | 30–40 | 1–2 |
| Ferret 5 | 750–800 | 10 |
| Guinea pig 6–8 | 500–800 | 85–90 |
| Rabbit 5–6 | 1000–7000 | 100 |
| Cat 13–17 | 3500–4500 | 110 |
| Dog 13–17 | 10 000–30000 | 200–500 |
| Rhesus Monkey 15–20 | 5000–12000 | 400–450 |
| Marmoset 8–12 | 250–600 | 25–35 |

**Table 12.5** Number of animal procedures in Great Britain in 2020. Reproduced from ref. 38 with permission from Understanding Animal Research, Copyright 2020.

| Species | Experimental procedures | % | Creation & breeding genetically altered animals | % | Total procedures (2020) | % | % Change from 2019 |
|---|---|---|---|---|---|---|---|
| Mice | 827 801 | 57.35 | 1 238 834 | 86.03 | 2 066 635 | 71.68 | −17.58 |
| Fish | 189 200 | 13.11 | 186 332 | 12.94 | 375 532 | 13.02 | −21.70 |
| Rats | 198 763 | 13.77 | 9847 | 0.68 | 208 610 | 7.24 | 21.94 |
| Birds | 123 157 | 8.53 | 1988 | 0.14 | 125 145 | 4.34 | −5.77 |
| Other mammals | 82 328 | 5.70 | 155 | 0.01 | 82 483 | 2.86 | −3.43 |
| Reptiles | 0 | 0.00 | 0 | 0.00 | 0 | 0.00 | 0 |
| Amphibians | 4399 | 0.30 | 2837 | 0.20 | 7236 | 0.25 | −1.90 |
| Primates | 2393 | 0.17 | 0 | 0.00 | 2393 | 0.08 | −16.04 |
| Cats | 146 | 0.01 | 0 | 0.00 | 146 | 0.01 | 11.45 |
| Dogs | 4340 | 0.30 | 0 | 0.00 | 4340 | 0.15 | 2.67 |
| Horses | 10 790 | 0.75 | 0 | 0.00 | 10 790 | 0.37 | 2.64 |
| Total | 1 443 317 | 50.06 | 1 439 993 | 49.94 | 2 883 310 | 100 | −15.23 |

mouse model. In addition, their smaller size and the abundance of genetic variances make mice often the preferred choice to rats. Generating complete knock-out, or conditional knock-out models is economical and a relatively straightforward process these days. Rats are the next obvious choice as laboratory species, mainly because of their size and the existence of a large bank of current and historical experimental evidence regarding their physiology, pharmacology and toxicology. Other rodents such as guinea pigs, gerbils, ferrets and hamsters are also frequently used, depending on their anatomical and physiological similarities with humans (Table 12.4). A good example of this is the use of guinea pigs, particularly within respiratory therapy, where similarities with humans in the anatomical and physiological composition of their lungs make this species an attractive choice for animal modelling. Lower species such as zebrafish are widely used for investigating development, genetics, immunity, behaviour, physiology and nutrition due to easy genetic manipulation, external fertilization, rapid development (~3 months, screening) and nearly transparent embryos.[40]

Larger species such as rabbits, dogs and sheep are also frequently used in toxicology studies, as well as to investigate particular physiological questions that cannot be addressed using mice and rats. Non-human primates are highly valued in biomedical research because of their genetic similarity to humans, which means they can be especially useful for testing the safety of new drugs and studying infectious diseases, and in neurophysiology, where they can be trained to respond to external stimuli and their CNS responses monitored or followed in some way.[41] However, their similarity to humans also raises specific ethical concerns about their use in scientific experiments and there has been a marked reduction in the number of non-human primates being used in research in the EU and US. Figures show that approximately 6000 were used in scientific procedures in the EU in 2011, compared with almost 10 000 in 2008.[42] Although there is more willingness to use non-human primates in the US some institutions are no longer using primates, such as the Harvard Medical School, which closed its affiliated primate facility in 2015 and the US National Institutes of Health announced recently that it would review all non-human primate research that it funds.[43] In general, the larger the animal, the fewer the numbers used in the experiment. Although in drug discovery settings more rats are used than mice, there is no particular statistical justification for this. A more likely explanation is that rats, being larger, allow for more parameters to be measured with greater precision. Rats are also a popular choice for safety and toxicology studies within the drug discovery environment, hence the current attraction of PKPD relationship assessment. The cross-over activity of compound series across the different species is also an important determinant in selecting species for animal model experiments. Ideally test compounds should exhibit similar pharmacology to humans in the chosen species.

#### *12.6.1.3 Gender Choice*

Historically, preclinical PD and disease mechanism efficacy model studies are mainly conducted in male animals. The reason for this has been that researchers fear that inclusion of male and females in the study design would lead to increased variability in the data through the oestrous cycle and associated hormonal changes.[44]

However, as clinical trials include both male and female patients and pathologies impact male and females differently, it would make sense from a translational perspective to design preclinical studies in a similar manner. Mogil and colleagues[45] have demonstrated that inclusion of females does not lead to increased variability and importantly that there are differences in pain thresholds between male and female experimental subjects. In order for efficacy studies to be published it is expected that both male and female subjects are included in the design,[45,46] unless there is good justification for not including both genders. For example, male rats are widely used to model streptozocin (STZ- induced diabetic polyneuropathy, as female rats show resistance to STZ diabetogenic effects.[47]

### 12.6.2 Selecting the Model

It is important to choose the species and strain that is appropriate for the model and research project. Table 12.6 lists the most commonly used mouse and rat strains and the associated disease mechanism models.

There is a large range of genetic strain types currently used for biomedical research, which can be divided into three main types:

- Genetically undefined "outbred" animals: each animal in this stock should be considered generally unique (*i.e.* there will be limited knowledge about its genotype), unless determined. Still used in some disciplines, but the use of these animals is considered less desirable by researchers these days due to their inherent variability and potential for genetic drift.
- Genetically defined "isogenic" animals: the most important factor regarding these strains is that their genotype is replicated across all individuals. Inbred strains are generally produced by more than 20 generations of mating between so-called "brother and sisters" and in many cases they represent clones of genetically identical material. These isogenic animals tend to exhibit phenotype uniformity when compared to outbred animals. There are over 600 inbred strains of mice and rats available worldwide. Nevertheless, about 80% of research is conducted using only the most popular 10 strains of isogenic animals (Table 12.6). It is important to emphasize that each strain has its own unique characteristics. Certain strains develop cancer naturally, such as (AKR/J) mouse strains, others are more prone to immunological phenotype (Table 12.6). A common approach is to choose a strain based on a particular research project. However, the most popular strains used in general research are BALB/C or C57BL/6 for mice, or Lewis and F344 for rats.
- Partially defined strains of animals (mutant and transgenic with an unidentified genetic background): only the genotype of the particular locus in these strains is usually defined. This is typical for transgenic animals that are bred with an undefined background in order to improve their survival rate. Potentially, use of these strains can create substantial challenges for data interpretation, since these animals can have genetic drift in their background strain genotypes and this can lead to modification of expression or functional redundancy of the gene of interest.

**Table 12.6** Most commonly used mouse and rat strains and the associated disease mechanism mode. Reproduced from ref. 1 with permission from the Royal Society of Chemistry.

| List of inbred strains of mice and rats with some of their phenotypic characteristics | | | |
|---|---|---|---|
| Mouse strains | Comments | Rat strains | Comments |
| BALB/C | Used for immunology and oncology models. Produce robust Th2 responses frequently used for asthma models. Resistant for diet-induced atherosclerosis. Frequently utilized for generating antibodies. | F344 | Used for general purpose, experimental autoimmune encephalomyelitis (EAE), oncology and autoimmunity. |
| C3H | Used in cancer and infectious disease area. | Lewis | Used for transplantation, induced arthritis/inflammation EAE and streptozotocin(STZ)-induced diabetes. |
| C57BL/6 | Most popular strain. Sensitive to pain and cold. Whole genome published. Convenient to create transgenic. | SHR | Hypertension research. |
| CBA | Used to study autoimmunity. Commonly used for leukaemia research also develop mammary tumours. | WKY | Control for SHR rats. |
| 129 | Many sub-strains available – used for targeted mutations. High incidence of teratomas | Brown Norway rats | Used for allergic respiratory and immunological research. |
| DBA/1 | Widely used for arthritis models. Susceptible to develop atherosclerosis once on artherogenic diet. | Dark Agouti | Used for EAE, arthritis and cardiovascular research. |
| C57BL/10 | Used in immunological research. Susceptible to ovalbumine but not to DNP-KLH. Susceptible to TSNB colitis and EAE. | WAG | Used in neuroscience, cancer and immunology research. |
| AKR/J | Used for cancer research and immunology. PVG Immunology research | SJL | Used for multiple sclerosis. Susceptible to EAE and muscular dystrophy. Immunocompetent but have elevated T cells number. |
| | | Sprague Dawley | Most widely used. Used for toxicology, safety reproduction and developmental testing. |

It is important to note that within each type there are individual strains and stocks of animals with specific characteristics. This increased complexity makes the investigator's task in selecting the correct strain quite a challenge. However, in some specific cases a particular strain, transgenic strain or even mutant is chosen due to its potentially desirable features or characteristics. For example, it is quite common for hypertension studies to use spontaneously hypertensive (SHR) rats since they have a propensity to develop hypertension and therefore provide a good phenotypic research tool. Furthermore, certain mouse strains seem to develop a particular type of tumour or grow tumours at a higher rate than other strains. A very popular mouse strain in the asthma research area is BALB/C, because of its propensity to develop robust and reproducible Th2 responses, which are considered one of the pathologies of the human disease. As good practice, however, it is generally desirable to use animals from defined isogenic stock.

Once the appropriate species and strain has been selected, it is possible that your model of choice may be induced or be a spontaneously naturally occurring pathology. The use of naturalistic or induced animal models is a current topic under debate and is prevalent in all areas of research, particularly in the field of chronic pain research, for example diabetes-induced polyneuropathy. Type 1 and 2 diabetes and the consequential neuropathy can be induced in animal models by genetic, chemical (STZ, alloxan, vacor, dithizone and 8-hydroquinolone) or dietary (high fat diet-induced and galactose-enriched) means. There are also a number of naturally occurring diabetic models, *e.g.* non-obese diabetic mouse model (NOD), Bio breeding (BB) rat, Long Evans Tokushima lean rat (LETL), New Zealand white rabbit, Keeshond dog, Chinese hamster and Celebes black ape (Macacca nigra).[48] As with other disease areas there are advantages and disadvantages to each, as well as limitations and these should be taken into careful consideration when selecting the model for interrogation. What should always be kept in mind is that the animal model, and endpoint, should accurately reflect the clinical situation as much as possible in terms of face, construct and predictive validity.

## 12.6.3 Objectives

The aims and objectives of the experiment must be clearly defined and achievable to ensure the experiment can be ethically justified based on the expected outcomes. Whilst these outcomes may not be achieved it is important to have a clear goal for the conducted experiment to ensure valuable data is gained and animals are not used unnecessarily without due consideration (see also Section 12.6.7 on Experimental Design). Additionally, defining a set of clear objectives for the study can help to ensure the data that is expected to be gained could not be achieved without the use of animals or with a lower order species (replacement). An experiment is usually designed to test a hypothesis, or differences between two variables, such as dose of a chemical used and an observed response. Alternatively, the objective of the experiment may be to explore a particular hypothesis, to formulate a new hypothesis, or simply to gather data for information purposes (*e.g.* dose ranging). Therefore, although formal statistical testing may be performed, it may not be the main objective of the study. No researcher should design an experiment without having a clear understanding of how the resulting data will be analysed.

A common mistake in designing *in vivo* experiments is correctly identifying the "experimental unit". Usually each animal or group of animals is considered the experimental unit. However, if, for example, the experiment is looking at changes in amount of consumption of different diet types then each "cage" of animals will become an experimental unit not the "individual" animals, as the amount of consumed per individual animal cannot be calculated. Conversely, if a particular cell type is isolated from animal blood or tissue and placed on culture dishes for different treatment, than each "culture dish" will be the experimental unit and not the animal the cell(s) originated from. To enable appropriate statistical analysis, experimental unit readouts must be robust and reproducible, and clearly defined from the outset.

### 12.6.4 Selecting the Endpoint

Study endpoints are the measurements or recordings (*e.g.* PD, behavioural, biomarkers and/or PK) that will be taken over the course of the study to provide data to support the study aims and objectives. Therefore, it is important to determine the aims and objectives before deciding on the endpoints to ensure that the data gained from these endpoints will allow the study to achieve the objectives.

#### *12.6.4.1 Primary Decision-making Endpoint: Outcome of the Study Based on the Results of this Endpoint*

The primary endpoint of a study is usually selected as the most important measurement that will determine if the null hypothesis is accepted or rejected, and determine if the primary objective has been achieved. In human clinical trials the primary endpoint is usually used to determine if research and further trials for a specific candidate should continue. Likewise, preclinically, the primary endpoint is the decision-making endpoint that the power analysis is conducted on (see Section 12.6.5) and decisions such as further screening/development of a candidate compound are made using. The primary endpoint should be selected as the most critical/valuable measurement that will be taken during the study.

#### *12.6.4.2 Secondary/Additional Endpoints: Nice to Have but Not Always Critical or Ethical Endpoints*

Secondary endpoints are additional (often nice to have) measurements to the primary endpoint of the animal study that may aid in decision-making processes. These may be alternative markers that are measured to support the findings of the primary endpoint, to assess changes in other measurements or monitor/observe for unexpected effects (*e.g.* toxicology, undesirable effects) that the treatment may cause. Some examples of secondary endpoints include:

- Integration of *in vivo* behavioural with *in vitro* and *ex vivo* biochemical, pharmacological data from each animal, thereby strengthening understanding of the relationship between mechanisms and complications, *e.g.* TRPV1 antagonism analgesia (primary *in vivo* endpoint) and TRPV1 antagonism reversal of vascular dysfunction complications (secondary *ex vivo* endpoints) in a model of diabetes-induced polyneuropathy.
- Monitoring/observing unexpected drug candidate effects (*e.g.* GLP acute and sub-chronic toxicology).
- Use of surplus tissues from animals for related/unrelated projects (sharing of tissues from same animals maximises data output, limiting animal use to a minimum).

Importantly secondary endpoints are not critical (primary objective) endpoints and although they provide additional information from the same animal, minimizing additional experiments (reduction) it would be unethical to lengthen the animal study to collect these secondary measures at a later time than the primary endpoint.

### 12.6.5 Powering a Study

The statistical power of an experiment is the probability of rejecting the null hypothesis when it is false. It is the probability (or chance) of achieving a statistically significant result when conducting a study given that, in reality, there is a real effect.[49] The power to detect a true effect (statistical power) requires that the experiment is large enough so that it is possible to obtain a reliable measurement of the within-group standard deviation and the treatment comparisons of interest.

Power analysis and the resource equation are the two main methods used for determining sample size. Power analysis should only be used to predict the properties of future studies and not used to assess the result of the current experiment.[49]

### 12.6.6 Controls

There are a number of control groups that should be considered and these include positive controls, which demonstrate that a change in the response being measured can be achieved, such as demonstrating a toxin can induce a pathology. Negative controls aim to demonstrate no change in the primary outcome of the study and can therefore highlight unwanted or unknown variables that may alter the results in other treatment groups. Additionally, there are vehicle controls that are used to ensure that excipients and vehicles that test compounds are dissolved or suspended in do not alter the measured variable and therefore confound the results. A sham control has broadly been defined as "a treatment or procedure that is performed as a control and that is similar to, but omits a key therapeutic element of the treatment or procedure under investigation".[50] Finally, a comparative control is a type of positive control where a treatment with a known effect is used to compare to the new treatments, such as using the current gold standard analgesic as a comparison in a pain study.

The use of control animals in preclinical experiments is a fine balance between reducing the number of false results (both positive and negative) and the number of animals used. Some controls are best used during the development and validation of a protocol, such as negative controls that will aid in identifying unknown variables but should not typically be used in protocols that are regularly repeated. Vehicle controls, however, are often used in all experiments to ensure the effects on a particular outcome can be attributed to the drug/treatment alone and not to the method it is delivered by. Therefore, it is important to consider the use of controls on an experiment-by-experiment basis and to ensure the data gained from them outweighs the ethical implications of using more animals in each experiment to gain this control data.

The use of control animals should always be to help reduce the occurrence of false positive and negative results and therefore improve the validity of the study results. Even so, whether it is ethical to use various types of controls has long been debated and there are both positives and negatives to their use. For all new protocols, the use of negative controls can be important to identify unknown factors that could affect treatment groups and therefore lead to an increase in either false positive or negative results. However, their continued use across multiple repeated trials may be called into question as excessive and therefore not confirmative to the 3Rs of reduction and refinement.

Alternatively, vehicle controls are more likely to be used in most studies to ensure that the changes can be attributed to the drug treatment alone and not to the vehicle or excipients.

The use of historical control data from previous data is useful if similar studies are done routinely so that the data can be compared for drift. However, since there are many factors that can account for variability within an *in vivo* study, for example seasonal influences, fluctuations in diet, microflora, personnel and methods of measurement, the need for a relevant control is important to the overall study design. However, it is important to consider the inclusion of appropriate controls carefully.

Wherever possible, researchers should always include one or more control groups which are untreated (satellite), treated with placebo or sham-treated animals. It is good practice to consider controls as treatment groups. If experiments are repeated frequently over time, controls should be monitored in order to understand fluctuation and trends. Analysing the data with time as a control chart (Manhattan plot or Shewhart chart) enables unusual results to be identified from natural variability and is generally considered a useful monitoring tool.[51–53]

## 12.6.7 Experimental Design

### 12.6.7.1 Randomization of Treatments and Groups

Treatments should be applied uniformly to all animals. Where possible, the experiment could be run over a block of time as a randomized block design, where there is one observation from each treatment group within a block, *e.g.* a "mini-experiment".

It is important to ensure that the treatment groups are evenly distributed across the study animals to remove variability between them. Typically, animals are procured either using an assigned identification number or using baseline data for the primary endpoint. Following this randomization through using a block randomization such as the Latin square method, a computer-generated number or other randomized event. However, where a more complex study design is employed, or the sample population has covariates that may affect the results randomization, a design that takes these into account may be needed. Randomization ultimately aims to ensure that variables that may affect the data are evenly distributed in each group to reduce their effects; however, it is still important to design the study so that the number of these variables is reduced where possible (see also Section 12.6.7.3 on Variability).

### 12.6.7.2 Double Blinding: Subjective and Objective Readouts

As far as possible, animals and samples should be coded so that operators are "blind" to the treatment group. Additionally, observers and testers should be blinded to the treatment the animal has received to ensure that this knowledge doesn't create bias in the results. This can be done by coding the animal's treatments and using separate operators to take any measurements from those who may provide the treatment to the animals. Additionally, it is most useful to employ objective measurements of an endpoint (where possible) to help to avoid subjective measurements, *e.g.* animals behaviour (Figure 12.8).

#### 12.6.7.3 Controlling for Variability

Controlling for variability within *in vivo* experiments is an essential part of the experiment. To design efficient experiments that produce meaningful quantification, researchers must have sufficient understanding of the biological variations between effect (signal) and natural variability (noise). Variability can be separated into two groups: "random" variability, which is mainly due to individual variability between animals, and "fixed" variability, such as animal sex, strain, diet, age and housing. The latter can be controlled by researchers. Increasing the signal-to-noise experimental window will result in an improvement in statistical significance and lead to a reduction in the number of animals used per experiment. The statistical significance test is mainly driven by the signal-to-noise ratio, hence if "noise" within the experiment is significant, the biological effect (of) the "signal" can be masked, making interpretation challenging.

#### 12.6.7.4 Group Sizes

The size of the groups used in preclinical studies that use animals has both ethical and statistical implications. To conform to the 3Rs regulations the number of animals in each experiment should be reduced as much as possible to avoid their excessive use. However, it is also important to ensure that there are enough animals in each group that a statistically significant difference can be detected, if one is present. A power analysis is the most common way to calculate the minimum number of animals that should be included in each group to balance the ethical and statistical implications. Power analysis assesses the mathematical relationship between the group size, standard deviation, effect size, statistical power, statistical test and significance level. This can therefore be used to calculate the appropriate number of animals per group (group/sample size estimation). Many statistical software packages have the ability to do these power calculations, *e.g.* SPSS, G power, InVivoStat (which can be freely downloaded at www.invivostat.co.uk). However, it is only a guide and needs to be adjusted on an experiment-by-experiment basis.[49]

## 12.7 During the Study

### 12.7.1 Animal Suppliers

Laboratory animal suppliers across the world are responsible for breeding the research animals, *e.g.* genetically engineered animals, rodents, rabbits, dogs, cats and primates, which they then sell to licensed establishments for scientific experimentation. The two most well-known in the UK are Charles River Laboratories and Harlan/Envigo. In 2010, the US Jackson Laboratory sold 2.9 million mice for a revenue of US$98.7 million.[54] It is also not unusual for pharmaceutical companies and universities to breed animals in-house. Although there is no clear rationale for animals from different suppliers to perform differently in behavioural tests, this is one variable that can and should be adequately controlled as this has been shown to impact on results. Studies have indicated differences in locomotor activity, object recognition and ethanol intake between animals of the same strain sourced from different suppliers.[55] This highlights the need for continuity in the sourcing of animals, even if it is the same strain and the need for repeating baseline testing if the supplier or strain are changed.

## 12.7.2 Animal Housing

Animals housed under optimal environmental conditions usually exhibit greater uniformity than animals housed under poorly controlled conditions. Bedding, diet (particularly for long-term studies) and physical environment can influence the outcome of experiments. Always procure bedding from reputable vendors that have been regularly vetted. Housing mice individually appears to increase variability in comparison to group housing. Current housing and enrichment practices conducted within the Biological Support Unit (BSU) at the University of Hertfordshire have greatly minimised or in most cases completely eradicated conflict between group housed male CD-1 and C57BL/6 mouse strains. The key to this seems to have been a combination of:

- Housing groups of up to three mice per cage, from between 21 and 27 days of age.
- Larger cage area to promote territorial zoning and hording.
- Dynamic enrichment options (providing choice and exercise).
- Staggered cage/enrichment cleaning regime (reduce the re-scenting stress).

### *12.7.2.1 Light/Dark Cycles and Nocturnal Animals*

Animals are usually housed in laboratories with controlled light/dark cycles, which allows for their adjustment based on the needs of the study. This is important for species such as mice and rats that are nocturnal and therefore typically less active during the light phase when most experiments are conducted. Additionally, as fields such as analgesia are moving towards assessment of naturalistic behaviours, consideration of when during the light/dark cycle measurements are taken should be considered. Disruption of the light/dark cycle, *e.g.* exposing animals to light at night, disturbs biological rhythms and has widespread physiological consequences due to mechanisms such as melatonin suppression, sympathetic stimulation and altered circadian clock gene expression.[56] Further, the impact of circadian biology on the timing, duration and frequency of dosing may be anticipated to have major effects on the efficacy and safety.[57] Attention to the lighting environment of laboratory animals and maintaining consistency of a light/dark cycle variable is imperative for study reproducibility.

### *12.7.2.2 Space Required and Enrichment*

Table 12.7 summarizes the basic requirements for good rodent housing and husbandry. Animal research care technicians at the University of Hertfordshire, in collaboration with a caging manufacturer, have recently designed rat "gang cages" that consist of multi-layered floors with a combined floor area of 11 620 $cm^2$,[58] (Figure 12.10). This new innovative system of rat gang caging allows stock rats to be housed in larger social groups, establish complex social hierarchies, enabling extensive natural foraging,

**Table 12.7** Basic requirements for good rodent housing and husbandry. Reproduced from https://www.nc3rs.org.uk/housing-and-husbandry-rodents with permission from the National Centre for the Replacement Refinement & Reduction of Animals in Research.

| |
|---|
| Be large enough to provide enough space for exercise and normal social behaviour. |
| Be designed with a minimum height of 18 cm, and preferably 26–30 cm or more. |
| Be well ventilated. |
| Have solid floors covered with an adequate depth of appropriate substrate (such as dust free Aspen wood chip, Megazorb or Alpha-Dri) for hygiene, comfort and to permit natural foraging and digging behaviour. |
| Contain sheltered areas for resting, security and managing social interactions. |
| Be softly lit and subject to a light/dark cycle. |
| Kept at a temperature range of 20–24 °C. |
| Socially housed and kept either in single sex groups or in stable breeding pairs or trios. |
| Provide objects to gnaw on (*e.g.* soft wood blocks, hard pellets, cardboard tubes) to prevent their teeth overgrowing. |
| Provide nesting material from a young age (*e.g.* paper strips, sizzle nest, nestlets) to enable nesting behaviour. |
| Provide access to playpens where they can exercise and socialize. |
| Provide at least one shelter (*e.g.* cardboard tube or plastic house) to encourage exploration and provide refuge. |
| A programme of acclimatization and handling will improve the rodent–handler relationship and reduce the stress of scientific procedures. |

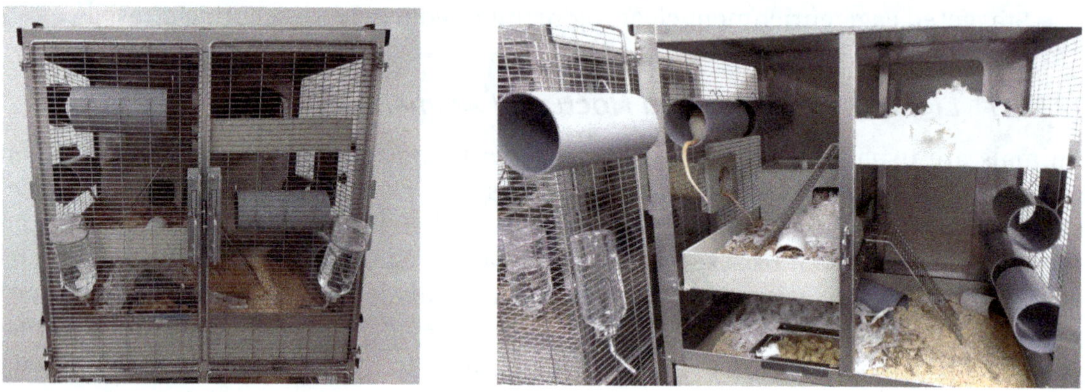

**Figure 12.10** Rat gang cage housing. Reproduced from ref. 58 with permission from David Clarke, Copyright 2018.

co-operative hoarding and nesting behaviours. The Royal Veterinary College (RVC) have since adopted this rat gang caging unit design and the University of British Columbia Animal Welfare Institute have acknowledged this new system,[59] demonstrating an international dialogue on best practice for animal research studies.

### 12.7.3 Animal Handling

When running behavioural pharmacology studies, a key part of the study is the familiarization/habituation process between the operator and the animal/subject to not only the handling but also the dosing and often (but not always) some of the behavioural procedures. This is another way to control for the inherent variability that can occur within *in vivo* pharmacology and toxicology.

### 12.7.4 Animal Weight and Age

The age and weight of each animal can influence the results it produces. For some studies the age or weight of the animal can be an important factor in the development of the model, such as age-related bone diseases.[60] However, in studies where these factors are not important to the development of the model, the variability of the age and weight of the animals in each study should be minimized. Additionally, the age and weight of the animals used in repeated studies should be kept consistent to avoid them becoming confounding factors that may introduce bias and added variability to the study results. Animals should be stratified by weight using randomized experimental design. Failing to do so can result in variability and create bias within the experiment.

### 12.7.5 Dosing

Administration of substances to laboratory animals is often a critical component of experimental design. Administered substances may include: infectious disease agents, various therapeutics, such as vaccinations, antimicrobials, pharmacologic agents, anaesthetics, and analgesics, chemical test agents, radiocontrast agents, electrolytes and other fluids and nutritive support.

Administration of substances to laboratory animals requires careful consideration, training and planning to optimize delivery of the agent to the animal while minimizing potential adverse events from the procedure, which could confound the results and lead to unintentional adverse effects on experimental animals.

Many different routes are available for administration of substances to all species of animal models used. An important factor in determining the route is whether the agent is being administered for a local or systemic effect. Routes such as intravenous or intraperitoneal that are outside the digestive tract (parenteral) usually lead to higher bioavailability than methods such as oral dosing that use the digestive tract (enteral). This is because parenteral routes avoid the first-pass effect of hepatic metabolism that can cause a breakdown of the agent, stopping it from entering the bloodstream. Additionally, the enteral absorptive processes can be unpredictable, which is avoided by parenteral administration. However, the most common route of administration in humans is oral dosing, therefore whilst parenteral routes are more predictable, enteral may more closely match the human dosing route.[61] For preclinical studies using the definitive model of choice prior to FTIH, the route, duration of administration and dose regimen must, at a minimum, conform to the proposed clinical protocol. The route of administration is not the only consideration that must be made, factors such as site of delivery, volume of administration and pH of the substance, amongst other factors, should be considered to refine the technique.[61]

### 12.7.6 Drug Formulation

Formulation development must consider not only the properties of the drug substance, but also the desired delivery system and the form of the final drug (drug discovery and development, technology in transition). Simultaneously with preclinical testing, a detailed physiochemical characterization of any NCE will take place. Commonly NCEs have poor water solubility causing difficulty in administering the NCE preclinically. Consideration of: (a) the correct approach to dissolve or suspend the NCE, (b) the excipients used, (c) the volume limits of the species and (d) logistics of transporting, creating and dosing the formulation.[62]

During the course of the drug discovery and development process, thousands of lead molecules will be screened to find potential candidate drugs. One of the hurdles that these lead molecules must overcome is solubility and a lack of it can cause NCEs with otherwise strong pharmacological activity to be dropped. A drug's bioavailability is directly correlated with its solubility, meaning NCEs with poor solubility may not be absorbed and distributed properly.[63] Preclinical formulators may employ strategies such as suspending the substance, adding slats to aid solubility or using cosolvents with the aim of overcoming poor solubility and increasing bioavailability.[62]

The project licence lays out the clear limits of dose volume of the species according to the chosen route of administration and will therefore dictate the acceptable dose volume and viscosity of the formulation. A compound that requires a highly viscous vehicle to carry it, will most likely require a wider needle diameter, thus reducing pressure on injection. However, a larger needle size will impact tolerability and animal welfare, *e.g.* greater injection pain.

## 12.8 After the Study

### 12.8.1 Statistical Analysis

The efficient use of statistics, both in terms of complex experimental design and powerful statistical analysis, can reduce the number of animals required[49] and therefore choosing the appropriate statistics for the study can contribute to the reduction and refinement of the study. Deciding on the specific statistical analysis used is a complex process and highly dependent on the specific study design. It is dictated by the aim and objectives of the study, the type of data (nominal, ordinal, discrete, continuous) and the types of observations used (repeated measures within the same groups or individual tests on different groups).[64] It can also be influenced by the number of experimental units in each group, which is the reason it is vital the statistical analysis for each endpoint is decided before the experimental design phase and used to structure the experiments rather than the other way around.

Selecting the wrong statistical test can not only lead to problems during the interpretation of the data, but can also cause an experiment to become invalid if statistical significance is not where there is a true difference (false negative) and goes against the 3Rs of reduction, as the experiment will likely have to be repeated or abandoned. This further highlights the need for a proper statistical and power analysis before a study is initiated as this helps to ensure that the data from a study can be properly analysed and if any changes are identified they will be significantly significant. This ultimately leads to better science being conducted and a reduction in animals used in scientific experiments by ensuring those that are used produce the best possible results. For more information on statistical analyses in preclinical research see ref. 1, 49 and 64.

## 12.8.2 Scientific Reporting

Results of animal research experiments are collected and analysed, and then shared with internal, commercial and academic communities, and the wider research community through reporting, usually *via* peer-reviewed publication. Scientific research progresses as hypotheses are further generated and tested, building on existing scientific findings. Such progress requires that scientific reporting is rigorous and that the findings are reproducible for decision-making. Although the use of open access journals has revolutionized biomedical research and contributed enormously to data sharing across and beyond the research scientific community, there is still substantial evidence showing that the reporting of *in vivo* data for biomedical research often fails to accurately describe research methods and, in some cases, fails to report results appropriately. Findings published can be irreproducible and unsound, although lack of reliability, validity and robustness of results (rigour) will be critiqued by any experienced and objective journal publisher or funding body peer reviewer. This in turn can have a range of implications for the entire research process and in some cases the reputation of the investigators and institutions involved. Kilkenny and colleagues in 2010 highlighted major unreported characteristics of animal experiments ranging from details about species, *i.e.* strain, sex, age, weight, to lack of clarity as to which statistical method had been used.[65] The NC3Rs launched its Animal Research Reporting *In Vivo* Experiments guidelines (ARRIVE), a checklist of recommendations, over a decade ago – maximizing the transparency, quality and reliability of scientific reporting of research involving animals, and enabling others to better scrutinise, evaluate and reproduce it.[65,66]

It is an ethical requirement and responsibility that scientists create and then follow their well-designed experimental protocols under authorised licence, to ensure the use of a minimum number of animals in providing valid results. Similarly, this responsibility should also apply to the scientific reporting of the valid legally compliant results. The majority of UK biomedical research institutes (currently 128) are signatories of the UK concordat on openness of animal research (2021)[67] and with similar transparency agreements in Europe (European Animal Research Association (EARA), 2021)[68] and New Zealand research institutes are committing to help the public understand more about animal research. It can be argued that the onus is on everyone involved (institute, individual, societies) to be integral and transparent in their scientific reporting in whatever form this takes. This can bring a diversity of ideas and values that could improve the quality of science, the credibility of animal researchers and the welfare of the animals in laboratories.[69] Further, a framework called Sharing Experimental Animal Resources, Coordinating Holdings (SEARCH) is freely accessible for researchers holding or requiring animal tissues to collaborate and share ethical samples reducing the need to generate new/additional animal models contributing to minimizing animal use (3Rs, reduction).[70]

A lack of scientific reporting due to unpublished (*e.g.* false negative, negative outcome, null hypothesis) or unpublishable results bias the biomedical literature, favouring positive *versus* negative findings and leading to duplicate studies that unnecessarily endanger animal and human subjects and waste resources. It is becoming increasingly recognized that the number of animals used does not necessarily lead to an improvement in the output, but in many cases merely illustrates the bad design of the experiment.

### 12.8.3 Unexplained Data Exclusions

It can be tempting to exclude an observation without any explanation, because it spoils an otherwise good result. In fact, excluded data points should be noted as well as the reason for the omission. Experimental outliers should be investigated in order to fully understand and improve the model.

## 12.9 Benefits and Downfalls of Animal Research Studies

### 12.9.1 What are the Benefits?

In the European Union (EU) a harm benefit analysis (HBA) is conducted to assess "whether the harm to the animals in terms of suffering, pain and distress is justified by the expected outcome" and whether the research "may ultimately benefit human beings, animals or the environment".[1] All proposed animal research experiments need to take into account the established harm/benefit analysis so that *maximum benefit* is derived from the data with minimum harm done to the protected species utilizing the NC3R principles.

Benefits can be considered as short, medium and long term. Short-term benefits usually encompass scientific benefits over the lifetime of the project, *e.g.* advance basic and applied understanding of animal/human disease, such as new target validation, proof of concept, guiding future dose selection of NCEs for clinical trials. Medium-term benefits will include promoting the benefits/significance of research findings to scientific and clinical communities to strengthen interdisciplinary and international collaboration, and public and commercial investment, paving the way for academic–pharmaceutical collaboration for patents and clinical trial development of novel therapies, procedures (*e.g.* surgical). Longer-term, patients and animals (veterinary medicine) may directly benefit and carers indirectly, which will have a positive social and economic impact by improving the health and wellbeing of people and animals. Without animal research there can be no PKPD modelling prediction of a safe starting dose for human clinical trials, meaning there would be no regulatory ethical clinical trials authorizations and no new medicine for human and animal health. Given the biological similarity, animals are susceptible to many of the same health problems as humans, *e.g.* cancer, diabetes, heart disease, obesity, and therefore benefit from many new medicines. Further, with a shorter life cycle than humans, animal models can be studied throughout their whole life span and across several generations, a critical element in understanding how a disease progresses and how it interacts with a whole, living biological system.

Animal research has been essential for numerous life-changing discoveries, from the rapid development of new vaccines (*e.g.* COVID-19), medicines, transplant procedures, anaesthetics and blood transfusions. Animal research (basic, applied and safety) has played a role in the prevention or symptomatic treatment of human conditions as diverse as tuberculosis, diabetes, polio, Parkinson's disease, depression, muscular dystrophy and high blood pressure. An animal research benefit relevant to everyone directly in 2021, is the technology for understanding how vaccines can use messenger ribonucleic acid (RNA) to get the body to fight viruses, which was developed in mice and patented more than 20 years ago at the University of Pennsylvania. It was licensed to vaccine developers in 2020 to rapidly develop the successful Pfizer/BioNTech and Moderna COVID-19 messenger RNA (mRNA) vaccines.[71] This novel vaccine technology is now being applied to human immunodeficiency virus (HIV), sickle cell disease and cancer. Millions of lives have been saved and wellbeing improved as a result of animal biomedical research.

### 12.9.2 What are the Limitations?

Success rates for NCE drugs in clinical development remain low, despite the human genome project and other molecular biology approaches having identified a large number of potential new drug targets based upon human target validation. Moreover, progress in the design of small molecule drugs (*e.g.* computer aided drug design) and the development of new biological drug formats such as Nanobodies®, has yielded a plethora of promising drug candidates addressing these potential new unprecedented targets.[72] As a consequence, a higher number of drugs interacting with less validated targets have entered clinical development during the last decade. However, this had led to a decline in the forward translation success rates (higher number of false positives) for drugs during clinical development. Limitations of animal models have been discussed in detail in Section 12.4.

## 12.10 The Future

### 12.10.1 Where Animal Research is Going/New Horizons

#### *12.10.1.1 Reverse Translation Transcriptomic and Proteomic Techniques*

Reverse translation transcriptomic and proteomic techniques are increasingly being applied to animal models to better understand disease-relevant pathways and mechanisms, and biomarkers to improve face and ultimately predictive validity. Omics/bioinformatics approaches are identifying differentially regulated genes and proteins, and relevant pathway associations from human diseased tissues and applying a similar animal omics approach to question whether animals have the same mechanisms/pathways and whether modulation of the mechanism/pathway also modulates mechanism/pathway-relevant biomarkers.

#### 12.10.1.2 *Directly Translatable Technologies in Small Animals*

The applicability of imaging techniques, such as PET, and functional magnetic resonance imaging (fMRI), within animals positions their use as a key translational biomarker in understanding the same processes from the clinic to the preclinical situation.[73] Despite the innate challenges associated with the various imaging techniques, particularly in small animals, this technology is still commonly used in rodents and considerable progress is continuing to be made in this field. For example, the identification of a core pattern of nociceptive-evoked events and brain regions activated in human pain imaging studies (somatosensory cortex, cingulate cortex, thalamus) are also activated in the majority of the rodent studies.[74,75] Moreover, pharmacological imaging in both rodents and humans shows overlapping activation patterns with pain and opiate analgesics. These studies have demonstrated a clear reduction in the pain-evoked activation of the brain regions associated with pain following opioid administration, thus demonstrating the translational nature of this methodology.

Quantitative electroencephalography (QEEG) can be used to profile CNS-active novel compounds on spectral power frequency bands in both animals and humans, providing a highly relevant translational biomarker platform. Furthermore, EEG has been applied to rodent mismatch negativity (MMN), a translational marker generated by a temporo-frontal network diminished in schizophrenic patients. Importantly QEEG is a technique that produces translatable and unbiased objective data to identify biomarkers of disease and guide strategic decision-making around dose prediction and PKPD relationships, as well as site and mechanism of action for a novel CNS penetrant test compound. Further development is needed to fully characterize the specific spectral EEG power changes/patterns in disease states that translate between animals and humans.

### 12.10.2 In What Ways are People Trying to Improve the Research?

#### 12.10.2.1 *Bidirectional Research*

Omics/bioinformatic approaches are being applied to human disease and animal disease models to focus on identifying the *right* target/mechanism/pathways. Deriving new targets/mechanisms from the human disease and showing they are relevant in the animal disease/mechanism model is key. This research strategy focuses on the first "R" in the five "R"s (the right target, the right patient, the right tissue, the right safety and the right commercial framework) of most important determinants of project success and pipeline quality.[30] This research approach should yield improved mechanism (rather than disease)-focused animal models that can demonstrate that a compound affects the target mechanism, give an understanding of the exposures required for efficacy of the mechanism and advance candidates to the clinic and the right patient group/sub-population more rapidly with a greater probability of success.

#### 12.10.2.2 *Improve Face Validity and Ultimately Predictive Validity*

Bidirectional research omics approaches will help improve mechanism/pathway face validity of animal models. Other approaches aim to remove the methodological *mismatch* of symptom face validity in animals *versus* humans, *e.g.* primary evaluation of chronic pain and analgesia in animals is oversimplified and can be argued not clinically relevant, given the huge failure rate of potential analgesics in patients.[4,76] Characterizing the impact of pain on ethological behavioural endpoints, *e.g.* anxiety- and depressive-like behaviour and objective endpoints (*e.g.* QEEG) are proving informative, with potential to improve the predictive value of these chronic pain animal models.[4,77]

## 12.11 Summary

We began this chapter by suggesting that the advancement of biomedical sciences is and has been substantially predicated on the thesis that animal physiology can be exploited to learn human biology. On the other hand, the use of animal models to advance novel pharmacological drug entities continues to be a challenge branded with a multitude of past failures. Thus the question should be asked, do animal models have a role in the drug discovery process at all? Some would default to a negative response, supporting a "glass half empty" philosophy with the mantra, "these animal models are not predictive".

We propose that pharmacology results from animal models needs to be placed into the context of both the specific scientific questions being asked and the conditions under which the data was generated. Moreover, we strongly advocate that these models, pathway biology PD, disease mechanism and toxicology, need to be integrated into a drug discovery platform geared at building confidence in the novel chemical/biological entities and the pathophysiological target. As described in this chapter, gaining a greater assurance around a new drug can be attained by an understanding of PKPD relationships and its target engagement in animals to directly estimate the PKPD, dose range to achieve optimal target engagement and PD response of disease-relevant mechanisms/pathways in humans. One caveat that needs to be considered when designing clinical trials is that the actual drug-target engagement and effective PD response achieved in healthy human volunteers (Phase I) may be different in the human disease population (Phase II/III) due to changes in target pharmacology, *e.g.* target desensitization, downregulation. For example, the anti-emetic NK-1 receptor antagonist, aprepitant, at clinically safe and tolerable doses, occupying and engaging >90% of its central target, is inefficacious in relieving ongoing pain in postherpetic neuralgia patients, despite convincing analgesic efficacy in animals.[3] Differences in the distribution and expression of NK-1 receptors is observed at supraspinal sites[78] and hence in certain disease states, *e.g.* neuropathic pain, even higher receptor occupancy (>90%) may be needed for clinical efficacy compared with emesis.

Fundamental in establishing a PKPD concept is an appreciation for the challenges of working with animals, which we have discussed in this chapter. Additional confidence in the target will be gained when disease mechanism/pathway models are anchored to a human translation platform, which incorporates the use of *in vitro* and/or *ex vivo* human diseased tissues (where possible), target proteomics and genomics to confirm its impact in patient population (bidirectional research). Caution should be used so as not to over-interpret results from animal models, given that they only serve as surrogates for complex and typically chronic human conditions (see Section 12.4 on Validity). Despite years of research, many diseases such as AD, depression, COPD and severe asthma still remain without curable treatment or known aetiology, perhaps suggesting that no single animal model will ever provide all the answers. There is still too much reliance on animals to find and validate mechanisms/pathways involved in human diseases (forward translation), particularly for CNS diseases, and hence the testing of mechanisms/pathways in animal systems that are not representative of human disease. We speculate how animal models will be used in the drug discovery and development process in the future and the focus must be on improving predictive validity using omic approaches and a bidirectional research strategy to identify disease-relevant mechanisms/pathways/objective biomarkers. Although few *in vivo* scientists are trained by UK universities undergraduate programmes, we are beginning to see an increase in academic–industry postgraduate knowledge exchange training and fellowship opportunities, some of which embed 3Rs training of graduate scientists. This will aid developing an effective, integrative, *in vivo* approach to drug discovery and development, as proposed in this chapter.

## 12.12 Hints and Tips

- Pharmacodynamic (PD) biomarkers are a critical tool in preclinical decision-making and lead compound prioritization, playing a pivotal role in mechanism of action, PKPD and translational studies.
- Animal models are essential within the research, drug discovery and development process, enabling identification and development of the PKPD profile of the compound under advancement.
- There are many different types of animal models used in the drug development cascade including pharmacokinetic (PK), pharmacodynamic (PD), disease, mechanism and toxicology models.
- The model selected should be simple, specific and robust for the pathway or target of interest.
- Validity of these models, including how they replicate the clinical signs (Face), onset of the disease (Construct) and predict effective treatments (Predictive) are key in selecting the optimal animal model.
- Ethical implications of using animals needs to be considered before undertaking *in vivo* research, closely following the 3Rs guidelines of replacement, reduction and refinement.[35]
- Before the study, careful thought should be given to the study design, endpoint, statistics, animal species, gender selection, dose route and the relevant regulatory requirements.[37]
- During the study, the handling of the animals, dosing techniques, animal supplier and optimal animal housing should be assessed to maximize the welfare and reliability of data.
- After the study, the results should be exposed to rigorous statistical analysis and responsible scientific reporting.
- Thought should be given to the translatability of *in vivo* data and the development of directly translatable technologies, to avoid over-reliance on animal data to find and validate mechanisms or pathways involved in human diseases.

## List of Abbreviations

**3Rs** Replacement, Reduction and Refinement
**AD** Alzheimer's disease
**ADME** Absorption, distribution, metabolism, and excretion
**ARRIVE** Animal Research Reporting *In Vivo* Experiments guidelines
**AUC** Area under curve
**AWERB** Animal Welfare and Ethical Review Body
**BB** Bio breeding
**BSU** Biological Support Unit
**CINP** Chemotherapy-induced neuropathic pain
**CIPN** Chemotherapy-induced peripheral neuropathy
$C_{max}$ Maximum attainable plasma concentration
$C_{min}$ Minimum attainable plasma concentration
**CNS** Central nervous system
**COPD** Chronic obstructive pulmonary disease
**COX-2** Cyclooxygenase-2
**DPP4** Dipeptidyl-peptidase-4
**EARA** European Animal Research Association
**EC50** Half maximal effective concentration
**ECG** Electrocardiography
**ED50** Effective dose for 50% of the population
**EEG** Electroencephalography
**FDA** United States Food and Drug Administration
**fMRI** Functional magnetic resonance imaging
**FST** Forced swim test
**FTIH** First time in humans
**GABA** Gamma aminobutyric acid
**GLP** Good laboratory practice
**HED** Human equivalent starting dose
**HIV** Human immunodeficiency virus
**IB** Investigational Brochure
**ICH** International Conference on Harmonisation of Technical Requirements for Registrations of Pharmaceuticals for Human Use
**IMPD** Investigational Medicinal Product Dossier
**LETL** Long Evans Tokushima lean rat
**LPS** Lipopolysaccharide
**MABEL** Minimum anticipated biological effect level
**MHRA** Medicines and Healthcare products Regulatory Agency
**MMN** Mismatch negativity
**MRI** Magnetic resonance imaging
**mRNA** Messenger ribonucleic acid
**MTD** Maximum tolerable dose
**NC3Rs** National Centre for the 3Rs
**NCEs** Novel chemical entities
**NK-1** Neurokinin-1
**NOAEL** No adverse effect level
**NOD** Non-obese diabetic mouse model
**NOEL** No observed effect level

| | |
|---|---|
| **PBMCs** | Peripheral blood mononuclear cells |
| **PD** | Pharmacodynamic |
| **PEL** | Establishment licence |
| **PET** | Positron emission tomography |
| **PGE2** | Prostaglandin-E2 |
| **PIL** | Personal licence |
| **PKPD** | Pharmacokinetic-pharmacodynamic |
| **PPL** | Project licence |
| **QEEG** | Quantitative electroencephalography |
| **RNA** | Ribonucleic acid |
| **RVC** | Royal Veterinary College |
| **SAD** | Single ascending dose study |
| **SCID** | Severe combined immunodeficient |
| **SEARCH** | Sharing Experimental Animal Resources, Coordinating Holdings |
| **SHR** | Spontaneously hypertensive |
| **SPF** | Specific Pathogen Free |
| **STZ** | Streptozocin |
| **TI** | Therapeutic index |
| $T_{max}$ | Time after dose administration to $C_{max}$ |
| **TRPV1** | Transient receptor potential vanilloid subtype 1 |

## References


1. M. Cicmil and R. L. McLeod, in *The Handbook of Medicinal Chemistry*, ed. A. Davis and S. E. Ward, Royal Society of Chemistry, Cambridge, 2015, pp. 310–335.
2. P. McGonigle and B. Ruggeri, *Biochem. Pharmacol.*, 2014, **87**, 162–171.
3. A. S. C. Rice and R. G. Hill, *Annu. Rev. Med.*, 2006, **57**, 535–551.
4. A. S. Fisher, M. T. Lanigan, N. Upton and L. A. Lione, *Front. Pharmacol.*, 2021, **11**, 2308.
5. K. Chiba, Y. Yanagawa, Y. Masubuchi, H. Kataoka, T. Kawaguchi, M. Ohtsuki and Y. Hoshino, *J. Immunol.*, 1998, **160**, 5037–5044.
6. S. Bingham, P. J. Beswick, C. Bountra, T. Brown, I. B. Campbell, I. P. Chessell, N. Clayton, S. D. Collins, P. T. Davey, H. Goodland, N. Gray, C. Haslam, J. P. Hatcher, A. J. Hunter, F. Lucas, G. Murkitt, A. Naylor, E. Pickup, B. Sargent, S. G. Summerfield, A. Stevens, S. C. Stratton and J. Wiseman, *J. Pharmacol. Exp. Ther.*, 2005, **312**, 1161–1169.
7. R. Krishna, G. Herman and J. A. Wagner, *AAPS J.*, 2008, **10**, 401.
8. N. R. Gavva, A. W. Bannon, S. Surapaneni, D. N. Hovland, S. G. Lehto, A. Gore, T. Juan, H. Deng, B. Han, L. Klionsky, R. Kuang, A. Le, R. Tamir, J. Wang, B. Youngblood, D. Zhu, M. H. Norman, E. Magal, J. J. S. Treanor and J.-C. Louis, *J. Neurosci.*, 2007, **27**, 3366–3374.
9. A. D. Medhurst, A. R. Atkins, I. J. Beresford, K. Brackenborough, M. A. Briggs, A. R. Calver, J. Cilia, J. E. Cluderay, B. Crook, J. B. Davis, R. K. Davis, R. P. Davis, L. A. Dawson, A. G. Foley, J. Gartlon, M. I. Gonzalez, T. Heslop, W. D. Hirst, C. Jennings, D. N. C. Jones, L. P. Lacroix, A. Martyn, S. Ociepka, A. Ray, C. M. Regan, J. C. Roberts, J. Schogger, E. Southam, T. O. Stean, B. K. Trail, N. Upton, G. Wadsworth, J. A. Wald, T. White, J. Witherington, M. L. Woolley, A. Worby and D. M. Wilson, *J. Pharmacol. Exp. Ther.*, 2007, **321**, 1032–1045.
10. N. Kafkafi, J. Agassi, E. J. Chesler, J. C. Crabbe, W. E. Crusio, D. Eilam, R. Gerlai, I. Golani, A. Gomez-Marin, R. Heller, F. Iraqi, I. Jaljuli, N. A. Karp, H. Morgan, G. Nicholson, D. W. Pfaff, S. H. Richter, P. B. Stark, O. Stiedl, V. Stodden, L. M. Tarantino, V. Tucci, W. Valdar, R. W. Williams, H. Würbel and Y. Benjamini, *Neurosci. Biobehav. Rev.*, 2018, **87**, 218–232.
11. P. J. Fitzgerald, J. Y. Yen and B. O. Watson, *PLoS One*, 2019, **14**, e0215554.
12. C. J. Woolf and R. J. Mannion, *Lancet*, 1999, 1959–1964.
13. M. M. Backonja, N. Attal, R. Baron, D. Bouhassira, M. Drangholt, P. J. Dyck, R. R. Edwards, R. Freeman, R. Gracely, M. H. Haanpaa, P. Hansson, S. M. Hatem, E. K. Krumova, T. S. Jensen, C. Maier, G. Mick,

A. S. Rice, R. Rolke, R. D. Treede, J. Serra, T. Toelle, V. Tugnoli, D. Walk, M. S. Walalce, M. Ware, D. Yarnitsky and D. Ziegler, *Pain*, 2013, **154**, 1807–1819.
14. A. Fisher, R. Magnusdottir, C. Chenu and N. Upton, in *IASP Congress 2016*, 2016.
15. S. M. Pritchard, S. Benham, A. Fisher, J. Cilia, N. Upton, C. D. Benham and L. A. Lione, *Proc. Br. Pharmacol. Soc.*, 2016, **18**, 183P.
16. S. Mishra, S. Bhatnagar, G. N. Goyal, S. P. S. Rana and S. P. Upadhya, *Am. J. Hosp. Palliat. Med.*, 2012, **29**, 177–182.
17. K. Budde, R. L. Schmouder, R. Brunkhorst, B. Nashan, P. W. Lücker, T. Mayer, S. Choudhury, A. Skerjanec, G. Kraus and H. H. Neumayer, *J. Am. Soc. Nephrol.*, 2002, **13**, 1073–1083.
18. E. Van De Steeg, R. Kleemann, H. T. Jansen, W. VanDuyvenvoorde, E. H. Offerman, H. M. Wortelboer and J. DeGroot, *J. Pharmacol. Exp. Ther.*, 2013, **347**, 635–644.
19. Rockville, *Guidance for Industry Estimating the Maximum Safe Starting Dose in Initial Clinical Trials for Therapeutics in Adult Healthy Volunteers Pharmacology and Toxicology Guidance for Industry Estimating the Maximum Safe Starting Dose in Initial Clinical Trials*, 2005.
20. D. R. Abernethy, J. Woodcock and L. J. Lesko, *Clin. Pharmacol. Ther.*, 2011, **89**, 793–797.
21. J. H. Duffus, M. Nordberg and D. M. Templeton, *Pure Appl. Chem.*, 2007, **79**, 1153–1344.
22. ICH: safety | European Medicines Agency, https://www.ema.europa.eu/en/human-regulatory/research-development/scientific-guidelines/ich/ich-safety, accessed 27 July 2021.
23. A. Nair and S. Jacob, *J. Basic Clin. Pharm.*, 2016, **7**, 27.
24. P. Willner, *Psychopharmacology*, 1984, **83**, 1–16.
25. L. Holcomb, M. N. Gordon, E. Mcgowan, X. Yu, S. Benkovic, P. Jantzen, K. Wright, I. Saad, R. Mueller, D. Morgan, S. Sanders, C. Zehr, K. O'Campo, J. Hardy, C. M. Prada, C. Eckman, S. Younkin, K. Hsiao and K. Duff, *Nat. Med.*, 1998, **4**, 97–100.
26. J. Götz and L. M. Ittner, *Nat. Rev. Neurosci.*, 2008, **9**, 532–544.
27. K. Mullane and M. Williams, *Biochem. Pharmacol.*, 2013, **85**, 289–305.
28. L. A. Lione, R. J. Carter, M. J. Hunt, G. P. Bates, A. J. Morton and S. B. Dunnett, *J. Neurosci.*, 1999, **19**, 10428–10437.
29. R. Sovner and N. Parnell-Sovner, *J. Clin. Psychopharmacol.*, 1989, **9**, 61–62.
30. D. Cook, D. Brown, R. Alexander, R. March, P. Morgan, G. Satterthwaite and M. N. Pangalos, *Nat. Rev. Drug Discovery*, 2014, **13**, 419–431.
31. J. T. Farrar, *Nat. Med.*, 2010, **16**, 1284–1293.
32. R. Baron, C. Maier, N. Attal, A. Binder, Di. Bouhassira, G. Cruccu, N. B. Finnerup, M. Haanpaä, P. Hansson, P. Hüllemann, T. S. Jensen, R. Freynhagen, J. D. Kennedy, W. Magerl, T. Mainka, M. Reimer, A. S. C. Rice, M. Segerdahl, J. Serra, S. Sindrup, C. Sommer, T. Tölle, J. Vollert and R. D. Treede, *Pain*, 2017, **158**, 261–272.
33. O. G. Berge, *Br. J. Pharmacol.*, 2011, **164**, 1195–1206.
34. ASPA 1986, https://www.legislation.gov.uk/ukpga/1986/14/contents, accessed 29 June 2021.
35. W. M. S. Russell and R. L. Burch, *The Principles of Humane Experimental Technique*, Butler & Tanner, London, England, 1959.
36. The 3Rs | NC3Rs, https://www.nc3rs.org.uk/the-3rs, accessed 27 July 2021.
37. Interactive 3Rs self-assessment tools launched | NC3Rs, https://nc3rs.org.uk/news/interactive-3rs-self-assessment-tools-launched?utm_campaign=July+2021&utm_medium=email&utm_source=govdelivery, accessed 27 July 2021.
38. Number of animals used in scientific research, https://www.understandinganimalresearch.org.uk/animals/numbers-animals/, accessed 27 July 2021.
39. Animal Research Numbers in 2019, https://www.understandinganimalresearch.org.uk/news/communications-media/animal-research-numbers-in-2019/, accessed 27 July 2021.
40. T. Teame, Z. Zhang, C. Ran, H. Zhang, Y. Yang, Q. Ding, M. Xie, C. Gao, Y. Ye, M. Duan and Z. Zhou, *Anim. Front.*, 2019, **9**, 68.
41. SCHER – Opinions (April 2009–March 2013) | Public Health, https://ec.europa.eu/health/scientific_committees/environmental_risks/scher_09-13/opinions_en, accessed 27 July 2021.
42. Scientific Committee on Health, Environmental and Emerging Risks (SCHEER) | Public Health, https://ec.europa.eu/health/scientific_committees/scheer_en, accessed 27 July 2021.
43. D. Cyranoski, *Nature*, 2016, **532**, 300–303.
44. N. Kokras and C. Dalla, *Br. J. Pharmacol.*, 2014, **171**, 4595–4619.
45. J. S. Mogil, *Nat. Rev. Neurosci.*, 2020, **21**, 353–365.
46. J. S. Mogil and A. L. Bailey, in *Progress in Brain Research*, ed. S. Ivanka, Elsevier B.V., New York, 2010, vol. 186, pp. 140–157.

47. R. N. Cortright, H. L. Collins, M. P. Chandler, P. W. R. Lemon and S. E. Dicarlo, *Physiol. Behav.*, 1996, **60**, 1233–1238.
48. F. Gao and Z. M. Zheng, *Exp. Clin. Endocrinol. Diabetes*, 2014, **122**, 100–106.
49. S. T. Bate and R. A. Clark, *The Design and Statistical Analysis of Animal Experiments*, Cambridge University Press, New York, 2014.
50. B. Horn, J. Balk and J. I. Gold, *J. Evidence-Based Complementary Altern. Med.*, 2011, 842767.
51. D. Scott and D. Firth, *J. Chem. Educ.*, 2019, 1037–1041.
52. M. F. W. Festing and D. G. Altman, *ILAR J.*, 2002, **43**, 244–257.
53. P. Gejdoš, *Procedia Econ. Financ.*, 2015, **34**, 565–572.
54. J. Keen, in *Animal Experimentation: Working Towards a Paradigm Change*, ed. K. Herrmaann and K. Jayne, Brill, Boston, 22nd edn, 2019, pp. 244–272.
55. A. A. Goepfrich, C. Gluch, C. M. Friemel and M. Schneider, *Physiol. Behav.*, 2013, **110–111**, 102–108.
56. K. M. Emmer, G. K. L. Russart, W. H. Walker, R. J. Nelson and A. Courtney DeVries, *Behav. Neurosci.*, 2018, **132**, 302–314.
57. B. Lemmer and M. Soloviev, in *Drug Discovery and Evaluation: Safety and Pharmacokinetic Assays*, ed. H. G. Vogel, J. Maas, F. J. Hock and D. Mayer, Springer Berlin Heidelberg, Berlin, Heidelberg, 2013, pp. 631–676.
58. D. Clarke and L. Ioannou, *Anim. Technol. Welf.*, 2018, **17**, 136–137.
59. I. J. Makowska and D. M. Weary, *ILAR J.*, 2020, 1–16.
60. L. F. Liu, W. J. Shen, M. Ueno, S. Patel and F. B. Kraemer, *BMC Genomics*, 2011, 212.
61. P. V. Turner, T. Brabb, C. Pekow and M. A. Vasbinder, *J. Am. Assoc. Lab. Anim. Sci.*, 2011, **50**, 600–613.
62. S. M. Shah, A. S. Jain, R. Kaushik, M. S. Nagarsenker and M. J. Nerurkar, *AAPS PharmSciTech*, 2014, **15**, 1307–1323.
63. R. Saka, P. Sathe, W. Khan and S. Dubey, in *Innovative Dosage Forms: Design and Development at Early Stage*, ed. Y. Bachhav, Wiley, 2019, pp. 119–153.
64. P. Mishra, C. M. Pandey, U. Singh, A. Keshri and M. Sabaretnam, *Ann. Card. Anaesth.*, 2019, **22**, 297.
65. C. Kilkenny, W. J. Browne, I. C. Cuthill, M. Emerson and D. G. Altman, *PLoS Biol.*, 2010, e1000412.
66. N. P. du Sert, V. Hurst, A. Ahluwalia, S. Alam, M. T. Avey, M. Baker, W. J. Browne, A. Clark, I. C. Cuthill, U. Dirnagl, M. Emerson, P. Garner, S. T. Holgate, D. W. Howells, N. A. Karp, S. E. Lazic, K. Lidster, C. J. MacCallum, M. Macleod, E. J. Pearl, O. H. Petersen, F. Rawle, P. Reynolds, K. Rooney, E. S. Sena, S. D. Silberberg, T. Steckler and H. Würbel, *PLoS Biol.*, 2020, **18**, e3000410.
67. Concordat on Openness on Animal Research in the UK | Openness in animal research, https://concordatopenness.org.uk/, accessed 27 July 2021.
68. Transparency Agreements | EARA, https://www.eara.eu/transparency-agreements, accessed 27 July 2021.
69. L. Carbone, *Anim*, 2021, **11**, 368, 2021, **11**, 368.
70. B. Morrissey, K. Blyth, P. Carter, C. Chelala, L. Jones, I. Holen and V. Speirs, *PLoS Biol.*, 2017, **15**, e2000719.
71. D. Laczkó, M. J. Hogan, S. A. Toulmin, P. Hicks, K. Lederer, B. T. Gaudette, D. Castaño, F. Amanat, H. Muramatsu, T. H. Oguin, A. Ojha, L. Zhang, Z. Mu, R. Parks, T. B. Manzoni, B. Roper, S. Strohmeier, I. Tombácz, L. Arwood, R. Nachbagauer, K. Karikó, J. Greenhouse, L. Pessaint, M. Porto, T. Putman-Taylor, A. Strasbaugh, T. A. Campbell, P. J. C. Lin, Y. K. Tam, G. D. Sempowski, M. Farzan, H. Choe, K. O. Saunders, B. F. Haynes, H. Andersen, L. C. Eisenlohr, D. Weissman, F. Krammer, P. Bates, D. Allman, M. Locci and N. Pardi, *Immunity*, 2020, **53**, 724–732.e7.
72. T. Denayer, T. Stöhrn and M. Van Roy, *New Horiz. Transl. Med.*, 2014, **2**, 5–11.
73. I. Tracey, C. J. Woolf and N. A. Andrews, *Neuron*, 2019, **101**, 783–800.
74. S. J. Thompson and M. C. Bushnell, *Neurosci. Lett.*, 2012, **520**, 131–139.
75. I. Tracey and P. W. Mantyh, *Neuron*, 2007, **55**, 377–391.
76. R. González-Cano, Á. Montilla-García, M. C. Ruiz-Cantero, I. Bravo-Caparrós, M. Tejada, F. R. Nieto and E. J. Cobos, *Neurosci. Biobehav. Rev.*, 2020, **113**, 238–261.
77. A. M. Cunha, J. Pereira-Mendes, A. Almeida, M. R. Guimarães and H. Leite-Almeida, *Neurosci. Biobehav. Rev.*, 2020, **119**, 101–127.
78. R. Hill, *Trends Pharmacol. Sci.*, 2000, **21**, 244–246.

# 13 Bioinformatics for Medicinal Chemistry

Emma Manners[a], Claire O'Donovan[a] and Maria J. Martin*[a]

[a]EMBL-European Bioinformatics Institute, Hinxton, UK
*E-mail: martin@ebi.ac.uk

## 13.1 Introduction

Twenty years have passed since the announcement on June 26, 2000 of the first draft of the human genome at a joint press conference between the US President Bill Clinton and the UK Prime Minister Tony Blair. The international research project Human Genome Project (HGP)[1] and the private company Celera Genomics[2] had published their findings in the *Nature* and *Science* journals, respectively. The HGP was launched in 1990 with the goal of sequencing the human genome for the first time and making the data freely available for all online. The rapid advances of sequencing technologies and the collaboration of international groups with more than 2800 researchers greatly accelerated the process going from 6% of the human genome sequenced to 90% in just the last two years. The HGP revealed that there are about 20 500 human genes which constitute the basic set of inheritable instructions for the functioning of a human being. This was a critical turning point in genomics and since then, there have been worldwide efforts to collect, organise and interpret genetic data and, with the dramatic reduction in the cost of sequencing, genomics now has a growing influence on human personalised health care. Genomics is defined as the study of the genome and in the fields of molecular biology and genetics, the genome is all genetic material of an organism. It consists of DNA (or RNA in RNA viruses – well-known entities in current times). In humans, the genome includes both the genes (the coding regions) and non-coding DNA as well as mitochondrial DNA. The coding regions are those sequences of DNA that carry the instructions to make proteins while the non-coding regions include introns, sequences for non-coding RNAs, regulatory regions and repetitive DNA. A gene/coding region is

The Handbook of Medicinal Chemistry: Principles and Practice, 2nd Edition
Edited by Simon E. Ward and Andrew M. Davis

Published by the Royal Society of Chemistry, www.rsc.org

transcribed or copied into a form known as "RNA". An intron is any sequence within a gene which is removed during this process. Sequences that are joined together in the final mature RNA are called exons. The complete set of RNA (also known as its transcriptome) is subject to some editing (cutting and pasting) to become messenger-RNA, which carries information to the ribosome,[3] a complex of ribosomal RNA (rRNA) and proteins that functions as the protein factory of the cell. mRNA carries this information as a sequence of four chemicals (known as "bases"), which are referred to as A, C, U and G (in DNA, T is found instead of U). The order of bases specifies the encoded protein; a set of three bases (a triplet "codon") corresponds to an amino acid within the final protein. The mRNA sequence is delineated by start and stop codons and the message (mRNA) translated into protein by the ribosome. During translation, transfer RNAs (t-RNAs) recruit and present amino acids to the ribosome. It is important to note that many proteins can be generated from one gene, depending on which exons are selected in the editing process. One of the major challenges for the HGP and subsequent efforts was to identify these coding regions and to distinguish between the exons and introns and how the multiple protein forms are generated in what is called alternative splicing. It is because of this complexity that the number of initially estimated human genes went from 100 000 to the current 20 500. Non-coding sequences make up 98% of the human genome and researchers are still discovering new functions and interactions between these sequences and the genes. Some examples of these efforts are the ENCODE[4] and the 1000 Genomes[5] projects. ENCODE, the Encyclopedia of DNA Elements, is an international collaboration of researchers funded in 2003 by the National Human Genome Research Institute (NHGRI) in the US with the goal to collect the functional elements in the human genome, both at the protein and RNA level and the regulatory elements that controls cells and how genes are "switched" on and off. The discovery and annotation of gene elements requires sequencing techniques and bioinformatic analysis tools which have developed rapidly in the last decade. These were key in performing a large number of sequence-based studies to map functional elements across the human genome, identifying protein-coding genes. The goal of the 1000 Genomes Project was to find most genetic variants with frequencies of at least 1% in the populations studied. It was the first project to sequence the genomes of a large number of people, to provide a comprehensive resource on human genetic variation. Genetic variation is the difference in DNA sequences between individuals within a population. Variation occurs in germ cells, *i.e.* sperm and egg, and also in somatic (all other) cells. Variations may be beneficial, harmful, or neutral. Data from both these projects was quickly made available to the worldwide scientific community through freely accessible public databases.

However, determining a genome is only the beginning of genomics. Once this is done, the genomic sequence is used to study the function of the numerous genes (functional genomics) which happens at the protein level.[3] Proteins are large biomolecules, consisting of one or more long chains of amino acid residues. Proteins do most of the work at the cellular level and are responsible for the function, structure and responsiveness of an organism to stimuli. They vary in their composition of amino acids, which is determined by the underlying DNA sequence of the gene. It is the amino acid sequence which in turn specifies how a protein folds into its 3D structure and gains its particular function. Variation in the underlying DNA therefore also has implications for the proteins which are produced within the cell. Some of the changes are benign, while others are detrimental to the health of the individual. Researchers are learning that nearly all conditions and diseases have a genetic component. Some disorders, such as sickle cell disease and cystic fibrosis, are caused by mutations in a single gene. The causes of many other disorders, however, are much more complex. Common medical problems such as heart disease, type 2 diabetes and obesity do not have a single genetic cause – they are likely associated with the effects of multiple genes (polygenic) in combination with lifestyle and environmental factors. Conditions caused by many contributing factors are called complex or multifactorial disorders.[6] To study this further and to understand its full implications, a multi-omics approach is needed. Genomics is an entry point for looking at the other omics sciences. The information in the genes of an organism, its genotype, is largely responsible for the final physical makeup of the organism, referred to as the "phenotype". However, the other omics and environment also have influence on the phenotype.[3] The next omic to the genome is the transcriptome which is the set of all RNA transcripts (both coding and non-coding) in an organism. The field of transcriptomics allows for the examination of whole transcriptome changes across a variety of biological conditions. The complete set of proteins in a cell is referred to as its proteome and the study of protein structure and function, and what every protein in the cell is doing is known as proteomics. The proteome is highly dynamic and it changes from time to time in response to different environmental stimuli. The goal of proteomics is to understand how the structure and function of proteins allow them to do what they do, what they interact with and how they contribute to life processes. Metabolomics is one of the newest omics sciences.[3] It is the systematic study of the small molecular metabolites in a cell, tissue, biofluid or cell culture media that are the tangible result of cellular processes or responses to an environmental stress. Collectively, these metabolites and their interactions within a biological system are known as the metabolome. Just as genomics is the study of DNA and genetic information within a cell, and transcriptomics is the study of RNA and differences in mRNA expression; metabolomics is the study of substrates and products of metabolism, which are influenced by both genetic and environmental factors.[7] Genomics and proteomics have provided extensive information regarding the genotype but convey limited information about the phenotype,[3] which is defined as the state of an organism resulting from interactions between genes, environment, disease, molecular mechanisms and chance.[8] Metabolomics is a powerful approach because metabolites and their concentrations, unlike other omics measures, directly reflect the underlying biochemical activity and state of cells/tissues. Because of this, metabolomics best represents the molecular phenotype.[7] A phenotype is any observable trait of an individual, such as height, while a clinical phenotype is used to describe how a disease presents in any specific individual.

The *transcription* of DNA into mRNA and *translation* of mRNA into proteins is central to molecular biology and studied in genomics, transcriptomics and proteomics. Whilst our DNA sequence ultimately determines protein structure, environmental and other influences on the transcription-translation process can be studied in epigenetics and epitranscriptomics (that investigate changes to DNA and RNA structure respectively that do not change the underlying nucleic acid sequences). In recent years, the influence of host-associated microorganisms, their genomes (the "microbiome") and their metabolomes has also received increased attention for the potential impact on health (Figure 13.1).

Combining all the omics is fundamental to understanding the relationship between the phenotype and the genotype, which in turn is critical for the development of personalised medicine and treatment. Again, it is not enough to understand the consequences of changes in one gene or its products. As mentioned before, many diseases are multifactorial and it is necessary to understand how the genome is operational at a systemic level in order to gain insight into the disease development pathways and possible treatments or prevention.

Systems biology is the study of biological systems in their entirety and usually involves computational and mathematical analysis and modelling to capture their full complexity. It can provide a powerful insight into the development of diseases and biological responses to stimuli such as drugs. Mathematical models are built upon granular omics data such as genomics, transcriptomics and proteomics information, which can be integrated using bioinformatics tools into a representation of more complex systems such as cells. Models based on quantitative kinetic data (concentrations of reactants/products) have predictive capacity and thus potential to inform drug discovery and development efforts.[9] The HGP is a collaborative project working in the field of genomics which has led to new studies in applied systems biology. One of the aims of systems biology is to model and discover properties of cells, tissues and organisms functioning as a system whose individual components and attributes have changed, such as in a disease state due to variation. It also led to insights into how variation is dispersed worldwide and the need for diverse population studies which informed the 1000 Genomes Project and related resources such as Finngen[10] and UK Biobank.[11] Having this ever-growing number of genomes from around the world has led to the development of genome-wide association studies (GWAS) which are used to detect variations in genomes, called single nucleotide polymorphisms (SNPs), that can be associated with a higher risk of a particular disease or condition. GWAS uses a phenotype-to-genotype approach, beginning with a specific phenotype that is associated with genetic variants across the genome.[12] Different from simple Mendelian diseases that result from an individual variant primarily in protein-coding regions in the DNA, the vast majority of SNPs that have been identified for multifactorial diseases map to

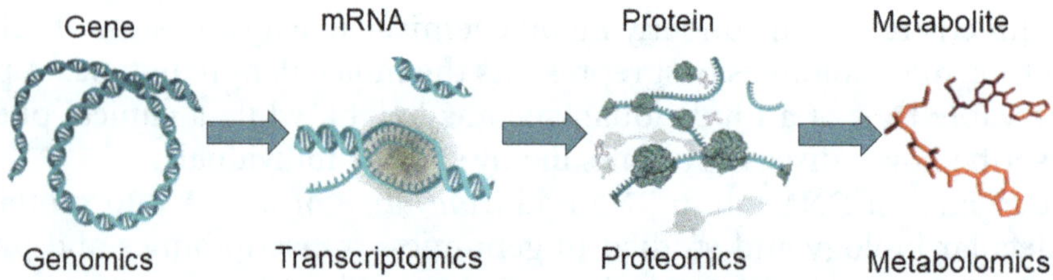


**Figure 13.1** Overview of the four major "omics" fields, from genomics to metabolomics. Image Credit: Metabolomics team (EMBL-EBI).

non-coding intergenic and intronic regulatory regions. SNPs altering the amino acids of protein-coding genes can drastically influence protein function, and play a vital role in disease pathophysiology. By contrast, regulatory SNPs (rSNPs) show modest effects that might modify gene function more subtly.[13] One of the strengths of GWAS is its unbiased whole genome nature, giving GWAS the ability to identify novel genes and pathways linked to common and complex conditions.[12] However, there are a number of challenges posed by the GWAS approach. The first of these is reaching a threshold of statistical significance for a particular gene/disease relationship due to the complexity of multiple comparisons testing (see Section 13.6 Hints and Tips). To be considered "GWAS significant", only those associations with a $P$ value of $<5 \times 10^{-8}$ are considered statistically significant.[12] Secondly, GWASs often fail to identify clinically relevant predictive associations and have difficulty explaining a significant portion of the predicted phenotypic heritability.[12] Thirdly, GWAS SNPs are predominantly common variants across the genome, while causative/functional polymorphisms may be in partial linkage disequilibrium with the genotyped SNPs, resulting in observed weak effects. Linkage disequilibrium refers to the fact that certain alleles may be inherited together and that the SNPs may not be independent. This is important, since non-random associations between SNPs can "tag" a region as relevant to disease; moreover, a rarer causal variant may exist within the tagged gene set. Finally, the vast majority of GWAS-significant SNPs are intergenic and identifying functional polymorphisms in intergenic regions is a particular challenge.[12] One alternative/complementary approach to GWAS to help with these challenges is the phenome-wide association study (PheWAS) which reverses the GWAS approach by starting with a genotype to test for associations over a wide spectrum of human phenotypes.[12] This again highlights the necessity to analyze the data across many different populations and at scale in order to connect SNPs with a particular disease or condition as the responsible variants will vary in different populations. With this vast and exponentially growing amount of multi-omics data being generated worldwide and the increasing research in systems biology, the approach of choice to collate, integrate and interpret this data is bioinformatics. The GWAS and PheWAS data highlights this effectively. To aid researchers with the significance challenge, the GWAS Catalog (http://www.ebi.ac.uk/gwas) was funded by the National Human Genome Research Institute to provide a consistent, searchable, visualisable and freely available database of SNP–trait associations, which can be easily integrated with other resources, and is accessed by scientists, clinicians and other users worldwide. All published GWAS studies are curated to extract the reported trait, significant SNP–trait associations and sample metadata (https://www.ebi.ac.uk/gwas/docs/about).[14] The PheWAS method was originally described using electronic medical record (EMR) data in the Vanderbilt DNA Biobank, BioVU,[15] but can also be applied to other richly phenotyped sets (https://phewascatalog.org). Platforms have been developed that integrate and display association statistics such as GeneBass (https://genebass.org/), an open-access tool built on UK Biobank data that reports exome association statistics. Here, associations between single-variant data and phenotypes can be visualised within a user-friendly split-screen interface starting from a gene or phenotype. In addition, the relevance of large-scale omics data to commercial drug discovery is exemplified by the involvement of pharmaceutical companies in the public-private UK Biobank[11] Exome Sequencing Consortium. Sequencing of the UK Biobank exome (200 000 sequences so far) coupled with longitudinal phenotypic data (from an unbiased population) provides a rich data source for the identification of new drug targets, enhanced understanding of causal mechanisms related to drug efficacy and unrelated phenotypes that may be linked to adverse events, a major cause of drug attrition.[16] The planned expansion of UK Biobank into proteomics data in "The Pharma Proteomics Project" will further increase the utility of the UK Biobank data. Having this online and publicly available curated data and associated tools is critical to advance research. Bioinformatics has accompanied the growth of omics science from the start. It has emerged as an interdisciplinary science that combines computer science, mathematics and statistics to analyze vast amounts of biological data, effectively extracting knowledge from data and facilitating fast advances on our understanding of biology and medicine and answering medicinal chemistry questions as listed below:

There is a need to develop treatments for Disease A; what questions might a medicinal chemist ask?

- What is known about the genetic basis of Disease A?
    - Is there a single causative gene?
    - Is Disease A polygenic and complex?
    - Is there GWAS or PheWAS data that links targets or pathways to the disease?
- What is known about the putative targets?
    - How do they function and is there potential to modulate the target(s) with beneficial effect?
    - What role does the target have in disease (metabolism, signaling *etc.*) and its cause (variation, altered expression *etc.*)?
    - What pathways include the target and can pathways be modulated independently?
    - Can the targets be prioritised?
- How "druggable" are these targets (do both small molecules and biologics have potential as drugs)?
    - Are compounds known to bind to the target? If so, what are the binding interactions?
    - How diverse is the chemical space?
    - How selective are compounds for the target *versus* related proteins?
    - Could potency, physicochemical or pharmacokinetic properties be improved?
- Do approved drugs for the target/disease exist?
    - What is the drug mechanism?
    - How efficacious are the drugs?
    - Are adverse effects known?
- Can systems data inform future drug development?
    - Is there data to show the wider impact of target modulation on an organism?
    - What is the contribution of individual differences to drug efficacy (is there pharmacogenomic data available)?
    - Is there potential for drug–drug interactions upon modulation of the candidate target?

## 13.2 From Genes to Drugs and Back Again: Past, Current and Future Perspectives on Omics Data in Drug Discovery

Disease can often be managed with medicines that replace or stabilise deficient proteins or enzymes (*e.g.* cystic fibrosis), control cell signalling and proliferation (*e.g.* cancers) or compensate for metabolic disorders (*e.g.* high LDL cholesterol). Many early drugs arose from phenotypic compound screens (that assessed the effect of a compound on a phenotype) using microbial natural products, which produced the desired biological effect but without knowledge of the mechanism. Target-based drug discovery began to dominate from the 1980s and was based on the principle that certain proteins (targets) can be modulated by small molecules to elicit a beneficial effect in disease. Current practice often incorporates elements of both strategies; for example, exploiting high-throughput target screens in relevant cell-lines.[17] Omics-driven strategies such as GWAS, PheWAS and metabolomics, as described above, offer alternative untargeted approaches that can reveal novel biological targets in complex diseases, whilst accounting for individual differences in the era of precision medicine.

To exemplify the progress in drug discovery through the application of omics approaches and informatics tools, the development of drugs for high LDL cholesterol will be considered and linked to resources containing relevant information. High LDL cholesterol is a risk factor for cardiovascular disease and can have a genetic cause or component, as seen in familial hypercholesterolemia (FH), but is also influenced by environmental factors such as diet.

### 13.2.1 Drug Discovery

The statins are a family of drugs used to treat high LDL cholesterol and reduce cardiovascular risk (Scandinavian Simvastatin Survival Study, 1994[18]) (Figure 13.2). Atorvastatin (Lipitor) is a "Blockbuster" drug and became one of the top selling drugs following its approval in 1996[19] and simvastatin features on the WHO List of Essential Medicines 2021.[20] Discovery of the statins was driven by the link between coronary artery disease and high LDL cholesterol, coupled with the elucidation of cholesterol biosynthesis which prompted target-based screens against the rate-limiting enzyme β-hydroxy β-methylglutaryl-CoA (HMG-CoA) reductase.[21] Compactin, a fungal metabolite, was the first confirmed HMG-CoA reductase inhibitor but was deemed too toxic for drug development.[21,22] Lovastatin, another fungal natural product, was identified in *Aspergillus terreus* extracts and became the first cholesterol-lowering drug in 1987.[21] Simvastatin and pravastatin, semi-synthetic derivatives of lovastatin, were subsequently approved in 1991 with fully synthetic statins achieving approved status over the following two decades (fluvastatin; 1993, atorvastatin; 1996, cerivastatin; 1997, rosuvastatin; 2003, pitavastatin; 2009). Rosuvastatin, the most potent member of the statin family, was rationally developed for increased selectivity for liver cells (the site of cholesterol biosynthesis). The increased hydrophilicity of rosuvastatin targets the drug to the liver, whilst metabolism is minimised, resulting in a longer lasting activity profile.[23] Subsequent

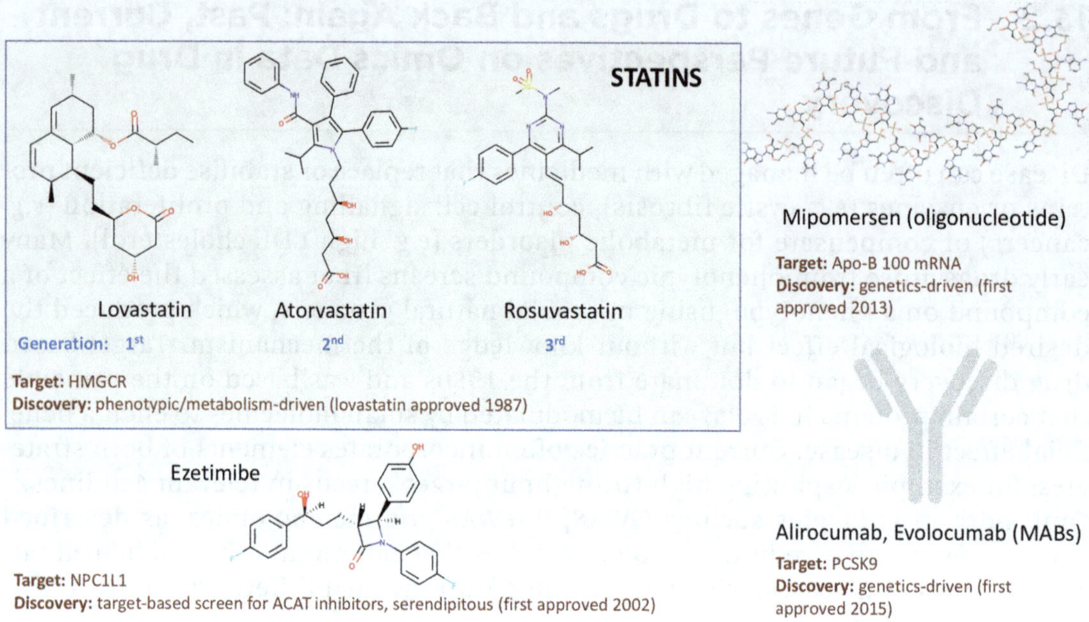


**Figure 13.2** Approved cholesterol-lowering drugs. Parts of this figure were derived from the ChEMBL website. Image Credit: ChEMBL.

crystallisation of the catalytic portion of HMG-CoA reductase bound to rosuvastatin explained the increased potency of rosuvastatin, which binds in the HMG-CoA binding site of HMG-CoA reductase through the same polar interactions as the natural substrate, but forms additional interactions with the enzyme through the sulfone group, resulting in tighter binding.[24] This crystallisation data was made freely available in the PDB database, which is one of the oldest bioinformatic resources available. Moreover, comprehensive protein target data is available through UniProt, and physicochemical and pharmacokinetic data for the statins is available through chemistry databases. The statins are an early example towards traditional target-based screens that require prior knowledge of the genes, pathways, proteins and/or metabolites underlying disease for compound screens against potentially druggable targets. Conversely, the discovery and approval in 2002 of ezetimibe, another LDL cholesterol lowering drug, was serendipitous and without a confirmed molecular target upon drug approval (Figure 13.2). Whilst the development of the statins and ezetimibe occurred in the pre-omics era, a bioinformatics strategy subsequently provided genetic support for the ezetimibe drug target as Nieman Pick C1 like 1 (NPC1L1) protein offering insight into the LDL cholesterol-lowering mechanism.[25,26] Furthermore, ongoing research on the statins has enhanced our understanding of their disease-impact as well as individual differences related to ADMET properties (as discussed below). Having this information on drug mechanism, biological context and ADMET properties at the start of a drug development programme using bioinformatics offers an improved starting point (Table 13.1).

In the post-genomics era, SNPs identified by GWAS may offer promising starting points for drug development. Familial hypercholesterolemia (FH) is monogenic disorder and

**Table 13.1** Data on the statin target *HMGCR*.

| Data type | Database accession/example data | Database |
|---|---|---|
| DNA | ENSG00000113161 | Ensembl |
| Variation | dbSNP:rs5908 (natural variant) | dbSNP |
| Protein (and proteomics) | P04035 | UniProt |
| Gene expression | ENSG00000113161 | Expression Atlas |
| Protein structure | 1DQA (HMGCR), 1HWL (HMGCR bound to rosuvastatin) | PDB |
| Pathways | R-HSA-191273 (cholesterol biosynthesis) | Reactome |
| Chemical biology | CHEMBL402 (HMGCR target) | ChEMBL |
| | **Drugs against HMGCR:** CHEMBL503 (lovastatin), CHEMBL1064 (simvastatin), CHEMBL1144 (pravastatin), CHEMBL2220442 (fluvastatin), CHEMBL1487 (atorvastatin), CHEMBL1477 (cerivastatin), CHEMBL1496 (rosuvastatin), CHEMBL1201753 (pitavastatin) | ChEMBL, FDA pharmacogenomic markers, dbSNP |
| | **Efficacy:** *e.g.* $K_i$ 0.9 nM for rosuvastatin (assayID: CHEMBL839925) | |
| | **Properties:** alog*P*: 2.4 (rosuvastatin), 4.59 (simvastatin) | |
| | **Pharmacokinetics, adverse effects:** Withdrawn drugs: CHEMBL1477 (cerivastatin, withdrawn in the US, 2001) Pharmacogenomic markers for statin-associated muscle symptoms:dbSNP:rs4149056 (SLCO1B1 variant 521C, identified by GWAS)[27] | |
| Systems | Enzymes involved in liver cell metabolism of atorvastatin: BIOMD0000000328 | BioModels |
| Integrated data | ENSG00000113161 | Open Targets, GeneBass |
| Alternative targets for cholesterol-related phenotypes | **Phenotype; HDL cholesterol** Targets include *LPL, APOC3* | GeneBass |
| | **Phenotype; Hypercholesterolemia** Targets include *PCSK9, NPC1L1* | Open Targets |

most cases are linked to variation in the low density lipoprotein cholesterol receptor (LDL-R) gene encoding the receptor responsible for uptake of cholesterol-containing LDL-C particles from the blood.[28] Interestingly, the efficacy of the statins is also partly mediated through upregulation of LDL-R (*via* inhibition of their direct HMGCR target) illustrating the importance of pathway knowledge and regulatory context in drug discovery. Variation in two other genes encoding Apolipoprotein B (ApoB) and Proprotein Convertase Subtilisin/Kexin type 9 (PCSK9) are also causal in FH. PCSK9 forms a complex with the LDL-R receptor facilitating its degradation and reducing LDL-R levels and subsequent uptake of plasma LDL cholesterol.[28] Variation in PCSK9 was first associated with FH in 2003 by sequencing,[29] and other gain-of-function mutations (causing higher plasma LDL cholesterol) and loss-of-function mutations (causing lower LDL cholesterol) have since been identified.[30] Just over a decade after variation in PCSK9 was first linked to LDL cholesterol level, the PCSK9-targeting monoclonal antibodies alirocumab and evolocumab were approved by the FDA for FH in 2015[31] and in 2020 the PCSK9 anti-sense inhibitor inclisiran was approved in Europe.[32] Mipomersen, an anti-sense oligonucleotide targeting ApoB, has also been FDA approved (Figure 13.2).[33] Recent genetic analyses (Mendelian randomisation) to identify targets associated with blood lipids and their causal relevance to coronary heart disease re-identified established LDL-C-lowering targets such as NPC1L1, HMGCR and PCSK9 that reduce CHD risk.[34] New targets were also identified and prioritised by methods that included a phenome-screen to assess potential mechanism-based adverse effects, which demonstrates the potential of genetic data for both the identification of new targets and preliminary safety evaluation. It remains to be seen whether new drugs for these and other targets will develop over the next few years. Significantly, omics data for cardiovascular disease was fundamental in teasing apart the contribution of various cholesterol-containing biomolecules and thus to the identification of new candidate drug targets.[35]

Cardiovascular disease is complex and multifactorial. High LDL cholesterol is one risk factor with associated drug targets but other clinical risk factors, such as obesity, may involve additional genes. The use of GWAS identified the fat mass and obesity-associated protein FTO (UniProt:Q9C0B1).[36] In contrast with the direct metabolic effect of the statins, *FTO*'s gene product FTO, an alpha-ketoglutarate-dependent dioxygenase, functions as a single-stranded RNA demethylase with an epitranscriptomic role (regulation of mRNA expression) that has been linked to obesity; however, the mechanism has not been fully elucidated (for example FTO could function *via* IRX3).[37] This highlights once again how important it is to be aware of changes across the omics that can directly affect the disease state or effectiveness of the treatment. Identification of FTO has prompted screens for small-molecule inhibitors as potential treatments for obesity-related diseases. A virtual screen of FDA-approved drugs (accessed from the ZINC database, https://zinc15.docking.org) against the FTO crystal structure (PDB:3LFM) led to the experimental confirmation of the approved drug entacapone (CHEMBL953) as an FTO inhibitor that improved body weight, glucose tolerance and adipose thermogenesis in mice.[38] Subsequent rational drug design based on the entacapone-FTO crystal structure (PDB:6AK4) produced an optimised compound (cpd-7, IC50 0.7 μM, PDB:6AEJ). In this obesity model, FTO-mediated demethylation of the downstream transcription factor FOXO1 (UniProt:Q12778), involved in regulation of gluconeogenesis, was proposed to form part of the anti-obesity mechanism, as informed by transcriptomics. The *FOX O1* is a challenging target but effective indirect modulation (reduced expression of its gene product Forkhead box protein O1) *via* inhibition of FTO was achieved.[38] FTO is also an oncogene, and inhibitors display potential for the treatment of acute myeloid leukaemia. Compounds with efficacy against a panel of human-derived cancer cell lines and *in vivo* mouse models have been synthesised.[39] In this case, transcriptomics indicated that FTO-mediated suppression of MYC, E2F and G2M signalling cascades and activation of apoptosis and p53 pathways may be involved. Patent data on FTO-targeted compounds as anti-obesity and leukaemia treatments (US-20180118665-A1 and WO2018157842, respectively) can be found in ChEMBLv29.

Emerging epitransciptomics drug targets such as FTO have relatively limited data at this stage, but the evidence that FTO may be druggable and the identification of inhibitors with favourable pharmacokinetic properties[39] demonstrates the potential for large-scale genome comparisons to reveal new target classes and the value of chemical and protein structure data for inhibitor screens. Rapid integration of new protein–ligand structures, transcriptomics and bioactivity data into open-access bioinformatics databases enhances the breadth of target data for the drug discovery effort. So far in this text, the bioinformatic resources cited include UniProt (proteins, https://www.uniprot.org), PDB (protein structure, https://www.ebi.ac.uk/pdbe/), Reactome (molecular networks, https://reactome.org), dbSNP (human variation, https://www.ncbi.nlm.nih.gov/snp/) and ChEMBL (bioactivity data for drug-like compounds, https://www.ebi.ac.uk/chembl/). All of these resources contain valuable information about the drug targets as described above and will be described in more detail in the next section.

### 13.2.2 Drug Development

Once a drug–target interaction has been established, bioinformatics strategies are also central to the drug optimisation and development process. The development of the statins, for example, provided a family of effective LDL cholesterol lowering drugs. However, fully understanding the individual differences in their efficacy, pharmacokinetics and adverse effects needs a broader range of omics investigations and could have avoided some of the problems seen in their side effects. Cerivastatin was withdrawn in the US in 2001 due to adverse effects. GWAS has also identified several pharmacogenomic markers potentially linked to statin biological response and subsequently a variant of the SLCO1B1 transporter (SLCO1B1 521C – db:SNP:rs4149056) has been highlighted as a biomarker for simvastatin myopathy[27] and included as a pharmacogenomic marker in the rosuvastatin prescribing information.[40,41] Environmental factors such as diet and concomitant drugs also influence statin effectiveness and pharmacokinetics, highlighting the importance of systems-based approaches that can also account for non-genetic factors.

## 13.3 Resources for Understanding Targets for Medicinal Chemistry

### 13.3.1 Genes, Proteins and Functional Genomics

Data on genes, proteins, small molecules and metabolites are collected, catalogued, managed and shared in a structured and freely accessible manner in bioinformatic life sciences databases. With this data being generated at such a large scale, these databases have become essential tools in bioinformatics serving a large and diverse base of global researchers from wet-lab biologists to computational bioinformaticians and medical scientists in both academia and industry. Our ability to understand biomedical processes based on genomic data is critically dependent on our knowledge of how individual proteins function and interact. Proteins provide an essential link between the genome sequence and the eventual phenotype as they are the primary effectors of the instructions encoded in our genomes and they and their products (including non-coding RNAs and metabolites) ultimately shape our cells, tissues, organs and bodies in response to our environment. Furthermore, knowing the biological targets (proteins) and their interaction with chemical compounds (both natural and synthetic) is essential in medicinal chemistry for understanding the effects of the drugs, their metabolism and potential side-effects.

The UniProt Knowledgebase (www.uniprot.org) is one of the most widely used biomolecular databases in the world and is ideal for discovering all known biology for a protein target.[42] UniProt was established in 2002 as a collaboration between the European Bioinformatics Institute (EMBL-EBI), the SIB Swiss Institute of Bioinformatics and the Protein Information Resource (PIR), bringing together expertise on protein research, biocuration and infrastructure under the umbrella of the UniProt Consortium. The UniProt Knowledgebase (UniProtKB)'s annotation of proteins is of exceptional quality. Expert biologists (biocurators) collect and evaluate multiple lines of evidence from text and figures from experiments in published literature in order to provide an accurate, reliable and ever-evolving description of protein function. Expert curation in UniProt is a well-defined process (https://www.uniprot.org/help/manual_curation) that has been refined over many years and continues to develop in response to community needs. A fully curated UniProtKB/Swiss-Prot record describes all known protein products of a given gene from a given species and provides a summary of published experimental data for each protein product. Protein products include those arising from alternative splicing and initiation codon and promoter usage, RNA editing and the proteolytic processing of peptide chains. No other resource provides such comprehensive curation of reference sequences from the genome through the transcript to the protein, and finally to the mature peptides – data that cannot be predicted from the genome. Annotation for each UniProtKB protein record includes a complete list of all relevant protein (and gene) names (including official names from protein nomenclature committees such as HGNC and the IUBMB Enzyme Nomenclature Committee [IUBMB-NC]), a complete description of all known functions (in free text form and using GO), enzymatic activities (EC numbers of IUBMB-NC), biochemical reactions (Rhea, https://www.rhea-db.org), pathways (GO, http://geneontology.org), interactions with small molecules such as ligands and cofactors (ChEBI), subcellular location and membrane topology (GO and UniProtKB controlled vocabularies), protein interactions and complexes (free text, GO and IMEx (https://www.imexconsortium.org)) and relevant diseases (OMIM, https://www.ncbi.nlm.nih.gov/omim). Curation of the protein sequence provides information on functional sites or regions such as domains, secretory signals, membrane anchors, and transmembrane regions. Links to family and domain records in InterPro (https://www.ebi.ac.uk/interpro/) and member databases provide up-to-date information into family classification and annotation. UniProtKB also includes functionally important post-translational modifications (currently linked to community standard vocabularies such as PSI-MOD (https://bioportal.bioontology.org/ontologies/PSIMOD) and RESID (https://proteininformationresource.org/resid/), and in future to ChEBI) and naturally occurring protein sequence variants (shortly to be described using HGVS nomenclature) of demonstrated pathogenic significance (to be standardised with respect to other resources such as ClinGen, https://clinicalgenome.org) and functional impact (to be standardised using VariO and other functional ontologies). The broad range of data and annotation types covered by UniProtKB – and links to the underlying genomic and transcript data – makes UniProtKB an ideal basis for the integrated analysis of genomic, transcriptomic, proteomic and metabolomic data. For medicinal chemistry, UniProt already provides the links between proteins and chemistry with well-established links to chemistry and drug resources, and standards like ChEBI and ChEMBL and plans to increase its integration with metabolomics data.

This comprehensive resource provides an excellent starting point to explore potential drug targets. To exemplify this, the original statin target, HMG-CoA reductase (3-hydroxy-3-methylglutaryl-coenzyme A reductase) is available as UniProt:P04035. This record provides extensive information on how the enzyme works, the substrates it catalyses and their products, the regulatory mechanism of action, important sites of function like the specific position in sequence of active sites, and phosphorylation and glycosylation sites, interaction partners and its role in the *R*-mevalonate biosynthesis, and provides links to the variant and structure information. Importantly, information on the less well-established targets, FTO (UniProt:Q9C0B1) and FOXO1 (UniProt:Q12778), implicated in obesity and cardiovascular disease, is also readily available and linked to other databases providing an excellent starting point for investigation of novel targets for drug discovery.

## 13.3.2 Reactions, Pathways and Metabolites

At the cellular level, life is a network of molecular reactions that enable signal transduction, transport, DNA replication, protein synthesis and intermediary metabolism. A variety of online resources capture aspects of this information at the level of individual reactions, such as Rhea, or at the level of reaction sequences spanning various domains of biology, such as KEGG (https://www.genome.jp/kegg/), MetaCyc (https://metacyc.org) or PANTHER (http://www.pantherdb.org).[43] Reactome collates this information in a curated database of human biological pathways that extends beyond metabolism to include biological processes such as cell signalling and DNA transcription. The database is hierarchical and builds upon individual reactions (*e.g.* from Rhea) to generate pathways, clusters and concepts. Over 50% of predicted human protein coding genes are included in the database v70, along with disease and drug mechanism annotations from the literature. Other drug-relevant information such as compound activation, transport and clearance, and impact of genetic mutations is also included.[43,44] The Reactome Knowledgebase systematically links human proteins to their molecular functions, providing a resource that functions both as an archive of biological processes and as a tool for discovering novel functional relationships in data such as gene expression studies or catalogues of somatic mutations in tumour cells.[43] An additional "disease" superpathway groups 484 annotations of disease counterparts of these normal cellular processes. These disease annotations include 1599 variant proteins and their post-translationally modified forms derived from 308 gene products, used to annotate 970 disease-specific reactions, tagged with 387 Disease Ontology terms (https://disease-ontology.org).[43] Reactome therefore provides an invaluable resource for drug discovery that can probe the wider context of disease or drug function and highlight this early in drug development.

Reactions and pathways relevant to the statin drugs are found in Reactome and details on the statin target HMGCR (R-HSA-9621345), enzymatic reaction (*via* Rhea 15 991) and cholesterol biosynthetic pathway (R-HSA-191273) are available (Figure 13.3).

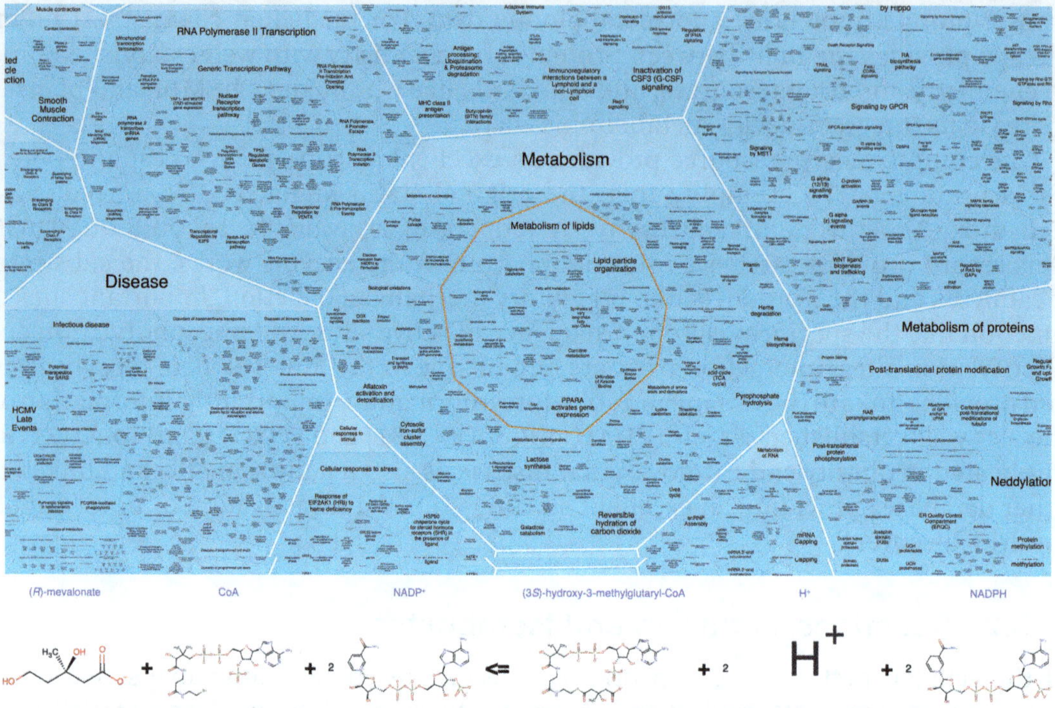


**Figure 13.3** Hierarchical pathway views of cholesterol metabolism (a. Voronoi visualisation). Taken from the Reactome website. Image Credit: EMBL-EBI. (b. HMG-CoA catalysed reaction). Taken from the Rhea website. Image Credit: Rhea, Swiss Institute of Bioinformatics.

Metabolomics is a relatively new field of omics technology that is primarily concerned with the global or system-wide characterisation of small molecule metabolites using technologies such as nuclear magnetic resonance, liquid chromatography and/or mass spectrometry. Because of its conceptual and technical overlap with many aspects of pharmaceutical research, metabolomics is now finding applications that span almost the full length of the drug discovery and development pipeline, from lead compound discovery to post-approval drug surveillance.[45] MetaboLights (https://www.ebi.ac.uk/metabolights/) is a global database for metabolomics studies, their raw experimental data and associated metadata. It is cross-species and cross-technique and covers metabolite structures and their reference spectra as well as their biological roles and locations. MetaboLights is the recommended metabolomics repository for a number of leading journals and ELIXIR, the European infrastructure for life science information. It offers user-submission tools and has strong reporting capabilities. It uses and further develops *de facto* standard formats where various components are encapsulated, such as the encoded spectral and chromatographic data, and associated information about the chemical structure, as well as metadata describing assays and the study as a whole. MetaboLights' semantic quality is based on various controlled vocabularies and ontologies linking data to existing resources such as ChEBI, Reactome, Rhea and BRENDA (https://www.brenda-enzymes.org). The team collaborates closely with major parties in world-wide metabolomics communities, such as the Metabolomics Society and the associated Metabolomics Standards Initiative (MSI) (https://www.ebi.ac.uk/metabolights/about). It has seen exponential growth in the last couple of years as the metabolomics field is rapidly evolving, in both the science and the technology. There have been as many submissions in the last year as there were in the previous eight years and while there are 3400 species represented in the MetaboLights database, there has been an increasing deposition of human and mouse data which now constitutes 50% of the studies, reflecting the use of metabolomics in clinical applications.[7] The MetaboLights team is working closely with its diverse user community (academia, industry, clinicians) to provide the highest quality of data and plans to build on the integrative work already achieved in UniProt for genomics, transcriptomics and proteomics to complement that data with experimental phenotype data for a fully comprehensive view of a particular gene, protein or disease. While it has nearly 2000 metabolomics studies from global researchers (USA, UK and China being the biggest submitters), it has plans to establish a data exchange collaboration with its American (Metabolomics Workbench) and Japanese (MetaboBank) colleagues to provide a truly global and comprehensive delivery in one resource. This will enable it to play its role with the other bioinformatic life science omics such as UniProt and ChEMBL to provide integrative and interpretable insights into health and disease and potential drug discovery.

### 13.3.3 Drugs, Targets and Biological Effects

Understanding how drugs interact with biological targets to mitigate disease is key to drug discovery. Chemistry databases provide valuable repositories of structured bioactivity data for drug discovery purposes and a number of open-access resources have been established based on deposited datasets (PubChem, https://pubchem.ncbi.nlm.nih.gov), literature and patents (ChEMBL, https://www.ebi.ac.uk/chembl/, SureChEMBL, https://www.surechembl.org/search/, BindingDB, http://bindingdb.org/bind/index.jsp) or with a specific focus on drugs (DrugBank (https://go.drugbank.com), Guide to Pharmacology (https://www.guidetopharmacology.org)) and drug pathways (PharmKB, https://www.pharmgkb.org). Each database (and others) contains a wealth of aggregated data and PubChem will be used to illustrate the diversity of chemical information and ChEMBL to illustrate how this information can be used in drug discovery.

PubChem[46] is a large database of chemical and bioactivity data that was founded in 2004 and is maintained by the U.S. National Center for Biotechnology Information (NCBI). The three linked databases that comprise PubChem include a dedicated "Substance" database for user-deposited data, a "Compound" database containing unique and standardised structures from the "Substance" database and BioAssay database containing associated bioactivity data. In October 2021, PubChem included 111M unique structures with 293M bioactivities against >95k target proteins. Compound data is extracted or deposited from multiple, varied sources. Individual compound pages are comprehensive and include a compound summary, diverse properties, spectral information, 2D and computationally generated 3D representations (for certain molecules), as well as vendor details and safety/handling information offering extensive chemical information in a single place. Bioactivity and therapeutic information spans targets, disease relevance, pharmacology and ADMET data, facilitating medicinal chemistry applications.

ChEMBL[47] contains bioactivity data for drug-like compounds. The original database was acquired by EMBL in 2008. The current version of ChEMBL (v29) contains bioactivity data manually extracted from over 81k documents covering the medicinal chemistry literature as well as selected patents; these patents are retrieved *via* a custom pipeline focused on data from underexplored targets. Inclusion of 180 deposited datasets and a subset of the PubChem database ensures broad coverage of relevant assays from both the academic and industrial settings. Overall, version 29 is comprised of 2.1M compounds that have been tested in 1.4M assays and provide 18.5M bioactivity data points against 14k established or potentially druggable targets.

The data in ChEMBL is primarily organised by "Compounds" and "Targets" which are linked through assays and annotated with available disease metadata. Compounds are mostly small molecules, but also include biotherapeutics (enzymes, proteins and cell lines), radioisotopes, oligonucleotides and oligosaccharides to fully reflect the breadth of approved therapeutics. Drug targets encompass proteins, nucleic acids and metabolites (molecular targets) but also cover higher level systems such as cells, tissues or whole organisms, which offer an insight into phenotypic and system-level effects. Before incorporation into ChEMBL, data undergoes several rounds of curation; compounds are rigorously standardised and represented by a range of computer readable standards (small molecules: molfiles, SMILES, InChi; biotherapeutics: HELM) and compound metadata is provided as a suite of calculated properties (*e.g.* Log$P$, molecular weight, structural alerts). Protein targets are included with their sequence, variation and drug binding site data and are further classified into relevant families, complexes and protein–protein interactions. Furthermore, mapping to UniProt provides a direct link to a dedicated and comprehensive protein resource. As a framework for drug–target–disease interactions, a subset of approved drugs and clinical candidates have been curated with established mechanisms and approved indications for use as a reference set.

Assays are central to medicinal chemistry and capture drug–target relationships by measuring the effect of bioactive compounds on genes, proteins or metabolites. Assays range from standard *in vitro* IC50s with a single purified protein to phenotypic screens such as those monitoring anti-proliferative effect on a cancer cell-line or glucose-lowering effect *in vivo*. To facilitate comparison across broadly similar assays, assays within ChEMBL are grouped into relevant types (*e.g.* binding, functional, toxicity) and common measurements such as IC50s are standardised. An effective drug must reach and bind its target(s) in an active form to elicit a beneficial biological response. Therefore, a wide range of assays covering pharmacodynamic and pharmacokinetic (ADMET) experiments are also included in ChEMBL. Furthermore, *in vivo* assays are classified into disease-relevant formats. Overall, combined measurements across binding, functional and ADMET experiments can provide a more complete picture of drug potency, toxicity and metabolism.

The availability of compound–target–disease interactions and relevant metadata in a single place supports large-scale comparisons, SAR analyses and target or toxicity prediction during drug discovery. Inclusion of structure/sequence similarity tools, target prediction models and ligand efficiency data into ChEMBL increases access to relevant drug discovery tools. Complementary data may be shared across databases to minimise duplication, and cross-referencing of ChEMBL to other dedicated chemistry, protein and metabolic resources, using the UniChem database mapping tool, enables bespoke queries that draw upon multiple resources to place drug-target relationships within the wider context of pathways or systems.

Medicinal chemistry information on the statin family of drugs is available in both PubChem and ChEMBL. As an example, rosuvastatin (CHEMBL1496, PubChem CID 446157) is annotated with structural and physiochemical data, curated with its therapeutic target HMGCR (CHEMBL402, PubChem gene 3156) and linked to potency measurements against a range of protein (and other) targets, as well as pharmacokinetic properties and safety data.

### 13.3.4 Systems Biology Resources and Drug Discovery

Drug efficacy and safety is rigorously evaluated during development and reported by regulatory agencies in open-access databases for drug approvals.[31] However, ongoing and evolving pharmacological research continues to improve our knowledge of the factors that could influence drug response. System-level models may more accurately reflect the pharmacokinetic and toxicity-related responses to drug exposure compared to *in vitro* data alone. Cross-domain and systems-level resources that include relevant individual factors (*e.g.* genetic variation affecting drug response) and clinical factors such as drug interactions can inform the pharmacokinetic and toxicity profile of existing drugs and feedback into the development of new compounds. Effective bioinformatics analyses include drug metabolism data (*e.g.* from PharmKB), enzyme inhibition activity (*e.g.* from ChEMBL and others) and potential drug interaction data (*e.g.* from DrugBank) at the earliest stage during drug development, and may offer an early insight into the potential role of individual differences in drug efficacy, pharmacokinetics and risk of adverse effects.[48]

As introduced earlier, computational models of multicomponent biological systems can provide a powerful insight into the development of diseases and biological responses to stimuli such as drugs. An example of a mathematical approach is BioModels (https://www.ebi.ac.uk/biomodels/), which is one of the most widely used model repositories covering diverse biological processes such as cell signalling and regulation, metabolism, stimulus-responses and genome-scale metabolism. The resource is open-access, searchable and, in November 2021, contains over 1000 manually curated, verified and standardised models produced in a range of formats with cross-references to relevant informatics resources to facilitate integration. Notably, human genome-scale metabolic models, such as the subset of 6750 models derived from clinical tumour samples, enrich the database with disease-relevant information.[9]

Drugs such as the statins are effective with now relatively few side effects as their mechanisms are better understood. The most common adverse effect is statin-associated muscle symptoms (SAMS) and risk is associated with increased exposure to statins (and their metabolites) potentially resulting from individual differences in drug uptake/transport and metabolism (pharmacokinetics). Models of the liver cell uptake and metabolism of atorvastatin[48] (BIOMD0000000328) in a panel of patient-derived hepatocytes highlighted the metabolic differences due to variation in the key metabolic enzymes CYP3A4 (UniProt:P08684) and UGT1A3 (UniProt:P35503). In addition, several GWAS studies[49] identified an SNP in the transporter SLCO1B1 521C (dbSNP:rs4149056) associated with adverse effects during simvastatin therapy and SLCO1B1 genotype is now a pharmacogenomic biomarker for rosuvastatin.[40,41] In addition to genetic factors, concomitant treatment with other drugs that modulate metabolic enzymes can alter overall exposure and subsequent risk of adverse effects and knowledge of these effects allows improved treatment.

### 13.3.5 Ontologies

Ontologies define database concepts, and the properties and relationships between entities. Ontologies enable shared definitions across multiple databases, such as metabolites as defined by ChEBI. Given the breadth of information relevant to the drug discovery process, using defined ontologies allows comparison and extraction of related chemical, biological and medical concepts from multiple resources. The European Bioinformatics Institute (EMBL-EBI) provide an Ontology Lookup Service (https://www.ebi.ac.uk/ols/index) for biomedical ontologies that allows users to identify ontologies relevant to their research area. Standardised disease concepts are essential for drug discovery informatics research and ontologies such the Medical Subjects Headings (https://meshb.nlm.nih.gov/search, U.S. National Library of Medicine) and MONDO Disease Ontology (https://mondo.monarchinitiative.org), for example, provide structured disease information. The Experimental Factor Ontology (EFO) (https://www.ebi.ac.uk/efo/) covers disease concepts but also captures broader experimental concepts found in EMBL-EBI databases such as the GWAS catalogue and Open Targets.

As an ontology example, ChEBI (https://www.ebi.ac.uk/chebi/) is a manually curated database and ontology of chemical entities of biological interest. There are two main subontologies, a chemical entity ontology that accounts for structural features and a role ontology that classifies entries according to their activity, function and/or applications.[50] Simvastatin is found within ChEBI (CHEBI:9150) alongside its standardised structural information and "biological" and "application" roles. The biological role records HMGCR inhibition and application role highlights its use as an anti-cholesteremic drug.

## 13.4 Harnessing Omics Data for Drug Discovery – The Open Targets Platform for Drug Target Identification and Prioritisation

Integration of public domain data enables target identification and prioritisation. One example is the Open Targets platform (https://www.opentargets.org).

Drug development remains costly and lengthy, with high attrition rates due to poor efficacy. Drug candidates supported by genetic evidence have a higher chance of success,[51,52] making it imperative to consider the omics evidence for the desired therapeutic effect at the earliest stage during development. To achieve this goal, skilled bioinformaticians can compile comprehensive data across multiple resources. However, publicly available platforms such as Open Targets collate the relevant information and provide an excellent starting point for new drug development initiatives accessible to the wider research community.

Open Targets[53,54] is a drug discovery platform focused on target–disease associations. Initially developed as part of public-private collaboration between the EMBL-EBI, WT Sanger and GSK in 2014, it has expanded to other pharmaceutical companies. Evidence for target–disease links is extracted by expert bioinformaticians from a broad range of omics data sources (including germline and somatic mutations from GWAS Catalogue and UK BioBank, expression data from Expression Atlas, drug data from ChEMBL *etc.*). Based on the strength of available evidence, target–disease associations are scored to provide sets of prioritised targets for individual diseases. Reliability is high due to manual curation and interpretation of GWAS evidence. A user-friendly interface displays relationships from a disease-centric view (to visualise targets associated with disease) or target-centric view (to visualise diseases associated with selected targets) alongside the original evidence. Programmatic access is available through an API and data dumps providing a versatile, well-maintained and structured open-access repository. Open Targets data has varied applications in drug discovery research, including modelling target–disease relationships,[55] new target identification[56] and drug repurposing.[57] In addition to the target validation tool, the Open Targets collaboration has also generated an unprecedented number of new oncology targets. Using CRISPR, a high-throughput and precision gene-editing tool, every gene in a panel of 300 cancer models (covering 30 cancer types) was disrupted. A priority list of 600 essential cancer genes was generated and integrated into Open Targets for focused anti-cancer screening programmes.[58] One of the newly identified targets, WRN, has since been crystallised[59] and the structure deposited in PDB (6YHR), facilitating rational drug design and illustrating the benefits of high-throughput experimental genetics approaches and the rapid integration of output data into open-access bioinformatics databases. Other integrated platforms are available, for example GeneBass which is built on UK Biobank data, offering the researcher a selection of drug discovery tools.

A query of Open Targets with hypercholesterolemia as a disease returned HMGCR as the top target followed by other targets that also have approved drugs (*e.g.* NPC1L1, PCSK9), as expected. With HMGCR as a query, top disease associations were lipid-related disorders (Figure 13.4). Using the GeneBass platform, a query with LDL cholesterol ("LDL direct") as a test phenotype, returned strongly significant associations with *PCSK9*, *APOB* and several other genes. Further exploration of phenotypes associated with the *PCSK9* gene using GeneBass provided lipid-related measurements such as LDL, Apolipoprotein B and cholesterol amongst the top associations supporting the known role of these targets in lipid-related disorders.

## 13.5 Conclusions and Predictions for the Future

In recent decades, nucleic acid sequencing technologies and high-throughput chemical screens have developed alongside bioinformatics tools that process their output. Researchers can use bioinformatics methods and databases in drug discovery to

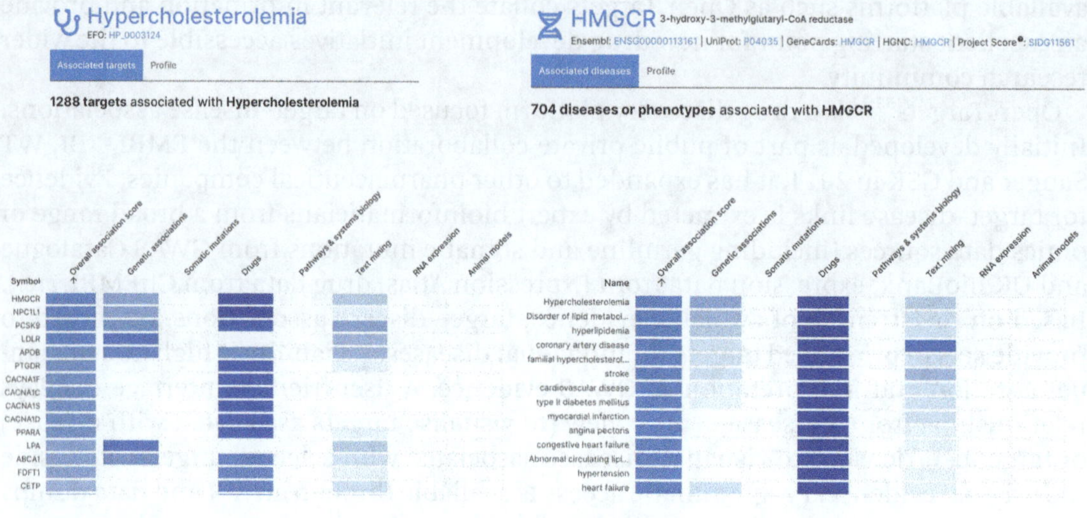

Figure 13.4 Open Targets disease-target associations (release 21.06). Image Credit: Open Targets.

extract relevant efficacy and toxicity data at the earliest stage and reduce the potential for costly attrition. In the future, increasing omics data will continue to improve our understanding of disease; from the global effects on a host to the changes occurring in a single cell. Improved understanding of systems biology may offer an insight into beneficial drug combinations that better modulate a disease-relevant pathway and may lead to more drugs that act on multiple targets. Fine-grained analysis of cells with technologies such as single-cell RNASeq and metabolomics tools can also improve our understanding of diseases. The development of safe drugs will likely be enhanced with increasingly relevant biological models and techniques, such as organ-on-a-chip.[17] Understanding this data in the context of our environment (including drugs) and combining dispersed data in a single place will remain valuable in drug discovery and development.

Precision medicine, informed by genome sequencing, is likely to have an increasing role in drug discovery and development. Variant-selective drugs illustrate the potential to generate compounds selective for disease (or resistance)-relevant mutations and highlight the importance of rapid whole genome sequencing. Moreover, newer drug types, such as gene therapies and anti-sense drugs, target nucleic acids directly. An interesting recent example is the combined genetic and metabolomic approach that delivered the first-in-class cancer drugs ivosidenib (approved 2018) and enasidenib (approved 2017). Their discovery built on somatic mutation analysis that identified the metabolic enzyme isocitrate dehydrogenase (IDH) as an oncogene; metabolomics tools revealed that gain-of-function mutations convert the enzyme to a producer of 2-hydroxyglutartate (2-HG), a novel oncometabolite.[60,61] More examples of precision drugs developed through multiple omics techniques are expected to follow.

## 13.6 Hints and Tips

### 13.6.1 Bioinformatics Skills and Tools

Bioinformatics skills are integral to the analysis of experimental omics data as well as the development of tools and resources that provide a starting point for drug discovery and development. The reciprocal nature means that the continued integration of new experimental data enhances databases which in turn feeds back into improved drug research.

### 13.6.2 Control of Gene and Protein Synthesis

Our phenotype depends on more than sequence alone; regulation of transcription and translation also has an impact. The levels of mRNA (from transcription of DNA) and proteins (from translation of mRNA) are influenced by many factors, such as secondary structure in nucleic acids, the rate of synthesis *versus* degradation, the action of regulatory proteins and the influence of environmental factors and metabolite levels.

### 13.6.3 Types of Genetic Variation

Genetic variation occurs in many forms, such as short insertions or deletions of DNA, duplications or inversions, all of which can influence our phenotype. GWAS is primarily focused on single nucleotide polymorphisms (SNPs) and their association with a higher risk of a particular disease or condition but can also include other variation types.

### 13.6.4 Targets with Limited Data

Proteins similar to the target of interest can be identified using a basic local alignment search tool (BLAST). The protein family, catalytic residues and structural features of identified proteins can be explored using the protein resources described in this text. Homology modelling is an approach that uses a similar protein (>30% sequence identity) to construct a 3D structure. Ligand docking experiments with the model can then inform screening experiments. SWISS-MODEL (https://swissmodel.expasy.org) is a freely available homology modelling resource.

### 13.6.5 Significance in GWAS Studies

A *P*-value of 0.05 is often used as a threshold for significance in single comparisons, this level accepts that 1 in 20 tests (5%) are false positives. Since GWASs assess the association of SNPs with phenotypic traits, multiple comparisons are performed to test 10s to 100s of thousands of SNPs simultaneously. Therefore, large numbers of false positives are expected with a *P*-value of 0.05. To be considered "GWAS significant", only those associations with a *P*-value of $<5 \times 10^{-8}$ are considered statistically significant; this provides a generally applicable and appropriate measure for modest sample sizes.[62] Nonetheless, there is scope to adjust the significance thresholds according to the experiment. The *P*-value of $<5 \times 10^{-8}$ was originally determined using a European population with a minor allele frequency (MAF) ≥5%. More stringent *P*-values may be required for less frequent variants (MAF <5%) and a series of alternative thresholds have been suggested.[63] Conversely, in large samples, a less stringent measure could be applied (*P*-value $<5 \times 10^{-7}$) to increase the power to discover significant associations with only a slight increase in false positives. Other methods to control false discovery rates may also be appropriate (*e.g.* Benjamini–Hochberg and Benjamini–Yekutieli corrections).[62] One final consideration is the multiple comparisons assume that each test is independent. Since sets of alleles may be inherited together, SNPs may not be independent and are therefore in linkage disequilibrium. Linkage disequilibrium is important since non-random associations between SNPs can "tag" a region as relevant to disease; moreover, a rarer causal variant may exist within the tagged gene set. A linkage disequilibrium threshold of LD $r2 < 0.8$ (meaning that SNPs are associated) was necessary for the *P*-value of $<5 \times 10^{-8}$ to remain valid.[63]

### 13.6.6 Large-scale Bioactivity Data

Large-screening datasets are valuable starting points in the identification of potential targets. Care should always be taken to understand the underlying data stored in repositories as well as appropriate interpretation and limitations. Bioactivity data may be sourced from multiple organisations and some variation is expected, even for similar assays. This can be problematic for targets with limited data where the significance of outliers is greater. Finally, data extraction and curation processes are often documented, and potential data validity warnings may be incorporated into databases to guide users.

### 13.6.7 Accessing Data in Repositories

A *web interface* is an interactive web page that provides a visual representation of data stored within a database.

*Application Programming Interfaces* (APIs) and *web services* may also be provided by a resource. An API is an interface, generally REST, with in-built functions and tools that allows users to interact with the service without the "presentation layer" of a web interface. APIs can also be used to log-in to a service or add/delete/update data. Web services are an example of an API that provide a means for direct computer–computer-based communication to retrieve data from a resource, *via* the internet, using structured, computer-readable instructions.

*Database downloads* ("database dumps") are copies of the underlying resource database which are often available in various formats. Databases can be downloaded in a local instance and more complex and bespoke queries performed using compatible database tools.

For more advanced data extraction, *programmatic approaches* using computer-readable code (such as Python) in a structured program (instructions) and can be used for data extraction, curation, analysis and/or integration pipelines using APIs or database dumps.

### 13.6.8 Bioinformatics language (Table 13.2).

For the beginner, a resource web interface (interactive web page) is often the best approach (Figure 13.5).

**Table 13.2** Bioinformatics language.

| Informatics language | | |
|---|---|---|
| Resources & repositories | • *Databases:* store raw data and associated annotations in a structured manner, using a database-specific vocabulary. Relational databases define the relationships between entities (such as proteins and ligands).<br>• *Accessions:* unique database-specific identifiers (accessions) are assigned to entities and used to retrieve associated information. Accessions may also be used to cross-reference between related resources. | *Advantages of structured repositories:*<br>• Consistency<br>• Defined searches<br>• Supports usability and FAIR principles (that data should be Findable, Accessible, Interoperable, Reusable) |
| Data structure | • *Database qualifiers*: define inter-relationships between database entities, such as the database table and column that stores the data points.<br>• *Ontologies:* define database concepts, and the properties and relationships between entities. Enables a shared definition across multiple databases, such as metabolites as defined by ChEBI. | |
| Data availability | • *Data access: via* an interface, API, web services, database dumps *etc.* (see Section 13.6, Hints and Tips).<br>• *FTP (file transfer process):* methods for transfer of large files.<br>• *Local host:* user computer that can be used to host and run bioinformatics packages. | |
| Data processing | • *Curation:* the process of checking, standardising, annotating and integrating data.<br>• *Data extraction:* retrieval of selected data in a desired format.<br>• *Programmatic analysis*: extraction or integration of data using defined computer languages to produce as program (structured instructions) for informatics analyses. | |

a

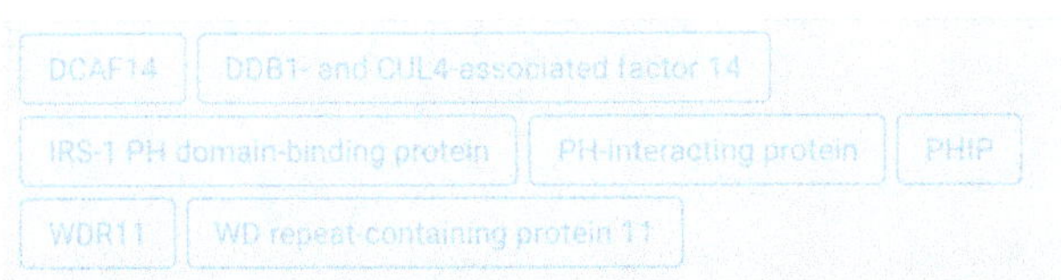


b

```
{
  'synonyms': ['DCAF14', 'DDB1- and CUL4-associated factor 14', ...]
}
```

**Figure 13.5** Synonyms for PH-interacting protein (CHEMBL2176773): (a) a visual representation from the ChEMBL (v29) interface, (b) web services output. Image Credit: ChEMBL.

## 13.7 Databases

(Table 13.3)

**Table 13.3** Example resources. A range of other resources can be found in relevant publications (*e.g.* ref. 64).

| Category | Database | Bioinformatic tools | Weblinks |
|---|---|---|---|
| DNA and RNA Sequences | INSDC<br>RefSeq<br>RNACentral<br>MgniFy | Sequence similarity search (Blast) | https://www.insdc.org<br>https://www.ncbi.nlm.nih.gov/refseq/<br>https://rnacentral.org<br>https://www.ebi.ac.uk/metagenomics/<br>https://blast.ncbi.nlm.nih.gov/Blast.cgi |
| Genes & Variation | Ensembl, Entrez Gene, ClinVAR, EGA, EVA, dbGAP, dbSNP | Sequence similarity search (Blast)<br>Sequence alignment (Kalign, MView) | https://www.ensembl.org/index.html<br>https://www.ncbi.nlm.nih.gov/gene/ |
| | | Compare a protein sequence to a genomic DNA sequence (GeneWise) | https://www.ncbi.nlm.nih.gov/clinvar/ |
| | | PhenGen, Ensembl VEP | https://ega-archive.org<br>https://www.ebi.ac.uk/eva/<br>https://www.ncbi.nlm.nih.gov/gap/<br>https://www.ncbi.nlm.nih.gov/snp/<br>https://blast.ncbi.nlm.nih.gov/Blast.cgi<br>https://www.ebi.ac.uk/Tools/msa/kalign/<br>https://www.ebi.ac.uk/Tools/msa/mview/<br>https://www.ebi.ac.uk/Tools/psa/genewise/<br>https://www.ncbi.nlm.nih.gov/gap/phegeni<br>https://www.ensembl.org/info/docs/tools/vep/index.html |
| Proteins | UniProt | Sequence similarity search (Blast, HMMER) | https://www.uniprot.org |
| | RefSeq | Sequence alignment (Clustal Omega, MAFFT, T-Coffee) | https://www.ncbi.nlm.nih.gov/refseq/ |
| | BRENDA | COBALT | https://www.brenda-enzymes.org<br>https://blast.ncbi.nlm.nih.gov/Blast.cgi<br>https://www.ebi.ac.uk/Tools/hmmer/<br>https://www.ebi.ac.uk/Tools/msa/clustalo/<br>https://mafft.cbrc.jp/alignment/software/<br>https://www.ebi.ac.uk/Tools/msa/tcoffee/<br>https://www.ncbi.nlm.nih.gov/tools/cobalt/re_cobalt.cgi |
| Protein families | InterPro<br>PFAM, SMART, PANTHER, PROSITE, TIGRFams, CDD | InterProScan<br>CDSearch | https://www.ebi.ac.uk/interpro/<br>http://pfam.xfam.org |
| | | | http://smart.embl-heidelberg.de<br>http://www.pantherdb.org<br>https://prosite.expasy.org<br>http://tigrfams.jcvi.org/cgi-bin/index.cgi<br>https://www.ncbi.nlm.nih.gov/Structure/cdd/cdd.shtml<br>https://www.ebi.ac.uk/interpro/search/sequence/<br>https://www.ncbi.nlm.nih.gov/Structure/cdd/wrpsb.cgi |

| | | | |
|---|---|---|---|
| Structures | PDBe | PDBeFold | https://www.ebi.ac.uk/pdbe/ |
| | SwissMODEL | PDBeMotif | https://swissmodel.expasy.org |
| | | VAST | https://www.ebi.ac.uk/msd-srv/ssm/ |
| | | | https://www.ebi.ac.uk/pdbe-site/pdbemotif/ |
| | | | https://structure.ncbi.nlm.nih.gov/Structure/VAST/vast.shtml |
| Proteomics | PRIDE, PeptideAtlas, ProteomicsDB, MASSIVE | GNPS MetExplore | https://www.ebi.ac.uk/pride/ |
| | | | http://www.peptideatlas.org |
| | | | https://www.proteomicsdb.org |
| | | | https://massive.ucsd.edu/ProteoSAFe/static/massive.jsp |
| | | | https://gnps.ucsd.edu/ProteoSAFe/static/gnps-splash.jsp |
| | | | https://metexplore.toulouse.inrae.fr/metexplore-doc/index.php |
| Gene Expression | Expression Atlas, GTEX | | https://www.ebi.ac.uk/gxa/home |
| | | | https://gtexportal.org/home/ |
| Chemical Biology | ChEBI | PDBeChem | https://www.ebi.ac.uk/chebi/ |
| | ChEMBL | UniChem | https://www.ebi.ac.uk/chembl/ |
| | SureChEMBL | PubChem Structure Search | https://www.surechembl.org/search/ |
| | MetaboLights | MetExplore | https://www.ebi.ac.uk/metabolights/ |
| | Rhea | Metaboanalyst | https://www.rhea-db.org |
| | PubChem | | https://pubchem.ncbi.nlm.nih.gov |
| | DrugBank | | https://go.drugbank.com |
| | Guide to PHARMACOLOGY | | https://www.guidetopharmacology.org |
| | Binding Database | | http://bindingdb.org/bind/index.jsp |
| | PharmGKB | | https://www.pharmgkb.org |
| | | | https://www.ebi.ac.uk/pdbe-srv/pdbechem/ |
| | | | https://www.ebi.ac.uk/unichem/ |
| | | | https://metexplore.toulouse.inrae.fr/metexplore-doc/index.php |
| | | | https://www.metaboanalyst.ca |
| Pathways | Reactome | | https://reactome.org |
| | GeneOntology | | http://geneontology.org |
| | MetaCyc | | https://metacyc.org |
| Integrated platforms & system-level data | GWAS catalog | Open Targets | http://www.ebi.ac.uk/gwas |
| | PheWAS catalog | GeneBass | https://phewascatalog.org/ |
| | Human Cell Atlas | | https://www.humancellatlas.org |
| | KEGG | | https://www.genome.jp/kegg/ |
| | BioModels | | https://www.ebi.ac.uk/biomodels/ |
| | | | https://www.opentargets.org |
| | | | https://genebass.org/ |
| Literature | PubMed | | https://pubmed.ncbi.nlm.nih.gov |
| | EuropePMC | | https://europepmc.org |

## Key References

These are the selected references:

M. R. Nelson, H. Tipney, J. L. Painter, J. Shen, P. Nicoletti, Y. Shen, A. Floratos, P. C. Sham, M. J. Li, J. Wang, L. R. Cardon, J. C. Whittaker and P. Sanseau, The support of human genetic evidence for approved drug indications, *Nat. Genet.*, **47**(8), 856–60, 2015.

Drug attrition due to poor efficacy is a costly problem in drug development. In this academic-industrial publication, a pipeline to review evidence for gene-trait associations (*e.g.* from GWAS data) was compiled and the likelihood of drug success evaluated. Drug mechanisms with genetic evidence had an increased chance of success.

D. Mendez, A. Gaulton, A. P. Bento, J. Chambers, M. De Veij, E. Félix, M. P. Magariños, J. F. Mosquera, P. Mutowo, M. Nowotka, M. Gordillo-Marañón, F. Hunter, L. Junco, G. Mugumbate, M. Rodriguez-Lopez, F. Atkinson, N. Bosc, C. J. Radoux, A. Segura-Cabrera, A. Hersey and A. R. Leach, ChEMBL: towards direct deposition of bioassay data, *Nucleic Acids Res.*, **47**(D1), D930–D940, 2019.

Biomedical resources are continually curated and enhanced resulting in frequent updates and addition of new features. Regular publications that summarise data content, access and improvements ensure that users remain familiar with the data structure and usage. This ChEMBL publication is an example of a periodic update that provides an overview of the database, recent updates and new features.

Z. Chen, M. Boehnke, X. Wen and B. Mukherjee, Revisiting the genome-wide significance threshold for common variant GWAS, *G3: Genes, Genomes, Genet.*, **11**(2), 2021.

Interpretation of GWAS studies and selection of an appropriate significance value can be challenging. This publication reviews methods for determining significance in GWAS experiments and confirms that $5 \times 10^{-8}$ is a generally applicable *P*-value but that there is potential to relax the threshold (and increase the discovery rate) for large studies under certain circumstances.

## Acknowledgements

We thank David Mendez for review and editing of the Hints and Tips "Accessing data in repositories" and Anna Gaulton for reviewing the text.

## References

1. International Human Genome Sequencing Consortium, Initial sequencing and analysis of the human genome, *Nature*, 2001, **409**, 860–921.
2. J. C. Venter and M. D. Adams, *et al.*, The sequence of the human genome, *Science*, 2001, **291**, 1304–1351.
3. International Service for the Acquisition of Agri-biotech Applications (ISAAA), Pocket K No. 15: 'Omics' Sciences: Genomics, Proteomics, and Metabolomics, *ISAAA*, [Online] 2021, https://www.isaaa.org/resources/publications/pocketk/15/default.asp.

4. ENCODE Project Consortium, The ENCODE (ENCyclopedia Of DNA Elements) Project, *Science*, 2004, **306**, 636–640.
5. 1000 Genomes Project Consortium, G. R. Abecasis, D. Altshuler, A. Auton, L. D. Brooks, R. M. Durbin, R. A. Gibbs, M. E. Hurles and G. A. McVean, A map of human genome variation from population-scale sequencing, *Nature*, 2010, **467**, 1061–1073.
6. MedlinePlus, What are complex or multifactorial disorders? [Online] 2021, https://medlineplus.gov/genetics/understanding/mutationsanddisorders/complexdisorders/.
7. K. Haug, K. Cochrane, V. C. Nainala, M. Williams, J. Chang, K. V. Jayaseelan and C. O'Donovan, MetaboLights: a resource evolving in response to the needs of its scientific community, *Nucleic Acids Res.*, 2020, **48**, D440–D444.
8. K. C. Cheng, S. R. Katz, A. Y. Lin, X. Xin and Y. Ding, Whole-Organism Cellular Pathology: A Systems Approach to Phenomics, *Adv. Genet.*, 2016, **95**, 89–115.
9. R. S. Malik-Sheriff, M. Glont, T. V. N. Nguyen, K. Tiwari, M. G. Roberts, A. Xavier, M. T. Vu, J. Men, M. Maire, S. Kananathan, E. L. Fairbanks, J. P. Meyer, C. Arankalle, T. M. Varusai, V. Knight-Schrijver, L. Li, C. Dueñas-Roca, G. Dass, S. M. Keating, Y. M. Park, N. Buso, N. Rodriguez, M. Hucka and H. Hermjakob, BioModels-15 years of sharing computational models in life science, *Nucleic Acids Res.*, 2020, **48**, D407–D415.
10. FinnGen, https://www.finngen.fi/en. [Online] 2021.
11. UK Biobank, *Biobank*, [Online] 2021, https://www.ukbiobank.ac.uk.
12. S. J. Hebbring, The challenges, advantages and future of phenome-wide association studies, *Immunology*, 2014, **141**, 157–165.
13. Q. Huang, Genetic Study of Complex Diseases in the Post-GWAS Era, *J. Genet. Genomics*, 2015, **42**, 87–98.
14. A. Buniello, J. A. L. MacArthur, M. Cerezo, L. W. Harris, J. Hayhurst, C. Malangone, A. McMahon, J. Morales, E. Mountjoy, E. Sollis, D. Suveges, O. Vrousgou, P. L. Whetzel, R. Amode, J. A. Guillen, H. S Riat, S. J. Trevanion, P. Hall, H. Junkins, P. Flicek, T. Burdett, L. A. Hindorff, F. Cunningham and H. Parkinson, The NHGRI-EBI GWAS Catalog of published genome-wide association studies, targeted arrays and summary statistics 2019, *Nucleic Acids Res.*, 2019, **47**, D1005–D1012.
15. Vanderbilt University Medical Centre, Department of Biomedical Informatics, Vanderbilt University Medical Centre, [Online] 2021, https://www.vumc.org/dbmi/biovu.
16. J. D. Szustakowski, S. Balasubramanian, E. Kvikstad, S. Khalid, P. G. Bronson, A. Sasson, ... and UKB-ESC Research Team, Advancing human genetics research and drug discovery through exome sequencing of the UK Biobank, *Nat. Genet.*, 2021, **53**, 942–948.
17. M. Leveridge, C. W. Chung, J. W. Gross, C. B. Phelps and D. Green, Integration of Lead Discovery Tactics and the Evolution of the Lead Discovery Toolbox, *SLAS Discovery*, 2018, **23**, 881–897.
18. Scandinavian Simvastatin Survival Study Group, Randomised trial of cholesterol lowering in 4444 patients with coronary heart disease: the Scandinavian Simvastatin Survival Study (4S), *Lancet*, 1994, **344**, 1383–1389.
19. The Lancet, Lessons from Lipitor and the broken blockbuster drug model, *Lancet*, 2011, **378**, 1976.
20. World Health Organisation, WHO model list of essential medicines – 22nd list, 2021. [Online] 2021, https://www.who.int/publications/i/item/WHO-MHP-HPS-EML-2021.02.
21. A. Endo, A historical perspective on the discovery of statins, *Proc. Jpn. Acad. Ser. B Phys. Biol. Sci.*, 2010, **86**, 484–493.
22. A. Endo, M. Kuroda and K. Tanzawa, Competitive inhibition of 3-hydroxy-3-methylglutaryl coenzyme A reductase by ML-236A and ML-236B fungal metabolites, having hypocholesterolemic activity, *FEBS Lett.*, 1976, **72**, 323–326.
23. M. Watanabe, H. Koike, T. Ishiba, T. Okada, S. Seo and K. Hirai, Synthesis and biological activity of methanesulfonamide pyrimidine- and N-methanesulfonyl pyrrole-substituted 3,5-dihydroxy-6-heptenoates, a novel series of HMG-CoA reductase inhibitors, *Bioorg. Med. Chem.*, 1997, **5**, 437–444.
24. E. S. Istvan and J. Deisenhofer, Structural mechanism for statin inhibition of HMG-CoA reductase, *Science*, 2001, **292**, 1160–1164.
25. M. W. Huff, R. L. Pollex and R. A. Hegele, NPC1L1: evolution from pharmacological target to physiological sterol transporter, *Arterioscler. Thromb. Vasc. Biol.*, 2006, **26**, 2433–2438.
26. J. Wang, C. M. Williams and R. A. Hegele, Compound heterozygosity for two non-synonymous polymorphisms in NPC1L1 in a non-responder to ezetimibe, *Clin. Genet.*, 2005, **67**, 175–177.
27. SEARCH Collaborative Group, E. Link, S. Parish, J. Armitage, L. Bowman, S. Heath, F. Matsuda, I. Gut, M. Lathrop and R. Collins, SLCO1B1 variants and statin-induced myopathy--a genomewide study, *N. Engl. J. Med.*, 2008, **359**, 789–799.
28. A. M. Moyer and L. M. Baudhuin, Genetic considerations in the treatment of familial hypercholesterolemia, *Clin. Lipidol.*, 2015, **10**, 387–403.

29. M. Abifadel, M. Varret, J.-P. Rabès, D. Allard, K. Ouguerram, M. Devillers, C. Cruaud, S. Benjannet, L. Wickham, D. Erlich, A. Derré, L. Villéger, M. Farnier, I. Beucler, E. Bruckert, J. Chambaz, B. Chanu, J.-M. Lecerf, G. Luc, P. Moulin, J. Weissenbach, A. Prat, M. Krempf, C. Junien, N. G. Seidah and C. Boileau, Mutations in PCSK9 cause autosomal dominant hypercholesterolemia, *Nat. Genet.*, 2003, **34**, 154–156.
30. Q. Guo, X. Feng and Y. Zhou, PCSK9 Variants in Familial Hypercholesterolemia: A Comprehensive Synopsis, *Front. Genet.*, 2020, **11**, 1020.
31. FDA, Novel Drug Approvals for 2015, *Drugs*, [Online] 2021, https://www.fda.gov/drugs/new-drugs-fda-cders-new-molecular-entities-and-new-therapeutic-biological-products/novel-drug-approvals-2015.
32. EMA. Leqvio, European Medicines Agency: Sciences Medicines Health. [Online] 2021. https://www.ema.europa.eu/en/medicines/human/EPAR/leqvio.
33. P. Hair, F. Cameron and K. McKeage, Mipomersen sodium: first global approval, *Drugs*, 2013, **73**, 487–493.
34. M. Gordillo-Marañón, M. Zwierzyna, P. Charoen, F. Drenos, S. Chopade, T. Shah, J. Engmann, N. Chaturvedi, O. Papacosta, G. Wannamethee, A. Wong, R. Sofat, M. Kivimaki, J. F. Price, A. D. Hughes, T. R. Gaunt, D. A. Lawlor, A. Gaulton, A. D. Hingorani, A. F. Schmidt and C. Finan, Validation of lipid-related therapeutic targets for coronary heart disease prevention using human genetics, *Nat. Commun.*, 2021, **12**, 6120.
35. D. Girelli, C. Piubelli, N. Martinelli, R. Corrocher and O. Olivieri, A decade of progress on the genetic basis of coronary artery disease. Practical insights for the internist, *Eur. J. Intern. Med.*, 2017, **41**, 10–17.
36. L. J. Scott, K. L. Mohlke, L. L. Bonnycastle, C. J. Willer, Y. Li, W. L. Duren, M. R. Erdos, H. M. Stringham, P. S. Chines, A. U. Jackson, L. Prokunina-Olsson, C.-J. Ding, A. J. Swift, N. Narisu, T. Hu, R. Pruim, R. Xiao, X.-Y. Li, K. N. Conneely, N. L. Riebow, A. G. Sprau, M. Tong, P. P. White, K. N. Hetrick, M. W. Barnhart, C. W. Bark, J. L. Goldstein, L. Watkins, F. Xiang, J. Saramies, T. A. Buchanan, R. M. Watanabe, T. T. Valle, L. Kinnunen, G. R. Abecasis, E. W. Pugh, K. F. Doheny, R. N. Bergman, J. Tuomilehto, F. S. Collins and M. Boehnke, A genomewide association study of type 2 diabetes in Finns detects multiple susceptibility variants, *Science*, 2007, **316**, 1341–1345.
37. S. Smemo, J. J. Tena, K.-H. Kim, E. R. Gamazon, N. J. Sakabe, C. Gómez-Marín, I. Aneas, F. L. Credidio, D. R. Sobreira, N. F. Wasserman, J. H. Lee, V. Puviindran, D. Tam, M. Shen, J. E. Son, N. A. Vakili, H.-K. Sung, S. Naranjo, R. D. Acemel, M. Manzanares, A. Nagy, N. J. Cox, C.-C. Hui, J. L. Gomez-Skarmeta and M. A. Nóbrega, Obesity-associated variants within FTO form long-range functional connections with IRX3, *Nature*, 2014, **507**, 371–375.
38. S. Peng, W. Xiao, D. Ju, B. Sun, N. Hou, Q. Liu, Y. Wang, H. Zhao, C. Gao, S. Zhang, R. Cao, P. Li, H. Huang, Y. Ma, Y. Wang, W. Lai, Z. Ma, W. Zhang, S. Huang, H. Wang, Z. Zhang, L. Zhao, T. Cai, Y.-L. Zhao, F. Wang, Y. Nie, G. Zhi, Y.-G. Yang, E. E. Zhang and N. Huang, Identification of entacapone as a chemical inhibitor of FTO mediating metabolic regulation through FOXO1, *Sci. Transl. Med.*, 2019, **11**, eaau7116.
39. Y. Huang, R. Su, Y. Sheng, L. Dong, Z. Dong, H. Xu, T. Ni, Z. S. Zhang, T. Zhang, C. Li, L. Han, Z. Zhu, F. Lian, J. Wei, Q. Deng, Y. Wang, M. Wunderlich, Z. Gao, G. Pan, D. Zhong, H. Zhou, N. Zhang, J. Gan, H. Jiang, J. C. Mulloy, Z. Qian, J. Chen and C.-G. Yang, Small-Molecule Targeting of Oncogenic FTO Demethylase in Acute Myeloid Leukemia, *Cancer Cell*, 2019, **35**, 677–691.
40. FDA, Table of Pharmacogenomic Biomarkers in Drug Labeling, *Drugs*, [Online] 2021, https://www.fda.gov/drugs/science-and-research-drugs/table-pharmacogenomic-biomarkers-drug-labeling.
41. Online, https://www.accessdata.fda.gov/drugsatfda_docs/label/2020/021366s042lbl.pdf.
42. UniProt Consortium, UniProt: the universal protein knowledgebase in 2021, *Nucleic Acids Res.*, 2021, **49**, D480–D489.
43. B. Jassal, L. Matthews, G. Viteri, C. Gong, P. Lorente, A. Fabregat, K. Sidiropoulos, J. Cook, M. Gillespie, R. Haw, F. Loney, B. May, M. Milacic, K. Rothfels, C. Sevilla, V. Shamovsky, S. Shorser, T. Varusai, J. Weiser, G. Wu, L. Stein, H. Hermjakob and P. D'Eustachio, The reactome pathway knowledgebase, *Nucleic Acids Res.*, 2020, **48**, D498–D503.
44. K. Sidiropoulos, G. Viteri, C. Sevilla, S. Jupe, M. Webber, M. Orlic-Milacic, B. Jassal, B. May, V. Shamovsky, C. Duenas, K. Rothfels, L. Matthews, H. Song, L. Stein, R. Haw, P. D'Eustachio, P. Ping, H. Hermjakob and A. Fabregat, Reactome enhanced pathway visualization, *Bioinformatics*, 2017, **33**, 3461–3467.
45. D. S. Wishart, Applications of metabolomics in drug discovery and development, *Drugs*, 2008, **9**, 307–322.
46. S. Kim, J. Chen, T. Cheng, A. Gindulyte, J. He, S. He, Q. Li, B. A. Shoemaker, P. A. Thiessen, B. Yu, L. Zaslavsky, J. Zhang and E. E. Bolton, PubChem 2019 update: improved access to chemical data, *Nucleic Acids Res.*, 2019, **47**, D1102–D1109.
47. D. Mendez, A. Gaulton, A. P. Bento, J. Chambers, M. De Veij, E. Félix, M. P. Magariños, J. F. Mosquera, P. Mutowo, M. Nowotka, M. Gordillo-Marañón, F. Hunter, L. Junco, G. Mugumbate, M. Rodriguez-Lopez,

F. Atkinson, N. Bosc, C. J. Radoux, A. Segura-Cabrera, A. Hersey and A. R. Leach, ChEMBL: towards direct deposition of bioassay data, *Nucleic Acids Res.*, 2019, **47**, D930–D940.
48. J. Bucher, S. Riedmaier, A. Schnabel, K. Marcus, G. Vacun, T. S. Weiss, W. E. Thasler, A. K. Nüssler, U. M. Zanger and M. Reuss, A systems biology approach to dynamic modeling and inter-subject variability of statin pharmacokinetics in human hepatocytes, *BMC Syst. Biol.*, 2011, **5**, 66.
49. J. P. Kitzmiller, E. B. Mikulik, A. M. Dauki, C. Murkherjee and J. A. Luzum, Pharmacogenomics of statins: understanding susceptibility to adverse effects, *Pharmgenomics Pers. Med.*, 2016, **9**, 97–106.
50. J. Hastings, G. Owen, A. Dekker, M. Ennis, N. Kale, V. Muthukrishnan, S. Turner, N. Swainston, P. Mendes and C. Steinbeck, ChEBI in 2016: Improved services and an expanding collection of metabolites, *Nucleic Acids Res.*, 2016, **44**, D1214–D1219.
51. M. R. Nelson, H. Tipney, J. L. Painter, J. Shen, P. Nicoletti, Y. Shen, A. Floratos, P. C. Sham, M. J. Li, J. Wang, L. R. Cardon, J. C. Whittaker and P. Sanseau, The support of human genetic evidence for approved drug indications, *Nat. Genet.*, 2015, **47**, 856–860.
52. E. A. King, J. W. Davis and J. F. Degner, Are drug targets with genetic support twice as likely to be approved? Revised estimates of the impact of genetic support for drug mechanisms on the probability of drug approval, *PLoS Genet.*, 2019, **15**, e1008489.
53. D. Ochoa, A. Hercules, M. Carmona, D. Suveges, A. Gonzalez-Uriarte, C. Malangone, A. Miranda, L. Fumis, D. Carvalho-Silva, M. Spitzer, J. Baker, J. Ferrer, A. Raies, O. Razuvayevskaya, A. Faulconbridge, E. Petsalaki, P. Mutowo, S. Machlitt-Northen, G. Peat, E. McAuley, C. K. Ong, E. Mountjoy, M. Ghoussaini, A. Pierleoni, E. Papa, M. Pignatelli, G. Koscielny, M. Karim, J. Schwartzentruber, D. G. Hulcoop, I. Dunham and E. M. McDonagh, Open Targets Platform: supporting systematic drug-target identification and prioritisation, *Nucleic Acids Res.*, 2021, **49**, D1302–D1310.
54. G. Koscielny, P. An, D. Carvalho-Silva, J. A. Cham, L. Fumis, R. Gasparyan, S. Hasan, N. Karamanis, M. Maguire, E. Papa, A. Pierleoni, M. Pignatelli, T. Platt, F. Rowland, P. Wankar, A. P. Bento, T. Burdett, A. Fabregat, S. Forbes, A. Gaulton, C. Y. Gonzalez, H. Hermjakob, A. Hersey, S. Jupe, Ş. Kafkas, M. Keays, C. Leroy, F.-J. Lopez, M. P. Magarinos, J. Malone, J. McEntyre, A. M.-P. Fuentes, C. O'Donovan, I. Papatheodorou, H. Parkinson, B. Palka, J. Paschall, R. Petryszak, N. Pratanwanich, S. Sarntivijal, G. Saunders, K. Sidiropoulos, T. Smith, Z. Sondka, O. Stegle, Y. A. Tang, E. Turner, B. Vaughan, O. Vrousgou, X. Watkins, M.-J. Martin, P. Sanseau, J. Vamathevan, E. Birney, J. Barrett and I. Dunham, Open Targets: a platform for therapeutic target identification and validation, *Nucleic Acids Res.*, 2017, **45**, D985–D994.
55. C. J. Proctor and G. R. C. Smith, Computer simulation models as a tool to investigate the role of microRNAs in osteoarthritis, *PLoS One*, 2017, **12**, e0187568.
56. I. Tachmazidou, K. Hatzikotoulas, L. Southam, J. Esparza-Gordillo, V. Haberland, J. Zheng, T. Johnson, M. Koprulu, E. Zengini, J. Steinberg, J. M. Wilkinson, S. Bhatnagar, J. D. Hoffman, N. Buchan, D. Süveges, arcOGEN Consortium, L. Yerges-Armstrong, G. D. Smith, T. R. Gaunt, R. A. Scott, L. C. McCarthy and E. Zeggini, Identification of new therapeutic targets for osteoarthritis through genome-wide analyses of UK Biobank data, *Nat. Genet.*, 2019, **51**, 230–236.
57. M. Khaladkar, G. Koscielny, S. Hasan, P. Agarwal, I. Dunham, D. Rajpal and P. Sanseau, Uncovering novel repositioning opportunities using the Open Targets platform, *Drug Discovery Today*, 2017, **22**, 1800–1807.
58. F. M. Behan, F. Iorio, G. Picco, E. Gonçalves, C. M. Beaver, G. Migliardi, R. Santos, Y. Rao, F. Sassi, M. Pinnelli, R. Ansari, S. Harper, D. A. Jackson, R. McRae, R. Pooley, P. Wilkinson, D. van der Meer, D. Dow, C. Buser-Doepner, A. Bertotti, L. Trusolino, E. A. Stronach, J. Saez-Rodriguez, K. Yusa and M. J. Garnett, Prioritization of cancer therapeutic targets using CRISPR-Cas9 screens, *Nature*, 2019, **568**, 511–516.
59. J. A. Newman, A. E. Gavard, S. Lieb, M. C. Ravichandran, K. Hauer, P. Werni, L. Geist, J. Böttcher, J. R. Engen, K. Rumpel, M. Samwer, M. Petronczki and O. Gileadi, Structure of the helicase core of Werner helicase, a key target in microsatellite instability cancers, *Life Sci. Alliance*, 2020, **4**, e202000795.
60. D. S. Wishart, Emerging applications of metabolomics in drug discovery and precision medicine, *Nat. Rev. Drug Discovery*, 2016, **15**, 473–484.
61. P. S. Ward, J. Patel, D. R. Wise, O. Abdel-Wahab, B. D. Bennett, H. A. Coller, J. R. Cross, V. R. Fantin, C. V. Hedvat, A. E. Perl, J. D. Rabinowitz, M. Carroll, S. M. Su, K. A. Sharp, R. L. Levine and C. B. Thompson, The common feature of leukemia-associated IDH1 and IDH2 mutations is a neomorphic enzyme activity converting alpha-ketoglutarate to 2-hydroxyglutarate, *Cancer Cell*, 2010, **17**, 225–234.
62. Z. Chen, M. Boehnke, X. Wen and B. Mukherjee, Revisiting the genome-wide significance threshold for common variant GWAS, *G3: Genes, Genomes, Genet.*, 2021, **11**, jkaa056.
63. J. Fadista, A. K. Manning, J. C. Florez and L. Groop, The (in)famous GWAS P-value threshold revisited and updated for low-frequency variants, *Eur. J. Hum. Genet.*, 2016, **24**, 1202–1205.
64. J. Paananen and V. Fortino, An omics perspective on drug target discovery platforms, *Briefings Bioinf.*, 2020, **21**, 1937–1953.

# 14 Translational Science

Outi Vaarala*[a,b], Sammeli Liikkanen[a] and Anu Moilanen[a]

[a]Research & Development, Orion Corporation OrionPharma, Espoo, Finland; [b]Clinicum, University of Helsinki, Helsinki, Finland

*E-mail: outi.vaarala@orionpharma.com

## 14.1 Introduction

Translational science is "the process of turning observations in the laboratory, clinic and community into interventions that improve the health of individuals and populations", as defined by the NIH National Center for Advancing Translational Sciences (NCATS).[1] Accordingly, translational science means that new therapies, medical procedures or diagnostics are created using scientific research, *i.e.* basic, clinical and population-based research as the starting point. Translational science aims to change the life of patients, treatment protocols and health policies.

Translational science can be divided into five phases, from the pre-clinical phase of discovery to the clinical phases of drug development, and ending with community-level outcomes (Figure 14.1).

The pharma industry is continuously challenged by the low probability of success and slow speed of drug discovery projects.[2–5] The success rate of drug development is less than 5%, and the time taken for discovery and development is on average between 13 and 15 years from target idea to launch of a new drug. During the different phases of translational science the level of confidence, *e.g.* in the drug discovery process, is tested, and the quality of the translational research is the only guarantee for the success of a project. Advances in translational science offer means to tackle the challenges, and the success factors for drug discovery are based on translational science (Table 14.1).

The first success factor emphasizes the importance of target identification and validation, which is the major focus in the pre-clinical phase of translational research. When translational research based on high-quality target identification and validation is the driver of project initiation, progression and closure, the probability of success in

The Handbook of Medicinal Chemistry: Principles and Practice, 2nd Edition
Edited by Simon E. Ward and Andrew M. Davis

Published by the Royal Society of Chemistry, www.rsc.org

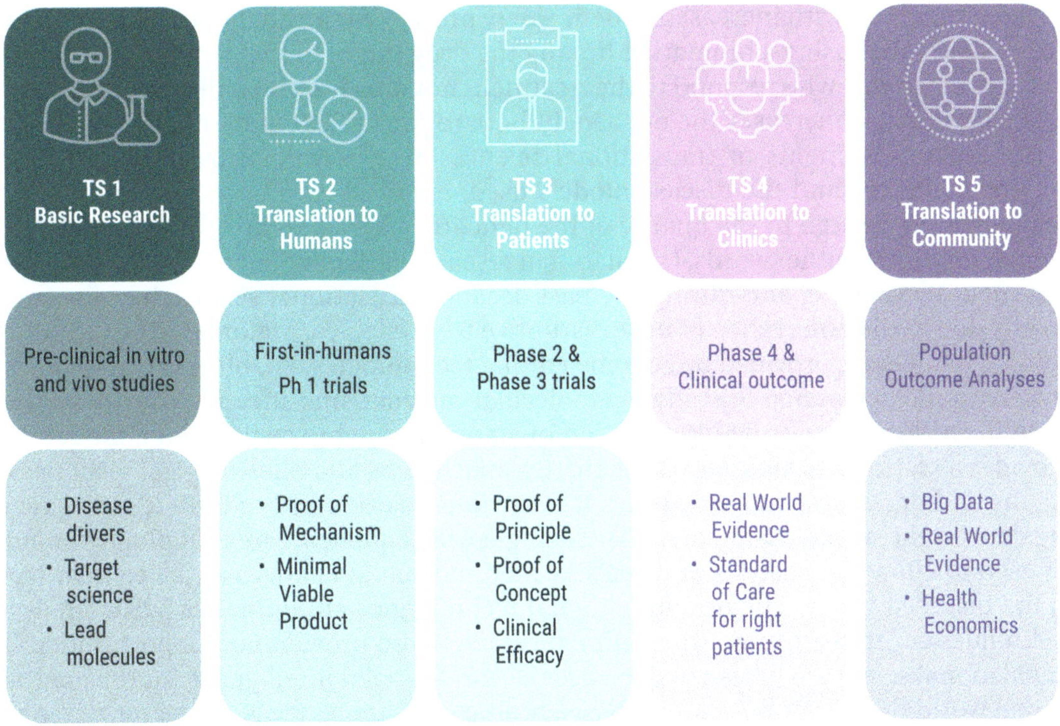
TS 1
Basic Research
TS 2
Translation to
Humans
TS 3
Translation to
Patients
TS 4
Translation to
Clinics
TS 5
Translation to
Community
Pre-clinical in vitro
and vivo studies
First-in-humans
Ph 1 trials
Phase 2 &
Phase 3 trials
Phase 4 &
Clinical outcome
Population
Outcome Analyses
• Disease drivers
• Target science
• Lead molecules
• Proof of Mechanism
• Minimal Viable Product
• Proof of Principle
• Proof of Concept
• Clinical Efficacy
• Real World Evidence
• Standard of Care for right patients
• Big Data
• Real World Evidence
• Health Economics

**Figure 14.1** Translational science transforms basic, clinical and population-based research into new therapies, bringing community-level health benefits, and can be divided into five phases with increasing level of confidence (proof of mechanism, proof of principle and proof of concept).

**Table 14.1** The success factors for drug discovery are based on high-quality translational research.

| Success factor | Key activities |
|---|---|
| The drug's target (pathway) is a disease driver | Drug discovery is based on a deep scientific understanding of the disease driver |
| The patient segment that benefits from the treatment is identified | Biomarkers (genetic, digital or biological), which are a link between the target and disease subtype, are identified and implemented in clinical trials to select patients |
| The line of sight from research to clinical development and population level outcomes is clear throughout the project | Increased collaboration between research, clinical development, business and patient advocacy groups |

drug discovery increases significantly. This phase of translational research is described in Section 14.2.

The second success factor is based on the identification of patients who respond to the developed treatment. Patient selection biomarkers provide a link between the target and the disease subtype. Biomarkers in translational science are discussed in Section 14.3.

Finally, understanding of the unmet clinical needs of patients, and the benefits and risks of the intervention at community level, needs to be clear from the early project to the post-marketing stage. A prime result of translational research is the development of targeted therapies with increased benefit-safety profiles for a patient population identified or diagnosed using a biomarker linking the drug target to the patients. The identification of patients who respond to the treatment not only improves the success rates of the trials, but also increases the net benefit both to the patient and to society.

The accomplishments of translational science are determined by the accuracy of the data collected and the disease models used, either *in vitro* or *in vivo*, and the key challenges are related to the quality of the data and translatability of the models into human disease. In other words, translational research is dependent on the technologies and models available, and during the past decade translational science has advanced greatly due to the emergence of new, disruptive technologies. Major advances in translational models are provided by genome editing technologies, enabling targeted modulation of gene expression to study the molecular mechanisms affecting the phenotype. Equally revolutionary is the introduction of an organ-on-chip translational model that provides a platform to simulate the activities, mechanics and physiological response of organs and organ systems. Nowadays it is obvious that instead of bulk RNA sequencing data on the whole tissue, new spatial single-cell sequencing methodologies should be used to allow the analysis of disease-related molecular changes at the cellular level in the diseased tissue. Furthermore, digital technologies and innovative data analysis techniques are transforming translational research and provide new opportunities for translational science. The use of data science and artificial intelligence for the analysis of real world-data from population-based studies or clinical trials opens new avenues for target ideas, biomarkers and patient stratification in drug discovery and development. The utilisation of data and data science means that we can provide sustainable treatments and medications that are based on real-world evidence.

It can be concluded that high quality of translational research is of utmost importance for drug discovery. The purpose of this chapter is to increase the understanding of the nature of translational science, and guide the practices used in drug discovery.

## 14.2 Target Science as a Starting Point for Drug Discovery

Translational science is the basis of modern drug discovery and development, which is built on molecular understanding of disease biology and the disease driver, *i.e.* the molecular mechanisms driving the disease phenotype. Analyses of success rates in drug discovery and development have demonstrated that the probability of success increases when the selection of the drug target is based on a deep understanding of the disease mechanism, and modulation of the target pathway by a drug is shown to affect the disease phenotype in *in vitro* and *in vivo* models, demonstrating proof of mechanism.[6–9]

The criteria for high-quality translational science in drug discovery are more easily achieved in therapy areas such as rare genetic diseases or oncology than in complex diseases, because the genetic disease association guides target identification.[10] This is clearly visible in the high success rate for drug discovery in rare genetic diseases[11] in which the genetic alteration causing the disease has been identified and reveals the target for drug discovery (Figure 14.2).

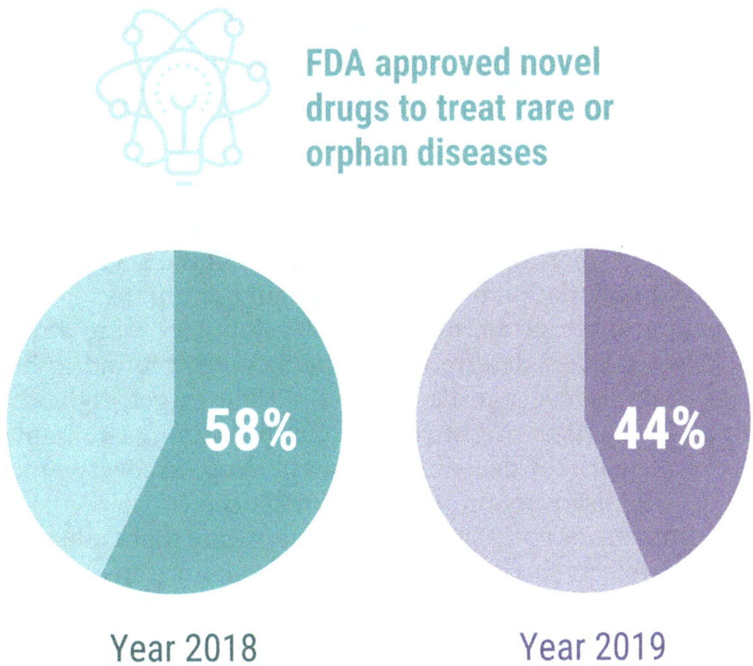


**Figure 14.2** Novel drugs to treat rare or orphan diseases show high approval rates by the FDA indicating the importance of understanding the disease driver, *i.e.* target pathway, as a starting point for drug discovery.

Also in oncology, when cancer-related genetic mutations driving tumor growth can be identified as a target for drug discovery, it becomes more straightforward. For example, mutations in the genes that encode fibroblast growth factor receptors (FGFRs) play a role in the development of several cancers, including urothelial carcinoma.[12] Genetic mutations of FGFR3 are found in the luminal subtype of muscle-invasive bladder cancer, and lead to ligand-independent constitutive FGFR signaling that contributes to oncogenesis.[13] The use of the tyrosine kinase inhibitor of FGFR1-4, erdafitinib, was associated with a tumor response in 40% of previously treated urothelial carcinoma patients,[14] and in 2019, the FDA approved erdafitinib for the treatment of patients with locally advanced or metastatic urothelial carcinoma with FGFR3 or FGFR2 genetic alterations.[15] Furthermore, the concept of the disease driver naturally leads to the subtyping of diseases according to the molecular disease mechanisms, which is the basis for selection of the therapy instead of disease severity or symptom profile.

The importance of target science in drug discovery and development is emphasized by analyses of success factors for drug discovery projects performed by pharma companies. When data from Phase 2 decisions for 44 programs were analyzed at Pfizer, it became obvious that the success of Phase 2 trials was determined by three major factors, *i.e.* solid data and understanding of the drug's exposure at the site of action, target binding and the functional pharmacological activity of the drug.[7] It was astonishing to see that in a large number of cases (43%), it was not possible to conclude whether the failure was really due to lack of efficacy or lack of adequate target modulation by the drug. As an example of this kind of situation, the authors describe a Pfizer clinical trial studying the therapeutic potential of the D3 receptor agonist PF592379 in the treatment of pain. Pre-clinical models of nociceptive pain supported the mechanism, and human PK data was encouraging. However, no efficacy of PF592379 on pain thresholds of patients with severe pain caused by osteoarthritis of the thumb was found in the clinical study. Because no evidence of modulation of the target of interest (*i.e.* the D3 receptor) at the site of action in the brain could be obtained, it remained unclear whether the failure was due to lack of pharmacological modulation of the D3 receptor or lack of the D3 receptor pathway in regulation of nociceptive pain in humans.

The success factors for drug discovery and development were analyzed by AstraZeneca too, and five technical determinants, the 5Rs, were found to be important in the evaluation of drug discovery projects, *i.e.* the right target, right tissue, the right safety, the right patient and the right commercial potential.[8] The implementation of the so-called 5R framework for decision-making in drug discovery projects improved the success rate of drug discovery projects in AstraZeneca.[9]

These examples from Pfizer and AstraZeneca demonstrate that evaluation of the potential of drug discovery projects should be based on high-quality translational research data. Pharma companies have developed frameworks to guide drug discovery and development activities in order to increase the productivity and speed of the projects. In Figure 14.3, the framework of OrionPharma is shown as a model to guide the decision-making for projects. This framework is used for drug discovery projects in both research and clinical phases.

The following guiding questions for the 5Ts provide the quality criteria for drug discovery programs and for go/no-go decisions (Boxes 1–5):

In conclusion, confidence about the target is the key to the success in drug discovery. In-house target validation is always needed; trusting just literature data is not enough since up to 60% of published pre-clinical data is not reproducible.[16] When it comes to target safety, there should be a relatively high bar for safety concerns to hinder project progression, even though safety risks are always present in drug discovery. Data providing confidence in the drug discovery project can be divided into experimental data packages (*e.g.* according to the 5Ts presented), which should be a prerequisite for drug discovery projects to progress.

As a case study of a drug discovery project built on strong target science, we discuss here the discovery of darolutamide for castration-resistant prostate cancer (CRPC). Androgen receptor gene aberrations were known to be associated with CRPC, and biological understanding of the androgen receptor as a disease driver suggested that novel androgen receptor inhibitors should be targeted to overcome the resistance mediated by both mutated and overexpressed androgen receptors.[17] The discovery of novel compounds that are able to modulate this biological mechanism, driving the development of castration resistance resulted in the identification of darolutamide. Cell-based transactivation assays demonstrated that darolutamide and its main metabolite keto-darolutamide are potent antagonists for overexpressed and mutated androgen receptors, which are commonly associated with CRPC.[18,19] Consistent with the observed target modulation, darolutamide inhibited cell proliferation of VCaP prostate cancer cells containing endogenous androgen receptor gene amplification and overexpressing androgen receptors. This mechanism of action translated to a significant anti-tumor activity in a

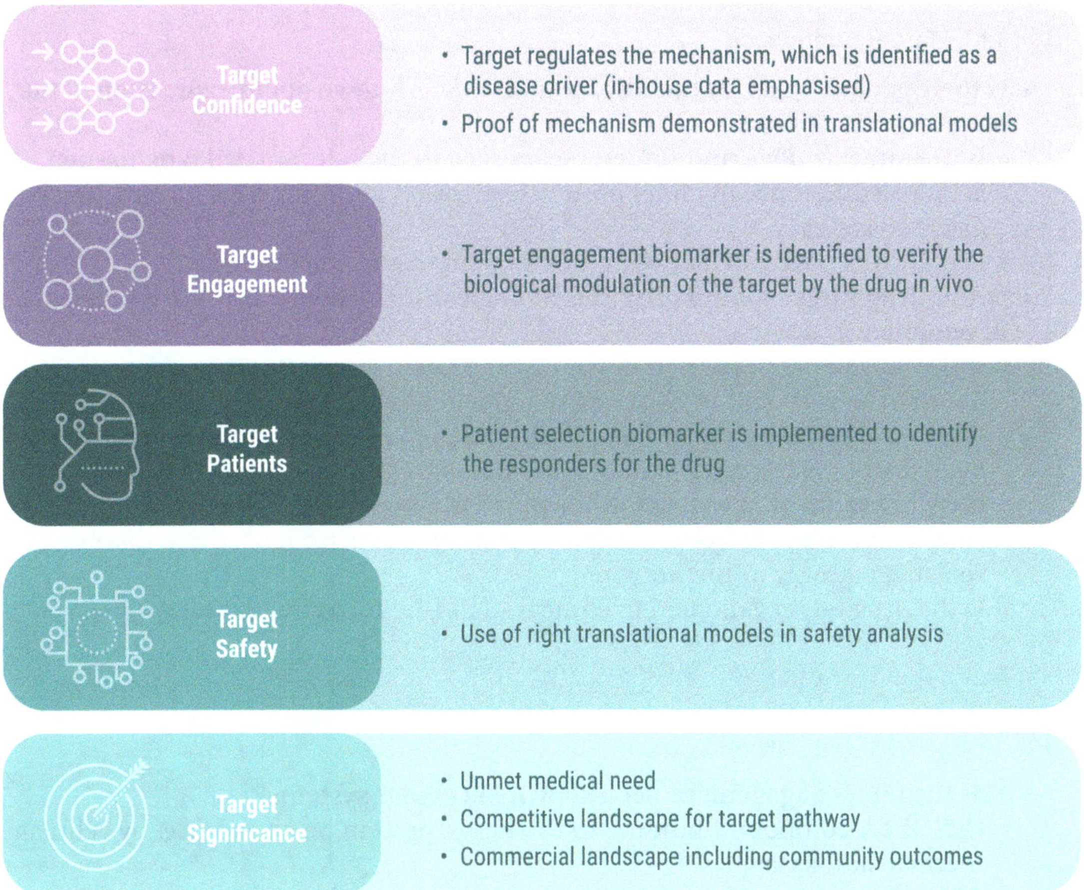


**Figure 14.3** Orion Pharma's 5Ts, to guide the evaluation of the potential of drug discovery projects, are based on translational research activities.

castration-resistant VCaP xenograft model.[18] In addition, *in vivo* efficacy has also been seen in other models, such as the LAPC-4, enzalutamide-resistant MR49F and bicalutamide-resistant KuCaP-1 models containing the AR wild type, F877L/T878A and the W742C mutations, respectively.[19,20]

Target engagement and biological response biomarkers in the darolutamide project are logically related to signalling downstream androgen receptors. In response to modulation of androgen receptor activity, darolutamide reduces the expression of androgen-stimulated target genes FKBP5, KLK3, KLK2 and TMPRSS2 in VCaP prostate cancer cells,[19] *in vitro*. Prostate-specific antigen (PSA), also known as kallikrein-related peptidase 3 (KLK3), is secreted by prostatic epithelial cells, and serum PSA levels are reported to be increased in prostate cancer due to the leakage of PSA into the circulation when the architecture of the prostate gland is disrupted. The rise in level of PSA is considered to indicate the progression of prostate cancer, and PSA is widely used as a dynamic response biomarker.[21] Darolutamide significantly decreased both PSA gene and protein expression in MR49F cells *in vitro* and

**Box 14.1 Target Confidence**

- **Is there genetic basis for the disease and what is known about expression of the drug target?**
  - Is the target (mRNA and protein) expressed in the relevant cell type/tissue?
  - Is there a difference in target protein expression and/or function in healthy *vs.* diseased states?
  - Is there a genetic link between the drug target and the disease?
- **Is the drug target modulating the biological mechanism driving the disease development?**
  - Is the mechanism of action of the target protein known?
  - Are there *in vitro* and *in vivo* disease models available for the disease?
  - Does recapitulation of the genetic alterations *in vitro* or *in vivo* reproduce the disease or treatment relevant phenotype?
  - Is there *in vitro* or *in vivo* data showing that target modulation with a tool (*e.g.* small molecule, antibody, siRNA or peptide) affects target activity, disease-associated pathway or phenotype?
  - Is the drug target validated in clinical trials (me-too or me-better drugs)?

**Box 14.2 Target Engagement**

- **Has the target engagement been shown in cellular systems?**
  - Can direct compound binding to the target protein be shown (*e.g.* by cellular thermal shift assay)?
  - Can cellular processes occurring downstream of binding be measured as a readout of target binding?
- **Does a drug bind to the target in the diseased tissue of the model organism?**
  - What methods can be used for measuring direct binding to the target in animal models (*e.g.* non-invasive imaging methods such as PET).
  - Can substrate and/or product changes be measured and used as a biological response biomarker?
  - Are there more distal readouts that are affected by the exposure to the drug?
- **What is the degree of target engagement and time on target required for efficacy?**
- **What is the accuracy of the pharmacokinetics/dynamics models?**

in subcutaneous MR49F xenografts in mice, an efficacious dose of darolutamide also significantly inhibited serum PSA levels.[22] In the dose-escalation portion of the Phase 1/2 ARADES trial, a PSA response (reduction of at least 50% in serum PSA) was noted across all of the six doses, while no dose-limiting toxicities were reported.[21] This data indicated that darolutamide had a sufficient exposure to demonstrate target engagement at a well-tolerated dose.

Box 14.3 Target Patients

- **Can the patients who respond to the treatment be identified with a biomarker?**
  - Does the biomarker provide a link between the target and the patients to be treated?
  - Can companion diagnostics be developed to aid in selecting or excluding patient groups for treatment (drug is only used in the patients with a biomarker)?
  - Can complementary diagnostic test be used to aid the benefit–risk decision-making (drug efficacy is increased in the patients with a biomarker)?

Box 14.4 Target Safety

- **What is known about the safety of the target in the preclinical models and in humans?**
  - Is the physiological role of the target protein known?
  - Does modulation of target function alter vital physiological responses in animals?
  - Is there safety margin *i.e.* difference between the effective dose and the dose that causes severe side effects?
- **What is known about the selectivity of the drug?**
  - Is the target protein amino acid sequence conserved between preclinical species and humans?
  - Are the potential off-targets of the drug known (toxic effects related to the compound hitting an unintended target)?
  - Does potential modulation of close family members or off-targets alter vital physiological responses in animals or humans?

Box 14.5 Target Significance

- **What is known about the unmet clinical need and the patient segment to be treated?**
  - Has the business case been evaluated?
  - Is it possible to get a patient organisation representative to the project team?
  - Has the impact of treatment on the quality of life been evaluated?
- **What is the competitive landscape?**
  - Is there understanding on the community level impacts including benefit/risk/cost aspects?
  - Is there understanding of the intellectual property (IP) space?
  - What are the predicted changes in the treatment due to the launch of new drugs for the same indication?

## 14.3 Target Identification

The start of target identification can be a genetic alteration associated with the disease. Genetics as the start of drug discovery is demonstrated by independent analyses revealing that the drug targets with at least one genetic association with the disease in Online Mendelian Inheritance in Man (OMIM)[23] or genome-wide association study (GWAS) catalogs[24] show better probability of success in the course of drug development (from 2.0% at the pre-clinical stage to 8.2% among approved drugs). Overall, it has been estimated that compounds whose target-indication has genetic support are twofold more likely to reach approval than those without genetic support.[25]

In the case of autosomal dominant disease, in which a disease-associated gene mutation is dominant and a single copy of the mutated gene is enough to cause the disease, the identification of the drug target is straightforward when the function of the gene is known and the target is considered druggable, *i.e.* the target can be modulated by available therapeutic modalities, *i.e.* small or large molecules, peptides, anti-sense oligonucleotides, mRNA or gene therapies.

In complex diseases, the path from a genetic association in a disease to a drug target identification and validation is complicated. Identification of the causal variants in GWAS-associated regions is needed for therapeutic target prioritisation. Understanding of the functional changes of the genetic variant is important, *e.g.* possible regulation of the expression of the gene itself or other genes localized on different chromosomes.[26,27] Target validation is extremely important to increase target confidence, *i.e.* the functional importance of the target and its modulation by the drug for the disease phenotype.

Data science-driven target identification has increasingly become the starting point for drug discovery.[28] Data science is used in the analyses of large, genetic studies to identify, *e.g.* genetic alterations associated with diseases, as discussed above. Data mining of genetic data sets is particularly useful when data is linked with other relevant data forms like primary care data or different patient-reported outcome questionnaires, as is the case with, *e.g.* UK Biobank,[29] Finnish FinnGen[30] and Generation Scotland.[31] The data mining of heterogenous data has become a more and more important tool for target identification and validation.

The concept of GWAS can be expanded from the use of genomic data alone into a phenome-wide association study (PheWAS), which includes the use of other omic datasets – such as epigenome, transcriptome, proteome, metabolome, interactome or pharmacogenome. These data sets are heterogeneous, often very large and contain data and information in various formats on different biological processes. Thus PheWAS requires a lot of data management effort and uses various modern data science techniques, such as machine learning. Analysis of these data sets enables the analysis of large populations in order to detect subpopulations and to develop various models, which can help in understanding different phenotypes, disease mechanisms and pathways. PheWAS can thus be used as a method to discover new target ideas, as well as in supporting existing drug discovery projects.

Proteomics-, metabolomics- and lipidomics-based databases can also reveal biomarkers associated with disease. When biomarkers, other than genetic, are used as a starting point for target identification, the approach requires a deep and thorough target validation to avoid the reverse causality phenomen, *i.e.* the biomarker is a consequence of the disease and not a disease driver. As an example, neutrophilic infiltration in the asthmatic lung (or in the blood of asthma patients) led to a program targeting neutrophils with a CXCR2 inhibitor, AZD5069, which decreased the neutrophil numbers and infiltration in the lung (*i.e.* target engagement achieved), but did not show efficacy in a Phase 2 trial.[32] Neutrophils are a biomarker of lung inflammation, but the results of the clinical trial questions the role of neutrophils in driving asthma.

It is also possible to have a phenotypic start for drug discovery. In phenotypic screening the defined phenotypic characteristics of the disease are measured in a cell line or an organoid model, in which screening of compounds reveals hit molecules affecting the phenotype. In this case, the target of the drug can be identified afterwards, and the mechanism of action studies are performed in disease models, *in vitro* and *in vivo*, to increase confidence. As an example, RVX-208 (apabetalone) was initially found in a phenotypic screen for compounds that enhanced ApoA-I mRNA expression in a human hepatocarcinoma cell line.[33] Its molecular target was not initially known. Later, binding assays and X-ray crystallography studies showed that RVX-208 binds to bromodomains of the BET (Bromodomain and Extra Terminal) family, competing for binding with an acetylated lysine. Experiments with small interfering RNAs (siRNA) further confirmed that BET family member BRD4 can induce ApoA-I mRNA.[34] Thus, the pharmacological activity of RVX-208 is accounted for by binding to the BET proteins. Apabetalone (RVX-208) has been developed by Resverlogix Corporation for the treatment of cardiovascular diseases associated with atherosclerosis.[35]

Target identification and validation processes based on target science and phenotypic screening are illustrated in Figure 14.4.

## 14.4 Processes and Methods of Target Validation

Target validation requires data demonstrating that the target is relevant to the disease, and a drug affects the target enough to change the disease phenotype. Importantly, target validation includes a mechanistic proof in appropriate disease models, which implies success for clinical drug development. An overview of target validation processes and methods is shown in Figure 14.5.

During the recent decade, an increasing number of potential drug targets have been identified using data mining approaches such as genetic association studies, studies of mRNA expression profiles and integrated screens of genomic alterations (*e.g.* DNA copy number changes, mutations, gene fusions) in human cancers. Additionally, functional genomic screens have enabled the screening of entire genomes to investigate functional consequences of altered gene expression.

However, as earlier discussed in Section 14.3, the biological importance of most of the genes identified in genomic studies remains unclear, and target validation studies are of utmost importance. Genetic association with diseases can be further validated as possible disease drivers in *in vitro* and *in vivo* models using, *e.g.* siRNA, tool molecules and genome editing tools (CRISPR/Cas9) to change gene expression and see the effects on phenotype. In all these experimental approaches, it is important to control

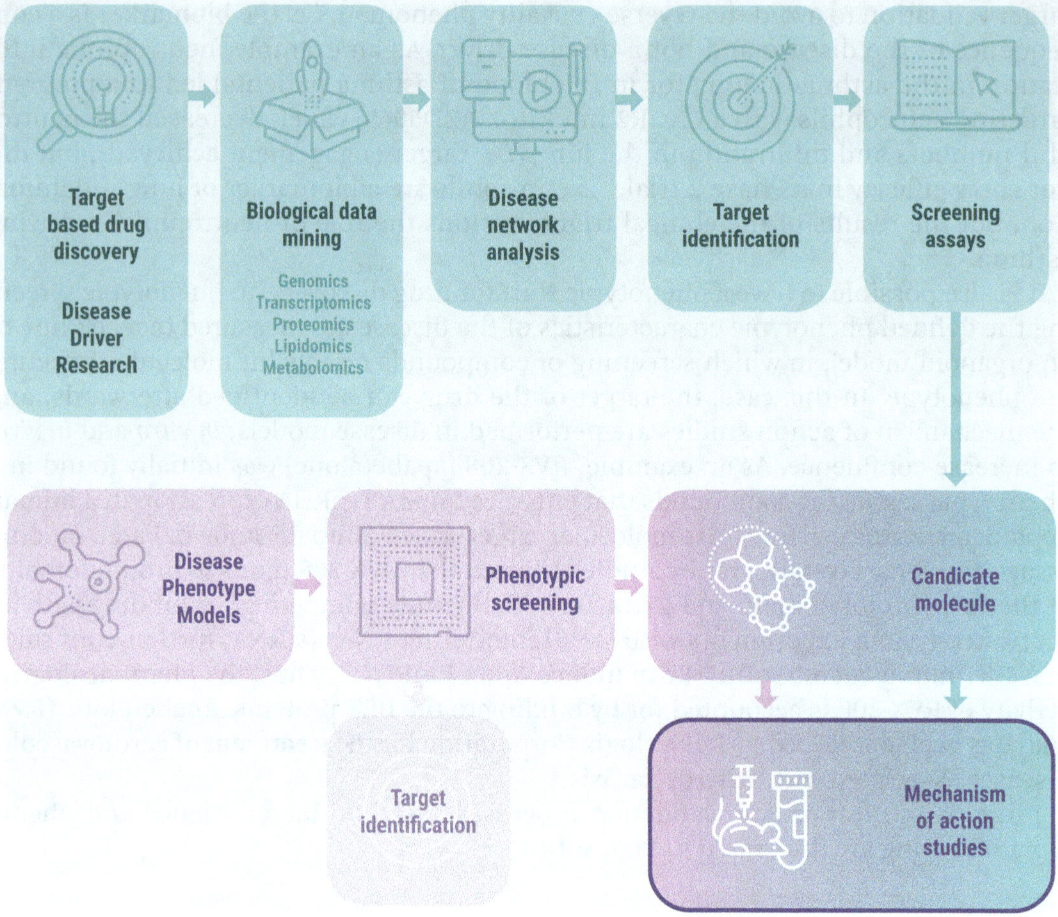


**Figure 14.4** Examples of target-based *vs.* phenotype-based drug discovery. In target-based drug discovery, target identification and validation is based on an understanding of the disease biology and drug discovery aims to find molecules that bind to the target in biochemical assays. The ability of the candidate molecules to modulate target function is then tested *in vitro* and *in vivo* models to demonstrate the functional effect on the disease phenotype. In phenotype-based drug discovery, molecules that affect the disease phenotype are identified and the target of the molecule and the mechanisms of action are identified afterwards.

the possible off-target effects, and thus it is best to use several different methods to modulate the identified target.

In oncology, amplified regions are common in human cancer genomes, but amplification events often include multiple genes. For successful target validation of a gene amplified in cancer, evidence is needed to demonstrate that the gene amplification is accompanied by the overexpression of the gene in tumor tissue.[36] In addition, functional correlation between clinical outcome and genomic alterations and overexpression needs to be demonstrated to indicate the clinical importance of the alteration. For example, androgen receptor gene aberrations commonly associated with castration-resistant prostate cancer include androgen receptor gene amplifications. Increased androgen receptor expression is a common feature in recurrent androgen receptor-amplified

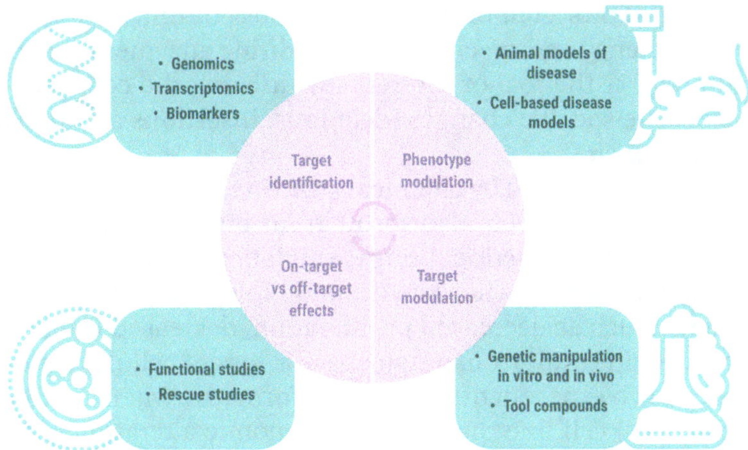


**Figure 14.5** An overview of target identification and validation processes and methods. Understanding the mechanism of action of a target is essential for the successful validation of a drug candidate. To establish the functional relevance of a potential target in cell-based disease models or animal models of disease, chemical compounds, RNA interference (RNAi), genetic knockdown and targeted protein degradation can be used to test the biological effect of target modulation and the possible off-target effects.

tumors, as compared with corresponding non-amplified primary tumors from the same patients.[37] Later studies have shown that elevated androgen receptor expression is sufficient to confer resistance to castration or anti-androgen therapy in xenograft models.[17] These findings have offered the rationale for development of novel second-generation anti-androgens that retain the ability to inhibit androgen receptor signalling in the presence of receptor overexpression. Three second-generation anti-androgens are currently approved by the FDA: enzalutamide, apalutamide and darolutamide.[38]

Knowledge of other genomic alterations such as gain-of-function mutations and chromosomal rearrangements can also help define the significance of a potential disease target as they may provide alternative mechanisms of gene activation. As an example, recent genomic studies have revealed the presence of several different kind of alterations in the genes encoding receptor tyrosine kinases such as EGFR, HER2/ErbB2 and MET. Many small-molecule inhibitors have been developed for treating cancers and other diseases caused by driving genomic alterations within receptor tyrosine kinases.[39]

Understanding the mechanism of action of a target is essential for the successful validation of a drug candidate. To establish the functional relevance of a potential target in a cell-based disease model, chemical compounds, RNA interference (RNAi), genetic knockdown and targeted protein degradation can be used in an attempt to produce the desired biological effect. The first robust functional genomic tool for site-specific downregulation of gene expression was RNAi that results in targeted degradation and subsequent repression of specific mRNA transcripts.[40] However, since highly active but target-specific small interfering RNAs (siRNAs) are difficult to develop, multiple siRNAs need to be constructed and tested to identify sequences that have minimal effects on off-target transcripts.

The discovery of the genome editing tools, especially clustered regularly interspaced short palindromic repeats and associated endonucleases (CRISPR/Cas9) gene editing in mammalian cells, allows gain-of-function and loss-of-function studies to be performed with high efficiency and specificity. Gene editing enzymes induce a site-specific double-stranded break at the loci of interest. By utilizing the cells' endogenous DNA repair mechanisms, site-specific changes (deletions, insertions and replacements) can be introduced to the cut site.

The cellular phenotypes caused by chemicals, siRNAs, shRNAs and CRISPR/Cas9-mediated gene editing can, however, also result from effects on their unintended targets (off-target activity). The functional target validation studies should, therefore, be interpreted with care, especially when the desired biological phenotype measured is a downstream readout (such as decreased proliferation, decreased viability or decreased tumor growth) and could result from a non-specific loss of cellular fitness.[41] Chemical inhibition or knockdown experiments are most informative when the tools do not have an effect in the diseased cell line that lacks the genomic alteration of the gene under investigation. In addition, rescue experiments can be set up to test whether the effects of a tool are on-target by making drug-resistant variants of targets. An expression vector encoding a target cDNA that is resistant to a drug can be used to test target-related toxicity of the drug. In siRNAs experiments, an expression vector that encodes an mRNA lacking the siRNA binding site of the target can be used by the introduction of synonymous mutations.[42] To further ensure that the result is due to an on-target effect, studies should be reproduced multiple times and under several conditions.

## 14.5 Biomarker Science

A biomarker is defined by the FDA as "a characteristic that is objectively measured and evaluated as an indicator of normal biologic processes, pathogenic processes, or pharmacologic responses to a therapeutic intervention". Biomarkers can be classified into pharmacodynamics biomarkers, predictive biomarkers and safety biomarkers.[42] Planning of the biomarkers should be initiated at an early stage of a drug discovery program to maximize the success of the project. Biomarkers are closely linked to the 5Ts framework (Table 14.1), where biomarkers are used to confirm target engagement, to identify target patients and to study target safety. Biomarkers help with critical go/no-go decisions and offer objective tools to recognize the factors indicating failure of the project, *e.g.* due to the lack of mechanistic link to disease phenotype or lack of modification of the target function.

Pharmacodynamic biomarkers are particularly important for the demonstration of proof of mechanism (PoM), proof of principle (PoP) and proof of concept (PoC), which are milestones in translational research, as illustrated in Figure 14.1. For PoM, it is crucial to show that the drug engages the target and modulates the target function, *i.e.* shows pharmacological effect. A PoM biomarker may be detected in blood and not necessarily in the diseased tissue, as the latter is often difficult to obtain in Phase 1 studies. As an example, when the drug target is a kinase, the dose-dependent inhibition of downstream phosphorylation can be demonstrated in the blood cells expressing the kinase. For many enzyme inhibitor therapies, a decrease in the downstream product can be used as a PoM biomarker, such as a decrease in blood testosterone for CYP17 inhibitor abiraterone targeting biosynthesis of androgens. A PoP biomarker is used to demonstrate the pharmacological effect in the diseased tissue, and should be measured in a subcohort in the clinical trial. It is also possible to measure a PoP biomarker in blood, such as in the case of anti-androgen therapy, in which prostate specific antigen (PSA) is used as a marker of pharmacological modulation of the target tissue when monitoring response to therapy in prostate cancer patients.[43] PoC is demonstrated as a pharmacological clinical efficacy, *i.e.* a drug-induced clinical change in the disease, and often this is only possible in the later phases of clinical trials. In the case of prostate cancer, the decrease in PSA is not enough to demonstrate PoC, but tumor shrinkage and increased progression-free survival are indicators for PoC. In many diseases, disease activation scores and/or imaging data of the diseased tissue can be used as PoC biomarkers.

Predictive biomarkers are used for the identification and enrichment of patients who respond to the treatment and, as discussed above, the use of patient stratification biomarkers significantly increases the probability of success in drug development.[42] It links the target modulation with the disease mechanism. In oncology, tumor gene mutations can be used for the selection of patients for treatments targeted to the pathways regulated by the genetic mutations and driving disease progression. As an example, poly(ADP-ribose) polymerase (PARP) inhibitors, which inhibit DNA repair mechanisms, are targeted to patients with homologous recombination DNA repair deficiency-associated genetic alterations, such as loss-of-function BRCA mutations, in their tumor tissue.[44] The tumor DNA can be analyzed in tumor biopsies or in blood where circulating tumor DNA is detected. The biomarkers for patient stratification may be genetic, biological or digital. Digital biomarkers are discussed in Section 14.6.

Safety biomarkers are used to detect signals of drug toxicity and these markers are very useful to prevent tissue damage or severe toxic side-effects. Usually the panel of safety biomarkers is large in Phase 1 and Phase 2 trials, including biomarkers for liver, cardiac and kidney toxicity. Inflammation-related biomarkers are also often included.

## 14.6 Digital Biomarkers

The use of digital means for collecting data delivers new opportunities for the invention of pre-clinical and clinical biomarkers for translational research.

Firstly, novel digital applications can be used to collect and analyze data from different instruments, *e.g.* high-throughput screening devices, microscopes, imaging devices and scanners, in order to develop new models for, *e.g.* diagnostic purposes. Secondly, different telemetry systems using implantable and/or external sensors provide, *e.g.* ECG, EEG, body temperature, glucose, heart rate variability data, in *in vivo* studies. Monitoring different parameters with, *e.g.* specialized cages, can be used in collecting data on metabolic parameters, behavior and physiology. The recent development of chronic neural interfacing implant systems has enabled longitudinal neural signal data to be collected using implanted electrodes. These data sources create new opportunities to develop pre-clinical digital biomarkers for monitoring disease progress and treatment response.

The advances in wearable and analysis technologies and methods have opened new possibilities to monitor patients in the clinical studies. We can detect directly or indirectly, *e.g.* how many times a night a prostate cancer patient needs to urinate or how many times a day a patient suffering from depression leaves the house. Novel data collection methods and data science algorithms for more objective and automated evaluation of symptoms and treatment response are transforming translational research. The field is quickly developing and at best the algorithms are developed using both physicians' and patients' own assessment of the symptoms in addition to the sensor-derived data. For example, measuring pain and the effect of a treatment has always been a challenge. Visual Analog Scale (VAS) scoring systems and electronic Patient Reported Outcome (ePRO) tools are highly subjective ways to measure pain, and more objective digital monitoring methods are under development.[45,46] In addition to the objectivity, digital health applications can offer a non-invasive opportunity to monitor disease progression and treatment response in diseases, where the present methods are expensive and require special hospital equipment, like PET or MRI methods in neurological diseases.

Different sensors, wearables and mobile devices allow the follow-up of vital and relevant biosignals such as heart rate variability, movement data, number of steps, sleep data and skin conductance, and then analysis and detection of clinically valid digital signals. The qualitative and quantitative analysis of biomarkers in sweat and saliva by biosensors in real-world settings is something that has emerged lately to support traditional clinical data collection. The use of different image recognition techniques in assessing, *e.g.* facial expressions, walking posture and gait is becoming more and more common in various indications in neurological diseases. For example, recognition of facial expressions has been researched in pain and various neurodegenerative diseases, both in animals and humans.[47–49] Biosensors can also be used as "electronic noses" in detecting the presence of different molecules in breath samples. This method has been used in asthma and lung cancer, but is not limited to respiratory diseases.[50–52] Furthermore, digital cognitive tests and games are used both as digital biomarkers and treatments for patients suffering from different neurological disorders.[53–55] These novel digital biomarkers can be used as clinically validated, complementary endpoints when: (a) diagnosing diseases at early stages, (b) monitoring the progression of diseases and (c) measuring the effect of therapeutic interventions, both with more traditional drug therapeutics and with so-called digital therapeutics (DTx).

## 14.7 The Role of Data Science and Real-world Evidence in Translational Science

The era of different digital devices, sensors and the internet, together with digitalization ("if it can be digitized, it will eventually get digitized") has witnessed an exponential growth of healthcare data being generated and analysed in recent years. According to IDC (www.idc.com) the healthcare part of the world's total data volume, the "datasphere", is growing faster than other industries at the moment. This massive amount of healthcare data opens enormous opportunities for different phases of translational research, but it may cause drawbacks if the data quality and relevance is not good. The integration and connection of various data sources and types in a meaningful way has become as valuable and important as the data itself. The one who has access to relevant data and is able to draw insights from it will succeed in the future.

Modern data science, including the use of different artificial intelligence methods, enables us to find and understand correlations and causalities in and between very complex datasets and data types. Machine learning applications can be used in all steps of drug discovery and development, but the challenges are related first to access to required and sufficient data, and later to the quality and relevance of that data. It is imperative that data is well curated and harmonized for analytical purposes. Compromised quality in the data always means compromised results, regardless of analytical capabilities. The vast majority of effort in translational data science is thus currently being put into data collection, management and curation phases, before actual analysis can happen.

Data science enables bidirectional workflows, where previous insights and learnings in the later phases of a process can be used in the earlier phases in predicting future outcomes. This is very a useful paradigm, especially in translational science, where the bidirectional workflow can be used to try to predict clinical outcomes from non-clinical data more accurately. This bidirectional workflow and use of predictive models can obviously be exploited within numerous different parts and phases of the research and development process, by always increasing the probability of success in the later phases of the process. By digitizing processes whenever possible and feasible (*e.g.* automated software-based analysis of high-throughput images or digital collection of patient-reported outcomes) and then analyzing these various data sets efficiently, we can also speed up the overall research and development process significantly. As an example, we can collect symptomatic data and adverse events from clinical study subjects by digital means. This allows us to analyze the safety data of, *e.g.* different study cohorts almost on-line, instead of retrospective data-analysis, a very powerful paradigm to speed up and enrich, *e.g.* the development process in oncology.

Real-world evidence can mean two different things. On the one hand it is: (i) collecting data from subjects in clinical trials by sensors and devices in real-world settings (individual level), but it also means (ii) collecting and analyzing various data sets and registries (population level). Furthermore, with the help of modern data science, the individual characteristics can be explored and analyzed against population characteristics in order to enable more stratified and personalized medication and treatment. The genetic, pathophysiological or symptomatic attributes of patients are better understood, and more accurate clinical phenotyping benefits clinical efficacy and safety, and enables faster clinical trials due to the smaller well-defined study population. The collection of real-world data from subjects gives novel access to longitudinal and more continuous data, all this outside of clinical settings, *i.e.* real world. This consequently opens up new opportunities for, *e.g.* diagnosis, monitoring and treatments.

## 14.8 Conclusions

It is obvious that translational science is the central function in drug discovery and development, and thus the capabilities for target selection and validation, pharmacokinetic and pharmacodynamic modeling, invention of biomarkers, data science and digital health investments, are crucial in pharma companies to build a successful pipeline. The technological and methodological advances have changed the area of translational science enormously during the last decade, including tools provided by data science and open databases for data-driven target identification. Target validation tools are diverse, allowing genetic modulation, chemical inhibition and protein degradation-based modulation of the target in various cell and animal models of the disease of interest. Biomarkers are not restricted to genetic or biological biomarkers, but expanded by digital biomarkers, which can be used for proof of mechanism, proof of principle and proof of concept, and safety studies, as well as for the identification of responders to the drug. These advances in the translational science are gradually being translated into better success rates in drug discovery and shorter times for drug development.

## 14.9 Hints and Tips

- Three factors that increase the probability of success in drug discovery and development: 1. Genetic link between the target and disease. 2. Available biomarker to detect target engagement and biological effect of target modulation. 3. Use of biomarkers to identify and select the patients who will most likely respond to the target modulation in the clinical trial (personalized medicine approach)
- Target identification and validation is the basis of drug discovery, and a key determinant of success. Use data science pro-actively to analyze available databases, including omics data providing a link between target and disease. Be aware of the reverse causality phenomen, *i.e.* the biomarker may be a consequence of the disease and not a disease driver.
- Be careful in selecting the right measures of target engagement and drug exposure in the relevant tissue – not only in pre-clinical models but also in the clinical development phases. A link between target engagement and drug exposure is an absolute requirement for the evaluation of the relevant biological and therapeutic effect. A study without a reliable biomarker of target engagement is a waste of time, money and effort. Even in the case of negative trial results, the understanding of the disease biology increases when we are able to conclude that drug exposure level was good enough to achieve the desired biological effect, but target modulation did not cause any therapeutic effect.
- Compounds are important in the evaluation of the mechanisms of action of a target, but always ensure the functional relevance of a potential target by using other means to modulate the target, such as RNA interferene, genetic knockdown and targeted protein degradation. This is crucial to increase target confidence and to understand the possible toxic effects. Off-target effects and other selectivity-related issues are always present when chemical compounds are used.
- Continue to evaluate target confidence, *i.e.* the relationship between the target modulation, mechanism of action and disease modulation throughout pre-clinical and clinical development. It is important to guarantee that you have the correct, reliable methods and markers and an open mind to follow the accumulating data. Earlier failure is always better and cheaper.
- Design and validate biomarkers at an early stage of drug discovery to maximize the success of the project: pharmacodynamic biomarkers, predictive biomarkers (to identify responders) and safety biomarkers. Do not forget the opportunities of digital biomarkers.

## Key References

https://ncats.nih.gov/
D. Cook, D. Brown, R. Alexander, R. March, P. Morgan, G. Satterthwaite, and M. N. Pangalos, *Nat. Rev. Drug. Discovery*, 2014, **13**, 419.
M. R. Nelson, H. Tipney, J. L. Painter, J. Shen, P. Nicoletti, Y. Shen, A. Floratos, P. C. Sham, M. J. Li, J. Wang, L. R. Cardon, J. C. Whittaker, and P. Sanseau, *Nat. Genet.*, 2015, **47**, 856.
M. Cully, *Nat. Rev. Drug Discovery*, 2015, **14**, 525.
E. Bradley, *Nat. Biotechnol.*, 2012, **30**, 596.

## References


1. https://ncats.nih.gov/.
2. M. Hay, T. D. W. Thomas, J. L. Craighead, C. Economides and J. Rosenthal, *Nat. Biotechnol.*, 2014, **32**, 40.
3. J. A. DiMasi, L. Feldman, A. Seckler and A. Wilson, *Clin. Pharmacol. Ther*, 2010, **87**, 272.
4. K. Smietana, M. Siatkowski M and M. Møller, *Nat. Rev. Drug Discovery*, 2016, **15**, 379.
5. C. H. Wong, K. W. Siah and A. W. Lo, *Biostatistics*, 2019, **20**, 273.
6. https://www.iqvia.com/insights/the-iqvia-institute/reports/global-oncology-trends-2019.
7. P. Morgan, P. H. Van Der Graaf, J. Arrowsmith, D. E. Feltner, K. S. Drummond, C. D. Wegner and S. D. Street, *Drug Discovery Today*, 2012, **17**, 419.
8. P. Morgan, D. G. Brown, S. Lennard, M. J. Anderton, J. C. Barrett, U. Eriksson, M. Fidock, B. Hamrén, A. Johnson, R. E. March, J. Matcham, J. Mettetal, D. J. Nicholls, S. Platz, S. Rees, M. A. Snowden and M. N. Pangalos, *Nat. Rev. Drug Discovery*, 2018, **17**, 167.
9. D. Cook, D. Brown, R. Alexander, R. March, P. Morgan, G. Satterthwaite and M. N. Pangalos, *Nat. Rev. Drug Discovery*, 2014, **13**, 419.
10. M. R. Nelson, H. Tipney, J. L. Painter, J. Shen, P. Nicoletti, Y. Shen, A. Floratos, P. C. Sham, M. J. Li, J. Wang, L. R. Cardon, J. C. Whittaker and P. Sanseau, *Nat. Genet.*, 2015, **47**, 856.
11. https://www.fda.gov/drugs/new-drugs-fda-cders-new-molecular-entities-and-new-therapeutic-biological-products/novel-drug-approvals-2020.
12. R. Dienstmann, J. Rodon, A. Prat, J. Perez-Garcia, B. Adamo, E. Felip, J. Cortes, A. J. Iafrate, P. Nuciforo and J. Tabernero, *Ann. Oncol.*, 2014, **25**, 552.
13. M. A. Knowles and C. D. Hurst, *Nat. Rev. Cancer*, 2015, **15**, 25.
14. Y. Loriot, A. Necchi, S. H. Park, J. Garcia-Donas, R. Huddart, E. Burgess, M. Fleming, A. Rezazadeh, B. Mellado, S. Varlamov, M. Joshi, I. Duran, S. T. Tagawa, Y. Zakharia, B. Zhong, K. Stuyckens, A. Santiago-Walker, P. De Porre, A. O'Hagan, A. Avadhani, A. O. Siefker-Radtke and BLC2001 Study Group, *N. Engl. J. Med.*, 2019, **381**, 338.
15. https://www.fda.gov/drugs/new-drugs-fda-cders-new-molecular-entities-and-new-therapeutic-biological-products/novel-drug-approvals-2019.
16. M. Baker, *Nature*, 2016, **533**, 452.
17. C. D. Chen, D. S. Welsbie, C. Tran, S. H. Baek, R. Che, R. Vessella, M. G. Rosenfeld and C. L. Sawyers, *Nat. Med.*, 2004, **10**, 33.
18. A. Moilanen, R. Riikonen, R. Oksala, L. Ravanti, E. Aho, G. Wohlfahrt, P. S. Nykanen, O. P. Tormakangas, J. J. Palvimo and P. J. Kallio, *Sci. Rep.*, 2015, **5**, 12007.
19. T. Sugawara, S. J. Baumgart, E. Nevedomskaya, K. Reichert, H. Steuber, P. Lejeune, D. Mumberg and B. Haendler, *Int. J. Cancer*, 2019, **145**, 1382.
20. H. Borgmann, N. Lallous, D. Ozistanbullu, E. Beraldi, N. Paul, K. Dalal, L. Fazli, A. Haferkamp, P. Lejeune, A. Cherkasov and M. E. Gleave, *Eur. Neurol.*, 2018, **73**, 4.
21. P.-O. Gaudreau, J. Stagg, D. Soulières and F. Saad, *Biomarkers Cancer*, 2016, **8**, 15.
22. K. Fizazi, C. Massard, P. Bono, R. Jones, V. Kataja, N. James, J. A. Garcia, A. Protheroe, T. L. Tammela, T. Elliott, L. Mattila, J. Aspergen, A. Vuorela, P. Langmuir, M. Mustonen and ARADES Study Group, *Lancet Oncol.*, 2014, **15**, 975.

23. https://www.ncbi.nlm.nih.gov/omim.
24. J. MacArthur, E. Bowler, M. Cerezo, L. Gil, P. Hall, E. Hastings, H. Junkins, A. McMahon, A. Milano, J. Morales, Z. M. Pendlington, D. Welter, T. Burdett, L. Hindorff, P. Flicek, F. Cunningham and H. Parkinson, *Nucleic Acids Res.*, 2017, **45**, D896.
25. M. Cully, *Nat. Rev. Drug Discovery*, 2015, **14**, 525.
26. J. Bryois, A. Buil, D. M. Evan, J. P. Kemp, S. B. Montgomery, D. F. Conrad, K. M. Ho, S. Ring, M. Hurles, P. Deloukas, G. Davey Smith and E. T. Dermitzakis, *PLoS Genet.*, 2014, **10**, e1004461.
27. C. Yao, R. Joehanes, A. D. Johnson, T. Huan, C. Liu, J. E. Freedman, P. J. Munson, D. E. Hill, M. Vidal and D. Levy, *Am. J. Hum. Genet.*, 2017, **100**, 985.
28. J. Vamathevan, D. Clark, P. Czodrowski, I. Dunham, E. Ferran, G. Lee, B. Li, A. Madabhush, P. Shah, M. Spitzer and S. Zhao, *Nat. Rev. Drug Discovery*, 2019, **18**, 463.
29. https://www.ukbiobank.ac.uk.
30. https://www.finngen.fi/en.
31. https://www.ed.ac.uk/generation-scotland.
32. P. M. O'Byrne, H. Metev, M. Puu, K. Richter, C. Keen, M. Uddin, B. Larsson, M. Cullberg and P. Nair, *Lancet Respir. Med.*, 2016, **4**, 797.
33. D. Bailey, R. Jahagirdar, A. Gordon, A. Hafiane, S. Campbell, S. Chatur, G. S. Wagner, H. C. Hansen, F. S. Chiacchia, J. Johansson, L. Krimbou, N. C. W. Wong and J. Genest, *J. Am. Coll. Cardiol.*, 2010, **55**, 2580.
34. K. G. McLure, E. M. Gesner, L. Tsujikawa, O. A. Kharenko, S. Attwell, E. Campeau, S. W. S. A. Stein, A. White, E. Fontano, R. K. Suto, N. C. Wong, G. S. Wagner, H. C. Hansen and P. R. Young, *PLoS One*, 2013, **8**, e83190.
35. S. J. Nicholls, K. K. Ray, J. O. Johansson, A. Gordon, M. Sweeney, C. Halliday, E. Kulikowski, N. Wong, S. W. Kim and C. G. Schwartz, *Am. J. Cardiovasc. Drugs*, 2018, **18**, 109.
36. T. Santarius, J. Shipley, D. Brewer, M. R. Stratton and C. S. Cooper, *Nat. Rev. Cancer*, 2010, **10**, 59.
37. M. J. Linja, K. J. Savinainen, O. R. Saramäki, T. L. Tammela, R. L. Vessella and T. Visakorpi, *Cancer Res.*, 2001, **61**, 3550.
38. I. Heidegger, M. P. Brandt and M. M. Heck, *Urol. Oncol.*, 2020, **38**, 129.
39. Z. Du and C. M. Lovly, *Mol. Cancer*, 2018, **17**, 58.
40. S. M. Elbashir, J. Harborth, W. Lendeckel W, A. Yalcin, K. Weber and T. Tuschl, *Nature*, 2001, **411**, 494.
41. W. G. Kaelin, *Nat. Rev. Cancer*, 2017, **17**, 425.
42. E. Bradley, *Nat. Biotechnol.*, 2012, **30**, 596.
43. M. J. Duffy, *Clin. Chem. Lab. Med.*, 2020, **58**, 326.
44. N. J. Curtin and C. Szabo, *Nat. Rev. Drug Discovery*, 2020, **19**, 711.
45. P. A. Healy, The Use of Behavioral Pain Assessment Tools and Pain Outcomes in Nonverbal Patients, *Honors Undergraduate Theses*, University of Central Florida, 2019, https://stars.library.ucf.edu/honorstheses/598.
46. H. Koskimäki, H. Mönttinen, P. Siirtola, H. L. Huttunen, R. Halonen, and J. Röning, Early detection of migraine attacks based on wearable sensors: experiences of data collection using Empatica E4, *Proceedings of the 2017 ACM International Joint Conference on Pervasive and Ubiquitous Computing and Proceedings of the 2017 ACM International Symposium on Wearable Computers*, 2017.
47. M. M. Sperry, Y. H. Yu, R. L. Welch, E. J. Granquist and B. A. Winkelstein, *Sci. Rep.*, 2018, **8**, 13894.
48. G. Bargshady, X. Zhou, R. C. Deo, J. Soar, F. Whittaker and H. Wang, The modeling of human facial pain intensity based on Temporal Convolutional Networks trained with video frames in HSV color space, *Appl. Soft Comput.*, 2020, **97**(Part A), 106805.
49. G. Mattavelli, E. Barvas, C. Longo, F. Zappini, D. Ottaviani, M. C. Malaguti, M. Pellegrini and C. Papagno, *J. Neuropsychol.*, 2021, **15**(1), 46–68.
50. C. Baldini, L. Billeci, F. Sansone, R. Conte, C. Domenici and A. Tonacci, *Biosensors*, 2020, **10**, 84.
51. W. Li, H. Liu, D. Xie, Z. He and X. Pi, *Sci. Rep.*, 2017, 7, 1969.
52. S. Dragonieri, V. N. Quaranta, P. Carratu, T. Ranieri and O. Resta, *Biomarkers*, 2019, **24**, 70.
53. S. H. Kollins, D. J. DeLoss, E. Cañadas, J. Lutz, R. L. Findling, R. S. E. Keefe, J. N. Epstein, A. J. Cutler and S. V. Faraone, *Lancet Digit Health*, 2020, **2**(4), e168–e178.
54. S. Adlakha, D. Chhabra and P. Shukla, *Chaos, Solitons Fractals*, 2020, **140**, 110192.
55. J. F. Vermeir, M. J. White, D. Johnson, G. Crombez and D. M. L. Van Ryckeghem, *JMIR Serious Games*, 2020, **8**, e18644.

# 15 Discovery Toxicology in Lead Optimization

Stefano Fontana*[a], Simone Braggio[a], Mauro Corsi[a], Rob Riley[b], Chris Strock[c], Jenifer Bradley[c], Caterina Virginio[a] and Paul Walker[b]

[a]Aptuit (Verona) Srl, an Evotec Company, Campus Levi-Montalcini, Via Alessandro Fleming 4, 37135 Verona, Italy; [b]Cyprotex Discovery Ltd, an Evotec Company, No. 24 Mereside, Alderley Park, Macclesfield, Cheshire, SK10 4TG, UK; [c]Cyprotex US, LLC, an Evotec Company, 313 Pleasant Street, Watertown, MA 02472, USA

*E-mail: stefano.fontana@evotec.com

## 15.1 Introduction

The cost impact of late-stage failures of drug candidates has motivated the pharmaceutical industry to develop, validate, and implement a more proactive testing paradigm, including an emphasis on conducting predictive *in vitro* and *in vivo* studies earlier. The goal of discovery toxicology is not to reduce or eliminate attrition, as is often misstated, but rather to reprioritize efforts to shift attrition of future failing molecules upstream in discovery. This shift in attrition requires additional studies and investment earlier in the candidate evaluation process in order to avoid spending resources on molecules with soon-to-be-discovered development-limiting liabilities.

## 15.2 *In Silico* Toxicology

*In silico* toxicology can be defined as the application of computational technologies to analyze and model available data in order to predict toxicological activity of substances from their chemical structure. It can be strictly a computer-based analysis of the relationship of chemical structure and toxicological activity (structure–activity relationship; SAR), or a simple structural alert identification and association with toxicity.[1–3] *In silico* toxicology methods such as computational toxicology, predictive quantitative

The Handbook of Medicinal Chemistry: Principles and Practice, 2nd Edition
Edited by Simon E. Ward and Andrew M. Davis

Published by the Royal Society of Chemistry, www.rsc.org

structure–activity relationship (QSAR) modelling of toxicity and predictive ADME-Tox are currently used in the pharmaceutical industry at the design stage, to help identify lead compounds with reduced toxicological potential risk.[4] In fact, being aware of potential toxicological issues early in the discovery process, can be very useful to prioritize chemical series at the hit identification stage or hopefully to fix these liabilities during lead optimization, (just as potency and pharmacokinetics properties are being optimized), before significant investment of time and financial resources are spent in clinical trials. The advantages of these methods are low costs, standardization, minimal equipment needs, and short time of execution (*i.e.* high throughput) and can hence be used as a pre-screen and to prioritize compounds for *in vitro* or *in vivo* assay testing.[5–7]

### 15.2.1 *In Silico* Toxicology Tools

A number of chemical–biological informatics-based tools and related software programs for toxicity prediction along with details of the algorithms have been described in various reviews.[8–15] Some of the more commonly used systems are listed in Table 15.1, along with a general brief description, availability and the biological endpoint they predict. Computational toxicology approaches are typically aimed at building toxicity databases, QSAR models and rule/descriptor-based methods, as well as classical ligand- and target-based techniques. Visualization tools combining QSARs models and systems biology and pharmacology pathway analysis[16] are also available. The choice of the modelling method can be influenced by many factors including: the size and the type of the dataset (few congeneric datasets or the diversity of the chemical library), the endpoint to be modelled and the decision process required. The common objective of all methods, however, is to attribute a toxicological indication/effect to a chemical structure.

### 15.2.2 Databases

Data collection is the most critical and time-consuming task. Toxicology heavily relies on the use of *in vivo* data obtained from a combination of *in vitro* and *in vivo* animal models, and human data, if available. If, however, the mechanism leading to toxicity is known, for example, in the case of the hERG potassium ion channel inhibition and subsequent QT interval prolongation, data from high-throughput screening (HTS) and high-content screening (HCS) methodologies alone can be used in place of *in vivo* data.[17–19] All the computational models employed in the field of toxicity prediction are based on the structure of existing, annotated ligands. Typically, scientists gather data from different sources: literature, patents, and, when available, from in-house programmes. Following several initiatives aiming at collecting information from legacy, unstructured systems (*e.g.* US National Toxicology Program Reports and literature) and integrating them into organized and searchable open-access databases,[20–26] more and more datasets are becoming available. Table 15.2 provides an overview of some of the publicly available, commercial databases and electronic data sources, including human health effects of substances, which are useful in risk assessment, safety evaluation, and hazard characterization. Accordingly, open sources of toxicity data are the first exploited

**Table 15.1** Most used computation systems for predicting toxicology alerts.

| System/ developer | Availability | Description | Toxicity endpoint prediction | Reference |
|---|---|---|---|---|
| MDL QSAR (MDL) | Commercial | Quantitative structure–activity and structure–property modelling system | Acute (oral) tox, hepatoxicity, nephrotoxicity, urinary tract toxicity, mutagenicity, carcinogenicity, skin sensitization and irritancy | 90 |
| HazardExpert (CompuDrug) | Commercial | Fragment, rule-based system | Mutagenicity, carcinogenicity, skin sensitization and irritancy, immunotoxicity and neurotoxicity | 91 |
| Derek (Lhasa Ltd) | Commercial | Knowledge-based expert system | Mutagenicity, carcinogenicity, skin sensitization and irritancy | 78 |
| ADMET Predictor (Simulations Plus Inc.) | Commercial | Modelling based on neural network | Hepatoxicity, mutagenicity, carcinogenicity, cardiac toxicity, allergenic skin and respiratory sensitization, phospholipidosis | 92 |
| Lazar (Freiburg University) | Freely available | Uses datamining algorithms to derive predictions for untested compounds from experimental training data | Chronic (oral) tox, hepatoxicity, mutagenicity, carcinogenicity | 93 |
| Leadscope (Leadscope) | Commercial | Integrates disparate sources of toxicity data, mines historical collections of public and proprietary toxicity data, builds predictive models, identifies analogues with toxicity data | Hepatoxicity, nephrotoxicity, urinary tract toxicity, neurotoxicity, genetic toxicity, carcinogenicity, reproductive toxicity, cardiac toxicity | 94 |
| MCASE/MC4PC (MultiCASE) | Commercial | Identifies molecular fragment with high probability of being associated with a toxic effect | Acute (oral) tox, hepatoxicity, nephrotoxicity, urinary tract toxicity, cytotoxicity, mutagenicity, carcinogenicity, teratogenicity, irritancy, maximum tolerated dose | 56 |
| TOPKAT (Accelrys) | Commercial | Uses cross-validated Quantitative Structural Toxicology Relationships (QSTR) models to assess various measures of toxicity | Mutagenicity, carcinogenicity teratogenicity, lethal dose, skin sensitization, chronic (oral) toxicity | 53 |
| OncoLogic (US EPA) | Freely available | Knowledge-based expert system | Carcinogenicity | 77 |

**Table 15.2** Publicly available and commercial databases and electronic data sources.

| Database/ developer | Availability/access | Description |
|---|---|---|
| Acutoxbase ("A-Cute-Tox" EU FP6 project) | Access restricted to project partners https://acubase.amwaw.edu.pl | For ~100 chemicals (50% drugs) available ~100 *in vitro* assays including general acute cytotoxicity, metabolism-mediated toxicity, biokinetics, and organ-specific toxicity; *in vivo*: ~2200 $LD_{50}$ values in rodents (rat and mouse) and other animals (*e.g.* guinea pig, dog) with various administration routes (oral, intravenous, *etc.*) compiled from published literature |
| ChemIDplus (US NLM) | Freely available http://chem.sis.nlm.nih.gov/chemidplus/ | Structure searchable toxicity data for ~130 000 chemical retrieved from TOXNET (Toxicology Data Network; http://toxnet.nlm.nih.gov |
| CEBS (US NIEHS) | Freely available http://cebs.niehs.nih.gov/ | *In vivo* data and acute dose on rat for a small number of known hepatoxicants |
| RTECS (Symyx Technologies) | Commercial: searchable through the Symyx Toxicity Database http://www.symyx.com/products/databases/bioactivity/rtecs/index.jsp and Leadscope Toxicity Database http://www.leadscope.com/databases/ | Structure searchable rat acute oral toxicity ($LD_{50}$) and acute inhalation toxicity ($LC_{50}$) data from published literature for ~7000 compounds (~4000 organic) |
| TerraBase databases | Commercial http://www.terrabase-inc.com/ | Several databases include rat and mouse $LD_{50}$ values for different product types (natural compounds, drugs, pesticides) |
| ZEBET (BfR ZEBET) | Freely available http://www.dimdi.de | Includes rat or mouse ($LD_{50}$) and cytotoxicity ($IC_{50}$) data for 347 compounds from the literature |
| MRTD Database (US FDA) | Freely available http://www.fda.gov/AboutFDA/CentersOffices/CDER/ucm092199.htm | MRTD (Maximum Recommended Therapeutic Dose) values for 1215 drugs from clinical trials, mostly by oral administration and daily treatments, (3–12 months), 5% of the drugs administered intravenously and/or intramuscularly) Includes structures Available from FDA and EPA DSSTOX |
| DSSTox | http://www.epa.gov/ncct/dsstox/index.html | Distributed Structure-Searchable Toxicity Database Network of downloadable, structure-searchable, standardized chemical structure files associated with toxicity |
| RepDose (Fraunhofer Toxicology and Experimental Medicine) | Freely available http://www.fraunhofer-repdose.de/ | Sub acute to chronic, oral, and inhalation data for ~700 publicly available chemicals in rat, mouse, and dog studies; also including structures, physicochemical properties and study designs |
| AERS (US FDA/CDER) | Freely available GuidanceComplianceRegulatoryInformation/Surveillance/AdverseDrugEffects/default.htm | US FDA/CDER Adverse Effects Reporting system of post-market safety surveillance for all approved drug and therapeutic biologic products |
| CEBS US NIH/NIEHS | Freely available http://cebs.niehs.nih.gov/ | Chemical Effects in Biological Systems Knowledgebase; integrates genomic and biological data (including dose–response studies) in toxicology and pathology |
| CERES (FDA) | Freely available http:www.fda.gov/ | Chemical Evaluation and Risk Estimation System Contains databases on toxicity of food ingredients, drugs, agro, and industrial chemicals, compound profiling, structural alerts, and QSAR-based toxicity predictions |

in computational modelling and *in silico* toxicology software programs. Furthermore, proprietary toxicity databases tend to offer promise for enhanced "predictive accuracy" or expanded chemical space of the representative molecular structures they contain compared to public databases. In addition, the aforementioned high-throughput capabilities developed and used by the pharmaceutical industry enable the attractive toxicological profiling approach to be pursued, using whole-cell and phenotypic assays (*i.e.* genotoxicity and metabolism modulation, hERG, cytochrome P450 3A4, Ames assay, and others).[27–31] Finally, the application of genomics techniques in toxicology, due to advances in sequencing technology, which allows whole-genome expression analyses for organisms used in toxicological tests, has led to the creation of a new discipline called toxicogenomics[32–34] that has proved to be very useful in prediction and interpretation of off-target effects.[35–37]

### 15.2.3 QSARs and Statistical Modelling

A toxicological QSAR model is a mathematical equation used to predict the toxicity of a new substance from a training set of chemicals with known toxicity and spanning a defined chemical space. It is usually specific to a single defined endpoint[38] (*i.e.* a specific biological target like hERG) or a defined toxic effect.[39,40] Accordingly, each model has a specific applicability domain, which is defined as a calculated region of chemical space of the training data set used to make the model,[41] where molecular features of compounds to be predicted are adequately represented. Consequently, toxicity of compounds falling outside the applicability domain cannot be reliably predicted. If the training set is large enough and diverse in molecular chemotypes, covering a huge chemical space, the model is termed global. If it is restricted to a set of congeneric compounds, it is termed local.[38–42] Global models are used especially by regulatory authorities that require assessment of diverse compounds that can present new structural classes.[43,44] The drug discovery industry also uses global models to broadly evaluate different chemical lead series in order to select the cleanest profile. Local models are built to address and hopefully solve toxicity issues in lead optimization as they are centred on the chemotype(s) of interest and hence are more specific and likely to be more accurate. For example, in global hERG models, lipophilic and positively charged compounds are in general predicted to be more potent hERG inhibitors compared with more hydrophilic neutral or negatively charged substances. However, most CNS drugs are lipophilic, carrying an ionizable amine. As such, a desirable model is able to predict within this unfavourable chemical space, the specific features that hinder hERG interaction in order to reduce this liability.

The most commonly modelled QSAR endpoints in toxicology are carcinogenicity and genetic toxicity, as these liabilities for a new drug under development (and its metabolites) can impede regulatory approval. In addition, genotoxicity and carcinogenic potential of a pharmaceutical is a critical regulatory milestone that cannot usually be tested in humans unless using very costly and time-consuming assays. In general, the aim of statistical commercial modelling software, such as Topkat 53 and Multicase[45,46] (see Table 15.1), is to utilize available data and automatically build models; however, these models would need to be carefully reviewed. Modelling techniques and structural descriptors have also to be carefully selected. A large number of independent investigations have been widely conducted by experts to assess the *in silico* QSAR/statistical modelling software products available in order to determine their performance for predicting carcinogenicity and mutagenicity. Those based on external validation methods are considered the most scientifically rigorous.[47–56] In general, the quality of predictions varies depending on many factors; among the most critical are applicability domain[41] and the complexity of the toxicological endpoint (*i.e.* the number of underlying mechanisms of action). Clearly, the more complex an endpoint, the more difficult it is to predict.[57,58] For example, the Ames test (salmonella mutagenicity assay that measures genetic toxicity; one of the mechanisms by which compounds can induce cancer) is a relatively simple assay because it involves a low number of underlying mechanisms, and many models with respectable accuracy exist.[60] By contrast, carcinogenicity, liver toxicity, and developmental toxicity are complex, with often multiple mechanisms involved, and as such prediction is considerably more difficult.[58–61] Hence, although they are useful in a few cases, the broad application of such predictions has been limited by the lack of accuracy. Clearly, from a regulatory reviewer's perspective of protecting public health, there is a need for models tuned for sensitivity (*i.e.* accuracy in predicting toxic compounds with a low number of false negatives) at the cost of specificity (accuracy in predicting non-toxic compounds with a low number of false positives). The focus, therefore, is on modelling simpler endpoints, such as off-target activity, to increase accuracy in prediction and hence application usefulness.

### 15.2.4 Human Knowledge-based Methods

Among the several approaches to predict the effects of small molecules from structure, human knowledge-based systems are distinct from statistical-based/machine learning approaches. These models rely on a set of predefined rules derived from specific examples, widely accepted within the scientific community to predict toxicity risk. These rules may suggest that the presence of a chemical feature in a molecule or a certain chemical class (*e.g.* heterocyclic amines, highly reactive groups such as aldehydes) provides a concern about the toxicity risk of a queried chemical.[62–66] Two of the most recognized systems using this modelling approach are the EPA's OncoLogic™freeware[67] and Lhasa Ltd's Derek for Windows (DFW) program. While the former only evaluates carcinogenicity, DFW has a knowledge base for predicting many toxicological endpoints, including carcinogenicity, mutagenicity, genotoxicity, skin sensitization and irritancy, teratogenicity, hepatotoxicity, neurotoxicity, and ocular toxicity. DFW is also fully integrated with a qualitative xenobiotic metabolism prediction program Meteor.[68] One of the problems associated with methods providing such structural alerts is the difficulty in using the identified fragments in medicinal chemistry for drug design purposes. Furthermore, the fragments are sometimes too small to unambiguously map onto a molecule. In addition, these structural rules are dependent on the reference set they are derived from and may, therefore, not be transferable from one chemical series to another. Consequently, although the information contained in these systems is considered reliable enough, these methods suffer from a lack of sensitivity.[26,56] The direct consequence is that many side effects are likely to be missed.

### 15.2.5 ADME-Tox Modelling

ADME-Tox modelling may provide a useful indication in order to address metabolic, pharmacokinetic, and toxicological issues related to drug disposition and fate, through *in silico* evaluation of individual or classes of compounds. These methods, such as expert systems and QSAR analysis,[69,70] enable millions of virtual molecules to be examined across a broad range of desired properties in lead identification and optimization. Some of these methods are based on simple and well-known rules for drug/lead/metabolite likeness, derived from physicochemical properties.[69,71–73] As part of these computational applications, either "off-the-shelf" products, or custom-built models, there is potential to identify properties of molecules that can be predicted to have "off-target" effects that can potentially have an impact on human health (*i.e.* hERG). Today the role of computational ADMET in helping to reduce the number of safety issues in the whole discovery phases is well recognized. However, the successful application of these simple approaches are often limited by the paucity of high-quality experimental data[74] and by the use of descriptors neglecting direct structural information about ADMET proteins. Hence, they can be of limited impact on drug design, especially in lead optimization. Accordingly, *in silico* methods based on the 3D structures of relevant proteins might add extra benefits to rule-based and/or statistical 2D methodologies.[75–77] This would provide understanding at the molecular level by analyzing ligand and/or protein interactions. To date, structure-based techniques have been rare in computational toxicology due to the lack of structural information for many drug targets, despite the increasing availability of databases in recent years containing protein X-ray coordinates. Docking experiments relying on target homology models and experimental SARs to propose binding pockets of ligands, can be inaccurate. Furthermore, application of docking-scoring methods to ADMET proteins is a challenging process because they usually have large and flexible binding cavities. An excellent review on structure-based ADMET, relating to metabolizing enzymes, including a list of ADMET proteins along with the available 3D structures from the PDB has been published.[75] It is also worth mentioning other promising *in silico* ADME-Tox approaches based on quantum mechanical/molecular mechanical (QM/MM) methods that are used to extract descriptors (*i.e.* HOMO, LUMO) to model the reactivity of compounds towards CYP isoforms and for predicting rates of reactions in drug metabolism.[78,79]

### 15.2.6 Application of *In silico* Tools in Lead Optimization

Knowledge/rule-based *in silico* "global" toxicity and structural/physico-chemical models are widely applied as filters in the lead identification phase. This approach usually allows the selection of developable and potentially clean chemical series. However, it is not guaranteed that these compounds are devoid of toxic effects, as these methods have low sensitivity[56] (*i.e.* as only known fragments/chemical groups responsible for toxicity are represented in the training set, see above). On the other hand, an overly restrictive application of these filters may result (especially for poorly tractable targets) in no, or too few chemotype compounds left, with the added risk of killing valuable leads.[74] It is often considered that toxicity can be de-risked during lead optimization.[80] It is, however, advisable to start a lead optimization programme with multiple, different varied chemotype chemical series, allowing some toxicology flags that need consideration during the optimisation process. Normally, little is known about toxicity issues of a new chemical class. Ideally, one would test all new compounds in every available *in vitro* profiling assay to identify potential off-target activities. However, because of cost and practicality aspects, only a few representative compounds (depending on the throughput of the assay) can be tested in a subset of assays. These are selected according to the knowledge of on-target relationships with the rest of the proteome (in particular with targets associated with adverse events) determined by sequence homology similarity and chemical connectivity (*i.e.* ligands in common). The latter information is provided by chemogenomics databases, which contain collections of cross-screening data from compounds tested on a diverse panel of assays spanning the druggable proteome. Interestingly, the two approaches (systems biology and chemoproteomics) do not always completely overlap, rather they provide complementary information. As for *in vitro* safety pharmacological profiling, only the more likely potential issues are usually studied (*e.g.* cytotoxicity, mitochondrial toxicity, genotoxicity, and transporter/ion channel liability, see Walker *et al.*, 2020 for further detail).[105] ADMET targets are finally added to the panel, among the most common are CYP interaction (inhibition or induction), plasma protein binding (PPB), and P-gp interaction. Once a single liability is identified, computational models are built using the most appropriate approach, depending on the available structural information on the target and data on ligands. As soon as a model has been built, any number of structures can be tested *in silico* in a very short time frame. For some of these targets, global models are also commercially available, but caution has to be used for their correct application (*i.e.* appropriateness of the applicability domain, see above). Local models, built using in-house data, around chemotypes of interest usually provide the best results. Clearly structure-based (docking) and pharmacophore approaches are preferred by medicinal chemists because they provide a better understanding of the recognition processes at a molecular level. "Local" QSAR models (only for congeneric series of compounds) can also be useful (provided that the chemical descriptors used are simple and meaningful from a physico-chemical point of view, rather than a combination of, sometimes "exotic", parameters). Among the most used statistical methodologies are MLRA (Multi Linear Regression Analysis) and PLS[81] (Partial Least Squares regression), the latter most suitable with high numbers of correlated dependent variables, or PLS-DA (Partial Least Squares regression-Discriminant Analysis) when the dependent variable is categorical. Model predictions need to be verified by testing key compounds with subsequent modifications as appropriate.

## 15.3 Target Selectivity

Regulatory requests to the pharmaceutical industry to improve preclinical safety testing have increased due to recent drug withdrawals.[82] Excellent and exhaustive guidelines to describe the identification of potential safety issues in discovery and development of novel drugs have recently appeared in the literature in response to high drug failure rates in the pharmaceutical industry.[83–86] Defining the risk of exposing humans to new drug candidates still depends on preclinical testing, which in many, but not all, cases predicts outcomes in humans accurately. Accordingly, understanding mechanisms of drug toxicity is an essential step toward improving drug safety testing by providing the basis for mechanism-based risk assessments. In a recent paper by Bowes and coauthors[87] it was reported that about 75% of all adverse reactions produced by novel drugs, are dose dependent and they can be predicted on the basis of their pharmacological profile. Drug interaction with off-targets might often be the reason for adverse reactions produced by a candidate compound when tested in animal or/and clinical studies. Therefore, the precise identification of the off-targets and their deep characterization are essential steps in modern drug discovery. The International Council of Harmonization (ICH) of Technical Requirements for Registration of Pharmaceuticals for Human Use (S7A)[88] document underlines recommendations for safety pharmacology studies applied to drug discovery and development. ICH S7A considers "secondary pharmacodynamics studies" as the mode of action and/or effects of a substance not related to its desired therapeutic target. The secondary pharmacodynamic studies are recommended but not a mandatory regulatory requirement. In drug discovery and development, *in vitro* pharmacological profiling is a term used to describe the investigation of the pharmacological effects of a drug at the molecular target distinct (off-target) from the intended therapeutic one.[89] This activity involves the testing of compounds against a panel of targets dissimilar from the intended therapeutic one. Off-target pharmacology may play a role in the prioritization of a particular chemical series during drug discovery and more importantly early risk assessment helps to avoid costly failures during the late phases of development. Structure–activity relationships can be explored within the chemical series. Moreover, computational and mathematical modelling can also be applied to optimize the molecule by moving away from the off-target activity at an early stage of drug discovery. Understanding the pharmacological profile of a drug is useful to interpret pharmacodynamics responses observed during *in vivo* preclinical efficacy and safety studies. In clinical trials there is the essential requirement for a drug to be safe and *in vitro* profiling aims to support an acceptable ratio between the benefit and the risk profile for a given therapeutic indication. Quite recent examples are fenfluramine and the fatty acid amide hydrolase inhibitor BIA 10-2474.

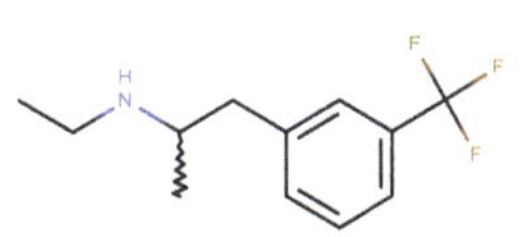

Fenfluramine

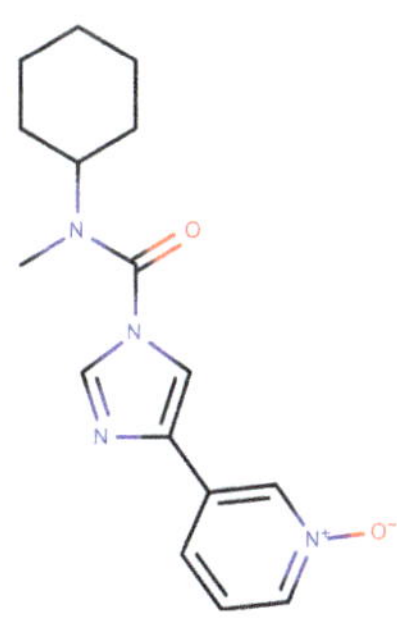

BIA 10-2474

Fenfluramine was originally marketed as an appetite suppressant for weight control and its efficacy was attributed to its agonism of 5-HT receptors. However, in 1997 fenfluramine was withdrawn from the market since it also induced heart valve disease and pulmonary hypertension. Indeed, it was discovered that whereas the clinically desired effect on appetite was related to the 5-HT2C receptor (primary target), the heart and pulmonary diseases were produced by agonism of 5-HT2B receptors (secondary target or off-target). The compound BIA 10-2474 was tested in a recent phase I clinical trial. It led to the death of one volunteer and produced mild-to-moderate neurological symptoms in four others.[90,91] These effects are suggested to have been produced by the compound acting on off-targets such as lipase enzymes.

Currently, regulatory guidance describing which targets should constitute the *in vitro* pharmacological selectivity panel does not exist, with the exception of the human-voltage gated potassium channel subfamily H member 2, also known as hERG, which is now considered obligatory by the FDA, together with other cardiac ion channels.[92] This allows for significant flexibility in the approaches and the number of targets a project may decide to evaluate.

### 15.3.1 The Target Panel for *In Vitro* Selectivity Evaluation

Specialized companies which screen for selectivity of novel chemical candidates exist and all have different types of solutions and different costs by offering small (fewer than 30 targets) to very large (more than 100 targets) target panels. It seems, therefore, that the decision on which panel is used for off-target characterization of a novel discovery compound will depend mostly on economic factors. However, in recent years, a new way of thinking has been introduced by pharmaceutical companies, with an approach that takes into account whether the characterization of the novel compound takes place in the lead generation/optimization or the clinical phases of the drug discovery process. Indeed, in the lead generation and optimization phases, the identification of off-targets is used to guide the optimization process, while in the candidate stage it is used to define the risk in going forward to clinical studies. Consequently, the composition of the panel should be different in the two situations. In addition, the primary target family and therapeutic area of interest always play an important role in the choice of target panels to be considered.

Hence, in the lead generation and optimization phases, pharmaceutical companies have now accepted that the screening for potential off-target activity can be carried out by a customized target panel made of approximately 30–50 targets.[93–95] Generally, a panel should encompass a broad array of target classes with several examples from GPCRs, ion channels, enzymes/kinases, nuclear receptors, epigenetic factors and transporters. As pointed out by other authors, the included targets become sentinels for potential targets of liability and the observed positive findings would require further evaluation within the target family. The advantage of such an approach in an early discovery phase is that the findings can immediately be transformed by the project into a dedicated SAR strategy to eliminate the liability of the off-target activity. The historical hit rate at a target or the potential risk associated with that target are generally taken into consideration when deciding which targets a panel should include. It is clear that no single panel has the ability to highlight all potential risks. Thus the mitigation of the development risk should be the final aim of the *in vitro* profiling. An example of a customized target panel used for projects dealing with CNS indications is listed below:

- Central benzodiazepine receptors ($GABA_A$),
- Opioid receptors (mu, k, delta),
- Serotonin receptors (5-HT2A, 5-HT2B, 5-HT3),
- NET, DAT, SERT,
- Cannabinoid receptors (CB1, CB2),
- MAO-B,

- Histamine H1 receptor,
- Dopamine D1 and D2 receptors,
- Phosphodiesterase PDE4,
- Neurokinin NK1 receptor,
- Alpha adrenergic receptors (alpha-1 and alpha-2),
- Beta adrenergic receptors (beta-1),
- Adenosine receptors (A2),
- Cyclooxygenase COX2,
- Muscarinic receptors (M1 and M2),
- L-type Ca channel,
- Nav1.5 channel,
- hERG channel.

The selected targets can potentially be indicators of drug abuse potential, convulsion, cognitive impairment, emetic and cardiovascular liabilities for compounds interacting with them (Table 15.3).

Two relevant factors still require consideration. First, whichever customized target panel is selected, the target assays should be robust enough for detecting both agonism and antagonism. Second, pharmacological species differences should be kept in mind when developing the assay and translating the results in animal or human studies (*e.g.* a clear pharmacological species difference exists, for instance, between human and mouse or rat NK1 receptors[96]).

Finally, for a novel candidate ready to be tested in clinical studies there is the general consensus that a large and sometimes very large panel of hundreds of potential off-targets is required to widely explore the selectivity of the compound. Projects targeting kinases generally require large off-target panels, since more than five hundred different kinases have been identified in humans.

## 15.3.2 Testing Strategies

Different technical approaches have been adopted for testing compounds on these targets. As deeply discussed by Bowes,[87] binding assays utilize purified preparation of membranes or proteins from recombinant or tissue sources expressing the target and a labelled high-affinity ligand that incorporates either a radioisotope or fluorescent probe. Test compounds are assayed for their ability (*e.g.* affinity) to displace the labelled ligand. Binding assays in their general configuration do not indicate if the test compound behaves as an agonist or antagonist. It is worth highlighting that allosteric ligands bind to a distinct site with respect to the natural ligand. Therefore, in a displacement format of radioligand binding assays, there is the potential to miss allosteric compounds since they do not displace the radioligand. On the contrary, allosteric ligands modify the structure of the receptor to prevent a functional response.

Functional assays measure activation, inhibition, or modulation of the activity of the target either expressed in a host cell or in a purified preparation. Assays for GPCRs rely on the measurement of secondary messengers (*e.g.* calcium, cAMP, IP3) β-arrestin recruitment and GTPγS-binding, to name some of them. For ion channels, technologies

**Table 15.3** Potential hazards produced by compounds acting on the following off-target panel.

| Target | Family | System | Agonism | Antagonism |
|---|---|---|---|---|
| Adenosine receptors A2 | GPCR | CNS<br>CV | Sedation<br>Vasodilatation | |
| Adrenergic α1, α2 receptors | GPCR | CV | Hypertension | Hypotension |
| Adrenergic β1 receptor | GPCR | CV | Tachycardia | Hypotension |
| D1 and D2 receptors | GPCR | CNS | Dyskinesias<br>Hypotension<br>Hallucination<br>Psychosis<br>Increased orgasmic intensity | Extra-pyramidal side effects |
| Muscarinic M1 and M2 receptors | GPCR | CNS<br>Peripheral<br>CV | CNS excitation<br>Gastrointestinal motility | Agitation<br>Hallucination<br>Memory impairment<br>Tachycardia |
| Opioid mu, k, delta receptors | GPCR | CNS | Dysphoria<br>Drug abuse | |
| H1 receptor | GPCR | CNS | | Sedation |
| 5-HT2A, 5-HT2B receptors | GPCR | CV<br>Peripheral | Vasoconstriction<br>Heart valve disease<br>Pulmonary Hypertension | |
| NK1 receptor | GPCR | CNS | Nausea | |
| Central benzodiazepine receptors (GABA-A) | Ion channel | CNS<br>Peripheral | Sedation | Muscular spasm Seizures Convulsions |
| L-type Ca channel | Ion channel | CV | | Hypotension |
| hERG channel | Ion channel | CV | | Arrhythmia<br>Torsade de pointes risk |
| Nav1.5 channel | Ion channel | CV | | Arrhythmia<br>Brugada syndrome |
| 5-HT3 | Ion channel | CV<br>CNS | Anxiety<br>Hypotension | |
| NET, DAT, SERT | Transporters | CNS | | Tachycardia<br>Drug abuse Seizures<br>Serotonin syndrome |
| MAO-B | Enzymes | CNS | | Dyskinesias Hallucination Hypotension |
| PDE4 | Enzyme | CNS<br>Peripheral | | Nausea |
| COX2 | Enzyme | CV | Hypertension<br>Cardiovascular risks | |

allowing automated electrophysiological measurement of channel activity when expressed in a host cell are used. Enzymes, including kinases, are assayed by measuring the product formed after their incubation with a specific substrate. Nuclear receptors are usually expressed in cells and tested in combination with gene reporters or by biochemical assays using time-resolved fluorescent resonance energy transfer (TR-FRET) technologies.

$pIC_{50}$ and $pK_i$ values are determined in binding studies (negative logarithm of the concentration of the test compound that displaces 50% of the labelled ligand; negative logarithm of the affinity constant of the test compound, respectively). $pK_i$ is derived from the $pIC_{50}$ value by applying the Cheng–Prussoff equation.[87] In functional studies, $pEC_{50}$ values (negative logarithm of the agonist concentration that produces 50% of the maximal response) or $pIC_{50}$ and $pK_B$ values (negative logarithm of the concentration of the antagonist/inhibitor that produces 50% inhibition; negative logarithm of the antagonist dissociation constant, respectively) are calculated. The $pK_B$ parameter can be derived by the use of competitive antagonist affinity from functional inhibition curves using the Gaddum, Schild, and Cheng–Prusoff equations.[97] Compound-related properties can significantly influence the results obtained. These include the physicochemical properties of the molecules, their colour and fluorescent properties, and equilibrium kinetics. Many assays are very rapid, for instance the calcium release in a FLIPR-based assay (*e.g.* a few seconds). In this assay a compound with slow onset kinetics may be underestimated in its activity if not enough time is allowed to reach equilibrium.

A point which generally creates discussion within the discovery project is the choice of the concentration of the compound to be tested against in the off-target panel. In the early profiling performed in the lead generation and optimization phases it is always recommended that the testing be performed at multiple concentrations to allow a direct and precise estimation of the compound activity (*e.g.* compound affinity, potency). This provides a faster and more reliable result than testing a single concentration. Of course this approach is more expensive if the off-target list is extensive, but the benefit of the approach is the early introduction in the project of a SAR strategy to reduce the potential liability risk of the lead series. A more balanced approach takes advantage of profiling a larger set of targets by using a single concentration (*e.g.* at lower cost) and then following up only the identified target hits with multiple concentrations of the test compound. The selection of a specific test concentration is an important step in the *in vitro* profiling. For the purpose of the single concentration approach, the standard accepted is generally 10 µM. However, there are several factors to take into consideration before selecting a concentration, for instance the expected free maximal exposure of the compound in humans. A hit is generally defined as a response that is equal or greater than 50% of the maximal response produced by a standard compound.

The *in vitro* profiling of enzyme inhibitors requires specific considerations. The determination of the $pK_i$ value of an enzyme inhibitor is of paramount importance to estimate the compound selectivity. However, for risk assessment, it is more important to define the safety margin under conditions similar to those expected in the cellular environment and in this respect the concentration of the substrate plays a big role. For kinases, many targets are run at [ATP] = $K_m$, whereas the cellular concentration of ATP is expected to be significantly higher in the cytosolic environment, in the range 1–10 mM.[98] Assuming the compounds are competitive in nature, when screened at [ATP] = $K_m$ there will be a high probability that many hits found are not physiologically relevant. However, profiling the same compounds at [ATP] = 1–10 mM may provide a more severe screen with hits more translatable to a cellular enzyme assay.

### 15.3.3 Data Interpretation

Potential leads and candidates should be prioritized based on the *in vitro* pharmacological profile, namely the selectivity for the primary target with respect to off-targets (*e.g.* secondary targets identified in the *in vitro* profiling). It is generally accepted that the greater the ratio between the compound activity for the primary target with respect to the off-target, the better it is for compound safety. However, it is very difficult to assess safety only from *in vitro* data. Complicating factors include species differences in receptor pharmacology, receptor distribution and density, access of the test compound to the active site, compensatory and synergic mechanisms, redundancy and plasticity of response systems. All of these can affect the outcome. As a rule of thumb it is suggested to contextualize such data with respect to the likely therapeutic concentrations of the test compound (non-protein bound or free $C_{max}$). If the ratio of the off-target activity measured *in vitro* is greater than 100× free $C_{max}$, it can generally be considered to represent no safety concern. Leads and candidates displaying lower values should be considered with prudence.

## 15.4 Cell Viability Assessment

The determination of cell viability has a fundamental role in all forms of cell culture. In toxicity assays, cell viability is the main purpose of the experiment; however, it can also be used to correlate cell behaviour to cell number. One of the most used cell viability assays using single endpoints is the 3-(4,5-dimethyl-2-thiazolyl)-2,5-diphenyl-2*H*-tetrazolium bromide (MTT) test.

The MTT cytotoxicity assay is a colorimetric method for determining the number of viable cells based on mitochondrial dehydrogenase activity measurement.[99] MTT is bio-reduced to formazan (coloured) by the intracellular dehydrogenase in living cells. The quantity of formazan that is directly proportional to the number of living cells in culture is measured spectrophotometrically. The assay is performed by adding test compounds at different concentrations to human prostate cancer (PC3) cells (or other cell lines) in a 96-well format. The MTT reagent is added directly to the cultured cells and after that an organic solvent is added to dissolve the insoluble purple formazan product into a coloured solution. The absorbance at 490 nm of this solution is quantified by a spectrophotometer. An internal standard is included in each assay for quality control. The effect of a series of standard compounds is reported in Table 15.4.

**Table 15.4** Compounds tested in the MTT assay in PC-3 cells. Compound potency, expressed as the negative logarithm of the compound concentration producing 50% reduction of cell viability ($pIC_{50}$) when tested in the MTT assay in PC-3 cells. The incubation time was 72 h at 37 °C.

| Test compound | $pIC_{50}$ |
|---|---|
| Taxol | 8.30 |
| Doxorubicin | 7.35 |
| 5-Fluoracil | 5.15 |
| Cisplatin | 4.60 |

As an alternative test to MTT, the adenosine triphosphate (ATP) monitoring system based on firefly (*Photinus pyralis*) luciferase can be used.[100] This luminescence assay is the alternative to colorimetric, fluorometric, and radioisotopic assays for the quantitative evaluation of proliferation and cytotoxicity of cultured mammalian cells. ATP monitoring can be used to assess the cytocidal, cytostatic, and proliferative effects of a wide range of drugs, biological response modifiers, and biological compounds. The major advantages are: high sensitivity, linearity, simplicity, fast results, and the lack of cell harvesting or separation steps. The assay is performed by adding test compounds at different concentrations to PC-3 cells (or other cell lines).

## 15.5 *In Vitro* Liabilities

From 1998–2008 most drugs withdrawn for safety reasons in US, European and Asian markets were either cardiotoxic, hepatotoxic, or neurotoxic.[101] This exemplified the need for establishing and implementing novel predictive safety assays, which are nowadays performed in earlier stages of drug development with the purpose of ensuring timely mitigation and also to proactively design safety into the molecules.[102] Here we focus on drug-induced liver injury (DILI), and cardiovascular and central nervous system toxicities, being the most common and impactful safety concerns.

### 15.5.1 Drug-induced Liver Injury (DILI)

Drug-induced liver injury (DILI) continues to be a major reason that drugs fail in clinical trials and is often the cause of drug withdrawals.[103] A large-scale comparison of safety liable compounds found preclinical animal models only predicted approximately 50% of the human DILI events attributed to these drugs.[104] As such, over the last decade the pharmaceutical industry has developed human-focused predictive *in vitro* strategies to aid risk assessment of hepatotoxicity in early drug discovery. This is evident by the large number of publications (>100; PubMed) in this field, culminating in comprehensive reviews of the *in vitro* assays and emerging DILI strategies from the pharmaceutical industry recently published (please see, *e.g.* Walker *et al.*, 2020[105] and Weaver *et al.*, 2020[106]).

These reviews include reference to attempts that have been made to minimize the discrepancies observed in *in vivo* DILI classifications within the literature[107] by creating the FDA's Liver Toxicity Knowledge Base (LTKB). This standardization allows comparison and alignment across published DILI strategies. It is clear that emerging trends are starting to coalesce, with multimechanistic assays, combined with organotypic 3D liver models, physiochemical descriptors, and evaluating data from *in vitro* assays with respect to *in vivo* (human) exposure being key. In order to improve further extrapolation and translation to clinical DILI risk analysis it is important to contextualize these parameters with human (unbound) exposure. Finally, modelling or Bayesian machine learning approaches should progress DILI prediction beyond binary endpoint analysis, advancing compound selection in drug discovery.[108]

## 15.5.2 Cardiac Liability

Cardiovascular toxicity remains a major cause of concern during preclinical and clinical development of drugs, as well as contributing to post-approval withdrawal of marketed drugs.[109] Amongst cardiac-related post-approval adverse events reported over the last 40 years, the majority are cardiac arrhythmias. Such data likely reflects the increased scrutiny around drug-induced QT interval prolongation and associated arrhythmias over the last decade.[110] Indeed, drug-related Torsade de Pointe (TdP), a potentially fatal arrhythmia characterized in the electrocardiogram (ECG) by a prolongation of the QT interval followed by a "twisting" of the waveform around the isoelectric line, accounted for one-third of all drug withdrawals between 1990 and 2006.[111]

There is a need to predict accurately the risk of drug-induced cardiotoxicity in preclinical and early clinical stages in order to avoid progressing drug candidates with a high-risk for cardiovascular toxicity into late clinical development and marketing approval phases.

### *15.5.2.1 Cardiac Function and Ion Channels*

The heart electrical activity determines its ability to beat and pump oxygenated blood successfully, and the overall electrical activity is determined by action potentials (APs) at the level of the cardiomyocyte. The sequential propagation of APs from the sinoatrial node to the ventricular muscle of the heart can be detected at the skin *via* the ECG (Figure 15.1).

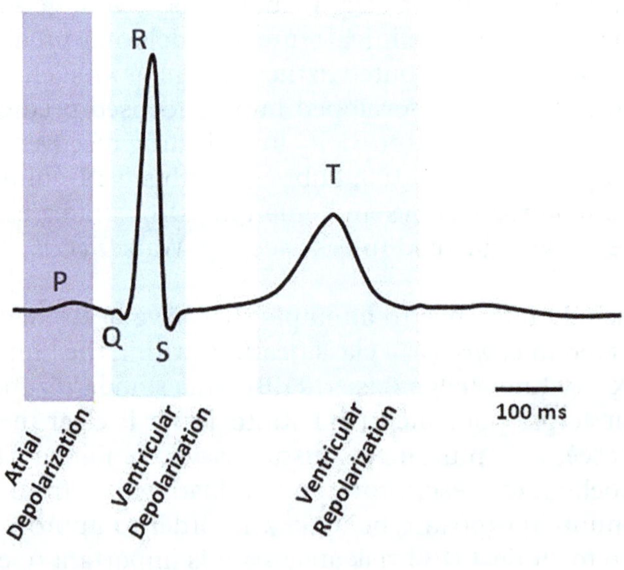


**Figure 15.1** Typical human ECG tracing of the cardiac cycle. The P wave, the QRS complex and the T wave are indicated by letters. The baseline of the electrocardiogram corresponds to the isoelectric line. Coloured shaded areas underline the phases of the electrical impulse propagation through the heart.

The cardiac AP is the electrical change across the membrane of the cardiac myocyte, and results from the sum of the activity of various ion channels. An ion channel is an integral transmembrane protein responsible for ion conduction across the cell membrane. In summary, the AP results from the balance between inward ($Na^+$ and $Ca^{2+}$) currents that depolarize and outward ($K^+$) currents that repolarize in the cardiac myocytes. In the cardiac AP five phases can be recognized (Figure 15.2):

- Upstroke (phase 0); large sodium current ($I_{Na}$) due to a rapid influx of $Na^+$ *via* opening of Nav1.5 channels.
- Early repolarization (phase 1); initiated by closure of Nav1.5 channels and activation of transient outward ($I_{to}$) and ultra-rapid ($I_{Kur}$) potassium currents *via* Kv4.2/4.3 and Kv1.5 channels, respectively.
- Plateau (phase 2); sustained by inward $Ca^{2+}$ current ($I_{Ca,L}$) due to L-type $Ca^{2+}$ channels (Cav1.2) and outward delayed rectifier $K^+$ currents *via* rapid hERG channel ($I_{Kr}$) and, in atrial cells, *via* ultra-rapid Kv1.5 ($I_{Kur}$).
- Late or final repolarization (phase 3); closure of Cav1.2 channels and activation of rapid ($I_{Kr}$) and slow outward rectifier ($I_{Ks}$) potassium currents *via* hERG and KCNQ1/mink channels, respectively, which brings the myocyte to the next phase.
- Resting state (phase 4); the resting potential is determined by inward rectifier $K^+$ current ($I_{K1}$) *via* Kir2.1 channels and is modulated by acetylcholine-regulated $K^+$ current ($I_{K,ACh}$).

### *15.5.2.2 Channels Causing the Greatest Potential Liabilities*

Functional alterations of one or more of the channels contributing to the AP lead to an abnormal ECG. Several mutation-associated cardiac diseases, such as atrial fibrillation, Brugada syndrome, cardiac conduction defects, long QT and short QT syndromes,

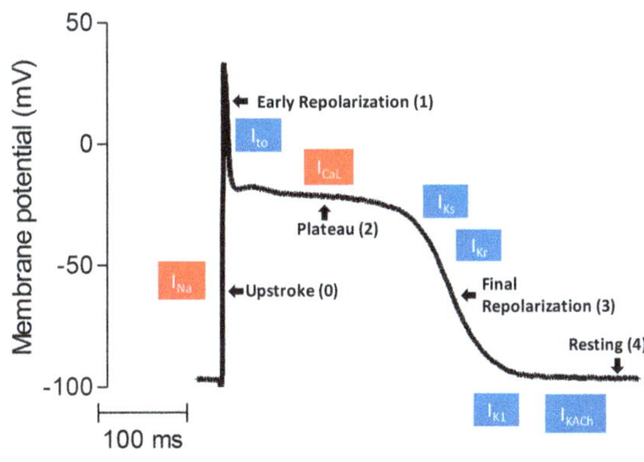


**Figure 15.2** Cardiac action potential recorded from a rabbit Purkinje fibre. The five phases are indicated by arrows. Action potentials are generated by the movement of ions through the ion channels present in the cardiac cells and indicated by red (inward currents) and blue (outward currents) boxes.

affecting $Na^+$, $K^+$, or $Ca^{2+}$ ion currents, have been described.[112] Such cardiac channelopathies may be clinically identified only by the presence of some characteristic ECG abnormalities.[113] Therefore, it is evident that drugs that modify the ECG parameters represent a major safety concern for pharmaceutical companies and regulatory agencies. Many compounds interact with cardiac ion channels, potentially leading to abnormal propagation of electrical action potentials through the heart tissue. This action is "designed into" antiarrhythmic drugs, but is often an unwanted side effect of non-cardiac drugs.

Historically, for drug development programmes that must establish cardiac safety profiles to achieve regulatory approval, the QT interval remains one of the most important ECG parameters. Prolongation of the QT interval is the consequence of an increased duration of AP due to a delay in repolarization that theoretically could arise from an increase in inward (depolarizing) current, or alternatively, from a decrease in outward (repolarizing) current. Hence, the interaction of the drug with even one ion channel contributing to the AP can result in a cardiac adverse event.

The cellular electrophysiological testing of drugs for cardiac safety tends to involve potassium channels, sodium channels, and L-type calcium channels, because the association of these channels with long QT syndrome is well established. The hERG channel is the most commonly tested ion channel for cardiac liability of new drugs because many drugs are linked to long QT syndrome mediated by hERG, presumably due to the structure of the channel which allows for promiscuous interactions with many different small molecules.[114] Examples of drugs withdrawn from the market between 1997 and 2002 due to an unacceptable TdP risk include astemizole and terfenadine (antihistamine drugs), cisapride (gastrokinetic drug), and thioridazine (antipsychotic drug). These were found to be hERG channel blockers.

For many years the only test of drug-induced channel blockade that was viewed as critical for cardiac safety by drug regulators was hERG (Figure 15.3), despite the fact that an ensemble of currents contributes to the AP (and the ECG) and extrapolating the net drug-induced effects on a range of channels based on measuring only one type of current can give false picture. Some drugs that are not proarrhythmic, such as verapamil (hypertension drug), phenobarbital (anticonvulsant drug), and ranolazine (antianginal drug), show positive results on hERG assay. A clear example of this is verapamil, a potent hERG blocker that does not cause QT prolongation, likely due to its concomitant blockade of the calcium current. Amiodarone is an example of a drug that affects multiple calcium and sodium cardiac currents (with higher sensitivity for late component over the peak component of $I_{Na}$) providing protection from proarrhythmia despite a hERG block.[115,116]

In 2005, the International Conference on Harmonization (ICH) released the guidelines S7B[117] and E14[118] that currently govern the cardiac safety landscape. S7B provides a non-clinical testing strategy to evaluate the potential for human pharmaceuticals to affect cardiac electrophysiology, with specific attention focused on ventricular repolarization. E14 addresses clinical evaluation of QTc (the QT interval "corrected" for the effects of heart rate) prolongation. These guidelines are focused on the hERG (as surrogate of proarrhythmia) and QTc interval, namely, the measurement of hERG current, the *in vivo* QT assay in an animal model and a trial examining the drug's effects on the QT interval of healthy volunteers. With evolving non-clinical and clinical data,

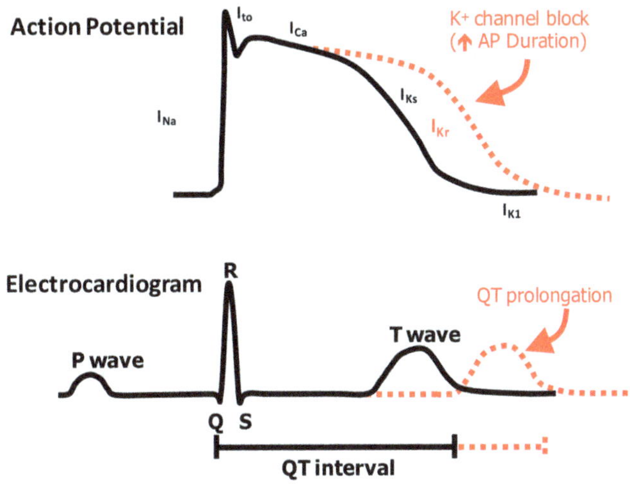


**Figure 15.3** Schematic representation of the effect of a hERG channel blocker on the cardiac action potential and on the ECG trace. The potassium channel block has the consequence of increasing the action potential duration and consequently prolonging the QT interval in the ECG recording.

it is appreciated that the hERG current block is one part of the whole picture related to proarrhythmic potential of non-antiarrhythmic drugs. The S7B and E14 guidelines have been successful since there have not been any withdrawals of marketed drugs for torsadogenic concerns since their adoption. However, they have had the consequence of promoting the perception that detection of even a small effect on hERG or mild QTc prolongation will result in adverse regulatory and commercial implications, impacting the pharmaceutical drug discovery pipeline by stopping the development of potentially valuable therapeutics.[119] This is why in 2013 the US Food and Drug Administration (FDA), the Health and Environmental Sciences Institute (HESI), and the Cardiac Safety Research Consortium (CSRC) presented a new paradigm for cardiotoxicity testing which is described in detail in Section 15.5.2.4.

#### *15.5.2.3 Binding vs. Functional Assays*

The gold standard for studying ion channel function and modulation is the manual patch clamp;[120,122] however, it is too slow and too expensive to be adopted in early phases of drug discovery. Alternative approaches with higher throughput and lower costs are binding, fluorescence, or flux assays, which represent an indirect readout of ion channel activity and as such are prone to false positives/negatives. The binding assay is not as informative as functional measurements because unless the sites at which test compounds interact with a channel are identical or strongly allosterically coupled to the region where the labelled probe binds, potential channel interactions can be missed. In a binding assay there is no possibility to identify compounds that interact with different functional states of the ion channel, so binding assay results do not necessarily correlate with functional activity.[121]

Although hERG binding assays (for example [$^3$H]-dofetilide or [$^3$H]-astemizole binding assays) have been used for many years, this approach is conceptually flawed when compared with profiling actives directly on hERG function. Many instances of hERG binding by drug candidates have yielded both false positive and false negative data during testing of novel structural series. False positives can be addressed by subsequent evaluation in a functional assay. However, false negatives can have disastrous programme consequences if the hERG liability is not detected until a potential preclinical candidate is profiled *in vivo*. The time wasted and lack of SAR information on the newly discovered hERG activity usually results in termination of development efforts. The use of hERG binding assays as the only support for medicinal chemistry is too risky, since alternatives exist for employing medium- and high-capacity functional hERG assay formats.[123]

Fluorescence assays by using ion-sensitive or voltage-sensitive fluorescent dyes can detect changes in intracellular concentrations of ions such as calcium or thallium (a permeable ion through potassium channels) or detect changes in membrane potential. Such assays show good correlation with patch clamp results, with the risk of false positives in the case of fluorescent compounds.

It is clear that assays directly measuring ion channel function are prone to fewer artefacts than those using an indirect measure, so that in the last two decades automated patch clamp instruments were developed in order to merge the quality of the manual patch clamp technique and the throughput of the other techniques mentioned. As a matter of fact, it is now widely applied to reduce the liability of compound series towards the hERG channel, as part of safety pharmacology assessment early during medicinal chemistry compound development,[119] as well as for the other aforementioned cardiac ion channels.

### 15.5.2.4 Comprehensive In Vitro Proarrhythmia Assays

In 2013 the US Food and Drug Administration (FDA), the Health and Environmental Sciences Institute (HESI), and the Cardiac Safety Research Consortium (CSRC) presented a new paradigm for cardiotoxicity testing,[124] the Comprehensive *in vitro* Proarrhythmia Assay (CiPA). The proposal is based on a comprehensive understanding of cardiac electrophysiology and the cellular mechanisms of TdP. To assess overall proarrhythmic risk, CiPA relies upon the testing of drugs on multiple human cardiac currents measured in heterologous expression systems, whose electrophysiological effects will then be integrated *in silico* by computer models reconstructing human cellular ventricular electrophysiology and confirmation of effects in a myocyte assay such as human stem-cell-derived cardiomyocytes. Evaluation of non-clinical *in vivo* models still remains part of the new paradigm. This upcoming new international cardiac safety paradigm may facilitate the use of non-clinical data as part of an integrated risk assessment strategy to inform clinical decision-making.

A comprehensive *in vitro* set of ion channel assays could explore drug effects on the isolated cardiac channels responsible for $I_{Kr}$, $I_{Ks}$, $I_{K1}$, $I_{Na}$ (fast and late), and $I_{CaL}$. Potency of current block ($IC_{50}$ values, the concentration of compound that inhibits 50% of the current) is of key importance and additional blocking mechanism characterization (for example voltage-, state-, use- or time-dependency) may be critical.[125]

Human stem-cell-derived cardiomyocytes, are suggested to be used to provide a cell-based integrated electrophysiological drug response, where the set of endogenously expressed channels produce a cardiac AP.[126,127]

The progress made by the CiPA initiative and other similar projects worldwide have led to the formation of an International Council for Harmonization (ICH) Implementation Working Group (IWG) to develop Questions and Answers (Q&As) for ICH S7B (non-clinical) and E14 (clinical) guidelines.[128]

### *15.5.2.5 Integrated Cardiovascular Risk Assessment Strategy*

A strategy to progress compounds and discharge cardiovascular risk can be put in place during the lead optimization phase and in later phases (Figure 15.4).

The identification of early warning signals is suggested by exploiting knowledge on the target and on the desired mechanism of action of compounds. Early, during

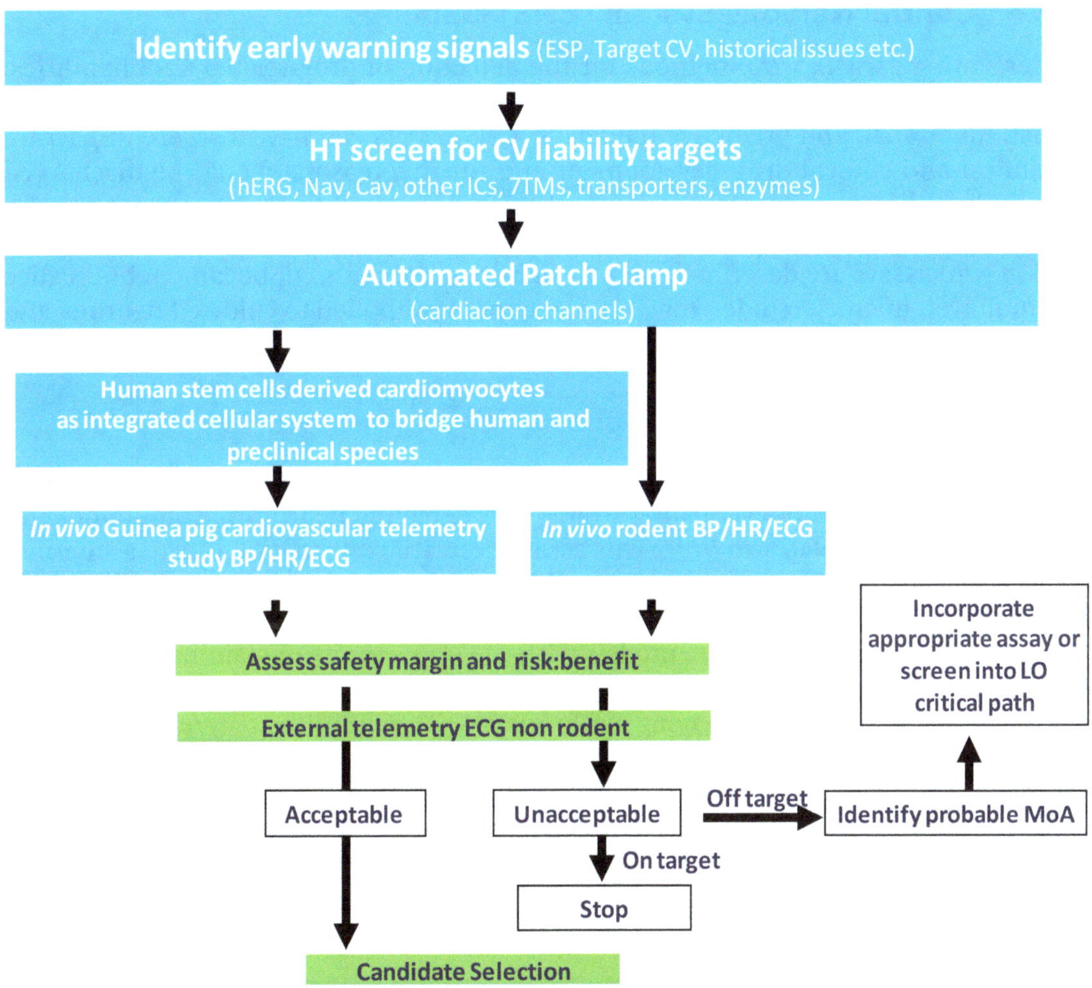


**Figure 15.4** Example of an integrated risk assessment strategy. Please note that the high-throughput (HT) screen for liability targets can be expanded outside the cardiovascular field, as described in the previous chapter. ESP = Early Safety Prediction, CV = Cardiovascular, HT = High Throughput, BP = Blood Pressure, HR = Heart Rate.

lead identification, the submission of compounds to *in vitro* pharmacological profiling against known cardiovascular targets, including cardiac ion channels, helps to discharge this cardiac risk, thereby decreasing drug discovery attrition. The testing of compounds in human stem-cell-derived cardiomyocytes, where the cardiac set of channels are expressed, allows evaluation of compound cardiac action potentials and helps to bridge between human and preclinical species such as guinea pig and rodents.

The functional assays for ionic currents in recombinant systems, for action potential in human stem-cell-derived cardiomyocytes and *in vivo* models, provide an integrated screening strategy to discharge cardiovascular risk for novel compounds in the drug discovery and development process.

### 15.5.3 Central Nervous System (CNS) Liability

Implementing early *in vitro* methods for the detection of drug-related CNS liabilities, such as seizures and off-target neurotoxicity, has been a challenge due to the lack of robust, functional, and predictive models.[129] CNS effects can have a severe impact on preclinical and clinical drug development and for this reason, should be discharged early in drug discovery. *In vitro* assays are therefore required to predict seizure/convulsive potential risk of new chemical entities.[130] Here, the most advanced and commonly used *in vitro* assays are described, such as neurite outgrowth, hippocampal brain slice and multiwell microelectrode array (MEA) technology applied to cultured neurons and induced pluripotent stem-cell-derived neurons.

#### *15.5.3.1 Neurite Outgrowth Assay*

The neurite outgrowth assay is a well-established high-content method that can be used as a high-throughput screening strategy for detecting neurotoxic compounds utilizing a cell imaging platform.[131,132] This assay is versatile due to its ability to accommodate many different cell types, such as multiple primary rodent cell types and human iPSC-derived neurons. Another positive aspect of this assay is the experimenter's ability to design chronic drug exposure models with the opportunity of staining many different CNS-related targets to determine morphological and developmental drug-induced changes. Most high-content imaging platforms have the ability to analyze multiple endpoints describing neurite structure and morphology, such as neurite length, neurite width, number of neurites per neuron/field/well, and both branch point and cross point statistics. Overall cell health can also be evaluated by analyzing endpoints pertaining to nuclei and cell bodies. In Figure 15.5, fCDI iCell neurons are plated in 384-well plates and treated with multiple concentrations of nocodazole, a positive control for decreasing neurite outgrowth.

#### *15.5.3.2 Hippocampal Slices*

Although it is high-throughput and informative, the neurite outgrowth assay is not able to detect chemical entities that disrupt electrophysiological neural network function

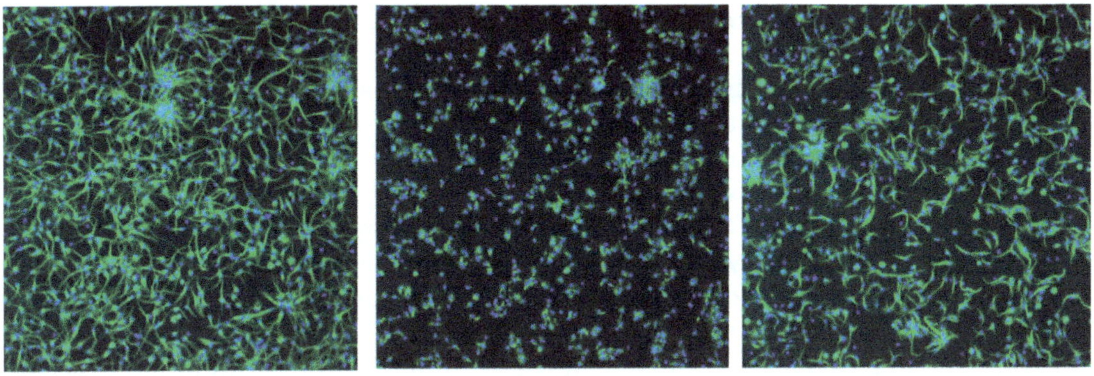


**Figure 15.5** Neurite outgrowth assay. fCDI iCell Neurons grown on clear bottom 384-well PDL coated plates with an additional pre-coating of laminin. The neurons were treated for 48 hours with multiple concentrations of nocodazole and vehicle control, DMSO 0.5%. After incubation with the compounds, the neurons were fixed, permeabilized, and stained with Hoechst 33342 (blue) and anti-Beta III Tubulin Antibody, Alexa Fluor® 488 (green).

or compounds that are exclusively pro-convulsant. A number of studies have demonstrated that hippocampal slices represent a predictable *in vitro* model to detect the effects of compounds associated with seizure induction in man.[133,134]

Even if it cannot be excluded that compounds could elicit seizures *via* mechanisms or targets not located in the hippocampus, hippocampal slices represent a useful *in vitro* model, as they retain a defined cytoarchitecture, and relevant receptors and constituents of the full brain system, including inter-area connectivity. This is of great importance, as the cause of seizures and epileptiform activity can be complex and interlinked with multiple hierarchical levels of the CNS.[135]

### *15.5.3.3 Multiwell Microelectrode Array (MEA)*

The gold standard for *in vitro* seizure prediction is the hippocampal brain slice assay.[132,136,137] This model, however, is relatively low-throughput, requires complex electrophysiological recording equipment, and its success relies on significant expertise and viable tissue preparations. Multiwell microelectrode array (MEA) technology provides the industry with a versatile platform for testing the effects on neural network functionality when exposed to a potential new drug entity.[138–144] This model has proven to be predictive of potential seizurogenic effects for compounds from different structural classes and for different targeted receptors.[138] MEA screening models are moderately high-throughput and have the ability to record the activity of any electrophysiologically excitable cell. Therefore, this technology can be utilized for CNS toxicity screening strategies. To date, both freshly isolated and cryopreserved rodent neurons grown on MEA plates have been successful in establishing robust and organized neural networks that are sensitive to the effects of neurotoxic and seizurogenic drugs. Cryopreserved rat cortical neurons mature into a robust neural network with spontaneous spike activity, organized bursting patterns and network synchrony. These neural networks are sensitive to a variety of compounds and can detect effects that cause decreases or increases in activity (spike or burst rate), compounds that cause increases in burst organization and network synchrony, and compounds that cause a deterioration in burst organization and network synchrony. These changes can be qualitatively observed by viewing the raster plots created in most MEA instrument software packages, or quantitatively assessed with analysis tools such as MATLAB (MathWorks), NeuroExplorer (Nex Technologies), or analysis modules provided with the instrument. Picrotoxin, a $GABA_A$ antagonist and known seizurogenic compound, causes an increase in activity, burst organization, and network synchrony at concentrations as low as 0.2 μM after treatment for 1 h. The raster plots in Figure 15.6 compare baseline activity in one well (configured with 16 electrodes) as compared to the activity in the same well after treatment with picrotoxin at a concentration of 10 μM with a 1 h incubation. A consistent pattern of regularized bursting with synchronicity across all electrodes is easily observed. The pattern of effect with picrotoxin is indicative of all $GABA_A$ antagonists, and in some cases, of compounds in different chemical classes.

Alternatively, compounds such as strychnine and NMDA that cause a deterioration in burst structure, a breakdown in network synchrony, a decrease in activity (spike rate, burst rate, or both) and a regularized pattern of isolated spikes, are also considered to have a seizurogenic pattern (Figure 15.7). This particular pattern is common with various known proconvulsant compounds, even though the targets or structures can be quite different.

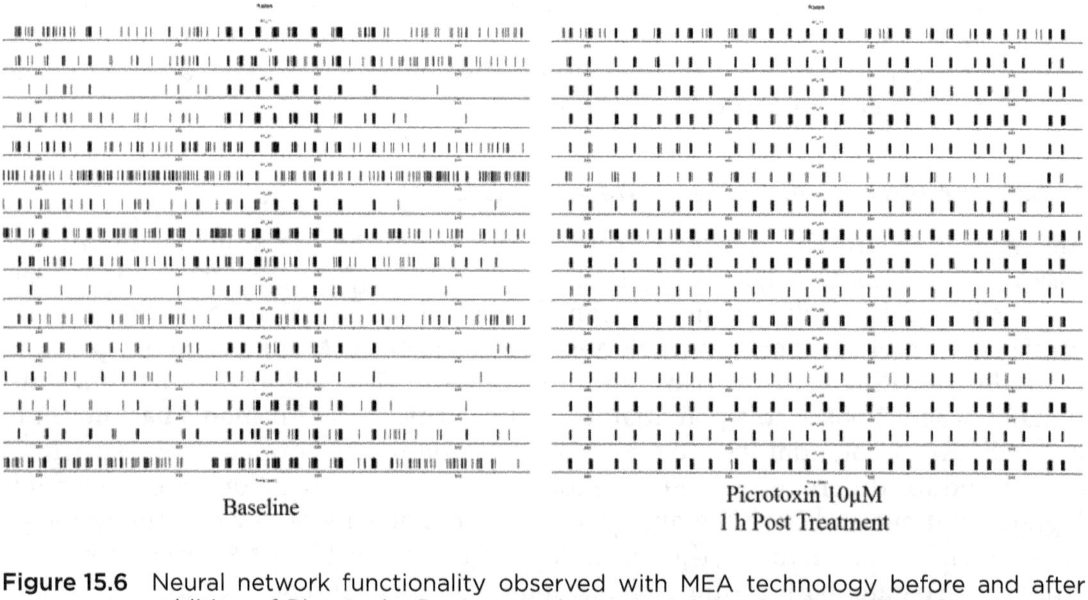


**Figure 15.6** Neural network functionality observed with MEA technology before and after addition of Picrotoxin. Representative raster plots of spike activity recorded for baseline and 1 hour post treatment with Picrotoxin at a concentration of 10 μM. Increases in activity, burst organization, and synchrony are observed.

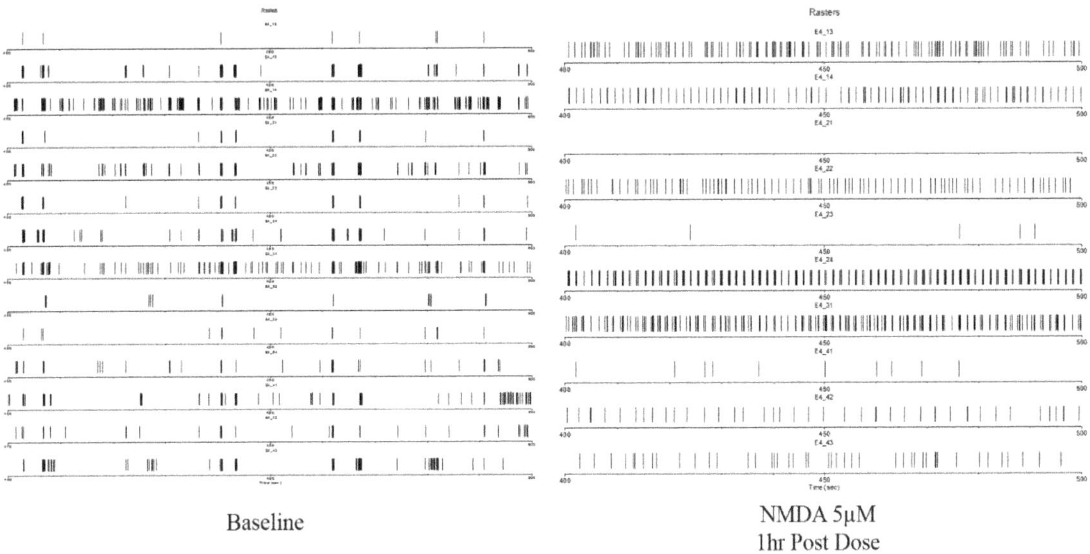


**Figure 15.7** Neural network functionality observed with MEA technology before and after addition of NMDA. The baseline raster plot shows an active well with regular bursting and observable synchrony with a considerable number of isolated spontaneous spikes. After the addition of NMDA at 5 μM for 1 h, the raster plot shows a complete change in firing pattern with most spikes occurring outside of bursts in a regularized pattern. There are fewer bursts and no network synchrony is occurring at all.

The two patterns of response described here have been clearly defined as seizurogenic in a rat cortical neuron model.[137] With the emergence in the *in vitro* testing of neuroactive and known proconvulsant compounds in MEA, there will be an increase in the understanding of these endpoint patterns *vs. in vivo* responses. This will allow for improved *in vitro* predictions much earlier in the drug discovery process enabling the advancement of safer molecules with less neurotoxic liabilities.

Commercially available human iPSC-derived neurons are becoming a viable option for MEA assay models.[145] When grown on MEA plates, some currently available cell types create an active neural network that organizes into a synchronous and robust phenotype that is mature enough for pharmacological testing. These cells have been shown to respond to seizurogenic compounds similarly to MEA models using rat neurons. Although some responses differ nominally from the rat neuron models, the responses are predictable, repeatable, and can be used to create a database of phenotypic responses for categorizing test article liabilities. The utility in screening with the hiPSC-derived neurons is the ability to test potential new drugs in a human cell model long before any *in vivo* safety studies commence, therefore bypassing the need to interpret or anticipate any cross-species deleterious effects. In addition to the availability of different types of human iPSC-derived neurons (*i.e.* GABAergic, glutamatergic, peripheral), the availability of neurons for specific disease models is becoming more abundant and will augment the robustness of this technology.

Overall, MEA neuronal screening models are a robust method for screening potentially neurotoxic and proconvulsant compounds early in the drug discovery process. These models can be used to compare different scaffolds or analogues to determine their relative safety. This will allow for the progression of safer molecules into animals. Alternatively, when seizures or other liabilities in animals are identified, this assay is often used to confirm and screen alternatives. This technology has the flexibility of using any electrophysiologically active cell type. Studies can be designed to screen for seizure potential, acute neurotoxicity, chronic neurotoxicity, developmental neurotoxicity, neural plasticity, and used for screening against specific disease models.

## 15.6 Drug–Drug Interactions

Polypharmacy is becoming a common practice around the world and is especially prevalent in elderly populations.[146,147] When multiple drugs are coadministered, they may lead to drug–drug interactions (DDIs) and result in toxicity or loss of efficacy. There have been a number of drugs notably withdrawn from the market because of DDI and this can cause significant ethical and economic problems for the pharmaceutical industry.[148–150] Additionally, it has been reported that with 76 000–137 000 cases a year, adverse drug reactions (ADRs) is one of the most common cause of deaths in hospitalized patients in the United States.[149] It has been found that the incidence of DDI-related ADRs was significant, and most of the events presented important clinical consequences. Because clinicians still have difficulty managing this problem, minimizing the factors that increase the risk of DDI-related ADRs is essential. For the pharmaceutical industry, a significant challenge in early drug discovery is the successful prediction of potential DDI in man using *in vitro* inhibition data.

### 15.6.1 Drug–Drug Interactions Mechanisms

DDIs can occur as a result of pharmacokinetic (PK) interactions, *i.e.* one drug affects the elimination or uptake of a comedicated drug by either inhibiting or inducing the enzymes or transporters that are responsible for the disposition of that drug, hence changing the PK behaviour of the comedication. A "perpetrator" is a drug that inhibits or induces enzymes or transporters and alters the PK of another drug, and a "victim" is a drug whose PK is changed by a perpetrator, leading to an effect on toxicity or efficacy.[151] Current DDI studies place a strong emphasis on the cytochrome P450 (CYP) enzymes, since they account for the clearance of about 45% of marketed drugs (Tables 15.5 and 15.6).[152] CYPs are mainly concentrated in the liver,[153,154] the major organ for metabolism of oral drugs. CYP enzymes are haeme-thiolate proteins that are responsible for the oxidative metabolism of a wide variety of xenobiotics. They comprise a superfamily of related enzymes that are grouped into families and subfamilies based on similarities in amino acid sequences. Currently, there are 18 superfamilies, 32 subfamilies, and 57 isoforms found in human P450s.[155,156] According to the regulatory guidelines, the inhibition potency, as a perpetrator, needs to be assessed for drug candidates against seven major CYPs, *i.e.*, 1A2, 2B6, 2C8, 2C9, 2C19, 2D6, and

3A4/5 (https://www.fda.gov/downloads/drugs/guidances/ucm292362.pdf, https://www.ema.europa.eu/en/documents/scientific-guideline/guideline-strategies-identify-mitigate-risks-first-human-early-clinical-trials-investigational_en.pdf http://www.pmda.go.jp/files/000228122.pdf).

Although CYPs are the most important class of drug-metabolizing enzymes,[157–160] there are increasing numbers of DDI cases due to interaction with non-CYP enzymes and transporters, such as UDP-glucuronosyltransferases (UGTs), P-gp, BCRP, OATPs, OATs, and OCTs.[161–164]

Major mechanisms of DDI are:

1. A compound may affect the effective plasma concentrations of other drugs taken concomitantly with the compound of interest, by inhibiting the metabolism of a coadministered drug. The affected drug thereby might have plasma concentrations higher than intended, leading to toxicity. A well-known case of inhibitory drug–drug interactions is the inhibition of the metabolism of terfenadine,[165] by the antifungal drug, ketoconazole, a well-known potent inhibitor of CYP3A4, the P450 isoform responsible for metabolism of terfenadine. Terfenadine is a prodrug, normally completely metabolized to its active form fexofenadine in the liver by CYP3A4. A number of patients developed fatal cardiac arrhythmia after they were administered both terfenadine and ketoconazole, owing to the elevated level of terfenadine, and its potent inhibition of the hERG channel.
2. If the parent drug is a CYP inducer, it may increase the clearance rate of concomitantly administered drugs which are metabolized by these CYPs. This may result in a decrease in the effective plasma concentrations of these drugs, thus decreasing their pharmacologic effects. The rifampin–birth-control pill interaction is an example of this type of drug–drug interactions. Rifampin is now known to induce

**Table 15.5** Known inhibitors and inducers of CYP isozymes.

| Enzyme | Inducers | Inhibitors |
|---|---|---|
| CYP1A2 | Cigarette Smoke, Phenobarbital, Ritonavir, Carbamazepine, Charbroiled Foods, Vegetables, Omeprazole | Enoxacin, Ciprofloxacin, Grepafloxacin, Fluvoxamine, Fluoxetine, Nefazodone |
| CYP2A6 | Barbiturates | |
| CYP2C9 | Rifampin, Carbamazepine, Ethanol, Phenytoin | Amiodarone, Fluvastatin, Fluvoxamine, Fluoxetine, Fluconazole, Miconazole, Metronidazole, Ritonavir, Sulfamethoxazole |
| CYP2C19 | Rifampin | Fluvoxamine, Fluoxetine, Ticlopidine, Ritonavir |
| CYP2D6 | Pregnancy | Quinidine, Fluoxetine, Paroxetine, Sertraline, Thioridazine, Cimetidine, Diphenhydramine, Haloperidol, Ticlopidine (Ticlid), Ritonavir |
| CYP2E1 | Ethanol, Isoniazid, Ritonavir | Cimetidine, Watercress |
| CYP3A4/5 | Carbamazepine, Dexamethasone, Rifapentine, Prednisone, Growth Hormone, Rifampin, Phenobarbital, Phenytoin, Troglitazone | Ketoconazole, Itraconazole, Erythromycin, Grapefruit Juice, Fluvoxamine, Fluoxetine, Diltiazem, Verapamil, Clarithromycin, Omeprazole, Ritonavir, Indinavir |

**Table 15.6** Known Cytochrome P450 substrates.

| Enzyme | Substrates |
|---|---|
| CYP1A2 | Amitriptyline, Betaxolol, Caffeine, Clomipramine, Clozapine, Chlorpromazine, Fluvoxamine, Haloperidol, Imipramine, Olanzapine, Ondansetron, Propranolol, Tacrine, Theophylline, Verapamil, (R)-Warfarin |
| CYP2A6 | Coumarin, Betadiene, Nicotine |
| CYP2C9 | Amitriptyline, Diclofenac, Demadex, Fluoxetine, Ibuprofen, Losartan, Naproxen, Phenytoin, Piroxicam, Tolbutamide, (S)-Warfarin |
| CYP2C19 | Amitriptyline, Citalopram, Clomipramine, Diazepam, Imipramine, Omeprazole |
| CYP2D6 | Amitriptyline, Betaxolol, Clomipramine, Codeine, Clozapine, Desipramine, Fluoxetine, Haloperidol, Imipramine, Methadone, Metoclopramide, Metoprolol, Nortriptyline, Olanzapine, Ondansetron, Paroxetine, Propranolol, Risperidone, Sertraline, Timolol, Venlafaxine |
| CYP2E1 | Acetaminophen, Caffeine, Chlorzoxazone, Dextromethorphan, Ethanol, Theophylline, Venlafaxine |
| CYP3A4/5 | Alprazolam, Amiodaron, Amitriptyline, Astemizole, Bupropion, Buspirone, Caffeine, Carbamazepine, Cerivastatin, Cisapride, Clarithromycin, Clomipramine, Codeine, Cyclosporine, Dexamethasone, Dextromethorphan, DHEA, Diazepam, Diltiazem, Donepezil, Doxycycline, Erythromycin, Estradiol, Felodipine, Fluoxetine, Imipramine, Lansoprazole, Lidocaine, Loratadine, Lovastatin, Midazolam, Nicardipine, Nifedipine, Omeprazole, Orphenadrine, Paroxetine, Progesterone, Quinidine, Rifampin, Sertraline, Sibutramine, Sildenafil, Simvastatin, Tacrolimus, Tamoxifen, Terfenadine, Testosterone, Theophylline, Verapami, Vinblastine, (R)-Warfarin |

CYP3A4 and oestrogen sulfotransferase, the two major pathways for the metabolism of birth control pill ingredients. Women of child-bearing age on the birth control pill experienced pregnancy owing to the induction of the drug-metabolizing enzymes for the active ingredients of the birth control pills.

3. Metabolites formed *via* CYP metabolism may be responsible for undesirable side effects, such as organ toxicity. Formation of reactive metabolic intermediates is one of the causes for drug toxicity. Oxidation to electrophilic intermediates or reduction to nucleophilic radicals that can attack DNA or RNA and induce carcinogenicity are two major reactions by which toxicity is exerted. Although many leads are abandoned early on in drug discovery due to toxic metabolite formation, presence of a toxic metabolite does not always imply toxicity in a given drug candidate, since there are other factors that can make the metabolite toxic or non-toxic. The presence of a toxic metabolite, however, raises a red flag, which must be examined extensively in subsequent (animal) toxicity studies.

Several of the drug-metabolizing enzymes, for example the CYP2 family, are polymorphic (having more than one variant of the gene). Although the CYP isozymes generally have similar functional properties, each one is different and has a distinct role (Table 15.7). This polymorphism forms a basis for inter-individual differences in the efficacy of drug treatment, side effects of drugs, and the toxic and carcinogenic action of xenobiotics. There is a wide variation in the expression, activity, and concentrations of different isozymes among individuals, species, and ethnic groups. The expression or the activity of these enzymes is influenced by factors such as species specificity, genetic

**Table 15.7** Examples of human polymorphic CYPs.[a]

| Enzyme | Major Variant Alleles | Mutation | Consequence | Caucasian | Asian |
|---|---|---|---|---|---|
| CYP2A6 | CYP2A6*2 | L160H | Inactive enzyme | 1–3 | 0 |
| | CYP2A6*3 | 2A6/2A7 conversions | Not known | 0 | 0 |
| | CYP2A6*4 | Gene deletion | No enzyme | 1 | 15 |
| | CYP2A6*5 | G479L | Defect enzyme | 0 | 1 |
| CYP2C9 | CYP2C9*2 | R144C | Reduce affinity for P450 reductase | 8–13 | 0 |
| | CYP2C9*3 | I359L | Altered substrate specificity | 7–9 | 2–3 |
| CYP2C19 | CYP2C19*2 | Aberrant splice site | Inactive enzyme | 13 | 23–32 |
| | CYP2C19*3 | Premature stop codon | Inactive enzyme | 0 | 6–10 |
| CYP2D6 | CYP2D6*2xn | Gene duplication/ multiduplication | Increased enzyme activity | 1–5 | 0–2 |
| | CYP2D6*4 | Defective splicing | Inactive enzyme | 12–21 | 1 |
| | CYP2D6*5 | Gene deletion | No enzyme | 4–6 | 6 |
| | CYP2D6*10 | P34S, S486T | Unstable enzyme | 1–2 | 50 |
| | CYP2D6*17 | T107I, R296C, S486T | Reduce affinity for substrates | 0 | n.d. |
| CYP2E1 | CYP2E1*2 | R76H | Less enzyme expressed | 0 | 1 |
| | CYP2E1*3 | V389I | No effects | <1 | 0 |
| | CYP2E1*4 | V179I | No effects | <1 | n.d. |
| CYP34A4 | CYP3A4*2 | S222P | Higher $K_m$ for substrates | 3 | 0 |
| | CYP3A4*3 | M445T | Unknown | 0 | <1 |

[a]n.d.: not determined (has a very high frequency among Black Africans and African Americans).

polymorphism, gender-hormonal control, age, disease, and environmental inducers (caffeine, cigarette smoke).

The variability associated with the CYP enzymes in each individual results in marked differences in response when the same drug and dose is administered to different individuals. Genetic polymorphism of CYP enzymes characterizes the general population into three groups:

A. Extensive metabolizers (EM): normal population.
B. Poor metabolizers (PM): individuals who inherit two inactive alleles (alternative forms of the gene) showing complete absence of enzyme activity.
C. Ultra-extensive metabolizers (UEM): individuals with one common allele and one amplified allele showing enhanced enzyme expression.

Ultra-extensive metabolism can cause therapeutic failure due to reduced bioavailability or lack of activation of the drug, whereas poor metabolism can lead to drug toxicity and sometimes death. For optimal drug therapy, the prescribing physician should have knowledge of the genetic makeup of the CYP enzymes in the patient.

The determination of the CYP enzymes responsible for the metabolism of new chemical entities (NCEs) and the identification of interactions with a specific CYP isozyme (*e.g.* inhibition or induction of that isozyme) can aid in predicting clinical drug interactions, and *in vitro* methods are commonly used to determine the CYP interaction potential of NCEs.

## 15.6.2 CYP-driven DDI Test Systems

*In vitro* studies are best suited to determine the types of clinical trials needed to assess potential DDIs. FDA guidelines suggest first using *in vitro* studies to assess the effect of drugs on metabolic pathways and if the results indicate possible DDIs, to follow up with *in vivo* assays. Well-established protocols are commonly used to determine the CYP-driven DDI potential of NCEs and there is a universally accepted strategy to use *in vitro* human liver-based experimental systems.[166,167]

The most widely used systems are discussed below in detail.

### 15.6.2.1 *Expressed Enzymes*

Advances in molecular biology have enabled the identification and characterization of a large number of individual CYP genes. Specific cDNA sequences for particular CYP isozymes have been cloned and expressed heterologously. These enzymes, which can be produced in large amounts to meet the increasing demand of screening assays for drug metabolism research, show catalytic properties comparable to those of human liver microsomes (HLMs). Resulting recombinant human CYPs are isolated in microsomal forms and are commercially available for CYP phenotyping, metabolic stability screening, metabolism or toxicity studies, and inhibitory potential evaluation. Moreover, since only one enzyme is present, non-selective substrates can be used. This system is particularly helpful for the study of polymorphic enzymes, for instance, as some UGT isoforms do not have selective substrate reactions available, recombinant enzymes are used to evaluate inhibition potencies. Heterologously engineered cells expressing individual enzymes can be used for metabolism or toxicity studies. Major drawbacks inherent to recombinant models are that concentrations of CYPs are far in excess of their relative amount in the human liver, and that secondary metabolism cannot be identified.

### 15.6.2.2 *Liver Microsomes*

Microsomes can be prepared easily from frozen liver tissues. They are highly enriched with membrane-bound enzymes such as the CYPs, UGTs, and flavin-containing monooxygenases (FMOs).[168] Their easy preparation and good long-term stability at − 80 °C make microsomes the most frequently used *in vitro* system in drug metabolism studies. Microsomes are isolated from liver cells by disrupting the cellular contents and centrifugation at 100 000 × *g*. The ability to phenotype microsomes greatly increases the utility of this system in the identification of the specific isozymes responsible. Metabolic information such as metabolic profiles, stability, metabolite identification, and kinetics can be obtained from microsomal systems. Microsomal incubations are most often used to obtain information on Phase I reactions. One disadvantage is that the information is not complete as from the cellular systems.

#### *15.6.2.3 Isolated Hepatocytes*

Cell cultures or cell suspensions can be used to study multiple aspects of drug metabolism, drug transport across cell membranes, cytotoxicity, and enzyme induction in an environment where enzymes and cofactors are present in normal physiological concentrations and cellular integrity is maintained. Human hepatocytes are primary liver cells that contain most of the drug-metabolizing enzymes and are considered to be more physiologically relevant than HLMs. Human hepatocyte suspensions contain cell membranes and maintain certain functional activities of uptake or efflux transporters.[169,170] The human hepatocyte assays used in drug discovery include suspensions, plated, and sandwich culture formats. For inhibition studies, the hepatocyte suspension format is most commonly used.[171] The assay design is similar to that of HLMs, but without the need for adding cofactors. In hepatocyte incubations, potential cytotoxicity needs to be monitored, especially at high test concentrations; indeed, cytotoxicity may sometimes be mistaken for "inhibition" due to reduced enzyme activity.

#### *15.6.2.4 Tissue Slices*

Tissue slices have certain advantages over other systems. With intact cell–cell junctions, normal hepatic cellular architecture is retained in the tissue. Since they contain the complete complement of drug-metabolizing enzymes with all the cofactors present in relevant concentrations, complete information on the metabolism reactions can be obtained. Liver slices can be easily and rapidly produced. In addition, liver slices are not exposed to proteolytic enzymes that can destroy important membrane receptors in the cell. Although liver slices do have utility in some drug metabolism studies, they have certain disadvantages. One drawback is the inadequate penetration of the medium. Liver slices cannot be cryo-preserved and they have a limited useful experimental period.

### 15.6.3 Drug-metabolizing Enzyme Inhibition

Enzyme inhibitors function in different ways. Competitive inhibitors compete with the substrate for the active site, *e.g.* fluvoxamine and caffeine for CYP1A2. Non-competitive inhibitors bind to the enzyme–substrate complex or to the haem group, *e.g.*, ketoconazole. The third type, irreversible inhibitors, inactivate the enzyme either by haem binding or protein binding.

Primary *in vitro* metabolic systems used in drug metabolism, to evaluate whether the drug in question would inhibit drug-metabolizing enzymes, involve hepatic enzymes or tissue preparations. The drug to be studied is incubated with recombinant enzymes, liver microsomes or hepatocytes in the presence of substrates of specific drug-metabolizing enzymes. The metabolic rate of these substrates in the presence and absence of the drug would allow one to estimate its inhibitory potential. Results are in general expressed as $IC_{50}$, the concentration leading to a 50% decrease in activity, or $K_i$, the inhibitory constant. Low $IC_{50}$ or $K_i$ values as compared with the intended plasma concentration would suggest a high potential for the drug to cause drug interactions with coadministered drugs, which are substrates of the affected enzyme.

In early drug discovery, *in vitro* CYP inhibition fluorescence assays[172] that are more amenable to high throughput may be used for initial screening purposes (Figure 15.8). Such assays provide critical information for evaluating, ranking, and/or eliminating compounds at the earliest stage of drug development. Validation of *E. coli*-expressed CYP enzymes as surrogates for their counterparts in pooled human liver microsomes[173] and also comparison of the kinetic properties of *E. coli*-expressed enzymes with liver microsomes on appropriate substrates have been reported,[174] comparing fluorescence-based CYP450 inhibition data generated using CYP enzymes (1A2, 2C9, 2C19, 2D6 and 3A4) expressed in *Escherichia coli* (Cypex bactosomes) or human lymphoblastoid cells (Gentest cDNA microsomes), and analyzing the prediction of these data sets toward DDIs using published clinical data on 68 marketed drugs.

Human liver microsomes are the most widely used *in vitro* metabolic models to assess the inhibition potential of drug candidates and, with the increase in number of NCEs due to combinatorial chemistry and high-throughput screening techniques, novel high-throughput liquid chromatography-mass spectrometry (LC-MS)[175] assays have been developed. A sensitive and rugged LC-MS/MS method was developed for a comprehensive *in vitro* metabolic interaction screening assay with an *N*-in-1 approach.[176] A cocktail, consisting of ten cytochrome P450 (CYP)-selective probe substrates with known kinetic, metabolic, and interaction properties *in vivo*, was incubated in a pool of

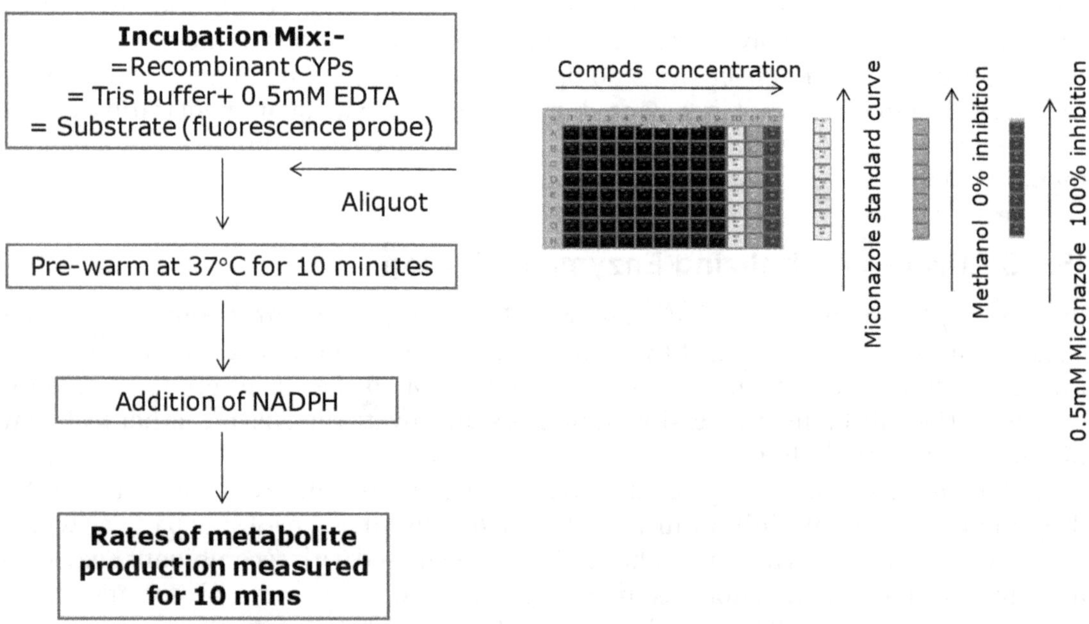


Figure 15.8 Incubation scheme for *in vitro* CYP inhibition fluorescence assay.

human liver microsomes, and 13 metabolites and internal standard phenacetin were analyzed in multiple reaction mode. Recently,[177] by integrating a RapidFire system with an API4000 mass spectrometer (RF-MS), a cytochrome P450 inhibition assay was developed and fully optimized on the system. The RapidFire is an integrated autosampler for ultrafast sample clean-up based on automated solid-phase extraction (SPE) and introduction to mass spectrometry. Compared with the classic liquid chromatography-mass spectrometry method, the RF-MS system generates consistent data with approximately 20-fold increase in throughput.

The lack of chromatographic separation of compounds, substrates, and metabolites can complicate data interpretation, but this occurs in a small number of cases that are readily identifiable. Overall, this system has enabled a real-time and quantitative measurement of a large number of ADME samples, providing a rapid evaluation of clinically important drug–drug interaction potential.

When a drug is converted to a reactive metabolite(s) by CYP enzymes, it may interact with them irreversibly and permanently inactivate their function. This is called mechanism-based inhibition (MBI).[178] By contrast, time-dependent inhibition (TDI) is characterized as time-variant, *i.e.* the inhibition potency of a compound for an enzyme changes with time.[179] Potential TDI mechanisms are: (1) a test compound is a mechanism-based inactivator and (2) formation of a more potent inhibitory metabolite. Metabolic drug–drug interactions resulting from TDI can display a delayed onset due to the time-dependence of inhibition and can persist even after the inhibitor has been eliminated, as enzymatic activity is only restored by *de novo* protein synthesis. Of those drugs currently on the market from various clinical categories that are associated with metabolism-dependent inhibition, most suffer from DDI.[180,181] Indeed, drugs such as astemizole, cerivastatin, cisapride, mibefradil, nefazodone, and terfenadine have been withdrawn from the market because of CYP-related DDIs.[182] All of these drugs inhibit CYP3A4, with the exception of cerivastatin, which is an inhibitor of CYP2C8. Given the importance of CYP inhibition to the developability and safety of new medicines, many pharmaceutical companies have implemented high-throughput assays to evaluate TDI early in the drug discovery process, in order to enhance the quality of development candidates and reduce attrition.[183–186] In general, in drug discovery studies, there are three different analytical approaches that are used for the study of CYP inhibition *in vitro*: liquid scintillation counting of radioactivity liberated during site-specific metabolism,[187] selective analysis of fluorescent metabolism,[188–190] and mass spectrometry.[191–193] Traditionally, the extent of inactivation of the test enzyme is determined from a decrease in the $IC_{50}$ after preincubation with the test compound. An "$IC_{50}$ shift" experiment consists of two $IC_{50}$ curves, one with NADPH and the other without, and both with test compounds in HLM during preincubation. Following preincubation, the probe substrate and the additional NADPH are added to both incubations to measure the enzyme activity remaining. If the $IC_{50}$ shifts to a lower value (left shift) in the presence of NADPH in the preincubation compared with the absence of NADPH, the compound is considered to be a TDI.[194] An $IC_{50}$ shift of at least 1.5-fold is generally considered to be a positive sign of TDI (Figure 15.9).[195]

Besides the $IC_{50}$ shift method, several other approaches have been developed to identify TDI, including the wash method, the dilution method, and the add method.[196–199]

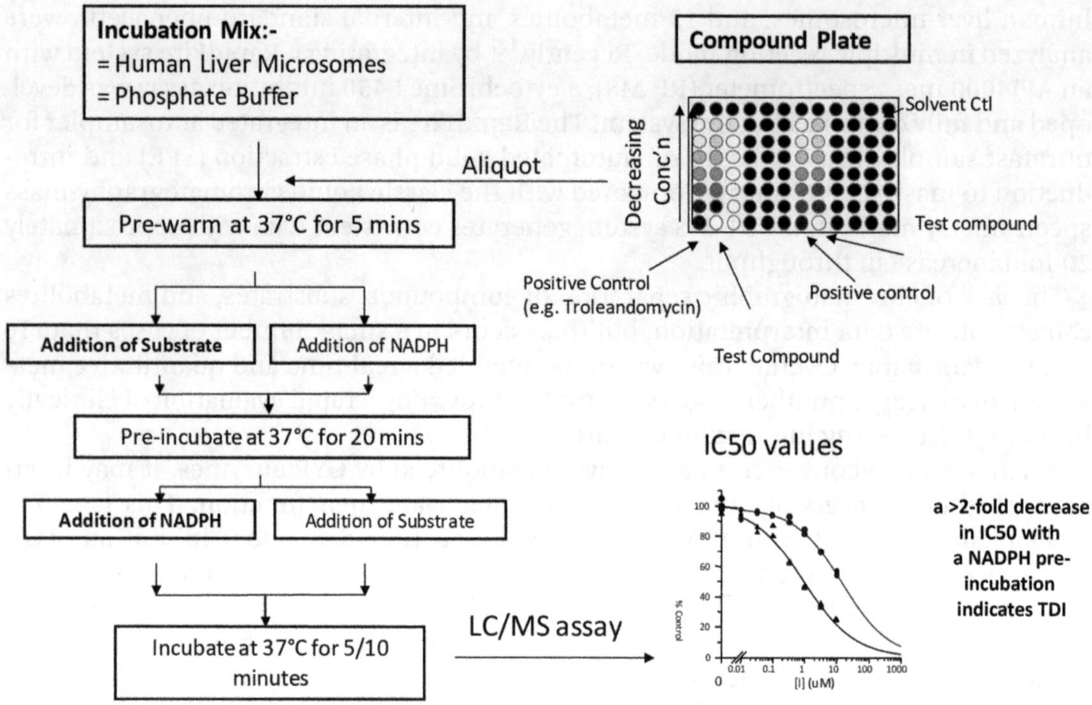


**Figure 15.9** Incubation scheme for "$IC_{50}$ shift" experiment for TDI assessment.

The wash method is less commonly used in drug discovery, as it is more labour-intensive and provides less accurate TDI parameters due to the loss of enzyme activity. The add method and the dilution method provide similar $k_{inact}/K_I$ values, although the $k_{inact}$ (maximal inactivation rate, 1/min) and $K_I$ (the concentration at which half of the maximal inactivation rate is observed, μM) are generally slightly lower in the add method than the dilution method.[197] The $k_{inact}/K_I$ is the efficiency of enzyme inactivation, similar to intrinsic clearance in the metabolic stability study.

## 15.6.4 Pathway Identification

Understanding which drug metabolism pathways are involved in the metabolism of a drug enables prediction of potential clinical DDIs, as well as prediction of potential variability in patient pharmacokinetics or pharmacodynamics due to genetic polymorphism or different expression levels. Some well-documented examples include the CYP3A4-catalyzed oxidation of terfenadine to carboxyterfenadine,[165] the CYP2D6-catalyzed *O*-demethylation of codeine to morphine,[200] CYP2C19-catalyzed oxidation of proguanil to cycloguanil,[201,202] and the CYP2C9-catalyzed oxidation of losartan to carboxylosartan.[203] In recent years, *in vitro* methods for determining which forms of CYP are involved in the metabolism of a given drug, so-called "CYP reaction phenotyping", have become firmly established. Reaction phenotyping can be generally described as a set of *in vitro* experiments with the overall goal of identifying the pathways responsible for the clearance of a new chemical entity (NCE) and, more specifically, to provide information that aids in characterizing an NCE as a victim of drug–drug interactions. Generally, pharmaceutical companies are looking for drugs with multiple routes of elimination, in fact, if any one route is impaired, the others can compensate.

In addition to CYP-mediated metabolism, several other enzymes, the most significant of which are the FMOs, can mediate the oxidative metabolism of various drugs and xenobiotics.[204] Less extensively studied, but potentially just as significant are polymorphisms and DDI involving other drug metabolism routes, such as UGT-mediated glucuronidation pathways.[205–207]

Currently, drug discovery capabilities in predicting clinical DDI for a drug candidate are adequate where the candidate drug is the perpetrator of DDIs (*e.g.* inhibitor of a drug-metabolizing enzyme like CYP3A4); while quantitative predictions of risk of DDI as victims are usually conducted relatively late in the drug development process. This is because definitive phenotyping a given reaction requires a thorough understanding of metabolic pathways, and radiolabelled drug or synthetic metabolite standards are usually not available early. However, it is often desirable to "screen" for desirable properties (*e.g.* multiple pathways) in drug discovery and lead optimization. Because radiolabelled material and authentic metabolite standards are not readily available in discovery, the approach of relative quantitation by assessing "substrate depletion" is typical at this stage. In a substrate depletion experiment, the amount of metabolism is assessed after various time points (*e.g.* 0, 5, 10, 20, 30, 45, and 60 minutes) by measuring how much substrate is remaining relative to that found at the initiation of the incubation. Since only the substrate is quantified, the amount of metabolism is equivalent to the sum of all metabolites formed. The rate of disappearance of parent or the rate of appearance of the metabolite(s), if known, is then monitored by appropriate analytical tools, frequently LC-MS/MS. By comparing the rates of metabolism across cell lines, one can then identify which enzymes are capable of metabolizing the lead compound.

Compared to measuring formation of metabolites, this approach is prone to potential underestimation of the determined parameters, especially for compounds with limited clearance. However, it has been shown that data generated from determination of parent disappearance *in vitro*, once processed with an extrapolation tool like SimCyp© can generate an acceptable prediction of the likely *in vivo* pharmacokinetic profile (about 85% success in the prediction).[208]

In drug discovery, perhaps the most common approach to reaction phenotyping is the use of cDNA-expressed enzyme systems, each expressing a different enzyme, to evaluate metabolism of lead compounds. For oxidative studies, the test compound is incubated with a panel of individually expressed recombinant human CYP enzymes (CYP1A2, CYP2A6, CYP2B6, CYP2C8, CYP2C9, CYP2C19, CYP2D6, CYP2E1, CYP3A4, and CYP3A5 in a typical panel) expressed in baculovirus-infected insect cell membranes. The incubation mixture typically contains the test compound at a final concentration of 1 μM or 10 μM. Ideally, pilot studies should be conducted to establish the concentration range for the test compound to ensure that substrate concentrations are in the linear range (well below the $K_m$ of the targeted enzyme). In practice, however, the evaluations are more commonly conducted in a screening format with two or three initial starting concentrations of test compound.

Various methods for scaling the results to predict *in vivo* drug clearance have been described, but for screening purposes, the usual approach is to use the following equation to calculate intrinsic clearances ($CL_{int}$) for each of the individually expressed enzymes based on the estimated turnover rate constants:

$$CL_{int\,x} = \left(\frac{k}{CYPx}\right) \text{per pmol of CYPx per mg microsomal protein}$$

where $CYP_x$ is the concentration of recombinant CYP enzyme in the incubation.

The contribution of an individual CYP enzyme to the overall oxidative metabolism of a drug candidate can be estimated as follows:

$$\%\text{Contribution by enzyme}_x = \frac{CL_{int\,x}\left(\mu\text{L per min per pmol rCYPx}\right) \times \text{Abundance}_x\left(\frac{\text{pmol}}{\text{mg protein}}\right)}{\sum CL_{int\,i}\left(\mu\text{L per min per pmol rCYPi}\right) \times \text{Abundance}_i\left(\frac{\text{pmol}}{\text{mg protein}}\right)}$$

A second approach to reaction phenotyping involves conducting incubations in hepatocytes, microsomes, or some other *in vitro* preparation using normal tissues as the enzyme source, but including selective chemical or immuno-inhibitors of specific enzymatic pathways. By performing a battery of incubations with various inhibitors, and comparing the relative rates of metabolism, one can identify which inhibitor reduces the overall metabolism to the greatest extent and thereby uncover the metabolic pathway that contributes the most to the clearance of a compound (Table 15.8).

The extent of inhibition is determined by comparing the extent of metabolism observed in the presence of inhibitors with the extent of metabolism observed in comparable incubations without inhibitors. This approach is generally preferred for experiments intended to deconvolute the contributions from various enzymes when multiple pathways are involved in metabolism of a compound. For compounds exhibiting low turnover, the use of specific inhibitors presents an additional challenge, since it may be very difficult to detect a decrease in an already very low metabolic rate. In such cases, monitoring for appearance of metabolite(s) is an option if the metabolic products are known. A chemically knocked down HLM has recently been introduced as a commercially available preparation, Silensomes™.[209] Silensomes™ are prepared by using mechanism-based inactivators to inactivate certain CYPs one by one in HLMs. Silensomes™ provide a convenient ("thaw-and-go") and more consistent source for reaction phenotyping without the need to add inhibitors for each experiment.[210]

**Table 15.8** Inhibitors used for microsomal reaction phenotyping incubations.

| CYP | Inhibitor |
|---|---|
| CYP1A1/2 | Furafylline |
| CYP2C9 | Sulfaphenazole |
| CYP2C19 | 3-Benzylnirvanol |
| CYP2D6 | Quinidine |
| CYP3A4 | Ketoconazole, Troleandomycin |

### 15.6.5 Drug-metabolizing Enzyme Induction

Several drug-metabolizing enzymes, for example CYP1A2, CYP2A6, CYP2B6, CYP2C9, and CYP3A4, can be induced. Enzyme induction is a relatively slow adaptive process that increases metabolic capacity, unlike direct enzyme inhibition, which is an immediate effect that decreases metabolic capacity. A drug-induced change in the expression of CYP genes is a key cause of issues in preclinical development and clinical DDIs. In particular, CYP induction can impact preclinical safety studies by reducing the exposure of the drug candidate, thus limiting the achievement of the exposure multiples expected by the regulatory agencies for the approval of a drug. CYP induction may increase the pharmacological effect of a drug. For example, upon coadministration of phenobarbital with alprenolol, the oral bioavailability of alprenolol is reduced by 45%. Despite the marked change in bioavailability, there is only a modest reduction in the pharmacological response. This observed effect can be attributed to β-adrenergic receptor activity of an alprenolol metabolite, 4-hydroxylprenolol, which is as potent as the parent. CYP inducers can indirectly cause cellular toxicity by increasing the rate of formation of toxicologically active products, such as stable metabolites or reactive intermediates. For example, CYP2E1 is responsible for the formation of *N*-acetyl-*p*-benzoquinoneimine (NAPQI), a toxic metabolite of paracetamol. Long-term ethanol consumption increases paracetamol hepatotoxicity, whereas acute or simultaneous ethanol and paracetamol consumption has limited or negligible toxicological effects. The time interval between ethanol consumption and paracetamol ingestion is key in terms of the observed toxicological consequences as ethanol is both an inducer and inhibitor of CYP2E1.

The major mechanism for CYP enzyme induction is *via* increased rates of transcription, which is mediated predominantly by the intracellular "nuclear hormone receptors" AhR, CAR, PXR, and PPAR (Figure 15.10).

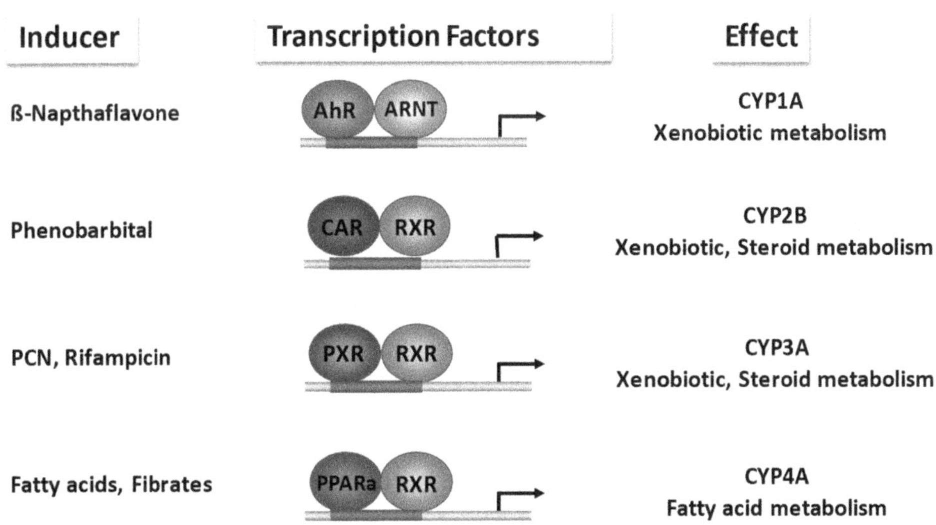


**Figure 15.10** Mechanism of CYP induction/regulation.

The mechanism of induction of CYP1A is based on increased protein synthesis, primarily initiated by the binding of the inducer to the Ah (aryl or aromatic hydrocarbon) cytosolic receptor (AhR). The activation of the constitutive androstane receptor (CAR) by translocation from the cytosol into the nucleus, mediates induction of CYP2B genes by phenobarbital (PB)-type inducers. The regulation of the CYP3A family of enzymes is complex, with marked species differences in the capacity of compounds to activate PXR and induce CYP3A in the liver. In addition, PXR agonists may induce intestinal CYP3A and the transcription of various genes for transporters.

Quantification of CYP induction in preclinical species is tested systematically as part of the toxicological safety evaluation and can be measured by ligand binding, reporter gene assays, mRNA levels (TaqMan®), protein, or catalytic end points.[211] Human-based assays involve the culturing of human hepatocytes in the presence of the drug tested at different concentrations and in parallel with known positive control compounds, *e.g.* rifampicin for CYP3A4, CYP2C9, and CYP2C19, phenobarbital for CYP2B6, and omeprazole for CYP1A2. Induction potential can be assessed by measuring the enzyme activity of model substrates determined by HPLC or LC-MS/MS, or by determining the protein or messenger RNA levels of drug-metabolizing enzymes, the latter using real-time quantitative reverse transcriptase polymerase chain reaction (qRT-PCR), commonly referred to as TaqMan® (Figure 15.11).

As these assays require gene and protein expression, human hepatocyte primary cultures represent the most appropriate experimental system. Cultured primary human hepatocytes represent the only proven *in vitro* experimental system for predicting the induction potential of metabolic enzymes and are considered by the FDA as the more realistic system for *in vitro* studies on CYP induction.

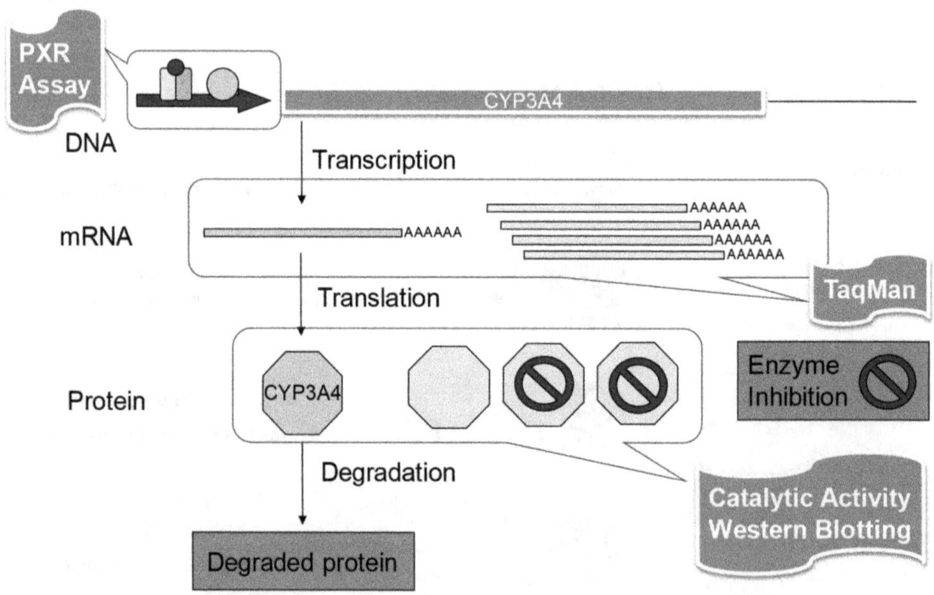


**Figure 15.11** Steps of regulation and type of measurements.

Several reporter cell lines[212,213] have also been developed as rapid screening assays allowing CYP induction to be evaluated early in drug development. It is generally believed that the results with these screening assays require confirmation with primary human hepatocytes.

### 15.6.6 Transporter-mediated Drug Interactions

In addition to the effects of drug-metabolizing enzymes on the pharmacokinetics of drugs, increasing attention is being given to transporters where emerging evidence indicates their important role in modulating drug absorption, distribution, metabolism, and elimination, as well as the historical importance of transporters in the development of drug-resistant tumours. Transporters, acting alone or in concert with drug-metabolizing enzymes, can affect the pharmacokinetics and/or pharmacodynamics of a drug and drug–drug interactions involving drug transporters, and genetic polymorphisms of drug transporters have been described (Table 15.9).[214,215]

Accordingly, methods allowing the rational prediction and extrapolation of *in vivo* drug disposition from *in vitro* data are also essential.

Many different drug transporters are expressed in various tissues, such as the epithelial cells of the intestine and kidney, hepatocytes, and brain capillary endothelial cells.[216–218] In recent years, a number of important transporters have been cloned, and considerable progress has been made in understanding the molecular characteristics of individual transporters. It has now become clear that some of these are responsible for drug transport in various tissues and they may be key determinants of the pharmacokinetic characteristics of a drug as far as its intestinal absorption, tissue distribution, and elimination are concerned.

**Table 15.9** Examples of transporter-mediated drug interactions.

| Interacting drug | Affected drug | Consequence | Fold changes in substrate plasma AUC |
|---|---|---|---|
| Quinidine | Digoxin | Digoxin exposure 1.7-fold increase | P-glycoprotein (P-gp, MDR1) inhibition |
| Rifampin | Digoxin | Digoxin exposure 30% decrease | P-gp Induction |
| Dronedarone | Digoxin | Digoxin exposure 2.6-fold increase | P-gp inhibition |
| Probenecid | Cephradine | Cephradine exposure 3.6-fold increase | Organic Anion Transporter (OAT) inhibition |
| Cimetidine | Metformin | Metformin exposure 1.4-fold increase | Organic Cation Transporter (OCT) inhibition |
| Cyclosporine | Rosuvastatin | Rosuvastatin exposure 7-fold increase | Organic Anion Transporting Polypeptide (OATP) inhibition & Breast Cancer Resistance Protein (BCRP) inhibition |
| Lopinavir/Ritonavir | Rosuvastatin | Rosuvastatin exposure 2-fold increase | OATP inhibition |

#### 15.6.6.1 Most Relevant Transporters for DDIs

Various transporters expressed in the small intestine are involved in the absorption of nutrients or endogenous compounds. Influx transporters expressed in gut, such as oligopeptide transporters (PEPT1), apical sodium-dependent bile acid transporters (ASBT), or organic anion transporting polypeptide-B (OATP) improve drug absorption,[219,220] while primary active efflux transporters, such as P-glycoprotein (P-gp) encoded by multidrug resistance gene (MDR1), multidrug resistance associated protein 2 (MRP2), or the breast cancer resistance protein (BCRP), are expressed in the brush border membrane of enterocytes and excrete their substrates into the lumen, resulting in a potential limitation of net absorption. P-gp modulates the absorption of many drugs because of its broad substrate specificity.[221] Multispecific transporters are expressed in the liver and kidney and play an important role in the elimination of many xenobiotics, acting as a detoxification system. Many drugs are excreted into the urine *via* organic anion and cation transport systems, expressed on brush border and basolateral membranes of renal tubular cells (PEPT2, OATs, OCT2, OCTNs).[222–224] As far as the liver is concerned, a wide variety of transporter families are known to be present at the sinusoidal and canalicular membranes and play a significant role in hepatobiliary excretion (Figure 15.12).[225–227]

Active transporters expressed on the sinusoidal membrane are responsible for the uptake of drugs from the blood into hepatocytes.[228] Primary active transporters (MDR1,

- OAT/Oat = organic anion transporter belonging to the SLC22 family
- OCT/Oct = organic cation transporter belonging to the SLC22 family
- **NTCP/Ntcp** = Na+/taurocholate cotransporting polypeptide belonging to the SLC10 family
- OATP/Oatp = organic anion transporting polypeptide belonging to the SLCO family (previously called SLC21)
- MDR1/Mdr1 = multidrug resistance protein (ABCB1)
- BCRP/Bcrp = breast cancer resistance protein (ABCG2)
- MRP2/Mrp2 = multidrug resistance-associated protein (ABCC2)
- BSEP/Bsep = bile salt export pump (ABCB11) all belonging to ABC-carrier proteins;
- *OA− = organic anion*
- *BS− = bile salt*
- *OC+ = organic cation*
- *DC− = dicarboxylate*
- *GSH = glutathione*

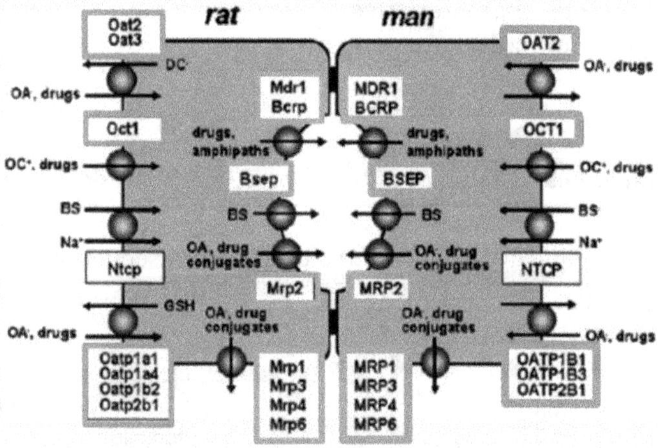


**Figure 15.12** Individual carriers in the hepatocyte which are involved in drug uptake and secretion.

MRP2, BSEP, BCRP) expressed on the canalicular membrane are involved in the biliary excretion of both parent drugs and their metabolites.[229,230]

Due to the broad substrate specificity of drug transporters, drug–drug interactions involving these transporters are very likely. Recently, both inhibition and induction of transporters have been implicated as one mechanism responsible for certain drug–drug interactions. P-gp inhibitors, such as quinidine and verapamil are known to increase plasma concentrations of digoxin because they block biliary and/or urinary excretion of digoxin *via* P-gp.[231,232] The hepatobiliary transporter of pravastatin has been shown to be carrier-mediated (OATP-C and MRP2).[233] This transporter is also expected to be involved in distribution to the liver, the main site of cerivastatin distribution, resulting in a drug–drug interaction between cerivastatin and cyclosporine during hepatic uptake. Recently, cerivastatin was withdrawn from the market because of severe rhabdomyolysis associated with cerivastatin–gemfibrozil combination therapy.[234]

P-gp may be involved in human drug–drug interactions associated with absorption. For example, the plasma concentration of talinolol is increased by coadministration of erythromycin.[235] In fact, erythromycin inhibits talinolol secretion from enterocytes into the lumen *via* P-gp, resulting in increased net absorption because of the lack of any significant metabolism of talinolol. Grapefruit juice and orange juice reduce oral bioavailability of fexofenadine, an OATP substrate, in healthy volunteers,[236] *via* inhibition of OATP-mediated drug uptake at the intestinal wall. Rifampin induces intestinal P-gp, resulting in reduced oral bioavailability of digoxin.[237] Since rifampin also induces intestinal MRP2, coadministration of rifampin is expected to increase secretion into the lumen of MRP2 substrates, such as glucuronide conjugates.[238]

#### 15.6.6.2 In Vitro Models to Study Transporter-related Drug–Drug Interactions

Many methods and models to study drug–transporter interactions *in vitro* have been and still are being developed. The optimal method of use depends on the specific research question, as well as on the physicochemical nature of the drug that is under investigation. *In vitro* transporter assays are usually carried out with either intact cells or isolated cell membranes over-expressing the transporter of interest. The advantage of *in vitro* assays is that they can be performed with relatively high throughput and low costs as compared to *in vivo* studies. In bi-directional transport assays polarized epithelial cells are cultured on so-called Transwell filter inserts that separate an apical and basolateral compartment. Using this approach, the effect of a specific transporter on the actual flux of a drug from the apical to the basolateral side of the cell monolayer and *vice versa* can be studied in detail. This experimental set up is the most widely used *in vitro* assay to investigate whether a drug is a substrate for a specific efflux transporter such as the ABC transporters P-gp, breast cancer resistance protein (BCRP), and the multidrug resistance proteins (MRPs) (Figure 15.13).

Alternatively, the influence of the drug on the transport of a model substrate can be assessed to evaluate potential drug–drug interactions. These assays are routinely performed using polarizing MDCKII (Madine–Darby Canine Kidney) cells that over-express the human version of the transporter of interest, and comparing the translocation of

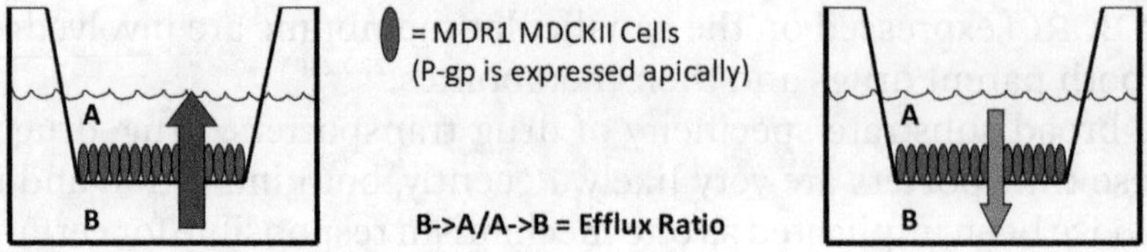


**Figure 15.13** Bi-directional transport P-gp assay.

the drug in these cells to that in mock-transfected MDCKII cells, which usually clearly indicates whether a drug is a substrate for the transporter of interest.

In addition to the cell lines transfected with a single human transporter, the human carcinoma cell line Caco-2 is used to study the transport of drugs in combination with inhibitors of the transporter proteins of interest. The advantage of this set-up is that Caco-2 cells are considered a good model for the translocation of drugs over the human intestinal epithelium, expressing considerable levels of a wider range of transporters (thus mimicking the *in vivo* combined effects of various transporters and cellular processes on drug uptake). The fact that Caco-2 cells express multiple transporters can in certain cases also be a disadvantage since inhibitors available for use in these studies show limited specificity.[239] However, for high-throughput screening of drugs for their transporter interaction potential this is a highly valuable and widely used model. A disadvantage of polarizing epithelial cells which express human transporters is that to study drug efflux, the drug should first enter the cells. Especially with very hydrophilic compounds this is often a problem, as passive diffusion over the cell membrane will hardly occur and active uptake transporters are necessary. Therefore, to study transporter interactions of drugs that cannot enter the cells described above, it is usually more useful to perform a study with inside-out vesicles expressing the efflux protein of interest. These vesicles can be prepared from almost any cell type (usually the insect cell line Sf-9 or, more preferably, human HEK293 cells) as well as from tissues such as liver or kidney that over-express the efflux transporter of interest. With this assay the active transport of a drug into the inside-out vesicles is studied (as the membranes are "inside-out", the studied efflux protein now transports its substrates towards the inside of the vesicles, where they are captured and can be detected). The tendency for transported compounds to diffuse back across the vesicular membrane limits their usefulness in substrate determination assays to low permeability compounds; however, because the cytoplasmatic side of the transporter is now directly accessible, the selection of an appropriate probe substrate allows the inhibition of the transporter to be measured for compounds of any permeability class. A big advantage of this transporter assay is that it is easily performed in a high-throughput setting. Furthermore, it is relatively fast (and less costly), as no cell culturing is needed for this assay. One limitation to the vesicular transport assay is the batch-to-batch variation. This can result from difference in transporter expression in the host cell lin,e as well as the percentage of inside-out vesicles formed during the membrane isolation procedure. Furthermore, the ability to cryopreserve a single large batch of membrane vesicles over a long time period allows for minimization of this variability across multiple transport experiments.

To study interactions of a drug with uptake transporters, various cell-based methods can be used. These models are ideally based on cell lines from human origin (*e.g.* HEK293 cells), as plasma membrane lipid composition can affect transporter function.[240] However, if not available, cells from other origins (*e.g.* CHO cells, MDCKII cells, or *Xenopus* oocytes) can also be used. The cells over-expressing the uptake transporter of interest (and their mock transfected controls) are plated on 24- or 96-well plates and incubated with the drug under investigation. The time- and concentration-dependent uptake of the drug and/or the effects of the drug on the uptake of a model substrate are subsequently analyzed. This is a very convenient way to study drug interactions with uptake transporters. One should, however, take into account that uptake transporters may need cotransport, antitransport or exchange of ions for their activity.

Although many *in vitro* assays are available nowadays to study drug transporter interactions, it is obvious that the effect of a transporter on the pharmacokinetics of a drug will not only depend on the direct interaction between a transporter and a drug. In the body many factors (*e.g.* metabolism, tissue distribution of the transporter, presence of endogenous compounds *etc.*) can influence drug transporter interactions. To gain insight into the *in vivo* effect of the drug transporter interactions, various models can be used. Combined with a wide range of analytical techniques such as imaging, microdialysis, and gall bladder/urinary bladder cannulations, these models provide highly useful tools to study the interactions between drugs and transporters *in vivo*. To study the *in vivo* influence of transporters on drug pharmacokinetics, pharmacodynamics, and toxicity, many mouse models have been generated recently. The most widely used model is the Mdr1a/1b (P-gp) knock-out mouse which has already been shown to be of great value for studies on the *in vivo* effect of the ABC transporter P-gp, for example to study the effect of P-gp on the brain penetration of drugs.[241] Especially in combination with cell lines expressing human or murine versions of this transporter, it appears quite possible to predict the effect of a transporter in the human situation. As there is a large overlap in substrate specificity between transporters, recently many transporter combination knock-out mice (mice lacking more than one transporter) have been generated, and can be used to study the relative *in vivo* effects of the transporters on the drug.[242] Still, although the tissue distribution and substrate specificities of ABC transporters in mice are in general quite comparable to those in humans, there are clearly species differences. To tackle this problem "humanized" transporter mice (mice in which the murine transporter is replaced by the human homologue) are also currently being generated.[243] In combination with transporter knock-out mice these are very useful models to study the interaction of drugs with human transporters *in vivo*. If the drug of interest has been shown to interact with a transporter *in vitro*, the effect of known modulators of this transporter on the pharmacokinetics of the drug under investigation (drug–drug interactions) can be determined in various animal models. A disadvantage of this type of interaction study is that the inhibitors are usually not very specific and may also influence other processes in the body. However, these studies are very useful to get an idea of possible transporter-related drug–drug interactions *in vivo*. A big advantage is that these studies can be performed in practically every animal model and therefore are easy to incorporate in the ADME studies routinely performed during drug development. With such studies one will not only add highly valuable data to standard

ADME study results, but also often provide better interpretations of the pharmacokinetic profiles found in animals. Furthermore, in combination with the *in vitro* studies described above, this will lead to better predictions of the situation in patients. However, despite all the available knowledge and techniques, it remains difficult to predict drug-transporter effects in the human body with absolute certainty. Research is currently ongoing to describe all these transporter-related processes in detail in an *in silico* model[244] and to investigate how data from the *in vitro* or *in vivo* transporter assays can be used as input data for this purpose. This will likely be highly useful for the prediction of internal drug levels and related effects in humans.

### 15.6.7 PBPK Modelling

Physiologically based pharmacokinetic modelling (PBPK) modelling and simulations are frequently applied to DDI prediction. PBPK models account for tissue volumes, blood flow, and other human physiological parameters. PBPK models divide the human body into several compartments and use kinetic information in and out of each compartment to model the absorption and elimination processes. They provide dynamic modelling of perpetrator and victim drugs to enable more accurate DDI prediction. Static models with the use of $C_{max}$ as inhibitor concentration [I] often over-predict DDI because it is assumed that the concentration of the inhibitor [I] is maintained at $C_{max}$ between dosing intervals and that there is no metabolism or elimination of the inhibitor.

While this model offers the worst-case scenario for DDI prediction, it is also not physiologically relevant because the concentrations of both perpetrator and victim change with time due to absorption, distribution, and elimination processes. Thus, considering a dynamic model with changing concentrations of both inhibitors and substrates at any given time is more optimal for DDI prediction.

PBPK takes into consideration both endogenous (drug-independent) and exogenous (drug-dependent) factors. These intrinsic factors include age, gender, race, disease status, genetics, and social behaviour (*e.g.* smoking and diet). Exogenous factors are drug-dependent, including the physicochemical properties of the drug that impact ADME, such as MW, $pK_a$, and $\log P$.

## 15.7 Phospholipidosis

Drug-induced phospholipidosis (DIPL) is an adverse side effect which can affect the registration of new drug entities. Phospholipidosis (PLD) is a lysosomal storage disorder where phospholipids accumulate in lysosomes, organelles essential in cellular biogenesis. Drug accumulation in lysosomes (lysosomotropism) is a known mechanism leading to PLD. Over 50 marketed drugs have been reported to induce PLD, these drugs are mostly cationic amphiphilic drugs (CADs), including antidepressants, antihistamines, antianginals, antibiotics, antimalarials, cholesterol-lowering agents, and other prescription drugs (Figure 15.14).[245] DIPL involves drug penetration through cellular membranes and once within the cell they are protonated in the acidic environments of lysosomes, becoming trapped, known as a lysosomotropic effect.[246] Drug trapping is followed by a gradual accumulation of drug–phospholipid complexes within the internal lysosomal membranes. The increase in undigested materials results in the abnormal accumulation of multilamellar bodies (myeloid bodies) in tissues. DIPL does not necessarily constitute toxicity, as the symptoms can resolve once the drug is stopped, but it is predictive of drug or metabolite accumulation in affected tissues that lead to liver, kidney, or respiratory failure. For these reasons, DIPL is of concern to the FDA, which in 2004 formed a DIPL Working Group to study the problem.[247] Currently, there are two prevailing hypotheses for the putative mechanisms involved in DIPL:

1. Inhibition of phospholipases due to binding of drug to substrate phospholipases,
2. Drugs bind to the phospholipids resulting in the formation of a complex that cannot be broken down by phospholipases.

The traditional method to evaluate DIPL is visual confirmation of myeloid bodies in tissues by electron microscopy, a time-consuming and labour-intensive technique, and/or quantitative PCR. More recently, fluorescent dyes have been employed to assess phospholipidosis in a high-throughput manner in cell lines[248] (*e.g.* in HepG2 or H9c2 cells) and a high-content imaging assay approach was established combined with *in silico* tools.[249] These assays determine DIPL by measuring the accumulation of specific fluorescent phospholipids (*e.g.* NBD-PE or HCSLipidTox™) in HepG2 cells treated with

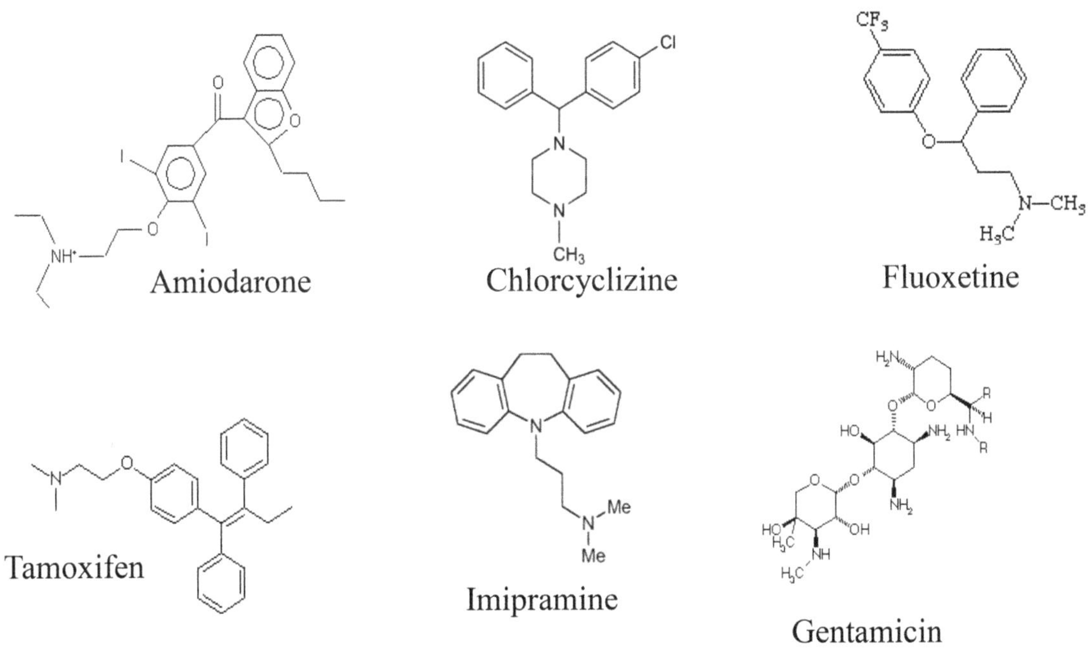


**Figure 15.14** Chemical structure of compounds inducing PLD. PLD is induced by drugs with a cationic amphiphilic (cationic lipophilic) structure (hydrophobic ring, hydrophilic side-chain and charged amine group).

increasing drug concentrations. When phospholipidosis is induced, the phospholipid does not get broken down and fluorescence accumulates in the cells. A cytotoxicity marker is run in parallel, such as Hoechst cell nuclear counts, to normalize the amount of accumulation to cell viability (Table 15.10).

A proposed screening strategy to progress compounds with phospholipidosis liabilities is shown in Figure 15.15.

Phospholipidosis is not considered to be a toxicity, but more likely an adaptive response; however, its presence should not be ignored as it is related to secondary damage to tissue structure or impaired function. The decision to progress the compound bearing DIPL potential should be taken on a case-by-case basis. For candidate selection

**Table 15.10** Examples of compounds positively or negatively associated with DIPL-inducing potential.

| | |
|---|---|
| No DIPL | Diazepam, 3-OH Gepirone, Gepirone, Buspirone, Valproic acid, 5-Phenoxybenzamine, Ketasarin, Almitrine, Haloperidol, Bufetolol, tetracycline |
| Positive in cell culture with low DIPL potency in animals | Mainserin, Propranolol, Cloсiguanil, Noxiptiline, Amitriptiline, Disobutamide, Promazine, Mesoridazine, Nortriptyline, Chlorpromazine, Maprotiline, Thioridazine |
| Positive in cell culture with PLD demonstrated in animals | Chlorcyclazine, Citalopram, Chlorphenteramine, Phentermine, Fenfluramine, Imipramine, Tilorone, Fluoxetine, Iprindole, Clomipramine, Triparanol, Mepacrine, Gentamycin, Erythromycin, Netilimicin, Azithromycin |
| Positive in cell culture with PLD demonstrated in humans and animals | Chloroquine, Amiodarone, Perhexiline, Desethylamiodarone, Tamoxifen, Gentamycin |

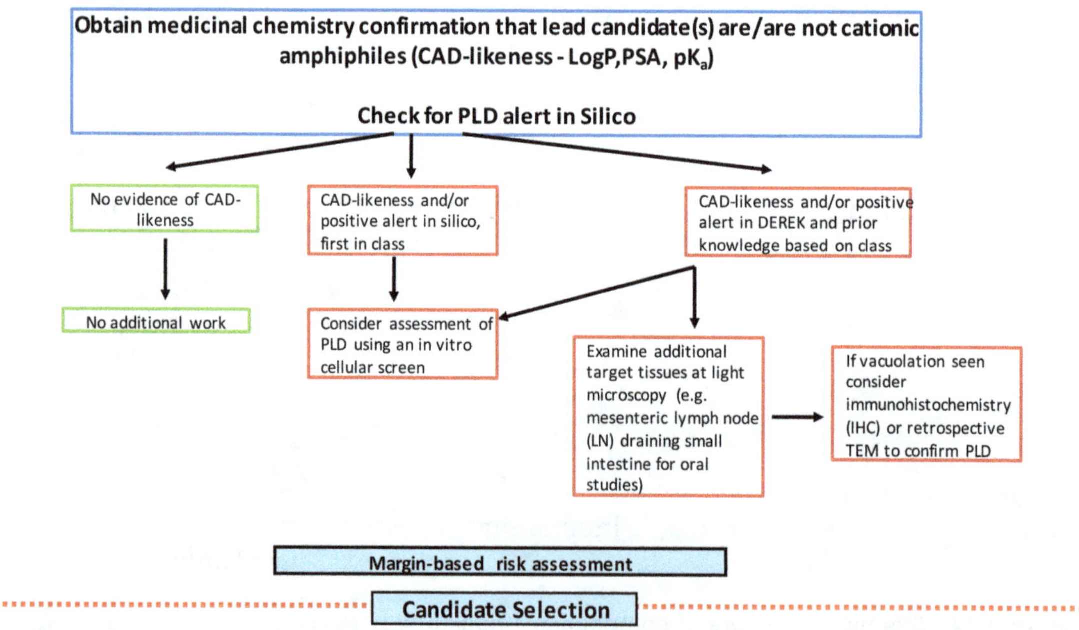


**Figure 15.15** Early screening strategy for phospholipidosis.

purposes the traditional standard margin-based risk assessment is used to reduce the attrition of safe medicines. Because the incidence and severity of DIPL increases with time, if present in short-term toxicology studies, a decision to anticipate longer-term toxicology studies should be taken, in order to assess the number of species affected, define the NOAEL, reversibility, and safety margins for clinical dosing. It should be finally noted that the occurrence of PLD accumulation in preclinical species does not necessarily predict its occurrence in humans and, conversely, phospholipid accumulation can occur in humans without any preclinical signal. For example, the PLD effects of 4,4′-diethylaminoethoxy hexesterol (coralgil) in the liver are different in humans, monkeys, and rats because of different drug metabolism.[250]

## 15.8 Phototoxicity

Phototoxicity (photoirritation) is a light-induced skin irritation response to a photoreactive chemical. Photoallergy is an immunologically mediated reaction to a chemical, initiated by the formation of photoproducts (*e.g.* protein adducts) following a photochemical reaction.

Safety testing of a new chemical entity (NCE) may include an assessment of acute phototoxicity, photoallergy, photogenotoxicity, and photocarcinogenicity.[251]

A photoreactive substance is defined as a chemical (or mixture of chemicals) which generates reactive chemical species following exposure to UV-visible light and as such this more likely to occur in substances or compounds that are topically applied or distribute sufficiently to light-exposed tissues (*e.g.* the skin and eyes). Clinically, phototoxicity results in exaggerated sunburn (erythema, increased skin temperature, pruritis, and oedema).

Drug-associated photosensitivity examples include tetracyclines, fluoroquinolones, sulfonamides, macrolides, betalactams, nitroimidazoles, and nitrofuranes.

The initial consideration for assessment of photoreactive potential is whether a compound absorbs photons at any wavelength between 290 and 700 nm (UVB; 290~320 nm and UVA; 320~400 nm). Light absorption is characterized by the molar extinction coefficient (MEC, also called molar absorptivity), which reflects the efficiency with which a molecule can absorb a photon at a particular wavelength (typically expressed as L $mol^{-1}$ $cm^{-1}$). This coefficient is influenced by several factors, including solvents. A compound that does not have a MEC greater than 1000 L $mol^{-1}$ $cm^{-1}$ at any wavelength between 290 and 700 nm is not considered to be sufficiently photoreactive to result in direct phototoxicity. Excitation of molecules by light can lead to generation of Reactive Oxygen Species (ROS), including superoxide anion and singlet oxygen *via* energy transfer mechanisms. Although photoreactivity can result in other molecular outcomes (*e.g.* formation of photoadducts or cytotoxic photoproducts), it appears that ROS are typically also generated. Thus, ROS generation following irradiation with UV-visible light can be an indicator of phototoxicity potential.[252]

A proposed phototoxicity screening paradigm to identify potentially phototoxic substances is described in Figure 15.16.

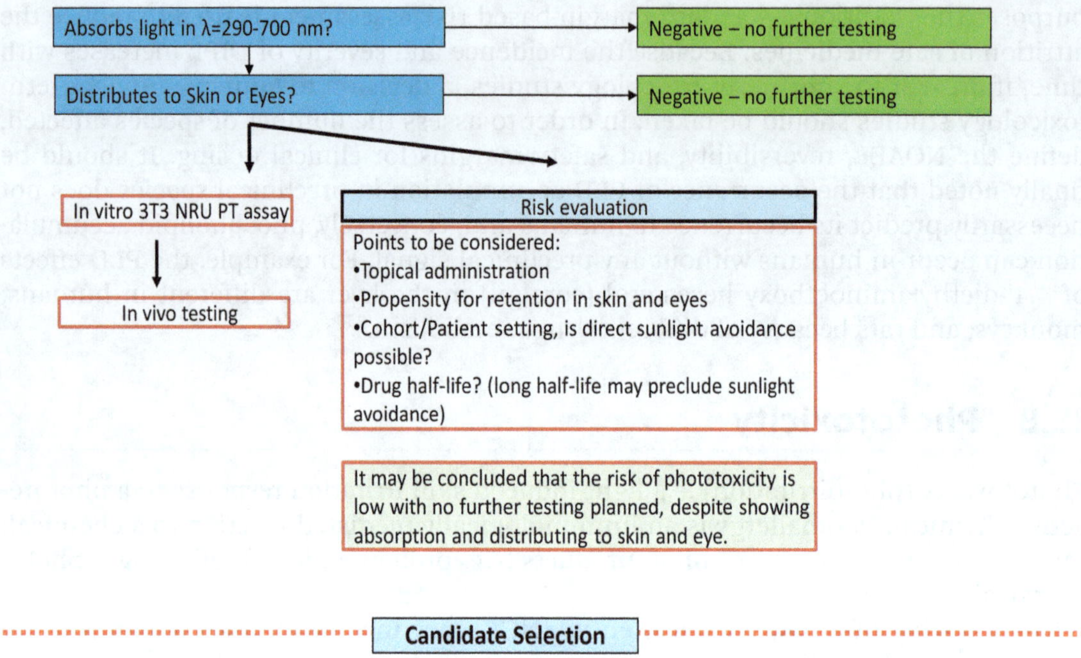


**Figure 15.16** Screening paradigm for phototoxicity.

The most widely used *in vitro* assay for phototoxicity is the 3T3 Neutral Red Uptake Phototoxicity Test (3T3 NRU-PT) for which an Organisation for Economic Co-operation and Development (OECD) guideline is available (No 432).[253] This is currently considered the most appropriate *in vitro* screen for soluble compounds. In addition to the 3T3 NRU-PT assay, erythrocyte photohaemolysis test, and phototoxicity test using a human 3-dimensional (3D) epidermis model are examples of alternative *in vitro* approaches.[254]

In terms of photogenotoxicity testing, the main objective is to make an assessment of the potential of a compound to turn into a photochemical carcinogen upon activation with UV or visible (sic solar-simulated) radiation. Several *in vitro* photogenotoxicity assays, such as the photo-Ames, photo-chromosome aberration (CA), and photo-comet assays have been described in the literature and are based on standard "dark" versions of regulatory assays used for genotoxicity assessment.[255]

However, it is recognised that *in vitro* photosafety assays (phototoxicity and photogenotoxicity) substantially over-predict human hazard.[256] As far as *in vivo* testing is concerned, no standardized study designs have been established. If an *in vivo* phototoxicity study has to be conducted, it is desirable to have some information about the pharmacokinetic profile of the compound before designing the study. This is to ensure that irradiation of the animals is conducted at the approximate time at which the maximum concentration of drug occurs after drug administration ($T_{max}$), and to assist in the selection of an appropriate study duration in relation to the intended clinical exposure. For species selection, models with both pigmented and non-pigmented animals are available. Generally, studies of a single day or up to a few days' duration of dosing are appropriate, using the clinical route of administration, if feasible. Single or repeated daily irradiations after dosing (around $T_{max}$) can be used. For these studies, a maximum dose level that complies with the recommendations for general toxicity studies is considered appropriate. Any identified phototoxicity reaction (erythema, oedema) should be evaluated regarding dose and time dependency, and if possible, the no observable adverse effect level (NOAEL) should be established.

It should also be mentioned that there are there are some limitations to the 3T3 NRU-PT assay as discussed, such as lack of IVIVE, as bioavailability and biokinetics cannot be modelled and the assay is not specifically validated for pharmaceuticals, as mentioned in the FDA International Harmonization Conference (ICH), S10 guideline (2015).[252]

In conclusion, the evaluation of a candidate with photoreactive potential should be based on experimental results, as well as a thorough risk assessment.

## 15.9 Genotoxicity

Genotoxins are chemical agents that directly or indirectly damage the DNA molecules within a cell, causing mutations, which is a major concern regarding the potential to cause cancer. Genotoxicity is often confused with mutagenicity as all mutagens are genotoxic, however, not all genotoxic substances have mutagenic potential. Genotoxicity encompasses mutagenicity (genetic mutations), clastogenicity (chromosomal aberrations), aneuploidy (a gain or loss of chromosome), and DNA damage (single- and double-strand breaks). Adverse genotoxic events can lead to hereditary changes in somatic cells or germ cells and are passed on to future generations. There are many cellular defence processes to prevent such effects, for example DNA repair mechanisms or cell-induced death (apoptosis); however, mutagenesis occurs when these cellular defence mechanisms fail.

In order to detect the range of possible chemical-induced DNA damage events that can occur, several bacterial, *in vitro*, and mammalian tests have been developed. During the early phase of development, high-throughput microplate-based assays can be utilized such us Fluctuation Tests (*e.g.* AMES MPF[257]) SOS umu Test (Umu operon reporter construct from the DNA damage response[258]) Greenscreen (GADD45 a reporter construct[259]) and automated *in vitro* micronucleus assay (HCS-MNT[260]) to screen high number of molecules. At the stage of lead optimization, assays detailed in the international (ICH) guidelines (ICH S2(R1)) are typically screened, including the Ames assay, micronucleus assay, chromosomal aberration test, the comet assay and *in vivo* toxicology tests.

Importantly, at these early stages, the test compound should be at the highest level of purity, to remove doubt that positive results are due to the presence of genotoxic impurities or contaminants.

### 15.9.1 Bacterial Tests

The bacterial test (Ames test) detects gene mutations. The Ames test uses amino-acid-dependent strains of *Salmonella typhimurium* and *Escherichia coli*, each carrying different mutations in various genes in the histidine (*Salmonella*) or tryptophan (*Escherichia*) operon.

In the standard plate incorporation assay at least five strains of bacteria are used (OECD TG471). These should include four strains of *S. typhimurium* (TA1535, TA1537 or TA97a or TA97, TA98, and TA100) and the strain *E. coli* WP2 uvrA or *E. coli* WP2 or *E. coli* WP2 (pkM101). The experiment is conducted in the absence and in the presence of metabolic activation (+/− S9).

To accommodate the need to carry out this critical test as soon as possible, industry has elaborated several versions of the Ames test (see Table 15.11), in order to reduce the requirement for test compound.[261,262]

However, the best approach is to use the five strains, in order to reduce the risk of facing mutagenicity issues during GLP studies. Pros and cons should be evaluated for selecting the reduced tests; *e.g.* knowledge of the chemical class *vs.* timelines.

## 15.9.2 *In Vitro* Mammalian Tests

There are several mammalian cell systems and each of them can address different end points. In Table 15.12 are listed the tests that are used for screening purposes; mammalian systems that are used for investigative purposes are not mentioned here. Experiments are performed both in the presence and in the absence of metabolic activation.[263–267]

The most used tests are reported in Table 15.12.

**Table 15.11** Different Ames test versions.

| Bacterial test | Strain | Notes | Compound |
|---|---|---|---|
| Ames 5 strains | *S. typhimurium* TA1535, TA1537, TA98, TA100 and *E. coli* wp2 *uvrA* (pKM101) | First choice, same strains that will be used in the GLP studies | 350 mg |
| Ames 2 strains | *S. typhimurium* TA98 and TA100 | Usually two strains of *S. typhimurium* are used, TA98 and TA100, able to detect the most frequent mutations, *i.e.* frameshift and base pair substitution, respectively<br>This test is also used in the genotoxic evaluation of impurities and of synthesis intermediates | 100 mg |
| Ames II | TA7001–TA7006 and TA98 | It is offered as a standardized kit with quality controlled bacterial strains, however it uses different strains to the GLP studies | 250 mg |

**Table 15.12** *In vitro* mammalian genotoxicity tests.

| Assays | System | Endpoint |
|---|---|---|
| Mouse lymphoma | Mouse lymphoma cell line | Gene mutation and chromosome aberration |
| *In vitro* mammalian chromosome aberration | Cell line, *e.g.* CHO (Chinese Hamster Ovary cell); CHL (Chinese Hamster line) | Chromosome aberration |
| | Primary human peripheral blood lymphocytes (HPLA) | Structural chromosomal damage and indications of numerical variations (*e.g.* polyploidy, aneuploidy) |
| Micronucleus test | Primary human peripheral lymphocytes or cell line (*e.g.* CHO) | Structural chromosomal damage |
| Comet assay | Primary human peripheral lymphocytes or cell line (*e.g.* CHO, MLA) | Single and double-strand breaks and alkali labile sites |

There are no strict criteria to select which particular mammalian test should be included in the lead optimization phase; however, the chromosome aberration (HLPA) or the *in vitro* micronucleus tests (MNT), alongside the AMES test, are the most standard preliminary assessments.

### 15.9.3 Evaluation of Results

Positive results in an Ames test are always a significant alert and should suggest deselecting the candidate. However, some considerations can be made when reviewing the result. A positive response can be both in the presence and in the absence of metabolic activation, or in one of the two conditions only. A more favourable outcome could be considered in an instance were the positive result is obtained in the presence of metabolic activation only, implicating a possible reactive metabolite. An analysis of the metabolite profile in the test system with the metabolite profiles in preclinical species or in human preparations may help determine the likely relevance of this finding. To explore this hypothesis, supplementary *in vivo* genotoxicity tests in liver can be considered (*e.g. in vivo* comet assay in liver or unscheduled DNA synthesis in the rat). Moreover, a new chemical entity that gives positive results *in vitro* in the presence of metabolic activation might not induce genotoxicity *in vivo* because the metabolite is not formed in humans, is formed in very small quantities, is metabolically detoxified or is rapidly excreted, greatly reducing the risk *in vivo*.

Scientific literature evidence indicates that *in vitro* assays may produce a false positive finding; as such any positive result should be evaluated on a weight of evidence approach. Factors to consider are, for example, the conditions of the experiments that do not occur *in vivo* (*e.g.* pH, osmolality, precipitates) or genotoxic evidence that occurs at high concentrations. In these cases, a weight of evidence approach indicates low likelihood of genotoxic potential and, assuming the subsequent battery of regulatory test are clean, then as standard, a single *in vivo* test only is considered. If there is not sufficient weight of evidence or mechanistic information to rule out the genotoxic potential, two *in vivo* studies are generally required, with appropriate endpoints and tissues, with an emphasis in obtaining sufficient systemic exposure to the test compound. Despite the importance of identifying mutagenic events, *in vivo* alternatives to determine the risk of compounds giving positive results in the Ames test are limited. The transgenic rodent assay[268] can be used to evaluate most tissues, but it is expensive and resource intensive, requiring 28 days of dosing. Recently the Pig-A assay,[269,270] that uses mutation in the phosphatidylinositol glycan-A (Pig-A) gene as the endpoint for *in vivo* mutations, has been proposed. However, this assay still requires validation work before routine and regulatory use.[270]

## 15.10 Early *In Vivo* Toxicology

There is a progression of complexity of the *in vivo* studies that are performed in lead optimization. They are aimed, step by step, to narrow down the candidate's properties. Each study is designed to answer to precise questions we pose and are essentially aimed to identify potential hazard and limiting toxicity early on. Moreover, the knowledge of the chemical class and the insight from the alerts resulting from *in silico* and *in vitro* work should also direct the inclusion of studies to explore potential pharmacodynamic issues.

The doses selected at this stage should be multiples of the pharmacologically predicted efficacies, in order to answer the question: are there severe toxicities or issues that preclude progression?

The selection of doses is driven by the pharmacological and pharmacokinetic properties of the candidates.

An example of a safety assessment cascade is given below:

1. Preliminary PK in rodent (preferably rat) and in a second non-rodent species (usually dog);
2. *In vivo* tox study, generally performed in one species (rodent) and in one sex (male).
3. Safety pharmacology studies targeted to investigate liabilities previously flagged or inherent to the chemical or pharmacological class (for example cardiovascular issues or convulsions).

Pharmaceuticals must be tested, except in exceptional circumstances, in rodents and non-rodents before and throughout the clinical phases of drug development programmes. For safety assessment purposes, species are chosen based on similarity to humans with regard to pharmacokinetic profile and, wherever possible, selected species should respond to the primary pharmacodynamic effect of the substance.

The first species used for PK or tox studies is a rodent, namely the rat. Rodents fall into the low neurophysiological evolutionary scale (*i.e.* have the least capacity to experience pain, distress, or lasting harm), are small in size, easy to handle, and require a limited amount of compound to be administered. The mouse is sometimes considered; however, this species is seldom used for regulatory tox studies, due to its small size and the high number of individuals necessary to allow adequate blood collection. During the lead optimization stage only the rodent species is generally explored. Non-rodents are rarely used, unless driven by previous experience, *e.g.* if the pharmacological receptor is only present in a particular species or previous experience has shown the rodent as non-predictive for a specific toxicity within a particular drug class.[271]

Should a second species be introduced, the default species is the dog, particularly the beagle, because of its size, tractability, and historical experience which makes the interpretation of toxicological findings easier.[272] Alternatively to the dog, the minipig, or rarely the ferret, is sometimes selected. Non-human primates (NHP) should be selected only as a last resort, being the nearest species to man in the evolutionary scale, which implies ethical considerations. For this reason any use of non-human primates must be specifically justified. Justification is based primarily on pharmacology when the target is known to be different in non-human primates *vs.* other species. Other considerations for selecting NHP are previous toxicological experience with compounds of that class, ability to achieve the required exposure, similarity to humans of important metabolic/biochemical processes (*e.g.* CYP450 structures or activities), specific pharmacological targets (*e.g.* COX-2 distribution in the kidney is similar in non-human primates and man, but different in dogs), or poor tolerability in other species (*e.g.* if emesis precludes achieving adequate systemic exposure).

### 15.10.1 Preliminary Pharmacokinetics

Pharmacokinetic (PK) studies are essential to translate the dose administered in terms of mg $kg^{-1}$ to the systemic exposure (AUC) following the process of absorption, distribution, metabolism, and excretion. Early *in vitro* and *in vivo* DMPK studies, typically available at the stage when a toxicity study is planned, are always used to help select the species, the doses, and the preliminary tox study design.

### 15.10.2 *In Vivo* Tox Study

Early tox studies study designs are usually simple, although able to ensure that potential hazards can be detected. A typical study design is shown in Table 15.13.

The active substance is typically administered for 7 days *via* the intended route of administration in humans, that is, in the majority of the cases, oral, intravenous, or inhalant.

A repeated administration of 7 days predicts most of the dose-limiting target organ toxicities observed in subsequent pivotal 4 week rodent studies. Target organs that may be missed are musculoskeletal toxicities observed with broad-spectrum matrix metalloproteinase (MMP) inhibitors, which may take 10–14 days to develop. Roberts *et al.*[272] report that at least 50% of the historical failures were attributable to target organ toxicities or to unexplained death that emerged within 14 days of repeat dosing.

Mortality or severe target organ toxicity at pharmacological exposure are preclusive of progression. The inclusion of three different doses is aimed to explore a range of margins; however, the preclinical safety margin (*i.e.* the ratio of the NOAEL – no observable adverse effect level – divided by the predicted human efficacious exposure level or exposure at the maximum anticipated dose in humans) will be defined with pivotal (GLP) toxicity studies that will be conducted at a subsequent stage.

In analyzing the findings of the studies, effects due to target organ toxicity, exaggerated pharmacology (primary pharmacology), or effects mediated by other (secondary) pharmacological targets should be identified.[273]

**Table 15.13** Early toxicity study design.

| Species | Rat |
|---|---|
| Sex | Male |
| Number of animals | 4/group |
| Groups | Vehicle, low, intermediate and high dose |
| Duration | 7 to 14 days |
| Observations | Clinical signs, body weight, clinical chemistry |
| Necropsy | Macroscopic examination |
| Microscopic examination of major organs | Adrenals, liver; lung; heart; kidneys; thymus; adrenals; testes; stomach if oral administration; injection site if IV administration; larynx if inhalation administration |

For each of these effects a risk assessment considering the nature of the finding and the safety margin should be made. As examples, alosetron (highly selective serotonin 5-HT3 antagonist), cerivastatin (statin), flosequinan (vasodilator), encainide (member of class 1C antiarrhythmic agents), and rofecoxib (COX-2 selective inhibitor) can be mentioned as agents posing issues related to primary pharmacology. Fenfluramine and dexfenfluramine (for obesity treatment), rapacuronium (neuromuscular blocking agent of nicotinic receptors), astemizole, and terfenadine (non-sedating H1 antihistamines), cisapride (gastrointestinal prokinetic motility agent), and mibefradil (long-acting calcium channel antagonist) can be quoted as agents posing issues related to secondary pharmacology.[274]

The need for toxicity studies in dogs or in other non-rodent species (see species selection) is less frequent and may be of help for new classes of agent with unknown toxicity; it is advisable to get toxicokinetics (TK) data at the maximum dose tolerated (MTD) before confirming suitability of the active substance. These studies can be non-terminal and aimed only to identify the MTD and the associated TK or may reflect the study design in the rat as described above.

## 15.10.3 Early Safety Pharmacology Evaluation

The scope of the safety pharmacology studies is to investigate the potential undesirable pharmacodynamic effects of a substance on physiological functions in relation to exposure in the therapeutic range and above. The regulatory core battery includes studies on the central nervous system, cardiovascular system, and respiratory system. Due to the rate of attrition, at early stages, the focus is the cardiovascular system and the central nervous system, while the respiratory system is investigated within the regulatory package of studies.

### *15.10.3.1 Cardiovascular (CV) Functionality*

One of the major causes of attrition during development are cardiovascular issues, particularly QT prolongation, and a big effort has been devoted to design early studies to set reliable stopping criteria. QT prolongation is an accessible, although imperfect, surrogate biomarker to gauge potentially fatal arrhythmias, notably Torsade de Pointes (TdP), an extremely rare but potentially lethal adverse drug effect.[275]

A CV attrition reduction strategy to progress compounds and discharge cardiovascular risk, which can be put in place during the lead optimization phase and in later phases has been discussed in Section 15.5.2.5 and is shown in Figure 15.4.

Early *in vivo* assessment of the haemodynamic and electrophysiological effects on the cardiovascular system are useful not only to confirm the significance of the *in vitro* data to detect cardiovascular safety with a chemical series, but also to predict the results of the IND-enabling GLP safety pharmacology studies, therefore reducing the attrition after development candidate selection. There are several models available, ranging from anesthetized to conscious (implanted or jacketed telemetry), using various species (rodents, guinea pigs, ferrets, dogs and monkeys).[276] Pharmaceutical R&D organizations conduct these early *in vivo* studies fit-for-purpose because all models have strengths and limitations. Anesthetized models are dosed by intravenous infusion requiring low amounts of material and do not cause pain or distress,[277] but might not correlate with effects in conscious animals, which could be more predictive of effects in the clinic.[278] In contrast, conscious models require larger quantities of material and are much more time- and resource-consuming.[279] Moreover, some models are not useful to detect electrophysiological effects relevant to humans, for example the rat that, not expressing the hERG channel, cannot be used for QT prolongation assessment.[280]

### 15.10.3.2 Nervous System Functionality

Early assessment of nervous system functionality is of value with highly potent compounds crossing the blood–brain barrier (BBB) or compounds that are flagged with potential convulsant properties (*e.g.* cannabinoid-1 antagonists, activators of the excitatory amino acids, $GABA_A$ receptor antagonists, 5-HT1B,1D receptor antagonists). Together with assessment of the chemical and therapeutic class, early target selectivity assays are able to identify potential hazards produced by compounds acting on off-targets receptors (see Section 15.3).

A proposed screening strategy to progress compounds with convulsant liabilities is shown in Figure 15.17.

The hippocampal brain slice assay for assessment of seizure liability[281] is an example of an *in vitro* test; *in vivo* studies include pentylenetetrazol-induced seizure in rats (PTZ)

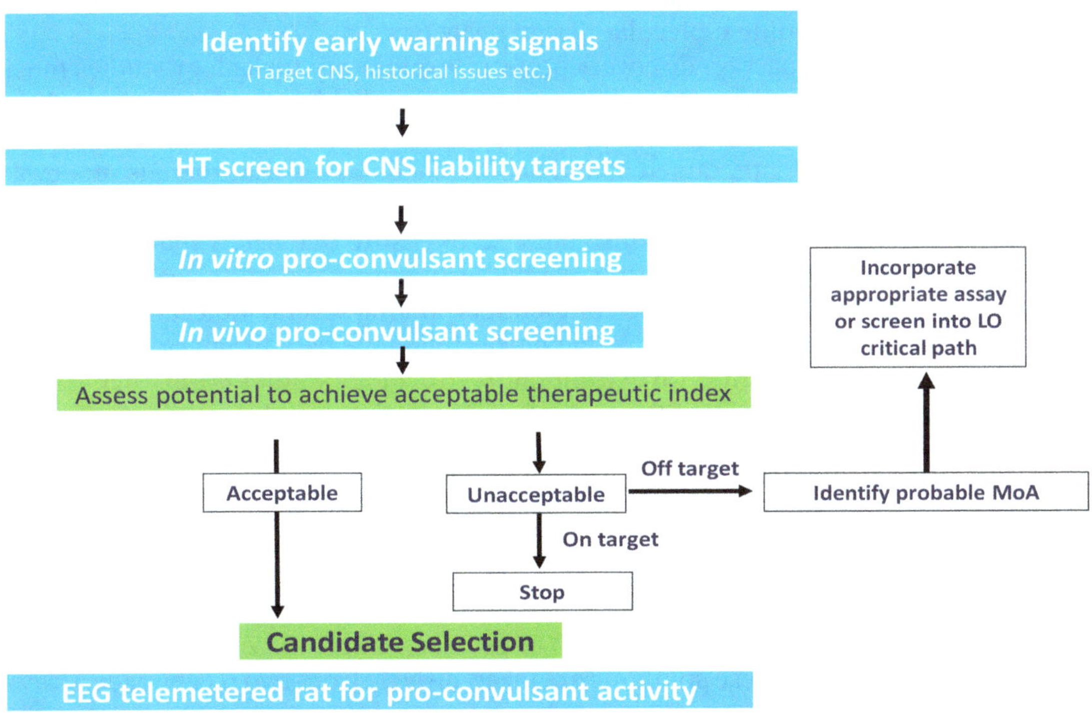


**Figure 15.17** Proposed screening strategy for compounds with potential convulsant liabilities.

or maximal electroshock seizure threshold (MEST) tests. PTZ is based on the continuous infusion of pentylenetetrazol and is a behavioural assessment in rats. MEST is based on a single corneally delivered electroshock and observation of tonic hind limb extension convulsions.

After candidate selection, telemetric electroencephalographic recording (EEG) in order to correlate PK/PD and interpret *in vivo* signs complementary to the timing of collection of TK metrics will complete the picture.

Undesired effects of drugs on the central and the peripheral nervous systems can also be detected with the neurobehaviuoral observation battery adapted from that first described by Irwin in mice[282] and subsequently modified as the neurologically based Functional Observational Battery (FOB). Behaviour represents the integration and integrity of the nervous system and it is generally considered a sensitive indicator, and perhaps the ultimate assay, of neuronal function.[283] A neurobehavioural observation battery consists of a series of observation/measurements, including home cage and open-arena observation, neuromuscular and sensory motor tests, and physiological/neurological measurements. As examples of read out, amphetamine induces a stimulation of the nervous system activities and marked hyperthermia, while chlorpromazine, diazepam, and clonidine induce depressive, anxiolytic, or sedative effects associated with hypothermia.

In the early stages this type of study is performed after single dose administration in male rats or mice.

In summary, early *in vivo* toxicology studies are not designed to generate an exhaustive assessment of the potential toxicological liabilities of compounds for humans. Rather, their main objective is to generate early data that may signal development-limiting toxicities and guide molecular design decisions.

To maximize their impact on discovery projects, exploratory toxicology studies must minimize compound requirements, since compound availability is almost always limited at these stages of the discovery process (usually <2 g). Moreover, these studies need to provide appropriate, targeted, and actionable data, *e.g.* that there is no development-limiting toxicity at insufficient margins. Therefore, several dosage levels are necessary to understand dose–response but also to ensure that safety margins can be appropriately estimated. Using multiple studies, exploratory rodent toxicology studies can also be used to select the best lead compound(s) among several molecules for a project through the generation of comparable *in vivo* tolerance data for all compounds. A recognized limitation and criticism of exploratory toxicology studies is that they cannot detect all toxic effects because of the short duration and reduced number of animals. The addition of more sensitive biomarkers or integration of new "omics" technologies to detect toxicity earlier could address this shortcoming in the next few years.

## 15.11 Hints and Tips

A summary of some specific hints and tips to use in optimization of discovery toxicology is given in Box 15.1. These solutions are taken directly from two recent papers[284,285] by respected scientists in three different pharmaceutical companies, which were consistent across the different organizations.

**Box 15.1 Optimisation Hints and Tips**

| Assessment core components | Target profile | Example evaluation tests |
|---|---|---|
| Selectivity/promiscuity | High selectivity/low promiscuity. Acceptable functional effects (agonist/antagonist) | Physicochemical risk profile; secondary pharmacology binding assays; target selectivity assays (*e.g.* kinase) |
| Intrinsic cytotoxicity | Not present or minimal | Primary hepatocyte viability |
| ADME/PK risk | Low intrinsic clearance; DDI not present or minimal | Metabolic stability; metabolic phenotyping; *in vitro* DDI studies; early dose to man and human PK prediction |
| | No/minimal reactive metabolite formation/covalent binding (burden) | Covalent binding/burden; metabolic profile (reactive metabolite formation) |
| | Acceptable distribution profile (tissue/cellular) | Transporter assessment; blood–brain barrier assessment; tissue accumulation assessment |
| Genetic toxicity (non-life threatening indications) | Eliminate mutagens and clastogens | Ames; *in vitro* micronucleus, GreenScreen, *etc.* |
| Target organ toxicity | Acceptable electrophysiological and haemodynamic cardiovascular profiles | Tissue specific models: CV (hERG, Na/K channels; human SC-derived cardiomyocytes, guinea pig, dog CV models) |
| | Minimize risk factors for DILI | Hepatic (mitochondrial toxicity, BSEP inhibition, 3D liver microspheres, hepatic organoids) |
| | Acceptable profile for therapeutic area indication | Target organ platforms (haematopoietic, renal, pulmonary, *etc.*) |

# Key References

Good general reading on general strategy for discovery toxicology:

D. M. Dambach, *et al.*, *Chem. Res. Toxicol.*, 2015, **29**, 452–472.
A. Eric and G. Blomme, *Chem. Res. Toxicol.*, 2016, **29**, 473–504.

*In silico* ADMET approaches in drug discovery

L. Michielan and S. Moro, *J. Chem. Inf. Model.*, 2010, **50**, 961.
M. P. Gleeson *et al.*, *Curr. Top. Med. Chem.*, 2011, **11**, 358.
G. Moroy, *Drug Discovery Today*, 2012, **17**, 44.

*In vitro* safety studies in drug discovery

J.-P. Valentin *et al.*, *J. Pharmacol. Toxicol. Methods*, 2018, **93**, 7–14. (Cardiac Safety).
J. S. Mitcheson, *Chem. Res. Toxicol.*, 2008, **21**, 1005. (Cardiac Safety).
T. R. Van Vleet *et al.*, *SLAS Discovery*, 2019, **24**(1), 1–24. (Off-Target Liability).
A. I. Grainger, M. C. King, D. A. Nagel, H. R. Parri, M. D. Coleman and E. J. Hill, *Front. Neurosci.*, 2018, **12**, 590. (Neurotoxicity).
A. Easter, M. E. Bell, J. R. Damewood Jr, W. S. Redfern, J. P. Valentin, M. J. Winter, C. Fonck, R. A. Bialecki, *Drug Discovery Today*, 2009, **14**(17–18), 876–84. (Nerotoxicity).
D. F. McGinnity, *et al.*, *Drug Metab. Dispos.*, 2000, **28**, 1327. (DDI).
R. J. Riley, K. Grime and R. Weaver, *Expert Opin. Drug Metab. Toxicol.*, 2007, **3**, 51–66. (DDI).
A. Ayrton and P. Morgan, *Xenobiotica*, 2001, **31**, 469. (DDI).
M. Kamber *et al.*, *Mutagenesis*, 2009, **24**(4), 359. (Mutagenesis).

*In vivo* exploratory toxicity studies
Non-Rodent Selection in Pharmaceutical Toxicology A "Points to Consider" document, developed by the ABPI in conjunction with the UK Home Office. August 2002.

J. A. Kramer, *et al.*, *Nat. Rev. Drug Discovery*, 2007, **6**(8), 636.
J. Hamdam *et al.*, *Toxicol. Appl. Pharmacol.*, 2013, **273**, 229–241

## References


1. J. Ashby, *J. Environ. Mutagen*, 1985, **7**, 919.
2. J. Ashby and R. W. Tennant, *Mutat. Res.*, 1988, **204**, 17.
3. J. Ashby and R. W. Tennant, *Mutat. Res.*, 1991, **257**, 229.
4. C. Merlot, *Drug Discovery Today*, 2010, **15**, 16.
5. J. R. Rabinowitz, *et al.*, *Environ. Health Perspect.*, 2008, **116**, 573.
6. D. Jacobson-Kram and J. F. Contrera, *Toxicol. Sci.*, 2007, **96**, 16.
7. P. McGee, *Drug Discovery Dev.*, 2005, **8**, 24.
8. G. M. Pearl, S. Livingston-Carr and S. K. Durham, *Curr. Top. Med. Chem.*, 2001, **1**, 247.
9. N. Greene, *Adv. Drug Delivery Rev.*, 2002, **54**, 417.
10. S. Ekins, *Biochem. Soc. Trans.*, 2003, **31**, 611.
11. R. Benigni and C. Bossa, *Curr. Comput.-Aided Drug Des.*, 2006, **2**, 169.
12. C. G. Mohan, *et al.*, *Mini-Rev. Med. Chem.*, 2007, **7**, 499.
13. W. Muster, *et al.*, *Drug Discovery Today*, 2008, **13**, 303.
14. F. Nigsch, *et al.*, *Expert Opin. Drug Metab. Toxicol.*, 2009, **5**, 1.
15. P. Szymanski, *et al.*, *Int. J. Mol. Sci.*, 2012, **13**, 427.
16. S. Ekins, *et al.*, *Drug Metab. Dispos.*, 2006, **34**, 495.
17. M. Jalaie and D. Holsworth, *Mini-Rev. Med. Chem.*, 2005, **5**, 1083.
18. E. Kerns and L. Di, *Drug Discovery Today*, 2003, **8**, 316.
19. J. Bajorath, *Nat. Rev. Drug Discovery*, 2002, **1**, 882.
20. A. M. Richard, *Chem. Res. Toxicol.*, 2006, **19**, 1257.
21. C. Yang, *et al.*, *Nat. Rev. Drug Discover*, 2006, **9**, 124.
22. A. M. Richard, *et al.*, *Nat. Rev. Drug Discover*, 2006, **9**, 314.
23. R. Judson, *et al.*, *Toxicol. Appl. Pharmacol.*, 2008, **233**, 7.
24. R. Judson, *et al.*, *Environ. Health Perspect.*, 2009, **117**, 685.
25. R. D. Benz, *Expert Opin. Drug Metab. Toxicol.*, 2007, **3**, 109.
26. C. Yang, *et al.*, *Toxicol. Mech. Methods*, 2006, **18**, 277.
27. W. Suter, *Curr. Opin. Chem. Biol.*, 2006, **10**, 362.
28. K. A. Giuliano, *et al.*, *Methods Enzymol.*, 2006, **414**, 601.

29. A. P. Li, *Chem.-Biol. Interact.*, 2007, **168**, 16.
30. A. P. Li, *Altern. Tierexp.*, 2008, **25**, 43.
31. C. Parng, *et al.*, *J. Pharmacol. Toxicol. Methods*, 2007, **55**, 103.
32. A. Oberemm, L. Onyon and U. Gundert-Remy, *Toxicol. Appl. Pharmacol.*, 2005, **207**, 592.
33. L. Suter, L. E. Babiss and E. B. Wheeldon, *Chem. Biol.*, 2004, **11**, 161.
34. W. B. Mattes, *et al.*, *Environ. Health Perspect.*, 2004, **112**, 495.
35. A. Bender, *et al.*, *ChemMedChem*, 2007, **2**, 861.
36. C. D. Scripture and W. D. Figg, *Nat. Rev. Cancer*, 2006, **6**, 546.
37. A. L. Hopkins, J. S. Mason and J. P. Overington, *Curr. Opin. Struct. Biol.*, 2006, **16**, 127.
38. R. Benigni, *et al.*, *J. Environ. Sci. Health, Part C: Environ. Carcinog. Ecotoxicol. Rev.*, 2007, **25**, 53.
39. W. Muster, *et al.*, *Drug Discovery Today*, 2008, **13**, 303.
40. N. L. Kruhlak, *et al.*, *Adv. Drug Delivery Rev.*, 2007, **59**, 43.
41. S. Weaver and M. P. Gleeson, *J. Mol. Graphics Modell.*, 2008, **26**, 1315.
42. M. G. Knize, *et al.*, *Environ. Mol. Mutagen.*, 2006, **47**, 132.
43. E. J. Matthews, *et al.*, *Toxicol. Mech. Methods*, 2008, **18**, 189.
44. C. Yang, *et al.*, *Toxicol. Mech. Methods*, 2008, **18**, 277.
45. G. Klopman, *Quant. Struct.*, 1992, **11**, 176.
46. E. J. Matthews and J. F. Contrera, *Regul. Toxicol. Pharmacol.*, 1998, **28**, 242.
47. S. K. Durham and G. M. Pearl, *Nat. Rev. Drug Discover*, 2001, **4**, 110.
48. G. M. Pearl, S. Livingston-Carr and S. K. Durham, *Curr. Top. Med. Chem.*, 2001, **1**, 247.
49. M. J. Prival, *Environ. Mol. Mutagen.*, 2001, **37**, 55.
50. P. D. Mosier and P. C. Jurs, *et al.*, *Chem. Res. Toxicol.*, 2003, **16**, 721.
51. R. D. Snyder, *Environ. Mol. Mutagen.*, 2009, **50**, 435.
52. R. D. Snyder, *et al.*, *Environ. Mol. Mutagen*, 2004, **43**, 143.
53. R. Benigni, *Chem. Rev.*, 2005, **105**, 1767.
54. K. B. Arvidson, *et al.*, *Toxicol. Mech. Methods*, 2008, **18**, 229.
55. J. Mayer, M. A. Cheeseman and M. L. Twaroski, *Regul. Toxicol. Pharmacol.*, 2008, **50**, 50.
56. L. G. Valerio Jr, *et al.*, *Toxicol. Appl. Pharmacol.*, 2007, **222**, 1.
57. I. V. Tetko, *et al.*, *Drug Discovery Today*, 2006, **11**, 700.
58. B. Simon-Hettich, *et al.*, *Toxicology*, 2006, **224**, 156.
59. E. J. Matthews, *et al.*, *Regul. Toxicol. Pharmacol.*, 2007, **47**, 136.
60. E. J. Matthews, *et al.*, *Regul. Toxicol. Pharmacol.*, 2006, **44**, 83.
61. F. P. Guengerich and J. S. Macdonald, *Chem. Res. Toxicol.*, 2007, **20**, 344.
62. M. Von Korff and T. Sander, *J. Chem. Inf. Model.*, 2006, **46**, 536.
63. P. Foggia, *et al.*, *Int. J. Pattern Recognit. Artif. Intell.*, 2006, **20**, 883.
64. R. Kho, *et al.*, *J. Med. Chem.*, 2005, **48**, 6671.
65. O. Llorens, *et al.*, *Int. J. Quantum Chem.*, 2002, **88**, 107.
66. B. Simon-Hettich, *et al.*, *Toxicology*, 2006, **224**, 156.
67. Y.-T. Woo and D. Y. Laiand, OncoLogic: A mechanism-based expert system for predicting the carcinogenic potential of chemicals, in *Predictive Toxicology*, ed. C. Hemla, CRC Press, Boca Raton, FL, USA, 2005, pp. 385–413.
68. C. A. Marchant, *et al.*, *Toxicol. Mech. Methods*, 2008, **18**, 177.
69. L. Michielan and S. Moro, *J. Chem. Inf. Model.*, 2010, **50**, 961.
70. M. P. Gleeson, *et al.*, *Curr. Top. Med. Chem.*, 2011, **11**, 358.
71. H. van de Waterbeemd and E. Gifford, *Nat. Rev. Drug Discovery*, 2003, **2**, 192.
72. P. D. Dobson, *et al.*, *Drug Discovery Today*, 2009, **14**, 31.
73. C. A. Lipinski, *et al.*, *Adv. Drug Delivery Rev.*, 2001, **46**, 3.
74. N. Bhogal, *et al.*, *Trends Biotechnol.*, 2005, **23**, 299.
75. G. Moroy, *Drug Discovery Today*, 2012, **17**, 44.
76. A. Vedani and M. Smiesko, *ATLA, Altern. Lab. Anim.*, 2009, **37**, 477.
77. L. Chen, *Drug Discovery Today*, 2012, **17**, 343.
78. C. M. Bathelt, *et al.*, *J. Phys. Chem.*, 2008, **112**, 13149.
79. R. Lonsdale, *et al.*, *J. Am. Chem. Soc.*, 2011, **133**, 15464.
80. H. Kubinyi, *J. Braz. Chem. Soc.*, 2002, **13**, 717.
81. S. Wold, *et al.*, *Chemom. Intell. Lab. Syst.*, 2001, **58**, 109.
82. CPMP/ICH/539/00. Note for guidance on safety pharmacology studies for human pharmaceuticals. S 7 A: Safety pharmacology studies – Step 5.
83. S. Jenkinson, *et al.*, *J. Pharmacol. Toxicol. Methods*, 2020, **14**, 106869.

84. J.-P. Valentin, *et al.*, *J. Pharmacol. Toxicol. Methods*, 2018, **93**, 7–14.
85. S. Bendels, *et al.*, *J. Pharmacol. Toxicol. Methods*, 2019, **99**, 106609.
86. T. R. Van Vleet, *et al.*, *SLAS Discovery*, 2019, **24**(1), 1–24.
87. J. Bowes, *et al.*, *Nat. Rev. Drug*, 2012, **11**, 909.
88. ICH Harmonised Tripartite Guideline, *Safety Pharmacology Studies for Human Pharmaceuticals S7A, Current Step 4 Version*, 8 November 2000.
89. S. Jenkinson, *et al.*, *J. Pharmacol. Toxicol. Methods*, 2020, **14**, 106869.
90. N. More, *Br. Med. J.*, 2016, **353**, i2956.
91. N. More, *Br. Med. J.*, 2016, **353**, i2727.
92. S. Whitebread, *et al.*, *Drug Discovery Today*, 2005, **10**, 1421.
93. S. Engberg, *et al.*, *Biochem. Pharmacol.*, 2007, 73, 259.
94. Y. Cheng and W. H. Prusoff, *Biochem. Pharmacol.*, 1973, **22**, 3099.
95. S. Lazareno and N. J. Birdsall, *Br. J. Pharmacol.*, 1993, **109**(4), 1110.
96. W. T. Bellamy, *Drugs*, 1992, **44**(5), 690.
97. J. J. Cali, *et al.*, *Expert Opin. Drug Metab. Toxicol.*, 2008, **4**(1), 103.
98. J. J. Zimmerman, A. V. S. A. Arnim and J. McLaughlinb, *Pediatric Critical Care (4th edn) Cellular Respiration*, 2011, ch. 74, p. 1058.
99. N. Ferri, *et al.*, *Pharmacol. Ther.*, 2013, **138**, 470.
100. J. S. MacDonald and R. T. Robertson, *Toxicol. Sci.*, 2009, **110**(1), 40.
101. H. British, *J. Pharmacol.*, 2011, **163**, 675.
102. J. Johansson, M. H. Larsson and J. J. Hornberg, *Curr. Opin. Toxicol.*, 2019, **15**, 99–108.
103. P. B. Watkins, *Clin. Pharmacol. Ther.*, 2011, **89**(6), 788–790.
104. H. Olson, G. Betton, D. Robinson, K. Thomas, A. Monro, G. Kolaja, P. Lilly, J. Sanders, G. Sipes, W. Bracken, M. Dorato, K. Van Deun, P. Smith, B. Berger and A. Heller, *Regul. Toxicol. Pharmacol.*, 2000, **32**(1), 56–67.
105. P. A. Walker, S. Ryder, A. Lavado, C. Dilworth and R. Riley, *J. Arch Toxicol.*, 2020, **94**, 2559–2585.
106. R. J. Weaver, E. A. Blomme, A. E. Chadwick, I. M. Copple, H. H. J. Gerets, C. E. Goldring, A. Guillouzo, P. G. Hewitt, M. Ingelman-Sundberg, K. G. Jensen, S. Juhila, U. Klingmüller, G. Labbe, M. J. Liguori, C. A. Lovatt, P. Morgan, D. J. Naisbitt, R. H. H. Pieters, J. Snoeys, B. van de Water, D. P. Williams and B. K. Park, *Nat. Rev. Drug Discovery*, 2020, **19**(2), 131–148.
107. M. Chen, V. Vijay, Q. Shi, Z. Liu, H. Fang and W. Tong, *Drug Discovery Today*, 2011, **16**(15–16), 697–703.
108. M. D. Aleo, F. Shah, S. Allen, H. A. Barton, C. Costales, S. Lazzaro, L. Leung, A. Nilson, R. S. Obach, A. D. Rodrigues and Y. Will, *Chem. Res. Toxicol.*, 2019, **33**(1), 223–238.
109. R. R. Shah, *Pharmacogenomics*, 2006, **7**, 889.
110. O. Campuzano, *et al.*, *Genet. Med.*, 2010, **12**, 260.
111. J. S. Mitcheson, *Chem. Res. Toxicol.*, 2008, **21**, 1005.
112. G. Guerri, G. Krasi, V. Precone, S. Paolacci, P. Chiurazzi, L. Arrigoni, B. Cortese, A. Dautay and M. Bertelli, *Acta Biomed.*, 2019, **90**, 20–29.
113. P. T. Sager, *et al.*, *Am. Heart J.*, 2014, **167**(3), 292–300.
114. C. A. Remme and A. A. M. Wilde, *Curr. Opin. Pharmacol.*, 2014, **15**, 53.
115. J. D. Moreno, *et al.*, *Circ. Res.*, 2013, **113**(7), e50–e61.
116. H. S. Karagueuzian, *et al.*, *Front. Pharmacol.*, 2017, **8**, 36.
117. ICH, Harmonised Tripartite Guideline S7B, Non-clinical evaluation of the potential for delayed ventricular repolarization (QT interval prolongation) by human pharmaceuticals. Step 4 Version, May 2005.
118. ICH, Harmonised Tripartite Guideline E14. Clinical evaluation of QT/QTc interval prolongation and proarrhythmic potential for non-antiarrhythmic drugs. Step 4 Version, May 2005.
119. K. Rae Chi, *Nat. Rev. Drug Discovery*, 2013, **12**, 565.
120. J. Heijman, *et al.*, *Curr. Opin. Pharmacol.*, 2014, **15**, 16.
121. S. Peng, *et al.*, *J. Pharmacol. Toxicol. Methods*, 2010, **61**, 277.
122. J. Ma, *et al.*, *Am. J. Physiol.: Heart Circ. Physiol.*, 2011, **301**, 2006.
123. E. Neher and B. Sakmann, *Nature*, 1976, **260**, 799.
124. O. P. Hamill, *et al.*, *Pflügers Arch.*, 1981, **391**, 85.
125. G. L. Kaczorowski, *et al.*, *Front. Pharmacol.*, 2011, **78**, 1.
126. C. Möller and H. Witchel, *Front. Pharmacol.*, 2011, **2**, 1.
127. C. D. Furberg and B. Pitt, *Curr. Controlled Trials Cardiovasc. Med.*, 2001, **2**, 205.
128. F. Estelle and R. Simons, *Ann. Allergy, Asthma, Immunol.*, 1999, **83**, 481.

129. Questions & Answers, 2018, Clinical and non-clinical Evaluation of QT/QTc Interval Prolongation and Proarrhythmic Potential (Concept Paper). International Council for Harmonisation of Technical Requirements for Pharmaceuticals for Human Use Available from: https://www.ich.org/page/safety-guidelines.
130. M. V. Accardi, M. K. Pugsley, R. Forster, E. Troncy, H. Huang and S. Authier, *J. Pharmacol. Toxicol. Methods*, 2016, **81**, 47–59.
131. A. I. Grainger, M. C. King, D. A. Nagel, H. R. Parri, M. D. Coleman and E. J. Hill, *Front. Neurosci.*, 2018, **12**, 590.
132. J. A. Harrill, T. M. Freudenrich, D. W. Machacek, S. L. Stice and W. R. Mundy, *NeuroToxicology*, 2010, **31**, 277–290.
133. B. L. Robinette, J. A. Harrill, W. R. Mundy and T. J. Shafer, *Front. Neuroeng.*, 2011, **4**(1), 1–9.
134. A. Easter, T. H. Sharp, J. P. Valentin and C. E. Pollard, *J. Pharmacol. Toxicol. Methods*, 2007, **56**(2), 223–233.
135. A. Easter, M. E. Bell, J. R. Damewood Jr, W. S. Redfern, J. P. Valentin, M. J. Winter, C. Fonck and R. A. Bialecki, *Drug Discovery Today*, 2009, **14**(17–18), 876–884.
136. A. W. L. Chiu, *Ann. Biomed. Eng.*, 2005, **33**, 798–810.
137. S. Authier, J. Arezzo, M. S. Delatte, M.-J. Kallman, C. Markgraf, D. Paquette, M. K. Pugsley, S. Ratcliffe, W. S. Redfern, J. Stevens, J.-P. Valentin, H. M. Vargas and M. J. Curtis, *J. Pharmacol. Toxicol. Methods*, 2016, **81**, 37–46.
138. A. Wahab, K. Albus, S. Gabriel and U. Heinemann, *Epilepsia*, 2010, **5**(3), 154–159.
139. J. A. Bradley, H. H. Luithardt, M. R. Metea and C. S. Strock, *Toxicol. Sci.*, 2018, **163**(1), 240–253.
140. E. Defranchi, A. Novellino, M. Whelan, S. Vogel, T. Ramirez, B. van Ravenzwaay and R. Landsiedel, *Front. Neuroeng.*, 2011, **4**(6), 1–12.
141. A. F. M. Johnstone, G. W. Gross, D. G. Weiss, O. H. Schroeder, A. Gramowski and T. J. Shafer, *NeuroToxicology*, 2010, **31**, 331–350.
142. M. Kreir, B. Van Deuren, S. Versweyveld, t A. De Bond, I. Van den Wyngaert, H. Van der Linde, H. R. Lu, G. Teuns and D. J. Gallacher, *Toxicol. Appl. Pharmacol.*, 2018, **346**, 45–57.
143. E. R. McConnell, M. A. McClain, J. Ross, W. R. LeFew and T. J. Shafer, *NeuroToxicology*, 2012, **33**, 1048–1057.
144. A. Novellino, B. Scelfo, T. Palosaari, A. Price, T. Sobanski, T. J. Shafer, A. F. M. Johnstone, G. W. Gross, A. Gramowski, O. Schroeder, K. Jügelt, M. Chiappalone, F. Benfenati, S. Martinoia, M. T. Tedesco, E. Defranchi, P. D'Angelo and M. Whelan, *Front. Neuroeng.*, 2011, **4**(4), 1–14.
145. A. M. Tukker, R. G. D. M. van Kleef, F. M. J. Wijnolts, A. de Groot and R. H. S. Westerink, *ALTEX*, 2020, **37**(1), 121–135.
146. K. Fattinger, M. Roos, P. Vergeres, C. Holenstein, B. Kind, U. Masche and P. J. Meier, *Br. J. Clin. Pharmacol.*, 2000, **49**, 158–167.
147. A. I. Shola and A. Adegboye, *Br. J. Pharm. Res.*, 2015, **8**, 43–54.
148. R. Diasio, *Br. J. Clin. Pharmacol.*, 1998, **46**, 1.
149. J. Lazarou, *et al.*, *J. Am. Med. Assoc.*, 1998, **279**, 1200.
150. S. A. Wrighton, *et al.*, *Drug Metab. Rev.*, 1993, **25**, 453.
151. C. Lu, *et al.*, *Biopharm. Drug Dispos.*, 2020, **41**(1–2), 3.
152. M. A. Cerny, *Drug Metab. Dispos.*, 2016, **44**, 1246–1252.
153. R. J. Riley, *et al.*, *Drug Metab. Dispos.*, 2005, **33**(9), 1304.
154. B. S. Kalra, *Indian J. Med. Sci.*, 2007, **61**(20), 102.
155. D. Mitschke, *et al.*, *Drug Metab. Dispos.*, 2008, **36**(6), 1039.
156. J. A. Willian, *Drug Metab. Dispos.*, 2004, **32**(11), 1201.
157. S. Fowler, *AAPS J.*, 2008, **10**(2), 410.
158. R. J. Bertz and G. R. Granneman, *Clin. Pharmacokinet.*, 1997, **32**, 210.
159. S. A. Testino Jr and G. Patonay, *J. Pharm. Biomed. Anal.*, 2003, **30**, 1459.
160. A. P. Li, *Drug Discovery Today*, 2001, **6**, 357.
161. Z. Du, G. Wang, Y.-F. Cao, C.-M. Hu, K. Yang, Y.-Z. Liu and Z.-Z. Fang, *Xenobiotica*, 2018, **48**, 452–458.
162. G. Englund, P. Lundquist, C. Skogastierna, J. Johansson, J. Hoogstraate, L. Afzelius and D. Projean, *Drug Metab. Dispos.*, 2014, **42**(3), 441–447.
163. B. T. Gufford, G. Chen, P. Lazarus, T. N. Graf, N. H. Oberlies and M. F. Paine, *Drug Metab. Dispos.*, 2014, **42**(10), 1675–1683.
164. N. Matsunaga, Y. Fukuchi, H. Imawaka and I. Tamai, *Drug Metab. Dispos.*, 2018, **46**, 680–691.
165. A. D. Rodrigues, *et al.*, *Drug Metab. Dispos.*, 1995, **23**, 765.
166. A. P. Li, *Curr. Top. Med. Chem.*, 2004, **4**, 701.

167. C. L. Crespi, *et al.*, *Anal. Biochem.*, 1997, **248**, 188.
168. D. Zhang, G. Luo, X. Ding and C. Lu, *Acta Pharm. Sin. B*, 2012, **2**, 549–561.
169. M. Li, H. Yuan, N. Li, G. Song, Y. Zheng, M. Baratta and Y. Lai, *Eur. J. Pharm. Sci.*, 2008, **35**, 114–126.
170. P. Lundquist, G. Englund, C. Skogastierna, J. Loeoef, J. Johansson, J. Hoogstraate and T. B. Andersson, *Drug Metab. Dispos.*, 2014, **42**, 448–458.
171. J. Mao, M. A. Mohutsky, J. P. Harrelson, S. A. Wrighton and S. D. Hall, *Drug Metab. Dispos.*, 2012, **40**, 706–716.
172. D. F. McGinnity, *et al.*, *Drug Metab. Dispos.*, 1999, **27**, 1017.
173. D. F. McGinnity, *et al.*, *Drug Metab. Dispos.*, 2000, **28**, 1327.
174. Li Di, *et al.*, *Int. J. Pharm.*, 2007, **44**(1), 1.
175. J. Ayrton, *et al.*, *Rapid Commun. Mass Spectrom.*, 1998, **12**(5), 217.
176. A. Tolonen, *et al.*, *J. Mass Spectrom.*, 2007, **335**(1–2), 960.
177. X. Wu, *et al.*, *J. Biomol. Screening*, 2012, **17**(6), 761.
178. S. Zhou, *et al.*, *Curr. Drug Metab.*, 2004, **5**, 415.
179. R. J. Riley, K. Grime and R. Weaver, *Expert Opin. Drug Metab. Toxicol.*, 2007, **3**, 51–66.
180. S. Zhou, *et al.*, *Clin. Pharmacokinet.*, 2005, **44**, 279.
181. K. M. Bertelsen, *et al.*, *Drug Metab. Dispos.*, 2003, **31**, 289.
182. L. C. Wienkers and T. G. Heath, *Nat. Rev. Drug Discovery*, 2005, **4**, 825.
183. A. Atkinson, *et al.*, *Drug Metab. Dispos.*, 2005, **33**, 1637.
184. E. S. Perloff, *et al.*, *Xenobiotica*, 2009, **39**(2), 99.
185. M. Kajbaf, *et al.*, *Drug Metab. Lett.*, 2010, **4**(2), 104.
186. N. Sekiguchi, *et al.*, *Drug Metab. Pharmacokinet.*, 2009, **24**(6), 500.
187. G. C. Moody, *Xenobiotica*, 1999, **29**, 53.
188. Z. Yan, *et al.*, *Eur. J. Drug Metab. Pharmacokinet.*, 2002, **4**, 281.
189. C. L. Crespi and D. M. Stresser, *J. Pharmacol. Toxicol. Methods*, 2000, **44**, 325.
190. T. Yamamoto, *et al.*, *Xenobiotica*, 2004, **34**, 87.
191. H. Yin, *et al.*, *Xenobiotica*, 2000, **30**, 141.
192. R. Weaver, *et al.*, *Drug Metab. Dispos.*, 2003, **31**, 955.
193. H. K. Lim, *et al.*, *Drug Metab. Dispos.*, 2005, **33**, 1211.
194. S. W. Grimm, H. J. Einolf, S. D. Hall, K. He, H.-K. Lim, K.-H. J. Ling, C. Lu and R. S. Obach, *Drug Metab. Dispos.*, 2009, **37**, 1355–1370.
195. L. M. Berry and Z. Zhao, *Drug Metab. Lett.*, 2008, **2**, 51–59.
196. Y. Chen, L. Liu, M. Monshouwer and A. J. Fretland, *Drug Metab. Dispos.*, 2011, **39**, 2085–2092.
197. M. Kosaka, Y. Kosugi and H. Hirabayashi, *J. Pharm. Sci.*, 2017, **106**, 2839–2846.
198. P. Zhao, K. L. Kunze and C. A. Lee, *Drug Metab. Dispos.*, 2005, **33**, 853–861.
199. A. Zimmerlin, M. Trunzer and B. Faller, *Drug Metab. Dispos.*, 2011, **39**, 1039–1046.
200. K. Hedenmalm, *et al.*, *Ther. Drug Monit.*, 1997, **19**, 643.
201. C. Funck-Brentano, *et al.*, *J. Pharmacol. Exp. Ther.*, 1997, **280**, 730.
202. D. J. Kazierad, *et al.*, *Clin. Pharmacol. Ther.*, 1997, **62**, 417.
203. K. A. Youdim, *et al.*, *Br. J. Clin. Pharmacol.*, 2008, **65**(5), 680.
204. S. B. Koukouritaki, *Pediatr. Res.*, 2002, **51**, 236.
205. C. Guillemette, *Pharmacogenomics J.*, 2003, **3**, 136.
206. E. Levesque, *et al.*, *Clin. Pharmacol. Ther.*, 2007, **81**, 392.
207. T. K. L. Kiang, *et al.*, *Pharmacol. Ther.*, 2005, **106**, 97.
208. K. A. Youdim, *et al.*, *Br. J. Clin. Pharmacol.*, 2008, **65**(5), 680.
209. Y. Parmentier, C. Pothier, A. Delmas, F. Caradec, M.-M. Trancart, F. Guillet and B. Walther, *Xenobiotica*, 2017, **47**, 562–575.
210. N. Murayama, K. Yajima, M. Hikawa, K. Shimura, Y. Ishii, M. Takada and H. Yamazaki, *Biopharm. Drug Dispos.*, 2018, **39**, 116–121.
211. T. Bjornsson, *et al.*, *J. Clin. Pharmacol.*, 2003, **43**, 443.
212. J. Raucy, *et al.*, *J. Pharmacol. Exp. Ther.*, 2002, **303**, 412.
213. G. Lemaire, *et al.*, *Biochem. Pharmacol.*, 2004, **68**, 2347–2358.
214. H. Kusuhara and Y. Sugiyama, in *Drug-drug Interactions*, A. D. Rodrigues, Marcell Dekker, Inc., New York, 2001, p. 123.
215. A. Ayrton and P. Morgan, *Xenobiotica*, 2001, **31**, 469.
216. M. Muller and P. L. Jansen, *Am. J. Physiol.: Gastrointest. Liver Physiol.*, 1997, **272**, G2185.
217. H. Koepsell, *Annu. Rev. Physiol.*, 1998, **60**, 243.
218. D. K. Meijer, *et al.*, *Nephrol., Dial., Transplant.*, 1999, **14**, 1.

219. V. H. Lee, *et al.*, *Adv. Drug Delivery Rev.*, 2001, **50**, S33.
220. G. A. Kullack-Ublick, *et al.*, *Gastroenterology*, 2001, **120**, 525.
221. H. Kusuhara, *et al.*, *J. Pharm. Sci.*, 1998, **87**, 1025.
222. G. Burckhardt and N. A. Wolff, *Am. J. Physiol.*, 2008, **278**, F853.
223. K. Inui, *et al.*, *Kidney Int.*, 2000, **58**, 944.
224. F. G. Russel, *et al.*, *Annu. Rev. Physiol.*, 2002, **64**, 563.
225. R. P. J. Oude Elferink, *et al.*, *Biochim. Biophys. Acta*, 1995, **1241**, 215.
226. M. Yamazaki, *et al.*, *Pharm. Res.*, 1996, **13**, 497.
227. K. N. Faber, *et al.*, *Adv. Drug Delivery Rev.*, 2003, **55**, 107.
228. P. J. Meier, *et al.*, *Hepatology*, 1997, **26**, 1667.
229. H. Kusuhara, *et al.*, *J. Pharm. Sci.*, 1998, **87**, 1025.
230. G. J. Hooiveld, *et al.*, *Eur. J. Pharm. Sci.*, 2001, **12**, 525.
231. J. Kovaril, *et al.*, *Clin. Pharmacol. Ther.*, 1999, **66**, 391.
232. A. Hedman, *et al.*, *Clin. Pharmacol. Ther.*, 1990, **47**, 20.
233. B. Hsiang, *et al.*, *J. Bio. Chem.*, 1999, **274**, 37161.
234. G. Alexandridis, *et al.*, *Am. J. Med.*, 2000, **109**, 261.
235. U. I. Schwarz, *et al.*, *Int. J. Clin. Pharmacol. Ther.*, 2000, **38**, 161.
236. M. Cvetkovic, *et al.*, *Drug Metab. Dispos.*, 1999, **27**, 866.
237. A. Johne, *et al.*, *Clin. Pharmacol. Ther.*, 1999, **66**, 338.
238. M. F. Fromm, *et al.*, *Am. J. Pathol.*, 2000, **157**, 1575.
239. N. H. Cnubben, *et al.*, *Expert Opin. Drug Metab. Toxicol.*, 2005, **1**, 219.
240. C. Hegedus, *et al.*, *Adv. Drug Delivery Rev.*, 2009, **61**, 47.
241. A. Aszalos, *Drug Discovery Today*, 2007, **12**, 838.
242. J. S. Lagas, *Mol. Interventions*, 2009, **9**, 136.
243. L. A. Stanley, *et al.*, *Drug Metab. Rev.*, 2009, **41**, 27.
244. F. Fenneteau, *et al.*, *Theor. Biol. Med. Modell.*, 2009, **6**, 2.
245. W. H. Halliwell, *Pathology*, 1997, **25**, 53–60.
246. J. A. Shayman and A. Abe, *Biochim. Biophys. Acta*, 2013, **1831**(3), 602.
247. B. R. Berridge, *et al.*, *Toxicol. Pathol.*, 2007, **35**, 325.
248. C. Bauch, S. Bevan, H. Woodhouse, C. Dilworth and P. Walker, *Toxicol. In Vitro*, 2015, **29**(3), 621–630.
249. P. Nioi, *et al.*, *Toxicol. Sci.*, 2007, **99**(1), 162.
250. T. Maurer, *Food Chem. Toxicol.*, 1987, **25**, 407.
251. Food and Drug Administration and HHS, International Conference on Harmonisation; S10 Photosafety Evaluation of Pharmaceuticals; guidance for industry; availability. Notice, *Fed. Regist.*, 2015, **80**(17), 4282–4283.
252. OECD Test No. 432: *In vitro* 3T3 NRU Phototoxicity Test.
253. S. Kim, K. H. Choi and J. Yun, *PLoS One*, 2018, **13**(5), e0196735.
254. A. M. Lynch, *et al.*, *Mutagenesis*, 2008, **23**, 111.
255. B. Henry, C. Foti and K. Alsante, *J. Photochem. Photobiol., B*, 2009, **96**(1), 57–62.
256. S. Fluckiger-Isler, *et al.*, *Mut. Res.*, 2012, **747**(1), 36.
257. Y. Oda, *Genes Environ.*, 2016, **38**(24), 18.
258. R. M. Walmsley, *Expert Opin. Drug Metab. Toxicol.*, 2008, **4**(6), 827.
259. M. A. Rodrigues, *Cytometry*, 2018, **93**(7), 706.
260. N. Flamand, *et al.*, *Toxicol. In Vitro*, 2001, **15**, 105.
261. M. Kamber, *et al.*, *Mutagenesis*, 2009, **24**(4), 359.
262. *Basic Mutagenicity Tests: UKEMS Recommended Procedures*, ed. D. Kirkland, 1990.
263. O. Östling and K. J. Johanson, *Biochem. Biophys. Res. Commun.*, 1984, **123**, 291.
264. N. P. Singh, *et al.*, *Exp. Cell Res.*, 1988, **175**, 1840.
265. E. Lorge, *et al.*, *Mutat. Res.*, 2006, **607**, 13.
266. M. Kirsch-Volders, *Mutagenesis*, 2011, **26**(1), 177.
267. Non-Rodent Selection in Pharmaceutical Toxicology A "Points to Consider" Document, Developed by the ABPI in Conjunction with the UK Home Office, August 2002.
268. V. Thybaud, *et al.*, *Mutat. Res., Genet. Toxicol. Environ. Mutagen.*, 2003, **540**, 141–151.
269. V. N. Dobrovolsky, *et al.*, *Methods Mol. Biol.*, 2014, **1105**, 205–221.
270. B. B. Gollapudi, *et al.*, *Mutat. Res., Genet. Toxicol. Environ. Mutagen.*, 2015, **783**, 23–35.
271. M. Pellegatti, *Expert Opin. Drug Metab. Toxicol.*, 2013, **9**(10), 161.
272. R. A. Roberts, *et al.*, *Drug Discovery Today*, 2014, **19**(3), 341.
273. J. A. Kramer, *et al.*, *Nat. Rev. Drug Discovery*, 2007, **6**(8), 636.

274. D. S. Smith and E. F. Schmid, *Curr. Opin. Drug Discovery Dev.*, 2006, **9**(1), 38.
275. W. S. Redfern, *et al.*, *Cardiovasc. Res.*, 2003, **58**, 32.
276. J. Hamdam, *et al.*, *Toxicol. Appl. Pharmacol.*, 2013, **273**, 229–241.
277. B. Van Deuren, *et al.*, *J. Pharmacol. Toxicol. Methods*, 2009, **60**, 11–23.
278. L. Hanson, *et al.*, *J. Pharmacol. Toxicol. Methods*, 2006, **54**, 116–129.
279. K. Derakhchan, *et al.*, *J. Pharmacol. Toxicol. Methods*, 2014, **171**, 509–522.
280. W. Mulla, *et al.*, *Front. Physiol.*, 2018, **9**, 1–11.
281. A. Easter, *et al.*, *Drug Discovery Today*, 2009, **14**(17–18), 876.
282. S. Irwin, *Psychopharmacologia*, 1968, **13**, 222.
283. E. Moscardo, *et al.*, *J. Pharmacol. Toxicol. Methods*, 2007, **56**, 239.
284. D. M. Dambach, *et al.*, *Chem. Res. Toxicol.*, 2015, **29**, 452–472.
285. A. Eric and G. Blomme, *Chem. Res. Toxicol.*, 2016, **29**, 473–504.

# 16 Toxicology and Drug Development

Ilona Bebenek*[a] and Owen McMaster[a]

[a]U.S. Food and Drug Administration, Division of Pharmacology/Toxicology for Infectious Diseases, 10903 New Hampshire Ave., Silver Spring, MD 20993, USA
*E-mail: ilona.bebenek@fda.hhs.gov

## 16.1 Introduction and Background

Drug development is a lengthy, multi-step process designed to characterize the safety and efficacy of drug candidates before being approved for marketing.[1] Phase 1 clinical trials typically provide safety, tolerability, and pharmacokinetic data for a drug following short-term administration in a small number of healthy subjects or patients. During a Phase 2 clinical trial, activity (*e.g.*, proof of concept) and safety are evaluated in a small number of patients. Finally, Phase 3 clinical trials involving many patients are conducted to provide more definitive efficacy and safety information. Progression through the range of clinical trials and ultimately to product approval depends on a series of risk *vs.* benefit analyses. A critical component of these analyses is the establishment of a toxicity profile. In addition to the human safety database generated during clinical trials, it is necessary to also consider non-clinical[†] data to support decision making. Providing this supporting information is the primary focus of non-clinical safety assessment. This safety assessment covers a broad range of scientific disciplines, including safety pharmacology, general toxicology, genetic toxicology, carcinogenicity, and developmental and reproductive toxicology. An understanding of drug metabolism and kinetics is also fundamental to non-clinical safety assessment.

A key assumption in drug development is that data obtained from non-clinical studies will be useful to inform human risk. When assessing the various safety related endpoints, *in vitro* and *in vivo* data is submitted to regulatory authorities to facilitate the decision making process. In some cases, non-clinical studies may supply the sole

[†]The term non-clinical instead of pre-clinical is used because this type of data may be generated prior to or during conduct of clinical studies.

The Handbook of Medicinal Chemistry: Principles and Practice, 2nd Edition
Edited by Simon E. Ward and Andrew M. Davis

Published by the Royal Society of Chemistry, www.rsc.org

source of safety data available to support the initiation of a Phase 1 clinical trial. As the clinical safety database is generated during development, non-clinical data helps support decision making in regard to conduct of additional clinical trials as well as the approval for marketing. Non-clinical studies will generally serve as the only source of information for endpoints that are not feasible and/or ethical to study in humans (*i.e.*, genotoxicity, carcinogenicity, developmental and reproductive toxicity).

To assist both regulators and sponsors of drug development, there are numerous guidance documents/guidelines that provide recommendations related to non-clinical drug development. Globally recognized guidelines are provided by the International Conference for Harmonization (ICH). Additional recommendations are provided by regional authorities such as the European Medicines Agency (EMA), Japanese Pharmaceuticals and Medical Devices Agency (PMDA), and the United States Food and Drug Administration (FDA). While guidance documents/guidelines provide recommendations on drug development and highlight current regulatory thinking, decisions are made on a case-by-case basis and require consideration of the best available science and weight of evidence approach.

## 16.2 Toxicology Testing

Standardized protocols exist for many studies conducted during drug development (*e.g.*, Organisation for Economic Co-operation and Development or OECD guidelines); however, sound scientific judgment must be exercised to maximize the utility of toxicology studies. When toxicology studies are conducted according to regulatory expectations (*e.g.*, good laboratory practices or GLP), there is added confidence that data are generated under appropriate conditions. However, exploratory or non-GLP studies are sometimes considered "fit for purpose" and, therefore, acceptable for regulatory purposes.

There are several important considerations for designing non-clinical studies. Of particular interest for *in vivo* evaluations is selection of appropriate animal models to maximize clinical relevance. Knowledge of a drug's *in vitro* metabolite profile or additional ADME information, as well as pharmacological target characteristics (*e.g.*, tissue expression profile) can provide a basis for comparing humans with the various non-clinical species. Historical experience for a particular drug class may also be informative in aiding species selection.

The route of administration used in non-clinical studies should, in general, mimic the expected clinical route. There may be instances where data from a second route of administration is needed. For instance, intravenous administration of a drug with low oral bioavailability can provide critical systemic exposure, resulting in detection of a potentially important clinical toxicity. Data from such a study will potentially provide safety data that could not be obtained otherwise.

Another critical factor in the design of non-clinical safety studies is the selection of doses. *In vitro* studies may include exposures to very high concentrations of questionable clinical relevance. Such a strategy is appropriate for assays intended to identify potential hazards *vs.* defining quantitative risk. *In vivo* studies may include doses yielding systemic exposure comparable to those expected in the clinic. However, these studies should also include higher doses in an attempt to increase the likelihood of detecting toxicity with potential clinical relevance.

In all non-clinical studies designed to characterize drug safety, it is important to determine whether effects are related to the drug or fall within the range of expected observations for a particular experimental model. The presence of a dose–response as well as statistical and/or biological relevance should all be taken into consideration when characterizing an effect as drug-related. An evaluation of relevance will be based on comparison with treated groups and appropriate control groups. Concurrent controls, cells or animals treated with a vehicle or inactive control article, are routinely included in the study design. In addition, historical control values are also an important source of data. When a value is deemed to be statistically significant but falls within the range of historical control values, the effect may be described as drug-related but possessing limited biological relevance. Here again, a case-by-case approach will be appropriate.

The following sections are intended to provide brief general descriptions of non-clinical toxicology studies routinely conducted during drug development. Focus is placed on the overall goal, endpoints evaluated, timelines for reporting, key sources of regulatory recommendations, and ultimate utility of the various non-clinical studies. A summary of the recommended non-clinical toxicology studies and timing for submission is provided in Table 16.1. Note that non-clinical development is conducted on a case-by-case basis so the actual studies conducted and timing may vary. For instance, sponsors may be asked to conduct embryo-fetal evaluations early for drugs in a class known to be associated with teratogenicity.

## 16.2.1 Safety Pharmacology

The goal of safety pharmacology studies is to characterize drug effects on vital physiological functions. Per ICH S7A,[2] a safety pharmacology testing battery should include extensive evaluations of central nervous system (CNS), cardiovascular, and respiratory parameters. Other organ systems (*e.g.*, kidney, gastrointestinal, *etc.*) may also be evaluated when appropriate. Measurement of multiple endpoints (*e.g.*, CNS assessments include numerous behavioral and functional endpoints) should be included to maximize the ability to detect adverse effects. *In vivo* studies are designed to identify effects over a dose range yielding exposures that exceed the expected clinical exposure. Each study is typically conducted in a single species. Cardiovascular assessments utilize telemeterized animals, allowing continuous measurement over a prolonged period (*e.g.*, 24 h). Telemetry is a powerful tool for identifying effects that may escape detection by less intensive sampling. In addition to the core battery of *in vivo* tests, an *in vitro* assay should be conducted to assess potential risks for inducing QT prolongation, a potentially serious effect associated with lethal cardiotoxicity. Regulatory recommendations concerning *in vitro* safety pharmacology studies are described in ICH S7B.[3]

Data from safety pharmacology studies can be used to calculate safety margins based on comparison with expected clinical exposure. The results can also be used to help select doses for additional non-clinical evaluations and identify parameters of concern that should be monitored during clinical trials. According to ICH M3(R2),[4] safety pharmacology studies should be submitted prior to Phase 1.

**Table 16.1** Recommended non-clinical studies.[a,b]

| Study | <Phase 1 | <Phase 2 | <Phase 3 | Marketing application |
|---|---|---|---|---|
| **Safety pharmacology** | | | | |
| - Cardiovascular | | | | |
| *In vitro* | ✓ | | | |
| *In vivo* | ✓ | | | |
| - Neurological | ✓ | | | |
| - Respiratory | ✓ | | | |
| **Genetic toxicology** | | | | |
| - Option 1 | | | | |
| Bacterial reverse mutation assay | ✓ | | | |
| *In vitro* mammalian cell assay | ✓ | | | |
| *In vivo* assessment | | ✓ | | |
| - Option 2 | | | | |
| Bacterial reverse mutation assay | ✓ | | | |
| *In vivo* assessment #1 | ✓ | | | |
| *In vivo* assessment #2 | ✓ | | | |
| **General toxicology** | ✓ | ✓ | ✓ | |
| **Developmental/reproductive toxicology** | | | | |
| - Fertility | | | ✓ | |
| - Embryo-fetal development | | | ✓ | |
| - Pre/post-natal development | | | | ✓ |
| **Carcinogenicity** | | | | ✓ |
| **Miscellaneous studies** | | | | |
| - Immunotoxicity | | | ✓ | |
| - Photosafety | | | ✓ | |
| - Abuse liability | | | ✓ | |
| - Local tolerance | | | ✓ | |

[a]Per ICH M3(R2).[4]
[b]Timing and scope of non-clinical studies may change during drug development.

## 16.2.2 Genetic Toxicology

Genetic toxicology studies are designed to establish a drug's potential to induce changes in the DNA sequence (*i.e.*, mutations) and consequently contribute to carcinogenicity in humans. Because of the correlation between genotoxicity and carcinogenicity, results from genetic toxicology assays are useful for understanding potential carcinogenic risks during the development phases. Similar to the safety pharmacology testing strategy, genetic toxicology testing utilizes a battery approach, as described in ICH S2(R1).[5] As the recommended assays are intended to identify potential genotoxic hazards, both *in vitro* and *in vivo* studies are performed using doses yielding exposures that may greatly exceed clinical exposure.

A bacterial reverse mutation assay, also known as the Ames assay, is performed to evaluate the potential to induce gene mutations *in vitro*. Additional *in vitro* studies in mammalian cells are used to detect structural chromosomal damage (*e.g.*, clastogenicity) and/or numerical chromosomal damage (*e.g.*, aneugenicity). Assays capable of investigating these critical endpoints include the mouse lymphoma assay and cytogenetic evaluations designed to identify chromosomal aberrations or micronuclei. An *in vivo* evaluation of chromosomal damage, most often micronuclei in peripheral blood or bone marrow from rodents, is also part of the testing battery performed. The combination of the Ames assay, an *in vitro* mammalian cell assay, and *in vivo* evaluation is referred to as Option 1. A second testing strategy (*i.e.*, Option 2) allows a sponsor to replace the *in vitro* mammalian cell assay with a 2nd *in vivo* endpoint. An example of a 2nd endpoint is the single cell gel electrophoresis assay (*i.e.*, Comet assay) in the liver. When positive results are encountered in any of the recommended assays, additional follow-up testing may be needed to further characterize genotoxic potential; results are evaluated in the context of all available data.

Genotoxicity data is used to determine whether or not clinical trials are safe to proceed. From a practical standpoint, the concept of safety margins does not apply to drugs that cause gene mutations or are considered true clastogens. In contrast, aneugenic compounds may be associated with a threshold (*i.e.*, exposure below which effects are not observed) and comparison with clinical exposure may allow for a margin of safety to be identified. Results from the Ames assay and an assessment of chromosomal damage in a mammalian system is typically submitted to support a Phase 1 study. Results from all components of the testing battery must be provided in advance of Phase 2 clinical trials. When a drug is approved for marketing, the genetic toxicology data is included in the label.

### 16.2.3 General Toxicology

The goal of general toxicology testing is to identify drug-related toxicity occurring in the whole animal. As such, these studies use high doses sometimes well above expected clinical exposures. Examples of criteria to limit the high dose include observations of a dose-limiting toxicity, maximum feasible concentration based on limits of solubility, saturation of systemic exposure, large differences in non-clinical exposure *vs.* the expected clinical exposure, or a limit dose (*e.g.*, 1000 or 2000 mg $kg^{-1}$ $day^{-1}$).[4]

The studies are wide in scope with regards to duration of dosing as well as the number and diversity of endpoints evaluated. Studies range from single dose to chronic studies of up to 9 months. To facilitate the use of a drug in clinical trials, general toxicology studies are evaluated throughout the development process. The studies are completed in a stepwise manner with initial clinical studies supported by short-term repeat dose non-clinical studies. Extended duration non-clinical general toxicology studies are required to support the initiation of longer-term clinical trials and submission of a marketing application (Tables 16.2 and 16.3). Specific recommendations regarding duration and timing of submission for general toxicology studies are provided in ICH M3(R2).[4] Following recommendations in ICH M3(R2) assures that the expected duration of non-clinical data is sufficient to cover proposed clinical dosing.

**Table 16.2** Non-clinical general toxicology studies needed to support clinical development.[a]

| Clinical trial | Non-clinical studies |
|---|---|
| ≤2 weeks | 2 weeks[b] |
| >2 weeks to ≤6 months | Equivalent to duration of clinical trial[b] |
| >6 months | 6 month study in rodent and 9 month study in non-rodent |

[a]Modified table from ICH M3(R2).[4]
[b]Studies should be conducted in both rodent and non-rodent.

**Table 16.3** Non-clinical general toxicology studies needed to support marketing approval.[a]

| Clinical use | Non-clinical studies |
|---|---|
| ≤2 weeks | 1 month[b] |
| >2 weeks to ≤1 month | 3 months[b] |
| >1 month to ≤3 months | 6 months[b] |
| >3 months | 6 month study in rodent and 9 month study in non-rodent |

[a]Modified table from ICH M3(R2).[4]
[b]Studies should be conducted in both rodent and non-rodent.

To maximize the potential to predict clinical risk, multiple endpoints are routinely evaluated in a rodent and non-rodent species. Observations and measurements routinely include changes in behavior/appearance, body weight parameters, food consumption, ophthalmoscopy, and electrocardiograms. Clinical pathology data is collected to help identify target organs of toxicity by monitoring changes in hematology, coagulation, clinical chemistry, and urinalysis parameters. Evaluations of organ weights and macroscopic tissue changes are useful; however, microscopic changes detected by histopathologic evaluation are often the definitive indicators of toxicity. Results of the various assessments are not viewed independently but are instead integrated. Overall, the most convincing evidence of target organ toxicity is consistency in effects detected by multiple endpoints (*e.g.*, hepatotoxicity indicated by both changes in clinical chemistry and histopathology).

Important outcomes from these studies include identification of target organs as well as establishment of the no-observable adverse effect level (NOAEL), no-observable effect level (NOEL), lowest observable adverse effect level (LOAEL), and/or maximum tolerated dose (MTD). Ultimately, the specific effect, severity, incidence, and reversibility (*i.e.*, persistence of an effect following a treatment-free period) will be considered to determine whether an effect is adverse or non-adverse. A 2016 working group of The European Society of Toxicologic Pathology, stated that "an adverse effect is a test item-related change in the morphology, physiology, growth, development, reproduction or life span of the animal model that likely results in an impairment of functional capacity to maintain homeostasis and/or an impairment of the capacity to respond to an additional challenge";[6] it is important to note that many other definitions of adversity exist.

Results from general toxicology studies can be used to guide clinicians when selecting endpoints to monitor in clinical trials. Another primary use of the data is generation of safety margins based on comparison of non-clinical and clinical doses or exposures. To support an initial clinical trial, safety margins are routinely based on body surface area conversion of the non-clinical NOAEL dose to the proposed clinical trial starting dose. Clinical trials are generally considered reasonably safe if the converted NOAEL dose is ≥10-fold the proposed clinical starting dose.[7] Note that larger or smaller safety margins may be appropriate, depending on the non-clinical toxicity profile observed. Larger safety margins may be warranted when a drug induces severe toxicity (including mortality), irreversible toxicity, or a non-clinical effect that is difficult to monitor clinically (*e.g.*, certain types of cardiotoxicity), or exhibits a steep dose–response curve. Lower margins of safety are sometimes acceptable for reversible toxicities and those that are more easily monitored in the clinical trial (*e.g.*, liver toxicity). A more refined method of calculating safety margins is to compare systemic exposures once both non-clinical and clinical data are available. In some instances, clinical data may be available for a Phase 1 study if clinical trials have been conducted in another country. Regardless of whether safety margins are calculated using dose, body surface area conversion, or systemic exposure, the information is important for risk assessment used in making decisions about the acceptability of clinical trials or marketing. General toxicity data is rarely included in the approved drug label.

## 16.2.4 Developmental and Reproductive Toxicology

Developmental and reproductive toxicology (DART) studies evaluate the ability of a drug to impact reproductive function in adult animals as well as development of offspring. While general toxicology studies can provide some limited information (*e.g.*, histopathological changes in reproductive organs), more focused studies are often needed. In general, DART studies should encompass observations through one complete life cycle (*i.e.*, from conception in one generation through conception in the following generation). Regulatory recommendations for these specific evaluations are described in ICH S5(R3).[8]

As part of the evaluation of developmental and reproductive toxicity testing, a study of fertility and early embryonic development (FEED study) is typically performed in the rat. The FEED study is designed to assess changes in mating behavior and fertility of adult animals, as well as effects on implantation and early stages of embryo development. An embryo-fetal development study (EFD study) is conducted to assess effects on maternal health as well as embryo-fetal development. Due to the severity of effects detected during embryo-fetal development (*e.g.*, malformations associated with teratogenicity), these studies should be evaluated in both a rodent and a non-rodent species, most likely the rabbit. Lastly, pre- and postnatal development (PPND) studies are designed to address potential effects on the pregnant and lactating female as well as embryo-fetal and pup development. Most often these studies are performed in the rat. In all studies, the timing and duration of dosing must correlate with the appropriate reproductive or developmental stage being evaluated. The doses evaluated in developmental and reproductive toxicology studies are determined by similar criteria to those used in general toxicology studies (*e.g.*, dose-limiting toxicity, maximum feasible concentration, saturation of exposure, *etc.*).

Developmental and reproductive toxicology data are used to guide design of clinical trials. While males and females can be included in early clinical trials without a specific assessment of fertility, clinical administration of drugs in women of child-bearing potential typically requires appropriate measures (*e.g.*, contraception) until embryo-fetal development data is available. The data from developmental and reproductive toxicology studies is also used to support regulatory decisions at the marketing stage and, if approved, is listed in the drug label. In general, evaluations of fertility and embryo-fetal development are needed prior to initiating Phase 3 clinical trials, while PPND studies can be submitted with the marketing application.

### 16.2.5 Carcinogenicity

Carcinogenicity studies are conducted to investigate the ability of a drug to induce tumors arising through both genotoxic and non-genotoxic mechanisms. Typically, carcinogenicity is evaluated in lifetime dosing studies in two rodent species because carcinogenicity is a multi-step process, usually requiring relatively long periods of time to develop. A lifetime study in rats or mice would include daily dosing, seven days a week for 104 weeks. Another option to fulfil the ICH requirement to assess carcinogenicity in a drug candidate is to conduct one 2-year rat study plus a shorter, 6-month study using a transgenic mouse model (typically Tg.rasH2) genetically modified to increase their response to carcinogens.[9] ICH has recently expanded the testing scheme by introducing an integrative approach that provides specific weight of evidence criteria that inform whether or not a 2-year rat study adds value in completing a human carcinogenicity risk assessment.[9] Regulatory recommendations for the need and conduct of carcinogenicity studies are included in ICH guidelines S1A,[10] S1B,[11] and S1C(R2).[12]

Endpoints of primary concern include animal health and tumor formation. Tumors are characterized through observation and palpation as well as macroscopic and microscopic pathology. To increase the likelihood of detecting a carcinogenic response, studies are conducted at doses that include the MTD, maximum feasible dose based on limits of solubility, saturation of systemic exposure, or at systemic exposures greatly exceeding the expected clinical exposure. In the US, the FDA provides guidance to drug companies with dose selection through its Executive Carcinogenicity Assessment Committee.[13] The statistical significance of any increase in tumours should be evaluated by both trend and pairwise comparisons to reduce false positives. Statistically significant increases in tumour incidence in rats are not always predictive of human carcinogenicity. This may occur if the relevant mode of action of the carcinogen does not operate in humans. For example, thyroid follicular cell tumors due to drugs that enhance the metabolism of thyroid hormones[14] or Leydig cell tumors due to drugs that increase luteinizing hormone.[15]

Genetic toxicology data serve as a surrogate to rodent carcinogenicity data during development, but carcinogenicity studies are most often submitted prior to marketing approval. If the drug is indicated for a serious or life-threatening illness, the carcinogenicity studies can be conducted after approval, as a post-marketing requirement. While carcinogenicity data can impact drug approval, the data are primarily used to inform prescribing physicians through the drug label.

### 16.2.6 Miscellaneous Studies

Drug development sometimes requires additional studies beyond the routine toxicity testing described above. The need to conduct special toxicity studies is dependent on both the drug development strategy as well as empirical non-clinical data collected in early development. When warranted, ICH M3(R2)[4] recommends the following studies should be conducted prior to Phase 3:

- Immunotoxicity studies to further evaluate the effects identified during standard toxicity testing, such as leukocytopenia/leukocytosis, granulocytopenia, granulocytosis, or alterations in immune system organ weights (*e.g.*, thymus or spleen).[16]
- Photosafety studies for drugs that absorb sunlight and distribute to tissues of concern (*i.e.*, skin and/or eye).[17]
- Evaluations of abuse liability for drugs affecting the central nervous system.
- Local tolerance studies for drugs administered through parenteral routes.

Routine toxicology studies may also be needed to demonstrate the safety of novel excipients,[18] impurities,[19–22] unique or important clinical metabolites, and in some cases, drugs administered in combination.[23] For drugs intended for use in pediatric populations, non-clinical juvenile toxicity studies in an appropriate species are sometimes informative. Juvenile toxicity studies can be informative in drugs that target organs that undergo significant postnatal development, such as joints, or to address the reversibility of a known toxicity.[24]

Bridging studies are useful to support a change in the route of administration or a new formulation. For instance, general toxicity should be evaluated for exposures occurring by the new route of administration. Bridging toxicity studies may also be recommended if reformulation results in significant changes to systemic exposure. A change in drug synthesis will likely have qualitative and/or quantitative effects on the impurity profile. As a result, bridging studies may be needed to qualify new impurities or those present at higher levels than previously encountered. Genotoxicity testing or QSAR evaluations may be conducted if new impurities are structurally related to known genotoxins or carcinogens.

The recommended timing for submitting data from these evaluations varies; however, the studies may be relevant at all stages of development.

### 16.2.7 Toxicokinetics

Toxicokinetic (TK) data characterize systemic exposures to drugs and relevant metabolites. Measurements of blood/plasma drug concentrations at various timepoints are routinely included in *in vivo* studies and provide a basis for understanding the relationship of exposure with administered dose. Following quantitative analysis, an area under the curve (AUC) can be obtained by applying non-compartmental modeling of the concentration *vs.* time data. The AUC is also used to compare doses used in toxicology studies to human doses, for example in the carcinogenicity section of the physician's prescribing information. Other examples of toxicologically useful parameters obtained during TK analysis are the maximum plasma concentration ($C_{max}$), time of maximum plasma concentration ($T_{max}$), and half-life ($t_{1/2}$).

TK data can add needed perspective to dose–response by helping differentiate between linear and non-linear dose–response, or identifying saturation of systemic exposure. Systemic exposure data is also useful for detecting potential differences between males and females as well as decreases (*e.g.*, from enzyme induction) or increases (*e.g.*, from accumulation) in exposure over time. TK data from developmental and reproductive toxicology studies can help understand the extent to which drug crosses the placenta or is transmitted during lactation. In addition to TK evaluations of the parent drug, characterizing systemic exposure to metabolites may also be justified. In most cases, metabolite measurements are limited to those accounting for a significant fraction of systemic exposure (*e.g.*, >10% of exposure to total drug-related material).[3] ICH S3A[25] provides regulatory recommendations on the conduct of TK evaluations.

## 16.3 Small Molecule Drugs *vs.* Biopharmaceuticals

Small molecule drugs are primarily organic chemicals that can cause toxicity through both target effects (*e.g.*, exaggerated pharmacology) and off-target effects. Biopharmaceuticals include proteins, peptides, and monoclonal antibodies derived from biotechnological processes. Because biopharmaceuticals have greater specificity than small molecules, toxicity concerns are generally restricted to target effects. Therefore, toxicity testing of biopharmaceuticals should be limited to animal models where the drug is active and there is relevant tissue expression of the target. The use of two species is recommended but one may be adequate if no other relevant species exist.[24]

Another important difference between small molecules and biopharmaceuticals that impacts toxicity testing is the potential for immunogenicity. Immunogenicity occurs when a protein elicits an immunologic response, potentially resulting in unintended clearance of the drug and/or toxicity. Rapid clearance of the drug can limit the utility of long-term dosing. In addition to evaluating toxicokinetics of the drug, monitoring antibody response is critical to understand exposure-response.

All the standard non-clinical safety studies described above are generally considered appropriate to support clinical development and marketing for small molecule drugs. This is not the case for biopharmaceuticals. As a result of the special concerns previously mentioned, some studies are not likely to provide relevant information. Unless an organic linker is included in the molecule, standard genetic toxicology testing is not appropriate. Likewise, carcinogenicity studies are not recommended unless a mechanistic concern exists. Of primary interest are *in vivo* studies that include safety pharmacology, general toxicity, and immunotoxicity endpoints. Developmental/reproductive studies may be appropriate in some cases. ICH S6(R1)[26] provides regulatory recommendations for biopharmaceutical drug development.

## 16.4 Regulatory Decision Making

The use of non-clinical toxicology testing to identify and characterize hazards is one component of regulatory decision making but these must be interpreted in the context of the potential benefit of the drug.

Risk:benefit comparisons are fundamental to decision making and occur throughout development. As drugs are developed for indications ranging from those intended to maintain quality of life to those that will treat life-threating conditions, decisions are made on a case-by-case basis. Certain non-clinical toxicities, for example the risk of a temporary loss of fertility in men, may be acceptable for serious and life-threatening indications such as tuberculosis, but would not be acceptable for drugs indicated for less serious conditions, such as for headaches, where there are numerous alternatives. The patient population who will be administered a drug (s) during a clinical trial is another important consideration. A safety liability, such as a cancer risk from a genotoxic drug may be deemed inappropriate for clinical trials involving healthy subjects, but may not be viewed as unfavorably for trials involving patients. Similarly, adult patients may be viewed differently than a pediatric population. The duration of dosing will also be considered when making regulatory decisions.

A proposal to initiate a first in human trial must be supported by the appropriate non-clinical data. *In vitro* and/or *in vivo* data describing the activity of a drug are usually submitted to provide an initial indication of potential efficacy. However, the most important consideration at this stage of development is non-clinical safety studies. Using non-clinical data, the regulatory agency will determine whether a proposed clinical trial is appropriate based on the toxicities observed and the duration of non-clinical testing. In the US, a drug will be deemed inappropriate for administration in humans under any conditions resulting in a full clinical hold. Alternatively, dosing may be allowed in humans but under more restrictive conditions than those proposed by the sponsor's protocol. This partial clinical hold may include a reduction in the starting dose, overall dose range, duration of dosing, or number of subjects. If deficiencies resulting in a clinical hold are related to non-clinical data, additional studies may be required to remove the hold and allow clinical development to proceed. Throughout the drug development process, non-clinical data helps supplement the clinical experience gained in clinical trials and may also contribute to a drug being placed on full or partial clinical hold.

Non-clinical toxicology data is also considered at the marketing application stage (*e.g.*, NDA or BLA) and plays a role in the regulatory decision to approve a drug and under what conditions. During the review phase of a marketing application, the sponsor and regulatory agency collaborate on the drug label. The drug label provides details on use of the drug (*e.g.*, indication, recommended dose, and duration, potential or known interactions with other drugs) as well as clinical and non-clinical safety data. Critical considerations for the non-clinical data include effects on pregnancy and lactation, mutagenicity, carcinogenicity, fertility, and other significant findings from animal studies. The non-clinical information serves to inform prescribing physicians of the hazards and risks associated with the drug.

## 16.5 Hints and Tips

1. *Safety Pharmacology*: Characterize effects on vital physiological functions including extensive evaluations of central nervous system, cardiovascular, and respiratory parameters. Additional organ systems (*e.g.*, kidney, gastrointestinal, *etc.*) may also be evaluated when appropriate.

2. *Genetic Toxicology*: Characterize potential to induce changes in DNA sequence (*i.e.*, mutations). Recommended testing includes an *in vitro* assay to evaluated gene mutations (*i.e.*, Ames assay) and assays to evaluate chromosomal damage *in vitro* (*e.g.*, chromosomal aberrations) as well as *in vivo* (*e.g.*, micronuclei).
3. *General Toxicology*: Characterize drug-related toxicity occurring in the whole animal. Studies are conducted in both a rodent and a non-rodent species to maximize the predictive potential. Toxicity is identified through observations and measurements such as changes in behavior/appearance, body weight parameters, food consumption, ophthalmoscopy, and electrocardiograms. Clinical pathology data is collected to help identify target organs of toxicity by monitoring changes in hematology, coagulation, clinical chemistry, and urinalysis parameters.
4. *Developmental and Reproductive Toxicology*: Characterize effects on reproductive function in adult animals as well as development of offspring. Important evaluations include fertility and early embryonic development, embryo-fetal development, and pre- and postnatal development.
5. *Carcinogenicity*: Characterize induction of tumors arising through both genotoxic and non-genotoxic mechanisms. Studies in wild-type rodents include dosing periods of 2 years while the alternative transgenic mouse study requires only 6 months of dosing.
6. *Miscellaneous Studies*: In some cases, it may be necessary to further characterize immunotoxicity, photosafety, abuse liability, local tolerance, as well as juvenile toxicity. Testing of important clinical metabolites and combination drugs may also considered.
7. *Toxicokinetics*: Characterize systemic exposure to drugs and relevant metabolites. Measurements of blood/plasma drug concentrations at various timepoints are routinely included in *in vivo* studies and provide a basis for understanding the relationship of exposure with administered dose.
8. *Adverse Effects*: Important conclusions from animal studies include the no-observable adverse effect level (NOAEL), no-observable effect level (NOEL), lowest observable effect level (LOEL), and/or maximum tolerated dose (MTD). A 2016 working group of The European Society of Toxicologic Pathology, stated that "an adverse effect is a test item-related change in the morphology, physiology, growth, development, reproduction or life span of the animal model that likely results in an impairment of functional capacity to maintain homeostasis and/or an impairment of the capacity to respond to an additional challenge"; it is important to note that many other definitions of adversity exist.
9. *Safety Margins*: Initial clinical trials are generally considered reasonably safe if the converted NOAEL dose is ≥10-fold the proposed clinical starting dose. A more refined method of calculating safety margins is to compare systemic exposure values once both non-clinical and clinical data are available. Larger or smaller safety margins may be appropriate depending on the non-clinical toxicity profile observed.

## Disclaimer

The views expressed are those of the authors. No official support or endorsements by the United States Food and Drug Administration are provided.

## Key References

ICH, *M3(R2) - Nonclinical Safety Studies for the Conduct of Human Clinical Trials and Marketing Authorization for Pharmaceuticals*, 2009.

- Provides comprehensive summary of regulatory recommendations addressing non-clinical development of small molecules.

ICH, *S6(R1) – Preclinical Safety Evaluation of Biotechnology-derived Pharmaceuticals*, 2011.

- Provides comprehensive summary of regulatory recommendations addressing non-clinical development of large molecules.

FDA, *Guidance for Industry: Estimating the Maximum Safe Starting Dose in Initial Clinical Trials for Therapeutics in Adult Healthy Volunteers*, 2005.

- Provides description of methods for calculating safety margins and rationale supporting more conservative approaches to clinical trials.

## Acknowledgements

The authors would like to thank Dr Mark W. Powley for his contributions to this chapter.

## References

1. L. A. Buckley, I. Bebenek, P. D. Cornwell, A. Hodowanec, E. C. Jensen, C. Murphy and H. N. Ghantous, *Int. J. Toxicol.*, 2020, **39**(5), 379.
2. ICH, Harmonised Tripartite Guideline S7A, *Safety Pharmacology Studies for Human Pharmaceuticals*, Step 4 Version, November 2000.
3. ICH, Harmonised Tripartite Guideline S7B, *Non-clinical Evaluation of the Potential for Delayed Ventricular Repolarization (QT Interval Prolongation) by Human Pharmaceuticals*, Step 4 Version, May 2005.
4. ICH, Harmonised Tripartite Guideline M3(R2), *Nonclinical Safety Studies for the Conduct of Human Clinical Trials and Marketing Authorization for Pharmaceuticals*, Step 4 Version, June 2009.
5. ICH, Harmonised Tripartite Guideline S2(R1), *Genotoxicity Testing and Data Interpretation for Pharmaceuticals Intended for Human Use*, Step 4 Version, November 2011.
6. X. Palazzi, J. E. Burkhardt, H. Caplain, V. Dellarco, P. Fant, J. R. Foster, S. Francke, P. Germann, S. Gröters, T. Harada, J. Harleman, K. Inui, W. Kaufmann, B. Lenz, H. Nagai, G. Pohlmeyer-Esch, A. Schulte, M. Skydsgaard, L. Tomlinson, C. E. Wood and M. Yoshida, *Toxicol. Pathol.*, 2016, **44**(6), 810.
7. Food, Drug Administration HHS, *Guidance for Industry: Estimating the Maximum Safe Starting Dose in Initial Clinical Trials for Therapeutics in Adult Healthy Volunteers*, July 2005.
8. ICH, Harmonised Tripartite Guideline S5(R3), *Guideline on Reproductive Toxicology: Detection of Toxicity to Reproduction for Human Pharmaceuticals*, February 2020.
9. ICH, *Addendum to the ICH Guideline S1B on Testing for Carcinogenicity of Pharmaceuticals*, May 2021.

10. ICH, Harmonised Tripartite Guideline S1A, *Guideline on the Need for Carcinogenicity Studies of Pharmaceuticals*, Step 4 Version, November 1996.
11. ICH, Harmonised Tripartite Guideline S1B, *Testing for Carcinogenicity of Pharmaceuticals*, Step 4 Version, July 1997.
12. ICH, Harmonised Tripartite Guideline S1C(R2), *Dose Selection for Carcinogenicity Studies of Pharmaceuticals*, Step 4 Version, March 2008.
13. MAPP 7412.1 Rev. 2 Management of CDER Executive Carcinogenicity Assessment Committee and Communication of Committee Proceedings, available at http://www.fda.gov/AboutFDA/CentersOffices/OfficeofMedicalProductsandTobacco/CDER/ManualofPoliciesProcedures/default/ht.
14. K. M. Wu and J. G. Farrelly, *Am. J. Ther.*, 2006, **13**(2), 141.
15. M. Murakami, S. Hosokawa, T. Yamada, M. Harakawa, M. Ito, Y. Koyama, J. Kimura, A. Yoshitake and H. Yamada, *Toxicol. Appl. Pharmacol.*, 1995, **131**(2), 244.
16. ICH, Harmonised Tripartite Guideline S8, *Immunotoxicity Studies for Human Pharmaceuticals*, Step 4 Version, September 2005.
17. ICH, Harmonised Tripartite Guideline S10, *Photosafety Evaluation of Pharmaceuticals*, Step 4 Version, November 2013.
18. Food, Drug Administration HHS, *Guidance for Industry: Nonclinical Studies for the Safety Evaluation of Pharmaceutical Excipients*, May 2005.
19. ICH, Harmonised Tripartite Guideline Q3A(R2), *Impurities in New Drug Substances*, Step 4 Version, October 2006.
20. ICH, Harmonised Tripartite Guideline Q3B(R2), *Impurities in New Drug Products*, Step 4 Version, June 2006.
21. ICH, Harmonised Tripartite Guideline Q3C(R5), *Impurities: Guidelines for Residual Solvents*, Step 4 Version, April 2021.
22. ICH, Harmonised Tripartite Guideline M7, *Assessment and Control of DNA Reactive (Mutagenic) Impurities in Pharmaceuticals to Limit Potential Carcinogenic Risk*, Step 4 Version, March 2017.
23. Food, Drug Administration HHS, *Requesting FDA Feedback on Combination Products: Guidance for Industry and FDA Staff*, December 2020.
24. Food, Drug Administration HHS, *Guidance for Industry Nonclinical Safety Evaluation of Pediatric Drug Products, Nonclinical Safety Evaluation of Pediatric Drug Products*, February 2006.
25. ICH, Harmonised Tripartite Guideline S3A, *Toxicokinetics: The Assessment of Systemic Exposure in Toxicity Studies*, Step 4 Version, October 1994.
26. ICH, Harmonised Tripartite Guideline S6(R1), *Preclinical Safety Evaluation of Biotechnology-Derived Pharmaceuticals*, Step 4 Version, June 2011.

# 17 Patents for Medicines

Paul A. Brady*[a] and Andrew Cook[b]

[a]Abel & Imray Patent Attorneys, 20 St Andrew Street, London EC4A 3AG, United Kingdom; [b]AstraZeneca, Global Intellectual Property, Eastbrook House, Shaftesbury Road, Cambridge CB2 8BF, United Kingdom
*E-mail: paul.brady@abelimray.com

## 17.1 Introduction

As pointed out by PhRMA, the leading US biopharmaceutical industry research company body, "Intellectual Property is the bedrock on which the development of new treatments and cures is built".[1] This viewpoint is reinforced by headlines in the financial pages of newspapers along the lines of "Patent cliff losses set to cost pharma $65bn by 2019"[2] and "Pfizer, Merck drop after Wall Street downgrades on 'patent cliff' and competition".[3]

This last comment regarding competition from generic companies is a key to the importance of patents. The costs of researching and developing a new medicine before it can be authorised for marketing are huge. Estimates for the cost of getting a medicine from the bench to the market place range from $1.3 billion to in excess of $2.5 billion.[4,5] In contrast, the cost of manufacturing that medicine is small, particularly when the active ingredient is a low molecular weight chemical entity – maybe the order of few dollars or even a few cents per unit dose.

In order to justify such huge up-front investments in R&D, investors will need to know that they will have a period of exclusivity to give them an opportunity to recoup some of that investment. Once there is competition from a "copycat" or generic version of the medicine, the price falls dramatically: a generic competitor who has not had to make the investment in the drug's development can operate profitably at a much lower sale price. As a result, the originator's market share of the sales of the medicine decreases dramatically, and without an initial period of exclusivity, any incentive to invest in innovation is undermined.

A typical illustration of the originator's investments and earnings for a drug is shown in Figure 17.1. In the figure, points below the $x$-axis represent investment (*i.e.* cost) and

The Handbook of Medicinal Chemistry: Principles and Practice, 2nd Edition
Edited by Simon E. Ward and Andrew M. Davis

Published by the Royal Society of Chemistry, www.rsc.org

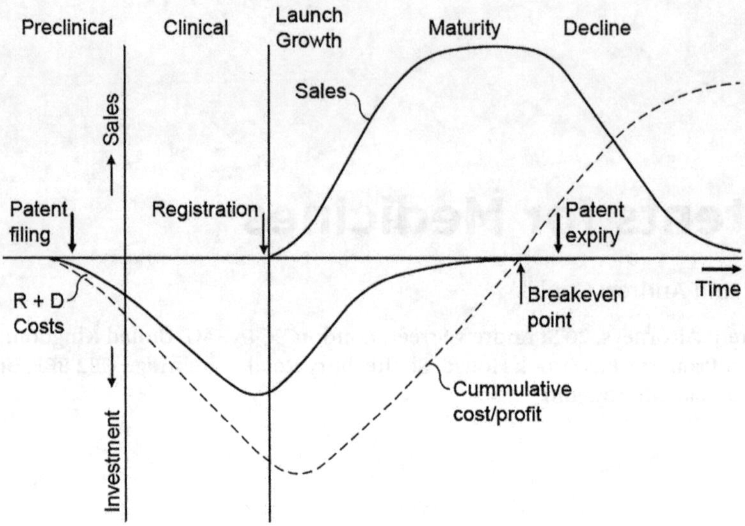


**Figure 17.1** Typical illustration of the originator's investments and earnings for a drug over its lifetime.

points above the *x*-axis represent income. Before registration, there is only expenditure and the area under the curve (*i.e.* the cumulative cost/profit) is entirely beneath the axis. Income to off-set the earlier expenditure only starts when the drug receives its registration, and the amount of time available to the originator company is limited by the timing of generic entry. A typical profile for sales figures of a medicine is shown in Figure 17.2. Annual sales grow steadily in the time after the product is placed on the market. However, once the patent expires, the originator's sales drop dramatically. It is not uncommon for sales to fall by over 80% within 3 months of the patent expiry. It is this drop in sales that prompts the decline shown in Figure 17.1.

All of the costs of the development of a drug must be recouped before the price collapse, and patents are the main tool that a drug originator has to maintain its exclusivity and thus delay the price collapse. Patents are therefore key to the viability of a drug development company as a business. It is vital that scientists working in drug discovery gain a good working knowledge of the patent system, both to avoid costly errors, and to help flag inventions when they are made. This chapter aims to give an insight into what patents are, what they can do, and how they are obtained and used. Beyond patents, there are further forms of market exclusivity, such as regulatory data exclusivity, and in some situations, such as when an old compound is first developed into a medicine or when an existing medicine is repurposed, those can be very important. They are discussed in Section 17.9.2 below.

## 17.2 What is a Patent?

A patent is an exclusionary right, and it gives its owner the right to exclude others from using the invention. It is important to note that a patent does not give its owner the right to practice their own invention; there may be other patents or impediments that

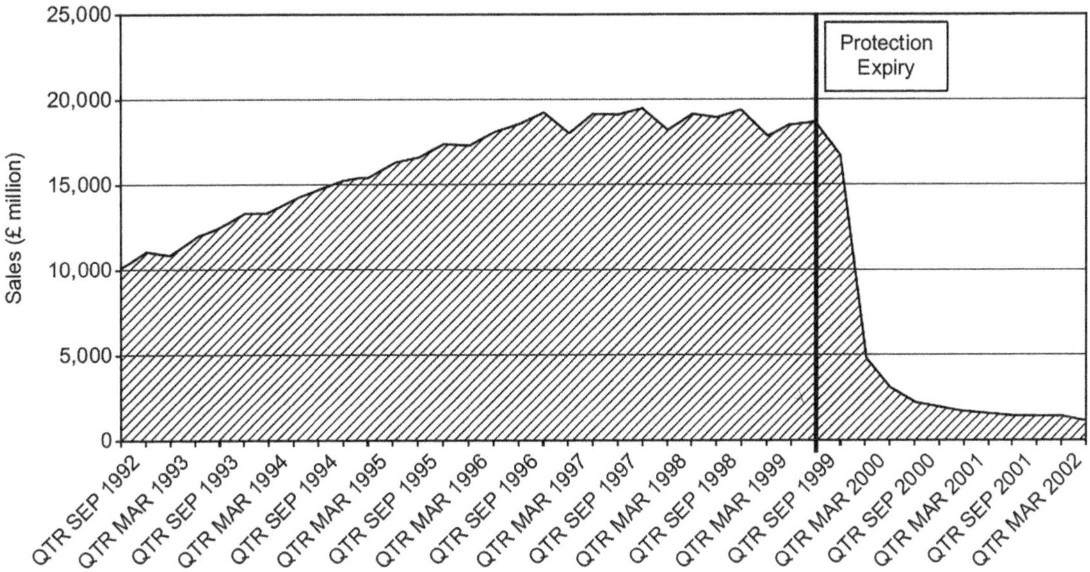


**Figure 17.2** Typical sales figures for a drug through the time of patent expiry.

prevent that. For example, a competitor may have a broad patent which protects an area where a later patent is granted. Patents are one of several rights collectively referred to as "Intellectual Property". Other forms of Intellectual Property include Trade Marks (names and logos applied to goods or services), Copyright (for creative works), Registered Design Right (for the appearance of articles), confidential information (including "know-how") and regulatory data exclusivity. These other rights are also important in the pharmaceutical industry, especially Trade Marks and regulatory data exclusivity, but they generally arise late in the drug discovery process or when a medicine is already on the market. However, patents are the most important rights for most organisations involved in drug discovery and development or drug manufacture.

Patents are granted for products (compounds, compositions, formulations, *etc.*) or for processes (routes of synthesis, methods of use). A patent for a product gives the owner the right to prevent others from making, using, offering for sale, or selling the invention defined by the patent claims in the country in which the patent has been granted and to prevent others from importing a product covered by the claims into that country. Where the invention relates to a process, the patent gives the owner the right to exclude others from using the claimed process or from using, offering for sale or selling in the country in which the patent has been granted, or importing, products made by that process.

Use of a patented invention without the permission of the patent proprietor is called infringement. The exclusive patent right is enforceable in a court of law, where the patent owner sues the infringer for patent infringement. More information on infringement is given in Section 17.8 below.

In general, policy makers and legislators are reluctant to grant monopoly rights: they can harm competition and they interfere with the operation of the free market. Patents are an exception to this general rule, and a patent constitutes a special "bargain" between an inventor and the state: in return for the inventor disclosing the invention to the public (all patent applications are published, generally 18 months after the first patent application is made for the invention), the inventor is granted a monopoly over the commercial use of the invention for a limited period (20 years in most countries). At the end of the patent term, the invention is available to the public for use. The period of exclusivity serves as an incentive to innovate and invent. This way, patents stimulate innovation and advances happen that would otherwise not happen. The net result is that technology progresses and humanity benefits.

The importance of the patent bargain was very recently highlighted by the UK's highest court, the Supreme Court, in *Unwired Planet International Ltd v Huawei Technologies (UK) Co Ltd*, a patent case concerning the alleged infringement of various telecommunications patents. In the Supreme Court's view:

> The starting point is the 'patent bargain' which promotes innovation and justifies the monopoly which a patent gives an inventor. The patent bargain is this: an inventor receives the reward of a time-limited monopoly of the industrial use of its invention in return for disclosing the invention and dedicating it to the public for use after the monopoly has expired.[6]

The principles behind patents apply across all fields of technology, and they are especially important in drug development: society as a whole requires medicines for diseases that are not yet adequately controllable. Without the availability of a period of market exclusivity, companies (and indeed charities and governments) could not invest the necessary, and large, resources needed to develop the next generation of medicines.

To ensure that the monopoly granted to an inventor is fair and commensurate to the inventor's contribution, it is necessary for the scope of the patent to be accurately defined and scrutinised. The scope of a patent is defined by its claims. A patent claim is a concise and precise definition of the invention, generally in a single sentence. The claims are usually found at the end of the patent specification, under the heading "claims". The claims are of central importance to a patent: it is the claims that are compared with what had been known before (the "prior art") in order to determine whether the grant of the patent is justified; and it is the claims that determine what competitors are not permitted to do. More information on claims is given in Section 17.4 below.

In some quarters, patents are perceived as being linked to secrecy. In fact, the opposite is true: the word "patent" is derived from the Latin "patens" meaning to lie open. This refers to how patents force open disclosure of technology, which might otherwise be kept secret. The lasting record of much of humanity's technology development of the last few centuries is to be found primarily in the patent literature. Patent publications thus form an important repository of information. More information on the patent literature and how to access it is given in Section 17.10 below.

For a more detailed treatment of patents for medicines than can be provided in this chapter, we recommend the book *Patents for Chemicals, Pharmaceuticals, and Biotechnology* by Grubb *et al.* which, at the time of writing is in its 6th edition.[7]

## 17.3 What Conditions Need to be Fulfilled in Order for a Patent to be Granted? Patentability

Patents need to be applied for *via* the national or regional patent office serving a particular country. Patent office officials, known as "examiners", carry out rigorous checks to determine whether or not all the requirements are met. If they are, then a patent is granted. In all countries, it is possible for a court to revoke a patent that has been granted, if it is later established that the requirements for patentability have not in fact been fulfilled.

Patents are granted by governments and the details vary somewhat from country to country. The following discussion gives broad-brush information applicable to most developed patent systems.

The statutes on patents set out that an invention must fulfil the following four criteria in order to be patentable. The criteria ensure that the inventor fulfils their side of the bargain in the "bargain" between an inventor and the state mentioned in Section 17.2 above and does in fact provide the public with a new invention. The invention must:

- be novel
- be inventive
- have industrial applicability
- not be specifically excluded from being protectable by a patent.

In addition, so that the public is in fact given all the tools and information needed to put the invention into effect and the patent applicant fulfils its obligations in the disclosure part of the "bargain", the specification for the patent application must:

- describe the invention sufficiently clearly and completely for the person skilled in the art to be able to put the invention into practice.

A patent which meets all of the requirements of the law is said to be "valid". Taking each of the above criteria in turn:

### 17.3.1 Novelty

An invention is novel if, at the date on which the patent application is filed, the invention is not in the state of the art. The state of the art is taken to be everything that has been disclosed to the public up to that date. Disclosures in any form must be taken into account. The state of the art thus includes not only printed publications and publications on the internet, but also oral disclosures, such as conference presentations or non-confidential discussions. Disclosure to the public can also occur by demonstrating a prototype or showing images in a video. There is no requirement for a disclosure to be generally known to workers in the field: an obscure disclosure, which might be in a foreign language, must also be taken into account.

The requirement for novelty flows from the requirement of the "bargain" mentioned in Section 17.2 above: if the invention was already known, then the inventor is not providing anything to fulfil their side of the bargain.

An important feature of novelty is that the inventor's own disclosure of their own invention is also part of the state of the art. An inventor's own disclosure before filing a patent application can thus compromise the novelty of an invention. It is thus crucial that an invention be kept confidential until a patent application is filed. Some countries, notably the US and Japan, provide a "grace period", a period in which inventors may publish their invention without damaging their own later patent application. A large number of countries (including most of Europe) have no grace period, however, so deliberate use of the grace period is not advised. Controlling disclosures prior to filing patent applications is a vital part of achieving effective patent protection across the world.

### 17.3.2 Inventive Step

In addition to possessing novelty, an invention must have an inventive step. An invention has an inventive step if it is not obvious over what was in the state of the art at the patent filing date. Referring again to the "bargain" mentioned in Section 17.2 above, the public should not be prevented from doing something that is a non-inventive variant of something that was already known. To use the often quoted example set out in the European Patent Office Guidelines for Examination, a machine for producing sausages, which consists of a known mincing machine and a known filling machine disposed side by side, is not inventive. It is instead a non-inventive combination of two "known devices or processes functioning in their normal way and not producing any non-obvious working relationship".[8]

Once it has been established what the state of the art comprises, the question of novelty should be a black and white one: "was something inside the patent claims disclosed before the patent filing date or not?". The question of inventive step is generally much more nuanced.

A large number of patent cases that reach the courts turn on the question of inventive step. The courts and patent offices have thus formulated tests in order to bring structure to the assessment so as to increase legal certainty for patent applicants and the public. The tests by the various authorities require a definition of the "person skilled in the art". Much has been written about this legal construct: they are taken to know everything that has ever been published or disclosed in other ways, but they have no inquisitiveness, and follow only very highlighted leads. In the case of Pfizer's patent covering the mechanism of action of Sildenafil (marketed under the trade mark Viagra ®) and other cGMP phosphodiesterase inhibitors in the treatment of erectile dysfunction, the person skilled in the art was described as follows by the UK High Court judge Mr Justice Laddie:

> The question of obviousness has to be assessed through the eyes of the skilled but non-inventive man in the art. This is not a real person. He is a legal creation. [...] He is deemed to have looked at and read publicly available documents and to know of public uses in the prior art. He understands all languages and dialects. He never

> misses the obvious nor stumbles on the inventive. He has no private idiosyncratic preferences or dislikes. He never thinks laterally. He differs from all real people in one or more of these characteristics.[9]

Thus, the "person skilled in the art" is not a single person that could ever exist, certainly not in a research or development role. In practice, it is necessary to gather evidence from the field of the invention regarding what was generally known to teams working in the relevant area, and then to impute that knowledge into the fictitious "person skilled in the art".

The European Patent Office (EPO) has probably the most rigid approach to the assessment of inventive step. This has become known as the "Problem and Solution Approach". The approach starts with identifying what is the single disclosure in the prior art that is the closest to what is claimed in the patent in question. Next, one has to see what the difference is between that disclosure and the claimed invention. Then one has to identify what technical effect that difference has, and whether that effect was plausible at the time of filing. That technical effect defines what the problem is that is considered to be solved by the invention (it may or may not be the same problem that the inventor actually thought they were working on). One then asks the question, "starting from the closest prior art disclosure, and trying to solve that problem, would it have been obvious to arrive at what is now claimed?".

Taking a chemical example: an inventor has devised a set of compounds with general formula (X) which have good activity at receptor Y. In the prior art, there is a compound (A) with structure similar to (X), but with a methyl group at a particular location where (X) has a phenyl group. The compounds (X) with the phenyl group have a higher affinity to receptor Y than compound (A) with the methyl group. One would then have to answer the question: starting from compound (A) and wishing to obtain a compound with higher affinity, would it be obvious to replace the methyl group in the compound with the phenyl group? The answer will depend on whether that replacement is known in other compounds to bring about the change in activity that has been found by the inventor.

This issue arose in the case of Olanzapine. Olanzapine is an anti-psychotic agent that is used in the treatment of schizophrenia. It has the following chemical structure:

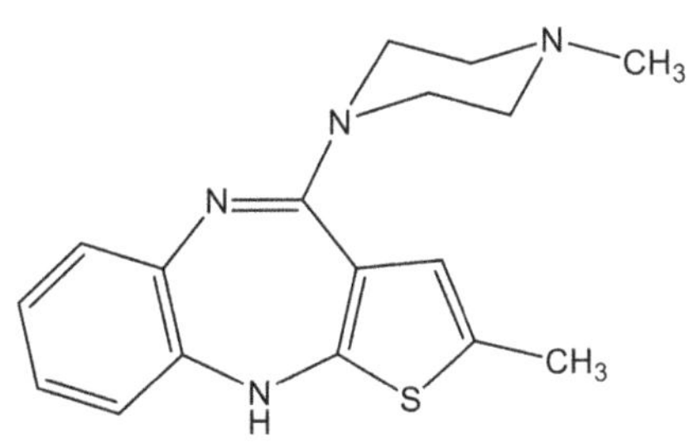


The validity of Eli Lilly's patent covering Olanzapine was challenged and the matter went to Court in the UK, with appeal to the Court of Appeal. In the case, a prior art journal publication was a report of an SAR study of potential neuroleptics and it included the disclosure of the general formula below.

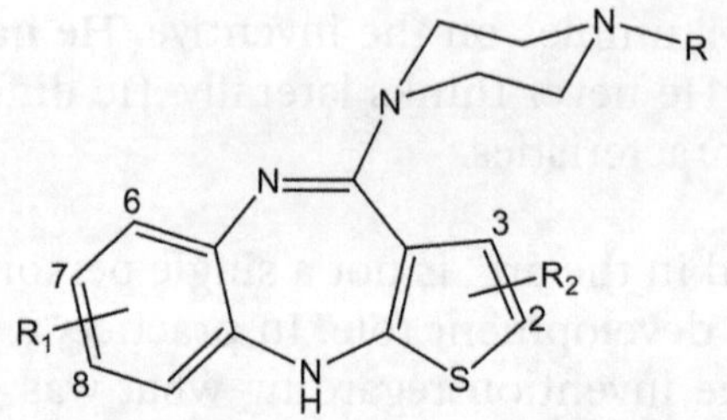

Olanzapine is the compound in which R is methyl, $R_1$ is hydrogen and $R_2$ is 2-methyl. The prior art publication included several example compounds in which R, $R_1$ and $R_2$ were varied, including the prepared and characterised example compound ("Compound 6") in which R was methyl, $R_1$ was hydrogen and $R_2$ was 2-ethyl. That is to say that Olanzapine differed from the published compound by the change of 2-ethyl to 2-methyl in the thiophene ring. The 2-methyl compound had good potency and low extra-pyramidal symptom side effects. Based on the description of the SAR in the paper and the skilled person's common general knowledge at the time, the UK High Court and Court of Appeal held that it was not obvious that the benefits would be obtained from the structural change that Eli Lilly made. The methyl compound (Olanzapine) was therefore held to be inventive and the patent was maintained as valid.[10]

An important factor in determining the answer is how predictable the field of technology is. If the field is highly unpredictable, then a finding that a compound has activity might very often be surprising, and hence supportive of inventive step. In a field that is unpredictable, it is all the more important that a patent applicant provides good evidence that the invention does indeed solve the problem. Generally, the evidence will be in the form of results of laboratory experiments. The better the evidence that the patent applicant can provide, the better will be the prospects of succeeding in demonstrating that the invention has an inventive step.

The EPO "Problem and Solution Approach" is perhaps the most rigid of the tests that have been developed. Slightly different tests are used in other places, sometimes giving similar results, and sometimes not. For a more extended analysis of inventive step treatment in different territories, see ref. 11 and 12.

The structured tests are of assistance when assessing inventive step and it is important that they are considered when one is writing a patent application. At the same time, it must be remembered that they are only helpful tests rather than the ultimate law itself, and so they must not be overly relied upon. Amongst other things, the tests evolve and can be overturned. A decade or more can pass between a patent application being written and a case coming to court. That is plenty of time for the approach on a particular matter to evolve. In general, a patent applicant puts themself in the best possible position by obtaining good data showing that the invention works well. Experiments comparing the invention side-by-side with what has been done before are especially useful. This sometimes involves making a different comparison from what would be done for an academic research paper: for a research paper, the important comparator to look at might be the "Gold Standard", or the current standard clinical treatment. To support inventive step in a patent application, the comparator should be the prior art compound or method that is closest in its features to what is being claimed. That compound or method from the prior art might be obscure, or it might not have achieved mainstream acceptance for other reasons, such as cost.

### 17.3.3 Industrial Applicability

An invention is considered to be capable of industrial application if it is made or used in any kind of industry. The concept of "industry" is interpreted very broadly, and includes essentially any commercial enterprise. In practice, and certainly in the field of drug discovery, essentially any invention will satisfy the industrial applicability requirement. In the early days of DNA sequencing, when certain sequences were determined but their function was not known, some patent applications for DNA sequences were refused under this heading. In 2011, the UK Supreme Court determined in the case of *Eli Lilly v. Human Genome Sciences* regarding a DNA sequence (for the gene for neutrokine alpha) that HGS's identification of the gene as being a member of the TNF ligand superfamily was adequate to show that the sequence had an industrial applicability, even though the assertion had not been supported by any wet laboratory work by the time the patent application was filed.[13] The requirement forces applicants and their patent attorneys to think about real-world uses of their inventions when formulating patent claims, but in general it is rarely a factor that actually interferes with being able to obtain a patent.

### 17.3.4 Exclusions

Certain forms of development are specifically excluded from patentability by the patent statutes for social or ethical reasons. The exclusion that most affects medicine is that most jurisdictions have a bar on the patenting of methods of medical treatment. The rationale for the exclusion is that patent law should not interfere with what a doctor can do when he or she is treating a patient.

In recognition of the fact that patents are key to the medical industry, many statutes make it clear that the exclusion does not prohibit the grant of a patent for a substance or composition for use in a method of treatment. This means that special wording must be used. In Europe, the use of a compound as a drug can be patented, but a patent claim must have the wording "compound X for use in the treatment of disease Y", rather than the more intuitive "method of treating disease Y by administering compound X". This may look like wordplay that subverts the exclusion in the statute, but that is not the case: the wording of the allowed claim makes it clear that it is the compound that is the infringement, thus making manufacturers and suppliers the potential infringers, rather than the doctor at the bedside carrying out the method.

In the US, methods of medical treatment are not excluded from patentability, and they are regularly granted by the US Patent and Trademark Office. The US patent statute deals with this matter in a different way, by exempting from the definition of patent infringement a medical practitioner's performance of a "medical activity" on a human or animal. The same end result of allowing doctors to treat patients how they see fit without a threat of patent infringement is thus achieved in the US in a different and, most would say, more logical way than in Europe.

In addition to methods of medical treatment, the excluded subject matter list for Europe also includes abstract concepts (discoveries, scientific theories or mathematical methods, and also methods for performing a mental act, playing a game, or doing business), or a program for a computer, and inventions the exploitation of which would be contrary to public policy or morality. This last category presents a bar to the grant of patent claims to a human being, in any stage of its development. In 2011, it was decided by the highest court in Europe that this includes human embryonic stem cells.[14,15] In certain areas of medical research, if patents are to be obtained, it is necessary to develop strategies to deal with this exclusion, for example by ensuring that any stem cells used are not derived from human embryos. The exclusion of computer programs should not be taken at face value: over the years, case law has developed to take account of the evolution of computers from simple mathematical machines that carry out abstract calculations to integral parts of modern technological devices with real-world technical effects. In practice, many software-based inventions are now patent-eligible.

### 17.3.5 Clarity and Sufficiency/Reproducibility

It is necessary for a patent application text to describe the invention with sufficient clarity and detail for the person skilled in the art to carry it out without having to use any inventive skill. The reason for this requirement is again linked to the "bargain" described in Section 17.2 above. If the patent applicant is to deserve the 20 year period of monopoly, the patent must describe the invention in such a way that at the end of the 20 year patent term, the public has full use of the invention and can put it into effect. The patent applicant is not allowed to keep important details secret. The standard of description is similar to that required for publication of a paper in a peer-reviewed journal.

For the preparation of chemical compounds, the sufficiency requirement is generally met if the patent application contains a description of the synthesis of specific example compounds. Usually, it is adequate to provide a single synthetic route but it is important that the descriptions start from compounds that are in the literature or are commercially available. For claims to compounds used in very specific treatments, the description should include details of how the treatment is carried out.

In the US, there is a particular requirement to disclose what the inventors consider at the time of filing the patent application to be the "best mode" of working the invention. The rationale behind the requirement is sound: it is a more rigorous onus on patent applicants to keep their side of the bargain described in Section 17.2 above. Until 2011, failure to disclose the "best mode" was a ground of invalidity or unenforceability of an issued patent. Significant attention therefore needed to be given to making sure that the best mode was described in a patent, and patent specifications in the pharmaceuticals area from before 2011 will therefore often include extensive descriptions of alternative synthetic routes, salts, or formulations. However, when US patent law was revised in 2011 with the passing into law of the "America Invents Act", failure to disclose the "best mode" ceased to be a basis for invalidating or rendering unenforceable an issued patent and the attention given to the requirement is now thus much reduced. It remains the case, however, that if a patent applicant leaves out pertinent information, then they risk not being able to make a narrowing amendment that they might later want to make. They also risk a competitor obtaining a patent on a narrow, but important, aspect of their invention.

The sufficiency requirement is particularly important in the case of certain biotechnological inventions. An antibody that has been raised by challenging the immune system of a laboratory mouse with a selected antigen may have very beneficial properties and may in principle be patentable. However, the isolation of a particular specific antibody can be a matter of chance, and a paper description alone will often not provide a skilled reader with everything they need to carry out the invention themself. To deal with this situation, there exist specifically approved International Depository Authorities which house and maintain samples of antibodies or other biological entities and make them available to members of the public who request them.

## 17.4 Anatomy of a Patent Specification

As will be apparent from the material above, patents are a specialised and complex field. Whilst it is possible for inventors to write and file their own patent applications, the drafting of a patent application is best carried out as a collaborative effort between the inventors and their patent attorney. Patent attorneys are scientists by background with specialised legal training. As a medicinal chemist, you will have significant involvement in the drafting of patent applications in your field. This section should provide some guidance as to what may be expected of you in that process.

The key part of a patent application is the "patent specification", which consists of a description and a set of claims, and in many cases figures. The claims will generally be written by the patent attorney, in close discussion with the scientists and often also a business manager. As a medicinal chemist, you will probably be involved mostly in the writing of the description. The writing of a patent specification has some features in common with the writing of an academic paper, but some important differences.

### 17.4.1 The Description

The description has several parts:

*Introduction*: this has to inform the reader of the technical field and background art. The technical field is important to direct the Patent Office Searcher to the correct area in which to carry out the search. The background does not need to be an analysis of the literature in the broad area of the invention, and it does not need to explain to the reader how the invention came about. It thus differs from the typical introduction to an academic paper. The introduction to a patent application should simply describe a small number of closest previous disclosures to show the prior art from which the invention is an advance. Ideally, this should include the "closest prior art" discussed in Section 17.3 above under inventive step, but that is not always known at the time of writing. The introduction may include a description of drawbacks or shortfalls of the prior art. Care needs to be taken in describing those shortfalls, as the new invention might well be an advance but not necessarily overcome all of the shortfalls in the prior art.

Before any patent searching has been carried out, the medicinal chemist will have a better idea of the background art than the patent attorney, and the medicinal chemist might thus often write the first draft of the introduction.

*Statement of Invention*: after the introduction, there follows a statement of invention. This is a re-stating of the main patent claim: "The invention provides compounds of formula (X)". That is followed by some statements setting out what is new and useful about the invention: "The compounds have high activity at receptor Y and they thus have use in the treatment of disease Z".

*Detailed Description*: this is the meaty part of the specification. Each aspect of the invention should be described in further detail. This includes setting out fall-back positions that are narrower than the main claims, in case something comes to light that means that the broadest claim cannot be pursued to grant. For the purposes of sufficiency of disclosure, the description also needs to explain how to carry out the invention. If there are alternative ways of carrying out the invention, the detailed description should include as many of them as possible. It is often also in a patent applicant's interest to disclose features here (for example combination treatments with other drugs) so as to put them into the public domain. When the patent application publishes, that disclosure prevents a third party from applying for a patent for those features.

*Worked Examples*: these follow the detailed description and they describe actual preparations and experiments that have been carried out. They serve in part to substantiate the sufficiency of disclosure. They also serve to provide evidence of the beneficial properties that underpin the inventive step of the invention. Generally, the medicinal chemist is the main author of the worked examples section.

*The Claims*: the claims define the invention; they define the monopoly that the applicant is requesting. They must be entirely clear and self-contained, they must not overlap with what is in the prior art, and everything within the claims must have the beneficial features that underpin the invention. The specific worked examples will have a strong bearing on inventive step, but the applicant actually provides more to the public than the specific examples; they may be opening up a whole new field or they may be providing a new class of compounds. Commensurate to the contribution to the art, the applicant is thus generally entitled to claim the invention more broadly than the specific worked examples: close variants can also be claimed. One of the most difficult elements in the drafting of a patent application is determining the best scope of claim to apply for. Features can be generalised, but everything in the claim must have the invention's beneficial features. The generalisation is thus constrained by what can reasonably be extrapolated from the data that has been obtained. At the same time, the whole of the scope must be novel and not obvious. This requires a complicated balance to be struck.

The patent application will contain several claims, so a broad and generalised first claim can be backed up by narrower claims. A patent can also contain claims in several different categories, for example a compound and its use. Categories of claims are summarised in the next section below.

### 17.4.2 Types of Patent Claim

Depending on the stage of the research, an invention can arise in various elements of a new medicine:

*Compound per se*: if a compound has never been made before, it is possible to claim the compound (and compounds similar to it) itself ("*per se*"). That claim covers the compound in any setting, in any form and for any use. In the US, this is called a "composition of matter" claim.

*Use in medicine (first medical use claims/methods of medical treatment)*: if a compound is known, but it has not previously had a use in medicine, then it is possible to claim the compound for use as a medicament (Europe, Japan and many other territories), or a method of treatment using the compound (US).

*Further uses in medicine (second medical use claims/second method of medical treatment)*: if a compound is known to have a use in medicine for the treatment of one (or more) conditions, and the compound is later found to have a use in the treatment of a second (or further) condition, then it is possible to claim that second use. The form of claim that is needed varies between countries: the claim can be to the compound for use in the treatment of that second condition (Europe), to the use of the compound in the manufacture of a medicament for the treatment of the second condition (Japan, China and many other territories), or to a method of treatment of the second condition using the compound (US).

*Salts or crystalline forms*: during drug development, new physical forms of the drug compound often need to be developed (such as polymorphs). Where several forms can exist and a new one is developed with beneficial and surprising properties, then the new form can be claimed in a patent.

*Composition claims and combinations*: a particular composition with particular excipients or with a particular other drug might be developed. If such a composition provides beneficial properties, the composition can be claimed.

*Dosage regimen claims*: if a clinical trial shows that a particular dosing regimen brings unexpected benefits, then such a regimen can, in many countries, be the subject of a patent.

*Synthetic processes*: improved methods of preparing compounds can be patentable.

In general, going down this list, the value of the protection decreases. This is for a combination of two reasons: the further one goes down the list, the more opportunities there are for a competitor to work around the claim, for example by devising an alternative route of synthesis; also in general the further one goes down the list the easier it is for a third party to challenge the inventive step of a claim. A drug development team puts itself in the best overall position by having a "portfolio" of patents covering various aspects of the final product. The later-filed patents for downstream developments may provide protection that is less secure than the first compound *per se* patent, but the later-filed patents have later expiry dates which may give them added value in practice.

## 17.4.3 Case Study (a): Typical Claims in a Pharmaceutical Patent

### *17.4.3.1 Small Molecule Drugs – Revlimid*

Lenalidomide is currently the world's highest selling small molecule drug. It is marketed by Celgene under the name Revlimid® for the treatment of multiple myeloma. It has the structure shown in Figure 17.3. It was first approved by the European Medicine Agency (EMA) in 2007 and by the US Food and Drug Administration (FDA) in 2005.

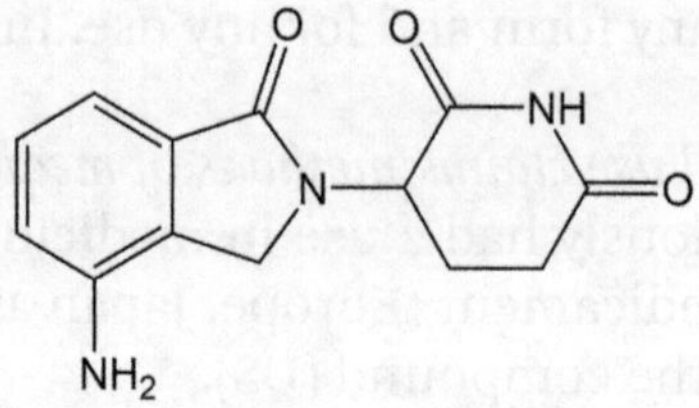

Figure 17.3 The structure lenalidomide, sold as Revlimid®.

The main patent protecting lenalidomide in Europe was EP0925294B. It expired on 24 July 2017, and its patent term extension will remain in force until 2022 (see Section 17.7.2 below for details of patent term extensions). The patent specification can be accessed for free over the internet from the Espacenet Database.[16]

Lenalidomide is 1-oxo-(2,6-dioxopiperidin-3-yl)-4-aminoisoindoline specifically disclosed in Examples 1 and 20 in the patent. As described above, it is not the examples that determine what is protected by the patent – it is the claims. In the patent, there are 6 claims, with claim 1 reading:

1. A 2,6-dioxopiperidine selected from the group consisting of
   (a) a compound of the formula:

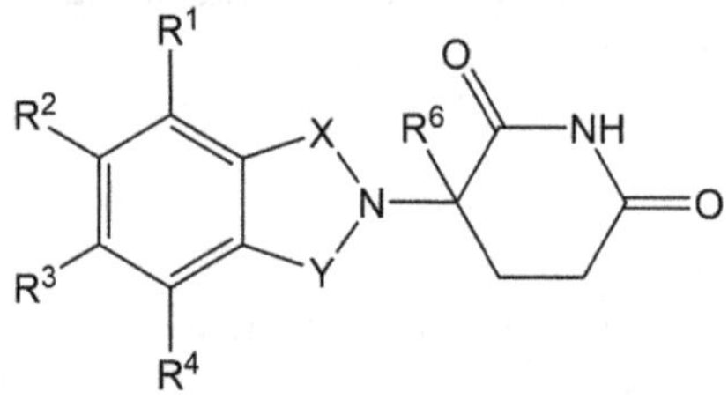

In which:
One of X and Y is C=O and the other of X and Y is C=O or $CH_2$;
One of $R^1$, $R^2$, $R^3$ and $R^4$ is $NHR^5$ and the others $R^1$, $R^2$, $R^3$ and $R^4$ are hydrogen;
$R^5$ is hydrogen or alkyl of 1 to 8 carbon atoms; and
$R^6$ is hydrogen, alkyl of 1 to 8 carbon atoms, benzyl or halo,with the proviso that $R^6$ is other than hydrogen if X and Y are C=O and $R^5$ is hydrogen;

   (b) the acid addition salts of said compounds which contain a nitrogen atom capable of being protonated.

Claim 1 does not refer to any other claims in the patent and is called an independent claim. It covers within its general formula not only the individual compounds exemplified in the patent application, but also compounds that are similar to them. A patent claim in which various parts of a structure are shown in a generalised way is often referred to as a Markush claim, named after the patentee in the first case of this type to be granted by the USPTO.[17] The patentee has specifically included in the claim acid addition salts that can be formed with the compound.

The next claims, claims 2 to 4, each refer back to claim 1 ("A compound according to claim 1, in which..."), and they introduce further limitations in the scope. These are referred to as "dependent claims" and they define the invention more narrowly. They are fall-back positions in case claim 1 should later be found to have a problem. Claim 3 is directed to single compounds selected from the examples. Specifically, lenalidomide is the second compound listed in claim 3.

Claim 4 reads:

4. A pharmaceutical composition comprising an effective quantity of a compound according to anyone of claims 1 to 3, for use in [sic] reduce levels of TNFα in a mammal.

Claim 4 thus relates to a pharmaceutical composition containing a compound of claim 1.

Claim 5 reads:

Use of (a) a compound of the formula

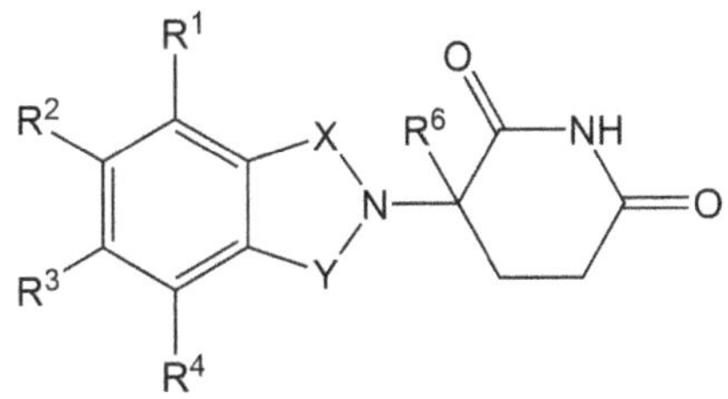


In which:

One of X and Y is C=O and the other of X and Y is C=O or $CH_2$;
One of $R^1$, $R^2$, $R^3$ and $R^4$ is $NHR^5$ and the others $R^1$, $R^2$, $R^3$ and $R^4$ are hydrogen;
$R^5$ is hydrogen or alkyl of 1 to 8 carbon atoms; and
$R^6$ is hydrogen, alkyl of 1 to 8 carbon atoms, benzyl or halo,

(b) the acid addition salts of said compounds which contain a nitrogen atom capable of being protonated, for preparing a medicament to reduce levels of TNFα in a mammal.

On the face of it, claim 5 looks it is directed to a method of manufacture. In fact, it is a second medical use claim and it covers the use of the compound in treatments for reducing levels of TNFα. The claim is present as a fall-back in case a prior art document comes to light which discloses a compound within the scope of the patent, but for a different use.

Claim 6 is a dependent claim that refers back to claim 5 and recites that the compound is one of the specific compounds listed.

It might seem that there is a lot of redundancy built in to the claims. Because the lenalidomide compound was new *per se* when the patent application was filed, the compound was claimed *per se* and the patent covers the compound in any composition and for any use.

Within the compound *per se* claims (claims 1 to 3), the broadest claim (claim 1) covers a group of compounds, and would catch "me-too" copies that a competitor might want to develop. Within the claim breadth, the most important compound to protect is the compound that has been taken to market, lenalidomide. That individual compound is therefore picked out individually in claim 3.

Despite the presence of the compound *per se* claims, it is important that the patent contains various different types of claims so that there are fall-back positions in case the compound *per se* claims should later be found to have a problem; in that situation, the additional different types of claim are necessary so that different infringers can be caught by the patent. The pharmaceutical composition claim, claim 4, would be infringed by somebody manufacturing tablets or capsules of lenalidomide. The second use claim, claim 5, would be infringed by somebody manufacturing the compound for use in reducing levels of TNFα in a patient.

#### *17.4.3.2 Large Molecule Drugs – Keytruda*

Pembrolizumab (Keytruda), MSD's immuno-oncology monoclonal antibody, is forecast to be the world's top selling drug by 2023.[18] The main patent protecting Keytruda in Europe is EP2170959B.[19]

As with lenalidomide, the patent claims provide focused protection around the drug molecule itself, although the claims look different because they are trying to capture relevant aspects of the antibody sequence, rather than aspects of the chemical structure. Claim 1 is an independent claim which reads:

1. An antibody or antibody fragment which binds to human PD-1, comprising:

light chain CDRs SEQ ID NOs: 15, 16 and 17 and heavy chain CDRs SEQ ID NOs: 18, 19 and 20;

wherein said antibody or antibody fragment blocks binding of human PD-L1 and human PD-L2 to human PD-1.

The CDRs, or complementarity-determining regions, are sections of the variable chains of an antibody which specifically bind to the target of interest (in this case PD-1). The CDRs largely determine the affinity of an antibody to a target, and small changes to the CDRs can have a dramatic effect on affinity. Here, in claim 1, the CDR sequences are narrowly defined by specific amino-acid sequences (sequences 15 to 20) which are listed in the body of the patent description, providing specific protection around the key binding regions of pembrolizumab.

As with lenalidomide, later dependent claims in the pembrolizumab patent introduce further limitations in scope, whether by being structurally limited to successively longer amino-acid sequences, or by being limited *via* both structural and functional features (*e.g.* binding affinity). In addition, both pharmaceutical composition and second medical use claims are included.

Therefore, although on the face of it, small molecule and large molecule patent claims may look very different, in reality they have a number of similarities. In essence, both sets of claims seek to address the same aim of providing a clearly defined and robust scope of protection around highly valuable commercial assets.

### 17.4.4 Case Study (b): The Importance of Experimental Data – Inventive Step

As mentioned above, it is a requirement for patentability that an invention has an inventive step; that is to say that it is not obvious over the published art at the filing date. In the life sciences, to demonstrate that a compound has an unexpected property, a patent applicant must almost always carry out an experiment and then present the resulting data in the patent application. Data are key to successfully demonstrating the presence of an inventive step.

This point was key in the recent decision of the European Patent Office's Board of Appeal concerning BMS's patent covering dasatinib, its leukemia treatment sold under the brand name Sprycel.[20] BMS's patent application contained a list of 580 example compounds, one of which was dasatinib. There were no structurally similar compounds in the prior art and the novelty of the claimed compound structures was not in doubt. Assays known to enable the identification of protein kinase (PTK) inhibitors were described in the patent application. However, the application contained no data or other evidence that the example compounds actually had PTK inhibitory activity. Without data to show that the claimed compounds had beneficial properties, the claims were vulnerable to being attacked for lack of inventive step.

It is common during the examination of patent applications at the EPO and the USPTO (and some other offices) to file additional data to show the examiner that a particular technical effect is present. In the dasatinib case, data was available that had been published after the patent filing date to show that dasatinib and other compounds were PTK inhibitors, and BMS filed that data during the EPO opposition. The Board of Appeal ruled, however, that post-filing data can only be used to corroborate something that had already been made plausible by the information in the patent application as originally filed. A small number of data points would most likely have been enough to make it plausible that the claimed compounds had activity. However, in the absence of any experimental data in the application as filed, the Board was not prepared to consider the invention as having been made plausible and the additional data was thus not permitted into the case.

Because the patent application did not contain any substantiating data and the patentees were not permitted to improve their position by filing data later, the inventive step was assessed on the basis of the application documents alone without any data to demonstrate that the compounds were indeed PTK inhibitors. With no data to substantiate the inventive step, the patent was revoked for lacking an inventive step. The case underlines the crucial role played in life science patents of data substantiating the inventive activity.

### 17.4.5 Case Study (c): The Importance of Experimental Data – Sufficiency

Another of the requirements in order for a patent to be granted is that the invention must be sufficiently disclosed. As recently confirmed by the UK Supreme Court in *Regeneron Pharmaceuticals Inc v Kymab Ltd*, one implication of this requirement is that patent claims cannot be so broad that they cover approaches which could not be put into practice at the date the patent was filed.[21]

The *Regeneron* case concerned Regeneron's UK patent describing improvements in the techniques available to use mice to generate antibodies which are suitable for treating humans. Previously, any attempt to generate human antibodies in mice would tend to make the mice sick, as the murine immune system recognised these humanised antibodies as foreign, thereby promoting an unwanted immune response. Regeneron's innovation was to recognise that by replacing only specific sections of the mouse antibody sequences with human versions (known as the V, D and J segments), the murine immune system would not recognise those insertions and therefore the mice would not become sick. This represented a significant step forward in antibody technology.

The problem for Regeneron was that at the time of their patent filing, the ability to engineer mouse antibodies was limited, and therefore only a small fraction of the claimed human sequence insertions could be carried out experimentally. In particular, it was not possible to replace all of the V, D and J segments with their corresponding human sequences, and in fact this did not become possible until over a decade after the filing. But it was this wholesale replacement of the V, D and J segments which was by far the most valuable aspect of the innovation, and indeed was the activity which Kymab had carried out.

The UK Supreme Court accepted that Regeneron's idea of replacing only specific segments of mouse antibodies with corresponding human sequences was highly innovative, and the court also accepted that Regeneron had shown at the time of filing that this could be done for at least some of those segments. But Regeneron could not show that this could be done for all of the specified segments, and therefore by seeking claims which would cover this broader aspect, the Supreme Court found that Regeneron had gone too far. In their view:

> ... the claim to a monopoly over the whole of that range went far beyond the contribution which the product made to the art at the priority date, precisely because mice at the more valuable end of the range could not be made, using the disclosure in the patents.

Accordingly, the Supreme Court decided to overturn the earlier decision of the UK Court of Appeal, and revoked Regeneron's patent for lack of sufficiency. In the Supreme Court's view, "patents are about products and processes, not pure ideas...", and for product claims in particular, "the contribution to the art is the product which is enabled to be made by the disclosure, not the invention itself". This case therefore underlines the importance of including enough experimental information in a patent to support the breadth of the claims being sought, and the potential risk which can result from seeking to over-stretch the extent of the monopoly.

## 17.5 Ownership and Inventorship

As patents are valuable pieces of property, it is important that they are owned by the body (generally a company) that needs to own them. This sounds simple, but it is surprising how often things can go wrong, and increasingly so in the current age of spin-out companies, virtual companies, joint-ventures and out-sourced research.

There are small variations from country to country, but in most jurisdictions, the first owner of an invention, and hence the patent rights in it, is the inventor or the group of co-inventors. Either by virtue of an employment contract, or by operation of the national law, an invention made by an employee who is employed to make inventions belongs to the employer. That is a relatively straightforward situation, though in corporate groups, it needs to be checked if the employing entity is actually the company that needs to own the patent rights. If a contract research organisation or an independent consultant is involved in the development of a product, then it is important that the contract with them includes an obligation to assign all patent rights to the company that engages them.

Given that ownership of a patent is determined by the inventorship, it is important that inventorship is determined properly. An inventor is a person who is the "actual deviser" of the invention. That is to say the person, or group of people, who came up with the invention that is being claimed. Inventorship differs from authorship on an academic paper: supervising research and providing resources for a laboratory does not constitute inventorship; nor does carrying out the laboratory work to show that an invention works, no matter how specialised or time-consuming the laboratory work may be. A rigorous approach needs to be taken to the determination of inventorship.

The US and some other countries (including China) have laws that restrict the ability of applicants to file patent applications for locally devised inventions abroad. These restrictions exist to prevent inventions relevant to national security from being disclosed in other countries. Early determination of inventorship is especially important if there is any involvement by somebody resident in the US, China, or another country with national filing restrictions in place. Taking the US as an example, if an invention is made by a person who was a resident of the US at the time of the invention being made, then the application must be first filed in the US, or a permit (a "foreign filing licence") must be obtained from the US Patent and Trade Mark Office (USPTO), before the application is filed in a country other than the US. If a foreign filing licence is not obtained, any subsequently granted US patent will be invalid and hence unenforceable unless the failure to procure the license was "through error". A foreign filing licence can be obtained from the USPTO on an expedited basis in around 3 days. In some other countries, there are criminal sanctions for failure to first file in the necessary territory.

Getting inventorship or ownership wrong can be very costly. It is always best to ensure that inventorship and ownership of patents are correct from the outset when all parties are on good terms and when the whereabouts of all relevant individuals are known. It can be problematic to sort out issues later on, particularly if a patent covers a valuable product. This can be a particular problem when patents are sold (assigned) to another company.

## 17.6 The Process for Obtaining a Patent

### 17.6.1 The National Nature of Patents

Despite their importance to international business, patents remain matters of national law. Ultimately, therefore, it is necessary for a company to have a separate national patent for an invention in each state in which patent protection is needed. Until recently, substantive requirements for patentability were also often very different in different territories. The TRIPS agreement (Agreement on Trade Related

Aspects of Intellectual Property Rights of 1994) went a long way to harmonising laws to a minimum standard. Some national differences remain, and it remains necessary for there to be a separate patent in each territory. The major downside to this fragmented national arrangement is that the patent specification needs to be translated into a large number of languages, and that litigation may need to be pursued in multiple jurisdictions.

In general, obtaining a patent in one's home market is not sufficient, and most organisations involved in medical research will want to obtain patents in several territories. Two long-standing international treaties facilitate the process of obtaining patents around the world: under the Paris Convention,[22] one can file a patent application in a first country, and then file corresponding applications in other countries within 12 months and claim for the later applications the filing date of the first country (known then as the "priority date"). The second international agreement is the Patent Cooperation Treaty (PCT). Under the PCT, one can file a single patent application for a large number of countries.[23] The PCT application can be filed in one language, in the applicant's home country and the claims are subjected to a high quality patent office search. A PCT application remains effective until 30 months from the priority date. At that time, it is necessary to decide which territories to pursue the patent in, and which not. A PCT application cannot itself become a granted patent; it is only after the application has been pursued in an individual territory that there can be a granted patent.

### 17.6.2 A Typical Application Process

A typical application process in the field of medicinal chemistry for a company based in the UK will thus be as follows:

- After discussion between medicinal chemists, business development manager and patent attorney, a decision is made to file a patent application.
- The application is then filed at the UK patent office. This filing date is the "priority date".
- 12 months later, if the invention remains of interest, a PCT application is filed. The PCT application may include additional material beyond what was in the original application (*e.g.* additional examples). The 12 month period is useful since often additional work is conducted in this period such that the invention is better exemplified and better understood by the time the PCT application is filed.
- A search is carried out by a patent office and the search report is sent to the applicant.
- At 18 months from the priority date, the PCT application is published.
- At 30 months from the priority date, it is necessary to enter the "national phase" in each country in which a patent is wanted.
- Over the following period (2 to 5 years), the application is examined by the various national patent offices. Providing no surprising unknown prior art documents come out of the woodwork, the patent should be granted in the various territories over this time scale.

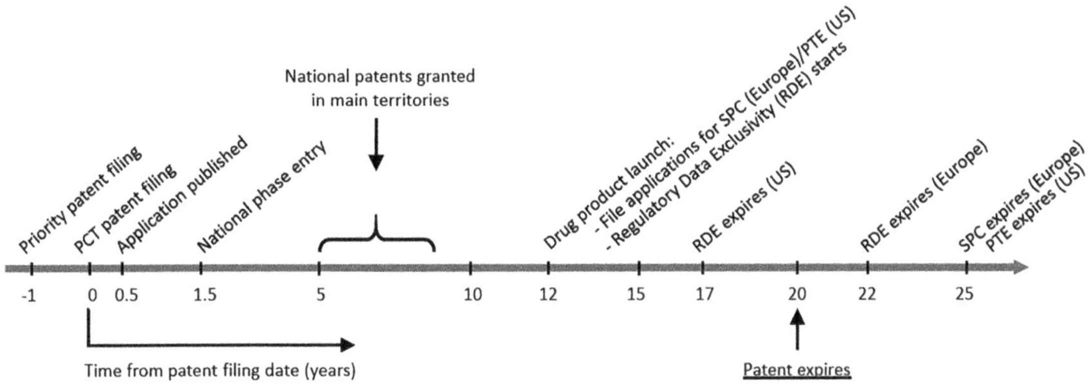


**Figure 17.4** A timeline showing the main events during the typical lifetime of a patent protecting a new medicine.

These stages of the patent application process are included in the example patent life timeline shown in Figure 17.4. The figure also includes the important time points at the later stages of the patent's life: expiry at 20 years from the filing date; patent term extension, which provides additional patent-like term when pre-marketing development and trials have taken a long time (discussed in Section 17.7.2 below), and Regulatory Data Exclusivity, which provides time-limited protection against third parties making use of the data obtained in the originator's clinical trials (discussed in Section 17.9.2 below).

Many observers are surprised that the patenting takes as long as it does: typically 4–6 years from filing to grant in the US, 5–8 years in Europe and 7–9 years in Japan. In almost every country, there are mechanisms by which the process can be accelerated if an applicant wants to do so. There is variation between technical fields, but it is often in applicants' interests for things to go slowly: every time the case advances a step through patent office prosecution, there tend to be costs; furthermore, when the patent is granted, the scope of the claims becomes fixed. If a product is still being developed, it can be useful if the claims could be changed to accommodate changes to the product, though it should be noted that it is not possible to add new material to a patent specification once it has been filed.

### 17.6.3 Costs

Costs are an important consideration for any organisation, and long-term budgetary planning is important for a patenting programme. Of course, the exact costs will vary from case to case, depending on the complexity. Considering the process described above, the typical costs for drafting and filing a "priority application" in the medicinal chemistry area are in the region of £5000–10 000. Filing a PCT application at the 12 month point typically costs around £5000, though there are page fees if the specification has more than 30 pages. If there is significant additional material, then the process of introducing that into the specification will also increase the costs.

The national phase entry at 30 months is the usually single largest cost point in the patenting process, often amounting to tens or even hundreds of thousands of pounds if a significant number of territories are to be covered. Thirty months as the national phase entry deadline was settled on as a compromise between providing certainty to third parties about whether there will be a patent in a particular territory, whilst allowing a patent applicant a reasonable amount of time to assess whether the invention will be sufficiently commercially successful to justify the national phase costs. In medicines research, 30 months can pass very quickly. Particularly for a small company, it is important to try and align this deadline with milestones in the development programme.

Larger corporations generally have defined sets of country lists for national phase entry and the appropriate list will be selected depending on the level of interest in the invention and its likely future value.

### 17.6.4 The National Phase: Examination of Patent Applications

In order to make sure that a patent application fulfils the requirements for patentability and disclosure described above in Section 17.3, most countries have a patent examination system in place. After an application enters the national phase in a particular country, it goes before an examiner at the national patent office. The examiner first carries out a search of the art (in some cases the search carried out previously in the PCT phase may be sufficient), and then writes a report to the applicant setting out whether or not the application fulfils the requirements. If it does not, then the examiner's report will explain why the application cannot be allowed and the applicant is given an opportunity to amend the patent claims and to provide arguments in favour of the claims. This correspondence between the patent office examiner and the applicant and their attorneys is known as "patent prosecution". It is usual that a patent specification is amended during this time. However, the applicant does not have a completely free hand when making amendments: the applicant is not allowed to introduce additional features or limitations not in the original disclosure. All amendments must be based on information contained in the application as originally filed.

Eventually, either the patent is granted in the country concerned, or the application is refused. If an application is refused by the patent office, the applicant has the opportunity to appeal to a higher court.

The patent prosecution process takes place in parallel in each country in which the applicant has applied for a patent. Some of this work is duplicative. On many occasions, different prior art is found by different patent offices, meaning that in the end the confidence in the validity of the patent is increased.

Having said above that patent applications remain national rights, in Europe, the majority of states (including all EU states, the UK and Switzerland) are members of the European Patent Convention and patents for those countries can thus be obtained at the European Patent Office (the EPO). Examination at the EPO takes place under a single procedure in English, French or German (at the applicant's choice). This avoids the duplication mentioned above within Europe. It is only after the "European Patent" has been granted that the patent splits into separate national rights, and the applicant needs to translate the text into local languages and decide in which European countries to have the patent in force.

In a move to further reduce costs and duplicated effort across Europe, 25 states of the European Union have signed an agreement to create a "European Patent with Unitary Effect"; a single patent that has effect across all of the 25 states involved. A second agreement was also reached between a similar set of countries to create a "Unified Patent Court", a single court in which European patents can be enforced for the whole of the territories involved. That will reduce the duplication that can currently take place when the same patent is litigated for the same infringement in multiple countries. Due to the exit of the UK from the EU in early 2020, European Patents with Unitary Effect will not have effect in the UK, and the UK will not be a part of the Unified Patent Court system. At the time of writing (in 2022), the European Patent with Unitary Effect is planned to start and the institutions of the Unified Patent Court are planned to open their doors in the first half of 2023. For up to date information on the progress of this, please see the websites of the appropriate government and private sector organisations.[24]

## 17.6.5 Strategic Aspects

It is seen from the process summary in Section 17.6.2 above that there are some key decision points in the process:

(1) The initial decision to file, and when to file

This is the one step in the application process that the applicant has complete control over. It is a decision that can be surprisingly difficult. The patent application will be strongest if it can contain as much experimental detail as possible and the results from advanced activity testing. Gathering that detail requires time and so leads to a later filing date. That needs to be balanced against the risk of a competitor making the same invention and filing a patent application before you do. That risk can be significant in a highly competitive area and an earlier patent filing date reduces that risk. In many situations, it can be necessary for inventors themselves to publicise the invention (for example in a collaboration with an academic institution or where a start up company needs to raise funding) and that makes it essential to file early.

When a structure–activity relationship is being explored, it can take some time from finding the first hit to identifying a clinical candidate. It is usual during such an exploration for several patent applications to be filed in succession as new structures are prepared and characterised. As patent applications are published 18 months after their priority filing dates, an important consideration when making the first filing is whether the programme is projected to have identified its clinical candidate in the 18 months from that first filing date. If a first, broad application is filed initially and a particular novel compound within the broad scope is later identified with especially beneficial properties, it can be possible to protect that novel compound in its own application. This is often referred to as a "selection invention" as the later compound is selected from within the original broad disclosure.

To be considered novel, a selection claim must generally encompass a selection from two prior lists. That is to say that, for at least two of the substituents in the selection claim, the claimed substituent must be a selection of one choice (or a very small number of choices) from a longer list in the broader earlier disclosed formula. For example if the earlier general chemical formula includes a "heteroaryl group" and says that a position can be substituted by "a natural amino acid", then a later claim that is limited to "pyrimidine" and substitution by "cysteine" should be considered to be a valid novel selection. This is on the basis that that combination of features together was not previously disclosed. In Europe, if the earlier formula has not yet been published, it is not a requirement to demonstrate that the later "selection" compounds have improved properties over the earlier compounds. In other territories, and certainly if the earlier formula has been published, it will be necessary to show that the selection compounds have some improved properties. The improvement can be in any relevant property; for example, stronger binding to a target, better stability or better DMPK. In practice, if the later compounds in the programme are more promising than the earlier compounds, then there will generally be an improved property that the applicant can point to. It is then important to include data from experiments that demonstrate that the improvement is seen for the selection compounds.

In most countries, perfectly valid selection patents are granted and they are fully enforceable. In some cases, the patentee can obtain a first broader patent covering a new class of compounds and then a second, narrower, patent that discloses and specifically claims the clinical lead compound. That way, the patentee has two compound patents, both of which cover the lead compound and that can put the patentee in a particularly strong position. In general, however, patents that are not "selection patents" have more clear distinctions from the prior art and, so, the stronger strategy is to aim not to have to rely on "selection patents" in this way.

(2) The decision at 12 months whether to proceed with a PCT filing

If the product development is going ahead well, then the PCT application should be filed. If the invention or the programme is not yet sufficiently advanced, the first priority application can be withdrawn, and a new priority application filed. This results in the application being re-dated, so it should be checked that there has not been any relevant publication in the intervening year that will compromise the validity of the patent. The third option, if the invention is no longer of any interest, is to abandon the application altogether. Proceeding with the PCT application at 12 months sets the application on the course for publication at 18 months.

(3) The national phase entry decision

The decision regarding which countries to proceed with for national phase entry at 30 months. This decision is very much determined by cost: how important is the project, and for which countries are the costs justified? The choice of countries is dictated mostly by the value that the medicine is likely to have in countries around the world. The major pharmaceutical markets of the USA, Europe, Japan and China tend to be the most important, but certain disease conditions, and hence, medicine demands, can have regional specificities. In addition, manufacture locations and supply-chain factors should be taken into account: a patent that covers a method of synthesis has most value in countries where significant pharmaceutical manufacture takes place. Major ports in Hong Kong, Singapore and Rotterdam make Hong Kong, Singapore and the Netherlands important locations for intercepting infringing goods in transit and those countries have value for patents that cover a drug that would likely be shipped in significant quantities.

(4) Further strategic aspects of portfolio development

Before a medicine can be authorised for administration to patients, many elements of the final product need to be developed: the drug compound structure, the best salt form, a suitable formulation that is stable and well tolerated, the optimised dosage and various other elements that will vary from case to case. As set out in Section 17.4.2 above, patent claim types are available to protect these different elements. It is important for the developer of the medicine to obtain as strong patents as possible to cover these technical advances that are made during the stages of the development process. Patents that cover the technical advances that are made during the later stages of the development process have particular importance as they have later expiry dates than the patents that cover the earlier stage work. Optimising the protection of these later technical advances requires close collaboration between the development team and the patent attorney, and particular attention to the publications of one's own patent applications. For example, if a lead compound is invented and a first application is filed to protect that compound *per se* and then salt development work later leads to the identification of a particularly advantageous salt, then it may be advantageous to file a patent application to cover the particular salt before the application disclosing the compound *per se* is published. By ensuring a strategic close coordination between the series of patent publications and the steps in the drug development process, the medicine developer can ensure that they build the best possible patent protection around the medicine that they bring to market.

## 17.7 The Patent after Grant

### 17.7.1 Maintenance

Once a patent has been granted, it is necessary to maintain it in force. In most territories, this is done by paying an annual renewal fee. There are two public policy reasons for governments insisting on annual fees: the first is that as part of the "bargain" between the state and the patentee, the monopoly should only be maintained if the patentee is actually making use of the invention. If the patentee is not using it, then the public should benefit from being able to use it before the 20 year expiry date. The second reason is that the annual renewal fees subsidise the costs of the patent office's search and examination operation. This enables the office to charge low up-front fees (thus facilitating access to the system), and it weights the cost of the patent system towards those who use it most, *i.e.* those patentees who maintain their patents in force the longest. Maintenance fees in most countries become more expensive as a patent progresses through its 20 year term.

### 17.7.2 Extension of Patents

The patent system is a single system that applies to all fields of technology. It does not take any account of the relative speeds of progress, or the different levels of investment needed in different fields. The 20 year patent term applies equally to a new shape of toilet brush as to a highly complex mobile phone or a specialised cancer treatment. In recognition of the fact that before a new pharmaceutical can be marketed, extensive trials are needed in order to obtain government approval (which can use up to 10 to 12 years of the patent term, or more), many countries have put in place patent term extension provisions for pharmaceuticals.

The exact mechanism for the calculation of the extension period and the method of implementation of the extension varies from country to country. In general, up to 5 additional years of patent-like protection can be obtained. In Europe, the extension is provided by a "Supplementary Protection Certificate" (SPC). It can be up to 5 years long, but has a maximum expiry date of 15 years from the first European marketing authorisation. It is not an extension of the whole patent; only the scope that covers the exact compound that is marketed. In the US, the extension is called a "Patent Term Restoration" and its duration is calculated on the basis of the time that the drug spends in pre-clinical and clinical regulatory review. Again, the extension cannot be more than 5 years, but the maximum expiry date is 14 years from the US marketing authorisation, so earlier than the 15 year European expiry. There are similar arrangements in Canada, Japan, Korea, Taiwan, the Russian Federation, Israel and Australia.

In the example shown in Figure 17.4 above, the drug received its authorisation 12 years from the patent filing date. In Europe, the full 5 year SPC term is then available; in the US, depending on the exact timings of the steps in the clinical trial work, the full 5 year period may also be available. The patent-like protection provided by the extensions will therefore expire at 25 years from the patent filing date.

These patent term extensions are of crucial importance to a drug development company since much of the income shown in Figure 17.1 is earned during the "maturity" phase and the maturity phase ends with the expiry of the patent (or its extension).

### 17.7.3 Challenges to Validity

It is a surprise to some observers that grant of a patent by a patent office does not constitute a guarantee of validity. Patent office examiners can work only on the basis of the documents and evidence that they have before them; their searches are limited to written literature, and they do not have facilities to repeat experiments. Examiners will not be able to find out if an invention was disclosed non-confidentially at a meeting, or if it does not actually work. Therefore, although patent office examiners do a good job, a patent that has been granted cannot definitively be assumed to be valid. A granted patent remains open to challenge after grant, either at a national patent office or before national courts.

## 17.8 Use of Patents

### 17.8.1 Infringement and Enforcement

The primary *raison d'être* of a patent is to keep competitors off the market and to preserve the patent holder's market exclusivity.

Infringement of a patent occurs if a third party uses a patented invention without permission of the patent owner. The patent owner has the legal right to stop the third party from carrying out the infringement. To assert this right, the patent holder must bring an action for infringement in the courts. The action is a civil action – in other words, it is the patent owner, rather than the state, that brings the action against the alleged infringer. In most countries, the case is heard before a technically qualified judge, although in certain countries, in particular the US, infringement actions may be heard before a jury. In the UK, the judges usually have a technical degree and then many years of experience arguing patent matters in the patents courts, both on behalf of patent owners and on behalf of alleged infringers.

The procedure and the costs of litigation vary tremendously between countries, with patent litigation in the US and to a somewhat lesser extent the UK, being very expensive.

In general, in the medicinal chemistry field, competitors are sophisticated companies and they know of the drug originator's patents. The existence of a patent will generally keep the competitor from launching a product until after the patent has expired (or, if the competitor considers the patent invalid, the competitor may challenge the validity). When infringement does take place, it is important to act quickly, so that the infringement can be stopped before the market price of the product drops. Often, there is a set of several patents protecting different aspects of a medicinal product. It is rare that the validity of a compound *per se* patent is challenged, but challenges are relatively common for formulation, use or pharmaceutical form patents.

In order to bring an action for patent infringement, the patent holder must identify who the infringer is, and what infringing acts they are carrying out. In a complex supply chain, this can be more difficult than one might expect: a drug being manufactured in India might be imported into Europe by a Greek company which passes it to a UK distributor who distributes the drug to pharmacists on behalf of a UK marketing authorisation holder that is headquartered in Monaco. If we have a UK patent, then we need to identify what in this chain is an infringing act in the UK, and who is carrying out that act. Most probably in this imaginary scenario, it would be the UK distributor and UK marketing authorisation holder that the patentee should bring the action against.

*Proving infringement:*

Once the infringing acts and the infringer have been identified, it is necessary to prove that an infringement has taken place. There are two parts to this. The first is gathering evidence of what acts have taken place. This might involve making test purchases and obtaining samples, or else obtaining copies of invoices or delivery notes showing what has taken place. Then, it is necessary to show that what is being sold falls within the claims of the patent.

*Claim interpretation:*
In general, it is usually a straightforward matter for the court to decide that a pharmaceutical patent is infringed. Where the invention concerns a product, defined by a general chemical formula (known as a Markush formula), it will usually be sufficient to show that the alleged infringement meets the definition for the particular generic formula. Often, the substance in question is specifically named in the patent, so there is little room for argument that the claims of the patent are infringed.

But occasionally, there is real doubt as to whether or not a product is covered by a patent claim. This requires the patent claim to be interpreted to determine what its scope is. In Europe, the statutes require a claim to be interpreted in such a way as to "combine a fair protection for the patent proprietor with a reasonable degree of legal certainty for third parties". To a very limited extent, a patent claim can sometimes be taken to cover so-called "equivalents". These are embodiments that are not within the literal reading of the claim, but that the court rules should be taken to fall within the scope of protection. In a landmark case between Actavis and Eli Lilly, the UK Supreme Court ruled in 2017 that in some circumstances, equivalents can be covered by a patent claim. In the case in question, a patent claim that recited pemetrexed disodium was ruled to be infringed by a potassium salt.[25] Whilst this Supreme Court ruling has general applicability, the circumstances in which equivalents can be taken to infringe a claim are very limited and it remains the case that equivalents cannot generally be relied on: it is always best to have a patent claim that explicitly covers all likely embodiments.

The question of claim interpretation also came to the fore in litigation between Pharmacia and Merck in the early 2000s concerning Merck's cyclo-oxygenase II (COX-II) inhibitor rofecoxib (Vioxx). In that litigation, Pharmacia sought an injunction against Merck, based upon their assertion that rofecoxib fell within the scope of the broadest claim in Pharmacia/Searle's patent EP0679157B,[26] which was directed to a compound of formula I:

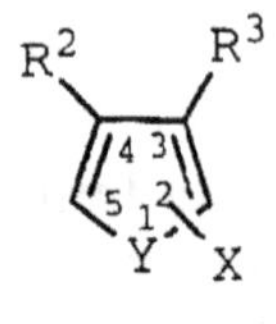


According to the claim, the definition of Y included O, the definition of X included –OH, and the definitions of $R^2$ and $R^3$ included aryl.

Merck's rofecoxib was a furanone, as shown in Figure 17.5. Pharmacia argued that although the structure drawn in the claim was of hydroxyfuran derivatives, the claim should be taken as including the corresponding furanones because hydroxyfurans tautomerise to furanones in water. The product that Merck proposed to sell was a dry tablet, but the compound would inevitably come into contact with water in the body once the patient took it. Pharmacia argued that the skilled person would realise that the tautomerisation would happen and would read the claim as including furanones. The structures of the keto and enol forms of rofecoxib are shown in Figure 17.5. Patents are addressed to the person skilled in the art and, in situations of factual doubt, the court

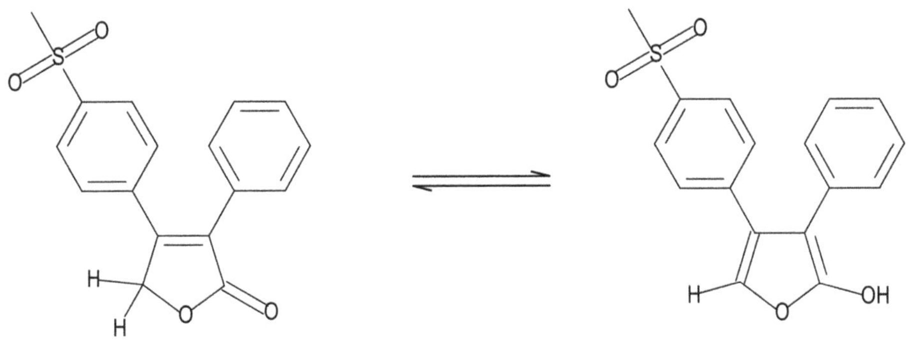


**Figure 17.5** The structures of the keto and enol forms of rofecoxib.

needs to be assisted by expert testimony to ascertain exactly what the person skilled in the art would understand the claim to mean.

Pharmacia therefore brought forward testimony from an expert from the field, an "expert witness". In an attempt to discredit Pharmacia's view, the defendants, Merck, brought forward testimony from their own expert witness. Pharmacia called on Professor Sir Jack Baldwin FRS, then head of the Dyson Perrins Laboratory in Oxford, and Merck relied on Professor Anthony Kirby FRS, then professor of bioorganic chemistry at Cambridge. The result was a fascinating match between two heavyweights of academic mechanism chemistry bringing their knowledge and experience to bear on a legal question.

A patent document is intended to be read by a person skilled in the art with a reasonable technical knowledge and understanding of the area. In this particular case, the skilled person was expected to have at least an undergraduate knowledge of organic chemistry – and so was expected to be familiar with keto–enol tautomerism. It was accepted by the parties that the proportion of furanone to enol in water at physiological pH was $6.3 \times 10^{10}:1$. Further, this overwhelming excess of keto to enol was known from undergraduate text books – so it could be expected to be part of the skilled person's "common general knowledge".

Professor Baldwin read the patent and its claims as referring to the keto tautomer as well as the expressly mentioned enol. Professor Kirby took a more literalist approach and interpreted the claim as limited to the enol form, to the exclusion of the keto form. At first instance, the judge favoured the literalist approach and held that keto forms were not included, and thus that Merck's compound did not fall within the claim.

However, Pharmacia appealed the decision to the Court of Appeal and, on appeal, this decision was overturned. The appeal judges were more convinced by Professor Baldwin's interpretation. The Court of Appeal took the view that the compounds of claim 1 are a class which are said to have activity in the body. In order to give fair protection to the patentee, it was reasonable to take into account the form in which the compound existed in the body. It was accepted that the enol form would exist in an inseparable equilibrium with the keto form, and that it was the composite that has the effect in the body. To restrict the claim to the minor tautomer would not appear to achieve any useful purpose so far as the patentees were concerned.

To construe claim 1 as covering the keto tautomer would not, in the Appeal Judges' view, prevent there being a reasonable degree of certainty for third parties. Of course third parties would appreciate that the keto form was not specifically mentioned. But they would know that that did not necessarily mean that the claim would be construed as limited to the explicitly mentioned compounds. If the contrary were the position, then claims to chemical compounds would have to be construed using too literal an approach. The skilled reader would also know that the inevitable result of using the enol was the formation of the other tautomer. They would therefore not be surprised if manufacture and sale of the other tautomer, which would form the enol in solution, would infringe. The Appeal Judges therefore concluded that claim 1 includes the keto form and so rofecoxib infringed.

Unfortunately for Pharmacia/Searle, the broad interpretation of the claim contributed to the finding that many compounds within the claim did not work, and thus that the claim lacked inventive step. The patent was therefore revoked. So, although the Merck compound had been found to infringe the claim, Pharmacia were not able to keep Merck's compound off the market.

## 17.8.2 Defences and Exemptions to Infringement

If a company is accused of patent infringement, what can it do?

### *17.8.2.1 Defence of Non-infringement*

The first line of defence to an allegation of patent infringement is to argue that the product or method in question does not fall within the claims of the patent. That is what Merck did in the case described above. In many cases in the pharmaceutical industry, it is a generic medicine copy that is alleged to be an infringement. In that case, there is little scope for arguing non-infringement, as the generic pharmaceutical compound will necessarily have to be the same as the originator's compound, and it is quite rare that an originator's patent does not cover its compound.

That said, the values at stake in the pharmaceutical industry can prompt some generic companies to try making arguments that most medicinal chemists would think have little chance of success: in a recent case in the US, a collective group of eight generic pharmaceutical companies argued that their generic versions of the drug pregabalin should not be held to infringe Pfizer/Northwestern University's patent US6197819 that covered the compound.[27] Pregabalin is sold by Pfizer under the name Lyrica® and it has the structure shown in Figure 17.6. It is approved for marketing as the single (*S*) enantiomer.

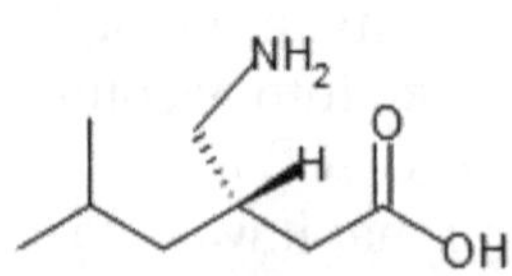


**Figure 17.6** The structure of pregabalin, sold as Lyrica®.

The patent claim in issue was directed to "4-amino-3-(2-methylpropyl) butanoic acid, or a pharmaceutically acceptable salt thereof". The generic companies argued that the claim did not specify that the compound is a single isomer and thus that it should only be considered infringed by a racemic mixture. The court disagreed with the generic companies and found the claim to be infringed by the single enantiomer compound.

#### *17.8.2.2 Counterclaim for Invalidity*

The next line of defence to an allegation of patent infringement is to counterclaim that the patent in question is not valid. This is what Merck did in the case described in Section 17.8.1 discussed above. This approach generally starts with carrying out a thorough search of prior art that can be raised against the patent. Documents or other disclosures that were not taken into account by the patent office when it granted the patent can be particularly useful here.

The case then needs to be made to the court to demonstrate which of the criteria for patentability are not fulfilled by the patent. The patent holder may request that the claims in the patent be narrowed once they have seen the case put forward by the counter-claimant. Very often, the validity of the patent will turn on inventive step: was it obvious to make the change in question at the time the patent application was filed? The two parties will bring together as much evidence as they can to show that it was, or was not, obvious to do that.

#### *17.8.2.3 Exemptions to Infringement*

Certain uses of a patented invention, even though not authorised by the patent owner, are nonetheless excluded from the definition of infringement. In the UK, acts done privately and for purposes which are not commercial are not infringements. The exemption that is most relevant to medicinal chemists is the experimental use exemption: acts that are "done for experimental purposes relating to the subject-matter of the invention".

The exemption needs to be treated with some caution. It does not mean that all uses of a patented invention in experiments is exempted. For example, if the patent relates to an assay system, capable of identifying new drug candidates for the treatment of a particular disease, then using such an assay without permission is almost certainly an infringement – the use is not in an experiment investigating the invention – rather it is a commercial use of the invention in an experiment, with the aim of identifying the potential new drugs.

In many countries (notably Germany and the US), the law is that carrying out a clinical trial falls within the experimental use exemption. However, there was considerable uncertainty around that in the UK and that uncertainty led to planning for clinical trial work being more onerous in the UK than in other countries due to the need to carry out a patent clearance in advance. In order to address this, a clarifying Legislative Reform Order was introduced in the UK in 2014. The Order makes it clear that "anything done in or for the purposes of a medicinal product assessment" is to be regarded as done "for experimental purposes relating to the subject-matter of the invention". This is a far-reaching exemption and covers essentially all steps of the drug development process, meaning that any clinical trial (including ancillary and preparatory work) can be carried out in the UK without patent infringement being a risk.

Lastly, a separate exemption was introduced in Europe in 2005 (including in the UK) which permits a generic company to do the studies necessary for getting a marketing authorisation for a generic product, before patent expiry.

In summary, certain experiments are exempted from patent infringement. The exemptions are quite specific and so it is not safe to assume that an exemption will apply. The clarification introduced in the UK in 2014 has made a significant difference to the treatment of clinical trial work in the UK.

### 17.8.3 The Consequences of Patent Infringement

If the court finds that a defendant's use of an invention is an infringement, then the patent holder will request that the court imposes one or more remedies, generally including:

- an injunction: a court order prohibiting any further unauthorised use of the invention during the lifetime of the patent.
- withdrawal of any product on the market and destruction of stocks.
- payment of damages, to compensate the patent owner for its lost revenue as a result of the unauthorised use of the invention.
- legal costs: the infringer may have to reimburse the patent owner for a substantial part of its legal costs in bringing the infringement action. Such costs can be extremely high. Each side in a major infringement action in the UK (which will usually involve a counterclaim from the infringer that the patent is invalid) will expect to incur well over £1 million in legal fees. In the US, where recovery of costs is relatively rare, each party's legal costs may well be over $10 million.

A special form of injunction merits a mention here: the preliminary injunction. Generic products are generally priced at a very substantial discount to the corresponding product of the originator. Unless it drops its price, the originator will rapidly lose market share to the generic. But if the originator drops its price, it is unlikely to be able to put it up again, even if following a successful patent infringement action, the generic product is withdrawn from the market. In these circumstances, the loss of revenue to the patent owner is impossible to quantify. Infringement actions generally take at least a year to come to court – if the generic drug were on the market for all that time, it would cause a dramatic change to the market place and a huge loss of earnings for the patent owner.

To avoid this situation, the patent owner will try to get an injunction immediately, and before the merits of the case are considered fully by the court. In the UK, an injunction obtained before a full trial is called a preliminary injunction. To be able to get a preliminary injunction, the patent holder must show the court that it has an arguable case for patent infringement and for patent validity, and that it would suffer unquantifiable damages by the infringement. In general, the patent owner must agree to compensate the alleged infringer for the loss suffered, in the event that the court eventually decides that the injunction should not have been granted.

A preliminary injunction is sometimes the most important remedy that a patent holder in the medicinal chemistry field will try to obtain.

### 17.8.4 Licensing

As discussed above, a patent does not give its owner the right to use the invention themself. Rather, it gives them the right to prevent others from using the invention commercially without their permission. A licence is, basically, the grant of permission to do things which, absent the licence, would be an infringement of the patent. A patentee is often said to be giving an "immunity from suit" when granting a licence.

A patentee (the licensor) and the person taking the licence (the licensee) may agree the terms of their licence to suit themselves, with one very important caveat: the terms of the licence must not be in breach of the law. Specifically, various laws exist which control monopolies and unfair competition, dealing with issues such as pricing, restrictive practices and cross-border trade. European Competition Law, which regulates (or, arguably, deregulates) trade between the member states of the EU is a complex subject and outside the scope of this chapter, but must always be taken into account when businesses operating in the EU enter into licence agreements. In addition to EU competition law, various national laws operate in similar areas, while in the US, these laws are called "anti-trust" laws. The European Commission's Directorate General for Competition has been particularly active in the pharmaceutical area.

Subject to this, any licence will be tailored to suit the particular situation. Common issues which arise in patent licence negotiations include the following:

The licence needs to clearly define what the licensee is allowed to do. It should define the permitted product, or process, or both. This can include everything within the scope of the claims of the patent, or it may be a narrower definition.

Subject to competition law, a licence may give permission to operate in a specific territory. For example, a patentee may wish to satisfy the whole market in their home territory, say Europe, themself, while raising revenue from licensing the technology in other territories, say the US. In this case the licence will contain a *territorial restriction*. Similarly, a patentee may wish to satisfy the whole market in a particular field of technology, but grant licences in other fields. If, for example, the invention is a pharmaceutical compound which can be used in either a cream for topical application, or in an injectable formulation for systemic use, they may choose to satisfy the whole market for one of these formulations themselves, while licensing the alternative use to others. In this case, the licence will contain a *field of use restriction*.

A licence can be a bare patent licence, *i.e.* include the grant of rights under a patent and nothing else. Many licences, however, include other things, for example the grant of rights to use confidential *know-how* belonging to the licensor, or the requirement for the patentee to provide technical advice and assistance.

*Exclusive* and *non-exclusive* are common terms in licence agreements, but can be misleading, because their precise definition differs from country to country. On the UK definition, if a licensor grants a non-exclusive licence, they remain free to grant additional non-exclusive licences to others, while if they grant an exclusive licence, they agree not to grant additional licences to others, and they are not free to commercialise the invention themselves. A *sole licence* is an agreement that the patentee will grant no further licences to others, but retains the right to commercialise the invention themself. A licence may or may not give the licensee the right to grant further licences, or *sub-licences*, to others.

*Payment* for the grant of a licence can be in many forms. It can be in the form of on-going royalty payments, or lump-sum payments, or a mixture of both, either form of payment being triggered by defined events. Possibly, no money at all changes hands: the licence may be *royalty-free*. A licence in which, rather than making payments, each party grants a licence to the other, is known as a *cross-licence*.

Finally, the *termination* clause is very important. This determines under what conditions one or both of the parties can terminate the licence. Bare patent licences usually terminate at the latest when the patent expires. If know-how is included, then a licence to use this know-how can continue for many years after patent expiry provided that the know-how still remains confidential.

Numerous other issues will arise, including the handling of disputes, action and responsibilities if third parties infringe or attack the patent, warranties and indemnities given by each party to the other, and regulation of liability. The prudent licensor always includes an audit clause in a licence, which gives them the right to appoint an independent auditor to inspect the books of the licensce to ensure that the correct payments are being made. Expert help in preparing a licence agreement is important.

### 17.8.5 The Patent Box

Until relatively recently, a patent has served only one purpose: to prevent competitors putting their products or services on the market (or at least to control the market by licensing). That remains the primary reason for any business to obtain patents. In addition, there came into force in the UK in 2013 a government tax initiative commonly referred to as the "patent box" which now provides UK businesses with an additional reason to obtain patents.[28]

The regime allows a business to pay corporation tax at the lower rate of 10% on net profits derived from a patented product. The profits can be made anywhere in the world, but to qualify for the lower tax rate, the organisation must have a patent in the UK (or a short list of other European countries), or be an exclusive licensee. The reason for the patent being needed is to demonstrate that the product from which the profits are derived is "innovative". There is no need to enforce the patent against competitors, and it does not matter if the patent is narrow and could be worked around.

The patent box regime is designed to encourage product development work in the UK. Similar regimes are in place in a small number of other countries, for example in the Netherlands. The regime in the UK was tightened in 2016 such that the tax reduction is only available where the research and development (R&D) expenditure required to develop that innovation also took place in the UK. The change has had full effect from 2021 onwards. The UK patent box was lobbied for by the UK pharmaceutical industry, and the take-up has been significant, with HMRC figures showing the value of the relief in 2016–17 exceeding £1 billion.[29] At the time of writing, the evidence is that the regime has helped medicinal chemistry businesses in the UK and encouraged their activities.

## 17.9 Generic Medicines and Hurdles to Generic Competition

An originator drug development company will often be keen to keep products from other drug originator companies out of its market patch. However, as mentioned in several places in this chapter, it is the generic pharmaceutical products that are the larger threat to an originator's business. Generic medicines thus merit special discussion.

### 17.9.1 What is a Generic Medicine?

Although precise legal definitions vary from country to country, in general a generic medicine is a medicine which is identical to that of the originator in terms of its active principle(s) and functionally equivalent in terms of its therapeutic profile, its safety profile and pharmaceutical form. To show functional equivalence for the therapeutic profile, a generic medicine must have bioequivalence with the original medicine. A drug is considered to be bioequivalent if there is no significant difference in the rate and extent to which the active moiety becomes available at the site of drug action when administered at the same dose under similar conditions. A generic company proposing to launch a generic medicine must provide proof (generally in the form of experimental evidence) that the proposed generic has bioequivalence with the original medicine. If the active is used and it has been shown to have bioequivalence, the safety equivalence is generally inferred, but it is necessary to keep a watch on that presumption after the generic product has started to be used in patients. A physician or pharmacist is permitted to substitute the generic drug when fulfilling a prescription for the originator compound.

Generic pharmaceutical companies have a very different business model to originator companies. They do not carry out research and development on new active ingredients. Instead, they focus all of their efforts on being able to efficiently manufacture and distribute pharmaceuticals. Generic pharmaceutical companies face direct competition from each other and from the originators, and so they operate under pressure for product price and quality. Generic pharmaceutical companies are important to healthcare organisations as they facilitate serving the healthcare needs of the population within the inevitable budgetary constraints.

A generic medicine is not always precisely the same as the originator medicine: it will contain the same active ingredient, but it may, for example, be in a different salt form or a different physical form. For example, Pfizer's calcium antagonist, Amlodipine (marketed under the name Norvasc®) is marketed by Pfizer as the besylate salt. It faced generic competition from the functionally equivalent product amlodipine maleate. Similarly, GSK marketed Paroxetine (under the name Paxil®) in the hemihydrate form, which was protected by a patent. The medicine containing anhydrous paroxetine hydrochloride was considered to be essentially the same by the medicines regulators, and so the generic product with anhydrous paroxetine hydrochloride could be substituted for GSK's product with paroxetine hydrochloride hemihydrate.

In general, there are three hurdles to generic competition for a medicine. The first is patents, as described in most of this chapter. Further hurdles are provided by regulatory data exclusivity and synthetic challenges.

### 17.9.2 Regulatory Data Exclusivity

In all the major pharmaceutical markets, including the US, Europe and Japan, the sale of prescription medicines is tightly regulated. The approval of a new medicine is only permitted after Phase III clinical trials have been carried out in patients, and demonstrated a satisfactory benefit-risk balance.

It is self-evident that once the originator has demonstrated a satisfactory benefit-risk balance to secure a marketing authorisation, it is not in the public interest that authorisation of generic versions of the medicine should require the generic company to repeat the same clinical trials as the originator to come to the market. Indeed, it would be highly unethical to carry out a further clinical trial and deny a control group of patients a treatment that we now know they would benefit from. Regulatory law makers in a number of countries have therefore struck a compromise between the needs of the originator pharmaceutical companies and the needs of the public by permitting companies to apply for a marketing authorisation for a generic medicine without repeating the originator's clinical trials. Instead, the competitor can rely on the safety and efficacy data generated by the originator. However, such use of the data by a competitor company is only permitted after a fixed period during which the originator has the exclusive permission to use the data. This is referred to as "Regulatory Data Exclusivity". Regulatory Data Exclusivity is a narrow, but strong, right. Unlike for a patent, it does not depend for its validity on any novelty or inventive step assessment; it is simply necessary for the trial to have been carried out. For as long as the Regulatory Data Exclusivity is in place, a third party cannot be granted a drug marketing authorisation. That constitutes an absolute bar to marketing the drug; the generic company does not have any option to launch "at risk", as they would in the face of a patent.

The period after which the loss of "Regulatory Data Exclusivity" occurs varies from country to country. In the US, it is 5 years from first US approval of a new small molecule drug. Although the specific rules are complex, in general no application for a marketing authorisation for a generic version of an originator's product – a so-called "abbreviated new drug application (ANDA)", as it is based only on limited bioequivalence studies – can be accepted by the FDA during this period. For "biologics" (proteins, nucleic acids, cells, tissues and other similar products), the period of data exclusivity in the US is 12 years from first US approval of the drug. When this legislation was introduced in 2010, the longer exclusivity period was believed to be necessary to properly incentivise the more costly and lengthy development of biologic medicines. It remains to be seen if the 12 year period was roughly right. That assessment will need to keep in mind that until 2010, there was no mechanism for the authorisation by the FDA of generic biologic medicines, meaning that for early biologics the originator had an essentially perpetual data exclusivity.

In Europe, for medicines first authorised after 2003, the competitor must wait until 8 years have elapsed before it can apply for a generic marketing authorisation. Further, the marketing authorisation of the generic medicine cannot take effect until 10 years after the first authorisation of the originator's version of the medicine in Europe. This applies to both small and large molecule drugs. In addition, if the originator gains approval for a new therapeutic indication in the first 8 years of marketing which brings significant clinical benefit over existing therapies, then the 10 year period before generic marketing can begin is extended by a further year. This combination of 8 years before a generic marketing application can be submitted, together with the further 2 years before marketing can begin delayed by a further 1 year in the event of a significant new indication is often referred to as the "8 + 2 + 1" rule for determining the earliest date when generic competition can begin in Europe.

In the example shown in Figure 17.4 above, the drug received its authorisation 12 years from the patent filing date. The US 5 year "Regulatory Data Exclusivity" will then expire at 17 years, so before the patent has expired. In contrast, the 8 + 2 year period for the European "Regulatory and Marketing Exclusivity" will expire at 22 years from the patent filing date, so after the patent has expired.

Given that a patent expires 20 years after filing (or up to 25 years if a patent term extension is available), whilst data exclusivity runs from the time of marketing authorisation, a medicine that reaches the market only very slowly may have a data protection period that goes beyond the date of patent expiry. In this situation, the timing of generic entry is determined not by the expiry date of the patent (and any relevant patent extensions) but rather by the availability of the abbreviated regulatory procedures. An example of this is the synthetic low molecular weight heparin derivative, Fondaparinux, marketed by Sanofi and then GSK as Arixtra®. In Europe, the patent protection for the active principle expired in January 2008, but the regulatory data protection period did not expire until March 2012, 10 years after the medicine was first approved. That meant that there was no possibility for a generic to enter the market until March 2012, despite the earlier patent expiry.

### 17.9.3 Technical Hurdles

The final hurdle to generic entry is the technical hurdle of synthetic complexity. This is illustrated, to some extent, by Fondaparinux. Fondaparinux is a pentasaccharide with the structure shown in Figure 17.7 and it is manufactured by a 57-stage process

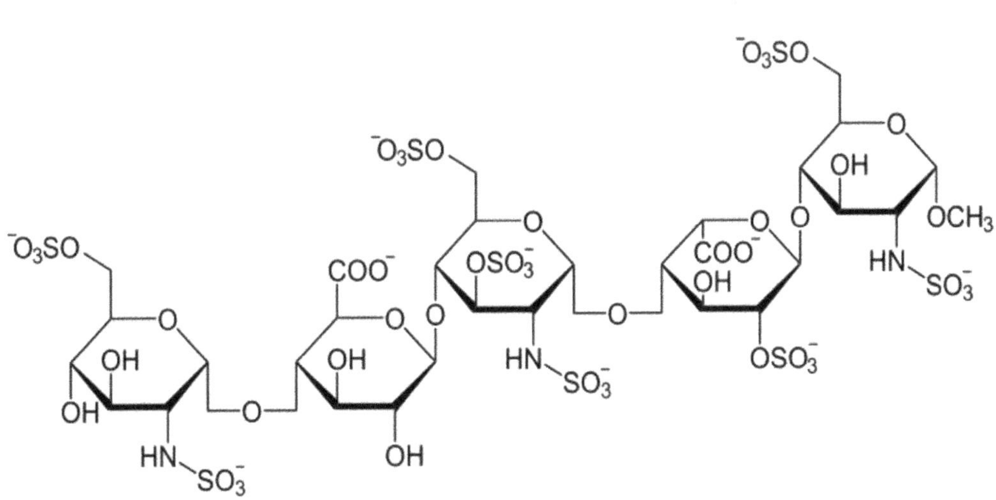

Figure 17.7 The structure of fondaparinux, sold as Arixtra®.

involving many difficult purification steps, as well as the introduction and removal of protecting groups.

Many thought that irrespective of the patent and regulatory hurdles to generic entry, the synthetic complexity would be an insuperable hurdle to overcome and that generic competition to Arixtra® would be unlikely. However, by 2011 a generic version of the medicine was developed by Alchemia and it is marketed in the US by Dr Reddy's Laboratories.

It is fair to say that technical difficulty is rarely a reliable hurdle to generic entry onto the market, though there are occasions when generic entry is delayed by technical issues. Medicine originators should not plan for that to occur, but rather treat it as an unexpected bonus if it does.

## 17.10 Patents as a Source of Information

The lasting record of much of humanity's technology development of the last few centuries is to be found primarily in the patent literature. Patent publications thus form an important repository of information, and they are available for free in paper form in various libraries and electronically over the internet. Patent specifications are quite dry and they generally do not tell as interesting a story as academic papers, but the information in them is necessarily complete and detailed, and they are well indexed and archived (at least for patents published in the last 30 or so years). They thus constitute a source of information that is highly beneficial to those engaged in medicinal chemistry research. Some gaps remain around older patents, but database providers have been catching up with back-filling their contents with older patents and that situation continues to improve. Machine translation has also improved significantly and translated versions of patents from most major languages can now be obtained rapidly that are at least intelligible, if not perfect.

The free on-line database with the broadest international coverage is Espacenet, operated by the European Patent Office. It is found here: http://worldwide.espacenet.com

Patent publications can be located in the database using keywords, inventor names, applicant company names and various other search criteria.

The USPTO operates a similar database, confined to US patent publications. It is found here: http://www.uspto.gov/patents/process/search

Google operates a database search interface. At the time of writing, its content is not yet completely global, but it covers all of the major territories (US, Europe, Japan, China, South Korea, PCT and several more) and the coverage is steadily growing. The search output is less structured than in the databases run by the patent offices, but it is perhaps more user-friendly for non-specialist users. It is found here: http://www.google.com/advanced_patent_search

To an extent, these free databases rely on the text of abstracts submitted by the patent applicants. They are thus not 100% reliable. There thus also exist pay-for-access databases, such as the Derwent World Patents Index® operated by Clarivate Analytics (formerly ThomsonReuters) (see https://clarivate.com/derwent/solutions/derwent-world-patent-index-dwpi/), and the CAplus database operated by CAS, the "Chemical Abstracts" division of the American Chemical Society (see: https://www.cas.org/content/references/patentcoverage). These databases include value-added abstracts and indexing. The commercial databases allow more complex search queries to be formed, as well as often allowing the keyword searches to be carried out through the claims or full text of patents. Further examples of such databases and systems include, STN (http://www.stn-international.de/en/productsservices/products-services), PatBase (https://www.patbase.com) and Questel-Orbit (http://www.questel.com).

Chemical Structure and Chemical Name searching is possible *via* more specialised databases. The CAS Registry database, produced by CAS, is searchable by structures and sub-structures. Searching of CAS Registry is available through STN (operated jointly by CAS and FIZ Karlsruhe), with its interface optimised for the more expert searcher user, and through SciFinder (operated by CAS), which is designed for academic chemists. Entry of structure search queries in the CAS Registry database is not straightforward, and specialised training and experience is generally needed to perform a reliable search. More limited structure-based searching can be done for free using, for example, the SureChem open database portal (https://www.surechembl.org/search/).

The databases mentioned above will provide lists of patent documents that disclose the requested information and allow access to the patent documents themselves. They do not provide up to date details of the status of a patent application: Has it been granted? Is it still in force? Has it been abandoned? For that information, it is necessary to look in the national patent registers. These are also available for free on-line, at the addresses given below. The language used in many of the databases necessarily contains much specialised legal phrasing, so it is recommended to consult a patent attorney before drawing important conclusions from these registry reports:

European Patent Office: https://register.epo.org/
UK IPO: http://www.ipo.gov.uk/types/patent/p-os/p-find/p-ipsum
Germany: https://register.dpma.de/DPMAregister/pat/einsteiger?lang=en
USPTO: https://patentcenter.uspto.gov/
Japan: http://www.jpo.go.jp/ and https://www.j-platpat.inpit.go.jp/

## 17.11 Summary

We hope that this chapter has given a general, if necessarily brief, introduction to the important role that patents play in medicinal chemistry. The main lessons that we hope you will take away are:

- Patents are crucial to medicinal chemistry as they allow the massive investment in product development to be recouped.
- A patent must be applied for and it constitutes a special bargain between a patent applicant and the state: in return for full disclosure of an invention, the inventor is granted a monopoly of limited duration (20 years). In some countries, patent term extensions of up to 5 years are available for patents that protect pharmaceutical inventions.
- During the monopoly period, the patent does not give the patent owner the right to use the invention, but it does give them the right to stop others using it commercially.

- Patent applications are examined by patent offices, but patent validity can be challenged after grant.
- Patents are enforced through the courts. Patent litigation is costly for both parties, so should only be undertaken after serious consideration. Instead of enforcing the patent, a patentee may grant a licence permitting another to use the invention in return for payment or some other benefit.
- In the current structure of the medicine development industry, many projects start in small companies and those companies raise funding or partner with other companies as the project progresses. Patents provide a company with a tradable asset that protects their drug candidate and gives commercial value to it as an asset. They hence enable investment in the progressive stages of a drug development project.
- Given the eventual importance of patents to a medicine development company, the strategy and approach to patents should be considered early in any drug development project.

**Hints and Tips**

- Patents are complicated and mistakes can be costly, so speak to a qualified patent attorney early in any project that will involve patents.
- A patent is a "deal" between an inventor and the state, an exclusionary right over the commercial use of the invention for a limited period in return for the inventor disclosing his or her invention to the public. A patent does not give the applicant the right to use his or her invention, but it does give them the right to stop others using it commercially.
- To be patentable, an invention must be novel, inventive, have industrial applicability and not be specifically excluded from being protectable by a patent. An important feature of novelty is that the inventor's own disclosure of his or her own invention is also part of the state of the art. It is thus crucial that an invention be kept confidential until a patent application is filed.
- The patent must also describe the invention sufficiently clearly and completely for the person skilled in the art to be able to put the invention into practice.
- A patent applicant puts themself in the best possible position by obtaining good data showing that the invention works well. Experiments comparing the invention side-by-side with what has been done before are especially useful. To support inventive step in a patent application, the comparator should be the prior art compound or method that is closest in its features to what is being claimed.
- Patent applications are examined by patent offices, but validity of a patent can be challenged after grant.
- A drug development team puts itself in the best overall position by having a "portfolio" of patents covering various aspects of the final product. The later-filed patents to downstream developments may be inherently less valuable than the first compound *per se* patent, but the later-filed patents have later expiry dates which give them added value in practice.

**Key References**

- P. W. Grubb, P. R. Thomsen, T. Hoxie and G. Wright, *Patents for Chemicals, Pharmaceuticals and Biotechnology*, Oxford University Press, UK, 6th edn, 2016.
- Much helpful information about patents is available on the websites of the UK IPO (https://www.gov.uk/topic/intellectual-property/patents) and the European Patent Office (https://www.epo.org).

## Acknowledgements

The authors acknowledge the assistance of Andrew MacGowan of mac eleven in the creation of Figures 17.1 and 17.2 and the advice of David Clark of Victor Green & Company in the compilation of the list of databases in Section 17.10. Many thanks are due to Sue Scott, Toby Thompson, Chloé Wildman, Philip French and Amelia Thompson of Abel & Imray for their helpful suggestions, drawing of chemical structures and thorough proof-reading.

## References

1. https://www.phrma.org/Advocacy/Intellectual-Property.
2. http://www.pmlive.com/pharma_news/patent_cliff_losses_set_to_cost_pharma_$65bn_by_2019_624492.
3. https://www.cnbc.com/2019/01/23/-pfizer-merck-drop-after-downgrades-on-patent-cliff-competition-.html.
4. O. J. Wouters, *et al.*, *JAMA*, 2020, **323**(9), 844–853.
5. J. A. DiMasi, *et al.*, *J. Health Econ.*, 2016, **47**, 20–33.
6. Unwired Planet International Ltd and another (Respondents) v Huawei Technologies (UK) Co Ltd and another (Appellants), Huawei Technologies Co Ltd and another (Appellants) v Conversant Wireless Licensing SÀRL (Respondent), ZTE Corporation and another (Appellants) v Conversant Wireless Licensing SÀRL (Respondent), [2020] UKSC 37, available at: https://www.supremecourt.uk/cases/docs/uksc-2018-0214-judgment.pdf.
7. P. W. Grubb, P. R. Thomsen, T. Hoxie, and G. Wright, *Patents for Chemicals, Pharmaceuticals and Biotechnology*, Oxford University Press, UK, 2016.
8. European Patent Office Guidelines for Examination, Part G, Chapter VII, Annex, Example 2, available at: https://www.epo.org/law-practice/legal-texts/html/guidelines/e/g_viia_2.htm#GLG_CVIIA_2.
9. [2000] EWHC Patents 49, available at: http://www.bailii.org/ew/cases/EWHC/Patents/2000/49.html.
10. Dr Reddy's Laboratories (UK) Ltd v Eli Lilly and Co Ltd, available at: https://www.bailii.org/cgi-bin/format.cgi?doc=/ew/cases/EWCA/Civ/2009/1362.html.
11. Comparative Study on Hypothetical/Real Cases: Inventive Step/Non-obviousness, Report by the Trilateral Initiative of the European Patent Office, the Japan Patent Office and the United States Patent and Trademark Office, 2008, available at: https://www.trilateral.net/sites/default/files/attachments/b6d4ad95-00be-446b-9cdf-25a96dda7c02/Comparative_Study_on_Cases_Inventive_Step.pdf.
12. L. Xiang, *J. Intellect. Prop. Law Pract.*, 2013, **8**, 539.
13. Human Genome Sciences Inc (Appellant) v Eli Lilly and Company (Respondent), 2011, UKSC 51, available at: https://www.supremecourt.uk/cases/docs/uksc-2010-0047-judgment.pdf.
14. Brüstle v Greenpeace eV; Court of Justice of the European Union Case C-34/10, available at: http://curia.europa.eu/juris/liste.jsf?language=en&num=C-34/10.
15. E. Callaway, *Nature*, 2011, **478**, 441.
16. EP0925294B is available at:http://worldwide.espacenet.com/publicationDetails/originalDocument?CC=EP&NR=0925294B1&KC=B1&FT=D&ND=4&date=19910130&DB=EPODOC&locale=en_EP.

17. US1506316 is available at: https://worldwide.espacenet.com/publicationDetails/originalDocument?CC=US&NR=1506316A&KC=A&FT=D&ND=3&date=19240826&DB=EPODOC&locale=en_EP.
18. http://www.pharmatimes.com/news/keytruda_to_be_top_drug_by_2023_1312064.
19. EP2170959B is available at: https://worldwide.espacenet.com/publicationDetails/originalDocument?FT=D&date=20131002&DB=EPODOC&locale=en_EP&CC=EP&NR=2170959B1&KC=B1&ND=4.
20. European Patent Office Board of Appeal Decision T488/16 can be found here: https://www.epo.org/law-practice/case-law-appeals/recent/t160488eu1.html.
21. Regeneron Pharmaceuticals Inc (Respondent) v Kymab Ltd (Appellant), 2020, UKSC 27, decision can be found here: https://www.supremecourt.uk/cases/docs/uksc-2018-0131-judgment.pdf.
22. The text of the Paris convention can be accessed on the website of the World Intellectual Property Organisation available at: http://www.wipo.int/treaties/en/text.jsp?file_id=288514. A current list of member states is available at: http://www.wipo.int/treaties/en/ShowResults.jsp?lang=en&treaty_id=2.
23. Information about the Patent Cooperation Treaty, including the text of the treaty itself is available at: http://www.wipo.int/pct/en/. A current list of member states is available at: http://www.wipo.int/pct/en/pct_contracting_states.html.
24. For up-to-date information about the see the website of the Unified Patent Court at: http://www.unified-patent-court.org/. Various private sector organisations are also providing up to date commentary, see for example http://www.bristowsupc.com/.
25. https://www.supremecourt.uk/cases/docs/uksc-2016-0197-judgment.pdf.
26. The specification of EP0679157B is available at: https://worldwide.espacenet.com/publicationDetails/originalDocument?FT=D&date=19971119&DB=EPODOC&locale=en_EP&CC=EP&NR=0679157B1&KC=B1&ND=4.
27. The specification of US6197819B is available at: http://worldwide.espacenet.com/publicationDetails/originalDocument?CC=US&NR=6197819B1&KC=B1&FT=D&ND=3&date=20010306&DB=EPODOC&locale=en_EP.
28. More information on the UK Patent Box is available at: https://webarchive.nationalarchives.gov.uk/20140102175714/http://www.hmrc.gov.uk/budget-updates/march2012/patent-box-tech-note.pdf.
29. For details, see: https://www.gov.uk/government/statistics/patent-box-reliefs-statistics/patent-box-relief-statistics-september-2021.

# 18 Target Validation for Medicinal Chemists

Matthew Thomas*[a] and Lorna Ewart[b]

[a]Boehringer Ingelheim Pharma GmbH & Co KG, Immunology and Respiratory Diseases Research Biberach, Birkendorfer Strasse 65, 88397 Biberach an der Riss, Germany; [b]Emulate Inc., 27 Drydock Avenue, Boston, MA 02210, USA
*E-mail: matthew_james.thomas@boehringer-ingelheim.com

## 18.1 Introduction

To validate a target is to provide sufficient evidence of a key role in disease pathobiology – indicating that modulation would confer therapeutic benefit. Yet within this broad definition, we find ambiguity which must be resolved to be successful in the drug discovery process. How much evidence is 'sufficient' and by when must key data be generated in support of the therapeutic concept? Validation of a target is an iterative process which evolves in sophistication together with drug discovery from initial identification, through hit finding and lead optimisation, until the concept is tested in patients (Figure 18.1). Yet how can we effectively identify 'losers' within a portfolio of projects and focus on 'winners' which will go on to help patients? Ultimately, we can only truly validate a target through positive clinical data generated with a selective therapeutic which effectively modulates the target, yet such an assertion is unhelpful to a drug discoverer considering a potential mechanism to pursue. Therefore we must ask ourselves several questions when considering a new target: Have we looked in the right place? What value might a drug for this target offer patients? How much evidence is sufficient to initiate drug discovery (and is some evidence more meaningful than others)? What level of risk are we willing to take in pursuit of this target? Can we generate a critical path of experiments to mitigate such risk? What considerations are important in the translational path of a new drug going into healthy volunteers, then ultimately patients?

The Handbook of Medicinal Chemistry: Principles and Practice, 2nd Edition
Edited by Simon E. Ward and Andrew M. Davis

Published by the Royal Society of Chemistry, www.rsc.org

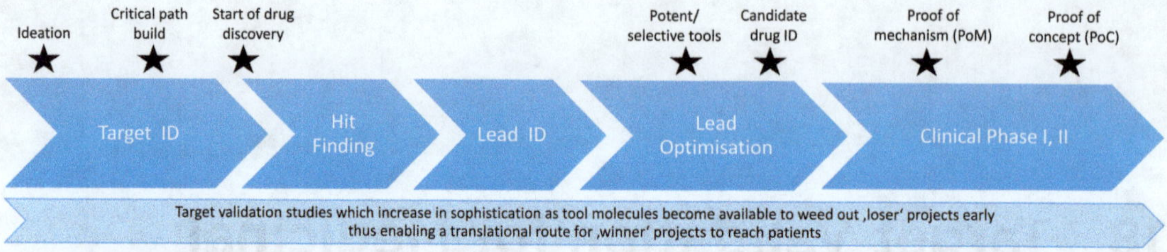


**Figure 18.1** Stages in the drug discovery process. Summary of stages in the drug discovery process from initial target identification through to clinical assessment. Validation of a target is an iterative process which evolves together with drug discovery and enhances our confidence in therapeutic benefit at each stage. The goal of a drug discovery team is to push attrition into earlier stages of the process, thus releasing resource to focus on 'winners'.

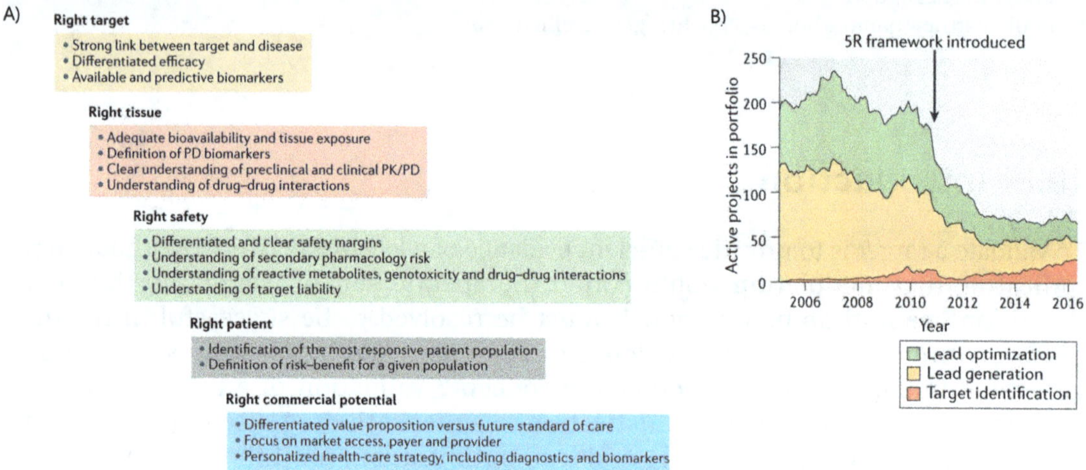


**Figure 18.2** AstraZeneca's 5 Rights for drug discovery. (A) Summary of the '5 Rights', which when implemented at AstraZeneca, increased clinical success of drug discovery projects. (B) The impact of the 5Rs framework on the balance of activity within the discovery portfolio – reducing the number of projects and pushing activity (and attrition) earlier in the drug discovery process.

Several large pharmaceutical companies provide guidance on target validation for their organisation and the industry as a whole, so as to bring attrition forward in the drug discovery timeline – failing early is a far more effective use of time and resources. AstraZeneca has championed the '5 Rights' for drug discovery which guided a profound strategic change for AstraZeneca (Figure 18.2A) – one which improved success rates from candidate drug nomination to phase III completion from 4% in 2005–2010 to 19% in 2012–2016. A consequential part of this change was a reduction in the number of active preclinical projects (by as much as 65%). In addition, the balance of activity dramatically changed. Before 2010, the target identification phase represented <10% of activity, with the remaining 90% split between lead identification and optimisation.

After 2010, these phases shared equal levels of activity – an indication of the need to improve/expand initial target validation (Figure 18.2B).[1,2] Pfizer's '3 Pillars' also provide a useful guide, yet refer more to feasibility by placing emphasis on mechanism of action and effective modulation of target.[3]

Importantly, target validation does not end with the initiation of drug discovery, yet continues throughout the project, benefitting from potent and selective large or small molecules which build our understanding of target modulation and how this might ultimately benefit patients. We can use the '5 Rights' principles to illustrate how an advancing drug discovery project can ask increasingly complex questions which build the validation package. The 'Right Target' requires evidence of 'strong disease linkage', 'differentiated efficacy' and 'available and predictive biomarkers'. Finding links to disease will be covered in some depth within this chapter, as will measures of efficacy – particularly in human patient cell systems. Initially this can be through genetic knockdown or target modulation with suboptimal tool molecules, yet as a project progresses – and the quality of tool molecules improve, especially to the point of candidate nomination – a greater understanding of the 'differentiated efficacy' can be achieved through more complex cell and *in vivo* systems. Such experiments also start to show whether we impact the 'Right Tissue' as we begin to understand pharmacokinetic/target engagement/pharmacodynamic (PK/TE/PD) relationships. As we draw closer to the clinic, a deep understanding of the 'Right Safety' profile is assessed – for a target to be truly validated, modulation must offer benefit to the patient, which can only be achieved with an appropriate therapeutic index (*i.e.* benefit outweighs any adverse effects). Finding the 'Right Patient' is an extension of target biomarker exploration initiated early in a project, yet will include identification of a responder population – likely *via* pathway biomarkers dysregulated in disease, yet responsive to modulation by the evolving therapeutic. The answers to these questions form preclinical predictions of a clinically valid target, with the ultimate proof demonstrated by phase III clinical trial data.

In this chapter we aim to provide a framework by which a drug discover can effectively ask questions key to novel target validation. We also hope to provide guidance on how to construct a critical path of experiments – each of which having the potential to de-validate the target. Equivocal data from these pivotal experiments would mean carrying far greater risk into drug discovery which must be mitigated as early as possible. Clear, positive outcomes in critical path experiments should provide sufficient confidence in the validity of a target to initiate drug discovery and the subsequent efforts to build on that understanding as the project progresses toward patients.

## 18.2 'Hide and Seq' – Searching for Novel Targets

The first critical step in any validation process is searching for a meaningful target. A target whose disregulation we hypothesise may be a driver of disease pathology, and whose modulation may provide a therapeutic effect with an acceptable safety margin. Evidence starts with the patient. It may come from genetics (GWAS or rare variant analysis) which highlight a potential association of genetic variants to prevalence of, or protection from disease. It may come from evidence the target is upregulated/downregulated/activated or repressed in disease as evidenced from disease tissue. It may come from pathway analysis comparisons (transcriptomics, proteomics and/or metabolomics) between healthy and diseased tissues which may point to a key target on the pathway. Evidence may also come from targeted perturbations in phenotypic disease-relevant cellular assays using genetics of pharmacological interventions. It may come from animal models which recapitulate some aspect of disease pathology. Ideally evidence builds from multiple sources. Validation seeks to provide data that our hypothesis is valid and may require increasingly complex model systems – from primary cells, cell co-culture, organoids, tissue slices, to whole organs and finally *in vivo* models. Each of these steps will be discussed further in the next sections.

### 18.2.1 Genetic and Epigenetic Factors

The first step in any validation process is searching for a meaningful target. Genetics may provide a very useful guide to finding the right target – the relative success of novel therapeutics which have a basis in observed genetic modifications is 2-fold greater than those which do not.[4,5] Different methods of identifying genetic mutations (or single nucleotide polymorphisms, SNPs) can reveal modifications of differing interpretation and value. Genome Wide Association Studies (GWAS) tend to reveal targets or pathways which influence biology in many individuals, albeit to a small degree. Such mutations are less likely to reveal specific target pathways yet provide an area of biology to further explore. As an example, research into schizophrenia indicates a strong genetic linkage with a child of two schizophrenic parents having a 40% likelihood of developing a form of the disease. Over the past decade, GWAS has revealed over 100 disease-linked mutations, yet their low odds-ratios (*i.e.* a low magnitude of disease association for a given allele) make downstream signalling networks and biologic consequences that lead to disease currently unfeasible to determine, and thus currently limits their application to novel target identification/validation.[6]

Rare variant analysis is needed to reveal polymorphisms with a profound impact on pathophysiology – a target pathway which affects fewer people but whose modulation has a higher chance of correcting pathology. An example of such a disease-linked mutation is alpha-1 antitrypsin mutations, which reduce protective effects on the connective tissue of the lungs from the elastase released by leukocytes. Through a rare loss of function mutation, when inherited homozygously it frequently leads to lung emphysema in adults.[7]

Yet which genes we express are not only controlled by DNA sequence – increasingly, epigenetic factors which control the accessibility of genes *via* environmental influences, are recognised as key to disease susceptibility.[8] Epigenetic players include histone modifiers, enzymes which alter DNA methylation and microRNAs, which are small, non-coding RNA molecules that can post-transcriptionally regulate gene expression. In recent years, advances in technology have enabled the mutated factors themselves to be considered as feasible targets. Examples in early clinical trials include gene replacement therapy for cystic fibrosis, sickle cell anaemia and congenital blindness, where a virus containing the healthy gene may be used to re-introduce functional protein to key cell populations.[9–11] Furthermore, the strong links between Hepatitis C Virus (HCV)-

associated liver disease and miR122 have triggered the development of inhibitory miR species or 'antagomir' therapeutics – currently in phase II studies.[12]

### 18.2.2 Exploiting 'Big Data'

We have witnessed a dramatic growth in molecular biology technology over the last two decades – phenomenal amounts of data are generated on a daily basis, such as transcriptomics, proteomics or metabolomics. Such data may be structured or unstructured but is collectively referred to as 'big data'. Within the field of 'big data', data scientists and bioinformaticians work to analyse and extract data that is too large or complex for more traditional data-processing tools and technologies. Such application increases our understanding of pathobiology – generating novel hypotheses for testing and/or identification of novel targets for validation. Many large pharmaceutical companies have invested in high-throughput 'target mining' where algorithms are used to find connection points in gene expression or proteomic data-sets, and thus identify potential targets for modulation. These data-sets can be visualised to generate network maps of health and disease. More recently, these maps can look beyond whole tissue, which only reveal net changes across an array of cell types, to 'Single Cell Seq' studies, which offer individual cell resolution. These new technologies facilitate target discovery and validation within cells, between cells and between tissues to more comprehensively validate novel targets[13,14] (see Figure 18.3).

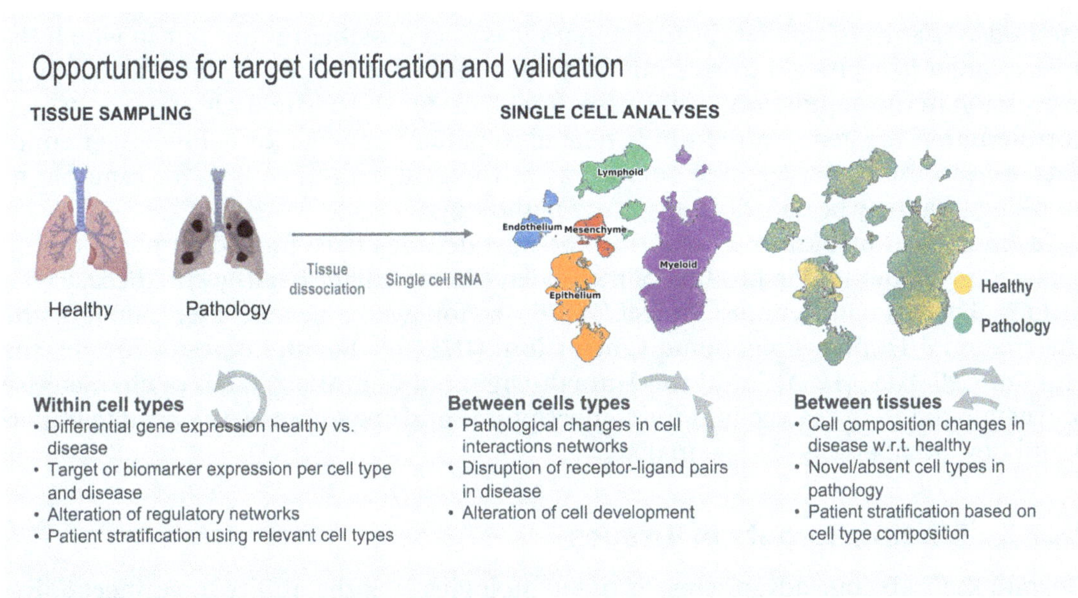


**Figure 18.3** Single cell seq in target identification and validation. How healthy *vs.* disease tissue sampling can be studied with single cell sequencing (shown as UMAP (Uniform Manifold Approximation and Projection for Dimension Reduction) plots) to reveal the pathobiology within cells, between cell types and between tissues.

Just at the beginning of this century, the Human Genome Project had farms of sequencing machines to decipher the human genome – by far the largest endeavour at the time at an estimated cost of $2.7 billion. Nowadays, democratisation of technology means that the same feat can be carried out in a single run of a modern sequencing machine for $5000 in just a few hours, which in turn has made it possible to sequence hundreds of thousands of individuals to explore human variation and its relation to phenotypic traits and genetic disorders. But not only has there been growth in DNA (genomics) or RNA (transcriptomics – that portion of the genetic code being transcribed into RNA at any one time in a cell), but other 'omic' technologies such as proteomics (that portion of the genome that is being translated into proteins at any one point in time) and metabolomics (the cell's metabolic profile at any one point in time) are increasingly used. Add to this the plethora of cell processes that had been transformed into the sequencing domain. For example ChIP-seq (chromatin immunoprecipitation sequencing), which identifies the genomic position of DNA or histone binding proteins, ATAC-seq, (assay for transposase accessible chromatin using sequencing), which detects open enhancer and promoter regions in the genome and high-throughput 3-C methods (chromosome conformation capture) that measures DNA proximity and allows the 3D reconstruction of the chromosomes in the nucleus, just to name a few. Together, these formidable and affordable data resources allow high-throughput measurements of putative drug targets, but how can they be effectively applied? Taking, for example, a new target candidate, these technologies can help us investigate changes between healthy and disease conditions at the protein, metabolite (if the target participates in a chemical reaction) and gene expression levels. Importantly, these data can be re-used for other target candidates or used for high-throughput mining of novel targets using machine-learning methods. Thanks to publicly available data it is also possible to find out in which tissues a target is expressed to rule out off-target effects, or we can explore variations in expression in the population. In the case of fatal diseases – particularly cancer – we can corroborate if the gene expression is related to patient survival, or using epigenomics data we can explore epigenetic alterations at the gene target, caused for example by smoking, that may be contributing to the pathology.

Technological breakthroughs during the past decades have fuelled large-scale projects to deepen our understanding of molecular biology under healthy and disease conditions. The Human Genome Project (HGP) was followed a decade later (2009) by the International Human Epigenome Consortium (IHEC).[15] For the current decade, the Human Cell Atlas (HCA)[16] and the Human Organoid Cell Atlas[17] seek to characterise and catalogue all human cells at the transcriptome and epigenome levels, and to understand how populations change in disease.

### 18.2.3 Finding Targets in Tissues

Despite their obvious advantages, 'seq' technologies lack the ability to connect a dysregulated target/pathway to complex disease features that are observed histologically (although recent advances in spatial transcriptomics may enable this in some tissues) and thereby build a picture of causality. Immunohistochemical (IHC) analysis of diseased tissues has been a fundamental target validation tool for decades, yet can have limitations based on reagent quality (*e.g.* antibody affinity), the number of markers assessed and throughput. More recently, IHC assessment has been advanced *via* multiplex methods (*i.e.* the sequential staining and stripping of antibodies on one tissue section) paired with computer-assisted image processing. An example of the utility of such systems can been seen in the oncology field, where a deep understanding of the complex tumour microenvironment is key to further development of novel immune-oncology targets. Where a simple score of CD3/8 T cell staining was previously considered prognostic for some cancers, we can now build a picture of many immune cell subtypes – where they are within the tumour and with what cell partners they are interacting. Staining for tumour-infiltrating immune cells (CD3, CD4, CD8, FOXP3 and CD68), immune checkpoint molecules (PD-L1, PD1, TIM3 and LAG3), and for identification of tumour cells themselves has recently been demonstrated in single formalin-fixed paraffin-embedded sections from gastric tumours – a test case for utility across an array of other tumours and similarly complex pathologic features.[18]

Modern technology has also impacted histological assessment – where previously the effectiveness of histological staining was dependent on the antibody affinity for or stain used to bind the target, techniques such as *in situ* hybridisation (ISH) bind genetic material (mRNA or DNA) within each cell to reveal expression/localisation of the target pathway. Chromogenic *in situ* hybridisation (CISH) enables you to gain genetic information in the context of tissue morphology using brightfield microscopy. DNA- and RNA-fluorescent *in situ* hybridisation (FISH) allows the detection of multiple gene locations/mutations (for DNA) or gene expression levels (for RNA) within cells or across tissues using fluorescence microscopy. Next-generation 'RNAscope' technology has improved signal-to-noise ratios to increase sensitivity – particularly useful when one is looking for rare cells. Furthermore, breakthroughs in spatial transcriptomics may be able to combine the unbiased power of RNAseq with tissue resolution of approximately 3–10 cells. Thus we can begin to combine our 'seq' technologies with methods which reveal disease pathobiology – a key element to the validation of novel drug targets.[19,20]

### 18.2.4 Starting with Quality Material

The effectiveness of any search for a novel target is dependent on the source and quality of the starting material. Patient material should be a priority in such searches, especially samples with a high degree of background information (including age, gender, disease subtype and severity, history of medication). It is important to note that tissue acquired *via* transplant is likely to represent end-stage disease and therefore must be aligned with the likely point of intervention conceived for the therapy. Furthermore, any sample should also be compared to a healthy control, which is relatively straightforward if your starting material is blood, yet more challenging if it is an organ. Using samples from animal models as a source for novel target mechanisms comes with significant risks in translatability to human. Although animal systems are a useful tool in drug discovery, they are a poor starting point, which we explore further in Section 18.6.

## 18.3 Phenotypic Screens – Search and Partial Validation in One System?

Phenotypic disease-relevant cellular assays are becoming more prevalent in modern drug discovery. Such assays modulate disease-relevant phenotypes without assuming a specific target or mechanism of action. Successful phenotypic assays often follow the 'Rule of 3': (1) clear linkage to the disease by using either human primary cells or induced pluripotent stem cells (iPSC), (2) the assay readout should be as close as possible to the disease pathobiology, (3) avoidance of exogenous stimuli to induce a disease phenotype to reduce the chance of identifying a stimulus- instead of disease-modifying mechanism.[21]

Phenotypic screens can be used for both pharmacological and genetic target identification and validation. Biologically annotated small molecule libraries (*i.e.* those which contain chemical matter known to modulate particular targets) can be used as a means to accelerate drug discovery research. This is based on the paradigm that similar receptors bind similar ligands.[22] For instance, to discover new kinase inhibitors, a library consisting of known kinase inhibitors may be screened in order to identify starting points for a medicinal chemistry optimisation programme.[23] On the other hand, chemically diverse, non-annotated libraries can also be used to screen for phenotypic changes in the relevant cell-based assays, although target deconvolution can be a long process and the affinity between the small molecule and its putative target needs to be shown.[24] One recent successful example aimed to discover a novel treatment for the genetic disorder Spinal Muscular Atrophy (SMA) – caused by a splice variant of Survival of Motor Neuron-2 (SMN2). Transcriptional profiling analysis of PNN1-46 SMA patient-derived fibroblasts were used in a screen to find modifiers of SMN2 splicing. The resultant chemical matter discovered led to risdiplam[25] – further details of which are discussed in Chapter 24.

### 18.3.1 Techniques to Modulate Gene Expression

With the development of RNA inhibitor (or RNAi) technology, high-throughput-based genetic target identification and validation in combination with phenotypic cell-based readouts became feasible, both in an arrayed and a pooled format. Modulating gene expression in cells has initially been achieved using RNAi technologies. RNAi-mediated gene repression relies on either transfection of synthetic (small interfering) siRNAs, plasmid-encoded (short hairpin) shRNAs or transduction of shRNA encoding viral particles (either as a simple stem loop or more recently an embedded (micro) miRNA backbone). However, RNAi reagents are frequently prone to off-target effects. Therefore, it is prudent to further validate hits from RNAi screens using orthogonal technologies such as CRISPR-Cas9 to exclude potential off-target activities responsible for the observed phenotype.[26]

CRISPR (an acronym for 'Clustered Regularly Interspaced Short Palindromic Repeats')-based technologies use an RNA-guided Cas9 endonuclease to drive genomic perturbation. The first functional genomic CRISPR-Cas9 screens used a fully active Cas9 endonuclease, which knocked out specific gene loci to evaluate the phenotypic effects of the deletions.[27,28] In these screens, Cas9-mediated gene knockouts are induced by endogenous DNA repair machinery repairing the double strand break. This is usually accomplished by non-homologous end joining, the cellular error-prone repair mechanism introducing short insertions or deletions (indels) at the repaired locus. The indels cause frameshift mutations which frequently lead to premature stop codons and thus functional gene ablation.[29] As the CRISPR-Cas9-based rate of gene deletion is rather high, homozygous gene deletions occur frequently and thus the impact of the perturbation on the phenotype is maximised. This is strikingly different from the RNAi-based approaches, which suppress gene expression but rarely reduce it entirely. Additionally, for loci where gene editing occurred successfully, the per cell and per (single guide) sgRNA impact on the relevant phenotype is very consistent, and again contrasts that of RNAi approaches, where individual shRNAs induce variable gene suppressions and thus quite variable phenotypic changes. This partiality in gene knock down and its associated phenotype may offer an opportunity in the evaluation of gene dosage effects – *i.e.* the degree of pathway modulation required for an effect, which is not feasible with CRISPR knockout screens.[26]

In addition to knocking out genes and evaluating the resulting phenotype, the CRISPR-Cas9 technology has been further developed to allow either transcriptional repression or activation of endogenous loci, known as CRISPRi for CRISPR inference or CRISPRa for CRISPR activation. CRISPRi and CRISPRa are both based on a nuclease-deficient or dead Cas9 protein (dCas9), which is used to specifically target individual promoter regions within the genome. For CRISPRi, the nuclease-deficient Cas9 sterically blocks transcriptional initiation and/or elongation, or is directly fused with a transcriptional repression domain, *e.g.* a KRAB zinc finger protein. For CRISPRa, various different fusion proteins of dCas9 with transcriptional activators have been described.[30] CRISPRi is more similar to RNAi than the CRIPSR knockout (CRISPRko) technology, and can be used to target genes or gene loci which are difficult to study by CRISPRko, *e.g.* amplified genomic regions as occurring in tumour cells.[31] CRISPRa enables something completely new to genomic-based screening, meaning gain-of-function analysis driven by gene expression from the endogenous locus. This should have a major impact on drug discovery, especially for diseases with complex cellular pathophysiology where target discovery and validation has proven challenging. In summary, CRISPRi and CRISPRa are promising tools for genetic target inhibition and activation, and together with RNAi-based and CRISPRko-based screening technologies are likely to become increasingly indispensable tools for target identification and validation.

### 18.3.2 Screening the Secretome

Moving away from phenotypes driven at the gene level, we can also consider cell–cell interactions that drive complex processes *via* a variety of secreted proteins that act on cell surface receptors. It is estimated that 3500 to 6000 proteins are actively transported out of the cell.[32] Having (complementary) cDNAs coding for secreted proteins cloned in expression vectors enables large-scale protein expression leading to the generation of secreted protein libraries that can be used for new target discovery in virtually all screening assays, and their permutations. Such protein libraries are available commercially or can be custom-made if additional features (tags) or expression methods are desired. The major advantages of using secreted protein are: (1) application of the protein to the cell culture does not involve stressing cells (in contrast to transfection and infection approaches), (2) the protein quantities can be dosed and also combined with additional test vehicles (neutralising antibodies, small molecules) to further focus the screen on the identification of desired outcomes, (3) protein mutagenesis can readily be performed to confirm validity of the results and identify functionality of protein domains.

Generation of secreted protein libraries involves a number of considerations, including tagging the proteins for detection, purification and expression in serum-free systems.[33] Libraries can be generated by simple transfection methods in cells with HEK293 cells being used the most frequently because they offer high transfection efficiency and protein expression levels. Each expression plasmid is used to transfect cells in one well of a 96- or 384-well plate and the exogenous protein is harvested in the supernatant of transfected cells and used without further purification. Levels of exogenous protein in the supernatant can be detected in the nanolitre range or lower. Protein purification is a complex, lengthy and costly process so scientists typically try to avoid it, but because cells are exposed to significant stress following DNA transfection, they can release factors that might affect the performance of the subsequent screening assay. Therefore it is advisable to test supernatants of cells transfected with control DNA.

Following hit confirmation using newly transfected cell supernatants, preliminary structural analysis of hit proteins can identify potential functional domains that can be mutated or deleted and re-expressed for additional functional analysis in the preferred assay system. These results provide additional confidence in the role of the hit proteins and pave the way to assess mode of action of the protein in the pathways that drive the functional response. Tagging proteins at this stage is also advisable in order to embark on studies aimed at identification of potential functional partners of the newly identified proteins. Protein pull-downs, fluorescence activated cell screening (FACS) analysis and other methods can be used to identify binding partners and can lead to extensive characterisation of the biological role of the newly identified proteins.

Secretome libraries of different formats and complexities have been used in phenotypic screens that led to successful identification of pigment epithelium-derived factor (PEDF) as a regulator of embryonic human stem cell pluripotency,[34] cytokines such as IL-34 and their receptors,[35] novel complement-binding proteins from *S. aureus* allowing immune evasion,[36] survival factors and anti-proliferative agents. Examples include fibroblast growth factor (FGF)16 – a candidate for cardiac regeneration and repair, and colony stimulating factor 1 receptor (CSF-1R) which was identified as a key regulator of tumour-associated macrophages (TAMS) which was developed as an antibody therapeutic.[37]

Overall, secreted protein libraries are valuable tools for identification of new targets and are ideally suited for application in phenotypic screens due to the ease of subsequent hit characterisation using recombinant technologies.[38]

## 18.4 Functional Cell Systems – Assessing 'Differential Patient Biology'

Modulation of a target rarely impacts one cell type and even if so, the consequences of modulation are even less likely to be restricted to that cell. The nature of a target pathway can only be truly revealed when a network of cells and interaction partners (*e.g.* extra-cellular matrix) is assembled within a test system. By enriching the environment in which cells act and react, including stimuli which are more representative of the physiological or pathophysiological situation, we increase the likelihood of observing a difference between healthy and disease cells. Once observed, this 'differential patient biology' can be explored for pathway activity and opens opportunities for modulation of targets within key pathways to return pathobiology toward health. Robust evidence of a target driving 'differential patient biology' can provide the core around which an extensive validation data package is built.

### 18.4.1 Co-culture Systems

Studies from the Medzhitov group elegantly demonstrate how certain cell types can form heterogeneous units, in which each cell partner provides support for the other. One such example is a fibroblast (structural cell) and a macrophage (immune cell), where the fibroblast senses environmental factors (*e.g.* physical space/proximity to other cells, or oxygen availability) which influences growth factor (colony stimulating factor) release to a neighbouring macrophage. The responding macrophage, in turn, releases another growth factor (platelet-derived growth factor) which supports the fibroblast.[39] And thus, pathobiology which involves these cells (*e.g.* remodelled/fibrotic tissue) would benefit from co-culture so as to capture the role of a target/pathway within this network of signalling.

Another example of co-culture needed for target validation is in the study of adaptive immune processes. Here, responsiveness of a system is reliant on stimulator cell (*e.g.* the antigen-presenting dendritic cell) and a responder cell (*e.g.* the T lymphocyte) as well as the immune status of the donor. Co-culture of immune cells from a single donor is favoured to avoid responses against 'non-self' antigens. This can cause practical challenges in isolation and preparation of some populations. For example, dendritic cells generated from blood monocytes take several days of differentiation, during which autologous T cells from the same sample must be preserved (usually frozen). Once paired, an *in vitro* response must still be initiated by loading of antigen into the presenting dendritic cell and is reliant on a corresponding T cell receptor – an indicator of immunity in the donor. Yet it is only when these elements are brought together that the signalling pathways which drive this immune synapse and the ensuing pathologic proliferation and cytokine production can be used to determine the role of the target of interest.[40]

Another important cell pairing to consider is that of structural cells (*e.g.* fibroblasts or pericytes) and barrier cells (*e.g.* epithelium or endothelium). Attempts to culture endothelial cells into a vessel have failed in the absence of a supporting pericyte.[41] Similarly, culture of alveolar type 2 cells – the source of gas-exchanging type 1 cells and therefore

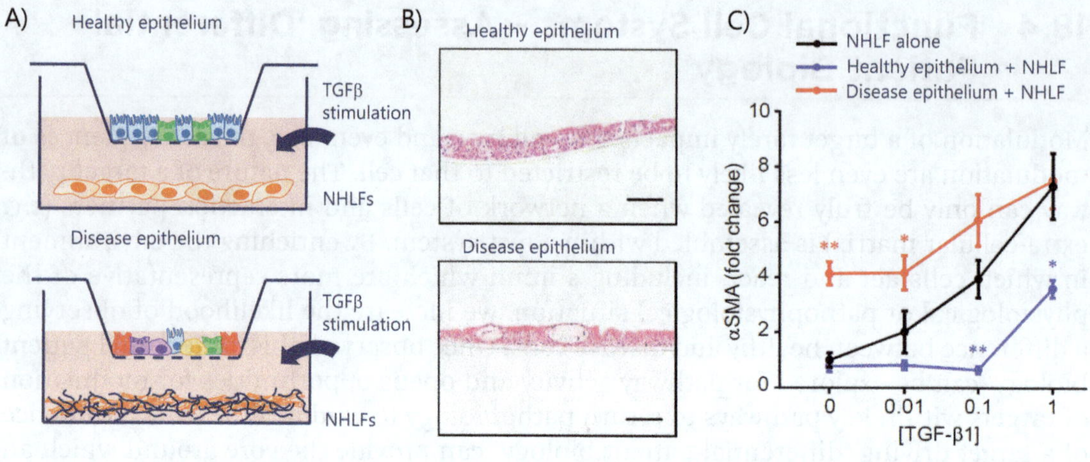


**Figure 18.4** Epithelial:fibroblast crosstalk. (A) Schematics of epithelial cells, cultured in inserts at an air–liquid interface from primary basal epithelium isolated from healthy or fibrosis patient lungs. Normal healthy lung fibroblasts (NHLFs) co-cultured in the wells below - stimulated with increasing concentrations of TGFβ. (B) H&E images of healthy *vs.* diseased (fibrotic) epithelium, showing fewer ciliated cells and more secretory populations. (C) Mono-culture NHLF response to TGFβ dose response (black), showing increased alpha smooth muscle actin - an indicator of fibroblast to myofibroblast transition. Fibrotic epithelium promotes fibroblast transition in the absence of TGFβ (red). Healthy epithelial co-culture protects fibroblasts from pro-fibrotic effects of TGFβ.

important in repair of alveoli – is far more effective with fibroblast co-culture.[42] Furthermore, we can observe a reciprocal influence of primary small airway epithelial cells (SAECs), grown at an air–liquid interface, together with fibroblasts (see Figure 18.4). When derived from healthy donors, epithelial cells exert a protective effect on fibroblasts challenged with a fibrosis-driving growth factor (TGFβ – transforming growth factor β). However, if derived from pulmonary fibrosis patient donors or conditioned with stimuli from fibrosis patients, SAECs can drive fibrotic transition in fibroblasts in the absence of stimulation.

Finding target mechanisms which can reverse the differential patient biology of diseased/conditioned epithelial cells may provide the key to effective repair of barrier tissues. The disruption of barrier integrity, whether between us and the outside world (gut or lung epithelium) or between our circulation and tissue (microvascular endothelium) is a common feature of disease. Attempts to model such processes acutely (*e.g.* inflammatory mediator release) or chronically (*e.g.* repair/fibrosis) is vital for the validation of new targets which can treat our most burdensome diseases.

### 18.4.2 Environmental Stimuli

Studying phenotypic and functional characteristics of primary patient cells is important, yet said features are also influenced by their culture environment. Extracellular matrix (ECM) is the network of collagen/fibronectin fibres and glycoproteins, which hold tissues together. The composition of ECM can vary greatly between and within organs and can be altered in disease – especially fibrotic diseases, which are characterised by the deposition of modified matrix as scarring. Scar tissue is stiff and will trigger mechano-sensing pathways in cells which sit within it. This can convert a normal healthy fibroblast into a collagen-producing myofibroblast, thus exacerbating the problem, or change the way a macrophage migrates – open, flexible matrix is navigated by amoeboid movement, in which the macrophage squeezes through the tissue, whereas stiff, dense matrix stimulates mesenchymal macrophage movement where enzymes are produced to dissolve holes through which the cell moves.[43] Furthermore, proteomic assessment of matrix content reveals profound differences between health and disease. The influence of matrix on cell behaviour was nicely demonstrated by Bitterman and colleagues, who compared the gene signature and phenotype of fibroblasts derived from healthy or fibrosis patients, cultured in matrix isolated from either healthy or fibrotic tissue.[44] The authors found that the source of the cells had surprisingly little influence on phenotype, yet the matrix in which they were cultured did – where healthy matrix conferred a heathy phenotype on disease-derived cells, and diseased matrix converted healthy cells to a fibrotic phenotype. Therefore, where possible, when designing a functional cell assay, a relevant matrix should be considered.

The sophistication of stimuli is also key to revealing differential patient biology. Assay systems which utilise a single mediator to stimulate a disease process tend to find inhibitors of that mediator – only useful in the rare situations in which a single mediator is the key disease driver. As an example, fibroblast cultures stimulated with TGFβ will transition to myofibroblasts, as assessed using staining for αSMA (alpha smooth muscle actin). Yet this effect is seen equally in cells isolated from healthy individuals or those suffering from tissue fibrosis. However, when an epithelial cell line is co-cultured with the fibroblasts and stimulated with low-level TGFβ (unable to stimulate change in the fibroblasts alone), then a cocktail of mediators released from the epithelium induces fibroblast transition. Importantly, it is only under these more sophisticated conditions that we can observe a difference in sensitivity in the responder fibroblasts – approximately 2-fold greater transition observed in diseased cells.

### 18.4.3 Organoids

Within the last decade, organoids have gained significant attention as cell systems to enable complementary study of targets in the drug discovery process. Organoids are self-organising, 3D culture systems with a high degree of similarity to human organs. By emulating human organ development that would be seen in the embryo, organoids are generated in the laboratory from either tissue or pluripotent stem cells. Consequently, organoids can be generated that are specific to an individual, bringing forward the possibility of personalised efficacy and safety, or precision medicine. It is now commonplace in the laboratory to re-program cells into induced pluripotent stem cells (iPSC) with much attention on the generation of neurons or cardiomyocytes in culture. But culture methods continue to evolve and now include several differentiation cues to recreate different stages of the human developmental process. As such differentiated iPSCs can aggregate to form an organ bud, that continues to develop into structures that have a high degree of similarity to the mature organ. Organoids from adult stem cells are simpler structures and can be derived from biopsies of the organ of interest, where accessibility is not limited. But they are usually only composed of epithelial cell types and, as discussed above, the importance of supporter cells such as endothelial cells is therefore lost from this approach.

Organoid formation essentially involves three considerations: firstly inclusion of activators or inhibitors of key signalling pathways that regulate development, secondly the media composition to enable terminal differentiation of cell types and lastly aggregating cells or embedding them in a 3D matrix to guide their expansion in 3D.

An early example of the potential value of organoids in greater disease understanding and therefore for further target validation is in the study of cystic fibrosis. This disease is genetic, with approximately 90 000 patients worldwide who suffer from a loss-of-function mutation in the gene which encodes cystic fibrosis transmembrane conductance regulator (CFTR), a critical chloride channel that controls fluid and electrolytes on the epithelial surface of the airway and intestine. It is now believed that there are nearly 2000 mutations in this gene, each of which lead to an increase in viscous mucus in the airway and gastrointestinal tract. Dekkers and colleagues took their knowledge of organoids and applied it to generate a functional, quantitative assay of CFTR using human and mouse primary intestinal organoids, which is now recognised as a landmark paper in the organoid field.[45] These investigators demonstrated that CFTR was also responsive to the adenylate cyclase activator forskolin, and when applied to intestinal organoids, CFTR was activated and caused a rapid swelling. Furthermore, organoids derived from patients with cystic fibrosis or from mice with the CFTR F580del mutant protein did not demonstrate a similar response, confirming the loss-of-function mutation. This elegant example shows how organoids could be a valuable tool in the target validation phase of drug discovery and beyond.

### 18.4.4 Microphysiological Systems

Microphysiological systems (MPS) are the next level of sophistication in creating a meaningful cell culture assay and present a unique opportunity to assign function to a novel target. MPS is an umbrella term that is used to describe any advanced cellular model that combines engineering with cell biology to exhibit 3D architecture, multi-cellular interactions, tissue–tissue interfaces or organ-level mechanical cues with Organ-Chip models also containing a dynamic fluid flow.[46–48] Each of these components have been shown to help recreate the unique microenvironment that cells are exposed to within the human body and in theory provide the preclinical scientist with a more predictive tool.

Tissue engineering has been around for decades, where early pioneers recognised that this approach would be transformational for drug discovery,[49] but the concept really took off following the seminal publication on lung-on-a-chip.[50] In this investigation, Huh and colleagues described the microfabrication of a device that contained two microchannels separated by a porous membrane. The membrane was coated with extracellular membrane and alveolar epithelial cells and pulmonary microvascular endothelial cells were coated on the top and bottom channels respectively, either side of the membrane. The epithelial cells were exposed to air to encourage full maturation whilst the endothelial cells remained submerged in medium. To emulate the intrapleural pressure changes caused during inspiration and expiration, a vacuum was applied to the chip, which stretched the membrane that separates the two channels. Whilst in this configuration, cells are thought to have the correct cues that enable them to maintain longer-term viability and functionality. Furthermore, the physiological nature of the system was nicely demonstrated by adding bacteria to the epithelial surface and neutrophils to the bottom vascular channel. Because the bacteria set off a local inflammatory reaction, fluorescently tagged neutrophils can be seen attaching to the endothelial cell layer and migrating through the vessel barrier to reach the epithelial surface, where they engulf the bacteria. Such sophistication demonstrates the superiority of these models for studying biological processes that until this point were not possible *in vitro*.

Earlier in the chapter we highlighted the need to understand the impact of a potential drug target in disease settings, as such an approach should contribute to a greater probability of success during clinical development. An elegant example of such target validation has been demonstrated with organ-chip technology, this time using a device microfabricated for cardiomyocytes[51] Wang and colleagues combined expertise in iPSC technology together with organ-chip engineering to study the pathophysiology of Barth syndrome, a rare X-linked cardiac myopathy resulting from a mutation in the Tafazzin gene. These mutations impact the acylation of a major phospholipid in the membrane of mitochondria, leading to short stature, an enlarged and weakened heart, weakness in muscles used for movement, and recurrent infections due to small numbers of white blood cells (neutropenia). Taking patient-derived iPSCs onto the chip, the team were able to demonstrate the reduced contractile stress generation, a distinct feature of the disease. However, if the same iPSCs were genome-edited using CRISPR or were treated with a modified RNA to correct one of the mutations, the contractile stress was returned to levels consistent with normal cardiomyocytes. This seminal study thereby demonstrates the value that organ-chip technology can bring to target validation.

It is widely anticipated that MPS will make a positive impact on the pharmaceutical industry, not least because these model systems are built with human cells, thus removing any interference coming from potential species differences but also increasingly important in an era when there is an ascendance of engineered molecules that do not cross-react with targets in animals. Despite this, the transition from academic research to drug discovery is slow, yet building momentum.[52]

### 18.4.5 Cell Source

When constructing and optimising more sophisticated culture systems, organoids or MPS, wherever patient cells are utilised, the issues of source, isolation procedures and variability must be considered. We now understand that the location of cells within a tissue is very important to their phenotype and function, and also the disease lesions are seldom uniform across an organ. Therefore sampling and isolation of patient cells requires consideration of the distribution of disease. For example, isolation of fibroblasts from a liver, kidney or lung usually requires that the cells 'grow out' of tissues cultured in a dish. Yet we now believe that significant pathobiology is driven by senescent cell secretions, which characteristically do not grow. Therefore, trying to understand/reproduce said pathobiology is not feasible with the vast majority of isolated fibroblasts. The heterogeneity within diseased organs is further complicated by the heterogeneity of disease between individuals. The pattern of biologic dysregulation in one patient may be different in some aspects to another, despite suffering from the same disease. These differences could be related to age, sex, ethnicity, severity or treatment regimen. Yet all of these factors may contribute to inconsistencies within a test system. Therefore, it is essential that the boundaries of variability for a test system are understood and that controls are included to manage changes in response window. For example, assessing changes in phenotype/function before and after stimulation with disease-relevant mediators can offer a percentage modulation from baseline, which can then be compared to other assays using different donors and a variable magnitude of response.

## 18.5 *Ex Vivo* Tissue Systems in Target Validation

Cell co-cultures, organoid and microphysiological systems, although able to reproduce many aspects of pathobiology, cannot hope to reproduce the complex network of interactions with cells and matrix established in an organ. Indeed, even when using patient-derived disease cells, the isolation process itself will impact the expression profile and subsequent morphology/function of the cells, thus eroding the utility of the system to faithfully reproduce 'differential patient biology'.

### 18.5.1 Precision-cut Tissue Slices

A technique which can mitigate some of these risks is precision-cut tissue slices (PCTS) which preserves organ microarchitecture and the plethora of different cell types (parenchymal, stromal, immune cells, *etc.*) in their physiological context. PCTS are viable tissue slices of a few hundred μm thickness and can be prepared from nearly every organ of mammalian species. Depending on the species, up to several hundred slices can be obtained from one donor and therefore this technique nicely complies with the 3R concept (reduction, refinement and replacement of animals in research), by reducing the number of animals or even by replacing them if human tissue is accessed.

One of the big advantages of using a tissue for target validation, is the ability to readout a complex, multi-factorial, multi-cellular process. Good examples of such use can be seen with Precision-Cut Liver Slices (PCLS), which can be exposed to a range of different stimuli to reproduce different liver diseases. Ethanol exposure leads to mega-mitochondria, a classical hallmark of Alcoholic Liver Disease (ALD). Exposure to a mixture of oleic and linoleic acids can simulate Non-Alcoholic Fatty Liver Disease (NAFLD). Furthermore, liver tumour slices co-cultured with matched immune cells can be used as a model of cancer-immune cell interactions.[53] Many other examples for lung diseases, including severe asthma and fibrosis have benefitted from PCTS.[54,55]

Despite the many advantages of PCTS as a technique, there are also potential artefacts to consider. The slicing process does trigger an injury response, which interferes with healthy biology for at least the first 2 days of culture. There are also limits to the longevity of PCTS culture, which results in a defined window within which experiments can be performed. When tested in gut, liver and kidney PCTS, culture led to common increases in inflammatory and fibrotic signalling, yet could retain differences between species-, organ- and pathology-specific gene regulation. Furthermore, the underlying pathology in human diseased PCTS endured, influencing biological processes like cytokine release.[56] Secondly, when working with human tissues from transplant, one has the option to study either healthy samples (which are rare) or diseased samples, yet because preservation techniques have been largely unsuccessful, the chances of comparing health *vs.* disease in a single experiment are virtually nil. Thus, studies are restricted to PCTS +/− stimuli, unless one uses animal tissue from *in vivo* models of disease *vs.* healthy controls.

### 18.5.2 Isolated Organs

An alternative to PCTS can be whole isolated organs from animals which not only retain cells and surrounding structures in appropriate balance, but can also incorporate blood flow and higher organ function as a means to validate targets reliant on circulation. For example, targets which impact the tone (constriction) of pulmonary vasculature, such as in pulmonary arterial hypertension (PAH), cannot readily be assessed in human systems due to the challenges of reproducing effective vessels from isolated human cells. Neither can such processes be reproduced *in vivo*, because changes to vessel tone by a validating tool are instantaneously compensated for by the baro reflex – changes in heart rate designed to normalise blood pressure. Therefore, we need to isolate the lungs (in this example, rat), using the heart as a hub for artificial blood flow (stopping the baro reflex).

In addition, the pathologically increased vascular tone characteristic of PAH is only apparent when the lung vasculature has been remodelled in response to chronic *in vivo* exposure to the alkaloid toxin monocrotaline AND perfused blood within the isolated lung has been derived from a hypertensive (monocrotaline exposed) rat. Novel targets can be tested for effective impact in such a system, especially where tools are of insufficient quality for full *in vivo* testing. An additional utility that can be assigned to some isolated organs or even rare *in vivo* settings is intra-vital microscopy. This technology uses a range of dyes to depict cells and signalling pathways to enable the real-time target observation/validation within complex physiologic processes. Examples include targets associated with oxidative stress, metabolism, cell chemotaxis and inflammation,[57,58] Yet, if we exclude the possibility of isolated human organ systems for testing, animal systems still retain the potential caveats in translation associated with all animal experiments.

## 18.6 *In Vivo* Novel Target Validation

*In vivo* models have been the source of new targets for decades, yet in recent years we have come to question such models as a starting point for drug discovery. However, when used appropriately, *in vivo* systems can be a valuable means to validate a target –

originally identified in patient material and as part of a package of data, including human/patient cell systems. Of vital importance is a detailed understanding of the signalling pathways and mechanisms at play in a disease model and how they translate to the human disease. Historically, this has been poor for some models. An example of poor translatability is the bleomycin model of pulmonary fibrosis. Literature analysis of the targets tested in the model compared to reflective clinical data indicate effective translation in just 24% of cases.

Yet this poor translational record is largely due to poor experimental design. The bleomycin model starts with an inflammatory phase which peaks at 5 to 7 days and lasts out to day 10, followed by an overlapping fibrosis phase which starts at day 7, peaking at 3 weeks. In many studies, treatment is initiated at the same time as bleomycin injury, thus the mechanisms inhibited are largely inflammatory, rather than anti-fibrotic *per se*. Therapeutic studies show a greater level of translatability for testing anti-fibrotic concepts. In addition, young mice are almost always used, which is in stark contrast to patients, who have a mean age of at least 60 within recent trials. This disparity was recently addressed by Birk *et al.* in a comparative *in vivo* study of young *vs.* old mice. This comparison revealed equivalent inflammatory and fibrotic phenotypes experienced in young and old animals, yet a less effective repair phase in aged groups. Direct comparison of gene profiles demonstrated a far greater overlap of signalling activity between older bleomycin-treated animals and patients (see Figure 18.5A and B).

It is with detailed analyses such as these, that an *in vivo* model can be appropriately designed – with knowledge that the target you wish to validate and the subsequent pathologic mechanisms you wish to explore, are represented in the animal as they are in the patient.

There are tactics by which truly human pathobiology can be modelled, to some degree, in animals. One example is the use of immune-compromised mice as recipients of a cancer xenograft from a patient. Such models can be used to assess the impact of chemotherapeutic agents and search for inhibitors directed toward a specific tumour-based mutation/mechanism. Unfortunately, what they cannot validate are modulators of the anti-tumour immune system.[59]

Finally, one key factor which must be considered in using an *in vivo* system to validate your target of interest is the potency, selectivity and pharmacokinetic/pharmacodynamics of the experimental tool. Interpretation of *in vivo* data in which a target modulator is used must account for the tissue exposures achieved and the number of pathways inhibited at said levels. A truly selective tool inhibitor is seldom available for a novel target, yet more value can be gleaned from an experiment with the assessment of direct effects on target (*e.g.* measures of receptor phosphorylation for a tyrosine kinase inhibitor). As discussed earlier, genetic models (*e.g.* CRISPR knockout or virally transduced animals) are an alternative to 'classic' *in vivo* pharmacology.

Targets which, when modulated, can return the phenotype and function of primary patient cells, can return normal biology to stimulated organoids, microphysiological systems or precision-cut tissue slices or can improve higher biologic functionality in isolated organs or whole animal disease models, have a far greater chance of modulating the complex pathobiology observed in patients. Yet, model systems are of little value (indeed, can hinder progress) if they do not represent the patient pathobiology

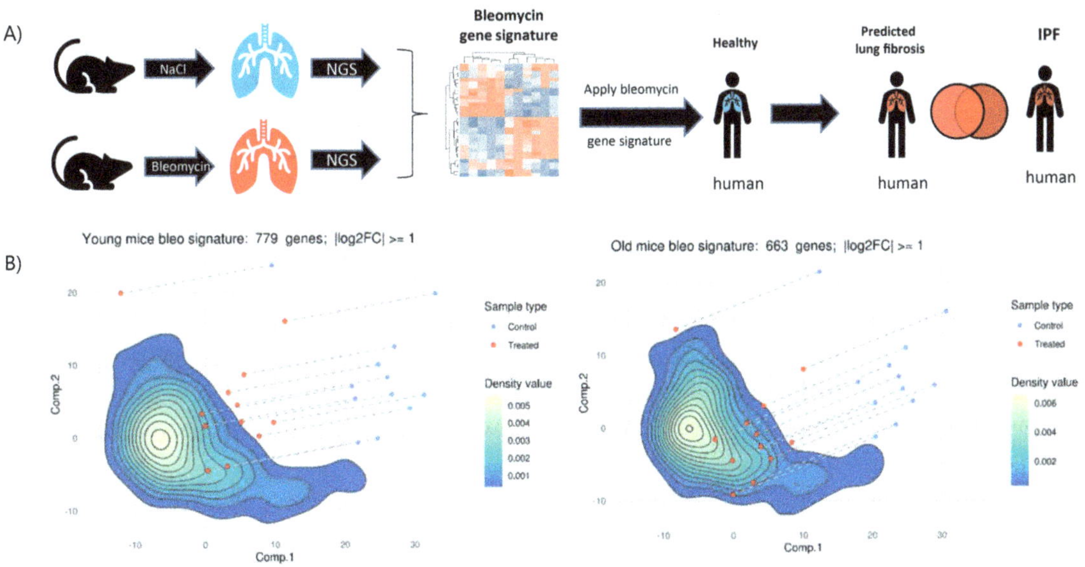


**Figure 18.5** Translational value of pulmonary fibrosis bleomycin model improved by analysis of aged mice *vs.* patients. (A) Graphical description of the *in silico* comparison model. Next-generation RNAseq gene patterns from bleomycin *vs.* control mice were used to generate a lung fibrosis signature, which was then overlayed onto IPF patients. (B) Old mice treated with bleomycin are closer to human IPF. Two principal component analysis density plots show human IPF gene signatures *vs.* young (left) and old (right) mice. The single blue dots symbolise the single gene signatures of control mice and red dots bleomycin-treated animals. Far more red dots in old bleomycin mice fall within the human IPF density plot, indicating a higher level of overlap in gene expression changes and therefore a greater level of translational value.

of interest. We can now assess the degree to which a test system translates to human disease by the overlay of gene expression profile between each. The overlay need not be complete – to anticipate complete recapitulation of a complex disease within any culture system is unrealistic. However, if one wished to validate a target related to, for example, oxidative stress in the gut, a focused pathway analysis of healthy *vs.* diseased gut Ox-stress machinery, overlayed with the model (+/− stimuli) can offer a measure of how useful said model is in the validation process. An example of such analysis is captured in Figure 18.5.

## 18.7 Preparing for Drug Discovery

The successful completion of the target validation phase of an emerging drug discovery concept is a critical inflection point in the lifetime of a project. At this milestone, additional resources from across a research organisation are folded into the project to expand upon the initial biology insights, and to identify and develop molecules for candidate selection and ultimately clinical prosecution.

It is vital at this time for the expanded team of drug discovery scientists to carefully consider, objectively, the external and internal challenges to the project and develop a custom, fit-for-purpose, drug discovery strategy to overcome those challenges. This strategy can provide the team with a critical path of experiments, needing focused resources from across the organisation, to accelerate the project to meaningful decision points.

### 18.7.1 Assessing Risk in Exploratory Portfolio

What must we know of a target/project and how much risk can be carried into drug discovery? How can management effectively assess risk across multiple projects within a portfolio? A simple framework is most effective which comprises key questions to sharpen the focus of the project team. Building on the '5 Rights' from AstraZeneca can again be used as an example:

*Right Target*: How robust is the link to human disease? Is there evidence of human genetic linkage? Do we find strong dysregulation on gene, protein and activity level co-localised with pathologic features? Have we demonstrated 'differential patient biology', returning functional consequences of dysregulation to normal with a genetic or pharmacologic tool? How closely does the test system(s) reproduce human pathobiology? What evidence is there that such effects are not achieved by standard of care therapies? And within all the systems explored, are there early indicators of biomarkers of target engagement and patient responsiveness? Based on an objective answer to the above question with considerations for the current and emerging external competitive pressures for those patients, a team can develop the biology strategy to further support and enrich the therapeutic concept (*e.g.* head-to-head testing of a genetic tool +/− leading standard of care therapy in your key human disease *in vitro* assay).

*Right Tissue*: What attributes must a molecule possess to deliver on the medical value proposition? Project teams often get seduced at this time to jump to considerations around molecular potency in a biochemical assay for an envisaged modality. This may ultimately be misleading though, as the crucial question relates to how much a molecule must interact with a target (potency/PD) and for how long in the needed location (PK) to achieve sufficient modulation of disease-relevant biology in patients to realise the full therapeutic potential. Within these considerations, target burden is also important and will likely require an understanding of target levels and turnover within disease. The results of this PK/PD relationship and impact on the human dose estimate requires careful preclinical experimentation and the required tools and approaches to develop this understanding generally begin immediately following the target validation phase. Hypothesis-based criteria for molecule attributes at this stage must be consistently challenged and refined based on the evolving biology and PK/PD understanding during the drug discovery process to ultimately reach a definitive human dose target for clinical interrogation and safety assessment.

*Right Safety*: What is known in terms of potential mechanism or target class safety considerations and what is the earliest opportunity to assess and identify hazards? The attrition rate for small molecule inhibitors due to an insufficient therapeutic index remains extraordinarily high.[60] Project teams should carefully consider selectivity requirements and a safety strategy to de-risk any known mechanism-based concerns. A 'discovery toxicology' assessment starts with a sound understanding of the target in 'normal' physiology.

Literature evidence is crucial for developing this understanding, but increasingly algorithms are being built to exploit 'big data' sets to elicit novel or previously undescribed pathways, that the intended target may be expressed within. Typically toxicologists try to establish whether gene mutations (either gain-of-function or loss-of-function) in the intended target lead to any undesirable effects. For example, a gain-of-function mutation in the ion channel Nav 1.7 is associated with an increased incidence of seizure, whereas a loss of function mutation can lead to pain insensitivity.[61] Data from transgenic mice are also valuable, especially if any adverse effects are seen in homozygous knockouts. The resulting assessment should indicate the potential for adverse effects and influence strategies to mitigate any concerns raised. For example, significant safety flags of chronic target modulation may be acceptable if studies show intermittent dosing can drive efficacy and reduce toxicity or whether local *vs.* systemic administration of the drug will be favoured. The safety of the drug itself will be assessed further, including potential drug–drug interactions, at far later stages of the drug discovery process.

*Right Patient*: Do we already know which patients might benefit most? Such information usually comes later in the project (especially for particularly novel targets), yet hypotheses based on mechanistic biomarker insights or from patients who are unresponsive to current therapies may lay the groundwork of this ongoing consideration. To build a strong translational path from the mechanism of your target through to the effects observable in *in vitro*/*in vivo* test systems, then finally linked to known disease progression biomarkers, constitutes massive de-risking for a project.

*Right Commercial Potential*: Is the unmet need clear and addressed by the therapeutic concept? Would the predicted benefit to the patient justify investment in the project? As the investment in a project at the point of drug discovery initiation is comparatively low, then such financial considerations are less pressing. However, a clear vision of how a successful therapy would change the treatment paradigm is an important 'guiding light' for the project team, with discussion of companion diagnostics and biomarkers becoming increasingly key as the therapeutic reaches patients.

### 18.7.2 Drug Discovery Transition

A depth in the understanding of all the above elements is unlikely to be available at the point of drug discovery initiation. The successful transition of a project will, in part, rely on the portfolio in which it sits. A balance of high-risk/high-reward projects together with lower risk opportunities is a sign of a healthy and robust exploratory portfolio. Where the risk lies can also vary and should be spread within a portfolio. High-risk strategies for modulation (*e.g.* gene therapy or less conventional chemical approaches, such as proteolysis targeting chimera (PROTAC) inhibitors) are better paired with lower risk targets for which the disease link is strong, yet previous strategies for modulation have failed. Alternatively, a high-risk novel target class for which less is known biologically might benefit from up-front feasibility studies to better enable the search for modulators (*e.g.* generating crystal structures or CRISPR knockout cells/animals).

Armed with a customised strategy for the drug discovery phase of a project, the team must remain open to confronting unexpected challenges that will arise over the course of the campaign. Successful drug discovery teams are those that can anticipate and mitigate risks upfront and directly confront new challenges and re-derive a project strategy once they arise.

## 18.8 Case Study: Platelet Derived Growth Factor as a Target for Pulmonary Arterial Hypertension

Many of the techniques/principles discussed in this chapter were used in the validation of platelet-derived growth factor (PDGF) as a target for pulmonary arterial hypertension (PAH) – a disease of increased lung blood pressure and structural remodelling of the lung blood vessels. Although vasodilator treatments had been available for PAH since the 1990s, it was becoming apparent in following years that a next generation of therapies which directly impacted the remodelling of vessels was needed. One key feature of PAH vascular lesions is the proliferation and migration of smooth muscle cells (SMCs). The association of various growth factors with fibrosis and SMC proliferation, including PDGF, had been previously indicated in other diseases, such as idiopathic pulmonary fibrosis.[62] Furthermore, Humbert *et al.* linked PDGF expression in lung biopsies to the development of PAH in HIV patients.[63] However, the first attempts to validate PDGF as a target came in 2005, using the monocrotaline model of PAH – a system which replicates SMC lesions well (yet other disease features less so). Schermuly *et al.* demonstrated increased survival and changes to vessel lesions in monocrotaline-treated animals when therapeutically treated with imatinib – an oncology tyrosine kinase inhibitor which targets growth factor receptors (PDGFR, c-kit and BCR-Abl).[64] In this study imatinib was also shown to functionally arrest the proliferation and migration of pulmonary artery-derived SMCs stimulated with PDGF.[65] Helpful as these data were, the link to human disease was still missing, until in 2008, gene expression studies of PAH patient pulmonary artery tissue showed increases in both ligand and receptor expression. Unfortunately, single cell technology was not available at the time, but IHC imaging of patient lung tissue revealed a more convincing causal association with the disease by demonstrating that the increased levels of both ligand and receptor were increased localised within concentric neo-intimal vascular lesions, characteristic of a PAH patient biopsy. Furthermore, phospho-PDGF receptor staining was increased and co-localised with smooth muscle cell proliferation – indicating that the pathway elements were not only present but active and directly linked to pathobiology. These data were complemented by patient-derived smooth muscle cell cultures confirming the inhibitory impact of imatinib, as was previously seen in rodent cells. Yet it was not until Takahashi *et al.* in 2016 that we could see functional evidence of PDGF-driven differential patient biology between PAH-derived *vs.* healthy SMCs in culture,[66] although equivalent PAH patient cell functional dysregulation had already been demonstrated for other target pathways, such as TGFβ a decade before.[67]

In 2005, greatly accelerated by the availability of an approved drug (for chronic myeloid leukaemia), a case study of imatinib compassionate treatment was published in a letter to the New England Journal of Medicine.[68] This indicator, together with the limited validation data generated thus far, triggered a phase II study of imatinib in PAH and a drug discovery campaign to explore more potent/selective chemical matter (potential for inhalation). Positive data in the phase II study were seen following *post-hoc* redistribution of treatment groups based on high *vs.* low pulmonary vascular resistance – a measure of lung vessel remodelling.[69] Further mechanistic understanding of imatinib efficacy was also undertaken, demonstrating efficacy in *in vivo* models of more complex pathologic features and the identification of cross-talk between PDGF signalling and serotonin pathobiology in trial-derived patient samples.[70] Although the subsequent phase III clinical study showed efficacy, registration was not pursued due to poor retention of patients on drug and insufficient biomarkers needed to identify treatment-responsive patients.[71] Improved chemical matter for the inhibition of PDGFR signalling through inhalation was created and published in 2016 but has yet to be developed for PAH or other associated diseases.[72]

There are several lessons to be learnt from this case study. As was so often the case in drug discovery of decades past, the potential role of PDGF was rationalised based on known function, then the hypothesis tested in an animal model before a more comprehensive picture of patient validation was established. Using more modern techniques and strategies, a more profound link to patient pathobiology would have been discovered far earlier, both decreasing the risk of the clinical programme and accelerating a parallel search for alternative chemical matter. Furthermore, it is unusual for a project to advance into the clinic with such agility – enabled by the availability of a suitable tool (imatinib). Yet despite this, it could be argued that a greater effort in linking mechanistic understanding from preclinical studies to the clinical design of the trials might have enabled registration. We knew from both preclinical and clinical studies that the mechanism of action for PDGFR inhibition was only observed chronically – requiring weeks to impact rodent models and months in patients – a timeframe in stark contrast to vasodilator therapies, whose effects were seen acutely. Had we built more robust preclinical methods of pathway activity (*e.g.* pPDGFR in blood), then translated such findings to patients, then responder patients could have been better identified. Furthermore, blinded assessment of target engagement could also have helped retention in trial – telling test subjects that at least the drug under trial was effective on the target pathway. It is tempting to postulate that, had we had access to more modern technology and better considered the translation of target validation studies to clinical trials, then imatinib and next-generation PDGFR inhibitors would be therapeutics available for today's PAH patients.

## 18.9 Summary

We have explored what it means to validate a novel target for drug discovery and the array of technologies available to identify suitable starting points. We have also explored how culture systems of mounting sophistication can be used to reveal the potential of a target to modulate patient pathobiology. The complementary use of *ex vivo* and *in vivo* systems, when sufficiently understood, can provide invaluable information in a validation package – a summary of pros and cons are captured in Table 18.1. We consider how the validation package for a novel target might be assessed for the initiation

**Table 18.1** Summary table: pros and cons of target identification and validation technologies. Here we provide the principal advantages and disadvantages of the technologies captured in this chapter. We indicate where such methods are more applicable to target identification or validation (not mutually exclusive) and also rank them in terms of impact (left to right) for drug target validation.

| | GWAS or RVAS | Patient tissue single cell seq | Immuno-histo-chemistry | *In situ* hybridization | Phenotypic screens |
|---|---|---|---|---|---|
| **Pros** | • Proven advantage to target success<br>• GWAS are broad<br>• RVAS are focused | • Advantage over bulk seq by associating expression with a cell type<br>• Can link cells to their progenitors | • Links target and potentially activity to disease-relevant lesions | • Links target expression and signalling patterns to disease-relevant lesions<br>• More expansive target range | • Can both identify and partially validate a target in x1 system<br>• Mid-high throughput |
| **Cons** | • GWAS rarely provide a target, but a direction to explore<br>• RVAS targets may serve relatively few patients | • Not all targets are regulated *via* transcription<br>• Some cells under-represented<br>• Data is not functional | • Reliant on quality of antibodies<br>• Limitations to the number of analytics | • Low throughput<br>• Reliant on known signalling networks for validation data | • Higher throughput system lacks complexity, thereby limiting output |

of drug discovery – using the '5 Rights' of drug discovery as an example framework. We also offer a case study – PDGFR inhibition for the treatment of PAH – in which elements of the validation concepts discussed were applied or omitted, and reflected, with the benefit of hindsight, upon consequences for this project.

The research tools available to drug discoverers have been subject to profound technological evolution in recent years, which has changed the way we validate novel targets and greatly expanded the target opportunities open to us. We now have the chance to greatly increase our confidence that modulation of a target will profoundly impact human disease – confidence which grows as we near the patients who will benefit. We all await the next wave of novel therapeutics aimed at revolutionising the treatment paradigm of the most challenging diseases – helping the patients of greatest unmet medical need.

## 18.10 Target Validation: Pro Tips

- Finding a genetic/epigenetic link between target and disease doubles the success rate of the therapeutic

| Isolated organs | *In vivo* models | Precision-cut tissue slices | Micro-physiological systems | Patient cell organoids | Patient cell co-culture systems |
|---|---|---|---|---|---|
| • Can model complex whole organ processes<br>• Can be extended to intra-vital microscopy to see function in real time | • Can model complex multi- organ processes<br>• Key to PK/TE/PD calculations later in a project | • Can model multi-cell processes in a system which retains higher structural relationships | • Emerging technology to model multi-cell culture with greater physiological cues (*e.g.* tissue stretch) | • Mid-throughput systems which model multi- cell interactions<br>• Emerging utility in personalized target validation | • Mid-throughput systems which reveal differential patient biology<br>• Highly adaptable<br>• Physiologic queues |
| • Restricted to animal biology<br>• Technically challenging<br>• Low throughput | • Restricted to animal biology<br>• Limited by tools (*i.e.* must be selective, potent and good PK) | • Damage response to cutting process and limited culture time<br>• Simultaneous healthy *vs.* patient experiments difficult | • Limited utility of primary and patient cells thus far<br>• Mid-low throughput | • Reliant on patient cells<br>• Lack many physiologic queues (*e.g.* air in lung organoids)<br>• Lack access to apical cells | • Reliant on access to patient cells<br>• Variations from donor to donor require effective controls |

- 'Big data' provides an invaluable resource for identifying targets, establishing disease linkage and deconvoluting the target mechanism
- Linking a target to disease pathology is more meaningful if changes reach beyond gene expression to include translation of protein, altered pathway activity and development pathologic features within cells and tissues
- Techniques to modulate a target must be carefully chosen – potent and selective pharmacologic tools are rarely available for a novel target; RNA methods are relatively quick, yet frequently partially active and may have off-target effects; CRISPR-Cas9 may soon become a 'gold standard' method to repress or activate target genes
- Phenotypic screens may offer both target identification and partial validation
- Functional cell systems used to assess 'differential patient biology' offer important information to a target validation package – if a human cell culture system has enough sophistication to show the difference between health and disease, then functional modulation of target leading to restoration of 'health' is key (advantages/disadvantages of test systems are shown in Table 18.1)
- Animal models are not a good starting point for target identification, yet can offer useful information on the modulation of the target within complex,

multi-organ pathology, yet ONLY when the degree of disease translatability has been assessed

- An effective target validation package relies on a 'critical path' of experimentation which reveals key gaps in our knowledge to reduce risk and build sufficient confidence to initiate drug discovery
- Target validation continues throughout the life of a project and should be guided by a framework of principles until therapeutic benefit is demonstrated in the clinic

## Acknowledgements

We wish to thank significant contributions from Dr Francesc Fernandez-Albert[a], Dr James Garnett[a], Dr Marc Kästle[a], Dr David Lamb[a], Dr Huy Le Quang[a], Dr Craig Miller[a], Dr Sergio Picart-Armada[a], Dr Fidel Rameirez[a], Dr Marco Schlepuetz[a], Dr Michael Schüler[a], Dr Heiko Stahl[a] and Dr Jaromir Vlach[a]
[a] Boehringer Ingelheim Pharma GmbH & Co KG

## References

1. D. Cook, D. Brown, R. Alexander, R. March, P. Morgan, G. Satterthwaite and M. N. Pangalos, *Nat. Rev. Drug Discovery*, 2014, **13**, 419–431.
2. P. Morgan, D. G. Brown, S. Lennard, M. J. Anderton, J. C. Barrett, U. Eriksson, M. Fidock, B. Hamrén, A. Johnson, R. E. March, J. Matcham, J. Mettetal, D. J. Nicholls, S. Platz, S. Rees, M. A. Snowden and M. N. Pangalos, *Nat. Rev. Drug Discovery*, 2018, **17**, 167–181.
3. P. Morgan, P. H. V. D. Graaf, J. Arrowsmith, D. E. Feltner, K. S. Drummond, C. D. Wegner and S. D. Street, *Drug Discovery Today*, 2012, **17**, 419–424.
4. M. R. Nelson, H. Tipney, J. L. Painter, J. Shen, P. Nicoletti, Y. Shen, A. Floratos, P. C. Sham, M. J. Li, J. Wang, L. R. Cardon, J. C. Whittaker and P. Sanseau, *Nat. Genet.*, 2015, **47**, 856–860.
5. E. A. King, J. W. Davis and J. F. Degner, *PLoS Genet.*, 2019, **15**, e1008489.
6. D. Avramopoulos, *Complex Psychiatry*, 2018, **4**, 35–51.
7. V. Tam, N. Patel, M. Turcotte, Y. Bossé, G. Paré and D. Meyre, *Nat. Rev. Genet.*, 2019, **20**, 467–484.
8. S. L. Berger, T. Kouzarides, R. Shiekhattar and A. Shilatifard, *Genes Dev.*, 2009, **23**, 781–783.
9. R. Khamsi, *Nature*, 2020, **583**, S12–S14.
10. A. Nowogrodzki, *Nature*, 2018, **564**, S12–S13.
11. J. Bennett, M. Ashtari, J. Wellman, K. A. Marshall, L. L. Cyckowski, D. C. Chung, S. McCague, E. A. Pierce, Y. Chen, J. L. Bennicelli, X. Zhu, G. S. Ying, J. Sun, J. F. Wright, A. Auricchio, F. Simonelli, K. S. Shindler, F. Mingozzi, K. A. High and A. M. Maguire, *Sci. Transl. Med.*, 2012, **4**, 120ra15.
12. E. Bonneau, B. Neveu, E. Kostantin, G. J. Tsongalis and V. D. Guire, *eJIFCC*, 2019, **30**, 114–127.
13. J. Paananen and V. Fortino, *Briefings Bioinf.*, 2020, 1937–1953.
14. T. Stuart and R. Satija, *Nat. Rev. Genet.*, 2019, **20**, 257–272.
15. H. G. Stunnenberg and M. Hirst, *Cell*, 2016, **167**, 1145–1149.
16. A. Regev, S. A. Teichmann, E. S. Lander, I. Amit, C. Benoist, E. Birney, B. Bodenmiller, P. Campbell, P. Carninci, M. Clatworthy, H. Clevers, B. Deplancke, I. Dunham, J. Eberwine, R. Eils, W. Enard, A. Farmer, L. Fugger, B. Göttgens, N. Hacohen, M. Haniffa, M. Hemberg, S. Kim, P. Klenerman, A. Kriegstein, E. Lein, S. Linnarsson, E. Lundberg, J. Lundeberg, P. Majumder, J. C. Marioni, M. Merad, M. Mhlanga, M. Nawijn, M. Netea, G. Nolan, D. Pe'er, A. Phillipakis, C. P. Ponting, S. Quake, W. Reik, O. Rozenblatt-Rosen, J. Sanes, R. Satija, T. N. Schumacher, A. Shalek, E. Shapiro, P. Sharma, J. W. Shin, O. Stegle, M. Stratton, M. J. T. Stubbington, F. J. Theis, M. Uhlen, A. van Oudenaarden, A. Wagner, F. Watt, J. Weissman, B. Wold, R. Xavier and N. Yosef, *eLife*, 2017, e27041.
17. C. Bock, M. Boutros, J. G. Camp, L. Clarke, H. Clevers, J. A. Knoblich, P. Liberali, A. Regev, A. C. Rios, O. Stegle, H. G. Stunnenberg, S. A. Teichmann, B. Treutlein, R. G. J. Vries and The Human Cell Atlas 'Biological Network' Organoids, *Nat. Biotechnol.*, 2021, **39**, 13–17.

18. J. Koh, Y. Kwak, J. Kim and W. H. Kim, *Cancer Res. Treat.*, 2019, **52**, 98–108.
19. C. Cui, W. Shu and P. Li, *Front. Cell Dev. Biol.*, 2016, 89.
20. A. P. Kann and R. S. Krauss, *Development*, 2019, **146**, dev179259.
21. F. Vincent, P. Loria, M. Pregel, R. Stanton, L. Kitching, K. Nocka, R. Doyonnas, C. Steppan, A. Gilbert, T. Schroeter and M. C. Peakman, *Sci. Transl. Med.*, 2015, **7**, 293ps15.
22. J. G. Moffat, F. Vincent, J. A. Lee, J. Eder and M. Prunotto, *Nat. Rev. Drug Discovery*, 2017, **16**, 531–543.
23. L. H. Jones and M. E. Bunnage, *Nat. Rev. Drug Discovery*, 2017, **16**, 285–296.
24. G. C. Terstappen, C. Schlüpen, R. Raggiaschi and G. Gaviraghi, *Nat. Rev. Drug Discovery*, 2007, **6**, 891–903.
25. H. Ratni, M. Ebeling, J. Baird, S. Bendels, J. Bylund, K. S. Chen, N. Denk, Z. Feng, L. Green, M. Guerard, P. Jablonski, B. Jacobsen, O. Khwaja, H. Kletzl, C.-P. Ko, S. Kustermann, A. Marquet, F. Metzger, B. Mueller, N. A. Naryshkin, S. V. Paushkin, E. Pinard, A. Poirier, M. Reutlinger, M. Weetall, A. Zeller, X. Zhao and L. Mueller, *J. Med. Chem.*, 2018, **61**, 6501–6517.
26. C. le Sage, S. Lawo and B. C. S. Cross, *SLAS Discovery*, 2020, **25**, 233–240.
27. T. Wang, J. J. Wei, D. M. Sabatini and E. S. Lander, *Science*, 2014, **343**, 80–84.
28. H. Koike-Yusa, Y. Li, E. P. Tan, C. V.-H. Mdel and K. Yusa, *Nat. Biotechnol.*, 2014, **32**, 267–273.
29. M. Jinek, A. East, A. Cheng, S. Lin, E. Ma and J. Doudna, *eLife*, 2013, **2**, e00471.
30. M. Kampmann, *Chem. Commun.*, 2017, **53**, 7162–7167.
31. A. J. Aguirre, R. M. Meyers, B. A. Weir, F. Vazquez, C. Z. Zhang, U. Ben-David, A. Cook, G. Ha, W. F. Harrington, M. B. Doshi, M. Kost-Alimova, S. Gill, H. Xu, L. D. Ali, G. Jiang, S. Pantel, Y. Lee, A. Goodale, A. D. Cherniack, C. Oh, G. Kryukov, G. S. Cowley, L. A. Garraway, K. Stegmaier, C. W. Roberts, T. R. Golub, M. Meyerson, D. E. Root, A. Tsherniak and W. C. Hahn, *Cancer Discovery*, 2016, **6**, 914–929.
32. M. Uhlén, M. J. Karlsson, A. Hober, A. S. Svensson, J. Scheffel, D. Kotol, W. Zhong, A. Tebani, L. Strandberg, F. Edfors, E. Sjöstedt, J. Mulder, A. Mardinoglu, A. Berling, S. Ekblad, M. Dannemeyer, S. Kanje, J. Rockberg, M. Lundqvist, M. Malm, A. L. Volk, P. Nilsson, A. Månberg, T. Dodig-Crnkovic, E. Pin, M. Zwahlen, P. Oksvold, K. von Feilitzen, R. S. Häussler, M. G. Hong, C. Lindskog, F. Ponten, B. Katona, J. Vuu, E. Lindström, J. Nielsen, J. Robinson, B. Ayoglu, D. Mahdessian, D. Sullivan, P. Thul, F. Danielsson, C. Stadler, E. Lundberg, G. Bergström, A. Gummesson, B. G. Voldborg, H. Tegel, S. Hober, B. Forsström, J. M. Schwenk, L. Fagerberg and Å. Sivertsson, *Sci. Signaling*, 2019, eaaz0274.
33. T. Battle, B. Antonsson, G. Feger and D. Besson, *Comb. Chem. High Throughput Screening*, 2006, **9**, 639–649.
34. R. Gonzalez, L. L. Jennings, M. Knuth, A. P. Orth, H. E. Klock, W. Ou, J. Feuerhelm, M. V. Hull, E. Koesema, Y. Wang, J. Zhang, C. Wu, C. Y. Cho, A. I. Su, S. Batalov, H. Chen, K. Johnson, B. Laffitte, D. G. Nguyen, E. Y. Snyder, P. G. Schultz, J. L. Harris and S. A. Lesley, *Proc. Natl. Acad. Sci. U. S. A.*, 2010, **107**, 3552–3557.
35. H. Lin, E. Lee, K. Hestir, C. Leo, M. Huang, E. Bosch, R. Halenbeck, G. Wu, A. Zhou, D. Behrens, D. Hollenbaugh, T. Linnemann, M. Qin, J. Wong, K. Chu, S. K. Doberstein and L. T. Williams, *Science*, 2008, **320**, 807–811.
36. L. Scietti, K. Sampieri, I. Pinzuti, E. Bartolini, B. Benucci, A. Liguori, A. F. Haag, P. L. Surdo, W. Pansegrau, V. Nardi-Dei, L. Santini, S. Arora, X. Leber, S. Rindi, S. Savino, P. Costantino, D. Maione, M. Merola, P. Speziale, M. J. Bottomley, F. Bagnoli, V. Masignani, M. Pizza, M. Scharenberg, J. M. Schlaeppi, M. Nissum and S. Liberatori, *Sci. Rep.*, 2016, **6**, 27996.
37. F. Harbinski, V. J. Craig, S. Sanghavi, D. Jeffery, L. Liu, K. A. Sheppard, S. Wagner, C. Stamm, A. Buness, C. Chatenay-Rivauday, Y. Yao, F. He, C. X. Lu, V. Guagnano, T. Metz, P. M. Finan, F. Hofmann, W. R. Sellers, J. A. Porter, V. E. Myer, D. Graus-Porta, C. J. Wilson, A. Buckler and R. Tiedt, *Cancer Discovery*, 2012, **2**, 948–959.
38. M. Ding, H. Tegel, Å. Sivertsson, S. Hober, A. Snijder, M. Ormö, P.-E. Strömstedt, R. Davies and L. H. Schiavone, *SLAS Discovery*, 2020, **25**, 535–551.
39. X. Zhou, R. A. Franklin, M. Adler, J. B. Jacox, W. Bailis, J. A. Shyer, R. A. Flavell, A. Mayo, U. Alon and R. Medzhitov, *Cell*, 2018, **172**, 744–757.e17.
40. R. V. Goddard, A. G. Prentice, J. A. Copplestone and E. R. Kaminski, *Clin. Exp. Immunol.*, 2001, **126**, 16–28.
41. H. Zhao and J. C. Chappell, *J. Biol. Eng.*, 2019, **13**, 26.
42. J. M. S. Sucre, C. S. Jetter, H. Loomans, J. Williams, E. J. Plosa, J. T. Benjamin, L. R. Young, J. A. Kropski, C. L. Calvi, S. Kook, P. Wang, L. Gleaves, A. Eskaros, L. Goetzl, T. S. Blackwell, S. H. Guttentag and A. Zijlstra, *Am. J. Respir. Cell Mol. Biol.*, 2018, **59**, 158–166.
43. V. Čermák, A. Gandalovičová, L. Merta, J. Fučíková, R. Špíšek, D. Rösel and J. Brábek, *Sci. Data*, 2018, **5**, 180198.

44. M. W. Parker, D. Rossi, M. Peterson, K. Smith, K. Sikström, E. S. White, J. E. Connett, C. A. Henke, O. Larsson and P. B. Bitterman, *J. Clin. Invest.*, 2014, **124**, 1622–1635.
45. J. F. Dekkers, C. L. Wiegerinck, H. R. de Jonge, I. Bronsveld, H. M. Janssens, K. M. de W. Groot, A. M. Brandsma, N. W. de Jong, M. J. Bijvelds, B. J. Scholte, E. E. Nieuwenhuis, S. van den Brink, H. Clevers, C. K. van der Ent, S. Middendorp and J. M. Beekman, *Nat. Med.*, 2013, **19**, 939–945.
46. S. N. Bhatia and D. E. Ingber, *Nat. Biotechnol.*, 2014, **32**, 760–772.
47. U. Marx, T. B. Andersson, A. Bahinski, M. Beilmann, S. Beken, F. R. Cassee, M. Cirit, M. Daneshian, S. Fitzpatrick, O. Frey, C. Gaertner, C. Giese, L. Griffith, T. Hartung, M. B. Heringa, J. Hoeng, W. H. de Jong, H. Kojima, J. Kuehnl, M. Leist, A. Luch, I. Maschmeyer, D. Sakharov, A. J. Sips, T. Steger-Hartmann, D. A. Tagle, A. Tonevitsky, T. Tralau, S. Tsyb, A. van de Stolpe, R. Vandebriel, P. Vulto, J. Wang, J. Wiest, M. Rodenburg and A. Roth, *Altex*, 2016, **33**, 272–321.
48. U. Marx, T. Akabane, T. B. Andersson, E. Baker, M. Beilmann, S. Beken, S. Brendler-Schwaab, M. Cirit, R. David, E. M. Dehne, I. Durieux, L. Ewart, S. C. Fitzpatrick, O. Frey, F. Fuchs, L. G. Griffith, G. A. Hamilton, T. Hartung, J. Hoeng, H. Hogberg, D. J. Hughes, D. E. Ingber, A. Iskandar, T. Kanamori, H. Kojima, J. Kuehnl, M. Leist, B. Li, P. Loskill, D. L. Mendrick, T. Neumann, G. Pallocca, I. Rusyn, L. Smirnova, T. Steger-Hartmann, D. A. Tagle, A. Tonevitsky, S. Tsyb, M. Trapecar, B. V. de Water, J. V. den E. Raaij, P. Vulto, K. Watanabe, A. Wolf, X. Zhou and A. Roth, *Altex*, 2020, **37**, 364–394.
49. L. G. Griffith and G. Naughton, *Science*, 2002, **295**, 1009–1014.
50. D. Huh, B. D. Matthews, A. Mammoto, M. Montoya-Zavala, H. Y. Hsin and D. E. Ingber, *Science*, 2010, **328**, 1662–1668.
51. G. Wang, M. L. McCain, L. Yang, A. He, F. S. Pasqualini, A. Agarwal, H. Yuan, D. Jiang, D. Zhang, L. Zangi, J. Geva, A. E. Roberts, Q. Ma, J. Ding, J. Chen, D. Z. Wang, K. Li, J. Wang, R. J. Wanders, W. Kulik, F. M. Vaz, M. A. Laflamme, C. E. Murry, K. R. Chien, R. I. Kelley, G. M. Church, K. K. Parker and W. T. Pu, *Nat. Med.*, 2014, **20**, 616–623.
52. L. Ewart and A. Roth, *Nat. Rev. Drug Discovery*, 2021, 327–328.
53. E. Palma, E. J. Doornebal and S. Chokshi, *Hepatol. Int.*, 2019, **13**, 51–57.
54. S. Switalla, L. Lauenstein, F. Prenzler, S. Knothe, C. Förster, H. G. Fieguth, O. Pfennig, F. Schaumann, C. Martin, C. A. Guzman, T. Ebensen, M. Müller, J. M. Hohlfeld, N. Krug, A. Braun and K. Sewald, *Toxicol. Appl. Pharmacol.*, 2010, **246**, 107–115.
55. H. N. Alsafadi, C. A. Staab-Weijnitz, M. Lehmann, M. Lindner, B. Peschel, M. Königshoff and D. E. Wagner, *Am. J. Physiol.*, 2017, **312**, L896–l902.
56. E. Bigaeva, E. Gore, E. Simon, M. Zwick, A. Oldenburger, K. P. de Jong, H. S. Hofker, M. Schlepütz, P. Nicklin, M. Boersema, J. F. Rippmann and P. Olinga, *Arch. Toxicol.*, 2019, **93**, 3549–3583.
57. L. Paes, D. Lima, C. Matsuura, M. D. G. de Souza, F. Cyrino, C. Barbosa, F. Ferrão, D. Bottino, E. Bouskela and P. Farinatti, *PLoS One*, 2020, **15**, e0218228.
58. R. R. Silvares, E. N. Pereira, E. E. Flores, V. Estato, P. A. Reis, I. J. Silva, M. P. Machado, H. C. Neto, E. Tibiriça and A. Daliry, *Int. J. Exp. Pathol.*, 2016, **97**, 266–277.
59. C. P. Day, G. Merlino and T. V. Dyke, *Cell*, 2015, **163**, 39–53.
60. M. J. Waring, J. Arrowsmith, A. R. Leach, P. D. Leeson, S. Mandrell, R. M. Owen, G. Pairaudeau, W. D. Pennie, S. D. Pickett, J. Wang, O. Wallace and A. Weir, *Nat. Rev. Drug Discovery*, 2015, **14**, 475–486.
61. E. C. Emery, A. P. Luiz and J. N. Wood, *Expert Opin. Ther. Targets*, 2016, **20**, 975–983.
62. J.-M. Vignaud, M. Allam, N. Martinet, M. Pech, F. Plenat and Y. Martinet, *Am. J. Respir. Cell Mol. Biol.*, 1991, **5**, 531–538.
63. M. Humbert, G. Monti, M. Fartoukh, A. Magnan, F. Brenot, B. Rain, F. Capron, P. Galanaud, P. Duroux, G. Simonneau and D. Emilie, *Eur. Respir. J.*, 1998, **11**, 554–559.
64. R. Capdeville, E. Buchdunger, J. Zimmermann and A. Matter, *Nat. Rev. Drug Discovery*, 2002, **1**, 493–502.
65. R. T. Schermuly, E. Dony, H. A. Ghofrani, S. Pullamsetti, R. Savai, M. Roth, A. Sydykov, Y. J. Lai, N. Weissmann, W. Seeger and F. Grimminger, *J. Clin. Invest.*, 2005, **115**, 2811–2821.
66. J. Takahashi, M. Orcholski, K. Yuan and V. de J. Perez, *FEBS Lett.*, 2016, **590**, 101–109.
67. M. Thomas, C. Docx, A. M. Holmes, S. Beach, N. Duggan, K. England, C. Leblanc, C. Lebret, F. Schindler, F. Raza, C. Walker, A. Crosby, R. J. Davies, N. W. Morrell and D. C. Budd, *Am. J. Pathol.*, 2009, **174**, 380–389.
68. H. A. Ghofrani, W. Seeger and F. Grimminger, *N. Engl. J. Med.*, 2005, **353**, 1412–1413.
69. H. A. Ghofrani, N. W. Morrell, M. M. Hoeper, H. Olschewski, A. J. Peacock, R. J. Barst, S. Shapiro, H. Golpon, M. Toshner, F. Grimminger and S. Pascoe, *Am. J. Respir. Crit. Care Med.*, 2010, **182**, 1171–1177.
70. L. Ciuclan, M. J. Hussey, V. Burton, R. Good, N. Duggan, S. Beach, P. Jones, R. Fox, I. Clay, O. Bonneau, I. Konstantinova, A. Pearce, D. J. Rowlands, G. Jarai, J. Westwick, M. R. MacLean and M. Thomas, *Am. J. Respir. Crit. Care Med.*, 2013, **187**, 78–89.

71. A. E. Frost, R. J. Barst, M. M. Hoeper, H.-J. Chang, R. P. Frantz, Y. Fukumoto, N. Galié, P. M. Hassoun, H. Klose, H. Matsubara, N. W. Morrell, A. J. Peacock, M. Pfeifer, G. Simonneau, V. F. Tapson, F. Torres, C. D. Vizza, D. Lawrence, W. Yang, J. M. Felser, D. A. Quinn and H.-A. Ghofrani, *J. Heart Lung Transplant.*, 2015, **34**, 1366–1375.
72. D. E. Shaw, F. Baig, I. Bruce, S. Chamoin, S. P. Collingwood, S. Cross, S. Dayal, P. Drückes, P. Furet, V. Furminger, D. Haggart, M. Hussey, I. Konstantinova, J. C. Loren, V. Molteni, S. Roberts, J. Reilly, A. M. Saunders, R. Stringer, L. Sviridenko, M. Thomas, C. G. Thomson, C. Tomlins, B. Wen, V. Yeh and A. C. Pearce, *J. Med. Chem.*, 2016, **59**, 7901–7914.

# 19 Lead Generation

Frank Narjes*[a], Garry Pairaudeau[b] and Dušan Petrović[c]

[a]Medicinal Chemistry, Research & Early Development, Respiratory & Immunology, BioPharmaceuticals R&D, AstraZeneca, 431 50 Gothenburg, Sweden; [b]Exscientia, The Schrödinger Building, Oxford Science Park, Oxford, OX4 4GE, UK; [c]Hit Discovery, Discovery Sciences, BioPharmaceuticals R&D, AstraZeneca, 431 50 Gothenburg, Sweden
*E-mail: frank.narjes@astrazeneca.com

## 19.1 Introduction

### 19.1.1 What Is Lead Generation and Why Do We Need It?

Most small molecule drug projects progress through three distinct phases:

- Target identification – the selection of a biological protein target that is hypothesised to modulate the disease of interest;
- Drug discovery – the creation of the active drug molecule with the desired balance of properties to progress into humans; and finally,
- Drug Development – testing that drug molecule in human clinical trials to ensure it is safe and efficacious.

Drug discovery is a complex and high-risk endeavour and most large organisations find it helpful to break the process down into several distinct phases. This allows them to visualise the portfolio, plan more effectively transitions from discovery into development and measure progress.

Lead generation (LG) is the process of identifying hit molecules that interact with the desired target and then undertaking limited optimisation of those hits to a point where there is high confidence that a drug candidate will be identified. During this period the project will hopefully identify high-quality chemical tools suitable for advanced cellular and *in vivo* studies, which help to strengthen the validation of the target and increase confidence in the proposed mechanism (Figure 19.1). This is a critical point in

The Handbook of Medicinal Chemistry: Principles and Practice, 2nd Edition
Edited by Simon E. Ward and Andrew M. Davis

Published by the Royal Society of Chemistry, www.rsc.org

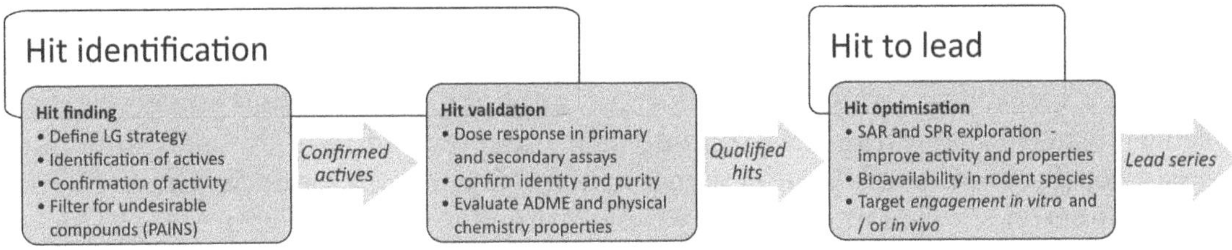


**Figure 19.1** Schematic representation of the lead generation process and its key activities.

> **Box 19.1 Helpful Definitions**
>
> A *hit* can be defined as a molecule which shows the desired activity (affinity or function) in a screening assay.
> A *qualified hit series* consists of a group of similar compounds, which are active on the target and demonstrate a structure-activity relationship (SAR).
> A *lead series* has a predefined level of activity, displays suitable physicochemical and pharmacokinetic properties, as well as the absence of toxic functionalities.

a drug discovery program, where choices that have a profound impact on the future of the clinical candidate are being made. A candidate drug needs to balance potency with pharmacokinetic properties and safety to be able to test the therapeutic hypothesis at a reasonable dose.[1] It is generally accepted that higher quality chemical starting points will enable faster progression and provide a greater chance of ultimately delivering a quality candidate drug (Box 19.1).

To ensure the identification of high-quality leads, a lead generation strategy will be defined at the outset of the project and will take into account all the available knowledge of the target. Based on the druggability or tractability assessment conducted at the target validation stage, a decision will have been made that target function can be modulated by a small molecule approach, and if an agonist or antagonist or a covalent mode of action (MoA), would lead to the desired therapeutic effect.[2,3] These factors will determine the choice of hit finding options to be applied to the target.

There is a significant portion of the human proteome that is not amenable to a small molecule approach, since many targets lack well-defined binding pockets or have no functional activity to modulate.[4] Other modalities such as peptides, antibodies, antisense oligonucleotides, or gene editing can be an option to tackle these so-called 'undruggable' proteins. In contrast to small molecules, peptides, and antibodies, which modulate protein function, oligonucleotides and gene editing work on the translational or transcriptional level, abolishing or enhancing production of the protein with all of its associated functions.[5] Of interest for the medicinal chemist is the discovery that degradation, as well as stabilisation of proteins can be accomplished with small molecules.[6] These can be complex natural products such as FK506, but also relatively simple structures, exemplified by lenalidomide (see Section 19.2.7). The degradation of target proteins, either by so-called molecular glues or heterobifunctional degraders, also known as proteolysis-targeting chimeras (PROTACs), has received a lot of attention from the drug discovery community.[7,8] There are expectations that these modalities will expand the 'druggable' target space for small molecule approaches. Other non-traditional applications for small molecule drug discovery, such as targeting RNA splicing or protein translation have also come into focus recently.[9–11] Most of these new mechanisms have been identified from phenotypic, cell-based screens and cannot yet be rationally designed, with the exception of heterobifunctional degraders. The choice of the modality or mechanism to target will thus affect the lead generation strategy and should be considered alongside the potential hit finding options.[12,13]

All of these considerations, choice of modality and MoA, will be part of the candidate drug profile, which a project team will define at the start of a project. In addition, it will describe the required properties (potency, pharmacokinetics, pharmacodynamics and safety) of the future candidate drug, and will provide line of sight for the duration of the discovery process.[14,15] The exact parameters will depend on the indication, the envisioned route of administration (oral, inhaled, or intravenous) and the location of the target.[16,17] This candidate drug profile will determine the parameters of the lead target profile and guide the selection of high-quality leads.

To provide a way to judge the quality of hits or leads, the concept of lead-likeness was introduced at the at the turn of the millennium.[18–20] This was a consequence of an observed decline in productivity in the pharmaceutical industry, due to attrition in the drug development phase, with poor compound properties being one of the reasons.[21]

As a result, drug-like property space was examined and several metrics were introduced to guide medicinal chemistry design.[22–26] Commonly, these focus on orally bioavailable molecules, and their property space is usually referred to as the rule of five (Ro5) space, but guidelines for inhaled molecules have also been summarised recently.[27] Several orally bioavailable drugs with properties lying outside the Ro5 space have been approved lately, or are currently in development; an example is the emerging PROTAC modality, and as a consequence, novel property limits have been proposed.[28,29]

The concept of lead-likeness asserts that a lead structure should be simpler and less complex than the envisioned drug candidate. This is grounded in the observation that potency and property optimisation of hits or leads invariably causes an increase in molecular weight and lipophilicity.[30,31] Excess lipophilicity is linked to poor physicochemical properties and metabolic as well as safety liabilities, which have been a major source of compound attrition in the past.[32]

Relatively simple compound quality measures have been developed, which quantify the contribution of size and lipophilicity of a molecule to target binding.[33,34] The most widely used are ligand efficiency (LE), which describes the binding efficiency per heavy atom, and lipophilic ligand efficiency (LLE or LipE), which is size-independent and describes the potency adjusted by lipophilicity.

$$\mathrm{LE} = (-2.3\ \mathrm{RT/No.\ of\ heavy\ atoms}) \times \mathrm{p}K_\mathrm{d}(\mathrm{pIC}_{50})$$

$$\mathrm{LLE} = \mathrm{pIC}_{50}(\mathrm{p}K_\mathrm{i}) - \log P(\log D)$$

There has been some discussion of the validity of these metrics, especially in the case of LE, but overall, they have seen increasing uptake in the medicinal chemistry community and been used in the discovery of a number of clinical candidates, and some examples are provided in this chapter.[35]

The major reason for compound attrition nowadays is associated with lack of efficacy and safety issues, whereas poor pharmacokinetics has become a minor contributor, thanks to the understanding and application of design principles for optimal molecular property space.[15,36] As a consequence, the demand on the attributes of a lead have risen continuously. In today's environment, a lead series not only needs to combine potency, good absorption, distribution, metabolism and excretion (ADME) properties with a relatively benign off-target profile, but in addition should demonstrate target engagement and the desired mechanistic and phenotypic response as an early indicator of efficacy.[37]

These experiments should be conducted in relevant cell assays with read-outs that link modulation of the target to the clinical hypothesis, since it will further strengthen the belief in the target and in the initially proposed mechanism of action.[38] It is dangerous to rely on biochemical or binding assays alone. An example is the PARP inhibitor Iniparib, which showed lack of efficacy in a variety of clinical trials. Later on it was discovered that the molecule achieved its antiproliferative effect by being redox-active.[37] For novel targets with unproven biology, high-quality leads are important to validate or de-validate its role in a given disease.[39]

Although lead generation describes the status of a molecule or chemical series, the transition from LG to lead optimisation (LO) is as much a function of confidence in the target hypothesis as it is in the chemical series. Traversing the lead generation phase of a project is about building trust that the project can deliver a clinical candidate.[40–43]

## 19.1.2 The Lead Generation Process

Historically, drugs were derived from natural products, and from the screening of distinct compounds for pharmacological activity in complex cell or *in vivo* models. These phenotypic approaches, although still in use, have been replaced by a more target-centric approach to increase the efficiency of the drug discovery process.[44]

Lead generation is a complex and multi-disciplinary endeavour, involving a variety of different skills, such as biology, medicinal, computational and analytical chemistry, as well as cheminformatics, which need to be combined in a project team to design a robust screening cascade and execute on it.[45]

Figure 19.1 provides an overview of the lead generation process and its key activities. The hit identification phase can be further segmented into two distinct activities:

1. Primary hit finding
2. Hit validation and characterisation.

Only qualified hits, which in addition to the desired potency present attractive physicochemical and pharmacokinetic properties will move into the hit to lead phase. In the following section we provide a general overview over these activities and will discuss the major hit finding options and the hit to lead process in more detail.

### 19.1.3 Hit Identification

All drug projects need to start from somewhere and hit identification is the process of identifying one or more well-characterised starting points for a drug project. Based on target knowledge, desired modality and MoA, and the available resources, a project team will elect the most appropriate strategy for hit finding.

The strategy employed to find chemical starting points will have a big impact on the course and outcome of a drug discovery project. There are different approaches available for hit identification, summarised in Table 19.1. They can be classified into knowledge-

**Table 19.1** Overview and key features of major hit finding approaches.

| Hit finding approaches | Description | Benefits | Limitations |
|---|---|---|---|
| Knowledge-based | Based on existing chemical matter, or approved drugs. | Fast and starting points may be high quality. | Need to differentiate and identify novelty, risk of getting scooped. |
| Focused screening | Knowledge of target class or ligand available and focussed, smaller libraries are screened. | Fast and cheap to run, high success rate for well-known target classes. | May lack novelty and risk of only finding what you already know. |
| High-throughput screening (HTS) | Unbiased screening of large compound collections in a miniaturised assay format. | Widely applicable *de novo* approach, identifies diverse hits; high chance of success. | Slow and expensive, often relies on simplified assays. |
| DNA encoded library screening (DEL) | Affinity selection from a library of DNA-tagged compounds in a single experiment. | Relatively rapid once the technology is established.<br>Access to greater chemical space compared to HTS.<br>Excellent for PROTACS | Limited to well-behaved soluble proteins, only measures affinity. |
| Virtual Screening (VS) | *In silico* libraries are evaluated against a pharmacophore model of known actives (ligand-based) or docked into the protein (structure-based). | Very fast and cost effective. Provides access to large chemical space beyond HTS collections and commercially available databases. | Requires significant skill, experience, computational resources, and high-quality models to be effective. |
| Fragment-based lead generation (FBLG) | Screening of less complex low molecular weight compounds (MW < 300). | Widely applicable method, identifies small optimisable fragments. | Usually requires crystal structure, screening at high compound concentration, and follow-up chemistry. |
| Phenotypic screen | Target-agnostic screening in cellular models or organisms.<br>Can be done in high-throughput format or with smaller annotated compound collections. | Identifies molecules with desired mode of action directly. | Highly sensitive to artefacts and identification of the molecular target requires significant effort post screen. |

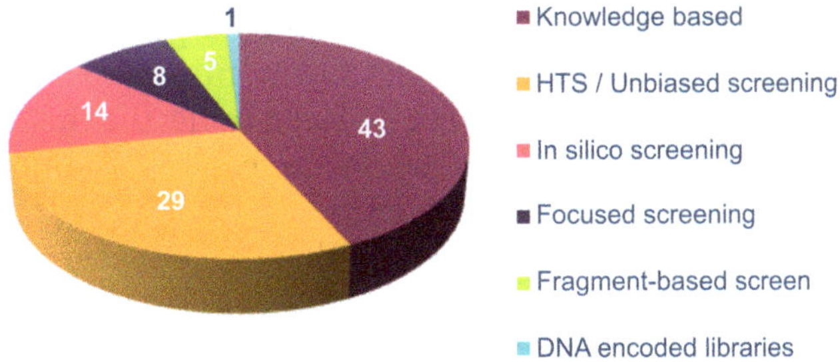


**Figure 19.2** Distributions of the six sources of lead generation strategies leading to clinical candidates published in the *J. Med. Chem.*, 2016–2017. Adapted from ref. 31 with permission from American Chemical Society, Copyright 2018.

based approaches, screening of diverse compound libraries or fragments, and *in silico* or computational approaches. Each of these has strengths and weaknesses and while it is possible to use a single hit finding method, it is more common that two or more are combined in a so-called integrated hit or lead generation strategy and run in parallel. The goal is to provide differentiated lead series from each approach to enhance the probability of success for the drug discovery project.[41,43,46,47]

An analysis of the strategies used for 66 clinical candidates published in the *Journal of Medicinal Chemistry* between 2016 and 2017 revealed that the majority (43%) of the programmes were based on known compounds, which was followed by screening approaches, with HTS, or random screening contributing 29%, followed by fragment-based screening. *In silico*, or structure-based design approaches took third place (Figure 19.2).[31]

However, as a result of the explosion of research into new biological mechanisms, genomics, and other target identification paradigms, the need for *de novo* hit finding approaches is likely greater now that it has ever been. There is a wealth of new, often unprecedented target opportunities that lack any quality chemical ligands or what chemical equity exists is of insufficient quality to launch a drug discovery effort.

In these cases, *de novo* hit finding is required, and this usually necessitates at least one, or a mixture of screening approaches:

- High-throughput screening (HTS) of a diverse screening collection[48]
- DNA encoded library screening (DEL)[49,50]
- Fragment screening or fragment-based lead generation (FBLG)[51]
- Virtual screening (VS)[52]
- Phenotypic screening.[53,54]

These *de novo* hit finding approaches will be discussed in more detail in Section 19.2.

## 19.1.4 Hit to Lead

Once a series of hits, or ideally multiple series of hits have been identified and validated, a project will move into the hit to lead phase. Unless the hit series already meets all the requirements, medicinal chemistry efforts are started with the goal to establish which of the series has the essential attributes to move into the LO phase. This can involve extensive SAR investigations to improve potency and ADME properties, show chemical scope within the series, and indicate its potential to deliver a molecule that could meet the candidate drug target profile. In the past, lead series might have been progressed based on affinity, selectivity, and maybe synthetic feasibility alone, but today a full data package is generated, which includes physicochemical and pharmacokinetic parameters, as well as off-target activities, the potential for toxicity, and the scope for optimisation. The novelty of the series, *i.e.*, can it eventually be patented, is another consideration. This stringent assessment serves to identify potential liabilities early on and avoid failure at later, more costly stages of the drug discovery programme or in the clinic.[40]

## 19.2 Hit-finding Approaches

The choice of hit finding approaches can have a profound influence on the final candidate molecule. High-quality starting points undoubtedly shorten the ensuing drug discovery phase, and it remains true that candidate molecules more often than not resemble the original hit series. However, there are pros and cons for each hit finding approach, which include time, cost, and suitability for the given target.

### 19.2.1 Knowledge-based Approaches

For many targets there is a significant corpus of knowledge in the literature and this information can be used to start a project. Here the rationale for a medicinal chemistry effort is to provide an improvement over already existing molecules or approved therapies, but the starting point can also be an endogenous ligand. These so-called knowledge-based approaches have developed significantly in recent years with improvements in computational methods and machine learning.

Figure 19.3 shows a recent example of a knowledge-based approach, where information from the clinic and preclinic was used to guide the design of the back-up candidate. This effort led to the discovery of Risdiplam, an orally bioavailable, CNS-penetrant drug, approved for the treatment of spinal muscular atrophy (SMA) in 2020 (see Chapter 24).[55] SMA is a disease caused by a mutation in the gene responsible for the production of survival motor neuron protein 1 (SMN1). Compounds **1** and **2** are so-called splicing modulators, which increase the protein levels of a related paralogue, SMN2, that under normal conditions is produced in a truncated, non-functional form.

The chemical series was identified from a cell-based screen, and compound **1** was the first to reach the clinic. It was stopped due to the potential for retinal toxicity observed in cynomolgus monkeys. To identify a viable back-up candidate the optimisation focussed on three areas:

- Increasing potency
- Reducing the basicity of the compound, which gave rise to a large volume of distribution, thought to be responsible for the risk for phospholipidosis and activity on the hERG channel
- Avoiding *N*-demethylation of the piperidine moiety, since the resulting metabolite is responsible for an off-target effect.

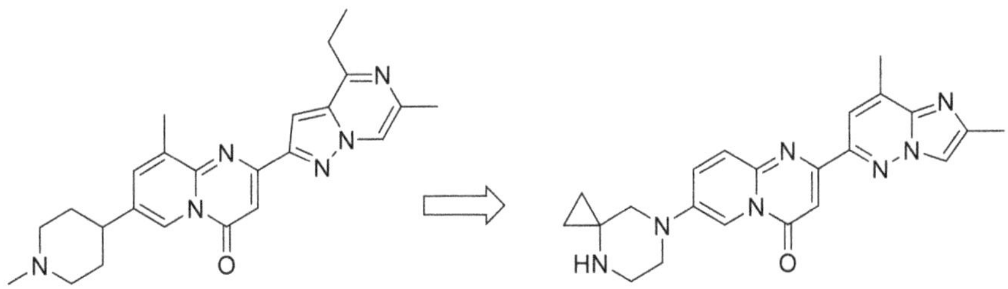

**1** (RG7800) **2** (RG7916) **Risdiplam**

| | **1** | **2** |
|---|---|---|
| SMN2 splicing $EC_{1.5x}$ (nM) | 23 | 4 |
| pKa (measured) | 10.9 | 6.8 |
| $V_{ss}$ rat (L/kg) | 29 | 3.1 |

**Figure 19.3** Optimisation of clinical candidate **1** leading to the approved drug Risdiplam (**2**).

Exchanging the heterocycle on the right-hand side of **1** to an imidazopyridazine led to a boost in potency, and also avoided the risk of phototoxicity. To identify a suitable replacement for the *N*-methylpiperidine, a virtual library was prepared to define compounds with the optimal combination of basicity, lipophilicity, and potency. This identified the piperazine contained in Risdiplam, which led to the desired reduction of basicity and lowered the volume of distribution.

### 19.2.2 High-throughput Screening

HTS remains the single most versatile and generally applicable method of identifying hits, particularly in cases where there is little known chemical equity or there is a strong desire to identify novel chemical matter.[48,56] HTS is usually conducted in a dedicated screening centres with extensive automation and specialist compound-handling capabilities. These are expensive facilities to construct and only viable for large pharmaceutical companies wishing to run many projects every year. Fortunately, there are a number of CRO facilities available, as well as not-for-profit and academic centres such as ESCU lab, UCLA MSSR, Sanford Burnham HTS centre and many others.

One of the key advantages of HTS is the ability to screen for functionally active molecules directly in either a cellular or biochemical setting and identify compounds with the desired MoA directly.[48,57] Historically, HTS has always focussed on screening the largest possible collection of molecules in a relatively simple assay. While there is still a place for this approach, in recent years some groups have moved away from bulk screening towards more iterative or focussed approaches.

Novartis have described a detailed evaluation and stratification of their collection into a series of layers. Compounds with the best physical properties, particularly permeability and solubility, along with the greatest structural and biological diversity are in the first layers. If a team only has time or capacity to screen a small set of compounds, *i.e.*, 50K or 125K, they can choose the first 1 or 2 layers. For maximum diversity, they can of course screen more, but this method provides a rational way to stratify the collection and cater to many different project requirements.[58] Using this new subset, a publication by Novartis describes a retrospective analysis of 34 HTS campaigns conducted in-house. An iterative screening approach, where the initial hits are used to select chemically and biologically similar compounds for the next iteration, showed improved efficiency over the bulk screening method. For example, screening only about ~1% of the compounds contained in Novartis' full screening deck, corresponding to roughly ~15 000 molecules, retrieved on average the top 0.5% of the most active compounds independent of the assay format, covering around 40% of the scaffolds.[59]

Employing machine-learning approaches, a retrospective analysis of HTS data from PubChem demonstrated that an iterative screening setup, evaluating about 35% of the screening collection over as few as three iterations has a median return rate of approximately 70% of the active compounds.[60] Application of this methodology will also save cost and time, or could allow the use of more complex assays. This approach should not be confused with a focussed screening approach, where a subset of the library, based on target class knowledge or chemical similarity is evaluated.

#### 19.2.2.1 Choice of Assay

In principle, any assay could be used for a high-throughput screen, but in reality, there are compromises to be made to achieve the required throughput in a reasonable period of time. Modern automated platforms are capable or conducting incredibly complex screens, reliably and reproducibly. However, the more complex the assay, the longer it will take to develop. In general it will likely be more susceptible to interference and risk of false positives. Whilst it may be possible to deconvolute complex screens with simpler assays downstream, this is paradoxical and it is usually pragmatic to start with the simplest assay format and then confirm translation with a more complex biologically relevant assay later. There is a vast number of assay technologies available to support hit finding, and these have been reviewed recently.[61]

Broadly, assays can be grouped in to three main categories:

- *Biochemical assays*: A wide range of biochemical assays are available for HTS.[61] Historically, radiochemical assays were often used. However, these have largely been replaced by fluorescence-based screening technologies, such as homogeneous time resolved fluorescence (HTRF), amplified luminescent proximity homogeneous assay (ALPHAscreen) or fluorescence polarisation (FP). The fluorescent read out can be susceptible to interference from coloured compounds or compounds possessing extended chromophores, but this can readily be controlled using a counter screen of an unrelated target. Recently, mass spectroscopy has become a popular endpoint. This read-out usually does not require a specific labelled ligand to be created and is therefore faster to develop.[62]
- *Affinity-based screens*: Several affinity-based methods have been used for high-throughput screening campaigns. These include affinity selection mass spectroscopy (ASMS),[63] calorimetric assays such as differential scanning fluorimetry (DSF)[64] and even cellular high-throughput screens using cellular thermal shift assays (CETSA).[65,66] They can be fast to run and often require little assay development but do not measure activity.

ASMS is an efficient high-throughput screening method, which has evolved from being a rarely used alternative to traditional HTS to an established technology for hit finding. Screening mixtures of molecules is possible, sometimes up to 500 compounds per well, and needs relatively small amounts of the target protein, which is incubated with the compound mixture. Target-bound ligands are directly identified after separation from non-bound ligands with high-resolution mass spectrometry (HR-MS).[62]

- *Cellular screens* are used extensively for membrane-bound targets such as GPCRs and ion channels that are challenging to express in the non-membrane-bound form. Technologies such as FLIPR (fluorescence imaging plate reader) which measure intracellular calcium using calcium-sensitive dyes, or other cellular messengers are widely used. These are good approaches, although care must be exercised as confirming target engagement can be challenging without a biophysical secondary screen. Screening in a cellular environment also ensures that the protein is in a more physiological situation and that the ligands are more relevant. In the case of phenotypic screening, typically human cell lines are used, and a biologically relevant end point is the read-out. Alternatively, high-throughput imaging, or high-content screening provides a valid alternative. Image-based profiling uses automated microscopy at single cell resolution and captures the morphology of the cell and its organelles, providing information on the biological process under investigation, which differs from the single point measurement (affinity or activity) which is frequently encountered.[67] Previously, only a small number of features were extracted from an experiment, but the increase in available computational power and machine-learning-based methods are now able to extract and analyse much more information. Applications include identifying disease-associated phenotypes, understanding disease mechanisms and predicting the activity or toxicity for a drug molecule.[68]

It may seem that one should always go for the most relevant cellular system every time, but there are big trade-offs with doing this. An HTS will screen millions of compounds, which could easily be 1000–2000 plates, even in a 1536-well format. The cost of reagents could be enormous. More importantly, the more complex the system the harder the assay is likely to be to develop, and it will take to achieve the exacting conditions of robustness needed for an HTS. Also, the greater the chance that the observed biological effect is due to other non-specific events or off-target activity. Finally, screening an intracellular target in a cell requires the compounds to be cell penetrant and to compete with the endogenous substrate. On balance, it is generally true that an HTS run with a simple biochemical assay is most suitable to a high-throughput campaign; complex assays are best reserved for later in the screening cascade.

The endpoint of an HTS screen is usually a binding event or inhibition in an assay at a single concentration.

#### 19.2.2.2 Screening Collections

What makes a good screening collection? Is an often-debated question. Most large pharma collections have evolved over decades through a combination of natural addition of compounds synthesised as part of ongoing drug project activities, combined with a mixture of acquisition from compound providers, and directed efforts to synthesise diverse libraries of compounds.[69–71] It has also been recognised that HTS screening collections might not be suited to address challenging targets, and broader chemical space might be required. Here, compound collections based around natural products or natural-product-inspired molecules, macrocycles, or peptides have been used, and there are several reviews available summarising these approaches.[72–74]

There are two critical components to be considered in any screening collection:

1. *Structural Diversity*: Chemical space is so huge that simply applying a strategy of making diverse molecules is a highly inefficient approach to finding hits and best reserved for DNA encoded library or virtual screens. The best screening collections contain a wide range of structural types and exploit motifs known to bind to biological targets. It is also helpful if the collection is comprised of many small related clusters of compounds, with 3–10 molecules per cluster, giving immediate SAR around a hit and adding confidence that a hit is real during the hit ID phase.[70] It is also generally recognised that low molecular weight, low lipophilicity lead-like compounds make the best starting points for drug discovery, as discussed in the introduction. They will generally offer more opportunity for optimisation, and there is also support for the idea that lead-likeness or lower molecular complexity increases the chance of finding hits.[75] Finally, a screening collection should not contain molecules likely to interfere with assays or react with the target, so reactive compounds, oxidisers, and coloured or fluorescent compounds should be avoided.[76,77]
2. *Compound Quality*: The actual physical quality of the compounds being screened is also an important criterion. Care should be taken during the preparation of the collection to remove metals or reactive intermediates during the later stages of chemical synthesis. A recent study demonstrated that many screens are exquisitely sensitive to metal contamination at very low levels in the screening sample.[78] In addition, compounds will likely be stored for long periods in DMSO and the physical quality and purity of the actual sample screened should be checked.

### 19.2.2.3 Working up the HTS

The evaluation of hits from HTS assays, where many structurally diverse compounds are tested, presents more challenges than for other more focussed screening efforts. The most critical phase of an HTS work up is determining which of the many compounds that have shown activity are actually interacting with the target through the desired mechanism of action, as opposed to interfering with the assay. Due to the large numbers of potential hits, a hit rate of 1% for a library of 1 000 000 molecules equates to 10 000 compounds. Efficient cheminformatic tools have been developed to triage the hit list, which are supplemented with empirical approaches, such as target and compound knowledge.[76–80]

The main reasons for a false positive signal are:

- Chemical features of the compound itself, which interfere with the assay signal. Typical examples are redox-active or fluorescent compounds, compounds containing reactive groups which react with the protein or the ligand, or compounds which lead to protein aggregation or unfolding.
- Simple errors in the assay which could arise from mechanical issues such as blocked tips, reagent problems, and contaminations. When an assay is run millions of times, even with the tightest control, there is a lot of opportunity for things to go wrong and the data should be approached with a healthy degree of scepticism.

As well as flagging potential structural features that may identify frequent hitters, companies that run many HTS campaigns have annotated their collections based on the number of times they have been active in previous campaigns.[81] Therefore they can identify potential interfering compounds that could be false positives in an unbiased way. Of course, when screening target classes such as kinases in collections with many previous kinase projects, compounds can be frequent hitters for very good on-target biological reasons. In order to overcome these challenges, great attention must be paid to designing the hit triage cascade. Running an HTS campaign should not be thought of as running a single assay but seen as a collection of assays that together will identify validated hits.

Figure 19.4 shows a simplified cascade. The basic principle is to remove compounds that act through interference mechanisms and confirm thoroughly that a compound binds to the desired target using more than one type of assay. Finally, to ensure that the molecule has the desired mechanism of action, ideally in a relevant cellular assay. HTS often requires compromises in the physiological relevance of the assays used, so it is critical to test that the hit series identified works in the desired setting. This can be a challenge if the hits do not have sufficient potency or physical properties to display cellular activity, in which case cycles of optimisation may be needed before a molecule can be tested. This is not unusual, but the project is at risk until the MoA has been confirmed. Once one or more active series of compounds have been identified, it is good practice to rescreen related molecules from the collection to ensure the maximum SAR has been found. Often the entire collection was not screened in the primary screen and there may be extra knowledge to be gleaned. Also at this point, any available commercial near neighbours should be purchased and passed through the screening cascade (sometimes referred to as 'SAR by catalogue').

Many people believe that a series is never fully confirmed until a small number of members have been resynthesised and the structural identity and purity confirmed. This is undoubtedly good practice.

## 19.2.3 DNA Encoded Library Screening

DNA encoded library technology (DEL), also referred to as encoded library technology (ELT), offers the possibility to screen large numbers of molecules, usually millions to billions, in a single experiment.[49,50] The idea to encode the identity of compounds with

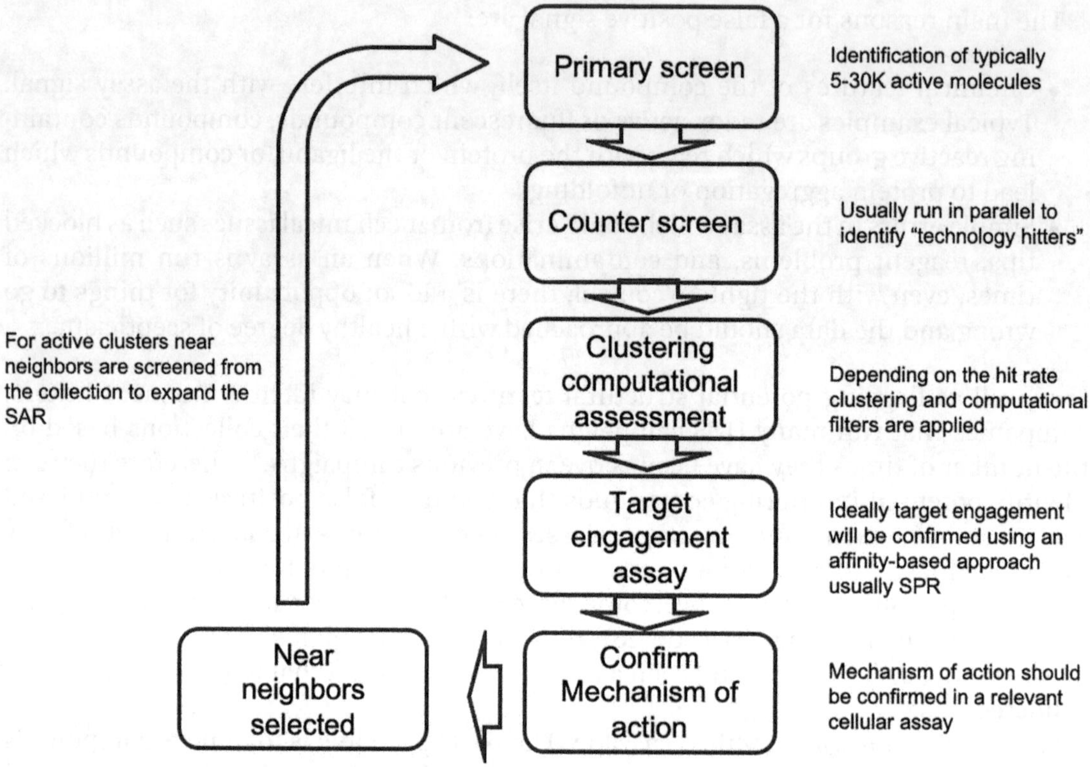


**Figure 19.4** Simplified screening cascade for HTS.

a DNA tag, published in 1992,[82] along with advances in DNA amplification and next-generation sequencing, has led to the wide adoption of this hit finding methodology, and resulted in the discovery of novel ligands and clinical candidates for a wide variety of protein targets.[49,83]

Different to HTS, where individual compounds are screened (one compound per well), in the majority of DEL experiments the whole library, which fits in a small test tube, is evaluated against a protein target and this can be done at a fraction of the cost and time compared to HTS. The identity of the compounds is encoded by a unique DNA tag, which is built during its synthesis. Screening is usually based on affinity selection, where the compound library is incubated with the immobilised protein target. Non-binding compounds are removed in a washing step, the binders are released from the protein, further enriched in additional selection cycles, and subsequently identified by amplification of the DNA tag's sequencing. It is also relatively straightforward to combine selection methods, and compare the enrichment profiles after selection. This way one can screen for a specific MoA by including known binders or select for specificity across closely related proteins.[84] An illustrative example is provided below in Figure 19.5.

The method is unbiased and can identify molecules binding to all potential sites on a protein. It is suitable for proteins with low druggability, where the lack of known binders or function might make the preparation of reagents for biochemical assays difficult. Compared to HTS compound collections, the larger library size allows a deeper

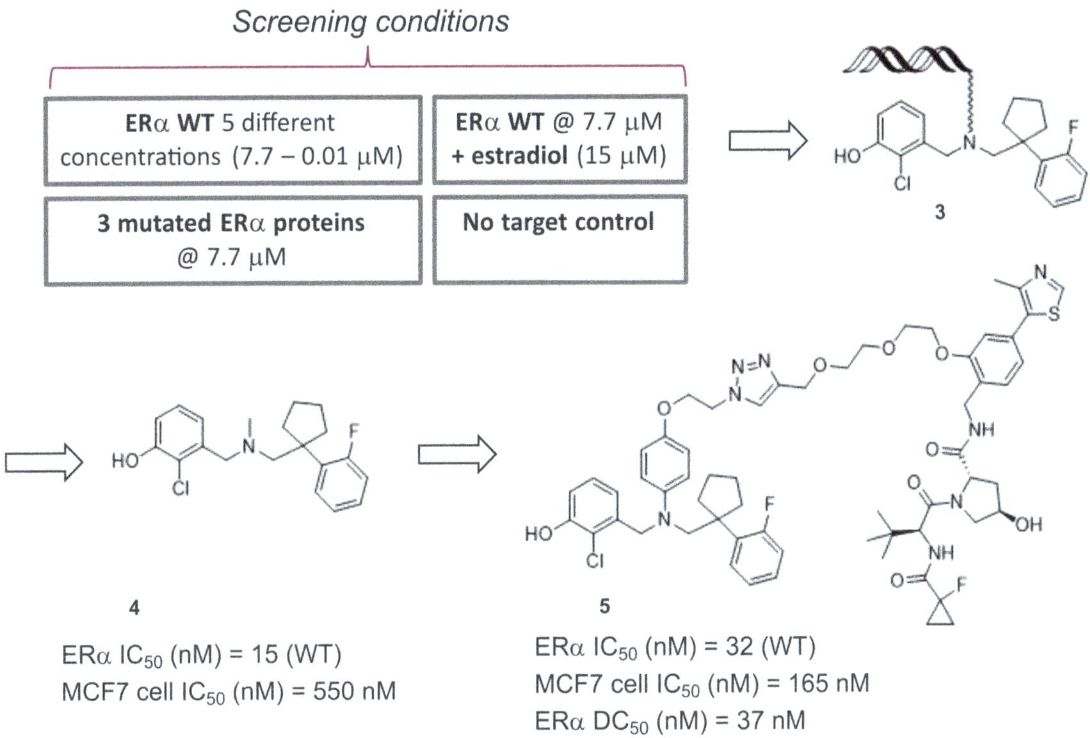


**Figure 19.5** Identification of ERα binder **3** by DEL screening under 10 different conditions and its use in the construction of heterobifunctional degrader **5**.

exploration of chemical space, which can lead to a higher number of hits. The presence of the DNA tag as well as the matrix used for immobilisation of the target can cause screening artefacts.

The majority of DEL applications rely on affinity screening on recombinant immobilised proteins, which limits its scope to proteins which can be expressed and purified in their native form. To expand the target space, specific techniques have been developed which permit screening of proteins in cell lysates and on the cell surface for membrane-bound targets.[85] For the latter, a relatively straightforward approach relies on overexpressing the target protein on the cell surface and using cells with normal expression levels as the control. A successful example was reported by researchers at GSK from screening of a triazine-based library on immobilised HEK293 cells, overexpressing the membrane bound Neurokinin-3 (NK-3) receptor, a GPCR of the tachykinin family. Potent antagonists of NK-3 were discovered, which showed selectivity against the related family members NK-1 and NK-2.[86] Since toxicity overexpression of certain proteins on the cell membrane can lead to cell death, another approach makes use of a reactive group on the DNA tag of the DEL. After the binding event, a covalent linkage of the DNA to protein target is established, which were expressed as tagged fusion proteins. This then allows copurification of the whole protein–compound–DNA construct after cell lysis. This method has also been applied to screen inside cells. Here, the highly polar DEL compounds were delivered into cells using a cyclic cell-penetrating peptide, conjugated to the DNA tag of each compound.[87] Very recently, researchers at Vipergen injected a DEL library of 194 million compounds into oocytes from a frog species and were able to find hits for three different targets under physiological conditions.[88]

One downside of DEL screening is that there is no compound storage available from which molecules can be ordered or purchased to confirm the activity. The hits identified from sequencing need to be prepared 'off-DNA' by traditional synthesis. Depending on the chemistry used to attach the first building block to its DNA tag, this attachment point is usually transformed into a smaller functional group. The DNA attachment point also presents opportunities for optimisation of physicochemical properties. Since the linker position is known, it can be used for the rapid construction of PROTACs, thus circumventing time-consuming SAR studies to find a suitable linker attachment point, as shown in Figure 19.5. Screening a DEL library of 120 billion compounds on different forms of the ligand binding domain of the Estrogen receptor alpha (ERα), including the wild-type and three gain-of-function mutations, identified **3**. It did not bind to the matrix, and binding could be competed by the presence of estradiol, suggesting binding in the orthosteric site of ER.[89] Compound **4**, where the linker was truncated to a methyl group indeed showed potent binding to all four ERα ligand binding domains. Using the DNA attachment vector, a phenyl piperazine was built off the central nitrogen, which was used to attach a known binder of the E3 ligase VHL, yielding PROTAC **5**, which demonstrated potent degradation of ERα.

DEL libraries rely on the concept of split and pool synthesis and libraries are typically synthesised in 2–4 steps from building block collections. Synthesis needs be compatible with the DNA tag, which limits the array of applicable synthetic methods to robust reactions which can be run under aqueous conditions, such as amide bond formation, cross-coupling reactions, nucleophilic substitutions, reductive aminations and certain heterocycle formations. There is a considerable effort underway to expand the synthetic toolbox for DEL libraries, and the application of novel synthetic methodology such as C–H activation and photoredox-based couplings has been reported.[90] It has been noted that DEL libraries are less lead-like compared to a well-curated HTS library. High compound numbers are achieved by using a large number of building blocks in the diversity step, and not all of these will be lead-like.[91]

### 19.2.4 Focussed Screening

Focused screening is in some ways related to knowledge-based approaches and *in silico* screening methods, which are discussed below. The number of compounds to screen is reduced by constructing subsets from highly annotated compound collections using a combination of different *in silico* approaches.[92] They have been built around several target classes, such as GPCRs, proteases, ion channels or kinases.[93–95] It is also possible to target a desired MoA, for example libraries with metal binding motifs for metalloproteases or histone deacetylases or libraries containing a covalent moiety. The advantages of a focussed screening approach are: the use of more complex assays for hit finding; reduced screening resources and cost; and the potential for rapid optimisation of the hits.

### 19.2.5 *In Silico* (Virtual) Screening

The main goal of virtual screening (VS) is to shortlist a large molecular database by applying various computational chemistry methods, thus enriching the selected subset with active molecules that will be screened in biological assays. To that end, VS can be used to find new chemical equity without any previous knowledge, starting directly from the structure of a target protein. However, any additional information on known active molecules from other hit finding approaches, enzyme substrates, compounds that trigger a given target as a side activity, or similar can be incorporated into the virtual screening workflow. Especially in the 'me too' and 'fast follower' programmes, VS can be initiated starting from known drugs or drug candidates for a given target. Common scenarios in VS include searching through the corporate databases of in-house available molecules, or through external supplier catalogues to pick compounds for acquisition. A significant part of the work is focussed on searching virtual libraries of either target-specific or general drug-like compounds that have not been synthesised yet, with a focus on making decisions which compounds to prioritise.

Typical pharma screening collections are at the order of few million compounds. Virtual libraries can be enumerated *in silico* using known chemical reactions and available building blocks, and often count $10^{10}$–$10^{15}$ compounds.[96–98] These would typically cover readily synthesisable molecules with drug-like properties, which if identified by a VS procedure – could be directly synthesised and tested in the biological assays. Even though they cover vast numbers of different chemotypes, often with many near neighbours to explore the SAR, the enumerated libraries are just a small subset of the theoretical chemical space of all drug-like molecules, which by some estimates is reaching $10^{60}$ compounds with up to 30 heavy atoms (C, N, O and S).[99]

From a technical perspective, VS methods can be classed as either ligand-based (LB) or structure-based (SB), depending whether they rely on the known ligands or the known protein receptor structures. Among the LBVS methods, pharmacophore modelling is one of the most commonly applied approaches. A pharmacophore identifies the most essential steric and electronic features needed to ensure productive molecular interactions and trigger a biological response with a target, and maps their arrangement in 2D or 3D space. Every atom or group in a molecule can be reduced to one or more pharmacophores, such as hydrogen bond donors or acceptors, positively or negatively charged groups, rings, aromatic moieties, hydrophobic systems, *etc.* For example, Figure 19.6A depicts a possible pharmacophore model based on the antiretroviral drug Efavirenz. Pharmacophore models can also be proposed based on the structure of a protein binding site, or even a protein–ligand complex. For example, the minimal pharmacophore for the kinase inhibitors can be developed from the structure of the kinase-ATP complex (Figure 19.6B). The essential pharmacophore is the hydrogen bond donor–acceptor–donor motif on a hydrophobic carrier, imitating the adenine interaction with the kinase hinge region (Figure 19.6C), as illustrated by Crizotinib binding to the ROS1 kinase. Once a pharmacophore model is developed and validated, large databases of on-the-shelf or virtual compounds can be analysed for the presence of the key features. A first pass through the pharmacophore model identifies a large population of molecules satisfying the critical features. These have the potential to be active against

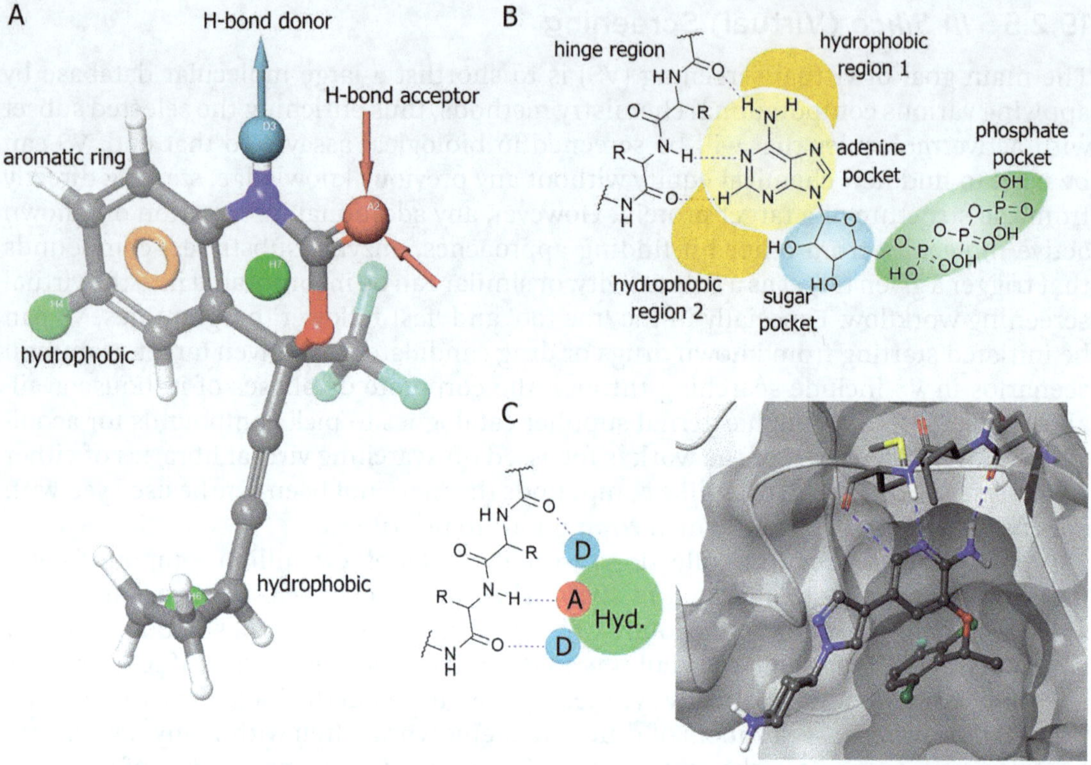


**Figure 19.6** Pharmacophore models in virtual screening. (A) Ligand-based pharmacophore model of the antiretroviral drug Efavirenz, a non-nucleoside reverse transcriptase inhibitor. (B) Structures of a protein–ligand complexes can be used to develop a pharmacophore model, *e.g.*, for a typical kinase ATP binding pocket. (C) The general ATP-site kinase pharmacophore and an example of Crizotinib, a potent kinase inhibitor, bound to the ROS1 kinase domain (PDB ID: 3ZBF).

the given target, and would then be refined using more compute-intensive processes, described later.

Another important concept in virtual screening is molecular similarity, typically quantified using the Tanimoto coefficient. Defined as the ratio of the intersection and the union of features of two molecules, Tanimoto coefficient can take values between 0 (for two molecules sharing no common features) and 1 (for two identical molecules). Such a Tanimoto similarity is often calculated in 2D using molecular fingerprints, as shown in Figure 19.7. Morphine and codeine are very similar molecules, with a Tanimoto coefficient of 0.8, and only a single point of difference at one of the hydroxyl groups. However, a Tanimoto score of 0.1 indicates that morphine and methadone are very different molecules, as can be directly observed from their molecular structures. As a synthetic opioid agonist, methadone acts on the same opioid receptors in the brain as morphine and similar opioid pain medications. In fact, shape and pharmacophore overlays in 3D point to a good similarity between these two molecules, where the phenyl rings and the basic nitrogen atoms overlap. Identifying molecules with a similar 3D shape to the known actives is an important LBVS method, where the underlying

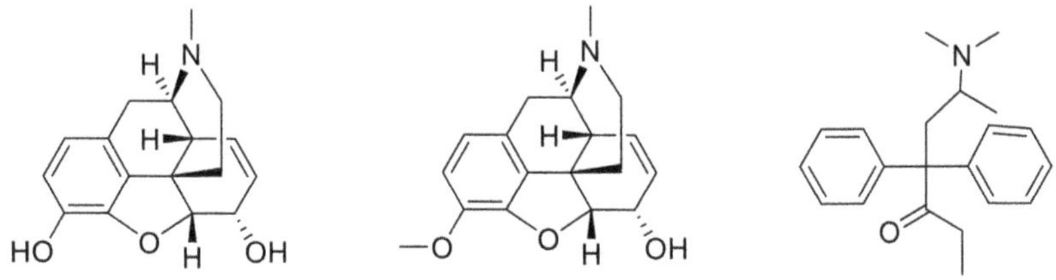


**Figure 19.7** Despite their low 2D similarity (Tanimoto coefficient of 0.1), morphine and methadone act on the same opioid receptors in the brain, due to their shape and pharmacophore similarity in 3D.

assumption is that two molecules with a similar 3D shape and pharmacophore feature arrangement will cause a similar biological effect on a target, even if their 2D similarity is rather low. Some of the shape similarity searching methods, such as Rapid Overlay of Chemical Structures (ROCS) can be applied for screening ultra-large chemical libraries to identify promising hits with novel chemotypes.[100] With the advantage of cloud computing, such a calculation can be parallelised over hundreds of graphical processing units (GPUs), comparing and screening billions of molecules in a matter of an hour.[96]

Structure-based methods, on the other hand, focus on predicting how a ligand binds into the protein binding pocket, and assess the affinity of their interactions. One of the most widely used SBVS methods is molecular docking, which consists of two phases. In the pose generation stage, docking algorithms explore internal conformational landscape of a ligand, as well as ligand positioning within the protein. Most often, protein conformation is kept fixed, which is one of the major limitations in docking. Even though some receptor flexibility can be incorporated by using multiple receptor structures, obtained from structures with multiple ligands, or through computational receptor sampling approaches such as induced fit docking, these are usually too computationally expensive for routine large-scale virtual screening runs. In the pose scoring phase, for each generated ligand pose, docking evaluates the binding and interactions (such as hydrogen bonds, $\pi$-stacking, ionic and van der Waals interactions), and quantifies the binding affinity. In addition to the productive interactions with the protein, docking penalises potential clashes between the receptor and a ligand, but also takes into account desolvation penalties. The process of ligand docking can be biased with the knowledge of a system. For example, if there is a key protein pharmacophore, ligands could be constrained to it using hydrogen bonds. Alternatively, known NMR NOE signals could be used as constraints. Docking algorithms can be massively parallelised for the assessment of hundreds of millions of compounds in make-on-demand virtual libraries, prioritising which compounds to select for synthesis.[101,102] As the size of a virtual library increases, docking entire collections is becoming cost prohibitive. To that end, machine learning and artificial intelligence can be employed as the active-learning docking protocols, which can significantly increase the throughput.[103]

Scoring functions used for evaluating ligand affinities are rather approximate, and due to the static nature of the protein during docking, the output is often rescored with an orthogonal technique. Physics-based methods, such as molecular dynamics (MD), are able to simulate the time-dependent behaviour of a protein–ligand complex. Although they are significantly more computationally expensive than docking, even short MD simulations have been shown to improve the hit rate in SBVS. Among MD techniques, free energy perturbation (FEP) simulations have become particularly important in drug design. Despite long simulation times and high computational cost, FEP can accurately predict potency and selectivity of hits across many structurally enabled targets, assisting a chemist in selecting only the most promising molecules for synthesis. Finally, with active-learning FEP methods, the simulation throughput increases at a fraction of the cost, enabling large-scale virtual screening efforts.[104]

Machine-learning approaches have been part of virtual screening for decades. For example, if biological data on the target of interest is already available for a diverse set of molecules, *e.g.*, from previous patent applications, quantitative structure–activity relationship (QSAR) models could be trained on these to distinguish between active and inactive molecules. Such a regression model can be used to quickly evaluate very large molecular databases. Furthermore, artificial intelligence (AI)-based methods such as active learning can be combined with docking and FEP calculations, as described earlier. In such applications, FEP simulations are run for a small number of compounds, and an AI model is trained on the results to predict the binding affinities for the remaining molecules in the database. After several rounds of active learning, a model can predict affinities with sufficiently high accuracy, even without running expensive FEP calculations for all the molecules. Finally, *de novo* design, or generation of molecular structures beyond what is captured in the enumerated virtual libraries is one of the AI applications gaining popularity. Such methods are often based on previously discussed techniques, such as ROCS or docking, aiming to identify novel molecules suitable for a given target, while often optimising physicochemical and metabolic properties.

In practice, VS campaigns rarely rely on a single computational method. Instead, if the program is fully enabled with known actives and protein structures, both LBVS and SBVS methods are combined to guide hit creation. The workflow normally starts with less expensive (computer time-consuming) ligand-based methods able to process larger chemical libraries, or AI-based generative efforts. After retrieving compounds with the predefined shape and pharmacophore, and filtering for the physicochemical and metabolic properties needed in the program, the remaining compounds are typically docked. Due to previously discussed limitations, docked hits are often rescored with an orthogonal computational method. With the modern hardware and cloud computing infrastructure, FEP is becoming the leading physics-based method to rescore ligands. Finally, after visual inspection of the top hits by a chemist, a number of compounds would be selected for acquisition or synthesis and further biological testing. In a recent study, a database of nearly 2 million on-the-shelf molecules was screened using ROCS, shortlisting 1700 compounds with high shape and pharmacophore scores to known urease inhibitors.[105] These molecules were docked to the enzyme binding site, and 10 compounds among the top 100 scored hits were selected for acquisition in such a way to cover multiple chemotypes. Biological testing confirmed three compounds with submicromolar $IC_{50}$ values against the target, providing good hits for further development.

### 19.2.6 Fragment-based Lead Generation

Fragment-based lead generation (FBLG), also sometimes called fragment-based drug discovery (FBDD) consists in screening simple, low molecular weight molecules, usually having less than 20 non-hydrogen atoms, against a drug target. This approach identifies binders with relatively weak potency, compared to hits from HTS or DEL libraries. Larger, lead-like molecules are derived from these in a subsequent step through medicinal chemistry efforts. This method has become increasingly popular, both in the pharmaceutical industry as well as in academic research laboratories, and is one of the major approaches for the generation of high-quality hits.[51,106,107]

Fragments are the ultimate lead-like molecules and calculations by Hann and colleagues have shown that fragments cover the same chemical space with fewer molecules than much larger HTS libraries.[108] Their low complexity enables them to bind to a greater number of protein sites, where they can establish well-defined interactions, whereas more complex ligands have less of a chance to interact with a given target. Another advantage of fragments is that they are able to bind to sites on proteins other than substrate binding sites. Targeting these secondary or allosteric sites can directly affect its biological function *via* an allosteric mechanism, or modulate interactions with other binding partners.[109]

Most pharmaceutical companies as well as academic laboratories use FBLG as part of their LG efforts. A major factor for its success has been the availability of information on the binding mode of the hit, either through NMR spectroscopy or X-ray crystallography enabling rational design of lead candidates from the fragment hits. This has resulted in several approved drugs and an ever growing number of clinical candidates, especially in the oncology area, where identified hinge binding fragments have been used with good success (Figure 19.8).[110]

The binding affinity of fragments is usually in the micro- to millimolar range, due to their small size, requiring screening at high compound concentrations and assay technology that is sensitive enough to detect these weak binding events. Biophysical

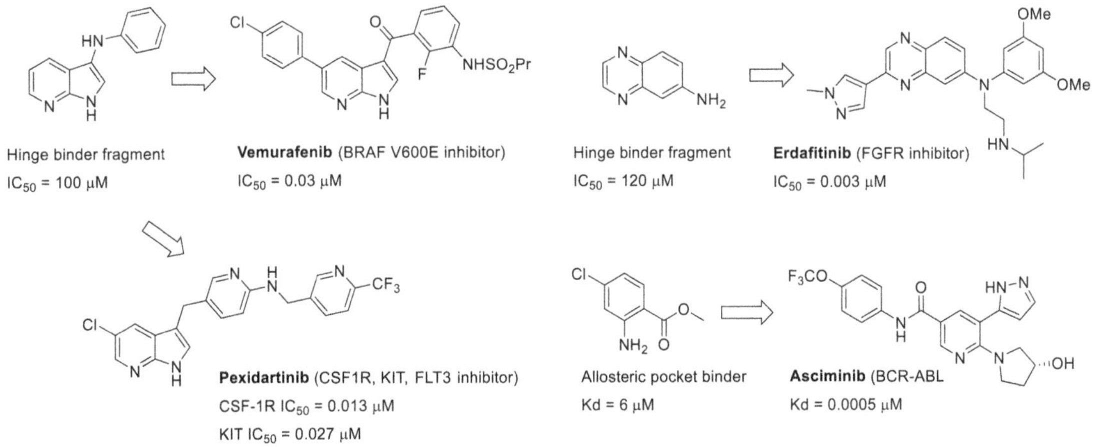


**Figure 19.8** Approved drugs obtained through FBLG efforts and their fragment starting points.

methods, such as NMR spectroscopy, surface plasmon resonance (SPR), thermal shift assays, mass spectrometry, or X-ray crystallography constitute the preferred screening methods. Also functional biochemical assays have been used, in a so-called high concentration screening format. The advantage is that these assays have a high throughput and generate a functional read-out, allowing for rapid generation of SAR.[107] Historically, NMR screening for fragment binding, pioneered by Fesik and co-workers (SAR by NMR), used proteins labelled with the NMR-active $^{15}N$ nucleus to monitor the protein signals for changes upon ligand binding. Another approach uses unlabelled protein and depends on magnetisation transfer pathways from either the protein itself or from bulk water to observe binding of the small molecule to the target of interest by monitoring its proton NMR.[51] More recently, $^{19}F$ NMR spectroscopy has gained widespread use, due to its high sensitivity and the absence of $^{19}F$ in proteins.[111,112] Machine-learning methods also begin to impact FBLG, with improvements in virtual screening approaches and automation for linking approaches being reported.[113,114]

High compound concentrations increase the risk for false positives and stringent counter screens need to be embedded in the screening cascade to confirm the initial activity. Often, more than one hit finding approach is used to confirm the activity, for example binding observed by NMR is followed up with an SPR assay. If the activity of the fragment hit is in the lower micromolar range, a functional assay might also be used.

Fragment libraries are orders of magnitude smaller compared to HTS decks. They need to be composed of compounds possessing high aqueous solubility to fulfil the requirement of testing at high concentrations. Rules for the construction of fragment libraries have been refined, and compounds contained in FBLG libraries usually adhere to the rule of three, meaning a molecular weight below 300, a clog*P* of three or less and equal to or less than three hydrogen bond donors or acceptors and rotatable bonds.[115]

Compound efficiency metrics, discussed in Section 19.1.1, are a critical component of any fragment campaign. Due to the often weak binding and polar nature, a ligand efficiency (LE) index is often used to rank hits. There are no strict guidelines, but a molecule with an LE value of 0.3 is viewed as a good starting point.

The biggest challenge in FBLG and the most time-consuming step is improving the binding affinity of the fragment hits and converting them into lead-like molecules. Three different strategies are employed in this process:

- *Fragment growing*, where atoms or functional groups are added to suitable positions.
- *Fragment merging*, where the hit is merged with features from other hits or known molecules.
- *Fragment linking*, where two or more fragment hits binding to adjacent sites in the protein are connected.

All of these approaches benefit from the availability of X-ray crystal structures, as mentioned above. A recent review looking at the approved drugs and clinical candidates resulting from FBLG found that fragment growing is by far the most widely used approach.[110] The key interaction between the fragment and its binding site are

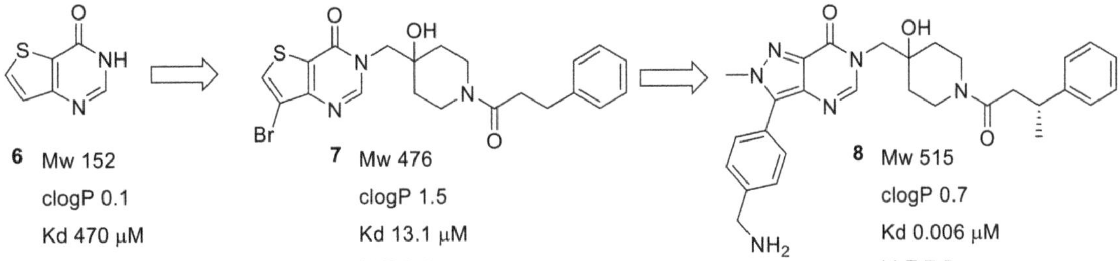

6 Mw 152 clogP 0.1 Kd 470 μM LLE 3.2

7 Mw 476 clogP 1.5 Kd 13.1 μM LLE 3.4

8 Mw 515 clogP 0.7 Kd 0.006 μM LLE 7.5

**Figure 19.9** Identification of fragment **6**, binding to an allosteric site on USP7, and its elaboration to compound **8**.

conserved during its elaboration into a lead, with the fragment presenting the 'minimal pharmacophore'.[116]

FBLG has played a key role in the discovery of allosteric inhibitors, which are often difficult to identify in HTS assays. To find inhibitors of the deubiquitinating cysteine protease USP7, a target involved in multiple oncogenic pathways, and where HTS has not yielded high-quality hits, scientists at Almac employed a fragment screen against the catalytic domain of USP7. Fragment **6** was identified from a library of 1946 molecules using surface plasmon resonance (Figure 19.9). Merging this fragment with the hydroxypiperidine part from a series of disclosed inhibitors led to compound 7 with measurable affinity for USP7, no redox liabilities and a good overall property profile. Further efforts culminated in compound **8**, a highly potent and selective USP7 inhibitor. These inhibitors bind to a previously undisclosed allosteric pocket on USP7, which is believed to prevent the catalytic activity by stabilising an inactive conformation.[117]

### *19.2.6.1 Covalent Fragments*

A recent noteworthy addition is the screening of covalent fragments to enable lead generation.[118–120] The renewed interest in covalent approaches to drug discovery, based on the approval of covalent kinase inhibitors such as Osimertinib or Ibrutinib,[121,122] has also led to applications of this approach in fragment-based drug discovery. While the approved drugs mentioned above, which target a reactive cysteine in the active site of the kinase, were rationally designed from a non-covalent binder, covalent fragments can be screened to identify new binding sites, or ligandable hotspots, which can subsequently be used as starting points for leads or tool compounds.[123] Advances in mass spectrometry and proteomics have allowed screening libraries of covalent fragments against whole cells to map the reactivity of all of its proteins, enabling the discovery and validation of novel targets.[119,124] Cysteine has been the target of most of the screening approaches, but progress has been made in addressing other potentially reactive amino acids such as lysine.[125] Principles and considerations in the design of electrophilic fragment libraries have been extensively reviewed.[126,127] An excellent example is the discovery of AMG-510, a covalent inhibitor of mutated KRAS(G12C) shown in Figure 19.10. Mutations in the RAS family are found in a variety of human cancers, but

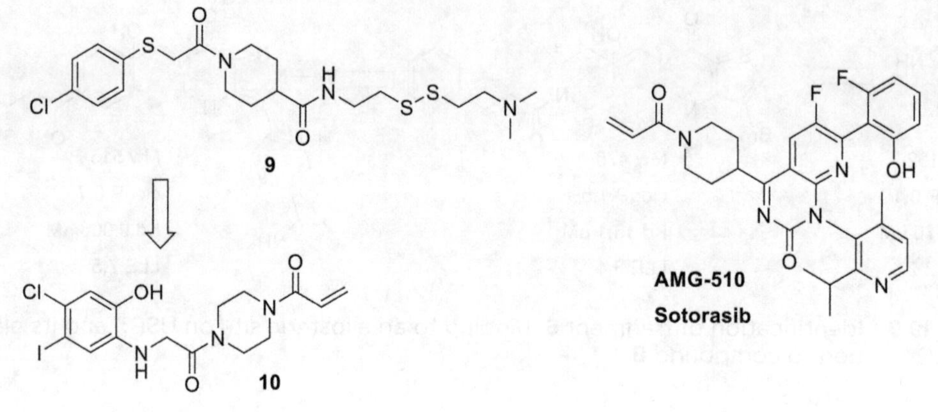

**Figure 19.10** Fragment-based KRAS(G12C) binders **9** and **10** and the approved covalent inhibitor AMG-510.

the small GTPases were considered undruggable due to the high affinity for its substrate GTP and the absence of other druggable pockets. Screening a small set of covalent fragments against mutated KRAS(G12C), revealed the formation of a new allosteric pocket upon irreversible binding of compound **9** to the mutated cysteine, as shown by an X-ray structure. The structural information was used to develop the covalent acrylamide-based inhibitor **10**, which inhibited RAS function in lung cancer cells.[128] This work has inspired several groups to start their own drug discovery programs. As a result, AMG-510 or Sotorasib was the first drug to be approved in 2021 for the treatment of KRAS(G12C)-mutated non-small cell lung cancer.[129]

### 19.2.7 Phenotypic Drug Discovery

In contrast to the target-based approaches described above, phenotypic drug discovery (PDD) approaches are target- and often mechanism-agnostic. Prior to the shift to target-based approaches, made possible by the progress in molecular biology, compounds were evaluated empirically in either cell or *in vivo* models believed to be linked to a certain disease.[130] Phenotypic screening approaches have led to the discovery of a variety of marketed drugs, for example Omeprazole for the treatment of gastroesophageal reflux disease,[131] Daclatasvir for chronic hepatitis C,[132] Ivacaftor for the treatment of cystic fibrosis[133] and more recently Risdiplam for the treatment of SMA[55] (see Figure 19.3).[56] Although PDD has never been completely abandoned, the risks and difficulties associated with it have led to the dominance of target-based approaches, but the realisation that diseases with complex underlying biology and limited mechanistic understanding, such as autoimmune or neurogenerative diseases, are difficult to address by a target-centric approach has brought PDD back into focus.[134,135] PDD promises to provide novel targets and/or novel mechanisms for these diseases, which are difficult to predict based on current knowledge, with the potential to lead to first in class drugs.[54] Technological advances in cell generation, imaging technology and bioinformatics have also greatly contributed to the resurgence of PDD.[136,137]

Despite these advances, the complexity of the screening systems, coupled with challenges in hit validation and target identification, make PDD a time-consuming and complex activity, requiring more up-front resources.[54,136,138] Compound libraries are typically screened in cell or *in vivo* systems believed to be of physiological relevance, evaluating physiological, morphological or pathway read-outs. Whole organisms, such as zebrafish, or specific states of parasites have been employed, but the use of cell-based systems is more common. Different from the less complex reporter cell lines typically used for higher throughput in project screening cascades, patient-derived cells, induced pluripotent stem cells, or 3D organoids, represent physiologically more relevant screening systems. However, their complexity can make it difficult to develop them into a robust and reliable assay system, fit for the screening of a larger number of compounds. Frequently, a compromise solution is used, where a subset of the compound collections, normally with annotated activities, can be screened. Whatever the chosen disease model, it was highlighted by Moffat that the endpoint of the assay system needs to be translatable to the clinic to make PDD a success.[54]

As for every hit identification campaign, but even more so for PDD, orthogonal read-outs, which can establish the validity of the hits are of prime importance. Hit triaging is even more complex for an unknown MoA. Apart from the false positives interfering with the assay technology, here compounds might produce a positive signal acting by an undesired MoA, for example cell toxicity. Several methods have been developed to facilitate hit triaging and have been reviewed recently.[138] Three key features for a successful PDD screening assay have been defined:

1. A relevant disease model.
2. Stimuli which produce a disease-associated response.
3. Read-outs reflecting the functional consequence of the disease.[138]

In the same review, the authors also advise against hit triaging based on structural attractiveness, as is often the case for target-centric approaches. All active compounds should be processed through the entire screening cascade to understand if they act through a potentially interesting MoA. Otherwise novel targets or interesting MoAs might be missed. An example is the discovery of Fingolimod, a first in class sphingosine 1-phosphate receptor (S1P) modulator, approved for the treatment of multiple sclerosis. It was derived from the fungal metabolite Myriocin, which based on its structural features would have been discarded in a normal hit triaging exercise (Figure 19.11A).[139]

The discovery of a small molecule inhibiting the production of proprotein convertase subtilisin/kexin type 9 (PCSK9), a protein that downregulates low-density lipoprotein receptor, is another illuminating example of uncovering novel biology. It is also a good example of how to run a high-throughput cellular screen of about 2.5 million compounds and identify a compound with borderline activity.[10] A phenotypic screen in CHO-K1 cells expressing a labelled form of PCSK9 identified R-IMMP as a cell-permeable compound which inhibited secretion of PCSK9 into the cell medium. Its $IC_{50}$ of 4.8 μM is close to the cut-off of the screening assay, and also of the follow-up assay. Thorough investigations into the MoA demonstrated that R-IMMP caused transcript-dependent inhibition of PCSK9 translation, and not decreased transcription (Figure 19.11B).

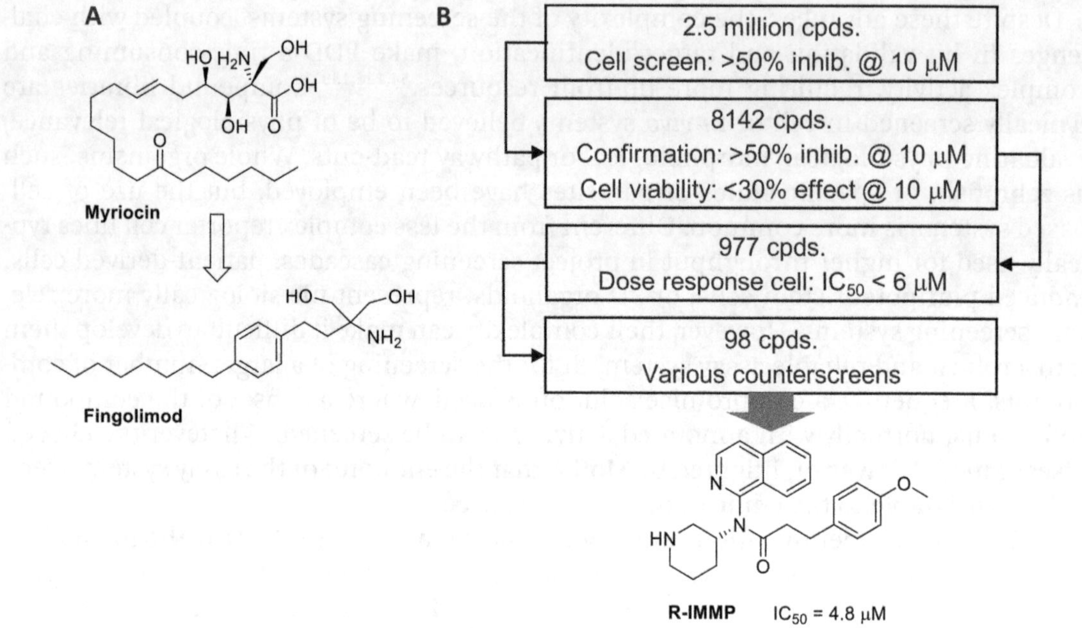


**Figure 19.11** (A) Structure of Fingolimod, an antagonist of the S1P receptor and the natural product Myriocin. (B) Schematic screening cascade for a phenotypic screen for the discovery of PCSK9 secretagogues and structure of hit R-IMMP.

Identification of the target, or the mechanism of action is not strictly required for further progression of the chemical equity, but is advantageous. It not only simplifies the registration of the potential drug, but also makes follow-up and further development of the hit series easier. Optimisation of hits based only on the phenotypic assay can be challenging endeavour. Distinct hit series might engage with different targets to modulate the same phenotype. Differences in cell permeability, solubility and target engagement of analogues can also make it difficult to derive well-defined structure–activity relationships and progress the series. Consequently, target deconvolution has a central role in PDD. Chemo-proteomic profiling or 'pull-down' experiments, which involves immobilisation of the hit compound on solid support *via* a linker and exposing it to cell lysates, has been widely used. Photoaffinity probes which react with the target have also been used, as well as the cellular thermal shift assay (CETSA).[140] The use of annotated libraries mentioned above helps in this respect, and might lead the project back to a target-centric approach.[136]

Phenotypic screening had a big role in the discovery of molecular glues, such as Lenalidomide or Pomalidomide, which after their discovery were developed without knowing the molecular target (Figure 19.12).[141] These imides bind to the E3 ubiquitin ligase cereblon and the complex with this newly formed interface can recruit novel substrates to the E3-ligase, which are ubiquitinated and degraded by the proteasome. A recent example of a successful screen for a molecular glue for the treatment of acute myeloid leukemia (AML) was reported by scientists at Biogen. They conducted a phenotypic screen of their cereblon modulator library against a panel of cell lines representing

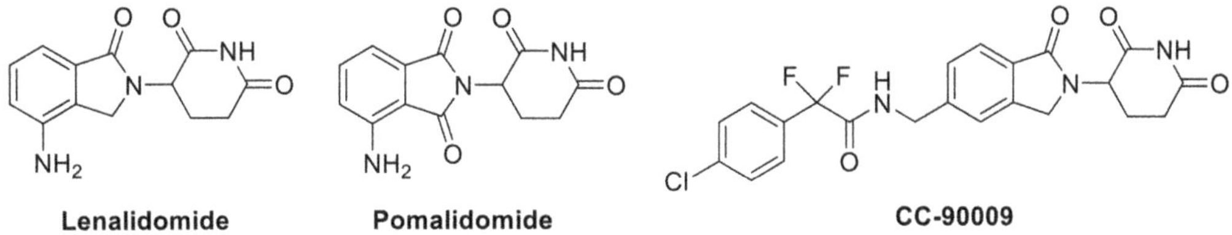


**Figure 19.12** Structures of molecular glues Lenalidomide and Pomalidomide, two approved drugs, and the novel clinical candidate CC-9009.

several genetic mutations characteristic for AML. This identified the clinical candidate CC-90009, which presents a different profile with respect to Lenalidomide or Pomalidomide, since it degrades the protein G1 to S phase transition 1 (GSPT1).[142]

## 19.2.8 Integrated Lead Generation Approaches

There are many examples of a single lead generation tactic being applied to great effect in a project scenario; however, many organisations now recognise the value of combining multiple approaches together. This has been described in a detailed review from GSK.[47] Different techniques may preference the identification of different types of hits or simply offer a back-up strategy to give different chemical series in case one fails. A popular strategy is to run a rapid hit finding approach at the start of the project once a small amount of protein is available, usually through virtual screening or affinity-based methods. Often some initial chemical matter can be identified to start a hit to lead campaign or at least be valuable in validating the screening cascade. Subsequently, this can be followed by a more comprehensive approach such as DEL or HTS. Fragment campaigns will complement any other hit finding approach and will almost always add value to an existing project. Chung *et al.* at GSK show the power of this approach in their optimisation of BET Bromodomain inhibitors.[143] Starting from a well-known benzodiazepine analogue **12**, originating from a phenotypic screen, they identified the critical acetyl lysine mimic from a crystal structure (Figure 19.13A). Based on this information, a fragment set enriched for potential acetyl lysine mimetics was screened. From this they identified multiple fragments, examples are compounds **13–16**, which were shown to bind to the acetyl lysine pocket by X-ray crystallography (Figure 19.13B).

Subsequent publications detail how this wealth of information was applied for lead generation. In one example, the weakly active isoxazole **13** was converted into lead **17** employing structure-based design (Figure 19.13C).[144] In the other example, the pyrimidone fragment **14** was used to substitute the metabolically labile phenol portion in compound **18**, previously identified from a DEL screen looking for novel BET inhibitors. Optimisation led to I-BET469, which possessed favourable pharmacokinetic properties, and was active in an *in vivo* model of inflammation (Figure 19.13D).[145]

In many organisations, it has become good practice to run a fragment screen alongside any structurally enabled project. The investment of time and effort is minimal, and the results are usually of benefit to the project. Knowledge-based approaches are also usually enriched with some *de novo* hit finding that offers a project team an additional,

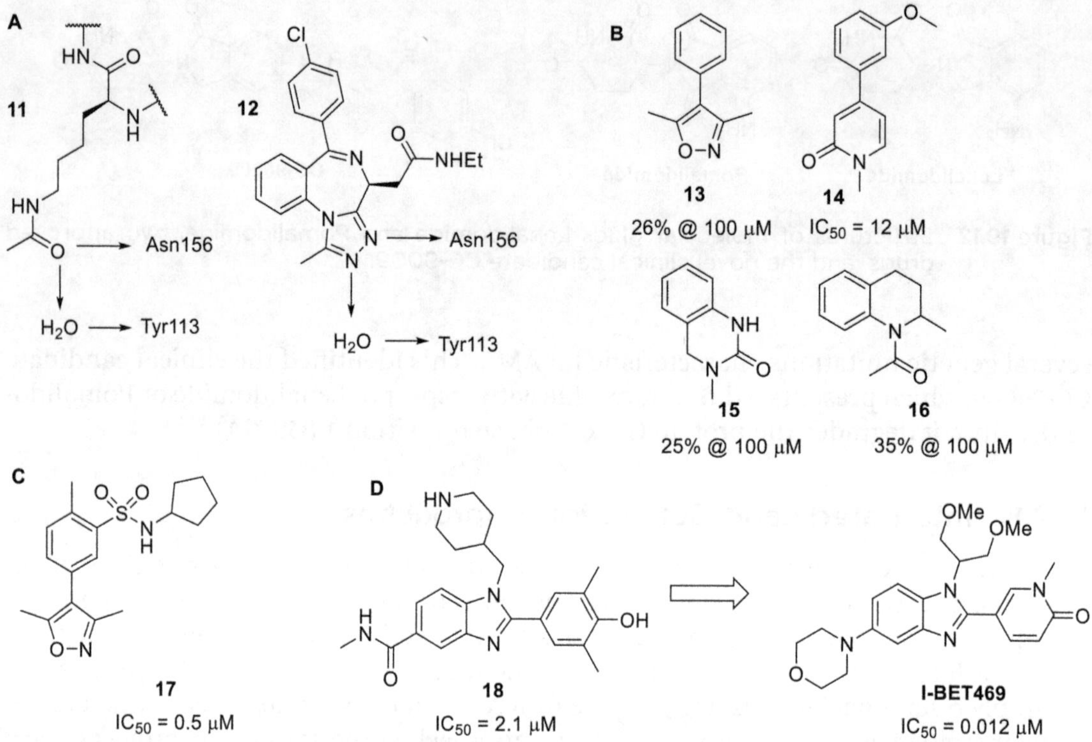


**Figure 19.13** (A) Schematic view of the interaction of acetylated Lys and **12** in the acetyl lysine pocket of BET proteins. (B) Fragments identified from a focussed screen. (C) Conversion of fragment **13** to lead **17**. (D) Use of fragment **14** for discovery of I-BET469.

novel structural motif that can either be integrated into the lead series during hit to lead or used as a back-up.

Thinking strategically about the risks in a project's primary hit finding approach will give an insight into the best tactics to mitigate those risks. A project rapidly advancing a single knowledge-based series would be well advised to have a backup DEL or HTS screen running along behind. And a project with a DEL output that may be slightly larger and more lipophilic than desired should look to a fragment campaign for supplementary chemotypes.

## 19.3 Hit to Lead

In the hit to lead (HtL) phase a thorough investigation of the validated hits or hit series will take place. The initial hit profiling is frequently done during the hit validation phase, and in companies with annotated screening collections, properties such as solubility and lipophilicity, as well as metabolic stability will already be known. Also similar compounds or near neighbours will have been tested during the hit validation stage. Since it is rare that hit series, coming directly out of the screen, fulfil the requirements of the lead target profile, optimisation by medicinal chemists will be needed. A more in-depth investigation of SAR is necessary to provide an understanding which motifs contribute to the observed activity, particularly for singletons or clusters containing only a few analogues. This is important for novel targets where no structural information of the binding mode is available. In addition, optimisation of potency, physicochemical and pharmacokinetic properties, as well as an investigation into off-target and safety liabilities, will take place. This effort is conceptually not different from work carried out during a lead optimisation campaign, but instead of improving a single molecule or series, the goal here is to evaluate several series in parallel and determine their strength and weaknesses. To do this in an efficient manner, parallel chemistry or library approaches are preferred at this stage, meaning that a synthetically challenging series might be down-prioritised, if more tractable options are available.

Integration of the SAR from integrated hit identification campaigns with several parallel tracks can lead to the design of novel hit series, as described above. To do this efficiently, a decision needs to be taken on which hit series should be included for further evaluation, which depends on the available resources, the synthetic accessibility, and also the quality and diversity of the starting points. A screening cascade with sufficient throughput needs to be available to enable an efficient design–make–test–analyse cycle.[146] It will not be too dissimilar to the one used during hit validation, but will be amplified with more secondary or counter screening assays and *in vivo* studies to determine pharmacokinetics and pharmacodynamics.

Automated workflows for physicochemical and metabolic properties have been implemented in most pharmaceutical companies to guarantee a rapid turnover of data.[147] It is also expected that automated screening and synthesis platforms will help in the efficient preparation and evaluation of hits.[148]

The overall goal of the effort is to deliver one, or better several, structurally diverse hit series with the following attributes:

- The SAR should not be driven by lipophilicity and should not be flat, or in other words, structural changes should have a notable impact on the activity of the molecule.
- The series should possess the required properties to enable pharmacokinetic and pharmacodynamic evaluation in pre-clinical models, which in a project aimed at oral administration are sufficient metabolic stability and oral bioavailability.
- Off-target and safety liabilities have been identified.
- The series is patentable.
- A plan for how the key liabilities might be addressed during the lead optimisation stage.

In the following we will present four case studies, which led to approved drugs or advanced clinical candidates and highlight some of the challenges that were encountered from the hit through the optimisation process.

The discovery of PT2385, an inhibitor of the transcription factor hypoxia-inducible factor-2α (HIF 2α), a key oncogenic driver in clear cell renal cell carcinoma (ccRCC), relied on prior knowledge of the binding mode of **19**. It binds in a hydrophobic cavity and blocks the function of HIF-2α. Structure-based design led to lead compound **20**, where several problematic features of **19**, such as the nitro group, the aniline linkage and the oxadiazole, were removed (Figure 19.14). The benzyl alcohol provided a boost in affinity and improved functional activity. Conformational restriction of the crucial hydroxyl moiety provided PT2385, which demonstrated proof of concept in patients with advanced ccRCC.[149] However, extensive metabolism resulted in poor pharmacokinetics and prevented its further advancement. This was addressed in the more potent back-up compound PT2977 (Belzutifan), which received FDA approval in 2021 for the treatment of certain kidney cancers.[150]

The discovery of a selective inhibitor of the TYK2 kinase BMS-986165 (Deucravacinitib), currently in phase 3 clinical trials for the treatment of psoriatic arthritis, is a good example for an HTS-derived lead generation programme showing that several hit series are an asset for successful project progression.

Several small molecule inhibitors of the Janus family of kinases (JAK), which are critical mediators of inflammation, have been approved for oncology indications. Achieving selectivity between the closely related family members JAK1-3 and TYK2 has been challenging, due to the high sequence homology of their catalytic domains. The lack of selectivity has led to a narrow therapeutic index. Targeting the pseudo-kinase domain of TYK2 was seen as a way to achieve high subtype selectivity and a greater therapeutic index.

An HTS campaign using a cellular reporter assay identified the imidazo[1,2-*b*]pyridazine **21** which could be optimised further to compound **22**, showing good functional potency and excellent kinase selectivity (Figure 19.15). Unfortunately, **22** exhibited poor metabolic stability and was a potent inhibitor of phosphodiesterase 4 (PDE4). A back-up programme looking for novel scaffolds identified nicotine amide **23**. This compound showed poor selectivity against the kinase domains of the other members of the JAK family and also against other members of the kinome, but was inactive against PDE4 and metabolically stable. The selectivity issue was solved by converting the amide to a methylamide. Deuteration was needed for metabolic stability. Further optimisation gave the highly selective lead **24**, which showed efficacy in an *in vivo* colitis model,[151] and led eventually to BMS-986165, which is a potent allosteric inhibitor of TYK2, with very high isoform and kinome selectivity. It is efficacious in several murine models of autoimmune disease, and was progressed as the first pseudokinase-directed inhibitor into clinical development as an oral treatment for autoimmune diseases.[152]

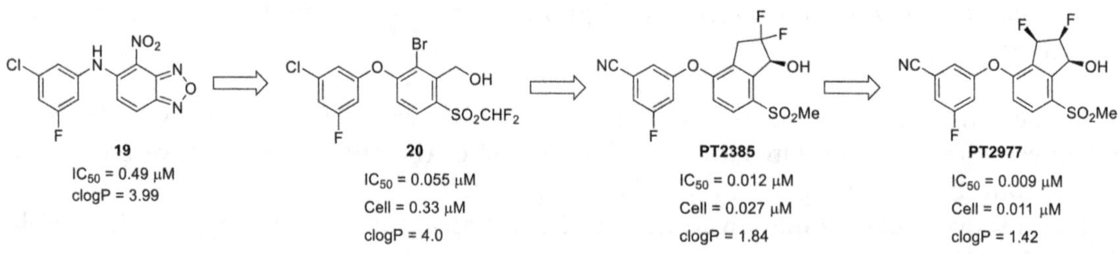


**Figure 19.14** The discovery of the HIF-2α inhibitors PT2385 and PT2977 from benzoxadiazole **19**.

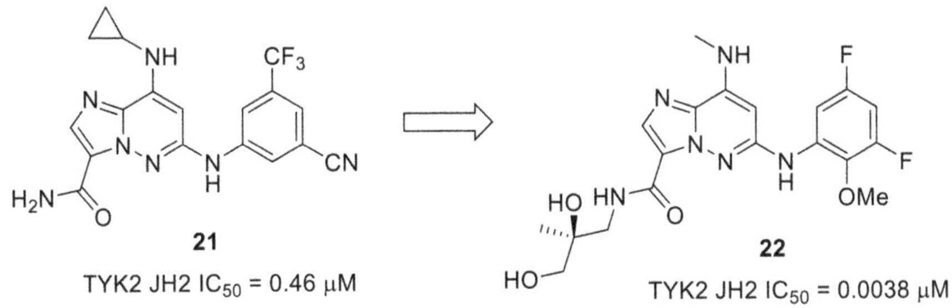

**21**
TYK2 JH2 $IC_{50}$ = 0.46 μM

**22**
TYK2 JH2 $IC_{50}$ = 0.0038 μM
cellular IFNα $IC_{50}$ = 0.16 μM

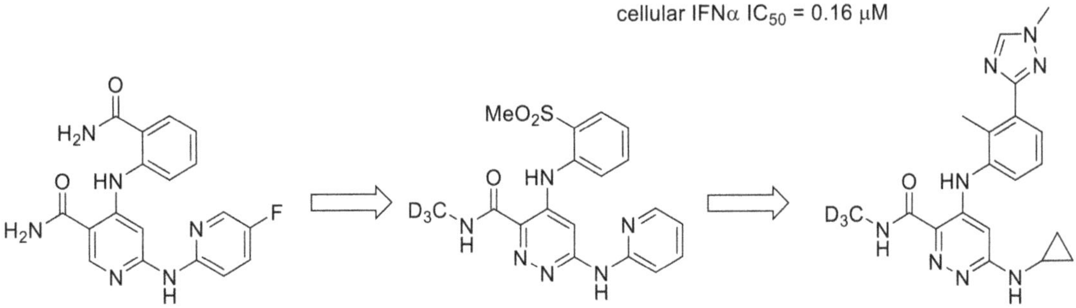

**23**
TYK2 JH2 $IC_{50}$ = 0.007 μM
cellular IFNα $IC_{50}$ = 0.37 μM

**24**
TYK2 JH2 $IC_{50}$ = 0.0005 μM
cellular IFNα $IC_{50}$ = 0.03 μM
human whole blood = 0.13 μM

**BMS-986165**
TYK2 JH2 $IC_{50}$ = 0.0002 μM
cellular IFNα $IC_{50}$ = 0.005 μM
human whole blood = 0.013 μM

**Figure 19.15** Development of an allosteric selective TYK2 inhibitor BMS-986165.

The discovery of PF-06650833, an inhibitor of Interleukin-1 receptor associated kinase 4 (IRAK-4), which is currently in phase 2 clinical trials for the treatment of rheumatoid arthritis, demonstrates some of the key features of a successful FBLG campaign.[153]

Screening of the Pfizer fragment collection against the kinase domain of IRAK4 using two assays, an NMR saturation transfer difference (STD) and in parallel a biochemical assay, identified several hits with dual activity. The activity was further confirmed in a functional NMR assay, measuring the conversion of ATP to ADP. Finally, modelling of the fragments into the ATP binding pocket of IRAK4 was used to identify potential hinge binding fragments, which were prioritised for co-crystallisation with the IRAK4 kinase domain. Carboxamide **25** emerged as a viable starting point, due to encouraging activity in an IRAK4 enzyme assay and good ligand efficiency (Figure 19.16). Based on the X-ray co-crystal structure, fragment **25** was grown into naphthalene **26**, which achieved nearly three orders of magnitude gain in potency with LE and LLE values comparable to **25**. For the further optimisation, care was taken to increase potency, while maintaining good ligand efficiency, by exploiting the shape of the ATP binding site with $sp^3$-rich fragments. This led to the quinoline **27**, with a more favourable LLE value compared to naphthalene **26**. Optimisation of cell potency and ADMET properties eventually led to the clinical candidate PF-06650833.

The discovery of Daclatasvir, a first in class orally bioavailable inhibitor of the hepatitis C virus (HCV) NS5A replication complex, highlights the importance of phenotypic

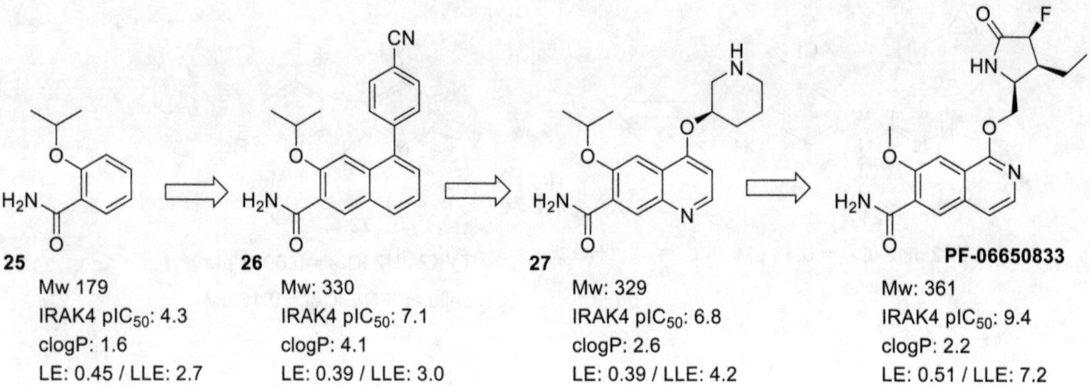


**Figure 19.16** Development of fragment hit **25** to lead **27** and clinical candidate PF-06650833.

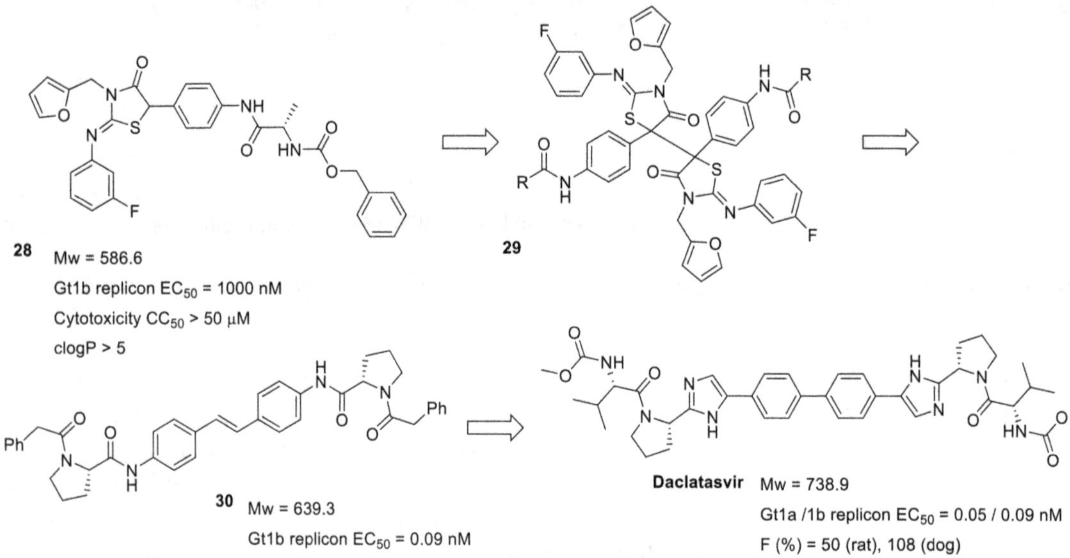


**Figure 19.17** Discovery of Daclatasvir from hit **28**, identified in a phenotypic screen.

screening for the discovery of novel targets and unexpected MoAs. It also showcases the development of a so-called beyond rule of 5 compound (Figure 19.17). A phenotypic screen in a cell assay using subgenomic constructs of HCV (HCV replicon) identified hydantoin **28**, a compound usually labelled as a frequent hitter, but it showed modest potency on genotype 1b replicon, without being cytotoxic. Selection of resistant mutants is an established way to identify the target in antiviral or antibacterial phenotypic screens. Here, resistant selection with **28** and a more potent derivative showed that the compounds acted through the viral NS5A protein, which has no ascribed enzymatic activity. During the optimisation efforts it became apparent that the hydantoin scaffold was unstable in both DMSO solution and in the medium of the cell assay. Eventually it was discovered that dimer **29** was responsible for the observed activity. Elimination of the hydantoin moiety led eventually to stilbene **30**, which displayed picomolar replicon activity, and from there to Daclatasvir, a pan-genotype inhibitor of HCV replication. It is used in combination with either inhibitors of the viral NS3 protease or NS5B polymerase to provide a cure for HCV infections.[132]

## 19.4 Conclusion

Lead generation is a critical phase of the drug discovery process and will have a profound impact on the time and likely success of the ensuing drug discovery project and resulting clinical candidates. A well-executed lead generation phase will result in multiple series of lead molecules that afford a choice of molecular scaffold and chemotype that can be optimised into a drug molecule. There are multiple hit finding approaches that can be employed, and the strategy and tactics will depend on the target and the capabilities and resources available. It is often beneficial to employ multiple approaches in parallel, however the temptation to 'throw the kitchen sink' at every target should be avoided. It is both costly and can result in long delays at the start of the project. With modern computational techniques, applications of virtual screening, *de novo* design coupled with well-judged use of experimental techniques can rapidly identify a good range of novel starting points for the majority of drug discovery projects.

## 19.5 Hints and Tips

- Defining an appropriate candidate drug profile is an important step to start lead generation. It will provide clarity on the modality, the MoA and provide a line of sight for the whole drug discovery process.
- Irrespective of pursuing a target-centric or a phenotypic approach, the establishment of biological assays of high quality and relevance to the target or phenotype under investigation is of critical importance for the success of any LG campaign.
- While success can be achieved using a single hit finding method, it is more common to pursue an integrated strategy, combining two or more approaches which complement each other. Thinking strategically about the risks in a project's primary hit finding approach will give an insight into the best tactics to mitigate those risks.
- The separation of true actives from compounds working by undesired mechanisms requires a combination of cheminformatics tools, a screening cascade with relevant assays and appropriate throughput and medicinal chemistry expertise in evaluating the hit series.
- Low molecular weight, low lipophilicity lead-like compounds make the best starting points for drug discovery.
- It is important to focus on the overall goal of a lead generation campaign, which is to deliver one or several structurally diverse series of high quality, which enable testing of the project hypothesis in pre-clinical models.

## Key References

Articles on lead-likeness and molecular complexity are always worth a read


- S. J. Teague, A. M. Davis, P. D. Leeson and T. Oprea, *Angew. Chem. Int. Ed.*, 1999, **38**, 3743–374.
- T. I. Oprea, A. M. Davis, S. J. Teague and P. D. Leeson, *J. Chem. Inf. Comput. Sci.*, 2001, **41**, 1308–1315.
- M. M. Hann, A. R. Leach and G. Harper, *J. Chem. Inf. Comput. Sci.*, 2001, **41**, 856–864.
- M. M. Hann, *MedChemComm*, 2011, 2, 349–355.
- C. P. Tinworth and R. J. Young, *J. Med. Chem.*, 2020, **63**, 10091–10108.


Reviews on LG strategies and tactics


- K. H. Bleicher, H.-J. Boehm, K. Mueller and A. I. Alanine, *Nat. Rev. Drug Discovery*, 2003, **2**, 369–378.
- P. Ettmayer, R. Schnitzer, A. Bergner and H. Nar, in *Comprehensive Medicinal Chemistry III*, ed. S. Chackalamannil, D. Rotella and S. E. Ward, Elsevier, Oxford, 2017, pp. 33–63.
- M. Leveridge, C.-W. Chung, J. W. Gross, C. B. Phelps and D. Green, *SLAS Discovery*, 2018, **23**, 881–897.


Impact of HTS and assay development on LG


- R. Macarron, M. Banks, D. Bojanic and *et al.*, *Nat. Rev. Drug Discovery*, 2011, **10**, 188–195.
- J. R. Born, V. K. Chenniappan, D. P. Davis, J. L. Dahlin, J. J. Marugan and S. Patnaik, *SLAS Discovery*, 2021, **26**, 1243–1255.


The success of FBLG is nicely described in these reviews


- A. Bancet, C. Raingeval, T. Lomberget, M. Le Borgne, J.-F. Guichou and I. Krimm, *J. Med. Chem.*, 2020, **63**, 11420–11435.
- I. J. P. de Esch, D. A. Erlanson, W. Jahnke, C. N. Johnson and L. Walsh, *J. Med. Chem.*, 2021.


A great article on ultra-large library docking


- J. Lyu, S. Wang, T. E. Balius, I. Singh, A. Levit, Y. S. Moroz, M. J. O'Meara, T. Che, E. Algaa, K. Tolmachova, A. A. Tolmachev, B. K. Shoichet, B. L. Roth and J. J. Irwin, *Nature*, 2019, **566**, 224–229.


Two key references for phenotypic screening


- F. Vincent, P. M. Loria, A. D. Weston, C. M. Steppan, R. Doyonnas, Y.-M. Wang, K. L. Rockwell and M.-C. Peakman, *Cell Chem. Biol.*, 2020, **27**, 1332–1346.
- J. G. Moffat, F. Vincent, J. A. Lee, J. Eder and M. Prunotto, *Nat. Rev. Drug Discovery*, 2017, **16**, 531–543.

## References


1. T. S. Maurer, D. Smith, K. Beaumont and L. Di, *J. Med. Chem.*, 2020, **63**, 6423–6435.
2. E. Perola, L. Herman and J. Weiss, *J. Chem. Inf. Model.*, 2012, **52**, 1027–1038.
3. D. Kozakov, D. R. Hall, R. L. Napoleon, C. Yueh, A. Whitty and S. Vajda, *J. Med. Chem.*, 2015, **58**, 9063–9088.
4. T. I. Oprea, C. G. Bologa, S. Brunak, A. Campbell, G. N. Gan, A. Gaulton, S. M. Gomez, R. Guha, A. Hersey, J. Holmes, A. Jadhav, L. J. Jensen, G. L. Johnson, A. Karlson, A. R. Leach, A. Ma'ayan, A. Malovannaya, S. Mani, S. L. Mathias, M. T. McManus, T. F. Meehan, C. von Mering, D. Muthas, D.-T. Nguyen, J. P. Overington, G. Papadatos, J. Qin, C. Reich, B. L. Roth, S. C. Schürer, A. Simeonov, L. A. Sklar, N. Southall, S. Tomita, I. Tudose, O. Ursu, D. Vidović, A. Waller, D. Westergaard, J. J. Yang and G. Zahoránszky-Köhalmi, *Nat. Rev. Drug Discovery*, 2018, **17**, 317–332.
5. E. Valeur, F. Narjes, C. Ottmann and A. T. Plowright, *Medchemcomm*, 2019, **10**, 1550–1568.
6. C. J. Gerry and S. L. Schreiber, *Nat. Chem. Biol.*, 2020, **16**, 369–378.
7. S. J. Hughes, A. Testa, N. Thompson and I. Churcher, *Drug Discovery Today*, 2021, 2889–2897.
8. M. Pettersson and C. M. Crews, *Drug Discovery Today: Technol.*, 2019, **31**, 15–27.
9. J. P. Falese, A. Donlic and A. E. Hargrove, *Chem. Soc. Rev.*, 2021, **50**, 2224–2243.
10. D. N. Petersen, J. Hawkins, W. Ruangsiriluk, K. A. Stevens, B. A. Maguire, T. N. O'Connell, B. N. Rocke, M. Boehm, R. B. Ruggeri, T. Rolph, D. Hepworth, P. M. Loria and P. A. Carpino, *Cell Chem. Biol.*, 2016, **23**, 1362–1371.
11. I. Alroy, W. Mansour, M. Klepfish and Y. Sheinberger, *Drug Discovery Today*, 2021, **26**, 786–793.
12. E. Valeur and P. Jimonet, *J. Med. Chem.*, 2018, **61**, 9004–9029.
13. M.-J. Blanco and K. M. Gardinier, *ACS Med. Chem. Lett.*, 2020, **11**, 228–231.
14. F. Bergström and B. Lindmark, *Drug Discovery Today*, 2019, **24**, 1237–1241.
15. D. Cook, D. Brown, R. Alexander, R. March, P. Morgan, G. Satterthwaite and M. N. Pangalos, *Nat. Rev. Drug Discovery*, 2014, **13**, 419–431.
16. J. Payandeh and M. Volgraf, *Nat. Rev. Drug Discovery*, 2021, **20**, 710–722.
17. N. C. Patel, *Bioorg. Med. Chem. Lett.*, 2020, **30**, 127503.
18. M. M. Hann, A. R. Leach and G. Harper, *J. Chem. Inf. Comput. Sci.*, 2001, **41**, 856–864.
19. T. I. Oprea, A. M. Davis, S. J. Teague and P. D. Leeson, *J. Chem. Inf. Comput. Sci.*, 2001, **41**, 1308–1315.
20. S. J. Teague, A. M. Davis, P. D. Leeson and T. Oprea, *Angew. Chem., Int. Ed.*, 1999, **38**, 3743–3748.
21. I. Kola and J. Landis, *Nat. Rev. Drug Discovery*, 2004, **3**, 711–716.
22. C. P. Tinworth and R. J. Young, *J. Med. Chem.*, 2020, **63**, 10091–10108.
23. P. D. Leeson, *Adv. Drug Delivery Rev.*, 2016, **101**, 22–33.
24. P. D. Leeson and B. Springthorpe, *Nat. Rev. Drug Discovery*, 2007, **6**, 881–890.
25. G. R. Bickerton, G. V. Paolini, J. Besnard, S. Muresan and A. L. Hopkins, *Nat. Chem.*, 2012, **4**, 90–98.
26. D. F. Veber, S. R. Johnson, H.-Y. Cheng, B. R. Smith, K. W. Ward and K. D. Kopple, *J. Med. Chem.*, 2002, **45**, 2615–2623.
27. E. Pasqua, N. Hamblin, C. Edwards, C. Baker-Glenn and C. Hurley, *Drug Discovery Today*, 2022, **27**, 134–150.
28. V. Poongavanam, B. C. Doak and J. Kihlberg, *Curr. Opin. Chem. Biol.*, 2018, **44**, 23–29.
29. S. D. Edmondson, B. Yang and C. Fallan, *Bioorg. Med. Chem. Lett.*, 2019, 1555–1564.
30. E. Perola, *J. Med. Chem.*, 2010, **53**, 2986–2997.
31. D. G. Brown and J. Bostrom, *J. Med. Chem.*, 2018, **61**, 9442–9468.
32. M. M. Hann, *MedChemComm*, 2011, **2**, 349–355.
33. A. L. Hopkins, G. M. Keserü, P. D. Leeson, D. C. Rees and C. H. Reynolds, *Nat. Rev. Drug Discovery*, 2014, **13**, 105–121.
34. M. D. Shultz, *Bioorg. Med. Chem. Lett.*, 2013, **23**, 5992–6000.
35. J. S. Scott and M. J. Waring, *Bioorg. Med. Chem.*, 2018, **26**, 3006–3015.
36. T. S. Maurer, M. Edwards, D. Hepworth, P. Verhoest and C. M. N. Allerton, *Drug Discovery Today*, 2021, **27**, 538–546.
37. J. Stefaniak and K. V. M. Huber, *ACS Med. Chem. Lett.*, 2020, **11**, 403–406.
38. T. B. Durham and M.-J. Blanco, *Bioorg. Med. Chem. Lett.*, 2015, **25**, 1004–1014.
39. M. E. Bunnage, A. M. Gilbert, L. H. Jones and E. C. Hett, *Nat. Chem. Biol.*, 2015, **11**, 368–372.
40. K. H. Bleicher, H.-J. Boehm, K. Mueller and A. I. Alanine, *Nat. Rev. Drug Discovery*, 2003, **2**, 369–378.
41. P. Ettmayer, R. Schnitzer, A. Bergner and H. Nar, in *Comprehensive Medicinal Chemistry III*, ed. S. Chackalamannil, D. Rotella and S. E. Ward, Elsevier, Oxford, 2017, pp. 33–63.
42. M. Furber, F. Narjes and J. Steele, in *The Handbook of Medicinal Chemistry : Principles and Practice*, ed. A. M. Davis and S. E. Ward, Royal Society of Chemistry, 2014, pp. 505–528.

43. J. Holenz and D. G. Brown, in *Lead Generation*, 2016, pp. 13–34.
44. J. Drews, *Science*, 2000, **287**, 1960–1964.
45. J. R. Born, V. K. Chenniappan, D. P. Davis, J. L. Dahlin, J. J. Marugan and S. Patnaik, *SLAS Discovery*, 2021, **26**, 1243–1255.
46. J. Holenz and P. Stoy, *Bioorg. Med. Chem. Lett.*, 2018, **29**, 517–524.
47. M. Leveridge, C.-W. Chung, J. W. Gross, C. B. Phelps and D. Green, *SLAS Discovery*, 2018, **23**, 881–897.
48. R. Macarron, M. N. Banks, D. Bojanic, D. J. Burns, D. A. Cirovic, T. Garyantes, D. V. S. Green, R. P. Hertzberg, W. P. Janzen, J. W. Paslay, U. Schopfer and G. S. Sittampalam, *Nat. Rev. Drug Discovery*, 2011, **10**, 188–195.
49. A. Gironda-Martinez, E. J. Donckele, F. Samain and D. Neri, *ACS Pharmacol. Transl. Sci.*, 2021, **4**, 1265–1279.
50. R. A. Goodnow, C. E. Dumelin and A. D. Keefe, *Nat. Rev. Drug Discovery*, 2017, **16**, 131–147.
51. D. A. Erlanson, S. W. Fesik, R. E. Hubbard, W. Jahnke and H. Jhoti, *Nat. Rev. Drug Discovery*, 2016, **15**, 605–619.
52. X. C. Yan, J. M. Sanders, Y. D. Gao, M. Tudor, A. M. Haidle, D. J. Klein, A. Converso, C. A. Lesburg, Y. Zang and H. B. Wood, *J. Chem. Inf. Model.*, 2020, **60**, 4144–4152.
53. N. Aulner, A. Danckaert, J. Ihm, D. Shum and S. L. Shorte, *Trends Parasitol.*, 2019, **35**, 559–570.
54. J. G. Moffat, F. Vincent, J. A. Lee, J. Eder and M. Prunotto, *Nat. Rev. Drug Discovery*, 2017, **16**, 531–543.
55. H. Ratni, M. Ebeling, J. Baird, S. Bendels, J. Bylund, K. S. Chen, N. Denk, Z. Feng, L. Green, M. Guerard, P. Jablonski, B. Jacobsen, O. Khwaja, H. Kletzl, C.-P. Ko, S. Kustermann, A. Marquet, F. Metzger, B. Mueller, N. A. Naryshkin, S. V. Paushkin, E. Pinard, A. Poirier, M. Reutlinger, M. Weetall, A. Zeller, X. Zhao and L. Mueller, *J. Med. Chem.*, 2018, **61**, 6501–6517.
56. J. Eder, R. Sedrani and C. Wiesmann, *Nat. Rev. Drug Discovery*, 2014, **13**, 577–587.
57. M. J. Wildey, A. Haunso, M. Tudor, M. Webb and J. H. Connick, in *Annual Reports in Medicinal Chemistry*, ed. R. A. Goodnow, Academic Press, 2017, vol. 50, pp. 149–195.
58. A. Schuffenhauer, N. Schneider, S. Hintermann, D. Auld, J. Blank, S. Cotesta, C. Engeloch, N. Fechner, C. Gaul, J. Giovannoni, J. Jansen, J. Joslin, P. Krastel, E. Lounkine, J. Manchester, L. G. Monovich, A. P. Pelliccioli, M. Schwarze, M. D. Shultz, N. Stiefl and D. K. Baeschlin, *J. Med. Chem.*, 2020, **63**, 14425–14447.
59. S. Paricharak, I. J. AP, A. Bender and F. Nigsch, *ACS Chem. Biol.*, 2016, **11**, 1255–1264.
60. G. H. S. Dreiman, M. Bictash, P. V. Fish, L. Griffin and F. Svensson, *SLAS Discovery*, 2021, **26**, 257–262.
61. S. A. Busby, S. Carbonneau, J. Concannon, C. E. Dumelin, Y. Lee, S. Numao, N. Renaud, T. M. Smith and D. S. Auld, *ACS Chem. Biol.*, 2020, **15**, 2636–2648.
62. D. G. McLaren, V. Shah, T. Wisniewski, L. Ghislain, C. Liu, H. Zhang and S. A. Saldanha, *SLAS Discovery*, 2021, **26**, 168–191.
63. R. Prudent, D. A. Annis, P. J. Dandliker, J.-Y. Ortholand and D. Roche, *Nat. Rev. Chem.*, 2021, **5**, 62–71.
64. K. DeSantis, A. Reed, R. Rahhal and J. Reinking, *Nucl. Recept. Signaling*, 2012, **10**, nrs.10002.
65. J. Shaw, M. Leveridge, C. Norling, J. Karén, D. M. Molina, D. O'Neill, J. E. Dowling, P. Davey, S. Cowan, M. Dabrowski, M. Main and D. Gianni, *Sci. Rep.*, 2018, **8**, 163.
66. M. J. Henderson, M. A. Holbert, A. Simeonov and L. A. Kallal, *SLAS Discovery*, 2020, **25**, 137–147.
67. J. Simm, G. Klambauer, A. Arany, M. Steijaert, J. K. Wegner, E. Gustin, V. Chupakhin, Y. T. Chong, J. Vialard, P. Buijnsters, I. Velter, A. Vapirev, S. Singh, A. E. Carpenter, R. Wuyts, S. Hochreiter, Y. Moreau and H. Ceulemans, *Cell Chem. Biol.*, 2018, **25**, 611–618.e613.
68. S. N. Chandrasekaran, H. Ceulemans, J. D. Boyd and A. E. Carpenter, *Nat. Rev. Drug Discovery*, 2021, **20**, 145–159.
69. A. Karawajczyk, F. Giordanetto, J. Benningshof, D. Hamza, T. Kalliokoski, K. Pouwer, R. Morgentin, A. Nelson, G. Müller, A. Piechot and D. Tzalis, *Drug Discovery Today*, 2015, **20**, 1310–1316.
70. C. Boss, J. Hazemann, T. Kimmerlin, M. von Korff, U. Lüthi, O. Peter, T. Sander and R. Siegrist, *Chimia*, 2017, **71**, 667–677.
71. M. Follmann, H. Briem, A. Steinmeyer, A. Hillisch, M. H. Schmitt, H. Haning and H. Meier, *Drug Discovery Today*, 2019, **24**, 668–672.
72. D. E. Scott, A. R. Bayly, C. Abell and J. Skidmore, *Nat. Rev. Drug Discovery*, 2016, **15**, 533–550.
73. C. Bechtler and C. Lamers, *RSC Med. Chem.*, 2021, **12**, 1325–1351.
74. A. G. Atanasov, S. B. Zotchev, V. M. Dirsch, I. E. Orhan, M. Banach, J. M. Rollinger, D. Barreca, W. Weckwerth, R. Bauer, E. A. Bayer, M. Majeed, A. Bishayee, V. Bochkov, G. K. Bonn, N. Braidy, F. Bucar, A. Cifuentes, G. D'Onofrio, M. Bodkin, M. Diederich, A. T. Dinkova-Kostova, T. Efferth, K. El Bairi, N. Arkells, T.-P. Fan, B. L. Fiebich, M. Freissmuth, M. I. Georgiev, S. Gibbons, K. M. Godfrey, C. W. Gruber, J. Heer, L. A. Huber, E. Ibanez, A. Kijjoa, A. K. Kiss, A. Lu, F. A. Macias, M. J. S. Miller, A.

Mocan, R. Müller, F. Nicoletti, G. Perry, V. Pittalà, L. Rastrelli, M. Ristow, G. L. Russo, A. S. Silva, D. Schuster, H. Sheridan, K. Skalicka-Woźniak, L. Skaltsounis, E. Sobarzo-Sánchez, D. S. Bredt, H. Stuppner, A. Sureda, N. T. Tzvetkov, R. A. Vacca, B. B. Aggarwal, M. Battino, F. Giampieri, M. Wink, J.-L. Wolfender, J. Xiao, A. W. K. Yeung, G. Lizard, M. A. Popp, M. Heinrich, I. Berindan-Neagoe, M. Stadler, M. Daglia, R. Verpoorte, C. T. Supuran and T. the International Natural Product Sciences, *Nat. Rev. Drug Discovery*, 2021, **20**, 200–216.

75. M. M. Hann and T. I. Oprea, *Curr. Opin. Chem. Biol.*, 2004, **8**, 255–263.
76. L. David, J. Walsh, N. Sturm, I. Feierberg, J. W. M. Nissink, H. Chen, J. Bajorath and O. Engkvist, *ChemMedChem*, 2019, **14**, 1795–1802.
77. J. L. Dahlin, D. S. Auld, I. Rothenaigner, S. Haney, J. Z. Sexton, J. W. M. Nissink, J. Walsh, J. A. Lee, J. M. Strelow, F. S. Willard, L. Ferrins, J. B. Baell, M. A. Walters, B. K. Hua, K. Hadian and B. K. Wagner, *Cell Chem. Biol.*, 2021, P356–P370.
78. J. C. Hermann, Y. Chen, C. Wartchow, J. Menke, L. Gao, S. K. Gleason, N.-E. Haynes, N. Scott, A. Petersen, S. Gabriel, B. Vu, K. M. George, A. Narayanan, S. H. Li, H. Qian, N. Beatini, L. Niu and Q.-F. Gan, *ACS Med. Chem. Lett.*, 2013, **4**, 197–200.
79. B. C. Duffy, L. Zhu, H. Decornez and D. B. Kitchen, *Bioorg. Med. Chem.*, 2012, **20**, 5324–5342.
80. J. B. Baell and G. A. Holloway, *J. Med. Chem.*, 2010, **53**, 2719–2740.
81. J. W. M. Nissink and S. Blackburn, *Future Med. Chem.*, 2014, **6**, 1113–1126.
82. S. Brenner and R. A. Lerner, *Proc. Natl. Acad. Sci. U. S. A.*, 1992, **89**, 5381–5383.
83. V. B. K. Kunig, M. Potowski, M. Klika Skopic and A. Brunschweiger, *ChemMedChem*, 2021, **16**, 1048–1062.
84. C. A. Machutta, C. S. Kollmann, K. E. Lind, X. Bai, P. F. Chan, J. Huang, L. Ballell, S. Belyanskaya, G. S. Besra, D. Barros-Aguirre, R. H. Bates, P. A. Centrella, S. S. Chang, J. Chai, A. E. Choudhry, A. Coffin, C. P. Davie, H. Deng, J. Deng, Y. Ding, J. W. Dodson, D. T. Fosbenner, E. N. Gao, T. L. Graham, T. L. Graybill, K. Ingraham, W. P. Johnson, B. W. King, C. R. Kwiatkowski, J. Lelièvre, Y. Li, X. Liu, Q. Lu, R. Lehr, A. Mendoza-Losana, J. Martin, L. McCloskey, P. McCormick, H. P. O'Keefe, T. O'Keeffe, C. Pao, C. B. Phelps, H. Qi, K. Rafferty, G. S. Scavello, M. S. Steiginga, F. S. Sundersingh, S. M. Sweitzer, L. M. Szewczuk, A. Taylor, M. F. Toh, J. Wang, M. Wang, D. J. Wilkins, B. Xia, G. Yao, J. Zhang, J. Zhou, C. P. Donahue, J. A. Messer, D. Holmes, C. C. Arico-Muendel, A. J. Pope, J. W. Gross and G. Evindar, *Nat. Commun.*, 2017, **8**, 16081.
85. T. Kodadek, N. G. Paciaroni, M. Balzarini and P. Dickson, *Chem. Commun.*, 2019, **55**, 13330–13341.
86. Z. Wu, T. L. Graybill, X. Zeng, M. Platchek, J. Zhang, V. Q. Bodmer, D. D. Wisnoski, J. Deng, F. T. Coppo, G. Yao, A. Tamburino, G. Scavello, G. J. Franklin, S. Mataruse, K. L. Bedard, Y. Ding, J. Chai, J. Summerfield, P. A. Centrella, J. A. Messer, A. J. Pope and D. I. Israel, *ACS Comb. Sci.*, 2015, **17**, 722–731.
87. B. Cai, D. Kim, S. Akhand, Y. Sun, R. J. Cassell, A. Alpsoy, E. C. Dykhuizen, R. M. Van Rijn, M. K. Wendt and C. J. Krusemark, *J. Am. Chem. Soc.*, 2019, **141**, 17057–17061.
88. L. K. Petersen, A. B. Christensen, J. Andersen, C. G. Folkesson, O. Kristensen, C. Andersen, A. Alzu, F. A. Sløk, P. Blakskjær, D. Madsen, C. Azevedo, I. Micco and N. J. V. Hansen, *J. Am. Chem. Soc.*, 2021, **143**, 2751–2756.
89. J. S. Disch, J. M. Duffy, E. C. Y. Lee, D. Gikunju, B. Chan, B. Levin, M. I. Monteiro, S. A. Talcott, A. C. Lau, F. Zhou, A. Kozhushnyan, N. E. Westlund, P. B. Mullins, Y. Yu, M. von Rechenberg, J. Zhang, Y. A. Arnautova, Y. Liu, Y. Zhang, A. J. McRiner, A. D. Keefe, A. Kohlmann, M. A. Clark, J. W. Cuozzo, C. Huguet and S. Arora, *J. Med. Chem.*, 2021, **64**, 5049–5066.
90. Z. Fan, S. Zhao, T. Liu, P. X. Shen, Z. N. Cui, Z. Zhuang, Q. Shao, J. S. Chen, A. S. Ratnayake, M. E. Flanagan, D. K. Kolmel, D. W. Piotrowski, P. Richardson and J. Q. Yu, *Chem. Sci.*, 2020, **11**, 12282–12288.
91. Y. Zhang and M. A. Clark, *Bioorg. Med. Chem.*, 2021, **41**, 116189.
92. A. M. Wassermann, L. M. Camargo and D. S. Auld, *Front. Pharmacol.*, 2014, **5**, 164.
93. S. L. Posy, M. A. Hermsmeier, W. Vaccaro, K.-H. Ott, G. Todderud, J. S. Lippy, G. L. Trainor, D. A. Loughney and S. R. Johnson, *J. Med. Chem.*, 2011, **54**, 54–66.
94. S. D. Bembenek, G. Hirst and T. Mirzadegan, *J. Chem. Inf. Model.*, 2018, **58**, 1434–1440.
95. J. Boström, *ACS Med. Chem. Lett.*, 2012, **3**, 769–773.
96. C. Grebner, E. Malmerberg, A. Shewmaker, J. Batista, A. Nicholls and J. Sadowski, *J. Chem. Inf. Model.*, 2020, **60**, 4274–4282.
97. Q. Hu, Z. Peng, S. C. Sutton, J. Na, J. Kostrowicki, B. Yang, T. Thacher, X. Kong, S. Mattaparti, J. Z. Zhou, J. Gonzalez, M. Ramirez-Weinhouse and A. Kuki, *ACS Comb. Sci.*, 2012, **14**, 579–589.
98. L. Ruddigkeit, R. van Deursen, L. C. Blum and J. L. Reymond, *J. Chem. Inf. Model.*, 2012, **52**, 2864–2875.
99. R. S. Bohacek, C. McMartin and W. C. Guida, *Med. Res. Rev.*, 1996, **16**, 3–50.
100. A. Kumar and K. Y. J. Zhang, *Front. Chem.*, 2018, **6**, 315.

101. J. Lyu, S. Wang, T. E. Balius, I. Singh, A. Levit, Y. S. Moroz, M. J. O'Meara, T. Che, E. Algaa, K. Tolmachova, A. A. Tolmachev, B. K. Shoichet, B. L. Roth and J. J. Irwin, *Nature*, 2019, **566**, 224–229.
102. B. J. Bender, S. Gahbauer, A. Luttens, J. Lyu, C. M. Webb, R. M. Stein, E. A. Fink, T. E. Balius, J. Carlsson, J. J. Irwin and B. K. Shoichet, *Nat. Protoc.*, 2021, **16**, 4799–4832.
103. Y. Yang, K. Yao, M. P. Repasky, K. Leswing, R. Abel, B. K. Shoichet and S. V. Jerome, *J. Chem. Theory Comput.*, 2021, **17**, 7106–7119.
104. F. Fratev and S. Sirimulla, *Sci. Rep.*, 2019, **9**, 16829.
105. M. Imran, S. Waqar, K. Ogata, M. Ahmed, Z. Noreen, S. Javed, N. Bibi, H. Bokhari, A. Amjad and M. Muddassar, *RSC Adv.*, 2020, **10**, 16061–16070.
106. G. M. Keserű and M. M. Hann, *Future Med. Chem.*, 2017, **9**, 1457–1460.
107. I. J. P. de Esch, D. A. Erlanson, W. Jahnke, C. N. Johnson and L. Walsh, *J. Med. Chem.*, 2021, **65**, 84–99.
108. A. R. Leach and M. M. Hann, *Curr. Opin. Chem. Biol.*, 2011, **15**, 489–496.
109. R. F. Ludlow, M. L. Verdonk, H. K. Saini, I. J. Tickle and H. Jhoti, *Proc. Natl. Acad. Sci. U. S. A.*, 2015, **112**, 15910–15915.
110. A. Bancet, C. Raingeval, T. Lomberget, M. Le Borgne, J.-F. Guichou and I. Krimm, *J. Med. Chem.*, 2020, **63**, 11420–11435.
111. N. S. Troelsen, E. Shanina, D. Gonzalez-Romero, D. Danková, I. S. A. Jensen, K. J. Śniady, F. Nami, H. Zhang, C. Rademacher, A. Cuenda, C. H. Gotfredsen and M. H. Clausen, *Angew. Chem., Int. Ed.*, 2020, **59**, 2204–2210.
112. J. B. Jordan, D. A. Whittington, M. D. Bartberger, E. A. Sickmier, K. Chen, Y. Cheng and T. Judd, *J. Med. Chem.*, 2016, **59**, 3732–3749.
113. H. Zhou, H. Cao and J. Skolnick, *J. Chem. Inf. Model.*, 2021, **61**, 2074–2089.
114. Y. Yang, S. Zheng, S. Su, J. Xu and H. Chen, *Chem. Sci.*, 2020, **11**, 8312–8322.
115. H. Jhoti, G. Williams, D. C. Rees and C. W. Murray, *Nat. Rev. Drug Discovery*, 2013, **12**, 644.
116. G. Chessari, R. Grainger, R. S. Holvey, R. F. Ludlow, P. N. Mortenson and D. C. Rees, *Chem. Sci.*, 2021, 11976–11985.
117. G. Gavory, C. R. O'Dowd, M. D. Helm, J. Flasz, E. Arkoudis, A. Dossang, C. Hughes, E. Cassidy, K. McClelland, E. Odrzywol, N. Page, O. Barker, H. Miel and T. Harrison, *Nat. Chem. Biol.*, 2018, **14**, 118–125.
118. E. Resnick, A. Bradley, J. Gan, A. Douangamath, T. Krojer, R. Sethi, P. P. Geurink, A. Aimon, G. Amitai, D. Bellini, J. Bennett, M. Fairhead, O. Fedorov, R. Gabizon, J. Gan, J. Guo, A. Plotnikov, N. Reznik, G. F. Ruda, L. Díaz-Sáez, V. M. Straub, T. Szommer, S. Velupillai, D. Zaidman, Y. Zhang, A. R. Coker, C. G. Dowson, H. M. Barr, C. Wang, K. V. M. Huber, P. E. Brennan, H. Ovaa, F. von Delft and N. London, *J. Am. Chem. Soc.*, 2019, **141**, 8951–8968.
119. W. Lu, M. Kostic, T. Zhang, J. Che, M. P. Patricelli, L. H. Jones, E. T. Chouchani and N. S. Gray, *RSC Chem. Biol.*, 2021, **2**, 354–367.
120. A. Keeley, L. Petri, P. Ábrányi-Balogh and G. M. Keserű, *Drug Discovery Today*, 2020, **25**, 983–996.
121. A. Abdeldayem, Y. S. Raouf, S. N. Constantinescu, R. Moriggl and P. T. Gunning, *Chem. Soc. Rev.*, 2020, **49**, 2617–2687.
122. F. Sutanto, M. Konstantinidou and A. Dömling, *RSC Med. Chem.*, 2020, **11**, 876–884.
123. A. M. Roberts, C. C. Ward and D. K. Nomura, *Curr. Opin. Biotechnol.*, 2017, **43**, 25–33.
124. C. G. Parker, A. Galmozzi, Y. Wang, B. E. Correia, K. Sasaki, C. M. Joslyn, A. S. Kim, C. L. Cavallaro, R. M. Lawrence, S. R. Johnson, I. Narvaiza, E. Saez and B. F. Cravatt, *Cell*, 2017, **168**, 527–541 e529.
125. M. E. Abbasov, M. E. Kavanagh, T.-A. Ichu, M. R. Lazear, Y. Tao, V. M. Crowley, C. W. am Ende, S. M. Hacker, J. Ho, M. M. Dix, R. Suciu, M. M. Hayward, L. L. Kiessling and B. F. Cravatt, *Nat. Chem.*, 2021, 1081–1092.
126. N. S. Troelsen and M. H. Clausen, *Chem. - Eur. J.*, 2020, **26**, 11391–11403.
127. T. Zhang, J. M. Hatcher, M. Teng, N. S. Gray and M. Kostic, *Cell Chem. Biol.*, 2019, **26**, 1486–1500.
128. J. M. Ostrem, U. Peters, M. L. Sos, J. A. Wells and K. M. Shokat, *Nature*, 2013, **503**, 548–551.
129. B. A. Lanman, J. R. Allen, J. G. Allen, A. K. Amegadzie, K. S. Ashton, S. K. Booker, J. J. Chen, N. Chen, M. J. Frohn, G. Goodman, D. J. Kopecky, L. Liu, P. Lopez, J. D. Low, V. Ma, A. E. Minatti, T. T. Nguyen, N. Nishimura, A. J. Pickrell, A. B. Reed, Y. Shin, A. C. Siegmund, N. A. Tamayo, C. M. Tegley, M. C. Walton, H.-L. Wang, R. P. Wurz, M. Xue, K. C. Yang, P. Achanta, M. D. Bartberger, J. Canon, L. S. Hollis, J. D. McCarter, C. Mohr, K. Rex, A. Y. Saiki, T. San Miguel, L. P. Volak, K. H. Wang, D. A. Whittington, S. G. Zech, J. R. Lipford and V. J. Cee, *J. Med. Chem.*, 2020, **63**, 52–65.
130. D. C. Swinney, in *Phenotypic Drug Discovery*, The Royal Society of Chemistry, 2021, pp. 1–19.
131. L. Olbe, E. Carlsson and P. Lindberg, *Nat. Rev. Drug Discovery*, 2003, **2**, 132–139.
132. M. Belema and N. A. Meanwell, *J. Med. Chem.*, 2014, **57**, 5057–5071.

133. F. Van Goor, S. Hadida, P. D. J. Grootenhuis, B. Burton, D. Cao, T. Neuberger, A. Turnbull, A. Singh, J. Joubran, A. Hazlewood, J. Zhou, J. McCartney, V. Arumugam, C. Decker, J. Yang, C. Young, E. R. Olson, J. J. Wine, R. A. Frizzell, M. Ashlock and P. Negulescu, *Proc. Natl. Acad. Sci. U. S. A.*, 2009, **106**, 18825–18830.
134. W. E. Childers, K. M. Elokely and M. Abou-Gharbia, *ACS Med. Chem. Lett.*, 2020, **11**, 1820–1828.
135. D. G. Brown and H. J. Wobst, *J. Med. Chem.*, 2020, **63**, 1823–1840.
136. M. Jörg and K. S. Madden, *RSC Med. Chem.*, 2021, **12**, 646–665.
137. S. Malandraki-Miller and P. R. Riley, *Drug Discovery Today*, 2021, 887–901.
138. F. Vincent, P. M. Loria, A. D. Weston, C. M. Steppan, R. Doyonnas, Y.-M. Wang, K. L. Rockwell and M.-C. Peakman, *Cell Chem. Biol.*, 2020, **27**, 1332–1346.
139. V. Brinkmann, A. Billich, T. Baumruker, P. Heining, R. Schmouder, G. Francis, S. Aradhye and P. Burtin, *Nat. Rev. Drug Discovery*, 2010, **9**, 883–897.
140. T. Friman, *Bioorg. Med. Chem.*, 2020, **28**, 115174.
141. P. P. Chamberlain, L. A. D'Agostino, J. M. Ellis, J. D. Hansen, M. E. Matyskiela, J. J. McDonald, J. R. Riggs and L. G. Hamann, *ACS Med. Chem. Lett.*, 2019, **10**, 1592–1602.
142. J. D. Hansen, M. Correa, M. Alexander, M. Nagy, D. Huang, J. Sapienza, G. Lu, L. A. LeBrun, B. E. Cathers, W. Zhang, Y. Tang, M. Ammirante, R. K. Narla, J. R. Piccotti, M. Pourdehnad and A. Lopez-Girona, *J. Med. Chem.*, 2021, **64**, 1835–1843.
143. C.-W. Chung, A. W. Dean, J. M. Woolven and P. Bamborough, *J. Med. Chem.*, 2012, **55**, 576–586.
144. P. Bamborough, H. Diallo, J. D. Goodacre, L. Gordon, A. Lewis, J. T. Seal, D. M. Wilson, M. D. Woodrow and C.-w. Chung, *J. Med. Chem.*, 2012, **55**, 587–596.
145. C. R. Wellaway, D. Amans, P. Bamborough, H. Barnett, R. A. Bit, J. A. Brown, N. R. Carlson, C.-w. Chung, A. W. J. Cooper, P. D. Craggs, R. P. Davis, T. W. Dean, J. P. Evans, L. Gordon, I. L. Harada, D. J. Hirst, P. G. Humphreys, K. L. Jones, A. J. Lewis, M. J. Lindon, D. Lugo, M. Mahmood, S. McCleary, P. Medeiros, D. J. Mitchell, M. O'Sullivan, A. Le Gall, V. K. Patel, C. Patten, D. L. Poole, R. R. Shah, J. E. Smith, K. A. J. Stafford, P. J. Thomas, M. Vimal, I. D. Wall, R. J. Watson, N. Wellaway, G. Yao and R. K. Prinjha, *J. Med. Chem.*, 2020, **63**, 714–746.
146. S. Harrison, B. Lahue, Z. Peng, A. Donofrio, C. Chang and M. Glick, *Future Med. Chem.*, 2017, **9**, 533–536.
147. J. Wernevik, F. Bergstrom, A. Noven, J. Hulthe, L. Fredlund, D. Addison, J. Holmgren, P. E. Stromstedt, E. Rehnstrom and T. Lundbock, *Assay Drug Dev. Technol.*, 2020, **18**, 157–179.
148. K. Gao, S. Shaabani, R. Xu, T. Zarganes-Tzitzikas, L. Gao, M. Ahmadianmoghaddam, M. R. Groves and A. Dömling, *RSC Med. Chem.*, 2021, **12**, 809–818.
149. P. M. Wehn, J. P. Rizzi, D. D. Dixon, J. A. Grina, S. T. Schlachter, B. Wang, R. Xu, H. Yang, X. Du, G. Han, K. Wang, Z. Cao, T. Cheng, R. M. Czerwinski, B. S. Goggin, H. Huang, M. M. Halfmann, M. A. Maddie, E. L. Morton, S. R. Olive, H. Tan, S. Xie, T. Wong, J. A. Josey and E. M. Wallace, *J. Med. Chem.*, 2018, **61**, 9691–9721.
150. R. Xu, K. Wang, J. P. Rizzi, H. Huang, J. A. Grina, S. T. Schlachter, B. Wang, P. M. Wehn, H. Yang, D. D. Dixon, R. M. Czerwinski, X. Du, E. L. Ged, G. Han, H. Tan, T. Wong, S. Xie, J. A. Josey and E. M. Wallace, *J. Med. Chem.*, 2019, **62**, 6876–6893.
151. R. Moslin, Y. Zhang, S. T. Wrobleski, S. Lin, M. Mertzman, S. Spergel, J. S. Tokarski, J. Strnad, K. Gillooly, K. W. McIntyre, A. Zupa-Fernandez, L. Cheng, H. Sun, C. Chaudhry, C. Huang, C. D'Arienzo, E. Heimrich, X. Yang, J. K. Muckelbauer, C. Chang, J. Tredup, D. Mulligan, D. Xie, N. Aranibar, M. Chiney, J. R. Burke, L. Lombardo, P. H. Carter and D. S. Weinstein, *J. Med. Chem.*, 2019, **62**, 8953–8972.
152. S. T. Wrobleski, R. Moslin, S. Lin, Y. Zhang, S. Spergel, J. Kempson, J. S. Tokarski, J. Strnad, A. Zupa-Fernandez, L. Cheng, D. Shuster, K. Gillooly, X. Yang, E. Heimrich, K. W. McIntyre, C. Chaudhry, J. Khan, M. Ruzanov, J. Tredup, D. Mulligan, D. Xie, H. Sun, C. Huang, C. D'Arienzo, N. Aranibar, M. Chiney, A. Chimalakonda, W. J. Pitts, L. Lombardo, P. H. Carter, J. R. Burke and D. S. Weinstein, *J. Med. Chem.*, 2019, **62**, 8973–8995.
153. K. L. Lee, C. M. Ambler, D. R. Anderson, B. P. Boscoe, A. G. Bree, J. I. Brodfuehrer, J. S. Chang, C. Choi, S. Chung, K. J. Curran, J. E. Day, C. M. Dehnhardt, K. Dower, S. E. Drozda, R. K. Frisbie, L. K. Gavrin, J. A. Goldberg, S. Han, M. Hegen, D. Hepworth, H. R. Hope, S. Kamtekar, I. C. Kilty, A. Lee, L.-L. Lin, F. E. Lovering, M. D. Lowe, J. P. Mathias, H. M. Morgan, E. A. Murphy, N. Papaioannou, A. Patny, B. S. Pierce, V. R. Rao, E. Saiah, I. J. Samardjiev, B. M. Samas, M. W. H. Shen, J. H. Shin, H. H. Soutter, J. W. Strohbach, P. T. Symanowicz, J. R. Thomason, J. D. Trzupek, R. Vargas, F. Vincent, J. Yan, C. W. Zapf and S. W. Wright, *J. Med. Chem.*, 2017, **60**, 5521–5542.

# 20 Lead Optimisation: What You Should Know!

Simon E. Ward*[a] and Andrew M. Davis*[b]

[a]Director of Medicines Discovery Institute, Cardiff University, Cardiff, CF10 3AT, UK; [b]Hit Discovery, Discovery Sciences, R&D, AstraZeneca, Cambridge, UK
*E-mail: Wards10@cardiff.ac.uk, andy.davis@astrazeneca.com

## 20.1 The Role of Lead Optimisation

As described in the various chapters within this book, the identification, clinical evaluation, and ultimate marketing of a drug molecule is a long and complicated process. To many looking from outside, it may seem to be so risky and convoluted that it is easy to understand why so many drug discovery programs fail.[1–4] This process is often represented as the classical chevron diagram in Figure 20.1 in which the start point is a formulation of a clinical hypothesis that modulation of target X will provide patient benefit in disease Y. Suitable chemical matter that can achieve the required target modulation is then identified, optimised to meet a target profile, then progressed through preclinical and clinical development to ultimately achieve regulatory approval as a new medicine.

This commonly used representation is however an over-simplification; the sequence is rarely linear, and the validation of the target is clearly informed by data that are generated during the non-clinical and clinical evaluation and development. Furthermore, this chevron representation tends to over-industrialise the idea of drug discovery, leading some people outside the field to regard this as a process akin to a production line, with inexorable progression from left to right requiring little more than budget and time. However, the process of designing and crafting a potential new drug molecule requires enormous creativity, experience, and perseverance. This is no more so than at the phase in the middle of these chevrons whereby the originating chemical matter or lead series is optimised to a single molecule, on which a development programme

The Handbook of Medicinal Chemistry: Principles and Practice, 2nd Edition
Edited by Simon E. Ward and Andrew M. Davis

Published by the Royal Society of Chemistry, www.rsc.org

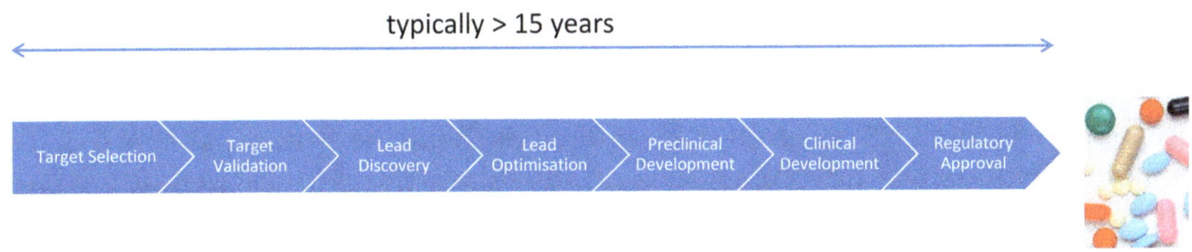


**Figure 20.1** Chevrons representing the stages of drug discovery.

costing potentially 100 s of millions of dollars will be based. This phase of lead optimisation is generally the main occupation of the medicinal chemist[5] and is a multidisciplinary effort that can last for many years for each individual target. As the optimisation progresses, and confidence increases that a molecule can be identified to start clinical development, then so does the value of the programme, both to the organisation conducting the research and to potential external investors or partners.

But the lead optimisation phase is more than finding the right molecule. During this period the project needs to build the biological rationale and strengthen the "platform of evidence", that modulation target x in patient population y will have an effect on the disease. The team will be considering assays and experiments that link the DMTA driving assays to the patient within translatable assays which may involve testing compounds in primary human tissue and mechanistic-based animal models (see Chapters 11 and 12). The project team will be building their clinical plan to provide evidence that the drug can not only meet a candidate drug target profile but also a therapeutic target profile. The project team needs to build confidence that the predicted clinical effect will be big enough and differentiated enough from standard of care that patients, payors, and regulators will find acceptable. The project may be proposing targeting a specific patient population that will be most likely to respond, and plans need to be matured to select those patients to demonstrate a differentiated effect. This will involve engagement with translational science, clinical, commercial, and regulatory colleagues. The team also needs to provide drug substance for those preclinical and clinical programmes, so engaging with process and pharmaceutical development colleagues as the programme starts to focus upon a compound shortlist is important for building a plan for the smooth progression of the project. The team will need to deliver a package of safety data that will support progression to clinical testing. All these threads must be woven together during lead optimisation such that the identified candidate drug and its ongoing development plan can be presented to gain investment in the ongoing project.

### 20.1.1 What is Obtained from Lead Identification: Assessing the Series

The start of lead optimisation usually begins with one or more series of compounds with a range of properties that give confidence they could be optimised to the final molecule. Confidence is gained, as it was once put to one of the authors, when you have all the right properties, just not in all the same molecule. Confidence is further gained by having a clear view of risks and gaps, and a chemical plan with scope to mitigate them.

Many of these properties are generic, but some are more specific. For instance, specific properties may depend on whether the programme is aimed at oral or topical treatment, whether once-a-day treatment is required or a more frequent dosing regimen is acceptable, whether CNS penetration is required or should be avoided, what is required for differentiation from the competition or standard of care, and what may be tolerated with respect to benefit *vs.* risk within the patient population.

At a high level, you (the team), are trying to deliver an effective low dose of a drug with a differentiated profile *vs.* other potential drugs at a suitable dosing frequency with acceptable margins to potential adverse safety liabilities, to test your target hypothesis in your targeted patient population.

Potency is a key generic property, as it is directly related to dose, which is often critical for device and formulation limitations, patient compliance and safety profile (higher potency and lower dose generally improves margins to safety liabilities). Metabolic stability is also a key generic property, affecting dose and dose frequency. A broad selectivity against off-targets, and an acceptable toxicological profile are also generically required, although different disease indications may have different tolerances to the safety profile. Controlling physical properties such as solubility and hydrophobicity is also important as these underlie many key features such as absorption, distribution, metabolism, and elimination, potency at your chosen target and key off-targets affecting the toxicological profile and safety window. One way of balancing these factors of potency and metabolism is to use dose predictions as a scoring function to measure progress.

Each individual project will also have a set of project-specific properties that will need to be optimised. Selectivity against closely related targets may be necessary, as well as generic selectivity against targets that cause common issues, *e.g.*, cardiac channels such as hERG (human cardiac potassium channel), $Na_V1.5$, $Ca_V1.2$, or phospholipidosis risk.[6,7] Metabolic stability should be in line with the desired dosing regimen. If the target is intracellular this will place additional demands on properties to ensure good cell penetration. If the compound acts on a receptor, it may be required, for example, to be a full or a partial agonist, an antagonist, or an allosteric modulator. If the compound is competitive with natural ligand, a high concentration of the endogenous ligand may provide an additional challenge on potency.[8] Many such questions need to be posed and answered before the journey from lead identification into lead optimisation commences. In addition, the series should be patentable or have the scope for patentability (unless other path to market or patient benefit is pursued) and will require advantages over any existing or competitor compounds both for patentability and commercial reasons. In short, the properties of a candidate molecule will need to fulfil a large range of demands, both specific and generic, and be tailored to the treatment and regimen envisaged, or demanded, by the targeted disease. This collection of properties that the candidate drug should be aimed at is commonly termed the candidate drug target profile.

### 20.1.2 Defining the Ultimate Candidate Profile

At the start of the lead optimisation phase, it is important to understand the parameters that make the ultimate target profile of the molecule. For most early projects, several of these parameters will be uncertain, due to an incomplete understanding of the pathway, mechanism, and link to the disease. It may not be clear what level of target engagement is required or what level of target or downstream functional efficacy will ultimately be required to show a clinical benefit. Furthermore, it is clear that these parameters cannot actually be fully defined until data are generated in the target disease setting and population, *i.e.*, initial patient trials, which lead to the need to manage a significant level of risk and uncertainty through the labour-intensive phases of lead optimisation and preclinical to early clinical development.

These challenges then require awareness during lead optimisation of what can be done to best manage these risks, and to maximise the chance of a successful proof of concept study in patients (*i.e.*, a clear result allowing either molecule/project progression or termination).[9]

Responding to this need, several major pharmaceutical companies have published retrospective analyses of their clinical projects which inform this thinking.

#### 20.1.2.1 Pfizer Pillars

Pfizer published an analysis of 44 projects that had reach a Phase II decision point.[10] From these projects, 32% were found to have achieved a clear, positive proof of concept result (*i.e.*, met their primary endpoint in the clinical study – generally being a positive efficacy measurement), 25% achieved a clear negative result, *i.e.*, lack of efficacy (with clear evidence of target engagement) or poor tolerability, but 43% were found to have not adequately demonstrated whether the mechanism was tested in the target study. This surprisingly high and clearly very resource-inefficient finding led to a further analysis of the project data. This led them to articulate fundamental data and knowledge needed from early stages of development, to assess whether a new medical entity (NME) has the potential to elicit a pharmacological effect and thereby test the mechanism of action in humans. These fundamental elements of data and knowledge were described as the 'three Pillars of survival'.

**Pillar 1: Exposure at the target site of action. Drug exposure at the target site of action is necessary to elicit a pharmacological effect over a desired time period**

Clearly, making sure that there is enough of the free drug at the target at the site of action to exceed the pharmacological potency for the desired period is a key objective. This can be determined by direct measurement of the drug concentration at the appropriate site in the body. This is not often possible, in which case measurement of free concentrations in blood can be used as a surrogate if enough confidence can be gained that the free drug hypothesis is valid (free drug concentrations at equilibrium are similar in all compartments). For some compartments this assumption may not be valid, for example targets in the brain where the blood–brain barrier may maintain a differential free concentration due to the action of efflux pumps. Confidence can be gained by the use of appropriate preclinical pharmacokinetic/pharmacodynamic PK/PD models, where measurement of drug concentrations in different compartments may be possible, and consideration of PBPK (physiologically based PK).[11]

**Pillar 2: Binding to the pharmacological target. Target occupancy is a prerequisite for expression of pharmacology and target modulation**

It is important to appreciate that just because high concentrations of molecule can be measured within the body, that this does not necessarily mean that there is the required concentration of the molecule at the molecular target(s) to drive occupancy (*i.e.*, at the specific, potentially intracellular, location). This requires a more direct measure of target engagement, for example using occupancy studies displacing labelled ligand (*e.g.*, PET[12]), or again indirect measures such as biomarker change in appropriate PK/PD studies.[13,14] Some confidence can be gained indirectly, if the binding properties and potency against the target are well understood (including potential impact of species differences in potency, polymorphisms, or other target phenotypes) combined with a high degree of confidence that adequate target exposure is being achieved (strong pillar 1 evidence). As well as occupancy, consideration should also be given to target binding kinetics and how this translates across *in vitro* and *in vivo* assays and species.

**Pillar 3: Expression of pharmacology. Functional modulation of the target is a prerequisite for expression of pharmacological activity to test the mechanism**

Again, it is the effect of the presence of the molecule at the target (not necessarily the fact that it is just present in the body) that is going to drive the required therapeutic benefit (*e.g.*, is the molecule driving/blocking the necessary downstream signalling pathways). This confidence will most likely come from measuring a downstream marker or physiological response from PKPD model or mechanistic models of disease.

These parameters were then adapted towards a risk management matrix in which projects could be assigned to one of four quadrants representing different levels of risk for progressing a project to a proof-of-concept clinical study, Figure 20.2. Projects where none of the risks could be mitigated or demonstrated represented a high-risk investment.

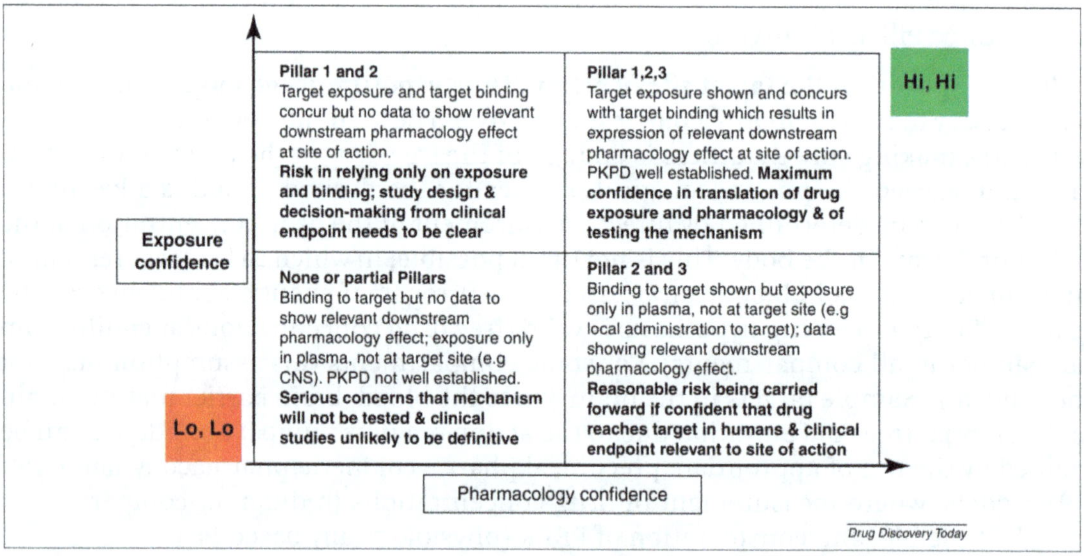


**Figure 20.2** Matrix of risk management based off the Pfizer 'pillars'. Reproduced from ref. 10 with permission from Elsevier, Copyright 2012.

### *20.1.2.2 AstraZeneca 'Rights'*

A similar analysis of development attrition at AstraZeneca reviewing projects from 2005 to 2010 covered 142 projects up to clinical testing in Phase II. For those that provided analysable data, it was clear that a lower than industry median percentage of AstraZeneca candidate drugs were reaching market. Projects were failing through preclinical and clinical development primarily due to safety findings (principally specific organ toxicity), and secondarily due to lack of efficacy. Further, projects with preclinical safety issues that were progressed often closed due to safety issues in the clinic, highlighting the need to pay attention to preclinical safety signals which rarely improve, rather becoming more problematic as the project progresses. A key conclusion was progression of molecules could have been stopped earlier through the application of more robust criteria. Compound properties could also limit the maximum potential dose, preclude the compound from achieving adequate exposure in the relevant tissue, or generate additional safety concerns (reducing the maximum dose that can be given). As for Pfizer, several projects were classified as efficacy failures as there was no way to determine target engagement of pharmacodynamic activity. A number of project failures were thought of as 'good failures', as they were able to demonstrate pharmacological engagement of the proposed mechanism but did not result in clinical efficacy, showing little doubt that the hypothesis was tested and that it was proven to be wrong. Conversely, projects which showed greater confidence in target validation (*i.e.*, more confidence in the role of the target in disease or genetic validation) were less likely to fail due to efficacy. Surprisingly, a number of Phase II project failures had not targeted the optimal patient population based on the scientific understanding of disease; rather clinical programs were driven by commercial value of the population. Higher confidence in patient selection was also a positive factor of Phase II success. Responding to the detailed analysis presented,[15,16] a fuller framework of principles was articulated, known as the 5 Rights, Table 20.1.

**Table 20.1** The 5-Rs framework. The 5Rs framework is used in AstraZeneca to assess the project at all governance decisions, from target selection onwards, with the questions being asked becoming more stringent as the project progresses.

| | |
|---|---|
| Right target | Strong link between target and disease<br>Differentiated efficacy<br>Available and predictive biomarkers |
| Right tissue | Adequate bioavailability and tissue exposure<br>Definition of PD biomarkers<br>Clear understanding of preclinical and clinical PK/PD<br>Understanding of drug–drug interactions |
| Right safety | Differentiated and clear safety margins<br>Understanding of secondary pharmacology risk<br>Understanding of reactive metabolites genotoxicity and drug–drug interactions<br>Understanding of target liability |
| Right patient | Identification of the most responsive patient population<br>Definition of risk-benefit for the given population |
| Right commercial patient | Differentiated value proposition *vs.* future standard of care<br>Focus on market access, payer, and provider<br>Personalised health-care strategy, including diagnostics and biomarkers |

Embedding the 3 pillars and 5-Rs thinking builds confidence in the project as the project progresses through LO. It can help chemists to build quality into the LO series and biologists to use your tool compounds to provide more confidence in forward translation by defining exposure effect relationships in human cellular and patient-derived tissue and animal mechanistic models of the disease. They can look for translatable biomarkers that can be measured preclinically that can also be used clinically.

### 20.1.3 Progressing into Clinical Development – Dose Selection

Several of the later descriptions within this chapter, and the various optimisation criteria highlighted, are essentially all targeting at one key ultimate parameter, namely the dose that will be used in humans in clinical trials and as an approved medicine; a dose that can be expected to drive significant efficacy while providing an acceptable margin to anticipated safety liabilities highlighted by preclinical safety studies and/or clinical experience. This dose size and frequency of administration are key to many aspects of drug safety, compliance,[17] and cost, as covered in several chapters within this book. It is worth emphasising that making the dose as low as possible[18] is the most effective way to minimise attrition during clinical development due to an unacceptable safety profile. Clearly then it is essential to develop early strategies and predictions to identify the target dose, and as with the various guidelines above, this can be challenging if the target is novel and there is limited understanding of the disease-target hypothesis.

An excellent description of the practical implementation is included in a 2020 review[19] which highlights several key concepts and potential pitfalls. Unsurprisingly, the dose required is a combination of its ADME, and pharmacology and physicochemical attributes, and whilst methods are well established to extrapolate to human PK characteristics, the extrapolation of PD, biomarker or *in vivo* pharmacology can be notoriously difficult. Three broad scenarios are presented which cover different levels of disease hypothesis understanding (Figure 20.3). Firstly, the ideal situation in which there is a very clear understanding of the nature of the disease and the degree of target modulation that is required to see clinical benefit (*e.g.*, reduction in microbe or parasite level) – panel A. The second-best situation – panel C – is where the direct link to the disease is not possible, but there is a clear rationale and link to a measurable surrogate marker.[20] The common third situation occurs for many novel targets where biomarkers have yet to be validated and the disease process or setting is such that the level of target inhibition required for clear clinical benefit is wholly or partly unknown. In this scenario, panel B, the pragmatic approach, is to aim for a clinical dose which achieves a high level of target modulation, without setting the bar unachievable high. Clearly, this bar will be adjusted as information develops through the project lifetime.

This thinking was then summarised with the seven most important considerations for a strategy to reduce dose size:[21]

1. Increase potency (affinity) against target
2. Decrease intrinsic clearance to increase AUCu/dose
3. Ensure efficient oral absorption

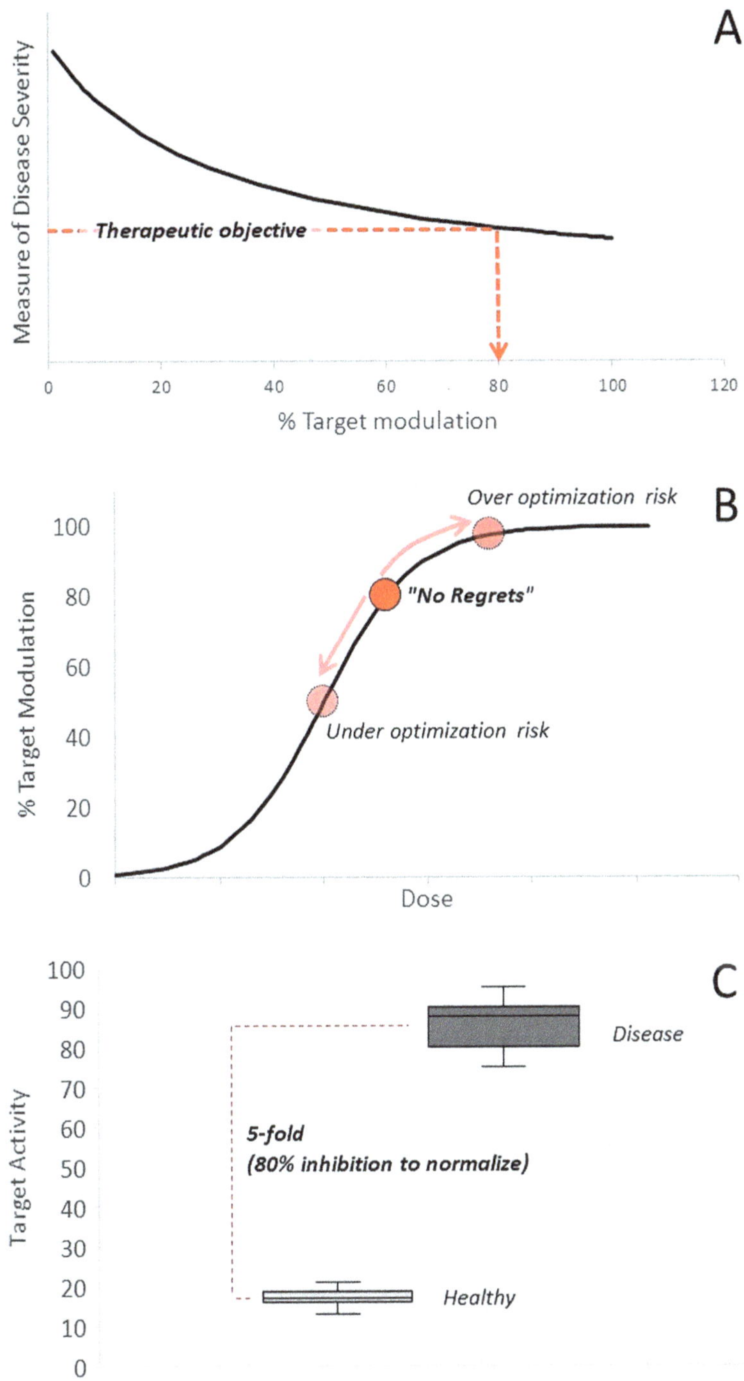


**Figure 20.3** Conceptual illustration of three approaches to a quantitative clinical objective in support of design. (A) 80% target modulation is targeted based on an understanding of the relationship between target activity and disease. (B) 80% target modulation is targeted based on a 'no-regrets' approach to ensuring that the mechanism will be tested in the clinic. (C) 80% target modulation is rationalised on the basis of data indicating that this is what's required to restore target activity to healthy levels. Reproduced from ref. 19 with permission from American Chemical Society, Copyright 2020.

4. Increase solubility
5. Increase dissolution by particle size reduction, *etc.*
6. Increase lipoidal permeability
7. Decrease efflux

and frequency:[22]

1. Decrease intrinsic clearance to lengthen half-life
2. Increase Vss to increase half-life

The same considerations apply to the required target concentrations, where an understanding of the pharmacokinetic profile of the molecule required to drive the target pharmacology to achieve clinical benefit will allow the project team to target specific a $C_{max}$ or $C_{min}$ or $C_{avg}$ (AUC/dose interval). Again, for novel mechanisms, these target values may not be clear – particularly when biomarkers are not easily available – and in these situations a pragmatic focus, such as defining $C_{min}$ as 75% target occupancy (in the absence of strong alternative hypotheses such as irreversible binders, knowledge of the time-course of downstream signalling *etc*). In a survey of 63 oral drugs across many therapy areas, most achieve 1–3-fold higher concentrations than the $XC_{50}$ at $C_{min}$.[23]

### 20.1.4 The Process of Optimisation

At the outset of lead optimisation, the project should have a well-considered candidate drug profile that it will aim for, Table 20.2. This is not a 'mindless checklist'; some demands that are not reached may be compensated by other properties that exceed the minimum standards set, and the ultimate molecule that is progressed into development will be the best balance of a series of compromises and informed guesses. For instance, some deficit in potency may be compensated for by an excellent half-life, and the various assumptions and estimates used are refined and revised as part of the progression towards clinical development. (The predicted dose to man is one way in which many of the factors can be balanced, *e.g.*, potency, stability, distribution, absorption rate). The 'process' of drug discovery is a journey of reducing risk – generating data that builds confidence in the disease-treating hypothesis and potential and reducing the risk that the target or chemical series will not succeed.

In the broadest terms, the rationale for setting a candidate profile up-front is to ensure that the properties of the final molecule will provide a compound that is of sufficient potency and selectivity, and whose pharmacokinetics allow a reasonably low dose which will interact potently with the target over the whole of the dosing period, without affecting undesired targets that will cause side-effects. Simplistically, it gives chemists designing and synthesising new molecules in the laboratory a target to aim for.

An ideal drug candidate will have sufficient:

POTENCY, such that the minimum concentration required to be maintained for efficacy is low (*e.g.*, less than 50 nM)

HALF-LIFE, such that the dose required to maintain $C_{min}$ does not produce a very much higher $C_{max}$ (*e.g.*, a $t½$ of 24 h will give a $C_{max}$–$C_{min}$ ratio of 2) for the dose frequency chosen

Table 20.2 Typical property characteristics for a drug candidate entering clinical evaluation.

| | | |
|---|---|---|
| Potency | Primary binding $IC_{50}$ | <5 nM |
| | Cell potency $IC_{50}$ | <20 nM |
| | Whole blood potency | <1 μM |
| Selectivity | *Versus* key related targets | >100-fold |
| | *Versus* large panel of diverse targets | <50% activity at 10 μM |
| | *Versus* key generic liabilities, *e.g.*, hERG | No target potency with 100× $C_{max}$ >30 μM |
| | Phospholipidosis $EC_{50}$ (mM) | $EC_{50}$ > 15 μM |
| Chemical properties | log*P*/log*D* 7.4 | Measured log*D* 7.4 <3.5 |
| | Aqueous solubility | >50 mM pH 7.4 buffer |
| | Light stability | Stable |
| | Intellectual property | Filed |
| DMPK *in vitro* | Human microsomes $CL_{int}$ (μL $min^{-1}$ $mg^{-1}$) | Measured |
| | Human hepatocytes $CL_{int}$ (μL $min^{-1}$ $10^{-6}$ cells) | Measured |
| | $P_{app}$ in CACO2 AB/BA (cm $s^{-1}$ × $10^6$) concentration response investigated | Good passive permeability $P_{app}$ >5 × $10^{-6}$ cm $s^{-1}$ |
| | Investigate OATP2B1, OATP1B1 and P-gp transport in MDCK cells | Good passive permeability no active absorption and no DDI |
| | PPB (% bound) | Measured |
| | Cb/Cp ratio | Measured |
| | Plasma stability | Measured |
| | CYP inhibition $IC_{50}$ (μM) | >10 |
| | *In vitro* cross species biotransformation | Measured |
| | CYP induction | $E_{max}$ <40% positive control or $EC_{50}$ > 10 mM |
| | Time dependent CYP inhibition | None |
| | Dose to man | <1 mg $kg^{-1}$ $day^{-1}$ |
| | Rat pharmacokinetics | *t*½ >2 h and bioavailability >30% |
| | *In vivo* dog pharmacokinetics | *t*½ >4 h and bioavailability >30% |
| | PK scaling to human | *In vitro in vivo* CL scaling in two species Predicts *t*½ suitable for desired dosing regimen *e.g.* 12–25 h for once-a-day |
| | Metabolite ID | Metabolites in preclinical species and human hepatocytes investigated –human metabolites qualified in preclinical species |
| | *In silico* genetic tox | Clean |
| | Five strain Ames | Clean with and without S9 fraction |
| Safety | Phototoxicity | No strong absorption 290-700 nM |
| | | Clean in 3T3 neutral red uptake phototoxicity assay |
| | Rat 14 d/28 d repeat dose | Acceptable margins for progression |
| | Dog 14 d/28 d repeat dose | Acceptable margins for progression |
| | Dog telemetry (Qtc) | 100× NOEL over predicted human free $C_{max}$ |
| | Maximum absorbable dose (MAD) | >Predicted dose to man |
| | Predicted fraction absorbed at predicted dose to man | >50% |
| Pharmaceutical properties | Crystallinity | Crystalline |
| | Thermal properties | No melt or other event <80 °C |
| | Hygroscopicity | <2% uptake at 25 °C/80% relative humidity |
| | Stability | >90% in solution formulation after at least day |

SELECTIVITY, such that toxicity (undesired pharmacology) is not seen until very much higher plasma levels than $C_{max}$ are achieved (*e.g.*, levels >10–100-fold above $C_{max}$ to give a safety margin of >10–100). This is illustrated in Figure 20.4 for the situation where modulation of target is continuously required above a minimum threshold level.

The minimum concentration required for efficacy ($C_{min}$) should be in line with that found in various preclinical studies and animal models (allowing for cross species potency differences), while the human pharmacokinetics should be predictable from that measured in at least two animal species, usually rat and dog (allowing for inter-species scaling), providing confidence in your prediction to the third species, human. Throughout the project, the profile of the candidate will change with additional information as more detailed biological understanding of the target and prospective patient population emerges. It may also be influenced by competitor compounds at the same or related targets or against the same disease population, which may mean new stricter targets or new targets are set for differentiation reasons. New criteria may be added such as regulatory authorities demanding better selectivity, or increased margins against toxicity. This target profile should be adaptable and evolving, but equally, if well-reasoned from the outset, the profile should not change so much that the ongoing optimisation is continually set towards new directions. A well thought through profile will act as a goal that the project team members will jointly focus on to deliver a suitable compound which meets those properties. Thus, the candidate profile becomes a key set of numbers to be attained.

It is also important to remember that, while the candidate profile may already contain quite a few demanding properties, when reaching the later stages of optimisation

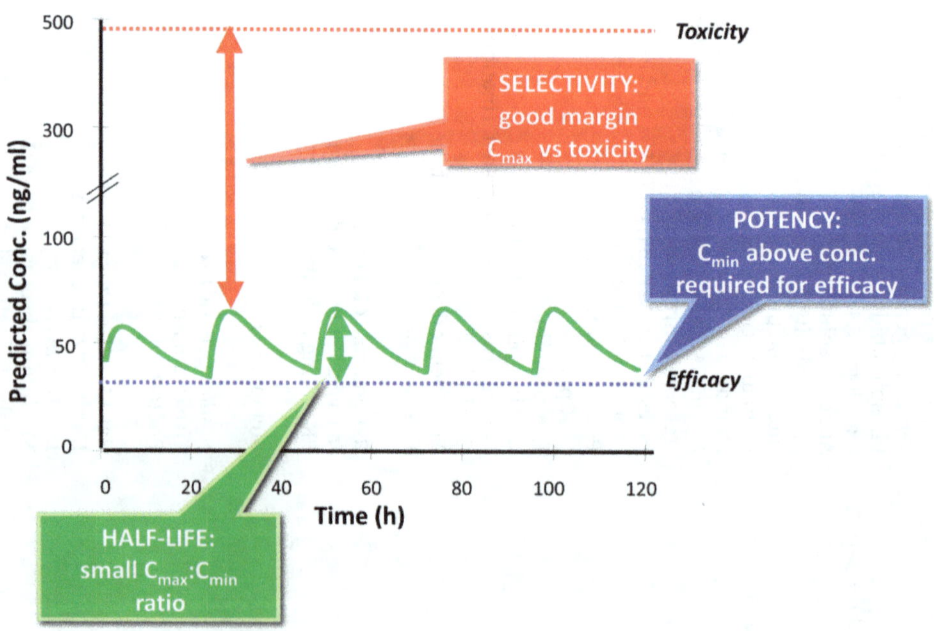


**Figure 20.4** Schematic showing the profile of an ideal drug molecule's concentration over time to be safe and effective.

as one learns more about the compound series, there may be a further extended range of properties that need to be satisfied. This extended range of criteria may not form part of the optimisation process but need to be tested before the final molecule is proposed as a candidate and taken into the expensive development phase. Thus, the profile of the candidate drug should encompass a set of properties, which if satisfied, will allow the clinical concept to be tested appropriately with a suitable molecule, by the required route of administration.

Once the prospective candidate profile is defined, the properties of the lead molecules identified should be measured against it to assess which properties need to be optimised. If the hit to lead phase has gone well, the lead compounds should have many of the desired properties already built in, but normally some of the required properties will be present in some molecules, and other properties in other molecules. Usually, it is not an easy job to combine all the required properties into a single molecule. The project will need to decide the main issues remaining in the compounds, and these will vary from project to project. Lead compounds do not usually have the potency required by the candidate, or if they do then it may be accompanied with an undesired property. For instance, it is common for early compounds that have high potency to also have high lipophilicity, leading to poor pharmacokinetics and physicochemical characteristics, while other examples in the same series may have lower lipophilicity and good pharmacokinetics, but much lower potency. This potency–lipophilicity relationship is well described, and it is the ratio of these two properties, described as lipophilic efficiency[24–26] (variously LLE or LipE), and more recently lipophilic metabolic efficiency (LipMetE)[27] that often needs to be improved. An early *in vivo* safety study may highlight important toxicologies to be mitigated during LO. Understanding the key deficiencies of the 'lead compounds' from the hit to lead campaign and the ability to change these undesired properties without adversely affecting any of the other good properties is key to making progress in the optimisation phase.

Often, chemical probes will be required during the project lifetime to either enable downstream assays or answer key questions regarding target validation or the clinical utility of the target.[28–32] It is important to emphasise that many of the properties required between a clinical candidate and a chemical probe may be similar (potency, selectivity, solubility, permeability *etc.*) but clearly others will be different (*e.g.*, the probe may require much greater selectivity but little attention is required for safety liabilities).

## 20.1.5 Screening Cascade

Once the candidate profile is defined and the deficiencies of the lead compounds are understood, the project needs an appropriate screening plan so that synthesis is directed towards compounds that could have the required properties of the ultimate candidate drug. Naturally not all properties are, or can be, measured at once, so the screening plan must be organised in order that key properties are measured at the right time, and on a reasonable number of compounds, to allow filtering of the best compounds for further testing, into the more expensive or time-consuming tests, such as rat pharmacokinetics or *in vivo* potency in a disease model. The assays present in the screening cascade will often represent a balance between the importance of the data to inform onward design *vs.* their in-house availability or external availability and cost.[33]

An effective strategy is often to profile early lead molecules as far as practical down the cascade of assays to identify potential series liabilities that may frustrate later attempts to identify a balanced candidate drug molecule – for example an off-target activity that proves impossible to separate from the target activity.

Clearly later, it is essential that all properties ultimately need to be verified on the actual candidate drug molecule. It should also be emphasised that profiling a wider set of properties is not merely stamp collecting but is part of evaluating and avoiding the risks of failure later in the development process. The extended testing cascades should be refined and tailored to the individual issues and challenges present in each unique project. A particular example of this pressure testing of series is early safety toxicology testing of suboptimal members of the series to avoid failures late in the screening cascade. This proactive early safety toxicology testing was prompted by expensive and resource-consuming failures of molecules in late safety testing. The reported data[34,35] shows that such safety front-loading has reduced the attrition due to idiosyncratic toxicity, and a greater proportion of late-stage failures are now due to insufficient efficacy. Whilst any later stage attrition is disappointing, reduced attrition due to toxicity at least allows more compounds to be progressed to man to test the concept of inhibiting the target in the disease, whereas late-stage toxicity failures are both costly, and mean the compounds fail prior to mechanism testing in man.

In compiling the screening cascade the project team should ensure that all tests are in place to ask and answer key questions. Are the screens relevant to the disease and route of administration? Is each assay in the right place in the cascade to enable fast filtering of compounds with the desired properties? Do the assays in the cascade form a translatable cascade, in that activity in the simpler higher-throughput assays higher up the cascade predict outcome in assays lower in the cascade. Is the availability and throughput for each assay fit for the place it occupies in the screening cascade? Is sufficient budget available or how can costs be managed? Should assays be set up in-house or outsourced? Compounds will stall in the progression sequence if a key assay delivers results too slowly for the screening plan or runs too infrequently. The screening cascade is critical to the project in providing the right data at the right time to allow the project to make critical decisions about compounds, to stop weaker compounds and progress stronger compounds. It also helps the project team to identify the drivers of the key properties and allows the project to run the iterative cycle rapidly. A screening cascade is often organised in screening tiers or waves, Table 20.3, where data in each wave is generated in parallel, the data from each wave used to inform the decision for progression to the next. Wave 1 provides enough data for an early dose to man prediction and a decision to progress to Wave 2 which is *in vivo* rodent PK. A decision from Wave 2 could be progression to a Wave 3 PD model in rodent if one exists and in parallel second species pharmacokinetics. Wave 4 could be into a more complex mechanism of disease model and key assays that select shortlist candidates, Wave 5 can profile the shortlist candidates to pick the compound nominated for further progression. In short, a well-planned screening cascade organises the discovery phase efficiently, and enables the project to rapidly identify a candidate drug with the right property profile.

**Table 20.3** Table depicting the typical organisation of screening assays in groups or waves.

| | | | |
|---|---|---|---|
| Wave 1 | Primary potency screen | Isolated enzyme/membrane prep binding/affinity | **DP1 progress to pharmacokinetics** |
| | Primary selectivity screen/s | Closely related targets | |
| | Microsomes and hepatocytes | *In vitro* DMPK stability/1st preclin species, usually rat | |
| | hPPB | % free | |
| | Log*D* | *n*-Octanol/water partition | |
| | Solubility | pH 7.4 solubility | |
| | hERG | Binding | |
| | P450s | Liability of problems for DDIs but also rat cassette PK | |
| | Early dose to human can be estimated in the above core data | | |
| Wave 2 | Rat PK iv and po | Check scaling *in vitro* to *in vivo*/absorption | **DP2 progress to pharmacodynamics** |
| | Cell activity assay | This may be Wave 1 for agonists | |
| | Cytotoxicity cell assay | Counter screen for cell activity and safety | |
| | Species crossover | Binding screen or cell screen – can we test PD *in vivo*? | |
| | Rat PPB/hum hepatocytes | Refined PK prediction | |
| | Metabolite id | Routes of metabolism | |
| | Caco-2 | Permeability and efflux | |
| | hERG electrophysiology | Functional hERG cell assay | |
| Wave 3 | Broader selectivity screening | Profiling and confidence in interpretating *in vivo* activity | **DP3 progress to disease model** |
| | Biological effect cell assay | Confirm translation to more relevant human cell | |
| | Solid state props | By now crystalline form ready for dog PK | |
| | PD model | *In vivo* efficacy, check PKPD predictions | |
| | *In vitro* safety | PLD, AHR bSEP MRP2 ion panel, AMES | |
| | Dog PK | Check scaling 2nd species | |
| | CYP induction | | |
| Wave 4 | Disease model | *In vivo* efficacy, maybe longer-term model | **DP4 progress to shortlist candidates** |
| | Check PKPD assumptions | | |
| Wave 5 | Refined dose to man | 14/28 day rat/dog | **DP5 CD selection** |
| | Further DMPK assessment | | |
| | Pharm dev assessment | | |
| | Pre-nomination Tox package | | |
| | *In vivo* tox | | |

## 20.1.6 Decision-making in the Screening Cycle

Once a suitable screening plan is in place the project must decide how best to run the plan. This will depend on many factors. How many compounds will be produced? Which tests are available to the project, and how often do they run? Who will evaluate the test results and choose which compounds to progress further? What is the critical data that will allow a compound to be progressed, and which value needs to be met? In whatever way a project is set up there needs to be a way for the project to decide which compounds to progress to the next level, or to analyse results and decide on actions to progress the project. To avoid prolonged debate around each individual compound it may be useful to set pre-determined progression criteria for the main decision-making assays.

### 20.1.7 Progression Criteria

Throughout the optimisation phase the project should have the candidate profile in mind as the final goal. However, at early stages, when the molecular properties are still some distance away, it may make sense to have looser progression criteria for moving a compound through the screening plan to understand all the molecule properties in a holistic way. For instance, some compounds in a series with insufficient potency should be advanced into rodent pharmacokinetics with a view to testing if the PK of the series is a strength or weakness. As the optimisation progresses and the properties are advanced toward those desired of the candidate drug, the progression criteria should be tightened, and ultimately coalesce with the candidate profile.

The project will need to decide which data to collect automatically on all molecules made, *e.g.*, primary potency, solubility, *in vitro* metabolism, measured log$D$. Some of this data can be key to the analysis of series to determine what are the drivers of specific properties, and where limits, *i.e.*, progression criteria, need to be drawn. On the other hand, many properties are now well predicted, and it may not make sense to collect all properties on all compounds, just because it is possible.

Equally, with easy access to tools for property prediction,[36–38] it makes no sense to make molecules with properties that are predicted to be bad. All compounds should be prepared to clearly address a question. Small, well-chosen arrays of each subtype are appropriate to explore property space, but the chemistry should be driven by molecules made to test a theory, and not just because one could easily synthesise 500 simple analogues.

### 20.1.8 Predicted Properties

It should be recognised that many properties of a molecule are fixed from the moment of conception. Furthermore, many of these properties are easily predicted (though not always correctly) and prior to synthesis the key properties should be predicted, and the molecule made only if the predictions are in an acceptable region. It is the defining of acceptable that may be problematic. Some will argue against rigidity in selecting compounds for synthesis solely on predicted properties; however, judicious choice of what to make can avoid difficult issues later. If a compound is predicted to be completely insoluble, why would you make it? Key physicochemical properties such as log$P$ and log$D$, p$K_a$ and solubility, QSAR and ML models are covered in Chapters 1, 3, and 6.

### 20.1.9 The Use of Colour to Simplify Decision-making

Once the project is in full throttle, many decisions will need to be made about the range of compounds that enter, and travel through, the screening plan. This can be simplified using colour in the results database. Looking at all the results for a compound, with the key results having their progression criteria coloured in a traffic light fashion, can make it easy to see when a compound passes all the relevant criteria and should be progressed. It is also very easy to see when a compound passes all criteria in the screening plan and is a potential candidate molecule. However, caution must be applied: the use of colour is powerful, and should be used carefully with appropriate judgment, especially at the boundaries of criteria. Nonetheless, the use of colour can streamline decision-making remarkably. Understanding when a possible candidate has been found is a key step for an optimisation project because it may change the nature of the following synthesis and testing from a hunting phase to a selection phase involving scale-up and a more detailed examination of a relatively small number of more focussed compounds.

## 20.2 Lead Optimisation – The Practicalities

### 20.2.1 Quality of Start Point is of Paramount Importance

In the same way as the most important decision in the drug discovery process is the selection of the correct target, the most important decision in the lead optimisation process is the very first decision, namely the selection of the chemical starting point itself. Whilst this is an obvious statement, there are several factors which drive initiation of medicinal chemistry activities, including the perceived priority, which can lead to optimisation starting on either poorly validated hits, or on molecules with a low probability of success of being able to be optimised into drug candidates. Given the resource that can be required to optimise from hit to lead to candidate and the momentum that can build up within a live project, it is vital that the resource is used effectively and applied along the correct trajectory.

Assuming the lead generation phase is complete, and the output appropriately validated, data should be generated to enable an appropriate selection of hit matter for a chemical start point. Typically, this should include data which is generated computationally and by high-throughput *in vitro* assays as well as examination by an experienced medicinal chemist. Additional early *in vitro* toxicology, wider selectivity and *in vivo* pharmacokinetics are informative at this stage, but their accessibility will be driven by the facilities and budget available.

Following this analysis, two common scenarios emerge:

1. A specific go/no-go criterion can be defined for an individual series. Typically, this could be to see if an undesirable structural feature can be removed, *e.g.*, removal of a carboxylic acid group to achieve CNS penetration or removal of a toxicophore such as a Michael acceptor.
2. A broad optimisation strategy is devised encompassing optimisation of several properties. The compounds required to be made should test specific hypotheses and should only be made if essential to answer that question (see Figure 20.5).

### 20.2.2 Starting Lead Optimisation: Identifying the Weaknesses

As with all aspects of drug discovery, the principle of 'the more information the better' applies, and often at the start of lead optimisation, there is insufficient data within the chemical class to allow effective use of QSAR or similar tools described in Chapter 6.

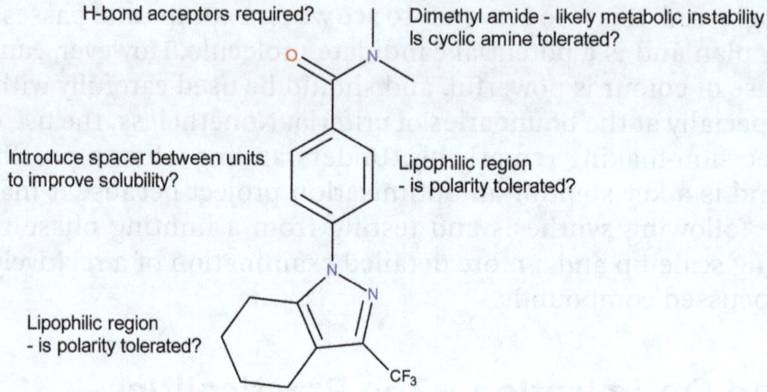


**Figure 20.5** Examples of early hit to lead questions. Lead obtained for AMPA receptor positive allosteric modulator project. Initial questions posed leading to first wave of analogues prepared or purchased.

Consequently, from any established lead, there are several initial avenues to gather additional data:

1. As above, the lead molecules should be characterised as extensively as resource/budget/facilities allow to maximise the chances of addressing key issues early on. Ideally this would include information on the kinetics and thermodynamics of the protein–ligand interaction.
2. If possible, structural data of the lead bound to the protein should be generated by X-ray crystallography. If unavailable, a computational model of the ligand bound to a homology model of the protein may provide some structural insight.
3. The structure–activity relationships for the lead should be developed by purchasing all related analogue structures (so-called 'SAR by catalogue').
4. Focussed small library sets (10–20 compounds) can be prepared around synthetically tractable areas of the molecule to generate additional SAR. Specifically, this would seek to generate several pair-wise comparisons to understand:
   - which features of the molecule are required for binding to target?
   - which physical property (measured or calculated) is driving the parameter in need of improvement?
   - if the project is in an area of pre-existing research, then clearly literature mining and pharmacophore generation from published SAR can drive new analogue design.

The output of this initial investigation should allow the medicinal chemist to prepare plans for the classical iterative cycle of design – synthesise – evaluate/test – analyse – allowing full lead optimisation to begin (see Figure 20.6).

### 20.2.3 Formulating a Strategy for Full Lead Optimisation

The principal challenge in lead optimisation is to recognise that the process requires optimisation of multiple parameters in parallel, and that a number of these parameters may be driven in opposing directions by the same underlying properties. The clearest

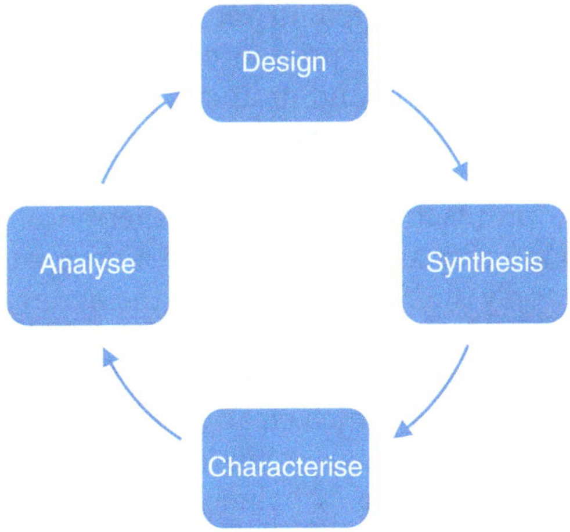


**Figure 20.6** Design cycle.

example of this is lipophilicity. It is apparent that affinity for the target can nearly always be achieved by increase in lipophilicity. However, it is equally apparent that increases in lipophilicity are associated with a reduction in overall drug-likeness and an increased chance of attrition.[34]

To this end, it is imperative to identify the underlying cause of the issue (*e.g.*, low solubility, poor distribution *etc.*) that requires optimisation, such as specific structural features, functional groups, or physicochemical properties. These observations will have been reinforced by the pair-wise comparisons and focussed library sets described above. The less data that is available, the more important it is to ensure that the analogues proposed cover a wider range of physicochemical space to be able to derive future hypotheses. Subsequent analogues should be used to refine these hypotheses, and data should be analysed for simple correlations between properties (*e.g.*, P450 3A4 inhibition and clog*P*; hERG affinity and $pK_a$ *etc.*) as well as multiparametric principal component analyses to identify trends between weighted combinations of several parameters.

However, in addition to these general principles, there are some additional common issues that are encountered in lead optimisation, for which a selection is discussed below.

## 20.2.4 Strategies to Optimise Common Parameters in Early Lead Optimisation

### *20.2.4.1 Target Affinity or Potency Vs Lipophilicity*

The affinity of the molecule for its protein target often dominates the early search for chemical starting points. This affinity is driven by a series of specific interactions which can be polar and non-polar in nature (for the simplest case of reversible non-covalent ligands). The various types of interactions as well as biophysical methods to characterise them are summarised in the excellent review by Stahl,[39] along with more recent specific updates on more focussed topics.[40–44]

Potency is very commonly the principal driver in early lead optimisation. When pursued in isolation from other molecular properties it has been blamed for the observed trends in increasing molecular weight and/or lipophilicity leading to compound-related attrition.[26,36] There are many hurdles to overcome during the process of drug discovery and development, and the balance of biological *vs.* physicochemical properties is the key to a successful lead optimisation strategy. Furthermore, given the unpredictable and challenging path to identify and then develop a drug candidate, it is imperative that medicinal chemists apply their skills to control the parameters and properties that lie within their control. One of the key parameters that all organic chemists are aware of, and that needs to transfer across to medicinal chemistry understanding is clearly $pK_a$ – in particular amine basicities, which clearly play a very significant role in the distribution and properties of the molecules prepared.[45]

Recognising the inherent challenge of balancing multiple parameters, many tools and indices have been adopted to assist the medicinal chemist in early lead optimisation. The simplest of these are the various modes of binding or ligand efficiency, which is most easily considered as a ratio of binding affinity or potency against a descriptor of molecular size:

$$\text{Ligand efficiency (LE)} = \frac{\Delta G}{n\text{Heavy Atoms}} \text{ or } \frac{\text{pXC50}}{n\text{Heavy Atoms}} \text{ or } \frac{\text{pXC50}}{\text{MWt}}$$

Calculating the ligand efficiency alongside the primary screening potency for each molecule is a powerful means of ensuring the efficiency of the optimisation process.[46,47] Furthermore, analysis of ligand efficiencies through optimisation campaigns indicates that they generally decrease, reinforcing the need to start with the most efficient chemical start point. In the same way that the physical properties of a molecule are fixed at the point of conception of the idea, the overall ligand efficiency of a chemical series is generally established from the ligand efficiency of its parent hits. Indeed, data supports the premise that the maximum ligand efficiency that can be achieved decreases with increasing molecular weight. This can be rationalised by considering that an ideal fit of ligand to protein is less likely as molecular complexity increases. The optimisation from leads to both Gefitinib and Sunitinib in Table 20.4 (adapted from content within *An Analysis of the Binding Efficiencies of Drugs and Their Leads in Successful Drug Discovery Programmes*[46]) illustrates the usual path, for which increasing molecular size was balanced with introduction of solubility and other properties leading to an overall decrease in efficiency of binding.

Notable exceptions to this can occur; however, a consideration of the first LE equation above should indicate that this requires increased $\Delta G$ for the same molecular size, *i.e.*, increase in $\Delta H$ or decrease in $\Delta S$. The former can be achieved by identifying additional polar or ionic protein–ligand interactions (as illustrated by Argatroban and Zanamivir in Table 20.4). However, it must be stressed that the design of additional polar interactions is challenging, even with the structural information provided by X-ray crystal structures of liganded proteins. A decrease in $\Delta S$ can be achieved by freezing the conformation of the ligand into its bioactive conformation to minimise entropic energy loss on binding, such as in Figure 20.7, which can equate to up to 5-fold increase in affinity per frozen rotation.

**Table 20.4** Example ligand efficiencies from lead to candidate drug. LE calculated as $pK_i$/HAC, where HAC = number of heavy, *i.e.*, non-hydrogen atoms.

| Lead | LE | $pK_i$ | Drug | LE | $pK_i$ | Drug name |
|---|---|---|---|---|---|---|
| Leads optimised to drugs with decrease in LE | | | | | | |
| 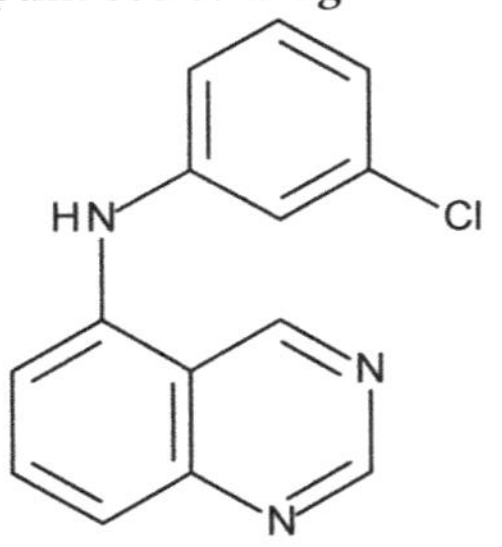 | 0.43 | 7.8 | 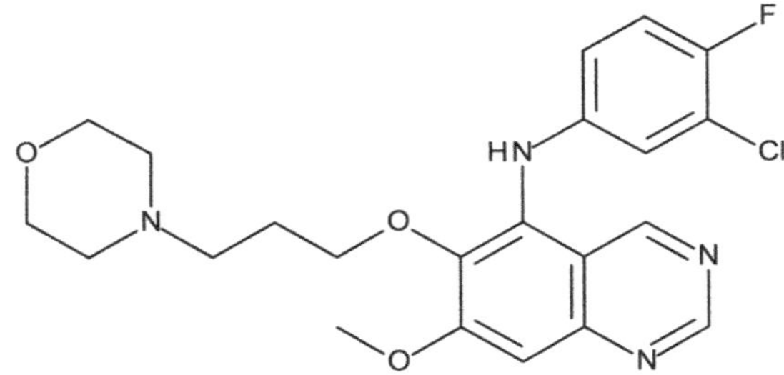 | 0,25 | 7.6 | Gefitinib (EGFR Tyr kinase) |
| 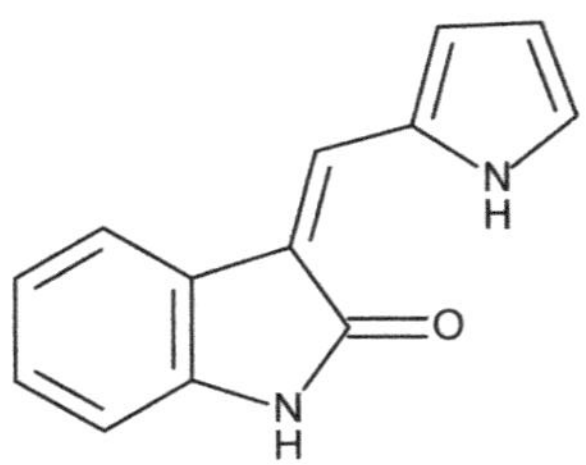 | 0.4 | 6.4 | 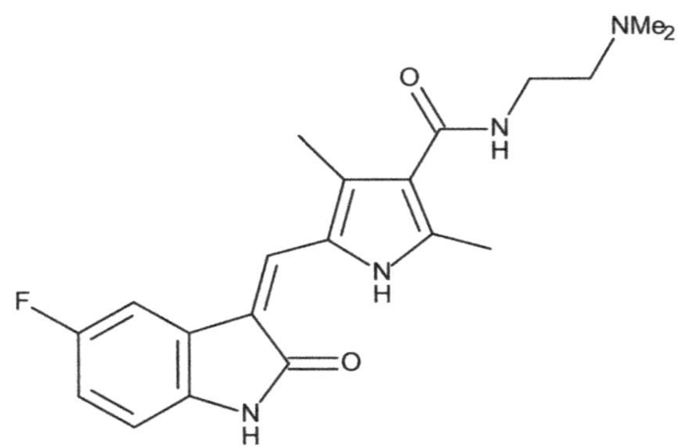 | 0.26 | 7.1 | Sunitinib (VEGF-R2 kinase) |

(*continued*)

**Table 20.4** *(continued)*

| Lead | LE | p$K_i$ | Drug | LE | p$K_i$ | Drug name |
|---|---|---|---|---|---|---|
| Leads optimised to drugs with increase in LE | | | | | | |
| 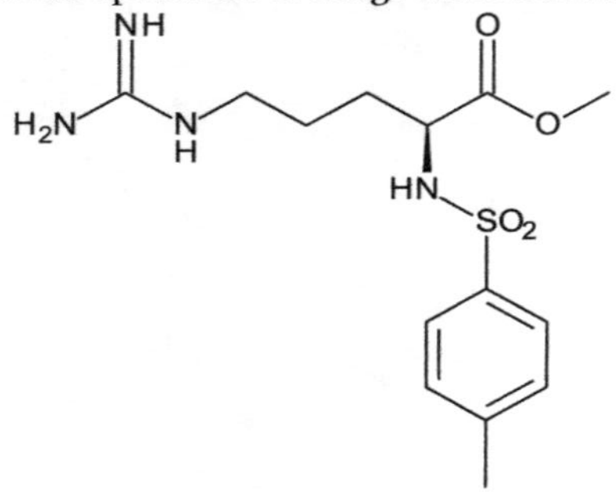 | 0.13 | 3.0 | 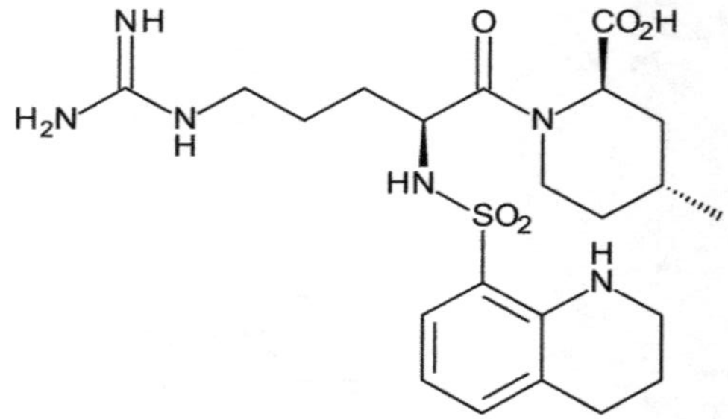 | 0.22 | 7.5 | Argatroban (thrombin) |
| 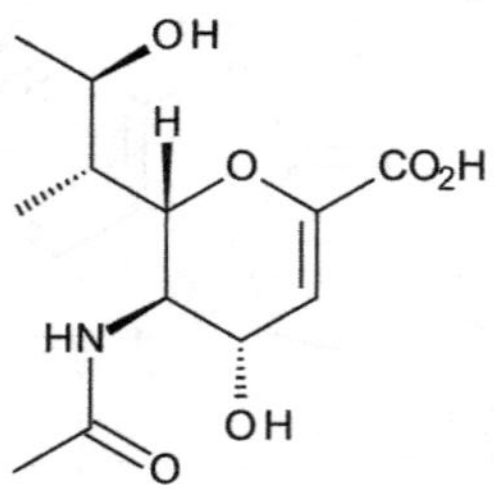 | 0.28 | 5.4 | 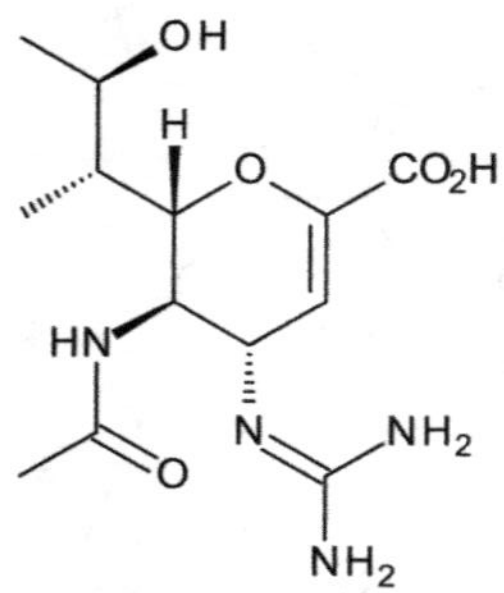 | 0.44 | 9.7 | Zanamivir (influenza neuraminidase) |

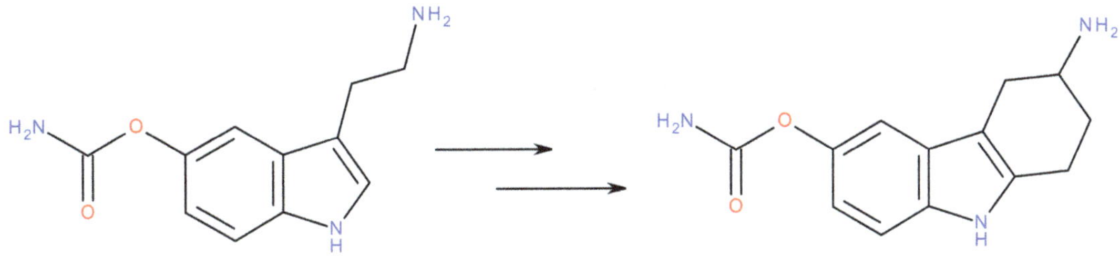


**Figure 20.7** Conformational restriction during lead optimisation.

In addition to the observations above, it is apparent that on average the potency of a drug is superior to that of its parent lead, however the ligand efficiency remains constant. This means that that the overall molecular size increases to achieve greater potency. Earlier chapters have stressed the importance of controlling lipophilicity in drug design, as it plays a major role in off-target and non-specific protein binding, phospholipidosis, solubility, toxicity, and countless other parameters. Together, this requires the medicinal chemist to be particularly aware of the impact on lipophilicity of the design strategy, and as such, the lipophilic ligand efficiency index is helpful:

$$\text{Lipophilic ligand efficiency (LLE)} = \text{pXC}_{50} - \text{clog}P\ (\text{or clog}D \text{ at pH 7.4})$$

This common and significant increase in lipophilicity over the course of an optimisation programme has been recognised as a probable contributor to current candidate attrition rates, although it is a parameter that can be controlled during the optimisation phase with scrutiny of both potency and lipophilicity of proposed and prepared molecules. The challenge to medicinal chemists is to design an optimisation path which improves potency and drug-like properties (potentially including an increase in molecular weight) but which does not overly increase lipophilicity. One way to do this is to optimise LLE. For instance, if a typical oral candidate has a potency of 1–10 nM, or in other words a $\text{pIC}_{50}$ of 8–9, and a typical log*D* of 2 for acceptable physicochemical properties, then the LLE of such a compound should be in the region of 6–7. Since early lead compounds will have lower potency, and possibly higher lipophilicity, starting LLEs are usually much lower, *e.g.*, in the region of 2–3.

### 20.2.5 Drop-off in Cellular Potency and Downstream Assays

One commonly observed issue is that the activity seen in isolated protein assays is not maintained through to cellular systems and onwards to *in vivo* models. The shift to a considerably more complex biological system inevitably introduces many other variables, and one objective of the target validation was to ensure that the targeted protein–ligand interaction is sufficient to drive the required biological effect in a whole organism. Nonetheless, two common parameters can often contribute to lower cellular rather than isolated protein efficacy. Firstly, solubility and permeability, which is required for the lead molecule to access intracellular protein targets or penetrate pathogenic invading organisms/cells. Clearly a molecule which is a potent inhibitor of a target mitochondrial enzyme, but which has low passive permeability will be unlikely to exert its required effect in cells. Furthermore, active efflux from the cell may result in even lower intracellular concentrations. Secondly, non-specific protein binding or non-specific tissue binding can restrict the levels of free drug which can bind to the target protein (as discussed in PK below). Fortunately, these parameters are easily accessed by a range of low-to-high throughput techniques in early lead optimisation. Two models of permeability are commonly employed:[48,49]

1. *PAMPA* (parallel artificial membrane permeability) comprises an artificial hexadecane membrane, across which the test compound can equilibrate, providing a derived apparent permeability for each compound ($P_{app}$).
2. *Caco-2* (colon adenocarcinoma cell line) comprises a confluent monolayer across which the test compound can equilibrate, and which importantly includes several transport proteins (additionally, transporter inhibitors, such as the P-gp inhibitor verapamil, can be included to assess transporter efflux). Compound permeation is measured by LCMS/MS and $P_{app}$ values are calculated. This model is used as a surrogate of intestinal absorption but clearly gives information additionally on general cellular permeability.

Whereas the PAMPA assay gives direct information about the intrinsic permeability of a compound, the Caco-2 assay, being an intact human cell system, gives additional information about the possible efflux of the compound by inherent transporters. Flow from apical to basolateral (AB) is governed by permeability, while flow from basolateral to apical (BA) includes both permeability and transporter effects. Thus Caco-2 generally gives more information. Optimisation away from active transport is frequently required to identify the candidate drug molecule, and whilst there has been considerable focus on PGP,[50] many other transporters exist, of which a subset require attention before committing to clinical evaluation (Table 20.5 below adapted from *Rational Approaches to Improving Selectivity in Drug Design*[51]).

Since plasma binding controls the free concentration in the plasma compartment, and hence the free concentration in all other compartments (if these are at equilibrium, but they are not always) it might seem useful to increase the free concentration

**Table 20.5** Known drug transporters along with their natural substrates.

| Transporter | Natural substrate | Drug substances |
|---|---|---|
| PEPT1 | Dipeptides, tripeptides | Ampicillin, temocapril, enalapril, midodrine, valacyclovir |
| PEPT2 | Dipeptides, tripeptides | Amoxicillin, cefadroxil, cefaclor, bestatin, valganciclovir |
| OCT1 | Organic cations | Zidovudine, acyclovir, ganciclovir, metformin, cimetidine |
| OCT2 | Organic cations | Memantine, metformin, propranolol, cimetidine, quinine |
| OAT1 | Organic anions | Quinidine, pyrilamine, verapamil, valproate, cephaloridine |
| OAT2 | Organic anions | Zidovudine, tetracycline, salicylate, methotrexate, erythromycin |
| OATP-A | Organic anions | Fexofenadine, rocuronium, enalapril, temocaprilat, rosuvastatin |
| OATP-B | Organic anions | Pravastatin, glibenclamide, atorvastatin, Fluvastatin, rosuvastatin |
| OATP-C | Organic anions | Benzylpenicillin, rifampicin, cerivastatin, pitavastatin, methotrexate |

available to engage the target. However, competing processes, such as metabolism, are increased, and, in general, optimisation of plasma binding (alone) for efficacy at decreased dose is not fruitful.[52–54]

However, addition of plasma protein or serum to cell assays to keep cells viable adds an artificial drug-binding sink, reducing the free drug concentration hence reducing the apparent potency of the compound. Such differences between isolated protein assays and cell assays should take account of such shifts, and free potencies should be calculated. Similarly in assays with high cell concentrations, non-specific membrane binding can lower the free drug concentration in the assay, and corrections for such non-specific binding can also be made.

Importantly, and beyond the detailed consideration possible here, differences in biological and pharmacological parameters can have a profound impact when progressing from isolated protein assays through to increasing cell, multicellular, organ, or whole-body studies. One of the most familiar situations is for competitive enzyme inhibitors, for which the concentration of the substrates or ligands can vary greatly from artificial test systems through to real-life situations. For instance, *in vitro* kinase assays are typically run at Km ATP concentrations, but *in vivo* concentrations of ATP (typically 1–5 mM) can result in significant shifts in apparent $IC_{50}$ and selectivity profiles.[55] Moving into more complex systems, such as organoid, organelle, and animal studies, differences in protein expression, dynamic regulation, and the nature of the experiment (*i.e.*, evoked/challenged responses) can all contribute to significant differences between assay readouts, and project teams should be alert to this potential disconnect.[56] GPCR-receptors and ion channels are particularly prone to complexities of functional activity varying considerably across assay systems, and instructive examples of this have been reported for many systems,[56] including 5-HT[57] and β3-adrenergic[58] receptors. Clearly, alternative modes of interaction, *e.g.*, irreversible inhibition, promoted degradation *etc.*, require complementary studies, particularly regarding resynthesis of protein, to understand the target potencies.[59]

## 20.2.6 Selectivity

It is important early in the drug discovery screening cascade to identify those protein targets that are likely to present undesirable off-target activities. These can be proteins that are closely related to the target protein or other proteins that are identified during wider screening. For the latter, it is important to characterise lead exemplars from each chemical series through a wide panel of enzymes, transporters, receptors, and ion channels to identify potential off-target liabilities which can then be included in the screening cascade. Clearly the specific design strategy required to achieve selectivity will depend on the profile being sought; however, a few general principles apply:

- *Conformational restriction.* In general, the more degrees of freedom open to a molecule, the greater the likelihood it will be able to interact with a wider range of biological targets.
- *Lower clogP.* In general terms, there is a correlation of increasing clogP with increasing promiscuity, and log$P$ >3 gives increased risk of off-target activity.[13]
- *Use the literature.* If an undesirable off-target activity is uncovered through cross-screening, this will inevitably be against a target for which there exists at least

one of protein structure, homology model, and/or developed SAR. All this information can be used to guide design of new molecules which will not bind to the undesired protein.

- *Make specific structural changes favourable to the target and unfavourable to the off-targets, while controlling log P.*

Additionally, several companies have shared data across this cross-screening panel set to identify the core set of cross-screening targets required, which provides a useful starting reference point for understanding the top-level risk of the off-target selectivity seen.[9,10]

### 20.2.6.1 Selectivity Vs hERG

In addition to the general selectivity mentioned above, considerable attention is focussed on ensuring molecules do not interact with the hERG potassium ion channel and cause potentially lethal disruption to cardiac rhythms. All drug discovery projects assess hERG binding at an early stage and, whilst the interpretation and follow-up studies are discussed in more detail elsewhere in this book, it is useful to review the main strategies for avoiding hERG inhibition. Optimisation away from hERG blockade can be achieved by lowering $\log P$, reducing the $pK_a$ of a basic nitrogen (or introducing a zwitterion) or by standard structural steric or electronic shape modification.[34,60] An analysis of the literature reported in 2008[7] identified that for molecules with $c\log P > 3$, the most successful strategy was to reduce $\log P$, with an average reduction of $0.8 \times$ hERG binding per log unit of $c\log P$ reduction. However, for molecules with $c\log P < 3$, then structural modifications such as to reduce $pK_a$,[45] introduce steric shielding of basic nitrogen, disrupt potential π-stacking interactions,[44] or replace basic amines with alternative solubilising groups is more successful. It should be stressed that not all hERG blockers are lipophilic molecules containing basic tertiary amines; however, analysis of a wide compound data set[61] identified that to have a 70% chance of achieving a hERG $IC_{50} > 10\ \mu M$ needs $\log D < 3.3$ for a neutral compound and $\log D < 1.4$ for a basic molecule.

Apart from its lethal effects on the heart, another difficulty with hERG inhibition is that historically selectivity against this channel *in vivo* has been over-estimated by measuring selectivity *in vitro*. It is apparent that effects on heart rhythm *in vivo* can occur at low levels of hERG inhibition, around $IC_{20}$, rather than the oft-quoted $IC_{50}$. Thus, margins to hERG activity are required to be higher than to other off-target activities.

### 20.2.6.2 Selectivity Vs Cytochrome P450 Inhibition

As many of the patients your candidate drug is intended to treat will be on other medications, and CYP450s are common metabolising enzymes for many drugs, potent inhibition of a CYP450, or substrates with a low Km, can be perpetrators of drug–drug interactions through inhibition of metabolism of co-administered drugs, or through induction of metabolism if your drug is a inducer of cytochrome P450s. Your drug could also be the victim of drug–drug interactions when administered with drugs that inhibit or induce P450s. Inhibition of P450 enzymes is typically screened initially against the

**Table 20.6** List of major P450 enzymes and their typical example substrates.

| CYP isoform | % Of total CYP | Typical substrate | Example substrate |
|---|---|---|---|
| 1A2 | 13% | Planar<br>Weak base | Caffeine |
| 2C9 | <5% | Weak acid | Ibuprofen |
| 2C19 | <5% | Neutral or weak base<br>2–3 H-bonding groups | Imipramine |
| 2D6 | 2% | H-bond acceptor at 5 Å from metabolic site | Imipramine |
| 3A4 | 30–70% | Promiscuous | Terfenadine |

five major metabolising isoforms (3A4, 2D6, 1A2, 2C9, 2C19). As the project nears nomination of preclinical candidates, it will also be important to understand a wider panel of inhibition potential against specific additional isoforms and subtypes as well as understanding which P450 enzymes are responsible for the metabolism of the parent drug (to predict future drug–drug interactions). Typically, molecules should have no or low inhibition of these enzymes; significant inhibition will lead to additional clinical drug–drug interactions during development and potentially restrict its label for administration. Each P450 enzyme has different, although overlapping, substrate requirements listed in Table 20.6 and advances in the structural determinations of these enzymes, coupled with the ability to use homology models to dock in leads, has allowed rational progress to design out a particular P450-driven interaction. As you reach your shortlist, you may wish to examine the likelihood your drug may induce the synthesis of P450s

Given that the major role of Phase I metabolism is to introduce polar functionality to enable Phase II conjugation and elimination, it should not be surprising that the cytochrome P450 (CYP) enzymes have broad affinity for lipophilic molecules. Therefore, probably the more commonly successful strategy is the lowering of log$P$ and/or altering the overall electronic structure (dipole moment *etc.*) of the molecule. Again, analyses of physicochemical data suggest that reducing log$P$ <3 reduces the likelihood of significant P450 inhibition. Furthermore, many specific functional groups/substructures are known to interact with CYP isoforms, and so can be avoided to reduce risk of P450 inhibition or interaction – Table 20.6. Unhindered neutral nitrogen acceptors, such as found in pyridines, and imidazoles tend to be potent CYP inhibitors due to chelation of the haem iron – but this liability can be mitigated by sterically crowding the nitrogen acceptor by α-substitution.[62]

## 20.2.7 Solubility

The most common complaint of screening biologists is that they have been given 'brick dust' to test, and poor solubility can also lead to false negatives in panel screening, and difficulties in increasing dose in safety studies. As such, optimisation of solubility is a key consideration (later chapters deal with possibilities in formulation and salt/polymorphic forms). Three main strategies are commonly employed:

1. Introduction of polar or ionisable groups such in Figure 20.8. This list is intended to be illustrative rather than exhaustive, however the options for introducing

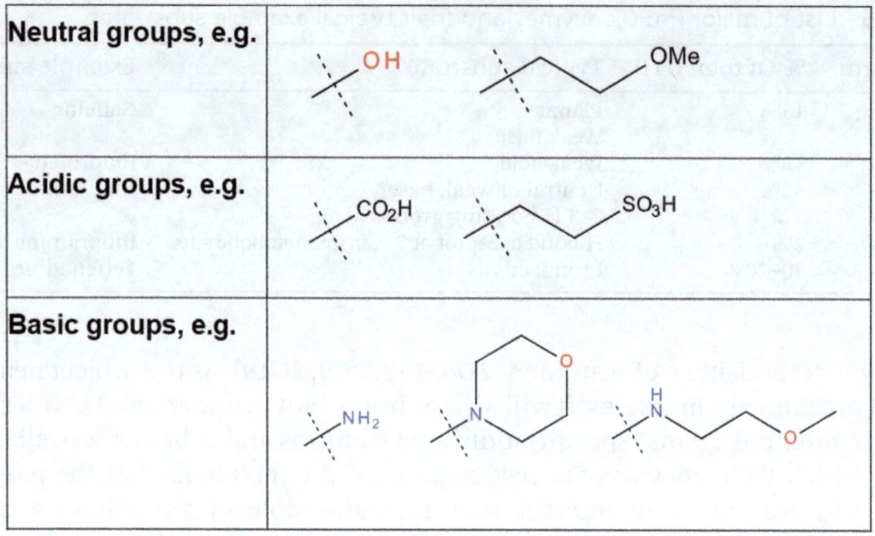


**Figure 20.8** Examples of structures with solubilising functionality.

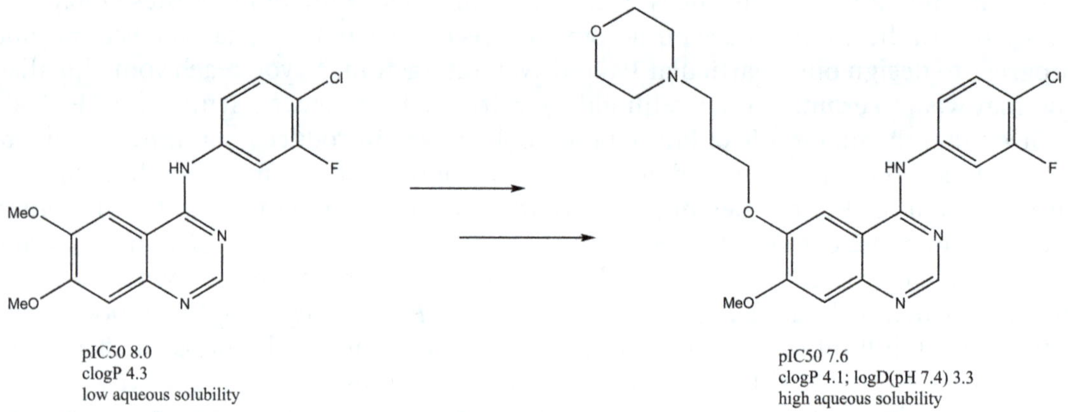


**Figure 20.9** Solubilising strategy to reach tyrosine kinase inhibitor Gefitinib.

neutral, polar or ionisable groups (with awareness of their p$K_a$s) should be clear to any trained organic chemist. For amines, an excellent resource of detailed p$K_a$ analyses for closely related amines is this 2007 review.[45]

By example, the lead optimisation of the tyrosine kinase inhibitor Gefitinib included a late-stage optimisation step in which a solubilising motif was appended to the quinazoline ring at a position known to be tolerant to substitution.[63] (Figure 20.9).

2. *Reduction in clogP* – either by introduction of polar functionality as above, or by removal of lipophilic groups. As a useful mnemonic, solubility decreases approximately 10-fold when log*P* increases by 1 unit. Over 45 000 compounds binned into solubility classes, high solubility was less likely once clog*P* >3.[61,64,65]

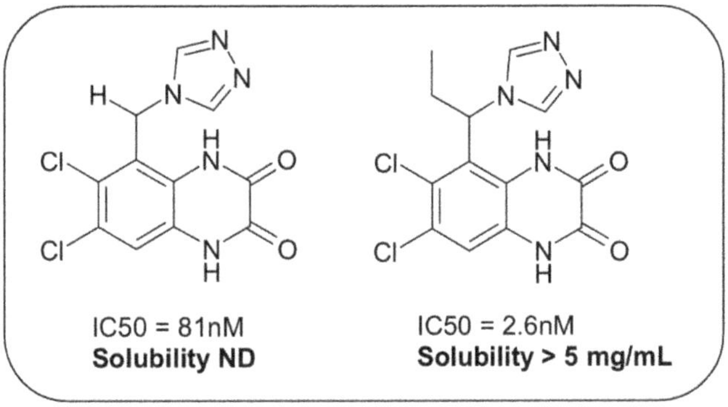


**Figure 20.10** Solubility increase achieved with disruption of crystal packing.

3. Disruption of crystal packing. For example, by introducing substituents to reduce planarity. As another useful mnemonic, solubility decreases by approximately 10× when melting point increases by 100 °C, or more specifically using the general equation reported (Figure 20.10).[66,67]

$$\log \text{Sol (aq.)} = 0.5 - \log P - 0.01(m - 25)$$

where m = melting point in °C

This means that a molecule with a melting point of 150 °C needs to have $\log P < 3.25$ to achieve aqueous solubility >100 μM.

The impact of solubility on the likely absorption of your candidate drug can be assessed by calculating the maximal absorbable dose. It is calculated by:

MAD = sol × $K_a$ × vol × $t$
sol = drug solubility in the <GI tract (mg $mL^{-1}$ at pH 6.5)
$K_a$ = the absorption rate constant (/min)
vol = the volume of fluid in the GI tract (250 mL for man)
$t$ = residence time (approx. 270 minutes for man)

If predicted human dose <MAD, one might anticipate good absorption in man which is not limited by solubility.

## 20.2.8 Metabolism

### *20.2.8.1 Relevance of Test System*

A commonly encountered problem early in lead optimisation is the need to make a molecule more metabolically stable. Metabolic instability is identified both using *in vitro* and *in vivo* experiments and as discussed in the screening cascade section, it is essential that the *in vitro* screening model is an appropriate surrogate for the *in vivo* profile. The example below illustrates this requirement. In the search for a clinical dopamine D3 receptor antagonist (Figure 20.11), the molecule under investigation was found to have good metabolic stability in microsomal preparations leading to moderate turnover *in vivo* and moderate bioavailability in both rats and dogs.[68] Human microsomal

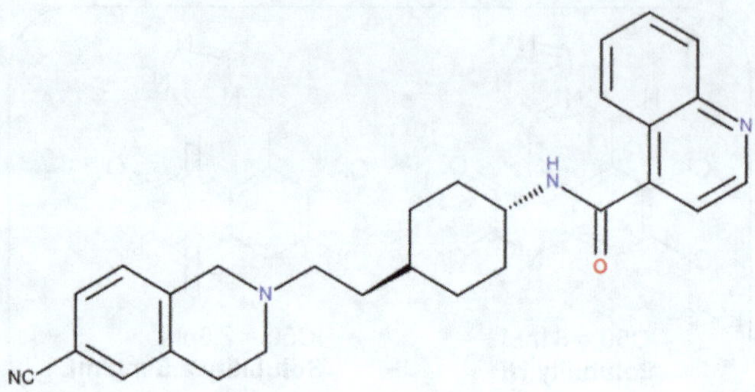

**Figure 20.11** Structure of D3 antagonist.

**Table 20.7** Evaluation of D3 antagonist candidate drug in cross-species pharmacokinetics. % LBF = % liver blood flow.

| | Microsomes $CL_i$ mL $min^{-1}$ $g^{-1}$ | Liver homogenate $CL_i$ mL $min^{-1}$ $g^{-1}$ | $CL_b$ (LBF) mL $min^{-1}$ $g^{-1}$ | $F_{po}$ % |
|---|---|---|---|---|
| Rat | 1.4 | <0.6 | 20 (85%) | 35 |
| Dog | <0.6 | <0.6 | 14 (31%) | 43 |
| Monkey | 1.7 | 9.9 | 58 (44%) | 2 |
| Human | 1.3 | 45 | ND | ND |

turnover was also low and so it was presumed that acceptable PK would be observed in man. However, a confirmatory primate PK study found the molecule to have high clearance and low bioavailability in contradiction to the microsomal stability data, creating uncertainty around the risk of progressing to clinical studies (Table 20.7). Analysis of *in vitro* systems with more metabolic competency, *i.e.*, hepatocytes, rather than microsomes, identified that hepatocytes had a good correlation with all *in vivo* data hitherto generated. Performing the same protocol with human liver homogenates showed the molecule was rapidly turned over and so would have led to a wasted clinical progression. Microsomes are only capable of Phase I metabolism, largely oxidative, and thus predict *in vivo* clearance well only when the *in vivo* metabolism is largely oxidative. Hepatocytes can perform both Phase I and Phase II metabolism, the latter involving conjugative metabolism, and thus better predict the whole metabolic process *in vivo*.

It is worth noting that in those cases where even hepatocyte metabolism does not predict *in vivo* clearance well, that other clearance pathways, *e.g.*, *via* renal or biliary excretion, may account for the increased total clearance observed. Where *in vitro* clearances predicted from hepatocytes do not predict the *in vivo* clearance, a thorough study of routes of clearance is warranted and an assessment of their relevance to man is made. Such non-scaling could be due to extra hepatic metabolism, renal or biliary clearance. Similarly, an unusual Vss for the ion class, or difference in unbound Vss across species may indicate transporter-mediated uptake – and further investigations and risk assessments are warranted to provide confidence in your prediction of volumes of distribution to man.

### *20.2.8.2 Clearance and Strategies to Improve Metabolic Stability*

Getting the right drug half-life is clearly important to establish the desired dosing regimen, and in particular the plasma concentration time course to maximise presence of drug above effective concentration at trough levels and minimising undesirable peaks. Depending on the indication, the target half-life may be short, moderate, or long, and this decision will be informed by detailed understanding of the target pharmacology and reinforced by appropriate PD studies. There are many excellent reviews which summarise these key principles and design opportunities.[19,69,70]

Pragmatically, to target the lowest possible dose of molecule to progress into clinical studies, optimisation strategies should focus on trying to:[19,71]

1. Improve target potency (or affinity) and target selectivity
2. Reduce intrinsic clearance $CL_i$ – and by doing so increase dose-normalised $[AUC]_u$. This will also reduce dosing frequency by increasing half-life (if Vss is unchanged)
3. Increase fraction absorbed (*i.e.*, improve solubility and permeability, reduce efflux, optimise physical form).

Of these, reduction of $CL_i$ by addressing metabolic soft spots can have a profound impact on the overall predicted dose level, and hence a significant proportion of early lead optimisation can be occupied by the need to improve the metabolic stability of the lead molecules.[72–74] There are many approaches to achieve this, the most used being:

1. *Reduction in lipophilicity*. Analysis of a set of molecules from Pfizer identified[7] that acceptably low *in vitro* metabolic turnover was more likely for molecules with $\log D$ $<3$, which can be rationalised by assuming that polar compounds are less likely to undergo Phase I metabolism. However, renal clearance of unchanged parent molecule increases up to 50% for compounds that are very polar, *i.e.*, with $\log D$ in the range 0 to −1.[18,75,76]
2. *Use of classical or non-classical bioisosteres*. This can be a direct replacement of a substituent which is the site of metabolism, for example replacing a hydrogen with a fluorine, or methyl with chlorine to block an oxidative Phase I metabolism, or replacing a metabolically labile peptide linkage with a non-classical isostere (examples in Figure 20.12;[77] readers are referred to the papers on tetrazoles[78] and oxadiazoles[79] as isosteres).
3. *Steric shielding*. Recognising that most metabolic processes are driven by enzymes operating as biocatalysts, we can learn from synthetic organic chemistry and appropriately modify our lead (or starting material) by introducing steric hindrance to slow the rate of reaction.
4. *Use metabolite rather than parent*. Progressing through lead optimisation it is necessary to know not only how much metabolic turnover is occurring but also what metabolites are being formed. Later in the process we also need to understand which are the major metabolising enzymes (to be aware of both drug–drug interaction potential in the clinic and of P450 genetic polymorphisms that exist in the wider population) and whether preclinical efficacy and toxicology species

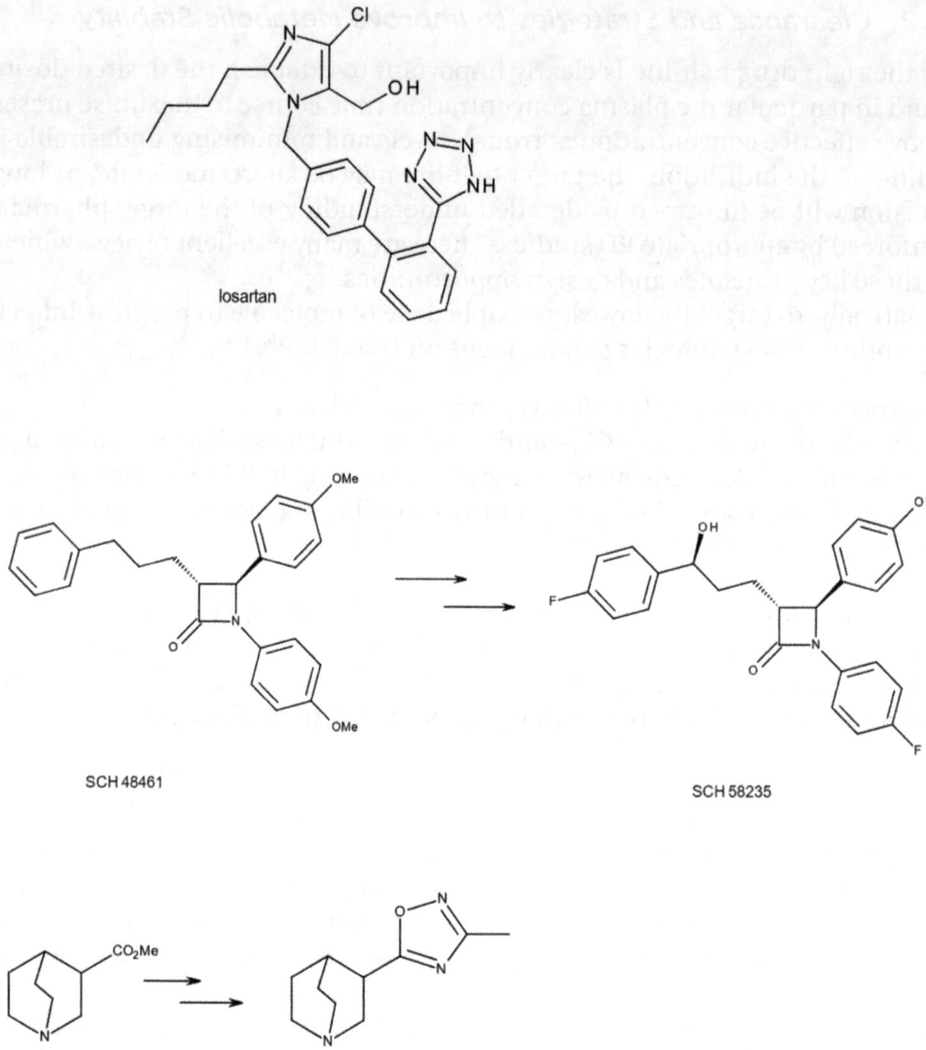


**Figure 20.12** Examples of metabolic blocking strategies: (i) replacement of a carboxylic acid with a tetrazole, as achieved in the hypertension drug losartan; (ii) various strategies implemented during optimisation of SCH 48461 to SCH 58235, including both blocking oxidative metabolism by introduction of a fluorine substituent and also preparation of the oxidised metabolite as a more stable entity. The combination of changes led to a decrease in $ED_{50}$ from 2.2 mg kg$^{-1}$ day$^{-1}$ to 0.04 mg kg$^{-1}$ day$^{-1}$ driven by improved pharmacokinetic exposure; (iii) replacement of a labile ester group with an isosteric oxadiazole motif.

produce the same metabolite profile as man (for appropriate toxicology evaluation). Commonly, simple metabolites also have affinity for the target protein, and sometimes this allows the metabolite to be progressed rather than the parent (see example in Figure 20.12), and also avoids the complexity of producing biologically active metabolites which would have to be extensively characterised and understood.

#### 20.2.8.3 Absorption

As for many of the preceding parameters, an analysis of 232 drugs by Topliss indicated that to achieve oral bioavailability ($F_{po}$) of greater than 80%, essentially all drugs had $\log D$ of between −2 and +3.[80] Further studies have suggested that optimal absorption is achieved at the range $\log D$ = 1–3, although specifically for rat $F_{po}$, a combination of polar surface area (PSA) and rotatable bonds gave a stronger correlation.[81]

Improving the fraction absorbed can be achieved by optimisation of solubility and permeability and minimising efflux. Clearly, as addressed in Chapter 23 on pharmaceutical development, there are many strategies around particle size, dissolution rates and formulations that can also provide significant enhancements.

#### 20.2.8.4 CNS Penetration

In addition to the barriers to achieving high levels of absorption there is an additional barrier involved with achieving high free concentrations of drug in the CNS. Many recent analyses have reiterated the need to focus on *free* concentration of drug in the brain and the ratio of the unbound fraction in brain *vs.* plasma rather than the traditional approach of simply measuring total brain concentrations and deriving brain/blood ratios. Additionally, the CSF drug concentration can sometimes be a surrogate for unbound drug concentrations in the brain, but these data can be misleading, particularly for drugs which are actively transported (P-gp at the blood–CSF barrier pumps into the CSF in contrast to P-gp at the blood–brain barrier).

In broad terms, to achieve appropriate distribution into the CNS, the optimal range of lipophilicity has been analysed to lie within the range $\log P$ 2–3/$\log D$ 1–3, maintaining a PSA <75 Å$^2$, and limiting efflux by tight control of H-bond donors. There are many exceptions to these approximations, but these criteria generally give good passive permeability, as well as minimising possible interactions with efflux proteins.[82]

### 20.2.9 Toxicity and Phospholipidosis

Whilst it is clearly challenging to give specific guidance on how to avoid a variety of toxicities which can halt progression of a molecule or series there are nonetheless some general observations that can be made:

1. *Aim for low overall dose*. Targeting a clinical dose of less than 1 mg kg$^{-1}$ day$^{-1}$ reduces the impact of toxicological issues, in particular hepatotoxicity. Even for reactive metabolites, a total dose of <10 mg has been reported to be acceptable.[35]
2. Avoid functional groups/substructures known to cause specific toxicities.[83,84]
3. *Reduce lipophilicity*. Analysis of Pfizer data indicated that $\log P$ <3 and PSA >75 Å$^2$ gives the lowest risk of non-specific toxicities.[7]
4. *Be aware of risk of phospholipidosis*. The combination of a basic nitrogen and lipophilicity is often required, either for mode of action or designed to balance potency and solubility. However, there is an increased risk of phospholipidosis. In other words, a molecule with a basic centre of p$K_a$ 9 needs $\log P$ <3 and, in general,

singly positively charged molecules require log$P$ <2.75 for lower overall risk of phospholipidosis.[84]

### 20.2.10 Pfizer MPO

To balance the seemingly impossible task of achieving good CNS penetration (clog$P$ 2–3; TPSA (topological polar surface area[85]) $\leq 75$ Å$^2$) in chemical space with low risk of unpredictable *in vivo* toxicity (clog$P$ <3; TPSA >75 Å$^2$), Pfizer have published a multiparametric optimisation tool which uses clog$P$, clog$D$ at pH 7.4, molecular weight, TPSA, HBD, and p$K_a$ to create a means of prioritising molecules for synthesis with an improved chance for CNS penetration. An active version of this calculator is available.[86]

When aiming to optimise a series of lead molecules towards a candidate drug many parameters require to be optimised in parallel, often in opposing directions. However, as described above, many of the parameters are dependent upon lipophilicity, which is a key property to control.[87]

## 20.3 The End Game: Choosing the Candidate Drug

### 20.3.1 Shortlisting

Once one compound is found that fits the screening plan view of a candidate molecule, the project will be able to rapidly synthesise a range of close analogues that all fit or come close to this standard. These compounds will all have subtly different properties. How does the project choose between them? One way is to assemble these compounds into a shortlist and test all these compounds in a stricter fashion to define the best overall compound. At this point there are two main things to check before committing to extensive animal safety studies.

Firstly, the key biochemical results (binding potency, cell potency, iso-enzyme potency, hERG potency, *etc.*) should be repeated enough times that the average result is secure, and will not change, *i.e.*, normally $n = 6$ repetitions will suffice if the results are not too variable. This is particularly important if selectivity criteria are set, *e.g.*, 100-fold selectivity over a related receptor, since the selectivity number is the quotient of two biochemically derived numbers, and even small changes to the primary numbers on retesting can turn a selectivity of 200-fold to one of 50-fold overnight! This is not as unlikely as one might imagine, since the screening plan will naturally select the compounds with the best selectivities on first testing. However, due to the inherent variability of biochemical screens, the best selectivities can arise from the best combination of outliers. Beware! On retesting the numbers will 'regress to the mean' and ultimately the selectivity may be reduced.

Secondly, the project will need to test the shortlisted compounds in a variety of other assays, not on the normal screening plan, to check their suitability as potential development candidates. Dependant on project and company this extended list of tests can be quite long, including simple tests such as CYP induction, whole animal tests for CNS effects, detailed predictions of human pharmacokinetics, safety toxicology studies, preformulation checks (crystallinity, hygroscopicity, thermodynamically most stable solid-state form, dissolution in simulated gastric fluids), and many others. One way for the project to assemble this data is to have a checklist for the data required at candidate drug nomination. A checklist is also very useful to review and update regularly thereafter, and for preparing the data package that will go to governance to get approval for taking the compound into clinical testing.

The use of such a checklist can help a project assemble a complex data package, check what data is already available, what is ongoing and what remains to be done.

### 20.3.2 Scale-up and Safety Testing

Shortlisting is also an effective way of preparing for the synthesis of the larger quantities that are needed during the extensive shortlist testing. The scale-up may require several phases, preparing, for example, batches for multiday rat and dog safety testing, 28-day GLP-standard rat and dog safety toxicology testing, and the large GMP-standard batch required for first time into human (FTIH) Phase 1 clinical testing.

All being well, the extended testing in the shortlisting phase will select the best compound from the shortlist (or at least leave at least one compound left to choose!) for nomination as a candidate drug. Hopefully the compound will come through the safety toxicity testing in rat and dog cleanly, or with sufficient margins to give confidence that dosing in man will be acceptable.

### 20.3.3 Back-up Approaches

The nature of drug discovery is an inherently difficult enterprise. Despite the best efforts of all in the industry to bring forward high-quality candidate drugs into clinical testing, where possible avoiding many of the known toxicities by early screening, the industry in general still suffers from high late-stage attrition. While the fraction of late-stage attrition due to late-appearing toxicity, or suboptimal pharmacokinetics has reduced in recent times, it still forms a part of clinical failure. Once a project has selected a candidate drug, it has been normal practice to search for a back-up compound that could replace the leading molecule should it fail in the clinic for toxicity or PK reasons. Because of the long timescales for feedback from the first compound in the clinic, many back-up compounds have been made without knowledge of any issue with the frontrunner. Therefore chemists, to anticipate problems developing with the first candidate molecule, searched for a back-up from a different structural class, rationalising that a different structure would be most likely to avoid any problems that might arise from the first compound. Thus, projects often made two or more candidate drugs with different structures which progressed into clinical testing in a sequential manner. Recently this strategy has been less favoured for several reasons:

1. The structural differences between the first and second candidates were often not as large as might have been hoped for at the outset, and the second compound failed for the same reason as the first.

2. Even when the structure was from a different series the second compound still failed for the same reason, because the deficiency was due to a common substituent, or a common physicochemical parameter.
3. It is costly and inefficient to have several clinical candidates aimed at the same target all going through clinical testing, even if staggered. Especially if they do not actually serve to replace a failure of the first candidate molecule.

It appears that the candidate family strategy often fails. However, it is also clear that the first molecule progressed into the clinic often does not become the drug, and only after a few candidate drugs have been through the cycle that the learning of these late-stage experiments can inform the project on how to prepare improved molecules that can go on to become successful drugs.

An alternative strategy might be to find the first candidate, then move resource off the project (to work on other targets). Only if, and when, the first molecule has an issue, would resource then be reapplied to discover a new improved molecule without the issue found in the first. This alternate strategy saves resource but may lose time (and dissipate experience).

Nowadays, to have a successful candidate drug, the organisation not only has to have the right molecule, but it should have the right animal data predictive of the disease state, the right safety profile, and the right clinical plan with the right biomarkers, aimed at delivering real benefit to the right patient segment, delivered at the right cost. All of this must be in place for the project's proposal to get its candidate drug accepted to progress into the next phase, that of clinical testing, where the organisation can have confidence in producing a meaningful clinical effect in patients.

## 20.4 LTC4S Inhibitor LO Case Study[88]

The arachidonic acid cascade forms a plethora of pro-inflammatory and pro-resolution lipid metabolites, including prostaglandins, thromboxanes, and leukotrienes, known to be involved in inflammation, bronchoconstriction, and pain. In particular, the cysteinyl leukotrienes (cysLTs, LTC4, LTD4, and LTE4) are strongly associated with asthma, as demonstrated by the clinical efficacy of cysteinyl leukotriene receptor 1 antagonists, montelukast, zafirlukast, and pranlukast, and the 5-lipoxygenase inhibitor, zileuton.

While these leukotriene modulators have reached the market, they have not achieved enough clinical efficacy to become the core of the asthma treatment pathway, which is dominated by short- and long-acting bronchodilators and increasing doses of inhaled corticosteroids, leading to oral steroids and biologic drugs for the most severe asthmatics. Still up to 50% of asthma patients remain uncontrolled on standard of care medication. With such a complex cascade, and clear unmet medical need, it remains an open question whether the optimum point to intervene in the leukotriene cascade had been found with the current drugs.

Montelukast, the archetypal cysteinyl leukotriene receptor antagonist (cysLTRec1) drug, blocks the action of LTD4 (and LTC4) at cysteinyl leukotriene receptor 1, but not the effects of LTC4 at its own receptor cysteinyl leukotriene receptor 2, nor the effects of LTE4 at its own putative LTE4 receptor. Zileuton blocks the complete synthesis of the cysteine leukotrienes and also LTB4, which has an equivocal role in asthma, but also blocks synthesis of LXA4, which has been shown to have a role in resolving inflammation (pro-resolution). Neither montelukast nor zileuton block the production of the pro-inflammatory eoxins, which, being products from the 15-lipoxygenase cascade are regioisomers of the cysteine leukotrienes, Figure 20.13.

Inhibition of the enzyme LTC4S may be a differentiated point to block the leukotriene cascade (Figure 20.13) as it would block the synthesis of LTC4, LTD4, LTE4, and EXC4, EXD4, and EXE4 while preserving LTB4 and pro-resolution LXA4.

Scientists from the Karolinska Institute, based on their history in leukotriene research and through a spinout called Biolipox (subsequently acquired by Orexo AB), began a project to discover potent selective inhibitors of LTC4S.

Dibenzoic acid (Figure 20.14) was identified as an $IC_{50}$ = 1.9 μM hit in a focussed screen of 400 commercially available compounds in an LTC4S enzyme assay. However, the hit suffered from poor physicochemical properties and was not active in the immediate downstream cellular assay. Rational design focussed on increasing potency and drug-like properties, which resulted in a monobenzoic acid which was potent in the LTC4S enzyme assay ($IC_{50}$ = 35 nM). By adding a methoxy substituent to the core pyridyl ring and extending the alkyl chain on the amine to a methyl cyclopropyl, the large 2-methoxy benzamide side chain could be removed, keeping potency in the LTC4S enzyme assay ($IC_{50}$ = 27.4 nM), improving physiochemical properties, and achieving activity in the PBMC cell assay ($IC_{50}$ = 46.7 nM).

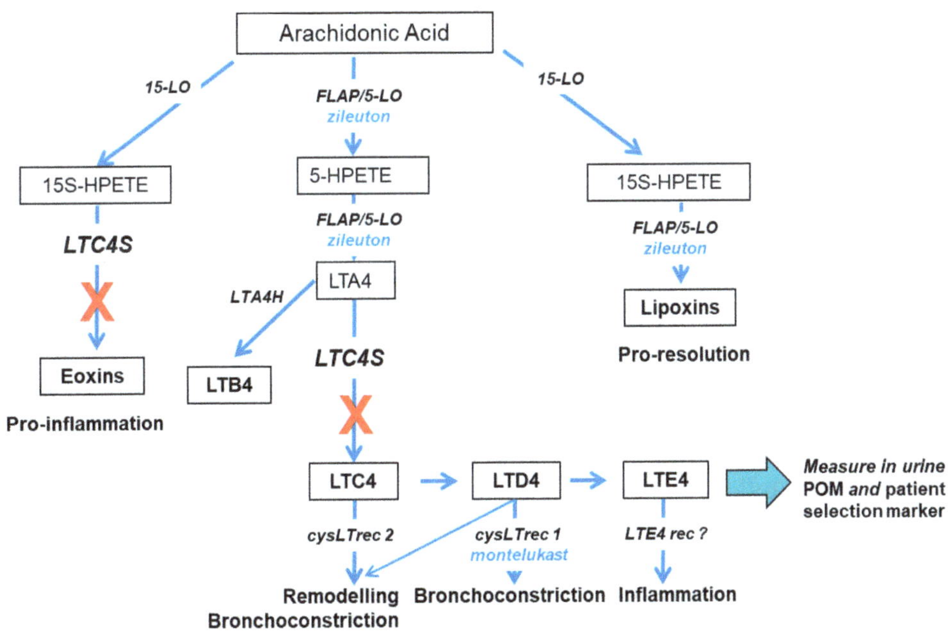


**Figure 20.13** Differentiation in the arachidonic acid cascade of an LTC4S inhibitor (marked with a red cross) compared to a cysteinyl leukotriene receptor 1 antagonist, montelukast, and a 5-lipoxygenase inhibitor zileuton.

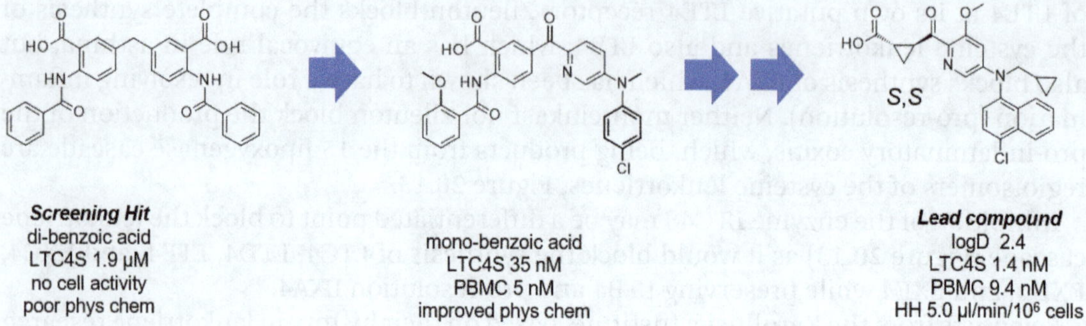


**Figure 20.14** The origins of the LTC4S inhibitor lead.

Having established cell potency, the focus was to further improve properties for oral administration. Exchanging the benzoic acid to a cyclopropane carboxylic acid further lowered lipophilicity to $\log D_{7.4}$ = 1.3, while retaining potency. The low lipophilicity of the cyclopropyl carboxylic acid allowed scope for a more lipophilic substituent on nitrogen and 4-chloronaphthyl was introduced. The most active S,S enantiomer further improved potency both in the enzyme assay $IC_{50}$ = 1.4 nM and in the PBMC assay $IC_{50}$ = 9.4 nM.

While the carbonyl was a concern as a site of metabolism, further studies showed the flanking cyclopropyl and the *ortho*-methoxy groups appeared to protect the keto function from reduction, minimising the overall hepatocyte $CL_{int}$.

The high potency of the lead compound, together with its reasonable stability in human hepatocytes, low percentage of keto reduction, and excellent aqueous solubility (576 µM @ pH 7.4) and permeability (Caco-2 apical–basal permeability at pH 6.5, 105 × $10^{-6}$ cm $s^{-1}$), prompted further profiling.

*In vivo* rat pharmacokinetics of the lead compound showed moderate clearance (12 mL $min^{-1}$ $kg^{-1}$) and an unusually high volume of distribution for an acid of 2.8 L $kg^{-1}$, suggesting some transporter-mediated uptake, yielding an effective half-life of 2.7 h. The rat oral bioavailability was 46%. The crossover of potency from human to rat was excellent, and it showed *in vivo* activity inhibiting cysteine leukotriene production in a calcium ionophore challenge rat model. Furthermore, the lead compound had no significant cytochrome P450 inhibition (>20 µM for CYP1A2, CYP2C9, CYP2C19, CYP3A4, and CYP2D6) and no significant hERG inhibition, and was negative in the five-strain Ames genotoxicity assays. With the series looking very attractive with scope for further optimisation, Orexo approached AstraZeneca to partner the project into the LO phase. AstraZeneca evaluated the project using the 5Rs framework (Table 20.1):

1. Right target looked a low risk with clinical efficacy already achieved with molecules acting above and below LTC4 on the pathway, although differentiated efficacy was a risk.
2. Right tissue was assessed as low risk, as an oral cell-permeable small molecule should inhibit LTC4S everywhere in the body, including the lungs, as the free drug hypothesis assumes the free concentration would be at equilibrium in all

compartments, which could be demonstrated with the right molecule in animal models.

3. Right safety was judged medium risk, as although no LTC4S inhibitors had been in man, molecules acting above and below LTC4 on the pathway had reached the market, albeit with safety flags. Zileuton leads to elevation in liver enzymes which require monitoring in the clinic, and montelukast had a label indicating a rare risk for suicidal ideation. Other compounds on the pathway (5-LO inhibitors) that had reached clinical development stages had reported signs of testicular toxicity in rats.
4. Right patients and right commercial were both the biggest opportunity and biggest risk for the project. The activity of the cysteine leukotriene cascade can be easily measured *via* the level of the stable end-product of the cascade LTE4 in urine. High urinary LTE4 (uLTE4) levels indicating a highly activated cascade can be measured in patients even on high dose steroids, and its levels correlated with the stability of a patient's asthma. The uLTE4 could be used as a personalised approach to identify the right patients most likely to respond to the treatment and even provide the potential for a complementary diagnostic for patient selection.
5. Right commercial posed a risk as two marketed and generic drugs already acted on this pathway, zileuton's use was limited by 4× day dose frequency and liver signals that required monitoring during clinical use, and hence was not widely used. However, montelukast, even with its modest efficacy, because of its a once-a-day dosing regimen, clean safety profile, and low cost posed a bigger commercial risk. An LTC4S inhibitor would always be compared to montelukast, unless evidence could be generated that an LTC4S inhibitor gave not only better efficacy but could work where montelukast had failed. So, the project needed to not only discover an excellent molecule, but also provide confidence in differentiation, evidence of a patient subgroup who might respond well to an LTC4S inhibitor (and ideally not respond to montelukast), and a clinical plan that managed the biggest project risk as early as possible.

Montelukast had never been tested in a selected patient population, and there was evidence from clinical challenge studies, as a competitive antagonist of LTD4, its efficacy may be attenuated in patients with a high cysteine leukotriene drive. The molecule would be tested in Phase 2 in a population most highly dependent on the mechanism, an extreme patient phenotype, identified by a composite biomarker of:

(a) high LTE4 showing an activated mechanism, (b) patients with high FeNO/eosinophil levels showing lung inflammation, and (c) who are likely to also be aspirin intolerant, a classic well-studied asthma subgroup who have high ulTE4 levels and nasal polyp phenotype, also a common feature of aspirin-intolerant patients. In this population the new inhibitor would be compared head-to-head with montelukast. Success here in demonstrating differentiated efficacy, would provide confidence in trialling in a broader population of aspirin-tolerant and aspirin-intolerant asthma patients who also possessed a similar composite biomarker and for life cycle management, in other cysteine leukotriene diseases.

The LO project vision became to develop a new personalised healthcare medicine bringing improved disease control to patients and physicians which treats cysteine leukotriene-driven inflammation and bronchoconstriction in patients with a highly activated cysteine leukotriene cascade.

But first, before a decision to enter LO was taken, the quality of the lead compound was fully assessed. To further evaluate the lead, the compound was progressed to a rat 7-day oral toxicology study at 30 and 300 mg $kg^{-1}$ (6 animals per group including controls, 3 males + 3 females) and was well tolerated at both doses. A complete histochemical assessment was undertaken, and unilateral sperm granulomas in the epididymal sperm duct were found in the high-dose male group of rats. These findings were attributed to potent inhibition of organic anion-transporting polypeptide 1B1 (OATP1B1) (0.6 μM) and/or other ATP-binding cassette (ABC) transporters, as these have been shown to protect sperm cells from xenobiotics. At the exposures achieved in the safety study, approaching 140 μM (~1 μM free) at $C_{max}$, OATP1B1 would have been inhibited.

A secondary pharmacology assessment in a panel of >150 *in vitro* radioligand binding and enzyme assays covering a diverse set of enzymes, receptors, ion channels, and transporters, found that the lead compound overall had a clean profile. However, it was a potent GABA-A-gated $Cl^-$ channel (rat cerebral cortex) binder with $IC_{50}$ = 0.074 μM. GABA-A receptor potentiators are anxiolytic, anticonvulsant, antihyperalgesic, sedative, could impair motor function, cause muscle relaxation, ataxia, dizziness, depression, and anterograde amnesia. Antagonists and negative allosteric modulators could be excitatory and pro-convulsant, and lead to seizures.

The chemistry team were confident they could mitigate the risks with the lead compounds with an LO strategy focussed upon maintaining high PBMC potency and low hepatocyte turnover, while reducing log*D* to reduce a general log*D*-driven toxicology risk, including the interactions with transporter proteins and GABA binding.

Ultimately, with confidence in the chemistry scope, and a 5Rs-based plan, interest and excitement in the project grew and the project entered LO.

The aims for the LO project stretched beyond just identifying the right molecule (right tissue, right safety) to provide evidence:

- An evolved LTC4S inhibitor could inhibit the cysteine leukotriene pathway and eoxin pathway, while not only preserving, but potentially even boosting pro-resolution LXA4 levels (right target)
- Build confidence in the size of commercially viable patient subset (right commercial)
- Develop a crisp clinical development plan to mitigate the montelukast differentiation risk (right patient)
- Create plans for a diagnostic to select patients which could be used in the clinical phases of the programme.

A screening cascade to mitigate the deficiencies of the lead compound was established, and assays conducted in parallel were defined as "waves", as previously described in Table 20.3.

Wave 1 contained the critical assays guiding compound design including LTC4S enzyme and PBMC cell potencies, physicochemical properties, metabolic stability, and

GABA binding. For compounds progressing to Wave 2, permeability and rat pharmacokinetics were included to explore *in vivo* pharmacokinetic properties and *in vitro* to *in vivo* scaling of clearance. Finally, in Wave 3, compounds were assessed for dog pharmacokinetics as a second pharmacokinetic species to provide additional confidence in predicting human pharmacokinetics. They were also assessed for efficacy in the rat lung calcium ionophore challenge PKPD model, in which the degree of inhibition of cysteinyl leukotriene production measured in rat bronchoalveolar lavage after calcium ionophore challenge was measured after oral administration of the LTC4S inhibitor. No preclinical disease model was used, as translatable models of asthma for interfering with the leukotriene cascade at this point did not exist, rather the PKPD model provided confidence in the time–concentration relationships between plasma levels and lung inhibition of LTC4S. For shortlisting potential clinical candidates, an integrated *in vitro* approach to risk-assess the potential for liver toxicity and idiosyncratic drug reactions in humans was undertaken. This consisted of assays addressing: (1) covalent binding of the parent compound or metabolites to human hepatocytes, (2) toxicity to transformed human liver epithelial 2 (THLE) cells with and without metabolic activation, (3) mitochondrial toxicity in HepG2 cells, and (4) inhibition potential against the human bile salt export pump (BSEP) and multidrug resistance associated protein 2 (MRP2). Additional safety liabilities were assessed through Ames assays, and pharmaceutical developability was assessed through crystallinity and melting points.

In a series of classic medicinal chemistry steps, focussing on potency, LLE and using the information from an X-ray structure of one of the lead molecules, the lead was optimised toward a candidate drug, Figure 20.15. Replacing the chloro-naphthyl of the lead molecule by 3-Cl phenyl lowered log*D* but lost potency and did not drastically improve human hepatocyte $CL_{int}$. Reducing log*D* did, however, have a clear effect on the GABA-A binding potency. Optimising the aniline by using knowledge of the X-ray, suggested a 5-F may be tolerated, which would also block a site of metabolism, and indeed 5-F

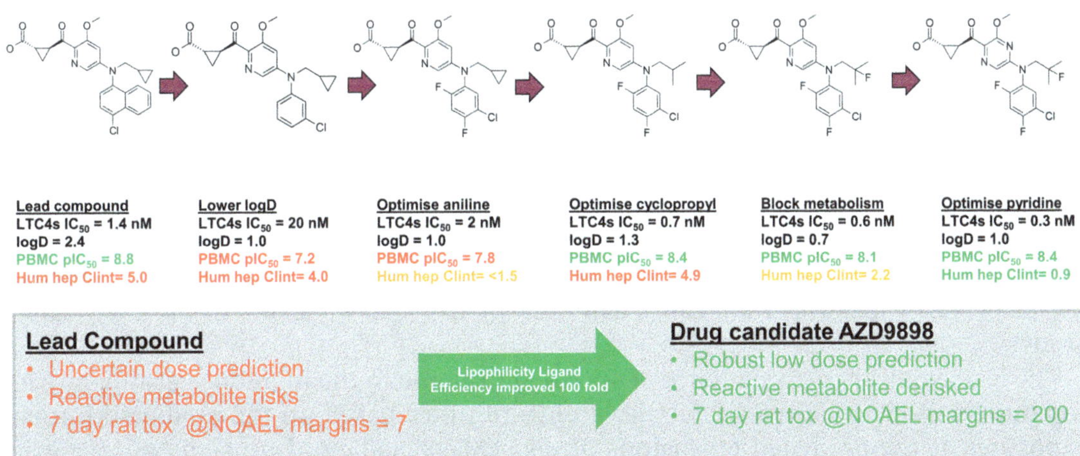


**Figure 20.15** Compound evolution towards the candidate drug.

improved both potency and reduced human hepatocyte $CL_{int}$. Opening the cyclopropyl to the isobutyl sidechain improved the shape match to the active site according to the X-ray modelling, removed a potential site for reactive metabolism (glutathione adducts had been seen for some homologues bearing the cyclopropyl sidechain), and resulted in an increased potency but introduced a further metabolic soft-spot. Fluorination blocked that metabolic site, reducing human hepatocyte $CL_{int}$ and lowering log$D$ further. Finally, the pyridine was replaced by pyrazine, which from the X-ray structure and QM calculations was predicted to have higher affinity to LTC4S. Indeed, the pyrazine core displayed a 2-fold increase in the LTC4S binding and PBMC potency compared to the pyridine matched pairs. AZD9898 proved to be potent, stable, clear of transporter interactions, GABA-A binding, and showed a good off-target selectivity profile.

AZD9898 showed a low turnover in human, monkey, dog, and rat hepatocyte incubations, which was also reflected in low plasma clearance observed *in vivo* in the preclinical species (<2% of liver blood flow). The unbound steady state volume of distribution (Vss) varied between rat and dog, which posed a risk for the prediction of the human volume of distribution. To increase confidence in predicting human Vss, the pharmacokinetics of AZD9898 was explored in a cynomolgus monkey in which the unbound Vss was found to be similar to the Vss of the dog. As that of the dog and monkey was more consistent, the human Vss estimate was based on these two species. AZD9898 had excellent pharmaceutical properties, being a non-hygroscopic crystalline anhydrate with a melting point of 129 °C, with no other thermal events. It showed no reactivity to glutathione and did not inhibit cytochrome P450 isoforms up to 30 μM. It displayed excellent selectivity in a panel of >200 *in vitro* radioligand binding and enzyme assays, covering a diverse set of enzymes, receptors, ion channels, and transporters. The only activity identified within 100× the human predicted $C_{max}$ was an interaction with GABA-A as a positive allosteric modulator at 24× the human predicted $C_{max}$. A positive allosteric modulator would enhance an endogenous response to GABA. No signs of GABA receptor potentiation were observed in any of the rat toxicology studies at up to 122 times the human predicted exposure, and the *in vitro* observation was assessed as a low risk for progression. Additionally, the compound had no activity below 33 μM in a panel of cardiovascular ion channels, hERG, kKV7.1, hKV4.3, hNav1.5, and hCaV1.2 showing >300× margins to human predicted free $C_{max}$, and was negative in a five-strain Ames genetic toxicology assessment. Taken together, these data demonstrated that AZD9898 was a highly selective LTC4S inhibitor with a low risk for off-target effects.

AZD9898 was evaluated head-to-head with the original lead compound in a 7-day rat toxicology study. In the study, doses were chosen so that AZD9898 achieved matching or greater exposures than those achieved by the lead molecule in the early safety study.

The lead again showed evidence of sperm granuloma in the high-dose group, providing margins to a no adverse effect level of 7–16 times based on the predicted human exposures at the predicted efficacious doses. AZD9898 showed no signs of rat testicular pathology and only adaptive changes in the liver due to cytochrome P450 induction, which were not judged as adverse, providing a 200-fold margin between the no adverse effect level and the predicted human exposure at the predicted therapeutic dose.

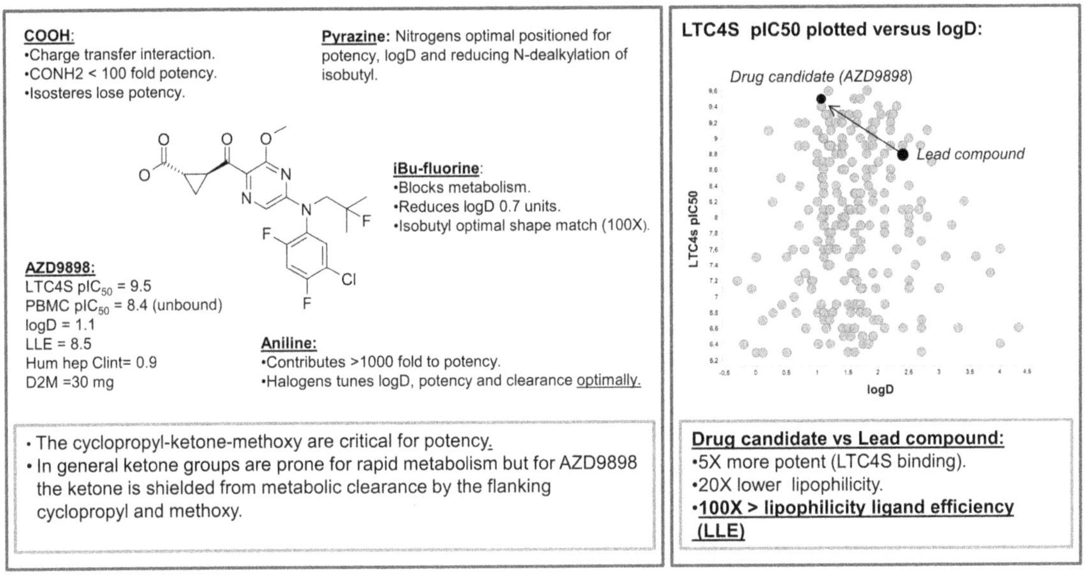


**Figure 20.16** Every atom of AZD9898 contributes to its candidate drug profile.

Finally, the compound showed only minimal effects at high margins in anesthetised guinea pig and dog telemetry cardiovascular assessment models. AZD9898 was selected for progression into preclinical development. Every atom contributes to its candidate drug profile is shown in Figure 20.16.

## 20.4.1 Pharmacological Profile of AZD9898

The PKPD relationship for *in vivo* LTC4S inhibition by AZD9898 was explored in a calcium ionophore challenge rat model, measuring inhibition of cysLT production in the lung following oral delivery. A dose–response experiment was first performed where the compound was administered 2 h prior to a terminal bronchoalveolar lavage with calcium ionophore A23187 followed by a time-course experiment where the challenge was done 0.5, 2, 6, and 24 h post a single dose and 0.5, 2, and 6 h after four days of daily oral dosing. The relationship between AZD9898 plasma concentration and reduction of cysLT in the BAL fluid across both experiments was well described by a sigmoid Emax model, suggesting that inhibition of leukotriene production in the rat lung was related to the instantaneous plasma level at the timepoint of the PD measurement, Figure 20.17.

While the PBMC assay proved a very robust cellular system in which to study LTC4S inhibition, to further explore the efficacy of AZD9898 in translational cell models, its potency was measured in $Ca^{2+}$-stimulated eosinophils, IgE-stimulated mast cells and $Ca^{2+}$-stimulated whole blood from healthy volunteers and asthmatic patients. The compound had the expected differentiated profile, inhibiting cysteinyl leukotriene production and eoxins, while preserving LTB4 and even boosting pro-resolution LXA4.

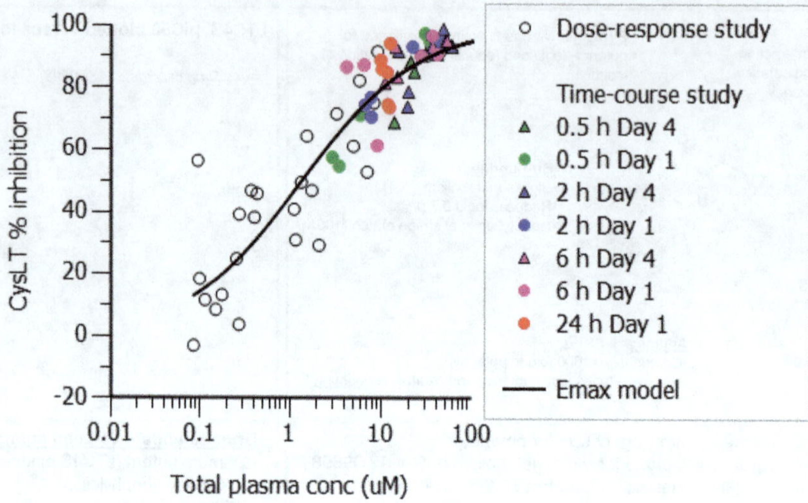


**Figure 20.17** Correlation of inhibition of cysLT production in rat lung stimulated by calcium ionophore to total plasma levels at the point of challenge. In the dose-response study, AZD9898 was administered orally 2 h prior to a calcium ionophore challenge *via* BAL. In the time-course study, the challenge was done 0.5, 2, 6, or 24 h post a single dose and 0.5, 2, or 6 h after four days of daily oral dosing at 3 or 10 mg $kg^{-1}$. Data across both studies were pooled and fitted to a sigmoid Emax model, yielding an $EC_{50}$ of 1.36 μM (CI 95%, 0.99–1.7), corresponding to an unbound $EC_{50}$ of 34 nM, which is within 5.2-fold of the free $IC_{50}$ measured in the human PBMC assay of $IC_{50}$ = 6.5 nM.

After correction for non-specific binding in each assay, free potencies for cysLT inhibition showed considerable variability, from 8 nM in zymosan-stimulated PBMCs, 22 nM in calcium ionophore-stimulated nasal polyp tissue from asthma patients, 38 nM in mast cells stimulated to produce cysLTs by anti-IgE, 38 nM in calcium ionophore-stimulated whole blood to 126 nM in $Ca^{2+}$-stimulated eosinophils. While changes in potency across cell assays can often be ascribed to artifacts of the assay setup, differences in non-specific binding leading to changes in free drug levels, and the "drive" in the system to be overcome by the inhibitor, comprehensive investigations could not explain the variability. As inhibition of the pathway can be measured very easily in the clinic, even after a single dose by monitoring LTE4 levels in urine (or plasma) the decision was taken to predict the human dose from the PBMC assay which showed the best precision with large *n* numbers, and assess an effective dose in the SAD phase in the Phase 1 clinical study.

## 20.4.2 Human Dose Predictions

The human effective dose at the steady state for AZD9898 was predicted, assuming a direct PKPD relationship in man, as was demonstrated for the rat in the calcium ionophore challenge model, and the requirement to maintain inhibition of at least 75% throughout the dosing period (free plasma concentration: 3 × PBMC $IC_{50}$, free).[23] The human PK parameters used to calculate a dose aiming to achieve the corresponding plasma concentration were a volume of distribution of 0.6 L $kg^{-1}$, predicted based on the average unbound volumes observed in the dog and cynomolgus monkey, and human clearance of 0.5 mL $min^{-1}$ $kg^{-1}$, estimated using a liver blood flow method. The predicted human effective half-life was 14 h, and assuming high and rapid absorption, the human predicted dose was 30 mg once a day. With the high permeability (Caco-2 $P_{app}$: 47 × $10^6$ cm $s^{-1}$) and solubility, the maximal absorbable dose[89,90] was calculated to be 10 g, suggesting a low risk for absorption limiting exposure at a 30 mg effective dose.

The compound progressed to 14-day non-GLP rat/dog safety studies. In rat, no testicular lesions were observed, as before, only an increase in liver weights, but with no associated liver pathology and a NOAEL of 14× human predicted exposures. This was classed as an adaptive change due to CYP P450 induction. However, surprisingly in dog, signs of testicular tubular degeneration were observed (NOAEL exposure 23-fold higher than predicted human). As this change was non-monitorable in clinical studies and reversibility was not demonstrated, an additional 10× safety margin was likely to be imposed, which meant exposures only up to 2.3× predicted therapeutic dose could be explored in Phase 1. The compound progressed to 14-day rat/dog GLP studies, with more males added in the dog dose groups and a 1-month recovery phase added to study reversibility. Similar testicular pathology was observed, and while some recovery was observed in the 1-month recovery periods, it was not complete, and the compound went forward into Phase 1 with the additional 10× safety cap.

With the uncertainties in potencies observed in *in vitro* cell assays, and the limited dose ranges that could be explored in the clinic, there was little room for error. If the effective human dose was significantly higher than 2.3 × 30 mg, a robust Phase 2 study could not be undertaken, as high enough doses to significantly block the pathway (>75% inhibition at $C_{min}$) could not be reached. To de-risk the testicular lesions, a 3-month dog study with 6-month recovery was recommended, but that would have required more drug substance than was available and would have delayed reaching the pivotal Phase 2 head to head study with montelukast – which was deemed a bigger risk to compound progression. As a result, the pivotal safety study was phased after Phase 2A. But as uLTE4 was such a facile biomarker of inhibition of the pathway, and inhibition of uLTE4 could be detected after even a single dose in healthy volunteers, the effective dose could be determined in the clinic. In healthy volunteers, cysLTs are continually produced from basal metabolism from the whole body, while in asthma patients, high cysLT levels are probably driven by their lung pathology. So, an additional SAD cohort of asthmatics with high uLTE4 was included in the Phase 1 studies so PKPD would reflect cysLT inhibition in the right compartment.

Meanwhile, the team sought evidence of the size of the potential patient population. The U-BIOPRED database[91] is a pan EU consortium that contains clinical and biomarker data across healthy volunteers, mild/moderate, and severe asthmatics. The analysis showed that a significant percentage of patients had high uLTE4 levels, particularly in the severe asthmatic cohort, Figure 20.18.

The 5Rs at the end of LO looked appealing (Figure 20.19). So based on its profile, AZ136AZD9898 progressed into Phase 1 clinical development. Overall, single doses were well tolerated, and no safety concerns were raised. Measurements of uLTE4 normalised to creatinine were included as a pharmacodynamic marker to evaluate inhibition of

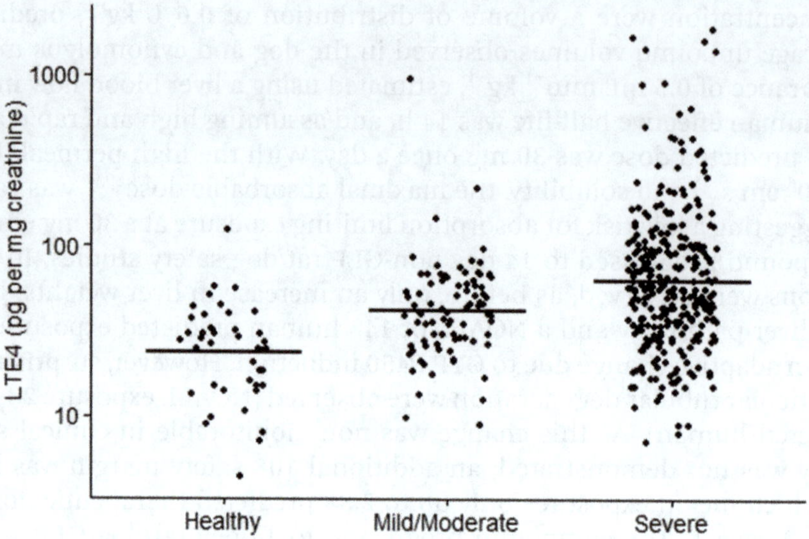


**Figure 20.18** Distribution of uLTE4 (pg mg$^{-1}$ of creatinine) with asthma severity from the U-BIOPRED database.

| Criterion | | Evaluation |
|---|---|---|
| Right target/ efficacy | Target | • Role of CysLT pathway is clinically validated in bronchial hyper-reactive patients (montelukast(CysLTR1 antagonist) and zileuton (5-LO inhibitor)<br>• AZD9898 completely blocks the CysLTs production in all tested in vitro and in vivo preclinical models.<br>• LTC4S inhibitors have shown to inhibit eoxins while preserving the lipoxins in vitro which have a role in inflammation resolution.**GAP:** Potency differences in artificial isolated cell assays which are not representative of the complex disease system. **Activity:** Continuing iinvestigation of compound potency in nasal polyp tissue from asthmatic patients where all cell types are represented |
| | Efficacy | • LTC4S inhibitor fully blocks the bronchoconstrictive and inflammatory effects of LTC4, LTD4 and LTE4 and the recently discovered eoxins, preserving resolution pathways, while LTRA antagonists such as montelukast only block LTD4. **GAP**: First in Class mechanism; clinical efficacy and differentiation of LTC4S inhibition remains to be demonstrated. **Activity:** Efficacy and differentiation from montelukast to be assessed in phase 2a study. |
| Right tissue/ right exposure | | • CysLTs production in the rat lung is inhibited following oral administration of AZD9898 (in the Rat Ca ion model) with a direct PKPD relationship (degree of inhibition and unbound plasma concentration).<br>• Excellent oral PK properties with high permeability, high oral availability and low clearance across all pre clinical assays studied. Low predicted dose once daily. **GAP:** Uncertainty in potency value used for dose-to-man prediction , may lead to higher required exposure would could increase DDI risk . **Activity:** uLTE4 measured in Ph1 program provides early target engagement marker to support human dose prediction. |
| Right patients / PHC | | • Asthma patients with activated CysLT pathway as identified by uLTE4, either alone or as a composite with other biomarkers. **GAP**: Identification of uLTE4 cut off. Link between uLTE4 or composite biomarker and clinical response to be established. **Activity:** Data mining of U-BIOPRED cohort. Access data and samples from other cohorts (BIOAIR, Korean cohort) to strengthen clinical evidence around uLTE4 and associated composite elements. Test uLTE4 and additional biomarkers in phase 2. |
| Right safety | | • No secondary pharmacology, genetic, reproductive or cardiovascular toxicity flags.<br>• **Testicular toxicity** with 5-LO inhibitors and structurally similar compounds. AZD9898 causes testicular tubular degeneration in dogs after 14 days. NOAEL 23-fold exposure margin over predicted human free AUC. Similar changes not seen in rats at exposures up to 228-fold higher than predicted human.<br>• Liver changes (liver weight increases, hepatocyte hypertrophy and vacuolation (fat), Cyp 2B and/or Cyp 3A seen in rats at $\geq$ 100 mg/kg for 14 days (exposure >80-fold higher than predicted human). NOAEL exposure >14-fold higher than predicted human. **GAP:** Risk of eroding safety margins with longer preclinical studies. **Activity:** 3 months tox studies in parallel with Ph1 (6 months recovery in dog study to fully evaluate testicular observations). |
| Right Commercial | | • Addresses an unmet need in patients with asthma inadequately controlled with SOC.<br>• Innovative, science-led precision medicine approach linked to a competitive value proposition vs. other add-on alternatives: Efficacy in symptom control and exacerbation prevention, safe and well tolerated, convenient once-daily oral posology.<br>Attractive upside opportunities (nasal polyps, expansion into populations in lower GINA control steps)<br>**Gaps:** Place in therapy hypothesis and unmet need yet to be validated. Validation of the strategy based on PHC to avoid price comparison with generic montelukast. **Activity**: Complete target product profile definition and validation with external expert input incl payer. Demonstrate the unmet need through RWE studies. |

**Figure 20.19** Evaluation of the project at the end of lead optimisation to the AstraZeneca criteria.

LTC4S. The pharmacodynamic data from the healthy volunteer SAD showed that, at the highest dose tested (45 mg), AZD9898 reduced uLTE4 levels for 14 h post dose with a maximum reduction at 6 h post dose. The magnitude and duration of the PD effect at a dose of 45 mg were lower than expected. Furthermore, modelling and simulation of data did not support that the required level of effect on uLTE4 inhibition could be reached (75% at $C_{min}$) and maintained, even with twice daily dosing. Therefore, the decision was made to stop the multipart Phase I study after the single dose phase. In humans, the *in vivo* potency appears lower than that predicted from the human PBMC assay and may lie closer to the *in vivo* efficacy observed in the rat PKPD model and mast cell assay. The patient SAD arm was not started.

In many ways this was a posterchild for a modern LO project. The 5Rs approach defined highlighted risks and opportunities in the initial evaluation and the plan to candidate drug. The translational data package, early safety studies, patient selection hypothesis, design of the Phase 1 programme and pivotal head-to-head Phase 2A clinical study were designed to address the biggest project risk. Early safety studies and full evaluation highlighted clear risks for the series and gave a focus for LO. The project took a classic LLE-based optimisation, focussing on physical properties potency, safety, and clearance – risks of scaling were investigated in detail during LO. A translational package strengthened the target rationale, which built support for the project as it progressed through LO. A robust personalised medicine opportunity was proposed. Uncertainties in potency seen across target cell assays could not be understood, even though great efforts were taken to identify assay technical differences underpinning the potency. The risk was apparent and carried forward into Phase 1, as a good target engagement biomarker existed to determine the effective dose to man. There was a plan to include patients in Phase 1 SAD to ensure PKPD in the right compartment was evaluated. Commercial differentiation from the generic montelukast was the main project risk, and although the inability to dose high enough to engage the target fully ultimately stopped the project, the project stepped forward with its eyes open, The project could have gone back and run the full 3-month dog study with 6-month recovery, which might have removed the additional 10× cap on dosing, but the portfolio had moved on and so the project was instead terminated.

## 20.5 Hints and Tips

- Multiobjective optimisation can be aided by some software tools like STARDROP http://www.optibrium.com/stardrop/
- Set a candidate drug profile to guide the optimisation process. It evolves with the project but provides a clear optimisation focus.
- A screening cascade should be established that can deliver a candidate drug matching the required drug profile and required drug dose.
- Using colour coding in results tables simplifies decision-making for compound progression.
- Breaking the potency-lipophilicity "correlation" is a common challenge in most LO programs.

- The properties of a molecule are fixed as soon as you have thought of it! So if you can predict the properties, and the molecule is predicted to be poor...why make it?
- Targeting a low dose reduces the impact of toxicological issues, as it, on average, improves safety margins. Targeting a dose <1 mg kg$^{-1}$ day$^{-1}$ is typical for an oral project. A dose <10 mg total can mitigate concerns over reactive metabolites, as the body burden is considered acceptable.
- Lead optimisation should focus on achieving the maximum concentration of drug within the biophase of the target and hence the smallest clinical dose. Optimisation should focus on increasing solubility, membrane permeability and reducing clearance and not on plasma protein binding as free drug concentration changes are counterbalanced by commensurate changes in drug clearance.

## Acknowledgements

The authors would like to acknowledge and thank Dr Stephen Connolly who co-authored this equivalent chapter in the first edition of this book.

## References

1. S. M. Paul, D. S. Mytelka, C. T. Dunwiddie, C. C. Persinger, B. H. Munos, S. R. Lindborg and A. L. Schacht, *Nat. Rev. Drug Discovery*, 2010, **9**, 203–214.
2. M. Abou-Gharbia and W. E. Childers, *J. Med. Chem.*, 2014, **57**, 5525–5553.
3. F. Pammolli, L. Magazzini and M. Riccaboni, *Nat. Rev. Drug Discovery*, 2011, **10**, 428–438.
4. I. Kola and J. Landis, *Nat. Rev. Drug Discovery*, 2004, **3**(8), 711–715.
5. W. J. Greenlee and M. C. Desai, *Curr. Opin. Drug Discovery Dev.*, 2005, **8**, 419–420.
6. J. L. Stevens, *Chem. Res. Toxicol.*, 2006, **19**, 1393–1401.
7. J. D. Hughes, J. Blagg, D. A. Price, S. Bailey, G. A. DeCrescenzo, R. v. Devraj, E. Ellsworth, Y. M. Fobian, M. E. Gibbs, R. W. Gilles, N. Greene, E. Huang, T. Krieger-Burke, J. Loesel, T. Wager, L. Whiteley and Y. Zhang, *Bioorg. Med. Chem. Lett.*, 2008, **18**, 4872–4875.
8. J. Hughes, S. Rees, S. Kalindjian and K. Philpott, *Br. J. Pharmacol.*, 2011, **162**, 1239–1249.
9. M. J. Waring, J. Arrowsmith, A. R. Leach, P. D. Leeson, S. Mandrell, R. M. Owen, G. Pairaudeau, W. D. Pennie, S. D. Pickett, J. Wang, O. Wallace and A. Weir, *Nat. Rev. Drug Discovery*, 2015, **14**, 475–486.
10. P. Morgan, P. H. van der Graaf, J. Arrowsmith, D. E. Feltner, K. S. Drummond, C. D. Wegner and S. D. A. Street, *Drug Discovery Today*, 2012, **17**, 419–424.
11. M. Rowland, C. Peck and G. Tucker, *Annu. Rev. Pharmacol. Toxicol.*, 2011, **51**, 45–73.
12. R. Arakawa, A. Takano and C. Halldin, *Neuropsychopharmacol. Rep.*, 2020, **40**, 114–121.
13. T. Tuntland, B. Ethell, T. Kosaka, F. Blasco, R. X. Zang, M. Jain, T. Gould and K. Hoffmaster, *Front. Pharmacol.*, 2014, **5**, 174.
14. J. M. Gallo, *Mt. Sinai J. Med.*, 2010, **77**, 381–388.
15. D. Cook, D. Brown, R. Alexander, R. March, P. Morgan, G. Satterthwaite and M. N. Pangalos, *Nat. Rev. Drug Discovery*, 2014, **13**, 419–431.
16. P. Morgan, D. G. Brown, S. Lennard, M. J. Anderton, J. C. Barrett, U. Eriksson, M. Fidock, B. Hamrén, A. Johnson, R. E. March, J. Matcham, J. Mettetal, D. J. Nicholls, S. Platz, S. Rees, M. A. Snowden and M. N. Pangalos, *Nat. Rev. Drug Discovery*, 2018, **17**, 167–181.
17. A. Sadosky, K. Srivastava, A. Arora, A. Kataria, J. C. Cappelleri and A. M. Peterson, *Patient Prefer. Adherence*, 2013, 419.
18. M. Chen, J. Borlak and W. Tong, *Hepatology*, 2013, **58**, 388–396.
19. T. S. Maurer, D. Smith, K. Beaumont and L. Di, *J. Med. Chem.*, 2020, **63**, 6423–6435.
20. C. Carini, A. A. Seyhan, M. D. Fidock and A. J. van Gool, in *Handbook of Biomarkers and Precision Medicine*, Chapman and Hall/CRC, 2019, pp. 2–7.

21. D. A. Smith, K. Beaumont, T. S. Maurer and L. Di, *J. Med. Chem.*, 2015, **58**, 5691–5698.
22. T. S. Maurer, D. Smith, K. Beaumont and L. Di, *J. Med. Chem.*, 2020, **63**, 6423–6435.
23. D. F. McGinnity, J. Collington, R. P. Austin and R. J. Riley, *Curr. Drug Metab.*, 2007, **8**, 463–479.
24. P. D. Leeson and B. Springthorpe, *Nat. Rev. Drug Discovery*, 2007, **6**, 881–890.
25. J. A. Arnott and S. L. Planey, *Expert Opin. Drug Discovery*, 2012, **7**, 863–875.
26. M. P. Edwards and D. A. Price, in *Annual Reports in Medicinal Chemistry*, 2010, vol. 45, pp. 380–391.
27. A. F. Stepan, G. W. Kauffman, C. E. Keefer, P. R. Verhoest and M. Edwards, *J. Med. Chem.*, 2013, **56**, 6985–6990.
28. H. Stark, *Expert Opin. Drug Discovery*, 2020, **15**, 1365–1367.
29. R. M. Garbaccio and E. R. Parmee, *Cell Chem. Biol.*, 2016, **23**, 10–17.
30. L. H. Jones, *Future Med. Chem.*, 2015, **7**, 2131–2141.
31. P. Workman and I. Collins, *Chem. Biol.*, 2010, **17**, 561–577.
32. J. Blagg and P. Workman, *Cancer Cell*, 2017, **32**, 9–25.
33. C. H. Emmerich, L. M. Gamboa, M. C. J. Hofmann, M. Bonin-Andresen, O. Arbach, P. Schendel, B. Gerlach, K. Hempel, A. Bespalov, U. Dirnagl and M. J. Parnham, *Nat. Rev. Drug Discovery*, 2021, **20**, 64–81.
34. P. D. Leeson and J. R. Empfield, *Annu. Rep. Med. Chem.*, 2010, **45**, 393–407.
35. R. A. Thompson, E. M. Isin, Y. Li, R. Weaver, L. Weidolf, I. Wilson, A. Claesson, K. Page, H. Dolgos and J. G. Kenna, *Chem.-Biol. Interact.*, 2011, **192**, 65–71.
36. J. A. Arnott and S. L. Planey, *Expert Opin. Drug Discovery*, 2012, **7**, 863–875.
37. M. Khan, I. Sylte, M. Khan and I. Sylte, *Curr. Drug Discovery Technol.*, 2007, **4**, 141–149.
38. J. G. Cumming, A. M. Davis, S. Muresan, M. Haeberlein and H. Chen, *Nat. Rev. Drug Discovery*, 2013, **12**, 948–962.
39. C. Bissantz, B. Kuhn and M. Stahl, *J. Med. Chem.*, 2010, **53**, 5061–5084.
40. B. R. Beno, K.-S. Yeung, M. D. Bartberger, L. D. Pennington and N. A. Meanwell, *J. Med. Chem.*, 2015, **58**, 4383–4438.
41. N. K. Shinada, A. G. de Brevern and P. Schmidtke, *J. Med. Chem.*, 2019, **62**, 9341–9356.
42. R. Wilcken, M. O. Zimmermann, A. Lange, A. C. Joerger and F. M. Boeckler, *J. Med. Chem.*, 2013, **56**, 1363–1388.
43. P. W. Kenny, C. A. Montanari, I. M. Prokopczyk, J. F. R. Ribeiro and G. R. Sartori, *J. Med. Chem.*, 2016, **59**, 4278–4288.
44. C. R. Martinez and B. L. Iverson, *Chem. Sci.*, 2012, **3**, 2191.
45. M. Morgenthaler, E. Schweizer, A. Hoffmann-Röder, F. Benini, R. E. Martin, G. Jaeschke, B. Wagner, H. Fischer, S. Bendels, D. Zimmerli, J. Schneider, F. Diederich, M. Kansy and K. Müller, *ChemMedChem*, 2007, **2**, 1100–1115.
46. E. Perola, *J. Med. Chem.*, 2010, **53**, 2986–2997.
47. A. L. Hopkins, G. M. Keserü, P. D. Leeson, D. C. Rees and C. H. Reynolds, *Nat. Rev. Drug Discovery*, 2014, **13**, 105–121.
48. J. Mensch, A. Melis, C. Mackie, G. Verreck, M. E. Brewster and P. Augustijns, *Eur. J. Pharm. Biopharm.*, 2010, **74**, 495–502.
49. J. M. Reis, B. Sinkó and C. H. R. Serra, *Mini-Rev. Med. Chem.*, 2010, **10**, 1071–1076.
50. S. A. Hitchcock, *J. Med. Chem.*, 2012, **55**, 4877–4895.
51. D. J. Huggins, W. Sherman and B. Tidor, *J. Med. Chem.*, 2012, **55**, 1424–1444.
52. X. Liu, M. Wright and C. E. C. A. Hop, *J. Med. Chem.*, 2014, **57**, 8238–8248.
53. X. Liu, C. Chen and C. E. C. A. Hop, *Curr. Top. Med. Chem.*, 2011, **11**, 450–466.
54. D. A. Smith, L. Di and E. H. Kerns, *Nat. Rev. Drug Discovery*, 2010, **9**, 929–939.
55. Z. A. Knight and K. M. Shokat, *Chem. Biol.*, 2005, **12**, 621–637.
56. T. Kenakin, *ACS Pharmacol. Transl. Sci.*, 2019, **2**, 9–17.
57. H. W. G. M. Boddeke, A. Fargin, J. R. Raymonde, P. Schoeffter and D. Hoyer, *Naunyn-Schmiedeberg's Arch. Pharmacol.*, 1992, **345**, 257–263.
58. S. Wilson, J. K. Chambers, J. E. Park, A. Ladurner, D. W. Cronk, C. G. Chapman, H. Kallender, M. J. Browne, G. J. Murphy and P. W. Young, *J. Pharmacol. Exp. Ther.*, 1996, **279**, 214–221.
59. T. S. Maurer, M. A. Tabrizi-Fard and H. L. Fung, *J. Pharm. Sci.*, 2000, **89**, 1404–1414.
60. Y. Kawai, S. Tsukamoto, J. Ito, K. Akimoto and M. Takahashi, *Chem. Pharm. Bull.*, 2011, **59**, 1110–1116.
61. P. Gleeson, G. Bravi, S. Modi and D. Lowe, *Bioorg. Med. Chem.*, 2009, **17**, 5906–5919.
62. R. J. Riley, A. J. Parker, S. Trigg and C. N. Manners, *Pharm. Res.*, 2001, **18**, 652–655.
63. A. J. Barker, K. H. Gibson, W. Grundy, A. A. Godfrey, J. J. Barlow, M. P. Healy, J. R. Woodburn, S. E. Ashton, B. J. Curry, L. Scarlett, L. Henthorn and L. Richards, *Bioorg. Med. Chem. Lett.*, 2001, **11**, 1911–1914.
64. A. P. Hill and R. J. Young, *Drug Discovery Today*, 2010, **15**, 648–655.

65. J. S. Delaney, *Drug Discovery Today*, 2005, **10**, 289–295.
66. Y. Ran, N. Jain and S. H. Yalkowsky, *J. Chem. Inf. Comput. Sci.*, 2001, **41**, 1208–1217.
67. M. Ishikawa and Y. Hashimoto, *J. Med. Chem.*, 2011, **54**, 1539–1554.
68. N. E. Austin, S. J. Baldwin, L. Cutler, N. Deeks, P. J. Kelly, M. Nash, C. E. Shardlow, G. Stemp, K. Thewlis, A. Ayrton and P. Jeffrey, *Xenobiotica*, 2001, **31**, 677–686.
69. D. A. Smith, K. Beaumont, T. S. Maurer and L. Di, *J. Med. Chem.*, 2018, **61**, 4273–4282.
70. A. J. Lucas, J. L. Sproston, P. Barton and R. J. Riley, *Expert Opin. Drug Discovery*, 2019, **14**, 1313–1327.
71. F. Broccatelli, C. E. C. A. Hop and M. Wright, *Expert Opin. Drug Discovery*, 2019, **14**, 221–230.
72. D. A. Smith, K. Beaumont, T. S. Maurer and L. Di, *J. Med. Chem.*, 2015, **58**, 5691–5698.
73. D. A. Smith, K. Beaumont, T. S. Maurer and L. Di, *J. Med. Chem.*, 2018, **61**, 4273–4282.
74. D. A. Smith, K. Beaumont, T. S. Maurer and L. Di, *J. Med. Chem.*, 2019, **62**, 2245–2255.
75. J. A. Arnott and S. L. Planey, *Expert Opin. Drug Discovery*, 2012, **7**, 863–875.
76. R. R. Miller, M. Madeira, H. B. Wood, W. M. Geissler, C. E. Raab and I. J. Martin, *J. Med. Chem.*, 2020, **63**, 12156–12170.
77. S. B. Rosenblum, T. Huynh, A. Afonso, H. R. Davis, N. Yumibe, J. W. Clader and D. A. Burnett, *J. Med. Chem.*, 1998, **41**, 973–980.
78. R. J. Herr, *Bioorg. Med. Chem.*, 2002, **10**, 3379–3393.
79. B. S. Orlek, F. E. Blaney, F. Brown, M. S. Clark, M. S. Hadley, J. Hatcher, G. J. Riley, H. E. Rosenberg, H. J. Wadsworth and P. Wyman, *J. Med. Chem.*, 1991, **34**, 2726–2735.
80. F. Yoshida and J. G. Topliss, *J. Med. Chem.*, 2000, **43**, 2575–2585.
81. D. F. Veber, S. R. Johnson, H. Y. Cheng, B. R. Smith, K. W. Ward and K. D. Kopple, *J. Med. Chem.*, 2002, **45**, 2615–2623.
82. Y. Lai, K. E. Sampson and J. C. Stevens, *Comb. Chem. High Throughput Screening*, 2010, **13**, 112–134.
83. J. Bowes, A. J. Brown, J. Hamon, W. Jarolimek, A. Sridhar, G. Waldron and S. Whitebread, *Nat. Rev. Drug Discovery*, 2012, **11**, 909–922.
84. A. J. Ratcliffe, *Curr. Med. Chem.*, 2009, **16**, 2816–2823.
85. S. Prasanna and R. J. Doerksen, *Curr. Med. Chem.*, 2009, **16**, 21–41.
86. T. T. Wager, X. Hou, P. R. Verhoest and A. Villalobos, *ACS Chem. Neurosci.*, 2010, **1**, 435–439.
87. N. C. Patel, B. Feng, X. Hou, M. A. West, P. E. Trapa, S. Sciabola, P. Verhoest, J. L. Liras, T. S. Maurer and T. T. Wager, *ACS Chem. Neurosci.*, 2021, **12**, 1007–1017.
88. M. Munck af Rosenschöld, P. Johannesson, A. Nikitidis, C. Tyrchan, H.-F. Chang, R. Rönn, D. Chapman, V. Ullah, G. Nikitidis, P. Glader, H. Käck, B. Bonn, F. Wågberg, E. Björkstrand, U. Andersson, L. Swedin, M. Rohman, T. Andreasson, E. L. Bergström, F. Jiang, X.-H. Zhou, A. J. Lundqvist, A. Malmberg, M. Ek, E. Gordon, A. Pettersen, L. Ripa and A. M. Davis, *J. Med. Chem.*, 2019, **62**, 7769–7787.
89. W. Curatolo, *Pharm. Sci. Technol. Today*, 1998, **1**, 387–393.
90. K. C. Johnson and A. C. Swindell, *Pharm. Res.*, 1996, **13**, 1795–1798.
91. D. E. Shaw, A. R. Sousa, S. J. Fowler, L. J. Fleming, G. Roberts, J. Corfield, I. Pandis, A. T. Bansal, E. H. Bel, C. Auffray, C. H. Compton, H. Bisgaard, E. Bucchioni, M. Caruso, P. Chanez, B. Dahlén, S.-E. Dahlen, K. Dyson, U. Frey, T. Geiser, M. Gerhardsson de Verdier, D. Gibeon, Y. Guo, S. Hashimoto, G. Hedlin, E. Jeyasingham, P.-P. W. Hekking, T. Higenbottam, I. Horváth, A. J. Knox, N. Krug, V. J. Erpenbeck, L. X. Larsson, N. Lazarinis, J. G. Matthews, R. Middelveld, P. Montuschi, J. Musial, D. Myles, L. Pahus, T. Sandström, W. Seibold, F. Singer, K. Strandberg, J. Vestbo, N. Vissing, C. von Garnier, I. M. Adcock, S. Wagers, A. Rowe, P. Howarth, A. H. Wagener, R. Djukanovic, P. J. Sterk and K. F. Chung, *Eur. Respir. J.*, 2015, **46**, 1308–1321.

# 21 Pharmaceutical Properties – The Importance of Solid Form Selection

Cheryl L. Doherty*[a], Amy L. Robertson[b], Nicola Clear[c] and Robert Docherty[†d]

[a]Medicines Research Centre, GlaxoSmithKline, Gunnels Wood Road, Stevenage, Hertfordshire, SG1 2NY, UK; [b]Chemical Development, Pharmaceutical Technology and Development, Operations, AstraZeneca, Macclesfield, SK11 2NA, UK; [c]Pharmaceutical Sciences, Pfizer Global R&D, Ramsgate Road, Sandwich, Kent, CT13 9NJ, UK; [d]School of Chemical and Process Engineering, University of Leeds, Leeds, LS2 9JT, UK
*E-mail: cheryl.x.doherty@gsk.com

## 21.1 Introduction

The selection of the commercial solid form is a key milestone in the development of any new chemical entity (NCE). It is critical not only from an active pharmaceutical ingredient (API) standpoint but also from a drug product performance and stability perspective. The regulatory landscape associated with the solid form of the API and dosage form development has already been described.[1,2] The issues associated with the formation of an unexpected solid form have been well documented and range from delays in the progression of a candidate through development (batch reworks, additional bioequivalence studies) through to product withdrawal in the most challenging circumstances. The most famous example of this is the antiretroviral drug ritonavir (Norvir) where a more stable, less soluble polymorph appeared during production reducing the dissolution of the capsule product.[3] This is not an isolated incident and, as highlighted in recent reviews there have, over the last two decades, been a number of product recalls due to ambiguous product performance as a result of unexpected solid state transformations.[4,5] The importance of the solid state features of a NCE to intellectual property has also been described extensively.[6,7] Pharmaceutical companies perform extensive experimental screening to prevent these issues occurring. Automation technologies have allowed expansion of the experimental space that can be routinely

[†]Retired from Pfizer.

The Handbook of Medicinal Chemistry: Principles and Practice, 2nd Edition
Edited by Simon E. Ward and Andrew M. Davis

Published by the Royal Society of Chemistry, www.rsc.org

covered, which is important when material quantity is limited.[8] Recently there has been increasing focus on utilising emerging computational structural methods to tailor the number of critical laboratory experiments.[9]

In 1987 the Nobel Prize for chemistry was awarded to Cram, Lehn and Pedersen for their work on supramolecular chemistry. Since then, publications[10,11] have charted the evolution of pharmaceutical materials science with solid form and particle engineering being core elements linking the final steps of the API design to drug product attributes. The challenge for the medicinal chemist and pharmaceutical scientist in tackling the crystallisation of highly complex chemical entities remains a significant one due to:

- Increasing molecular complexity resulting in a complicated solid form space that needs to be understood and evaluated.
- Multiple conformational degrees of freedom can result in complex solid form structures and consequently significant barriers to crystallisation.
- Different solid forms may have considerably different chemical or physical stabilities and biopharmaceutical properties.
- Anisotropic external particle morphologies with different crystal faces exhibiting different surface chemistry, and interactions with solvents and impurities.

Physico-chemical properties of a NCE that impact product performance and product robustness are strongly influenced by the solid state structure of the drug substance (Figure 21.1). The formation of different solid state structures (salt, co-crystal and polymorph) provides the pharmaceutical scientist an opportunity to mitigate undesirable properties by switching to an alternative stable crystal form. Product performance can only be assured when the NCE is delivered to the patient in a chemically and physically stable solid form. In this chapter we will link new academic research to the best

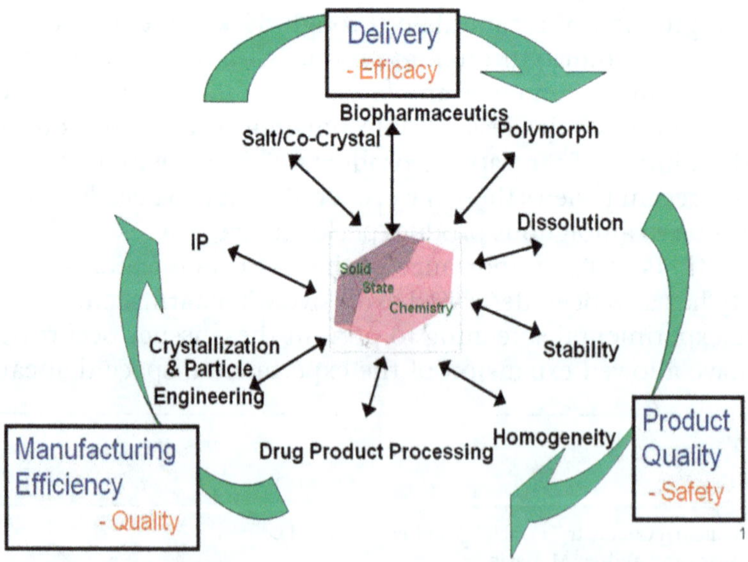


**Figure 21.1** The importance of the solid state in impacting product safety, efficacy and quality.

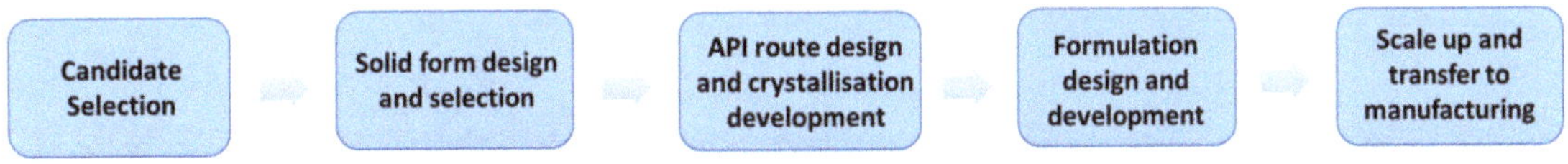


**Figure 21.2** A brief overview of pharmaceutical development activities.

current industrial practices that medicinal chemists and pharmaceutical scientists can apply in selecting the optimal solid form, to enable the rapid advancement of NCEs into medicines.

A typical workflow for the key pharmaceutical development activities is shown in Figure 21.2. The timing and sequencing of these work packages is determined by the desired final dosage form, the complexity of the API, the therapeutic area, project timelines and will also be dependent on company best practices and the position of the candidate in the portfolio.

## 21.2 Solid State Chemistry

### 21.2.1 Crystallography

Crystals are formed when atoms or molecules are arranged into ordered three-dimensional (3-D) arrays. The resulting crystalline systems can be described by defining

(i) The item to be repeated (the motif)
(ii) The way in which it is repeated (symmetry operations).

In the crystal structures of organic materials, the motif is the molecule, the lattice describing the scheme of repetition is a 3-D array and the unit cell is the smallest repeating unit within this 3-D structure. The unit cell is fully described by six lattice parameters, comprising three lengths of the unit cell ($a$, $b$ and $c$) with the three inter-axial angles ($\alpha$, $\beta$ and $\gamma$). Unit cells range from the highly symmetrical cubic ($a = b = c$ and $\alpha = \beta = \gamma = 90°$) through to the lower symmetry monoclinic and triclinic systems ($a \neq b \neq c$ and $\alpha \neq \beta \neq \gamma$) favoured by drug molecules.[12]

These systems can be further refined in terms of the symmetry elements present. The various rotation, translation and inversion operations together form 230 possible combinations that are known as space groups. The symmetry exhibited by a unit cell is reflected in both the arrangement of molecules in the internal crystal structure and in the physical and chemical properties of the resulting macroscopic crystal. Symmetry is evident in properties such as crystal growth rates and crystal shape and surface chemistry.

A deeper understanding of grown crystal habit can be made by reference to the internal crystal structure. Miller indices (*hkl*) are used to describe planes within the crystal lattice, defining the orientation of the surface in relation to the underlying crystallographic unit cell. This is demonstrated for lamotrigine[13] (Figure 21.3) where the (110) face shown in the predicted morphology cuts the $a$ and $b$ axes one unit cell from the origin and runs parallel to the $c$ axis. This provides an important link between modern

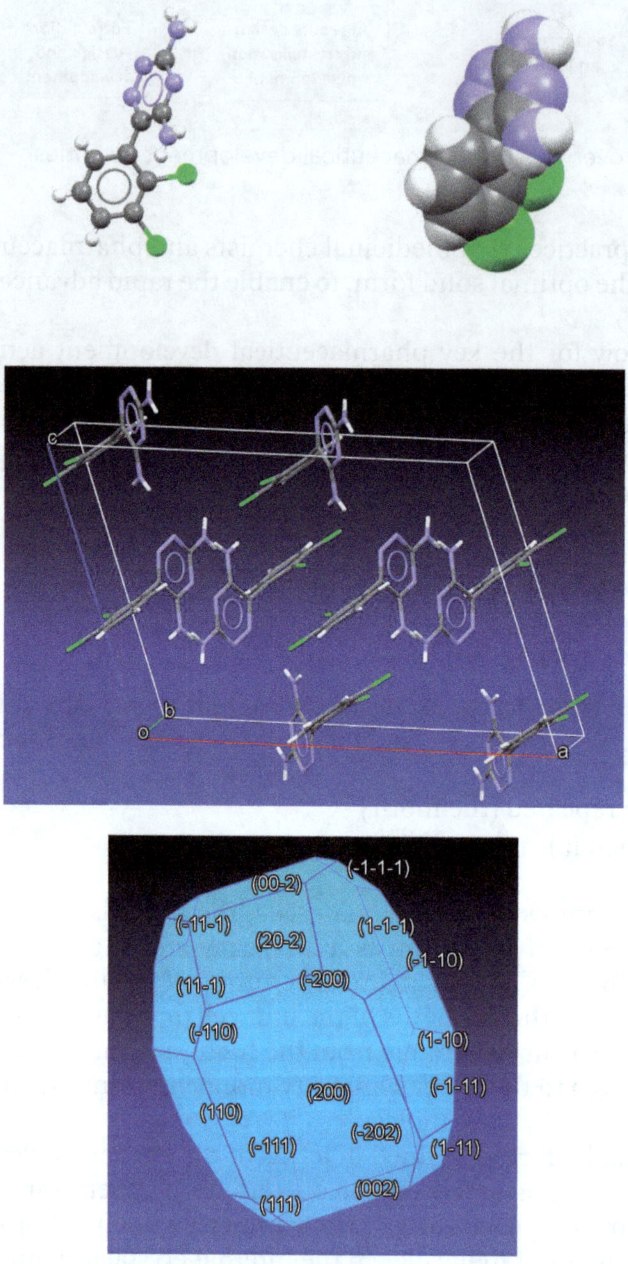


**Figure 21.3** The molecule, the crystal chemistry and the crystal morphology of lamotrigine. The molecular structure of lamotrigine (top) is shown in ball and stick and space-fill. The crystal packing of lamotrigine (middle) contains one unit cell in the *a*, *b* and *c* directions. Each unit cell contains eight lamotrigine molecules. The crystal morphology (bottom) shows the observed crystal faces labelled with the corresponding Miller indices.

structural crystallography and classical morphological crystallography, allowing the process chemist or pharmaceutical scientist to relate the internal molecular structure with the chemical functionality on the external surface structure.

The most common solid state chemistry analytical technique is X-ray powder diffraction (XRPD), which examines the angular dependence of X-rays when scattered from crystal lattice planes. This technique provides a definitive fingerprint of the solid state structure and probes the crystallinity and structural integrity of the packing arrangement. The position, intensity and width of the peaks are directly linked to the unit cell dimensions, molecular contents and quality of the crystal lattice.

XRPD is routinely used to define the form being isolated, the consistency of the crystallinity of the material and as a baseline for the solid state structure for any solubility determination.[14]

### 21.2.2 Crystal Chemistry and Crystal Packing of Drug Molecules

Molecules can essentially be regarded as impenetrable systems whose shape and volume characteristics are governed by the molecular conformation and the radii of the constituent atoms. The atomic radii are essentially exclusion zones in which no other atom may enter except under special circumstances, such as bonding. Figure 21.3 (top) shows a comparison between a ball and stick and van der Waals (space-fill) representation of lamotrigine.

The structures and crystal chemistry of molecular materials are often classified into different categories according to the type of intermolecular forces present.[15] A number of factors are of particular importance in assessing the influence of intermolecular bonding on the physicochemical properties of organic solids[16] including:

- the size and shape of the molecular entities that make up the structure
- the strength of the intermolecular interaction
- the distance over which the interaction exerts an influence
- the extent to which the interaction is directional or not.

Organic molecules in general and drug molecules in particular are found in a limited number of low symmetry crystal systems. These tendencies are reflected in an analysis of the Cambridge Crystallographic Database (CSD)[17] where the vast majority of the organic structures reported prefer the lower symmetry triclinic, monoclinic and orthorhombic crystal systems,[18] making the CSD a valuable resource to explore and understand the pharmaceutical solid state. Recent analyses of in-house pharmaceutical crystal structure databases alongside approved drugs in the CSD have confirmed these observations. They also demonstrated the increasing size and complexity of modern drug candidates, which will lead to more frequent complex solid form behaviour in future.[19]

### 21.2.3 Intermolecular Interactions, Crystal Packing Energies

The energy and direction of interactions between molecules together govern the solid state properties of drug materials. The development of atom–atom intermolecular potentials made it possible to interpret intermolecular packing effects in organic crystals in terms of interaction energies.[20] The basic assumption of this method is that the interaction between two molecules can be considered to simply consist of the sum of the interactions between the constituent atom pairs.

$$E_{\text{latt}} = 1/2 \sum_{k=1}^{N} \sum_{i=1}^{n} \sum_{j=1}^{n'} V_{kij} \tag{21.1}$$

The lattice energy $E_{\text{latt}}$ (or cohesive energy) for molecular materials can be calculated by summing up all the interactions between a designated central molecule and all the surrounding molecules. Hence, if there are $n$ atoms in the central molecule and $n'$ atoms in each of the $N$ surrounding molecules then the lattice energy can be calculated using eqn (21.1).[20]

Each atom–atom interaction pair ($V_{kij}$) consists of an attractive and repulsive dispersive interaction which can be described by a van der Waals representation, together with an electrostatic interaction and a hydrogen bonding potential. The use of these potentials has been validated by comparing the theoretical values with experimentally measured lattice energies (sublimation enthalpies).[21] A particular advantage of the calculated energy is that it can be broken down into specific interactions along particular crystallographic directions and further partitioned onto the constituent atom–atom and/or group contributions. This allows a profile of the important interactions to be built, linking the intrinsic molecular structure with the crystal packing in families of compounds. The increased understanding has allowed the design of molecular features to disrupt crystal packing and therefore enhance solubility, such as by disrupting the planarity of molecules, influencing hydrogen bonding or aromatic intermolecular interactions.[22,23] These approaches engage medicinal and pharmaceutical scientists at an early stage to facilitate optimisation in the design of molecular features.

### 21.2.4 Crystallisation Solubility, Supersaturation and Metastable Zone

The crystallisation process can be viewed as a two-step process involving the dissolution of the API, and then changing some attribute of the system, such as temperature, solvent composition or volume to induce crystallisation. At a given temperature and pressure there is a maximum amount of solute that can dissolve in a given amount of solvent. When this maximum is reached, the solution is said to be saturated. The amount of solute required to make a saturated solution at a given condition is the equilibrium solubility.[24]

During crystallisation the molecules must de-aggregate from their solvated state and self-assemble, aligning structural elements such as conformation and intermolecular interactions in order to enable the production of a stable 3-D ordered array of molecules. This highly time-dependent event makes crystallisation essentially a kinetically driven process dependent on supersaturation. Supersaturation occurs when the solute concentration exceeds the equilibrium saturation at a given temperature, giving a metastable solution and implying that crystallisation will ultimately occur, albeit after time has elapsed.[24] The region between the saturation curve and this unstable boundary is called the metastable zone, and it is within this that all crystallisation activities normally occur. If we plot concentration *versus* temperature behaviour we find three regions, Figure 21.4:

- a stable solution where crystal growth is not favoured
- a metastable region where the solution is supersaturated to a degree and where crystallisation will take place after a time
- an unstable region where the solution is more supersaturated and where spontaneous crystallisation with no time delay is expected.

The crystalline form that is obtained can be controlled by manipulation of the crystallisation process to tune nucleation, crystal growth and phase transformations. Although the process of nucleation is still not fully understood, a review by Davey *et al.*[25] highlighted the key steps involved in the formation of aggregates of molecules, some of which reach critical size, at which point they become stable and subsequently grow to form crystals. In a polymorphic system, the situation can be more complex. It is assumed that a number of different types of aggregate may exist in solution. Each type of aggregate is connected by competing equilibria and may subsequently develop into one or more different polymorphic forms. It is important to note that at any given temperature and pressure only one polymorphic form is stable. In a monotropic system only one polymorph is stable over a given temperature range. In an enantiotropic system one polymorph is stable below a determined transition temperature and the other is stable above it (Figure 21.4). Recent advances in spectroscopic techniques including FTIR, Raman, UV-Vis and NMR, along with synchrotron X-ray techniques combined with computational techniques are increasing our understanding of these complex processes.

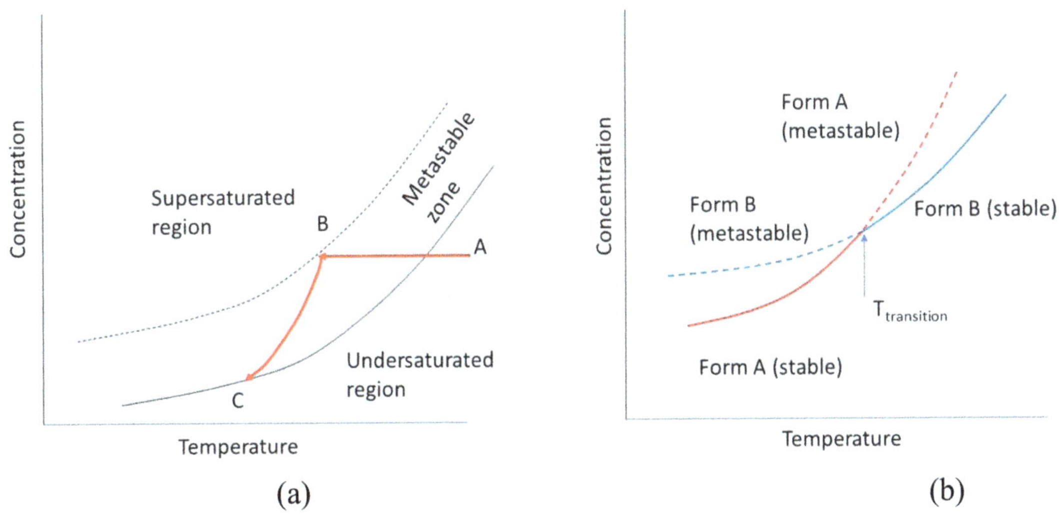


**Figure 21.4** (a) A schematic of the metastable zone. Cooling from A to B, crystallisation occurs spontaneously at B leading to a decrease in concentration as crystallisation proceeds to C (de-supersaturation). (b) Solubility curves for an enantiotropic system.

When developing any crystallisation process it is important to identify the solubility in the system and where an enantiotropic system is present ensure that the transition temperature is identified to develop a robust scaleable crystallisation and isolation process.

### 21.2.5 Pharmaceutical Polymorphs and the Solid State

Structural diversity in pharmaceutical solids arises from both the molecular conformations available in drug structures and from the broad range of intermolecular interactions possible, as described in Section 21.2.2. These different structural types are captured in Figure 21.5 for paracetamol.

The accessible structural types represent both a challenge to control and ensure a robust product, but also an opportunity to engineer a solid form that can enable a drug candidate with suboptimal properties to move forward into development and ultimately to a product. Key aspects are:

- *Amorphous.* Amorphous forms are disordered arrangements and are chemically and physically metastable with respect to their crystalline counterparts. They present an opportunity as they can be more soluble than the crystalline version, but are generally less stable.
- *Parent molecules, co-crystals and salts.* By manipulating the solid state packing through the addition of co-formers, properties such as melting point, lattice energy and solubility can be altered. The proton transfer in a salt changes the structure of the molecule, including conformation and electronic structure. This alters both

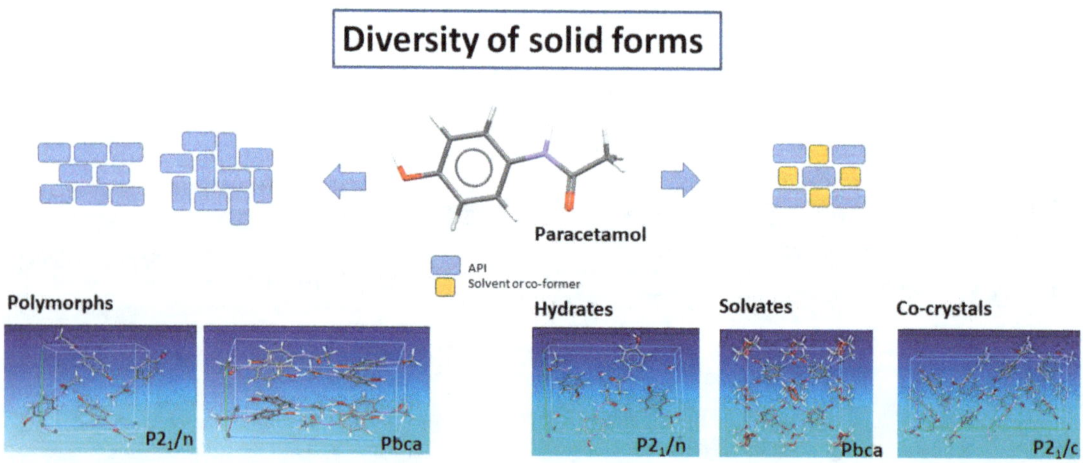


**Figure 21.5** The solid form landscape for paracetamol, including polymorphs, solvates and co-crystals. The schematic links the geometrical features discussed in Section 21.2.1 (blue bricks in different arrangements) with the crystal chemistry of drug molecules described in Section 21.2.2 (hydrogen bonds and molecular packing). The propensity to form these diverse set of structures is a combination of the molecular shape packing (density) and the degree of satisfaction of different intermolecular interaction patterns (lattice energy).

the solid state packing and the solvation properties of the drug species, enabling a greater change in solubility.

In Section 21.3 we will describe the current screening and selection practices used in industry to attempt to optimise the physical form and properties at the interface of medicinal chemistry and pharmaceutical development.

### 21.2.6 Polymorphism, Thermodynamic Stability and Solubility

Polymorphism, for the purposes of the present discussion, is the existence of a compound in at least two different crystal packing arrangements. Multi-component forms of that compound differ in composition and are therefore not considered to be true polymorphs.

In general for molecular materials, it is their intrinsic desire to closely pack in the solid state that is the single biggest driving force towards selected structural arrangements. For complex molecular materials, such as drug molecules, the need to form complex H-bonding arrangements can override this desire.[15] Weaker interactions such as C–H::::::O=C bonds and other polar interactions are probably not primary drivers in the packing arrangements but are often found to be optimised within this primary architecture, thereby providing some additional stabilisation to the 3-dimensional structure. Recent publications have importantly demonstrated that aromatic interactions in the crystal during nucleation can be sufficiently significant to drive the packing in the final solid form.[26]

The formation and behaviour of polymorphs is determined by the relative free energy of the different structures and the kinetic barriers to their formation and inter-conversion. The polymorph with the lowest free energy (lowest lattice energy) under a given set of conditions will be the most stable and therefore generally preferred for pharmaceutical development. Particular properties such as density, melting point, solubility and mechanical properties can all be impacted by different solid state structures. The solid form selection is made by balancing the relative suitability of these factors for the accessible solid forms of a desired drug product.

The influence of polymorph stability on solubility can be understood by considering two polymorphs A and B, where B is the more stable form. The solubility of a given molecule is ultimately a balance between the energy of solvation (how much the molecule likes to be in a solvent environment) and the lattice energy (how much the molecule likes to be in the solid state).[27] For a given drug candidate the energy of solvation is a molecular property and constant in a given solvent. Given B is thermodynamically more stable at room temperature it will have a stronger lattice energy than form A and hence will have a lower relative solubility. Differential scanning calorimetry (DSC)[28] is a thermal method to determine melting point and enthalpy of melting (sometimes referred to as enthalpy of fusion). The solid state structure that has the larger enthalpy of fusion for a given compound tends to be the most stable polymorphic form, for monotropic systems. As an example, published data for two polymorphs of chloramphenicol palmitate[29] show that form A is the most stable, with the highest melting point (by only 6 °C), the greatest heat of fusion (which is a surrogate measurement of the lattice energy) and less than half the solubility of form B. It should be noted that the energy difference between the polymorphs of 3.8 kcal mol$^{-1}$ is not unusual and neither is the significant 2-fold change in solubility. It is worth noting that most pharmaceutical compounds exhibit multiple polymorphs. In general, polymorph pair solubility ratios that are equal to or less than 2-fold are not uncommon, but there are also numerous instances of 5- and 6-fold solubility changes, especially for larger drug molecules.

## 21.3 Industry Practises

### 21.3.1 Salt Screening and Selection

The predominant reason for identifying salts of NCEs is to overcome any undesirable chemical or physical properties of the free acid/base. This may include poor solubility in bio-relevant media, exposure limiting dissolution rate, chemical instability and poor mechanical properties. Due to the additional electrostatic intermolecular interactions salts often achieve excellent crystallinity, good isolation, purification and stability. In the case of enantiomeric compounds, optical resolution can be achieved by diastereoisomeric salt formation in order to obtain high enantiomeric purity. An overview of acceptable salts and development factors that influence this selection process has been covered elsewhere.[30] A summary of the key development criteria is given in Table 21.1.

**Table 21.1** Properties which may be assessed during solid form selection for a standard oral dosage form. These are examined in a systematic approach as described in Table 21.3. In the case of other dosage forms, the balance of the criteria maybe refined. For a parenteral dosage form, the solubility and chemical stability in solution of the API may over ride other criteria. For a dry powder inhalation dosage from compatibility with lactose is likely to be a key selection criterion.

| | |
|---|---|
| Safety – generally stable under conditions of isolation, purification and storage | Salt is precedented for route of administration, frequency of use and dose<br>Chemical stability (*e.g.* hydrolysis, oxidation, photolysis)<br>Excipient compatibility<br>Thermal behaviour (decomposition, phase transitions)<br>Purity – good purge of key impurities through final step<br>Tendency to form unwanted solvates |
| Efficacy – timely and complete dissolution of dose administered | Aqueous solubility<br>Common ion effect on solubility<br>pH solubility profile<br>Crystallinity<br>Melting point<br>Particle size distribution and crystal habit and dissolution rate |
| Quality – ease of manufacture to ensure consistent product attributes. | Hygroscopicity – no change of hydrate state under storage conditions<br>Degree of polymorphism/landscape – ease to secure desired form in API manufacture<br>Physical stability to milling, micronisation and compaction<br>Acceptable powder flow and mechanical properties for tablet and capsule production<br>Absence of corrosiveness |

Most pharmaceutical compounds contain acidic or basic functional groups and the majority of these will ionise allowing salt formation. It is estimated that around half of all NCEs are utilised in dosage forms as salts.[31] A wide variety of organic and inorganic anions and cations are used in forming salts of drug compounds, and different sets of counter-ions are precedented for different routes of administration. While final selection of the most suitable salt former involves assessment of an extensive range of physical and chemical properties, the primary concern is that potential counter-ions must not exhibit any adverse physiological effects, so the safety of the counter-ion selected in the proposed dosage form regime is of critical importance. The most frequently used salts, their precedence in different delivery routes and the maximum precedented doses, have already been described (Table 21.2).[32]

When designing a salt screen there are some important factors to consider. For pharmaceutical compounds it is expected that there should be a $pK_a$ difference ($\Delta pK_a$) of 2 to 3 units[30] between the compound and its potential salt former to ensure robustness of the resultant salt form. Constraining the selection of counter-ions by using this approximation ignores the potential impact that solvent and temperature can have on possible salt forming reactions.

When designing a salt screen for multi-basic or multi-acidic compounds and counter-ions, the potential stoichiometries should also be considered. Even for mono-basic or mono-acidic compounds, multiple salt stoichiometries may be achieved. Similarly, when screening for salts of a chiral API, unique solid forms may be achieved by the use of single enantiomer salt formers. For example, a compound may form a salt with L-tartaric acid that meets all development selection criteria, whereas the D-tartrate salt is non-ideal, with poor crystallinity and high hygroscopicity.

The physical properties of the candidate salts must be assessed, which requires comprehensive characterisation of selected salts and their polymorphs or hydrates. This is extremely demanding in terms of experimental effort,[33] making it impractical to attempt characterisation of all aspects of every potential salt form. As a result, salt selection is typically carried out using a tiered approach. After selected characterisation at each level, a decision is made as to whether the salt proceeds to the next tier. The range of potential salts is, therefore, progressively narrowed down. The depth of characterisation increases from one level to the next, allowing a substantial number of salt forms to be investigated while minimising experimental effort. Table 21.3 shows a schematic representation of a possible multi-level salt selection process.

The importance of having a robust salt selection process from a development standpoint was lately highlighted with the partial breakdown of the hydrochloride salt of prasugrel back to its free base and the impact that had on the bioavailability, manufacturing

**Table 21.2** Partial list of common pharmaceutically acceptable counter-ions.

| Anions | Cations |
|---|---|
| Acetate, besylate, bromide, chloride, citrate, fumarate, gluconate, iodide, isethionate, lactate, malate, maleate, mesylate, methylsulfate, napsylate, nitrate, pamoate, phosphate, succinate, sulfate, tartrate, tosylate | Calcium, magnesium, meglumine, potassium, sodium, tromethamine, zinc |

Table 21.3 Multi-tier evaluation of potential salt forms.

| | Properties | Techniques |
|---|---|---|
| Tier 1 | Crystallinity | Optical microscopy |
| | Crystal form | Powder XRD |
| Tier 2 | Thermal properties and thermal behaviour (decomposition, phase transitions, de-solvation) | Differential scanning calorimetry (DSC), thermogravimetric analysis (TGA) |
| | Hygroscopicity, hydrate/solvate formation | Dynamic vapour sorption (DVS) |
| Tier 3 | Polymorph and hydrate screening | Powder XRD, Raman microscopy, DSC |
| | Aqueous and pH solubility | Powder XRD of solubility residues |
| | Chemical stability testing (*e.g.* hydrolysis, oxidation, photolysis) | HPLC |
| | Accelerated physical stability testing | Powder XRD, DSC |
| Tier 4 | Humidity/temperature induced changes in crystal form | Environmental powder XRD |
| | Influence of processing conditions (*e.g.* milling, micronisation, compaction) on solid form | Powder XRD, DSC, DVS |
| | Compatibility with excipients | HPLC |

process controls, shelf life and efficacy of the product.[34] A good understanding of potential risks and challenges allows design of an experimental programme that underpins manufacturability and ensures a robust product.

## 21.3.2 Co-crystal Screening

Co-crystals are defined as neutral multi-component systems having extended molecular networks formed through strong H-bonding patterns. Components of a pharmaceutical co-crystal include at least one API and one or more ligand (co-former), all of which tend to be neutral and solid at room temperature and atmospheric pressure.[19,35] The current regulatory landscape for pharmaceutical co-crystals[36,37] shows that co-crystals are considered not as new API, but are classified to be similar to a polymorph or solvate. Co-formers considered for use in a new medicine must be safe and generally will appear on the US FDA "Substances Added to Food"[38] list or be approved as "Generally regarded as safe" (GRAS).[39] The appeal of co-crystals in pharmaceutical solid form development is that they offer a pathway for altering the solid-state properties of non-ionisable API where salt options may be limited. There is also increasing evidence that co-crystals may have other attractive development attributes with lower tendency to form solvates/hydrates.[35,40] Co-crystals provide opportunities to:

- Deliver crystalline material when salts are not an option
- Reduce the requirement for sophisticated formulation technology as co-crystals can be progressed largely within the same operational development paradigm as salts
- Provide additional purity control options for the final form
- Enhance solid form stability, dissolution rates and oral bioavailability of the NCE.

Co-crystal formation between an API and ligand(s) relies on complementary, non-covalent interactions such as H-bonds, van der Waals, $\pi$–$\pi$ stacking and electrostatic interactions. Research on hydrogen bond motifs led to guidelines for the design of molecular assemblies.[16] These rules can also be applied to the targeted design of co-crystals, while taking broader aspects into consideration such as crystallisation kinetics and thermodynamic properties.[40] Experimentally, co-crystal screening uses many of the same methods as employed for salt screens. As well as traditional solution-based approaches to making co-crystals, other areas such as eutectic-based thermal screening and liquid-assisted grinding are proving fruitful.[41,42]

The ability of co-crystals to modify solubilities, dissolution rates and stabilities has also been described. The fluoxetine HCl : succinic acid (2 : 1) co-crystal shows an approximate 3-fold increase in intrinsic dissolution rate relative to fluoxetine HCl.[43] The photostability of furosemide was also successfully improved in nicotinamide co-crystals.[44] The further combination of multiple APIs into a single drug–drug co-crystal is so far a fairly uncommon strategy, but is attracting increasing interest. It can be challenging to identify suitable APIs with complementary mechanisms of action that can also be successfully co-crystallised in a therapeutically appropriate stoichiometry. However, where this can be achieved, the strategy offers potential advantages in drug delivery, reducing the pill burden and improving patient compliance.[45]

Co-crystals have been shown to offer a viable solid form alternative for pharmaceuticals so co-crystal screening is now widely performed. However, it is most commonly used where there are challenges with the parent, such as when the parent solid form landscape is complex and/or the API is non-ionisable. The physical stability of co-crystals in the drug product is also less well understood than for salts. In the last decade, increasingly successful translation of co-crystals through formulation processes and at manufacturing scale has led to some co-crystals becoming final commercial products.[46,47]

### 21.3.3 Polymorph Screening

The importance of polymorphism to the pharmaceutical industry can, in the views of most experts, be traced back to reviews by McCrone[48] and Byrn.[2] The temporary withdrawal of the protease inhibitor ritonavir 20 years ago[3] highlighted the potential impact of the appearance of a more stable polymorph on solubility, dissolution and ultimately bio-availability. The more recent appearance of a new polymorph in the rotigotine trans-dermal system[49] resulted in snowflake patterns in the patch which also proved to be a previously undiscovered thermodynamically more stable polymorph. The subsequent regulatory discussion and concerns for the efficacy of the patch highlighted the need for continued vigilance in screening for polymorphs.[4]

The possible impact on product manufacturing robustness, product development timelines and the potential need for repeated clinical and stability studies means that most pharmaceutical companies have incorporated solid form selection and screening programs and practices within their development strategies. In this section we will outline the key elements of screening practices and the appropriate timing of these activities during drug development. For medicinal chemists/development scientists the key questions are:

- What form(s) will my molecule crystallise in?
- How often, and under which conditions, do these forms appear?

- What will be the impact on biopharmaceutics and manufacturability?
- How many experiments are needed to ensure robustness?

These questions are difficult to give definitive answers to, but recent reviews in this area suggest that the vast majority of pharmaceutical compounds do exhibit multiple polymorphs.[50,51] They also show that hydrates are more prevalent for salts, and polymorphs are more likely for non-salts. Early screening is focused on the definition of the form being used and how to ensure consistent delivery of that form with the early route chemistry. Screening at this point will be typically targeted towards identifying the stable form and on building an early awareness of the potential forms that are accessible. These screens are essentially slurries in solvents with suitable solubility to facilitate the transformation from a given metastable solid state structure to a potentially more stable structure.[52] The rate of such solvent mediated transformations is driven by solubility in the selected solvents. This solvent mediated phase transformation starts with the dissolution of the metastable polymorph to produce a solution supersaturated with respect to the stable form. This is then followed by the nucleation and growth of the new more stable phase from this solution. Competitive slurries are also used to clarify relative stability relationships in polymorphic systems. In these cases, seeds of multiple known polymorphs are slurried together and the system will turn over to return the most stable solid form at a specified temperature over a period of time. The number of solvents used, the temperature and the duration of the experimental screening are often company practice dependent. A number of publications have articulated these principles but have also highlighted that these slurries are not a panacea for polymorph screening, as there are caveats that can reduce the effectiveness of the screen:[4,5]

- Small solubility differences between polymorphs may limit the transformation.
- A lack of solubility/stability in preferred solvents may limit the screen design.
- Solvation of a particular molecular functionality might limit the H-bonding or conformation that could be adopted, preventing a more stable structure emerging.
- Trace amounts of impurities that might inhibit the more stable form appearing.

In the later stages of development there is a commensurate increase in the effort to find polymorphs and solvates of the API and to link this emerging information to the product and process design and overall development strategy. Screens at this stage are designed to find all polymorphs to ensure a comprehensive understanding of the solid form space, the potential impact on the commercial manufacturing process and to inform the intellectual property strategy. This will involve a variety of crystallisation experiments and physical stability investigations of the bulk drug in different humidity and temperature ranges, in addition to consideration of the mechanical properties of the material. These screens will underwrite final process solvent variations, temperature excursions and the impact of impurities. Given the pivotal importance of the correct polymorph, the industry continues to enhance screening practices through both better informed screen design[53] and applied high-throughput technologies.[8]

Whilst much progress has been achieved, it is worthy of note that a number of recent papers highlight the challenges of accommodating a late stage polymorph appearance on a fast moving candidate.[54,55] In the first case, a more stable polymorph of LAB687, a candidate for the treatment for high cholesterol, was found after small changes in the impurity profile of the API occurred, during synthetic chemistry refinement and optimisation. In the second, changes to solvent and processing conditions for the cancer treatment axitinib led to accessing a higher energy conformation with more favourable intermolecular interactions, resulting in a more stable polymorph. In both cases the clinical plan had to be refined to incorporate the new form into the overall development programme. Given the potential regulatory and intellectual property impact, research on product processing-induced transformations is only likely to increase, given the issues highlighted.[4]

The exact timing of this work can be candidate/dosage form-dependent and dictated by the overall development strategy. For example, an inhalation candidate is likely to have these challenges addressed earlier, as would candidates being fast tracked in the oncology therapeutic area due to a desire to lock down the key elements of the API attributes prior to pivotal clinical studies.

### 21.3.4 Hydrate Screening

Hydrates are the most common type of solvate observed in pharmaceutical solid forms. As with polymorphs, it is known that a hydrated solid form of a drug can have a significant negative impact upon bioavailability.[50] It is also possible for the presence of water in the crystal structure to lead to chemical and physical instability, which may result in undesirable chemical reactivity with the excipients present in a solid dosage form. However, a greater understanding of the solid state chemistry of these systems has led to increased recognition that hydrates can also offer a viable and valuable route to a developable product.[56] Screening is typically performed to find stable hydrates that are viable as a commercial form, as well as to identify transient or metastable hydrates that might be accessible during manufacture or downstream processing. As the stability of a hydrate in the solid state depends on both the temperature and partial pressure of water and, in solution, on the temperature and water activity, a range of different experiments must be attempted to identify all such forms.

Dynamic vapour sorption is a key technique for assessing API hygroscopicity, examining water uptake as a function of relative humidity.[28] This approach may also be used to screen for potential hydrate formation, identifying the key conditions for anhydrous–hydrate transitions. The method may not be relied upon to prepare hydrates for all new API, since conversion to a hydrated form may be a kinetically slow process. The anhydrous form may also need dissolution and recrystallisation steps in order to incorporate water molecules into a new, low-energy, hydrate crystal structure, and high humidity alone may be insufficient to rapidly ensure this rearrangement.

One way to try to overcome these kinetic barriers to hydrate formation is to recrystallise or slurry in water. However, the drug molecule may have insufficient aqueous solubility to make this practicable. As in the case of polymorph slurry screening, it is essential that the API has sufficient solubility to allow the dissolution and recrystallisation of the new hydrated form. An alternative approach is to utilise organic solvent–water mixtures, of known water activity ($a_w$), to enhance the solubility of the drug candidate. Eqn (21.2) relates water activity to relative humidity:

$$\text{Relative humidity} = [a_w] \times 100 \tag{21.2}$$

Recrystallisation or slurry equilibration[57] have therefore become standard components in industrial screens for hydrated forms and, in practice, multiple solvent/water systems of high water activity, would be investigated. The formation of thermodynamically stable hydrates by this technique is reported to have a high success rate.[58] In addition, equilibration at multiple temperatures for these slurry conversions develops understanding of the anhydrous–hydrate phase diagram,[59,60] which is a useful tool when assessing the risk of isolation of the incorrect phase, or a solid form change during downstream processes.

This section has described typical practices and has highlighted that not all solid forms are obtainable using a single experiment type, making it necessary to screen multiple methods to fully characterise the hydrate–anhydrate transformations within a system. This has been demonstrated for the eleven solid forms of gandotinib, which were not all accessible from solution crystallisation.[60]

For the case where an anhydrous form is developed, if hydrated forms are identified, it is important to consider their potential impact upon bioavailability, stability or other physicochemical properties that may be affected by an anhydrous–hydrate conversion. In contrast, if a hydrate is to be the commercial solid form developed then this is also true for a hydrate–anhydrous conversion. In such cases it is important to ensure the secondary processing and stability aspects have been considered, as well as the control of hydrated state during API production.[61]

### 21.3.5 Amorphous Forms

As discussed in Section 21.2.5, amorphous forms are metastable with respect to their crystalline counterparts; however, for biopharmaceutical or manufacturability reasons they may be selected for commercial development, either as the free form or as a salt. As the complexity of small molecule NCEs increases, the challenges of crystallising the material increases and the option of a crystalline form may not exist. Examples of marketed drug products containing amorphous API include Crestor (rosuvastatin calcium), Accupril (quinapril hydrochloride) and Accolate (zafirlukast).

Amorphous materials have different physical properties to their crystalline counterparts, including higher solubility, faster dissolution rate and they are usually more hygroscopic. The uptake of water may lead to the crystallisation of some materials and care must be taken to identify this risk during the development of the manufacturing and downstream processes.[62] The glass transition temperature ($T_g$), commonly measured by DSC, is a key physical characteristic of any amorphous form and is the temperature at which there is a major change in the properties of the material. The $T_g$ is the point where the molecules exhibit a change in mobility: below the $T_g$ the solid is in the glassy state and will be brittle, above the $T_g$ the solid becomes rubbery. Amorphous APIs are usually in the glass state and differences in properties may exist between batches due to variations in preparation and storage.[63]

Amorphous forms can be prepared by direct precipitation from solution, spray drying, freeze drying and supercritical fluid precipitation. XRPD is commonly used to determine if a material is crystalline or amorphous. As described in Section 21.2.1 the position, intensity and width of the peaks in the PXRD are directly linked to the structure and ordering of the drug structure within the crystalline lattice. For an amorphous material with no ordering, the PXRD trace produces no sharp defined peaks and typically a broad diffraction trace, as shown in Figure 21.6.

The benefits of this technique include small material requirements and short measurement times. However, XRPD measures the long-range order and the absence of this is taken to indicate amorphous material rather than directly measuring a specific property of amorphous material. Recent advances have been made in the use of X-ray sources to measure pairwise distribution functions (PDF) of amorphous material.[64,65] This measures both the diffracted and diffuse X-ray scattering, allowing the investigation of the non-crystalline signals of the diffraction patterns and measuring the probability of finding a pair of atoms separated by a specified distance. This allows differences between samples of amorphous materials to be identified. Spectroscopic techniques including infra-red, Raman and solid state NMR are also used to characterise amorphous materials; broad and less resolved peaks are obtained by all three techniques.[66]

One of the challenges with amorphous material, is the risk of crystallisation during preparation, isolation, drying, downstream processing and storage. This must be carefully monitored during development to identify conditions under which crystallisation may occur.[80] In addition it is important that the correct packaging and storage conditions are used during the lifetime of the product to ensure the material remains amorphous. Managing an amorphous form through development is a major undertaking, given the inherent propensity for chemical instability and the potential for crystallisation on longer-term stability, impacting the bioavailability.

A detailed workflow covering each of the key solid form development activities described so far in this section is shown in Figure 21.7.

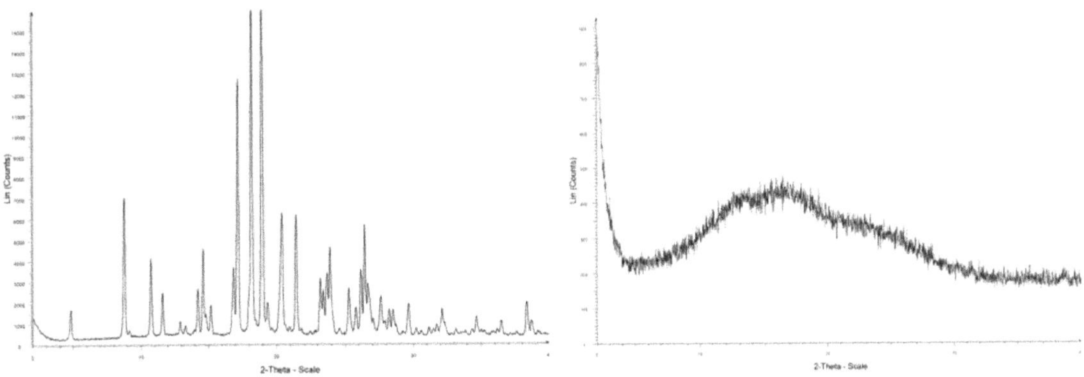


**Figure 21.6** Comparison of crystalline (left) and amorphous (right) X-ray powder diffraction patterns for verapamil hydrochloride.

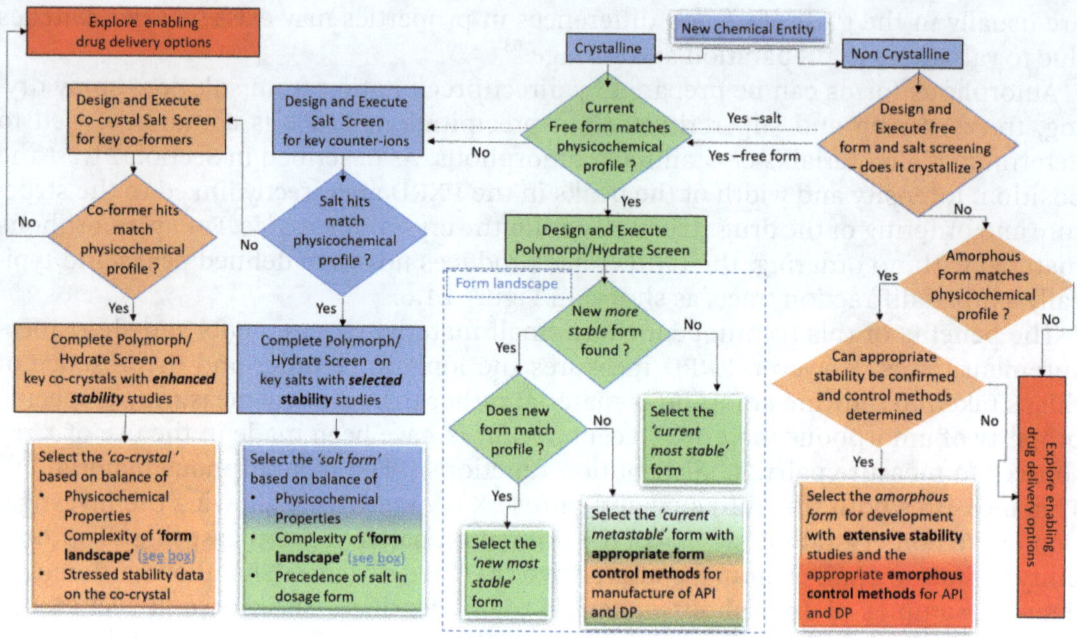


**Figure 21.7** A high-level flowchart to be used in conjunction with Figure 21.1 and Table 21.2. The decision tree is designed to enable the medicinal chemist and pharmaceutical scientist to build on the details in the chapter to both explore the potential solid state landscape and to guide the experimental and computational work to target the optimal solid form for commercialisation. The colour coding is an attempt to help the reader through balancing safety, efficacy and manufacturing requirements of the proposed active ingredient and dosage form. Green and blue represent more established standard workflows, whilst orange and red represent options with increased complexity, risk and/or enhanced potential regulatory scrutiny. For "match physicochemical profile", a decision is made by the team as to whether the properties of the form/salt identified are consistent with the proposed route/nature of delivery *etc.* The "Form Landscape" box captured in the blue dashed lines would also be applicable to the salt and co-crystal workflows, but is not reproduced fully in those workflows to avoid an overly complex picture.

## 21.3.6 Manufacturability and Particle Engineering

As part of the form selection process manufacturability needs to be considered. A manufacturing process to consistently crystallise the selected form, often at a tonnage scale, with the desired purity and particle properties is required to deliver a commercial drug product. This is typically achieved using a batch process, although in recent years there have been developments in the area of continuous crystallisation, avoiding the requirement for scale up and delivering consistent particles due to localised control of the supersaturation throughout the process.[67]

The typical API isolation process consists of a number of stages:

- Crystallisation
- Filtration
- Drying
- Particle size reduction (milling).

Each of these unit operations has a cost and yield loss associated with it. The common methods for crystallisation are: cooling, anti-solvent, reactive (including salt and co-crystal formation) and distillate or evaporative crystallisations. The selection of the appropriate method is often dependent on the degree of solubility of the NCE in suitable organic solvents, while the efficiency of the crystallisation process, and its scale up and robustness, determines the critical quality attributes of the resulting crystals, including purity, polymorphic form, crystal size and shape. Seeded cooling crystallisations are typically the most scaleable batch processes, whereas anti-solvent and reactive crystallisations are mixing dependent and can be challenging to scale consistently. The final process for crystallising the desired form must also be sustainable, limiting the use of solvent and excessive process time and ultimately becomes a balance between obtaining the desired crystals and having sensible solvent volumes and processing times.

The polymorphic form and purity are critical quality attributes in the crystallisation of an API, while the size and shape of the crystals have an impact on the downstream processing and manufacturability of the final dosage form. Needle morphologies often lead to challenges in isolation as they can block (commonly known as blinding) the filter leading to increased filtration times and typically exhibit poor flow properties, leading to challenges in downstream manufacturing processes. Crystal size, and size distributions, are also important. Crystal size is linked to bioavailability and can lead to issues with content uniformity in low dose formulations. Particle size distributions need to be controlled and consistent between batches to prevent issues with downstream processing and meet the API specifications that underpin the drug product performance.

In recent years there has been a drive to control the particle size through the crystallisation process rather than have an additional milling stage post drying, as this leads to a reduction in the number of unit operations with the associated yield loss, and a reduction in the manufacturing costs. Particle control can be achieved through controlling certain parameters during the crystallisation process, *e.g.* seed size and loading, cooling rate. High shear wet milling (HSWM) can be applied as part of the crystallisation process. This can be used *in situ* to reduce the particle size and is often used in combination with temperature cycles to control and modify the crystal shape. An example of the application of these techniques is in altering the particle width and length of an API with a needle morphology.[68] By using a combination of HSWM and temperature cycling it is possible to improve the bulk density and flow properties of a material.

After the crystallisation of the desired form and particle the material is isolated and dried. Isolation at scale is typically carried out in agitated filter dryers (AFD) or centrifuges, followed by drying in potentially a wide range of technologies. During both of these unit operations care has to be taken to preserve the form, size and morphology of the crystals. Attrition or agglomeration of the particles are common issues and can lead to problems with downstream processing either due to smaller particles or lumps causing issues with flow and content uniformity. Particular care has to be taken with hydrated forms to prevent dehydration to a different crystalline form or amorphous material during these stages of processing. During the development of both isolation and drying processes the form, particle size and morphology needs to be monitored.[69]

### 21.3.7 Computational Solid Form Design

Selection of an appropriate pharmaceutical solid form for development, previously based wholly on experimental output is now commonly enhanced with computational structural tools. The robustness of the solid form to meet safety, efficacy and manufacturing requirements is covered in ICH regulatory guidelines. In the guidelines the risk is defined as a combination of the probability of occurrence and the severity of the impact[70] and is consolidated specifically into a decision tree on polymorphs.[71] The first two decision points on this framework remain the key questions that need to be addressed.

- Decision Point 1: PROBABILITY – "can different polymorphs be formed?"
- Decision Point 2: IMPACT – "do the forms have different properties?

To achieve a greater definition of probability of a new form appearing, structural tools ranging from quantum chemistry analysis[72] and H-bonding statistics[17] to full polymorph prediction[73] can be applied either individually or in combination.

Recent developments in theoretical chemistry mean that from molecular knowledge 3D structure optimisation can occur and charges can be visualised on the van der Waals surface. These can be used to quantitatively describe the relative strength of the hydrogen bond donors and acceptors.[9] The Cambridge Crystallographic Data Centre (CCDC) has for the last 50 years consolidated organic crystal structure information and distilled this knowledge into tools and software that is routinely applied to drug design.[74] The Logit model[75] carries out a statistical analysis of hydrogen bonding patterns for a given structure. It identifies potential patterns which are compared to those in known crystal structures in order to rationalise the physical form stability. The approach has been successfully used to rationalise the observed thermodynamic stability ranking for polymorphs of lamotrigine,[76] crizotinib[9] and flunixin.[77] Full interaction maps are a further refinement[78] which provide a visualisation demonstrating the preferred geometries for intermolecular interactions in the form of a colour density plot. The data is drawn from observed geometries from a wide selection of pre-defined functional groups brought together to tailor a single visualisation, specific to the molecule and conformation. Full interaction maps have been successfully used to assess polymorph stability.[79]

Energetic and statistical analysis of the conformational landscape for flexible APIs has also been used to identify a high risk of conformational polymorphism.[80] Added value has been further demonstrated leveraging combined studies which incorporate multiple methods from this structural toolbox; to rationalise polymorphs,[81] improve the screening hit rate for co-crystals[82] and predict hydrate formation.[83]

The *ab-initio* generation of reliable solid state structures by computational methods based only on the molecular structure remains a major scientific goal. Computational crystal structure prediction (CSP) has been a rapidly growing field for more than 20 years.[73] Significant progress has been made on addressing early challenges in the field, including molecular flexibility, charged species and temperature-dependant contributions.[84,85] The CCDC have hosted a series of blind tests since 2000, demonstrating the rapid improvements in both accuracy and in the increasingly API-like nature of the test candidates.[86] The most recent of these in 2016 showed the successful CSP for salts and polymorphic systems from the pharmaceutical industry.[84] Retrospective studies from multiple groups have elegantly rationalised observed polymorphism for a number of interesting and pharmaceutically relevant systems.[87,88] Recent improvements in the computer hardware and algorithms have brought the accuracy and speed of calculations for typical candidates, in size and flexibility, into scope for candidates under active development.[89] Through comparing the computationally predicted solid form landscape with the experimentally known solid forms on a new candidate, it is possible to guide the solid form screening work needed. Where the predicted and experimentally obtained forms are both consistent and energetically distinct, the project can be progressed rapidly with high confidence in the stability of the polymorph. Otherwise, more expansive screening should be undertaken to mitigate the risk that the most stable form has not been found. The application of these tools and technologies has allowed the rapid acceleration of an oncology candidate to commercial launch.[9]

While CSP seeks to identify potential polymorphs and their relative stability, the answer to the question of whether a molecule can or will crystallise remains elusive. Recent publications began to address this[90,91] using machine learning (ML) approaches and achieved predictions with 75–80% accuracy. Despite using different approaches and data sets, the studies identified the number of rotatable bonds and the atomic connectivity as the most important molecular descriptors. In both of these studies the analysis was based on a small range of crystallisation conditions and did not take into account the effects of impurities, solvent compositions and properties, and variations in the range of crystallisation conditions. In an attempt to broaden the analysis Ghosh *et al.*[92] in 2019 used data from approximately 11 000 crystallisation experiments and 88 APIs to investigate ML approaches to predict crystallisation propensity. In addition to the features identified in the previous studies, molecular weight, chirality and the number of hydrogen bond acceptors were also identified as key molecular descriptors.

The crystallisation of drugs from the amorphous state also remains problematic, as captured in a short review of this area.[93] A challenge exists for the pharmaceutical industry in two scenarios, the first where amorphous material is required and understanding how to prevent crystallisation is important and the second when molecules are first synthesised and an understanding of how to crystallise the material is required. It is expected that the application of ML approaches to this area will continue to increase and further work is required to look at incorporating crystallisation conditions and increasing the size of the training datasets to improve the accuracy and relevance of the predictions. Although large amounts of data on crystallisation experiments exist across the industry, the collation of this into training datasets remains a large and challenging task. There is a need for enhanced crystallisation models and although a relatively high success rate was achieved in the published studies to date, the complexity of the glass formation of amorphous materials and the factors which affect this are not yet well enough understood to be able to predict which molecules will not crystallise.

Further progress has been made in the field of predicting the aqueous solubility of crystalline drug molecules.[94] Prediction of the intrinsic solubility of crystalline drug molecules allows early control of the quality of progressed candidates. A definitive accurate and comprehensive approach to predicting solubility has proven elusive. There have, however, been a number of semi empirical attempts to probe the changes in solubility as a function of structural changes in NCE structures in specific classes,[22] as well as systematic approaches to looking at matched molecular pairs to determine improved solubility as a function of small structural changes and inferred crystal packing disruption.[95] This has been further interrogated by efforts to describe the relative impact of molecular solvation and crystal packing on solubility[96] and examination of sublimation and hydration properties as a function of structural modifications.[97]

This section has demonstrated the tools which allow structural modifications to be tailored in order to improve the physical properties of the solid form. It has also highlighted the ways in which a comprehensive and computationally enhanced screening process can enable the solid form landscape of a new NCE to be fully understood, allowing rapid product design.[98]

## 21.4 Integration Within the Early Clinical Phases of Development

### 21.4.1 The Changing Drug Product Design Paradigm

Over the last two decades, significant progress has been made in defining relationships between the API properties and the formulation design aspects of new products. Examples of established progress include:

- API particle size distributions and content uniformity[99]
- API particle size distributions and flow,[100] mechanical properties[101]
- API particle size and dissolution[102]
- Crystal brittleness, milling behaviour and particle size reduction.[103]

Models have been built that allow the pharmaceutical scientist to explore the impact of particle size variation on dissolution rate and bioavailability. The Biopharmaceutics Classification System (BCS)[104] is used to define four classes of compounds based on the solubility and permeability of the compounds. Permeability is a molecular property, but solubility and dissolution rate are related to the internal structure and particle size distribution/surface area, respectively. A substance is considered highly soluble when the highest dose is soluble in less than 250 ml across the pH range 1 to 7.5. A compound is highly permeable when the extent of absorption in humans is greater than 90% of an administered dose compared to an intravenous reference dose. The four classifications are shown in Figure 21.8. API attributes are likely to have the biggest impact on classes II and IV. More recently this was built upon where the interaction between permeability and solubility, and the impact of using simulated gastric fluids in measuring solubility has brought greater definition to the impact of solubility and dissolution rate for BCS II and IV compounds.[105,106]

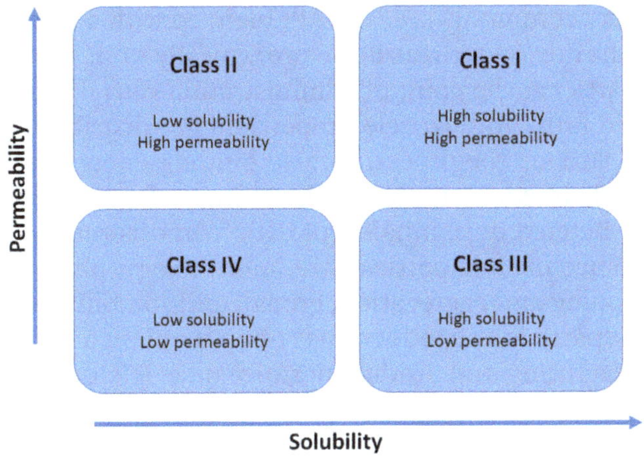


**Figure 21.8** The Biopharmaceutics Classification System.

## 21.5 Different Requirements for Dosage Form Types

The factors which influence formulation selection are wide ranging and encompass scientific consideration of the NCE physical properties, the proposed dosage form, the stage of development and overall project investment strategy. Typically, the most thermodynamically stable crystalline solid form is the preferential form for drug product development, and this is independent of the route of administration or dosage form type.

Although the greatest numbers of drug therapies are presented as oral medications, non-oral drugs are developed for a variety of reasons: to overcome high first pass metabolism, reduce side effects and/or enhance local efficacy. Examples include steroids which are delivered locally in smaller doses through inhalation, nasally and topically, decreasing inflammation without inducing harmful side effects seen by higher systemic concentrations. Non-oral dosage forms most commonly exist as solutions, suspensions or powders and can be delivered by different routes into the body.

For solution formulations a key consideration is to ensure the drug remains fully dissolved, as well as physically and chemically stable over the drug product shelf life.[107] It is important to ensure the API will not precipitate a more stable form, which could ultimately limit the dose achievable in a set volume. Therefore, a thorough understanding is required of the physical chemistry of the molecule, followed by the careful selection of buffer and counter-ion components, all to ensure less soluble *in situ* salts do not form/precipitate in the formulation.

Consistent suspension product performance relies on particles retaining the initial characteristics (size, shape, surface chemistry and amorphous content) over the product shelf life. Changes in particle size distribution within the suspension formulation can be due to dissolution from small particles and recrystallisation on to larger particles (Ostwald ripening), or agglomeration due to primary particles interacting. These are common issues for suspension-based products that can be linked back to solid form attributes including surface chemistry, amorphous content and crystallinity.

Inhaled drug delivery commonly sees the API blended with a carrier excipient (usually lactose), to bulk out the dosage form as doses are typically <1 mg. The API powder is then dispersed from the carrier at the point of administration *via* a dry powder inhaler device (DPI).[108] The API solid form and particle properties (size distribution, number of fines, amorphous content, surface roughness, lactose binding energy) all have the potential to impact the respirable fraction and hence the efficacy of the product. An alternative to a DPI is a pressured metered dose inhaler (pMDI).[109] In this the solid form and particle properties of importance include particle size, morphology, physical and chemical stability, particle partitioning and aggregation, growth and solubility within the propellant.

For many products, particle size reduction is often required to deliver suitable particle properties for manufacturing and product performance. Historically this was delivered by milling or micronisation; however, *in situ* high shear wet milling (Section 21.3.6) can replace dry milling, reducing the number of unit operations, provide tight particle size control and remove the risk of amorphous content in the milled material. For very small particles, *e.g.* for inhalation, dry micronisation techniques are still required due to the challenge of isolating small particles at the end of a crystallisation process. Different solid forms of the same API will behave differently during size reduction. This can be related to solid form properties, including melting point, compressibility and brittle fracture index.[103] The end result may be different degrees of amorphous content, which in turn could impact product performance and the shelf life achievable. Recent advances in technologies have replaced traditional formulation processes such as wet granulation, with dry processes such as roller compaction and continuous direct compression (CDC). A benefit of CDC is a reduction in the number of unit operations resulting in cost and sustainability savings. Dry processes have different requirements for particle properties, *e.g.* improved flow properties for continuous direct compression.[110] This has led to the development of new particle forming methods, including spherical agglomeration,[111] in which agglomerates of a specific size are generated after the API has crystallised.

## 21.6 Integration of Enabling Formulation Strategies

Drug development is a technically complex, inter-disciplinary, high risk, high cost business operating within an increasingly challenging environment. The industry employs a variety of different strategies in order to manage development costs whilst keeping a healthy product pipeline. During drug development, the project team continually assess the candidate progression, usually against four key factors;

- Confidence in efficacy
- Confidence in safety
- Confidence in development
- Medical needs.

These factors impact the scale and timing of the solid form selection process; ranging from comprehensive screening and solid form selection early in development with a high cost associated, through to a smaller package of work to select a form suitable for early trials. The latter option delays a more comprehensive screening until more data on the NCE safety and efficacy is known, which may lead to reformulation work being required later in the development process if the solid form selected for commercial development needs to be changed.

Influencing the physicochemical properties and hence solid form options for a molecule is a delicate balance and trade-off between optimisation of potency, selectivity and pharmacokinetics. The optimum time for the pharmaceutical scientist to engage with a project team is before lead series selection. Here a vast range of structural options are still in play and a combination of rapid solubility and stability screening can help direct the chemist towards more favourable series. Engagement in understanding solid form (and if crystalline material can be obtained) should ideally start before predictive pharmacokinetic studies commence, especially if the API is low solubility (BCS class II or IV). Although the most stable form may not be identified at this point, the ability to conduct an *in vivo* exposure study with a suspension of crystalline API *versus* a solution will provide a good indication of the solubility and or dissolution challenges facing molecule progression. In parallel to completing efficacy, safety and pharmacokinetic studies, the pharmaceutical scientist will assess the compounds "developability" for both early clinical and commercial requirements. Factors including the dosage form type and projected dose, the API synthetic complexity, solubility, stability, solid form and drug product processability will be assessed. For an oral compound, with appropriate solubility *versus* dose, the properties highlighted in Table 21.4 would give the pharmaceutical scientist some confidence in ease of further development at the pre-clinical compound selection stage.

However in reality this is often not achievable due to lack of appropriate API, time or solid form complexity, and usually a risk is carried forward into early development. One of the most common reasons for lack of crystalline material prior to first in human studies is a lack of purity. The purity required for pre-clinical safety and efficacy studies is usually around 95–98%, whereas these levels of impurities can often have a negative impact on crystal growth, making even the best crystallisation attempts futile.

Due to the general increase in more potent lipophilic molecules in development, there has been a parallel growth in enabling formulations to address poor solubility. Table 21.5 shows which molecular physical and chemical properties are amenable to which technology.

There are a number of enabling technologies that can be employed to move a drug forward when solid form design is not successful or possible. The selection is based on physical properties of the NCE and the requirements of the final dosage form. These include:

**Table 21.4** Key criteria for acceptable physical properties.

| | |
|---|---|
| Crystallinity | Crystalline |
| Melting point | >125 °C |
| Hygroscopicity | Non-hygroscopic (<3% moisture uptake over 0–90% RH) |

**Table 21.5** The compatibility of API physical and molecular properties with oral low solubility enabling formulation approaches.

| Formulation options | API physical/molecular properties |
|---|---|
| **Co-solvent systems** | Utility generally increases with increasing log*P* and decreasing melting point |
| **Micellisation** | |
| S-SEDDS (supersaturable self- emulsifying drug delivery system) | log*P* 1–4, solubility in ethanol, PEG |
| SEDDS (self-emulsifying drug delivery system) | log*P* > 4, solubility in triglycerides |
| **Complexation** | |
| Cyclodextrins | Rings with low substitution or aliphatic chains without nearby bulky groups |
| **Particle size reduction** | |
| Nanosuspension | Crystalline, $T_m$ > 125 °C, low aqueous solubility |
| Micronisation | Crystalline, $T_m$ > 125 °C |
| **pH adjustment** | |
| (*In situ* salts) | Acids of p$K_a$ < 9; bases of p$K_a$ > 4 |
| **Solid dispersion** | $T_m$ < 220 °C; $T_g$ > 70 °C, log*P* 2–8, solubility in methanol/acetone > 10 mg mL$^{-1}$ |

- *Particle size reduction*[112]
  - When considering whether particle size reduction will provide suitable enhancement, the rule of thumb is that the particle size diameter should be less than the solubility in µg ml$^{-1}$. To achieve particle sizes <15 µm micronisation is required. The importance of particle size distributions on dissolution and on oral absorption has been discussed elsewhere.
- *Self-emulsifying drug delivery systems (SEDDS)*[113,114]
  - In some cases NCEs can have properties that allow them to be dissolved in surfactants or mixtures of surfactants, lipids and co-solvents. Upon contact with water the mixtures form micelles and emulsions. This enhances solubility and the percentage absorbed.
- *Solid dispersions*[41,115]
  - Solid dispersions are amorphous API composites stabilised by common excipient polymers. They can significantly increase the oral absorption of low solubility drugs. Whilst the quasi stable form of these amorphous (high energy) solids can provide enhanced exposure, from an oral dosage form perspective, the metastable nature of this state can present challenges in terms of reproducibility and longer-term physical stability.
- *Supersaturable formulations*[116,117]
  - This is described as a spring and parachute concept, salts, co-crystals or self-emulsifying drug delivery system (SEDDs) formulations are used to create the initial supersaturation or spring, this state is then maintained for longer *in vivo* by the parachute, usually a second excipient that is a crystallisation inhibitor.
- *Pro-drugs*[118]
  - Pro-drug strategies that improve solubility are not that common because of the additional synthetic complexity and costs. Despite this, there are a number of examples where this has been applied successfully.

- *Nanoparticles*[119,120]
  - The use of nanoparticle technology is an emerging area. The particle size of the NCE is reduced to nano rather than micro size through the use of techniques such as ball or fluid energy milling or supercritical fluid processes. The reduction in particle size leads to an increase in solubility and rate of dissolution, thereby increasing the bioavailability.

A comprehensive overview of these and other strategies to address low solubility in drug discovery and development has been published.[121]

## 21.7 Future Outlook

Section 21.3.7 highlighted developments in computational methods that enhance our understanding of the solid form landscape and optimise experimental screening. Of these, CSP in particular has improved in speed and accuracy to the extent that it can now be used proactively to provide a "virtual screen", before any synthetic effort has been expended.[87,89] Modern methods are now able to successfully handle real NCE systems in terms of size, flexibility and salts, making this a viable route for many small molecule candidates. It is worthy of note that there are a wave of new elegant computational technologies emerging as foundation elements for the development and manufacture of advanced pharmaceutical particulate products. Recent examples illustrate the prediction of both crystal surface/solvent interactions and the enhancement of solubility as a function of particle size and morphological change.[122] The application of machine learning "big data" models are also showing utility in co-crystal design[123] and crystallisability prediction, offering similar promise.[85,90]

When it is not possible to improve the particle properties of an API through changing the solid form, optimisation of the crystallisation process or milling co-processing may provide an alternative route. A recent publication by the IQ consortium[124] reports on the types of co-processed materials that may be considered and highlights areas where the regulatory strategy needs to be established to allow these techniques to be progressed to commercial manufacturing processes.

The physical characteristics of the API solid form ultimately have the potential to affect the safety, efficacy and manufacturability of the product being designed and manufactured. The emergence of a range of computational tools, coupled to state of the art characterisation technologies, has allowed a greater range of desirable particle attributes to be accessed and understood in terms of product performance. Harnessing this capability and applying it to new sophisticated small-scale materials testing and institutionalised product design rules, has led to the creation of a "design by first intent" strategy for solid forms with tailored physicochemical attributes and functionality.

## References

1. W. H. DeCamp, *Am. Pharm. Rev.*, 2001, **4**, 66.
2. S. R. Byrn, R. R. Pfeiffer and J. G. Stowell, *The Solid State Chemistry of Drugs*, Academic Press, New York, 1982.

3. S. R. Chemburkar, J. Bauer, K. Deming, H. Spiwek, K. Patel, J. Morris, R. Henry, S. Spanton, W. Dziki, W. Porter, J. Quick, P. Bauer, J. Donaubauer, B. A. Narayanan, M. Soldani, D. Riley and K. McFarland, *Org. Process Res. Dev.*, 2000, **4**, 413–417.
4. D. Erdemir, A. Lee and A. Myerson, *Curr. Opin. Drug Discovery Dev.*, 2007, **10**, 746–755.
5. A. W. Newman and R. Wenslow, *AAPS Open*, 2016, **2**, 2.
6. W. Cabri, P. Ghetti, G. Pozzi and M. Alpegiani, *Org. Process Res. Dev.*, 2007, **11**, 64–72.
7. J. Bernstein, *Polymorphism in Molecular Crystals*, OUP Oxford, Oxford, 2nd edn, 2020.
8. R. A. Storey, R. Docherty and P. D. Higginson, *Am. Pharm. Rev.*, 2003, **6**, 100–105.
9. Y. A. Abramov, *Org. Process Res. Dev.*, 2013, **17**, 472–485.
10. C. C. Sun, *J. Pharm. Sci.*, 2009, **98**, 1671–1687.
11. J. Elliott and B. Hancock, *MRS Bull.*, 2006, **31**, 869–873.
12. F. C. Phillips, *An Introduction to Crystallography*, Longmans, London, 3rd edn, 1963.
13. B. Sridhar and K. Ravikumar, *Acta Crystallogr., Sect. C: Cryst. Struct. Commun.*, 2009, **65**, o460–o464.
14. N. K. Thakral, R. L. Zanon, R. C. Kelly and S. Thakral, *J. Pharm. Sci.*, 2018, **107**, 2969–2982.
15. J. D. Wright, *Molecular Crystals*, Cambridge University Press, Cambridge, 1st edn, 1987.
16. M. C. Etter, *Acc. Chem. Res.*, 1990, **23**, 120–126.
17. R. Taylor and O. Kennard, *J. Am. Chem. Soc.*, 1982, **104**, 5063–5070.
18. R. Docherty and W. Jones, in *Organic Molecular Solids: Properties and Applications*, CRC-Press, London, 1997.
19. M. J. Bryant, S. N. Black, H. Blade, R. Docherty, A. G. P. Maloney and S. C. Taylor, *J. Pharm. Sci.*, 2019, **108**, 1655–1662.
20. D. E. Williams, *J. Chem. Phys.*, 1966, **45**, 3770–3778.
21. S. Lifson, A. T. Hagler and P. Dauber, *J. Am. Chem. Soc.*, 1979, **101**, 5111–5121.
22. J. A. Cisneros, M. J. Robertson, B. Q. Mercado and W. L. Jorgensen, *ACS Med. Chem. Lett.*, 2017, **8**, 124–127.
23. M. A. Walker, *Bioorg. Med. Chem. Lett.*, 2017, **27**, 5100–5108.
24. R. Davey and J. Garside, *From Molecules to Crystallizers*, Oxford University Press, Oxford, 2000.
25. R. J. Davey, S. L. M. Schroeder and J. H. ter Horst, *Angew. Chem., Int. Ed.*, 2013, **52**, 2166–2179.
26. A. J. Cruz-Cabeza, R. J. Davey, S. S. Sachithananthan, R. Smith, S. K. Tang, T. Vetter and Y. Xiao, *Chem. Commun.*, 2017, **53**, 7905–7908.
27. D. J. W. Grant and T. Higuchi, *Solubility Behavior of Organic Compounds*, Wiley Interscience, New York, 1990.
28. H. G. Brittain, *Physical Characterization of Pharmaceutical Solids*, Taylor & Francis, Boca Raton, 1st edn, 1995.
29. A. Koda, S. Ito, S. Itai and K. Yamamoto, *J. Pharm. Sci. Technol., Jpn.*, 2000, **60**, 43–52.
30. P. H. Stahl and C. G. Wermuth, *Handbook of Pharmaceutical Salts*, Wiley-VCH, Weinheim, 2002.
31. C. Saal and A. Becker, *Eur. J. Pharm. Sci.*, 2013, **49**, 614–623.
32. G. S. Paulekuhn, J. B. Dressman and C. Saal, *J. Med. Chem.*, 2007, **50**, 6665–6672.
33. S. M. Berge, L. D. Bighley and D. C. Monkhouse, *J. Pharm. Sci.*, 1977, **66**, 1–19.
34. https://www.accessdata.fda.gov/drugsatfda_docs/nda/2009/022307s000_CrossR_P12.pdf (8 October 2020).
35. C. B. Aakeroy, M. E. Fasulo and J. Desper, *Mol. Pharm.*, 2007, **4**, 317–321.
36. https://www.fda.gov/downloads/Drugs/Guidances/UCM281764.pdf (8 October 2020).
37. http://www.ema.europa.eu/docs/en_GB/document_library/Scientific_guideline/2014/07/WC500170467.pdf (8 October 2020).
38. https://www.fda.gov/food/food-additives-petitions/substances-added-food-formerly-eafus (8 October 2020).
39. https://www.fda.gov/food/food-ingredients-packaging/generally-recognized-safe-gras (8 October 2020).
40. W. Jones, W. D. S. Motherwell and A. V. Trask, *MRS Bull.*, 2006, **31**, 875–879.
41. A. Newman, *Org. Process Res. Dev.*, 2013, **17**, 457–471.
42. H. Veith, M. Schleinitz, C. Schauerte and G. Sadowski, *Cryst. Growth Des.*, 2019, **19**, 3253–3264.
43. S. L. Childs, L. J. Chyall, J. T. Dunlap, V. N. Smolenskaya, B. C. Stahly and G. P. Stahly, *J. Am. Chem. Soc.*, 2004, **126**, 13335–13342.
44. R. Teraoka, T. Fukami, T. Furuishi, H. Nagase, H. Ueda, C. Tode, R. Yutani, S. Kitagawa and T. Sakane, *Chem. Pharm. Bull.*, 2019, **67**, 940–944.
45. X. Wang, S. Du, R. Zhang, X. Jia, T. Yang and X. Zhang, *Asian J. Pharm. Sci.*, 2020, **16**, 317.
46. M. A. E. Yousef and V. R. Vangala, *Cryst. Growth Des.*, 2019, **19**, 7420–7438.

47. S. A. Ross, D. A. Lamprou and D. Douroumis, *Chem. Commun.*, 2016, **52**, 8772–8786.
48. J. Haleblian and W. McCrone, *J. Pharm. Sci.*, 1969, **58**, 911–929.
49. https://www.ema.europa.eu/documents/scientific-conclusion/neupro-h-c-626-ii-24-epar-scientific-conclusion-variation_en.pdf (8 October 2020).
50. M. Pudipeddi and A. T. M. Serajuddin, *J. Pharm. Sci.*, 2005, **94**, 929–939.
51. A. J. Cruz-Cabeza, S. M. Reutzel-Edens and J. Bernstein, *Chem. Soc. Rev.*, 2015, **44**, 8619–8635.
52. C.-H. Gu, V. Young Jr. and D. J. W. Grant, *J. Pharm. Sci.*, 2001, **90**, 1878–1890.
53. N. Blagden and R. J. Davey, *Cryst. Growth Des.*, 2003, **3**, 873–885.
54. M. Prashad, P. Sutton, R. Wu, B. Hu, J. Vivelo, J. Carosi, P. Kapa and J. Liang, *Org. Process Res. Dev.*, 2010, **14**, 878–882.
55. A. M. Campeta, B. P. Chekal, Y. A. Abramov, P. A. Meenan, M. J. Henson, B. Shi, R. A. Singer and K. R. Horspool, *J. Pharm. Sci.*, 2010, **99**, 3874–3886.
56. S. M. Reutzel-Edens and A. W. Newman, in *Polymorphism: in the Pharmaceutical Industry*, 2006, pp. 235–258.
57. H. Zhu and D. J. W. Grant, *Int. J. Pharm.*, 1996, **139**, 33–43.
58. Y. Cui and E. Yao, *J. Pharm. Sci.*, 2008, **97**, 2730–2744.
59. M. D. Ticehurst, R. A. Storey and C. Watt, *Int. J. Pharm.*, 2002, **247**, 1–10.
60. D. E. Braun, J. A. McMahon, R. M. Bhardwaj, J. Nyman, M. A. Neumann, J. van de Streek and S. M. Reutzel-Edens, *Cryst. Growth Des.*, 2019, **19**, 2947–2962.
61. P. A. Basford, K. R. Back, M. Cram, R. Docherty, R. J. Davey and A. J. Cruz-Cabeza, *Cryst. Growth Des.*, 2019, **19**, 7193–7205.
62. V. Andronis, M. Yoshioka and G. Zografi, *J. Pharm. Sci.*, 1997, **86**, 346–351.
63. A. Newman and G. Zografi, *Mol. Pharmaceutics*, 2020, **17**, 1761–1777.
64. S. J. L. Billinge, *Philos. Trans. R. Soc., A*, 2019, **377**, 20180413.
65. J. P. Boetker, V. Koradia, T. Rades, J. Rantanen and M. Savolainen, *Pharmaceutics*, 2012, **4**, 93–103.
66. A. W. Newman and S. R. Byrn, *Drug Discovery Today*, 2003, **8**, 898–905.
67. C. J. Brown, T. McGlone and A. J. Florence, in *Continuous Manufacturing of Pharmaceuticals*, ed. P. Kleinebudde, J. Khinast and J. Rantanen, John Wiley and Sons Ltd, Hoboken, NJ, 1st edn, 2017, pp. 169–226.
68. D. Wilson, M. Bunker, D. Milne, A. Jawor-Baczynska, A. Powell, J. Blyth and D. Streather, *Powder Technol.*, 2018, **339**, 641–650.
69. S. Ottoboni, C. J. Price, C. Steven, E. Meehan, A. Barton, P. Firth, A. Mitchell and F. Tahir, *J. Pharm. Sci.*, 2019, **108**, 372–381.
70. https://database.ich.org/sites/default/files/Q9%20Guideline.pdf (8 October 2020).
71. https://database.ich.org/sites/default/files/Q6A%20Guideline.pdf (8 October 2020).
72. Y. A. Abramov and K. Pencheva, in *Chemical Engineering in the Pharmaceutical Industry:R&D to Manufacturing*, ed. D. J. a. Ende, John Wiley & Sons Inc, 2010.
73. S. L. Price, in *Polymorphism in Pharmaceutical Solids*, 2nd edn, 2016, pp. 52–75.
74. C. F. Macrae, I. Sovago, S. J. Cottrell, P. T. A. Galek, P. McCabe, E. Pidcock, M. Platings, G. P. Shields, J. S. Stevens, M. Towler and P. A. Wood, *J. Appl. Crystallogr.*, 2020, **53**, 226–235.
75. P. T. A. Galek, F. H. Allen, L. Fabian and N. Feeder, *CrystEngComm*, 2009, **11**, 2634–2639.
76. P. T. A. Galek, E. Pidcock, P. A. Wood, I. J. Bruno and C. R. Groom, *CrystEngComm*, 2012, **14**, 2391–2403.
77. M. C. Dávila-Miliani, A. Dugarte-Dugarte, R. A. Toro, J. E. Contreras, H. A. Camargo, J. A. Henao, J. M. Delgado and G. Díaz de Delgado, *Cryst. Growth Des.*, 2020, **20**, 4657–4666.
78. P. A. Wood, T. S. G. Olsson, J. C. Cole, S. J. Cottrell, N. Feeder, P. T. A. Galek, C. R. Groom and E. Pidcock, *CrystEngComm*, 2013, **15**, 65–72.
79. A. V. Vologzhanina, A. V. Sokolov, P. P. Purygin, P. N. Zolotarev and V. A. Blatov, *Cryst. Growth Des.*, 2016, **16**, 6354–6362.
80. A. J. Cruz-Cabeza and J. Bernstein, *Chem. Rev.*, 2014, **114**, 2170–2191.
81. N. Feeder, E. Pidcock, A. M. Reilly, G. Sadiq, C. L. Doherty, K. R. Back, P. Meenan and R. Docherty, *J. Pharm. Pharmacol.*, 2015, **67**, 857–868.
82. B. Sandhu, A. McLean, A. S. Sinha, J. Desper, A. A. Sarjeant, S. Vyas, S. M. Reutzel-Edens and C. B. Aakeroy, *Cryst. Growth Des.*, 2018, **18**, 466–478.
83. C. J. Tilbury, J. Chen, A. Mattei, S. Chen and A. Y. Sheikh, *Cryst. Growth Des.*, 2018, **18**, 57–67.
84. A. M. Reilly, R. I. Cooper, C. S. Adjiman, S. Bhattacharya, A. D. Boese, J. G. Brandenburg, P. J. Bygrave, R. Bylsma, J. E. Campbell, R. Car, D. H. Case, R. Chadha, J. C. Cole, K. Cosburn, H. M. Cuppen, F. Curtis, G. M. Day, R. A. Di Stasio Jr., A. Dzyabchenko, B. P. van Eijck, D. M. Elking, J. A. van den Ende, J. C. Facelli, M. B. Ferraro, L. Fusti-Molnar, C.-A. Gatsiou, T. S. Gee, R. de Gelder, L. M. Ghiringhelli,

H. Goto, S. Grimme, R. Guo, D. W. M. Hofmann, J. Hoja, R. K. Hylton, L. Iuzzolino, W. Jankiewicz, D. T. de Jong, J. Kendrick, N. J. J. de Klerk, H.-Y. Ko, L. N. Kuleshova, X. Li, S. Lohani, F. J. J. Leusen, A. M. Lund, J. Lv, Y. Ma, N. Marom, A. E. Masunov, P. McCabe, D. P. McMahon, H. Meekes, M. P. Metz, A. J. Misquitta, S. Mohamed, B. Monserrat, R. J. Needs, M. A. Neumann, J. Nyman, S. Obata, H. Oberhofer, A. R. Oganov, A. M. Orendt, G. I. Pagola, C. C. Pantelides, C. J. Pickard, R. Podeszwa, L. S. Price, S. L. Price, A. Pulido, M. G. Read, K. Reuter, E. Schneider, C. Schober, G. P. Shields, P. Singh, I. J. Sugden, K. Szalewicz, C. R. Taylor, A. Tkatchenko, M. E. Tuckerman, F. Vacarro, M. Vasileiadis, A. Vazquez-Mayagoitia, L. Vogt, Y. Wang, R. E. Watson, G. A. de Wijs, J. Yang, Q. Zhu and C. R. Groom, *Acta Crystallogr., Sect. B: Struct. Sci., Cryst. Eng. Mater.*, 2016, **72**, 439–459.
85. M. Yang, E. Dybeck, G. Sun, C. Peng, B. Samas, V. M. Burger, Q. Zeng, Y. Jin, M. A. Bellucci, Y. Liu, P. Zhang, J. Ma, Y. A. Jiang, B. C. Hancock, S. Wen and G. P. F. Wood, *Cryst. Growth Des.*, 2020, **20**, 5211–5224.
86. J. P. M. Lommerse, W. D. S. Motherwell, H. L. Ammon, J. D. Dunitz, A. Gavezzotti, D. W. M. Hofmann, F. J. J. Leusen, W. T. M. Mooij, S. L. Price, B. Schweizer, M. U. Schmidt, B. P. van Eijck, P. Verwer and D. E. Williams, *Acta Crystallogr., Sect. B: Struct. Sci., Cryst. Eng. Mater.*, 2000, **56**, 697–714.
87. M. Mortazavi, J. Hoja, L. Aerts, L. Quere, J. van de Streek, M. A. Neumann and A. Tkatchenko, *Commun. Chem.*, 2019, **2**, 1–7.
88. L. S. Price, J. A. McMahon, S. R. Lingireddy, S.-F. Lau, B. A. Diseroad, S. L. Price and S. M. Reutzel-Edens, *J. Mol. Struct.*, 2014, **1078**, 26–42.
89. S. L. Price, D. E. Braun and S. M. Reutzel-Edens, *Chem. Commun.*, 2016, **52**, 7065–7077.
90. J. G. P. Wicker and R. I. Cooper, *CrystEngComm*, 2015, **17**, 1927–1934.
91. R. M. Bhardwaj, A. Johnston, B. F. Johnston and A. J. Florence, *CrystEngComm*, 2015, **17**, 4272–4275.
92. A. Ghosh, L. Louis, K. K. Arora, B. C. Hancock, J. F. Krzyzaniak, P. Meenan, S. Nakhmanson and G. P. F. Wood, *CrystEngComm*, 2019, **21**, 1215–1223.
93. B. C. Hancock, *J. Pharm. Sci.*, 2017, **106**, 28–30.
94. P. Jain and S. H. Yalkowsky, *Int. J. Pharm.*, 2010, **385**, 1–5.
95. A. G. Leach, H. D. Jones, D. A. Cosgrove, P. W. Kenny, L. Ruston, P. MacFaul, J. M. Wood, N. Colclough and B. Law, *J. Med. Chem.*, 2006, **49**, 6672–6682.
96. C. M. Wassvik, A. G. Holmen, C. A. S. Bergstroem, I. Zamora and P. Artursson, *Eur. J. Pharm. Sci.*, 2006, **29**, 294–305.
97. G. L. Perlovich, *Mol. Pharmaceutics*, 2014, **11**, 1–11.
98. S. L. Price and S. M. Reutzel-Edens, *Drug Discovery Today*, 2016, **21**, 912–923.
99. S. H. Yalkowsky and S. Bolton, *Pharm. Res.*, 1990, **7**, 962–966.
100. M. P. Mullarney and N. Leyva, *Pharm. Technol.*, 2009, **33**, 126, 128–130, 132–134.
101. C. C. Sun, H. Hou, P. Gao, C. Ma, C. Medina and F. J. Alvarez, *J. Pharm. Sci.*, 2009, **98**, 239–247.
102. K. C. Johnson and A. C. Swindell, *Pharm. Res.*, 1996, **13**, 1795–1798.
103. L. J. Taylor, D. G. Papadopoulos, P. J. Dunn, A. C. Bentham, N. J. Dawson, J. C. Mitchell and M. J. Snowden, *Org. Process Res. Dev.*, 2004, **8**, 674–679.
104. G. L. Amidon, H. Lennernaes, V. P. Shah and J. R. Crison, *Pharm. Res.*, 1995, **12**, 413–420.
105. J. M. Butler and J. B. Dressman, *J. Pharm. Sci.*, 2010, **99**, 4940–4954.
106. K. Sugano, *Expert Opin. Drug Metab. Toxicol.*, 2009, **5**, 259–293.
107. S. Murdan, in *Aulton's Pharmaceutics*, ed. M. E. Aulton and K. Taylor, Elsevier, 5th edn, 2018, pp. 407–416.
108. A. H. de Boer, P. Hagedoorn, M. Hoppentocht, F. Buttini, F. Grasmeijer and H. W. Frijlink, *Expert Opin. Drug Delivery*, 2017, **14**, 499–512.
109. N. Roche and P. N. R. Dekhuijzen, *J. Aerosol Med. Pulm. Drug Delivery*, 2016, **29**, 311–327.
110. S. Chattoraj and C. C. Sun, *J. Pharm. Sci.*, 2018, **107**, 968–974.
111. K. Pitt, R. Pena, J. D. Tew, K. Pal, R. Smith, Z. K. Nagy and J. D. Litster, *Powder Technol.*, 2018, **326**, 327–343.
112. D.-M. Oh, R. L. Curl, C.-S. Yong and G. L. Amidon, *Arch. Pharmacal Res.*, 1995, **18**, 427–433.
113. W. N. Charman, *J. Pharm. Sci.*, 2000, **89**, 967–978.
114. C. W. Pouton, *Adv. Drug Delivery Rev.*, 1997, **25**, 47–58.
115. C. Leuner and J. Dressman, *Eur. J. Pharm. Biopharm.*, 2000, **50**, 47–60.
116. P. Gao, B. D. Rush, W. P. Pfund, T. Huang, J. M. Bauer, W. Morozowich, M.-s. Kuo and M. J. Hageman, *J. Pharm. Sci.*, 2003, **92**, 2386–2398.
117. P. Gao, M. E. Guyton, T. Huang, J. M. Bauer, K. J. Stefanski and Q. Lu, *Drug Dev. Ind. Pharm.*, 2004, **30**, 221–229.
118. P. Ettmayer, G. L. Amidon, B. Clement and B. Testa, *J. Med. Chem.*, 2004, **47**, 2393–2404.

119. J. K. Patra, G. Das, L. F. Fraceto, E. V. R. Campos, M. D. P. Rodriguez-Torres, L. S. Acosta-Torres, L. A. Diaz-Torres, R. Grillo, M. K. Swamy, S. Sharma, S. Habtemariam and H.-S. Shin, *J. Nanobiotechnol.*, 2018, **16**, 71.
120. R. Kumar, S. V. Dalvi and P. F. Siril, *ACS Appl. Nano Mater.*, 2020, **3**, 4944–4961.
121. H. D. Williams, N. L. Trevaskis, S. A. Charman, R. M. Shanker, W. N. Charman, C. W. Pouton and C. J. H. Porter, *Pharmacol. Rev.*, 2013, **65**, 315–499, 185 pp.
122. R. B. Hammond, S. Jeck, C. Y. Ma, K. Pencheva, K. J. Roberts and T. Auffret, *J. Pharm. Sci.*, 2009, **98**, 4589–4602.
123. D. Wang, Z. Yang, B. Zhu, X. Mei and X. Luo, *Cryst. Growth Des.*, 2020, **20**, 6610–6621.
124. L. Schenck, D. Erdemir, L. Saunders Gorka, J. M. Merritt, I. Marziano, R. Ho, M. Lee, J. Bullard, M. Boukerche, S. Ferguson, A. J. Florence, S. A. Khan and C. C. Sun, *Mol. Pharmaceutics*, 2020, **17**, 2232–2244.

# 22 The Medicinal Chemistry and Process Chemistry Interface

William R. F. Goundry*[a] and Jeremy S. Parker*[a]

[a]Early Chemical Development, Pharmaceutical Sciences, R&D, AstraZeneca, Macclesfield, United Kingdom
*E-mail: william.goundry@astrazeneca.com, jeremy.parker@astrazeneca.com

## 22.1 Why is the Medicinal Chemistry–Process Chemistry Interface Important?

The interaction between Medicinal Chemistry and Process Chemistry is hugely important for the overall success of drug projects. As the number of compounds under consideration in a project reduces to single digits and larger quantities of material are required, work that can be done collaboratively between the two groups aids Medicinal Chemistry in preparing material for early toxicology studies and allows Process Chemistry to start early on deliveries for late toxicology, clinical and formulation development studies. Thus, ensuring a positive and constructive relationship between the two groups should be a key focus as part of the strategy for any Drug Project. This is particularly important in the current era, with the extensive use of external partners for Medicinal Chemistry (Contract Research Organisations [CROs]) and Process Chemistry (Contract Development and Manufacturing Organisations [CDMOs]), making early engagement and planning even more important due to the number of groups involved.

### 22.1.1 Strategic Differences Between Medicinal Chemistry and Process Chemistry Syntheses

Both Medicinal Chemistry and Process Chemistry use synthetic chemistry to construct molecules, but there are differences in the focus for the two groups.

The Handbook of Medicinal Chemistry: Principles and Practice, 2nd Edition
Edited by Simon E. Ward and Andrew M. Davis

Published by the Royal Society of Chemistry, www.rsc.org

Medicinal Chemistry is initially looking for chemistry that allows rapid access to a diversity of targets, ideally allowing the variability to be introduced as late as possible in the synthesis, using approaches such as Late Stage Functionalisation (LSF). The chemistry initially only needs to be capable of delivering small amounts of material for screening, thus low yields, chromatography and use of expensive intermediates or reagents is acceptable.

Process Chemistry focus is on delivering robust and scalable synthesis, with the ultimate goal of delivering chemistry that supports commercialisation. The chemistry should be safe, efficient and reproducible.

At the interface between the groups, as larger amounts of material are required, the efficiency of both the synthetic route and processes need to be considered and improved. The stage at which these points need to be addressed will vary depending on the chemistry used and the amount required. For some projects Medicinal Chemistry introduces improvements to support early studies, whereas for other projects the initial chemistry can be scaled up to support early clinical studies. There is no formal definition as to when improvements need to start to be introduced, but the closer the cooperation between Medicinal Chemistry and Process Chemistry, the easier it is to consider the merits of the current chemistry, evaluate these against the criteria laid out in Section 22.1.2 and then make changes which match the requirements of the project at that time.

## 22.1.2 What Constitutes a Good Process Chemistry Synthesis?

Process chemists are often asked to provide factors that define a good synthesis. The SELECT[1] (Safety, Environment, Legal, Economic, Control, Throughput) criteria provide a good basis for considering factors that define a route that is suitable for scale-up and eventually commercialisation.

### 22.1.2.1 Safety

A synthesis that can be operated safely on scale-up is a key criteria for Process Chemistry. Specific safety issues, including explosivity of reagents or intermediates, exothermic events, gas evolution, and handling of flammable or pyrophoric reagents need to be manageable. Similarly, protecting the health of staff when working with toxic materials needs to be assured.

### 22.1.2.2 Environment

This criterion considers the sustainability or environmental impact of the synthesis. There is now significant focus on this important topic, and the environmental impact of the synthesis, typically measured by the PMI[2] (Process Mass Intensity), is something that clearly measures the merits of the synthesis. As well as considering the amounts of materials that are used in a synthesis (measured by PMI), the relative 'greenness' of reagents, solvents, methodologies and technologies are now also carefully considered and again used to judge the merits of the synthesis.[3]

#### 22.1.2.3 Legal

The synthesis needs to ensure freedom to operate, ideally by having patent protection for the intermediates and methodologies/technologies used. Syntheses where new patents can be generated offer advantages with the introduction of new intellectual properties and thus extended protection of product exclusivity.

#### 22.1.2.4 Economy

Ultimately, a synthesis will need to meet a Cost of Goods[4] (CoGs) target, which will be based on dose, cost of the final drug (including formulation) and selling price. A synthesis that meets this requirement will be a must for a project, but the relative cost of different syntheses provides a measure of the economic merits of the options. In general, more cost-effective routes involve fewer steps, are more convergent, use cheaper raw materials and have higher throughput (see below).

#### 22.1.2.5 Control

A synthesis with good control is essential for scale-up. Ensuring that individual steps are robust and reproducible within defined parameter ranges is critical, as well as the synthesis involving stable intermediates. Minimising impurities is also important, both by having chemistry that minimises formation, and by having control points such as crystallisation of intermediates. Raw materials and reagents should be available reliably on a scale with established specifications.

#### 22.1.2.6 Throughput

The throughput of a synthesis defines the amount of material that can be manufactured in a set unit of time. A range of factors affect this criterion, including chemical yield, cycle time for individual steps and volume of process solvents. More convergent synthetic routes have a significant impact on throughput, allowing simultaneous processing of parallel arms.

Each of these factors should be considered for the synthesis of an individual drug molecule, and the framework provides a good starting point for identification of issues that need to be resolved as larger amounts of material are delivered. However, some of the commonest issues that a medicinal chemist should be aware of are listed below.

### 22.1.3 Early Signs of Potential Issues

#### 22.1.3.1 Safety Concerns

Use of energetic reagents or intermediates (for example azides) poses significant issues on scale-up. There are similar issues with large-scale use of toxic or highly toxic reagents.

#### 22.1.3.2 Patent-protected Intermediates

Intermediates specifically included in a published patent can be used in early studies, but longer term cannot be used for commercial manufacturing campaigns without agreement and obtaining licences. This can cause significant challenges where there aren't clear alternative approaches to final compounds that use non-patented intermediates.

#### *22.1.3.3 Poor Availability of Raw Materials or Reagents*

Sourcing of raw material for small-scale work is typically easy using a catalogue supplier, but when larger amounts are needed, securing material (including of the right quality) can be a significant challenge. Similarly, some reagents are challenging to source on a larger scale (for example some of the newer ligands for transition metal catalysis), requiring identification of alternatives.

#### *22.1.3.4 Unstable Intermediates*

Unstable intermediates don't just impact the amount of final material from a synthesis, but also produce impurities that can be challenging to remove as scale increases.

#### *22.1.3.5 Low/Unpredictable Yields*

Low yields reduce throughput and are a particular issue for later steps, as much larger amounts of material need to be brought through the early parts of the synthesis. Unpredictable yields can also be challenging, as the potential variability requires large contingencies to ensure final target amounts are delivered.

#### *22.1.3.6 Long Linear Sequences*

Scale-up of long linear sequences typically results in low throughput, and even with good yields for individual stages, the overall yield of the synthesis can be low (for example, a 10-step synthesis with 80% yield per step results in an overall yield of only 10%).

#### *22.1.3.7 Late-stage Transition Metal Cross-couplings*

The use of transition metal cross-couplings late in a synthesis can result in high levels of metal impurities in the final compound, which is an issue for both toxicology and clinical studies. This can be addressed by step-reordering or by using metal 'scavengers', but this can add complexity to the synthesis.

## 22.2 Collaboration Opportunities at the Medicinal Chemistry–Process Chemistry Interface

With all the considerations listed above, setting up an early and focussed collaboration between the medicinal chemist and the process chemist is hugely important for the success of drug projects.

Early appointment of a process chemist to track and advise the project is a good step. This individual can review ongoing synthetic work and can advise on issues related to SELECT and more broadly.

As the list of potential compounds shortens, if there are common intermediates that will support the preparation of compounds, this can be a fruitful area of practical collaboration. Improving the synthesis of these molecules helps the medicinal chemist prepare larger amounts of materials for early toxicology studies, and allows the process chemist early engagement with the project chemistry, and an opportunity to develop and improve the synthesis in preparation for later campaigns. When the list of potential compounds is reduced to a handful, work from both groups on the remaining candidates provides equivalent benefit across all the synthetic work.

Finally, ongoing involvement of the medicinal chemist following transition to Process Chemistry can have benefits. This can include providing insight into experimental work completed in early stages of the project, or information about scientific improvements identified by Process Chemistry that can be incorporated into ongoing Medicinal Chemistry programmes.

In this section we outline some of the key areas where collaboration is important to the project transition, including some which represent opportunities to accelerate a project's development.

## 22.2.1 Provision of Information

A free exchange of information between the two groups is vital to ensure that a project transitions smoothly into the scale-up phase. Historically this would have been through the use of hand-typed reports, transcribing information from handwritten notebooks. A physical folder of reports and key information, including analytical data, was then passed on with the project. As industry adopted information technology, the same approach remained, but with a computer-based shared folder. Now, nearly all companies and other institutions work with electronic lab notebooks (ELNs), from which information can be taken directly, allowing the process chemist to see every time a reaction was tried by the medicinal chemist and what the outcome was.

The medicinal chemist has a key duty to ensure that their ELN write-ups conform to the FAIR (**F**indable **A**ccessible **I**nteroperable **R**eusable) data principles:[5]

- *Findable*: The experiment has the correct metadata or hashtags to allow it to be easily found.
- *Accessible*: The early chemical development team can easily access the data – this is not always the case as they may have different ELNs.
- *Interoperable*: Raw data that could help the process chemist is linked to the experiment (*e.g.* NMR FID files; HPLC files) in a format that can be interrogated.
- *Reusable*: There is sufficient information that the processes can be accurately repeated.

The medicinal chemist can greatly help the later development teams by authoring more detailed experimental write-ups (including visual observations, timings of operations, internal reaction temperatures, *etc.*). As well as the obvious experimental details it is useful to record:

- *Raw materials*: both cost and availability to help avoiding long lead times.
- *Solid state*: information on physical properties and crystallinity of compounds.
- *Analytical*: details of existing methods and data on the impurities they've detected.

### 22.2.2 Sustainability

While the medicinal chemist will strive to make new drugs using any available chemistry possible, the development functions have key objectives to make new medicines using sustainable green chemistry. Processes must be developed to minimise the amount of resources and energy consumed, while striving to reduce waste to the lowest level possible. All too frequently, in the name of advancing a compound quickly, non-sustainable processes are scaled-up to meet compound demands. Therefore, the earlier in a project's life that wasteful steps and reagents can be eliminated the better. The medicinal chemist has a key role in making green chemistry part of their mindset and making those early changes. Every time they use an environmentally damaging reagent, they can really help the process chemist by considering the mantra: Replace! Reduce! Recycle!

Often a company's key expertise in sustainability will be aligned to the development function. Good collaboration is required for medicinal chemists to access this expertise, and this should be discussed with process chemistry colleagues at an early stage. A simple example is solvent selection for a process.[6] Many pharma companies now have solvent selection guides to allow the substitution of damaging solvents for greener alternatives. These guides are backed up by *in silico* modelling to help predict the best solvent.

### 22.2.3 Process Safety

Process safety evaluates all processes that involve handling, using, storing, moving or manufacturing highly hazardous chemicals. Initial discovery research can begin on a very small scale, where it is easier to handle energetic and toxic reagents. It is not uncommon to see azide reagents being used, with routes that utilise highly energetic intermediates. As the chemistry is scaled up, process safety becomes increasingly important. A key time point for process safety is at the start of the Medicinal Chemistry–Process Chemistry interaction; while the demand for the final compound may be only 20 g, for a long linear route this may mean earlier stages are conducted on a >100 g scale. Typically, process safety expertise is based in a development function, so good collaboration is key to safe early scale-up. An example is shown in Scheme 22.1 where an intermediate building block, 2-(4-isopropyl-1*H*-1,2,3-triazol-1-yl)acetic acid, was formed on a gram

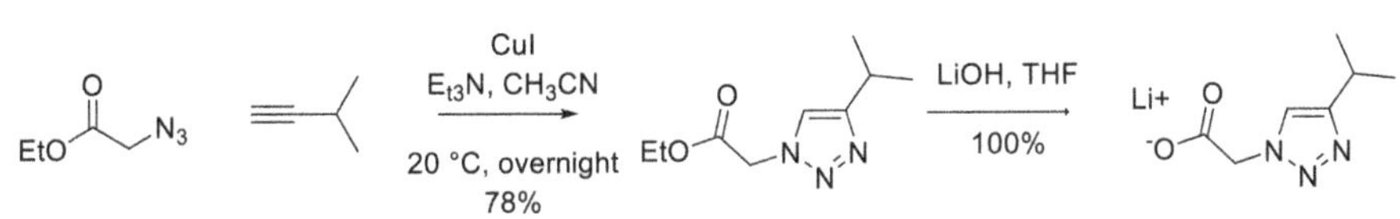


**Scheme 22.1** Initial synthesis of 2-(4-isopropyl-1*H*-1,2,3-triazol-1-yl)acetic acid.

scale in a two-step reaction from ethyl azidoacetate and 3-methylbut-1-yne.[7] The project team worked with their process safety team and identified that azidoacetate is a potential explosive; additionally, there was a risk of forming explosive copper azides in the reaction mixture. The team needed to find a way to make the synthesis safe and their solution is described in Section 22.2.5.1.

### 22.2.4 Route Design

Often the best approach to address both safety and sustainability is to develop a new route. Medicinal chemists should have an active dialogue with process chemists, so that the need for a new route can be identified and proactively worked on.[8] Where a shortlist of compounds is still under consideration, it can help to identify a key common intermediate for which a new route can be developed. Route design for a project is not down to a single person or a small local team; companies now use virtual meetings and internal social media platforms to allow input into the route design exercise by all of their scientists globally. This gives medicinal chemists the potential to influence the routes of all projects progressing.

For the antibody–drug conjugate payload tesirine, discovery scientists at Spirogen collaborated with AstraZeneca early development chemists to develop a new route.[9] Tesirine is a highly potent molecule, and the use of high potency manufacturing conditions represents a significant cost. The route was redesigned with a late stage ring closure, which minimised the number of high potency steps required. This made the manufacture safer, while reducing the cost of goods by ~60% (Figure 22.1).

### 22.2.5 Process Design

Often discovery routes are sufficient for early delivery and do not need immediately changing. As part of the Medicinal Chemistry–Process Chemistry interface, projects can be prepared for scale-up through early identification of key individual steps requiring improvement using process design. This may be through the application of specialist technologies or skillsets including Flow Chemistry, High Throughput Experimentation, Biocatalysis, Photocatalysis and Crystallisation/Solid State. One way to facilitate this is to have specialists embedded in the discovery group taking the lead on, for example, biocatalysis. For the ceralasertib project (AZD6738) AstraZeneca used this model of

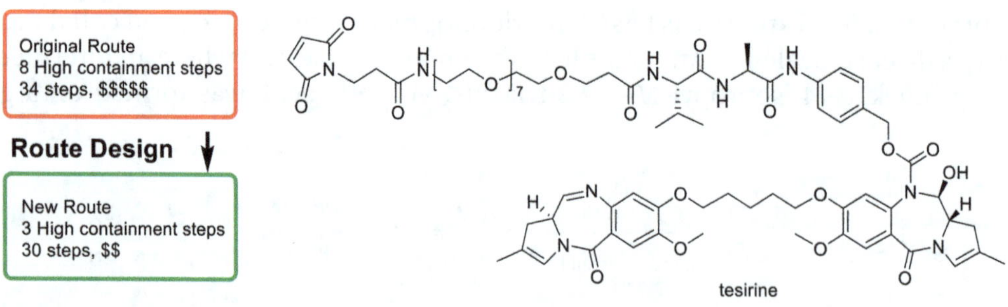


**Figure 22.1** Revised synthesis of tesirine.

embedded specialists, identifying opportunities to apply biocatalysis and flow chemistry to the medicinal chemistry route.[10] The process team then had a head start on applying these technologies for subsequent deliveries. This collaboration model does not work for all technical approaches, as some of the areas require a critical mass of specialists who reside in development functions.

#### *22.2.5.1 Flow Chemistry*

Flow chemistry can be used in process design to overcome a range of issues, including impurity formation and process safety challenges. A flow chemistry solution was used to overcome the process safety risks with the formation of 2-(4-isopropyl-1*H*-1,2,3-triazol-1-yl)acetic acid outlined in 22.2.3.[7] Isolation of hazardous intermediates was avoided and the risk was further minimised by inline FT-IR monitoring of the azide species involved (Scheme 22.2) The continuous method was used for the multi-hundred grams manufacturing of the triazole which was used for further elaboration into drug substance to support pre-clinical studies.

#### *22.2.5.2 High Throughput Experimentation (HTE)*

High Throughput Experimentation (HTE) is broadly defined as the workflow of running multiple reactions in parallel. The reactions are rationally designed to answer specific chemical questions, including: probing mechanism, reducing impurities and increasing yield. A HTE screen of a step represents a significant investment of time and resource in a single stage, and you might expect this effort to be applied at a late phase when a project has a greater chance of success. However, a 2019 survey of six of the top pharmaceutical companies highlighted that Process Chemistry HTE groups favoured an early engagement with projects in the pre-clinical phase.[11] Here the use of HTE can influence route selection and embed more sustainable processes in the project from the first deliveries.

Most commonly used to support catalytic steps, HTE is now being applied more broadly to any steps where there are a wide range of materials and conditions to be screened. Scientists at Bristol-Myers-Squib applied a HTE approach to rapidly screen and develop the conditions for an azide reduction (Scheme 22.3).[11] The initial conditions for the reduction used tin(II) chloride, but it proved challenging to remove the toxic tin salts and the yield was only 75%. A 96-well plate was used to screen 14 different reducing agents across five different solvents, identifying sodium bisulfite in water as

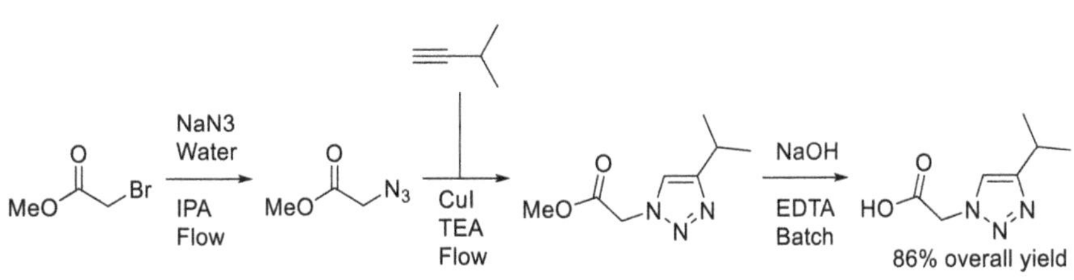


**Scheme 22.2** Flow synthesis of 2-(4-isopropyl-1*H*-1,2,3-triazol-1-yl)acetic acid.

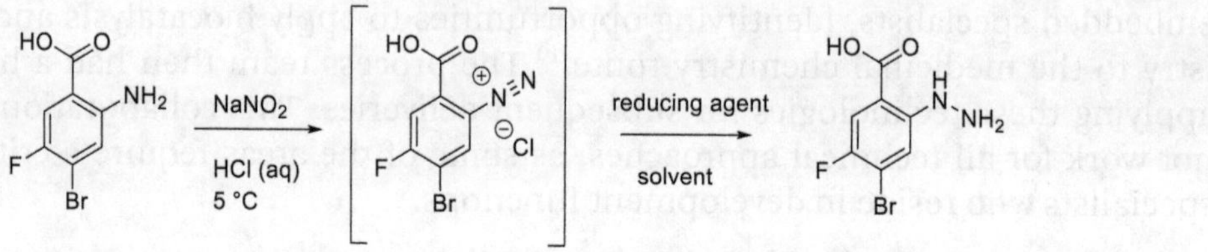


**Scheme 22.3** HTE optimisation of an azide reduction.

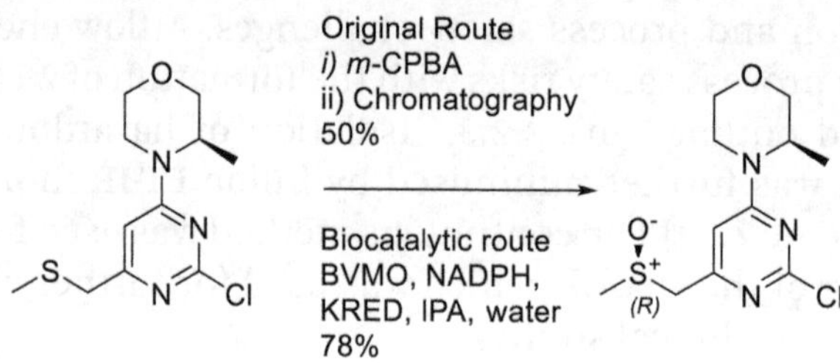


**Scheme 22.4** Introduction of a biocatalytic oxidation as part of the route to ceralasertib.

the most promising option. Following further optimisation, these conditions were used for >100 kg scale batches, giving the hydrazine product in 85% yield.

### 22.2.5.3 Biocatalysis

Biocatalytic processes represent one of the best ways to deliver sustainable pharmaceutical production and their inclusion in drug substance manufacture is becoming more commonplace.[12] It can take some time to develop a biocatalytic process, particularly if this requires directed evolution to develop a new bespoke enzyme, so process chemists need to engage as early as possible in a project to support biocatalysis screening.[13]

During the discovery phase of the ceralasertib project (AZD6738), an opportunity was spotted to replace a non-stereoselective chemical oxidation with biocatalysis (Scheme 22.4).[14] An embedded specialist screened 129 commercially available Baeyer–Villiger monooxygenases, identifying hits that gave the desired (*R*,*R*) diastereomer. A further, more focused, screen gave confidence that the transformation would be viable for scale-up. The hit was passed to the Process Chemistry team who were able to develop the process in time for the first clinical manufacture on a kilogram scale (Scheme 22.4).

### 22.2.5.4 Photocatalysis

The number of visible-light-mediated transformations has grown exponentially in the past decade and now represents a routine and well-established methodology. Alongside its growth within academic research has been its broad adoption in medicinal chemistry, with visible-light-mediated methods used to facilitate previously challenging disconnections, allowing access to increased chemical space. The scale-up of these reactions presents fundamental challenges when compared to classical reactions, due in part to the limitations of photon penetration into the reaction solution. While there are currently few documented

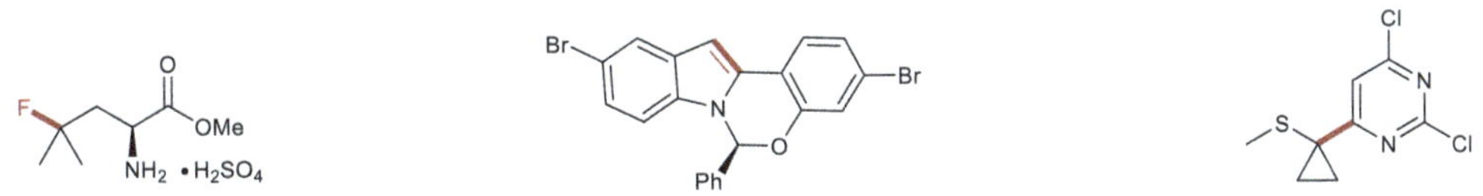

C-H fluorination: **45 g, 90% yield** — *key fragment of odanacatib*

Indoline oxidation: **86 g, 85% yield** — *core of elbasvir*

Minisci radical addition: **83 g, 31% yield** — *core of ceralasertib*

**Figure 22.2** Scale-up application of photocatalysis.

applications at production scale, a number of successful applications have been reported at scales relevant to the supply of pre-clinical manufacture and the transition from medicinal to process chemical development. For example Merck have demonstrated the synthesis of key intermediates for both odanacatib and elbasvir using flow chemistry, with AstraZeneca applying the same technology to access the core of ceralasertib *via* a visible-light-mediated Minisci reaction (Figure 22.2).[15–17] More recently, Merck have outlined a workflow for scaling visible-light reactions to multi-kg scale, which looks to represent a clear path to facilitate the transition from medical- to process-scale manufacture.[18]

### *22.2.5.5 Crystallisation/Solid State*

Advances in purification technology mean that crystallisation is seldom practiced in medicinal chemistry. While there is an obvious focus on the crystallinity and polymorph of the final drug substance, good crystalline intermediates are also highly important. Crystallisation of an intermediate represents a good control point to reject impurities. It is also generally easier to store a crystalline solid, as they tend to have greater stability than intermediates held in solution. The medicinal chemist can help by highlighting any crystalline intermediates or indeed the lack of them! If working on a large enough scale this can include the shape of the crystals and the bulk properties of the material, both of which can affect how well a solid flows and filters on scale.

## 22.3 Emerging 21st Century Challenges

Pharmaceutical companies are increasingly taking on more complex target molecules, allowing them to tackle previously undruggable targets. These 'New Modalities' include:

- Functionalised peptides
- Oligonucleotides
- Polymer–drug conjugates
- Antibody–drug conjugates

Special attention needs to be paid to these new modalities, and it is imperative that the medicinal chemists engage with the process chemists at a much earlier stage. These projects can have long multi-step routes with very low overall yields. This can mean starting the early steps of the synthesis on a multi-kilo scale just to make a few grams. As a result, the projects can have a long lead time for drug substance, with cost of goods and volumes

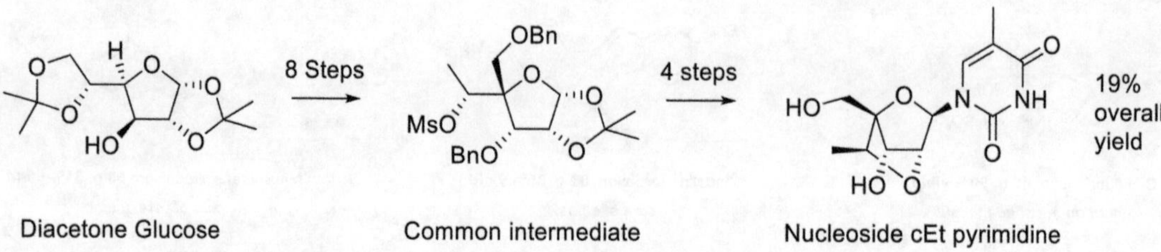


**Figure 22.3** The improved route to the nucleoside cEt pyrimidine.

of waste that are both extortionately high during the discovery phase when compared to traditional small molecules. Additionally, since the molecules are large and flexible, they are not crystalline, resulting in difficult purification and isolation. Many pharma companies are developing specialist teams to deal with these new modalities.

Antisense oligonucleotide drug projects at AstraZeneca required constrained ethyl (cEt) nucleosides as a key building block (Figure 22.3).[19] During early discovery, the route to the cEt nucleoside pyrimidine was 23 steps in 8% overall yield, with a similar synthesis and yield for four other required bases. A process chemistry team was assigned at a very early stage to develop a shorter, more sustainable, cost effective route. They developed a new route that was only 17 steps with a yield of 19%. The route has a common intermediate that could be used to synthesise the other bases.

## 22.4 Concluding Remarks

Effective collaboration between Medicinal Chemistry and Process Chemistry provides a key opportunity to accelerate drug projects and ensure a smooth transition between the discovery and development phases. As well as tackling key issues, such as safety and sustainability, a focus on improving science and seamlessly applying emerging technologies helps both groups achieve their goals.

## 22.5 Hints and Tips

- The quicker one can introduce effective chemistry into any programme, the faster it will go and the cheaper it will be.
- Be alert to tell-tale signs of potential future problems (safety concerns, long linear sequence, poor/variable yields/reagent availability *etc.*).

## Key References

For a general introduction to Chemical Development:

- Practical Process Research and Development a guide for Organic Chemists' Neal Anderson, Academic Press 2012
- On Chemistry, 5 On process chemistry, Colin Thomson, Graham Robinson, SCI-Ink Ltd 2013

For an understanding of the main issues of sustainability facing Chemical Development:

ACS Green Chemistry Institute Pharmaceutical Roundtable https://www.acsgcipr.org/

For the latest advances and publications in the field of process chemistry see:

Organic Process Research & Development https://pubs.acs.org/journal/oprdfk

For an overview of FDA guidance documents see Food and Drug Administration web site, Guidance documents, in particular, the section on Investigational New Drug (IND) Application.

## References

1. M. Butters, D. Catterick, A. Craig, A. Curzons, D. Dale, A. Gilmore, S. P. Green, I. Marziano, J.-P. Sherlock and W. White, *Chem. Rev.*, 2006, **106**, 3002–3027.
2. C. Jimenez-Gonzalez, C. S. Ponder, Q. B. Broxterman and J. B. Manley, *Org. Process Res. Dev.*, 2011, **15**, 912–917.
3. S. G. Koenig, D. K. Leahy and A. S. Wells, *Org. Process Rev. Dev.*, 2018, **22**, 1344–1359.
4. P. Basu, G. Joglekar, S. Rai, P. Suresh and J. Vernon, *J. Pharm. Innovation*, 2008, **3**, 30–40.
5. M. D. Wilkinson, M. Dumontier, I. J. J. Aalbersberg and G. Appleton, *et al.*, The FAIR Guiding Principles for scientific data management and stewardship, *Sci. Data*, 2016, **3**, 160018.
6. L. J. Diorazio, D. R. J. Hose and N. K. Adlington, Toward a More Holistic Framework for Solvent Selection, *Org. Process Res. Dev.*, 2016, **20**, 760–773.
7. S. Karlsson, C. Cook, H. Emtenäs, K. Fan, P. Gillespie and M. Mohamed, Development of a Safe Continuous Manufacturing Route to 2-(4-Isopropyl-1*H*-1,2,3-triazol-1-yl) acetic acid, *Org. Process Res. Dev.*, 2017, **21**, 1668–1674.
8. P. Cornwall, L. J. Diorazio and N. Monks, Route design, the foundation of successful chemical development, *Bioorg. Med. Chem.*, 2018, **26**, 4336–4347.
9. A. C. Tiberghien, P. W. Howard, W. R. F. Goundry, M. McCormack and J. S. Parker, An Alternative Focus for Route Design for the Synthesis of Antibody–Drug Conjugate Payloads, *J. Org. Chem.*, 2019, **84**, 4830–4836.
10. W. R. F. Goundry, K. Dai, M. Gonzalez, D. Legg, A. O'Kearney-McMullan, J. Morrison, A. Stark, P. Siedlecki, P. Tomlin and J. Yang, *Org. Process Res. Dev.*, 2019, **23**(7), 1333–1342.
11. S. M. Mennen, *et al.*, The Evolution of High-Throughput Experimentation in Pharmaceutical Development and Perspectives on the Future, *Org. Process Res. Dev.*, 2019, **23**, 1213–1242.
12. J. P. Adams, M. J. B. Brown, A. Diaz-Rodriguez, R. C. Lloyd and G.-D. Roiban, Biocatalysis: A Pharma Perspective, *Adv. Synth. Catal.*, 2019, **361**(11), 1615–4150.
13. J. L. Porter, R. A. Rusli and D. L. Ollis, Directed Evolution of Enzymes for Industrial Biocatalysis, *ChemBioChem*, 2016, **17**(3), 1439–4227.
14. W. R. F. Goundry, B. Adams, H. Benson, J. Demeritt, S. McKown, K. Mulholland, A. Robertson, P. Siedlecki, P. Tomlin and K. Vare, Development and Scale-up of a Biocatalytic Process to form a Chiral Sulfoxide, *Org. Process Res. Dev.*, 2017, **21**(1), 107–113.
15. S. D. Halperin, D. Kwon, M. Holmes, E. L. Regalado, L.-C. Campeau, D. A. Dirocco and R. Britton, Development of a Direct Photocatalytic C–H Fluorination for the Preparative Synthesis of Odanacatib, *Org. Lett.*, 2015, **17**(21), 5200–5203.
16. H. G. Yayla, F. Peng, I. K. Mangion, M. McLaughlin, L.-C. Campeau, I. W. Davies, D. A. Dirocco and R. R. Knowles, Discovery and mechanistic study of a photocatalytic indoline dehydrogenation for the synthesis of elbasvir, *Chem. Sci.*, 2016, **7**(3), 2066–2073.
17. M. A. Graham, G. Noonan, J. H. Cherryman, J. J. Douglas, M. Gonzalez, L. V. Jackson, K. Leslie, Z.-Q. Liu, D. McKinney, R. H. Munday, C. D. Parsons, D. T. E. Whittaker, E.-X. Zhang and J.-W. Zhang, Development and Proof of Concept for a Large-Scale Photoredox Additive-Free Minisci Reaction, *Org. Process Res. Dev.*, 2020, **25**(1), 57–67.
18. E. B. Corcoran, J. P. McMullen, F. Levesque, M. K. Wismer and J. R. Naber, Photon Equivalents as a Parameter for Scaling Photoredox Reactions in Flow: Translation of Photocatalytic C–N Cross-Coupling from Lab Scale to Multikilogram Scale, *Angew. Chem., Int. Ed.*, 2020, **59**(29), 11964–11968.
19. H. Blade, D. Bradley, L. Diorazio, T. Evans, B. R. Hayter and G. P. Howell, Modular Synthesis of Constrained Ethyl (cEt) Purine and Pyrimidine Nucleosides, *J. Org. Chem.*, 2015, **80**, 5337–5343.

# 23 Clinical Drug Development

Maarten Kraan*[a]

[a]AM-Pharma, Netherlands
*E-mail: m.kraan@am-pharma.com

## 23.1 Introduction

Clinical research on the effects of therapeutic interventions is probably as old as medicine itself; in documents of the old Greek masters such as Hippocrates, systematic approaches to study the effects of medicines in human disease are already documented. Since then, there have been evolutions and revolutions, but especially in the second half of the 20th century, systematic clinical studies of the benefits and risks of drug-related interventions in human disease have developed rapidly. This evolution was driven by:

1. The call for evidence-based medicine by patients, prescribers, payers, and health authorities. The challenge at hand in designing clinical development plans is how to predict in a relatively small and well-controlled sample size what the benefit and risks of a therapeutic intervention will be when used in the general population. This is relevant for the benefits as well as the risks and on the latter, one relevant example has been the completely unexpected side effects from thalidomide when used on a large scale by pregnant mothers for the indication it was registered for.[1]
2. A second important catalyst of change in the clinical part of drug development in recent decades has been the industries ever-declining success rates. Significant effort has been placed on understanding the various items' contribution to the current challenges, such as cycle time, probability of technical success/risk, value, and cost. Depending on the therapy area and type of drug, clinical development can now take as much 25 000 patient years and 20 years and still can have a significant post-registration commitment, increasing even further the amount of data generated on a therapeutic intervention.

The Handbook of Medicinal Chemistry: Principles and Practice, 2nd Edition
Edited by Simon E. Ward and Andrew M. Davis

Published by the Royal Society of Chemistry, www.rsc.org

3. A third important and very exciting promoter of change in the past decades has been the discovery and development of targeted medicines where the biological or genetic makeup of the patient/disease will determine the efficacy of the applied treatment. In this case, the therapeutic intervention is frequently connected to a diagnostic procedure as well. Most examples are found in the treatment of malignancies based upon the mutations driving the tumour growth, such as BRAF or BRCA mutations, and of rare genetic diseases such as Wilson disease, achondroplasia or Duchenne muscular atrophy.

In this chapter the focus will be on clinical trials in drug development, primarily designed to acquire data on the safety/tolerability and efficacy of pharmaceutical interventions related to health/disease. Clinical trials can also be used for non-pharmaceutical interventions, devices, and diagnostics but are considered out of context for this chapter.

## 23.2 Types of Clinical Trials

The definition of a clinical trial is wide; hence they can be categorized using a variety of approaches:

1. A simple classification is twofold, according to the intentions of the investigator.
   (i) In an *observational* trial, the aim is primarily to observe specific elements of disease, this can also include standard of care treatment. Data are generally generated on the outcome of the disease or symptom over a certain period. An example is a study comparing the incidence and prevalence of allergic diseases in children growing up in a big city compared to children growing up on a farm, aimed at understanding how these very different environments influence the immune system.
   (ii) In an *interventional* trial, the investigator applies a specific treatment or intervention. This can be done as a single intervention applied in all subjects, but in these clinical trials there is usually a control group that can be either with or without active treatment. When the choice is made that active treatment is given to the control group, this can be standard of care, or a so-called active comparator. In the case of an active comparator, the investigator uses a specific second drug intervention to compare the investigative compound to, this comparator usually has a treatment effect that is in the same category as the investigational compound. To increase the rigor and strength to come to a high-quality conclusion of the interventional trial and hence confidence in the data when no active treatment is given to the control group, the patient is given a fake dose without active ingredient, a so-called placebo. The use of placebo was introduced to correct for expectation bias, where the patient/health care provider are expecting a benefit or risk and will unconsciously respond to that expectation.

- Within these interventional trials there are some more relevant subcategories; when the patients are aware of what treatment he/she receives it is called an open-label investigation. As mentioned previously about the introduction of placebo, knowledge of treatment can influence the outcome, as for example the investigator and/or patient expect one of the studied compounds to be better/different than the other. Hence, a further maturation of the interventional trial is blinding of the groups involved, this implies the patient is not aware of which treatment arm they are exposed to. This will improve the reliability and reproducibility of the investigation, since the patient is not aware of whether the active treatment or the control treatment is used. This blinding has been demonstrated to significantly improve the quality and reliability of a study since it addresses the so-called expectation bias, where the patients anticipate the expected effects of the intervention. For further standardization, the investigator and staff can be blinded for the treatment as well. This is usually done by pre-packaging the medication, not allowing visual identification of the doses, or by using an independent pharmacist where local preparation is required. This is called a double-blind clinical study. When the study treatment is blinded and the two comparative treatments are very different, for example comparison of an intravenous with an oral treatment, a double dummy is applied, in that case there is an active and a placebo which are identical in colour, shape, taste, and overall appearance, enabling maximal control of the bias that either patient, investigator, or staff can identify what treatment is administered to the patient. To further control the variability between the various relevant clinical and demographic parameters, patients can be randomized, by assigning them randomly to the treatment options, hence the variations between the various groups can be controlled. In conclusion, the best controlled and most rigorous interventional clinical trial is the prospective, placebo controlled, double dummy, randomized trial. The last step can be stratification: if there is the expectation that some variables (such as, for example, age) are very relevant, the assignment of study medication is controlled to make sure there is a equal distribution over the relevant subgroups.

2. A second categorization is based upon what data are used, existing or new data. This is relevant in situations where the forward/prospective generation of a new data set is not needed/possible or good-quality existing data can be used. These types of clinical trial, that investigate data that are already generated are called retrospective; for example, a hospital that wants to know how patients with a pneumonia were treated over the past ten years. The challenge with retrospective trials is that the data used can be of variable quality or the circumstances under which they are acquired were subject to bias, which can significantly influence the outcome/conclusions of the trial without the investigator being aware of it.
3. A third approach is to categorize trials towards the projected outcome of the trial.
   (i) Prevention trials will measure the difference between two groups where an intervention is aimed to prevent the occurrence of either a disease or alternatively of a sign or symptom of a disease. An example is the assessment of whether the use of statins interfering with the lipid metabolism is effective in the prevention of stroke or myocardial infarction.

(ii) Screening trials are designed to detect disease in a certain population. For example, the trials that were done to study effect of mammography for early detection of breast carcinoma in women.
(iii) Closely related are diagnostic trials where the aim is to test the ability of a method to detect a certain diagnosis measure or the effect of a (biological) probe on detecting a disease state or diagnosis. An example is the use of PAP smears to demonstrate the sensitivity and specificity to predict cervical cancer.
(iv) The most traditional of all are the treatment trials. Here two interventions aimed on interfering with a disease state are compared.
(v) Quality of life trials are designed to measure changes in the impact of a disease state on the quality of day to day living. For example, measuring the impact of COVID-19 infection on daily life activities, returning to work/school/*etc.* comparing the infected and those not infected.
(vi) Compassionate use trials or expanded access trials provide partially tested, unapproved medicines to a small number of patients who have no other realistic options. Usually, this involves a disease for which no effective therapy exists, or a patient who has already attempted and failed all other standard treatments. Usually, case-by-case approval must be granted by both the regulatory bodies on the applicability and the pharmaceutical company on a patient-by-patient basis for such exceptions.

## 23.3 Phases of Drug Development

Traditionally drug development has been categorized in phases, largely determined by the type of data to be generated over the clinical maturation of the medicine in the period before commercialization. Since many therapy areas still follow this paradigm, it will be discussed first in this section. In the past decade, a new development has emerged, so called phase-less development. This was the response to the development of medicine for rare disease and oncology, where exposure of healthy volunteers was not ethical or relevant and/or there was a very small patient population and will be discussed later in this section as well.

1. **Phase 0 studies**
   This is traditionally a study in patients where no unregistered investigational product is used, and patients are either subject to standard of care or to a compound that is already registered to be used in that disease and the application is done within the label, as approved by the health authorities. The study readout can be almost anything, but most widely used is a symptom, biomarker, or any other signal of biological relevance. With the growing realization in the medical community that disease heterogeneity will have a direct effect on how pharmaceuticals will work on human disease, there is with increasing frequency a strong need/demand to study pathways and biosignals in humans. In the pre-clinical phase of drug development there is still a frequent use of animal models touching upon

elements of disease. However, we have learned in recent history that these have a limited translatability to human disease and hence there is a need to translate these signals to humans or to identify them. The purpose of these exploratory clinical trials in Phase 0 is to study the disease to be targeted; the aim can be to understand variables influencing outcome or response, or to develop biomarkers *etc.* An example is a study in rheumatoid arthritis, where two registered novel therapies with a distinct mechanism of action are compared to understand how these differences are detectable and how the immune system is modulated over time.

2. **Phase 1/First in man studies**

   This is traditionally the first step after completion of the non-human studies. The aim of this phase is to demonstrate the safety and tolerability of the investigational products and consequently this is the phase that humans are exposed to the investigational product for the first time. This can be done in either healthy volunteers or in patients. The choice is usually made based upon the expected profile of the drug, where especially tolerability drives the choice to go directly into patients (oncology). Alternatively, the choice to go into patients can be driven by the fact that the target is only expressed in diseased humans. The disadvantages of going directly into patients are co-morbidities and other treatments. At the end of this phase there should be clarity on the relation between the dose administered and the safety and tolerability, allowing a dose to be chosen for the next phase aimed on determining the efficacy of the intervention. Most programmes will already try to capture effects on the targeted disease, but they are usually only exploratory of nature.

   (i) Before human subjects can be dosed, a comprehensive package of non-human studies needs to be completed. These studies are all designed to study the pharmacology of the investigational product as much as possible with regards to its kinetic properties (half-life, distribution, and elimination) potential mutagenicity and teratogenicity, effects on fertility, and especially effects of supra-therapeutic doses over a significant period.

   (ii) The first study of a new investigational product is usually a single rising dose programme. Based upon the pre-clinical data, a dose-escalating programme is built, where the purpose is to find the maximally tolerated dose based upon clinical parameters. Although the route of administration can be both enteral and parenteral, the route chosen is usually the route preferred for the product when on label. The doses used during this phase are calculated using a framework established by regulators, based upon decades of drug research.[2] In summary, usually no adverse effect levels (NOAL) from the relevant animal studies are converted to the human equivalent dose (HED) using standard factors. Using sound scientific judgment, a safety factor is applied to the HED from the most appropriate species to arrive at the maximally recommended safe dose (MRSD). This process is meant to define the upper limit of recommended starting doses and, in general, lower starting doses can be appropriate. In the past decade there have been two major events (TeGeneRo[3] and cannabis[4]), where volunteers faced serious health challenges because the compound under investigation had an unexpected deleterious impact on the biological system with the doses used. These events have further reinforced the framework of careful transition from non-human GLP studies to human testing, aiming to detect the potential negative impact before entry into humans. Examples are careful choice of starting dose based upon a variety of factors such as:

- novelty of the agent
- biological potency
- mechanism of action
- degree of species-specificity of the agent
- dose–response curves of biological effects in human and animal cells
- dose–response data from *in vivo* animal studies
- pharmacokinetic and pharmacodynamic modelling
- calculation of target occupancy *versus* concentration
- calculated exposure of targets or target cells in human *in vivo* effective dosing

Once in humans, the dosing and escalation schedules have been adjusted, including calculation of the minimal acceptable biological effect level (MABEL), sentinel dosing, and reducing the number of volunteers or patients exposed when adjusting the dose levels. Other factors, such as the ability to assess target engagement warrant a diligent set of experiments in the pre-clinical phase.

(iii) After completion of the single rising dose programme, it is usually followed by a multiple rising dose programme, and frequently these are combined in a single investigation. Exceptions can generally be found in programmes with large molecules where half-life can be up to 21 days, hence a single administration results in a durable exposure. On designing such a programme, the rules of rising multiple doses are followed, which implies that the projected maximal dose is subject to higher scrutiny. Objectives in this phase are usually safety and tolerability, but there is usually a strong component of clinical pharmacology where target engagement is demonstrated. The term target engagement is used to define whether the potential medicine is interacting with the projected target. The types of target engagement used have changed quite dramatically over the past decades: where it originally was proof that the compound pharmacologically engaged the target (for example that a compound binds to the targeted receptor) it has evolved to proof that compound has meaningful biological effect (for example, that a drug for the treatment of HIV reduces the viral load, or an immune-oncology drug selectively changes the cell populations involved in the tumour environment). This has put more stress on the pre-clinical phase of development since this requires that patient-derived tissues are included much earlier to create the assay platform needed; the upside was that the platform of evidence matures much earlier and hence the probability of success (PTS) of the compounds once they have entered the clinical phase has improved significantly.

3. **Phase II studies**

In this phase the aim is demonstrate that the investigational product has a meaningful effect on the targeted disease. The questions addressed are best captured in the following principles: (1) proof of mechanism, evidence that the compound hits the projected target, (2) proof of principle, evidence that the compound changes the relevant disease biology after engaging the target, and (3) proof of concept, evidence that the disease responds to the compound in a meaningful way. These questions are usually answered in the first set of experiments, or Phase IIa. After these principles are addressed, there is commonly a Phase IIb, where the primary aim is to establish a dose. These studies serve two key purposes, first is to support internal decision making in the company developing the asset, and help design the Phase III programme, and second to facilitate discussions with regulators on the optimal design for the label-generating studies.

4. **Phase III studies**

   In this phase the investigational product has proven to be able to influence the targeted disease and needs to demonstrate a robust safety/benefit profile in the target population. Generally, this phase is used to generate the data that establish the label of the product, *i.e.* the data that are used by the sponsor to negotiate with the various health authorities on what claims can be made towards what effect the medicine will have upon the targeted disease.

   Health authorities are highly interested in the benefit the investigational compound creates in relation to the risk it poses to the individual; the latter is frequently crucial since some significant safety effects are not easily detected in the relatively small population exposed. For that reason, there is an increasing demand for sizable studies to make sure enough patients are exposed. Another crucial item is variability (between geographies for example) and hence health authorities frequently request two identical Phase III studies to be executed in parallel. In the past decade, a second stream of studies has been started during this phase as well, that are studies to demonstrate the value mainly aimed towards health care providers such as insurance companies, or governmental bodies such as the national institute (NICE) in the UK that are trying to distribute limited resources towards those health interventions that drive most value.

   (i) Many choices need to be made/options to be considered here. This phase is dominated by the four cornerstones, risk, time, value, and cost. Weighing of these four trade-offs needs to be made, where changes in one of these elements commonly impacts the others. For example, if a certain risk identified in Phase II is mitigated, there is usually an increase in cost and a delay in the timeline, which shortens the time on the market with patent protection, *i.e.* value.

   (ii) When the asset is developed for an indication that is not classified as orphan or rare, the sponsor is frequently asked by the health authorities to execute two parallel identical global trials to support the label claim, in order to control the heterogeneity of disease, which has been frequently observed in the past and caused a change in the risk to benefit profiles after commercialization compared to what was observed in the development phase. Another question that can be asked by the health authorities is to include two doses in the Phase III programme to be compared on risk and benefit if there are still questions after completion of Phase II. Since this will significantly increase the size of the trial it is usually avoided by optimizing the Phase II design, in close collaboration with the regulatory bodies. Finally, regulatory authorities usually require a significant number of patients (commonly 500 or more) to be treated for a significant period (commonly 1 year) before accepting the safety data set. There are, of course, indications/diseases where this is not possible.

5. **Phase IV studies**
   (i) This is the phase after the right for commercialization has been established. In this phase, two dominant themes dictate the data that need to be generated: (1) the need of the commercial organization to make sure the potential of the now approved drug is utilized and (2) the increasing need of regulators to understand the benefit/risk profile when the drug is exposed to a wider population not limited by stringent inclusion and exclusion criteria.
   (ii) When changes in the formulation (for example a switch from an intravenous administration to oral) are considered after commercialization, a whole new set of pre-clinical and clinical studies is required, as it is very likely considered a new drug by the regulatory and other authorities.
   (iii) When changes are made in the manufacturing and/or formulation of a drug (for example switching to a controlled release formulation) the extent to which pre-clinical and clinical studies need to be repeated depends on the specific situation and will be done in close discussion with the regulatory and health authorities.
6. **Phase-less drug development**
   Driven by rare oncological and orphan diseases, there has been an increasing number of medicines that have been tested in the last decades without using the traditional phases of development as discussed earlier in this section. This was catalyzed by the fact that there is a very small target patient population in combination with the observation that efficacy signals can be obtained early and in only a few patients. In addition, there is frequently no standard treatment available and/or the expected treatment effect is sometimes so specific that the traditional control/placebo patients are replaced by historical controls. The understanding that several molecular pathways are altered in cancer as a result of gene mutations and protein modifications with a result of abnormal activation of intracellular signal transduction (examples are BRCA, HER, PI3K/Akt/mTOR, BRAF, MEK), affecting cell proliferation, apoptosis, cell de-differentiation, and cell migration. Considering these molecular alterations has resulted in the development of molecules able to selectively bind to molecular targets only present on the surface of/in the tumour cells. In the early '90s was the discovery and development of the first selective tyrosine kinase inhibitor, imatinib mesylate (Glivec®), a specific competitive inhibitor of ATP, directed to the fusion protein BCR-ABL typical of patients with chronic myelogenous leukaemia and acute lymphoid leukaemia that are Philadelphia chromosome-positive. Many molecules have followed since. The first targeted programme with a monoclonal antibody started in 1992 with trastuzumab (Herceptin®) a monoclonal antibody directed toward the mutated HER2/neu receptor of breast cancer; registration was achieved in 1998 and since then many constructs have followed.

## 23.4 Targeted Drugs/Companion Diagnostics and Biomarkers

1. The increased knowledge of the biology underlying disease has allowed clinical drug development to focus on those patients where the biological driver of the disease can be identified before the treatment is initiated. This will dramatically improve the likelihood that the treatment will have a meaningful effect on disease progression or outcome, and hence has important implications on the clinical development. Areas where these have been most impactful in the past decades are in oncology and in (orphan) diseases, both in relation to a genetic mutation. Firstly, it has allowed the identification of patients at risk *via* testing the presence of the relevant mutation (examples are BRAF, MEK, BRACCA, Wilson) and hence excluding those that do not have this mutation and will not respond to targeted therapy. Secondly it has reduced the need for traditional phasing of drug development, shortening the clinical trial period, and thirdly it has reduced the number of patients that need to be studied since the target population is more homogenous.
   (i) When a companion diagnostic is considered, this needs to be implemented from the pre-clinical stage of development to make sure the biological signal used is incorporated into all phases of clinical development. In addition it requires a separate discussion and dossier with the competent authorities besides the clinical and CMC discussions. The most important reason is that the biological signal (for example the presence of mutated BRAF in melanoma as diagnostic for a BRAF-targeted drug such as encorafinib) has a relation to the observed clinical, pharmacological, and toxicological effects in patients with and without the targeted diagnostic marker.
2. Biomarkers have been equally important in drug development over the past decades and can be distinguished in various categories.
   (i) Markers of target engagement used during the pre-clinical and early clinical stages to determine whether the intervention established its primary mode of action in the biological system. In the pre-clinical phase these are mostly purposely built assay systems or animal models, but in the complex clinical systems they still need to perform, which has proven to be a serious challenge. An example is the ability of an IL-6r targeted construct to bind and neutralize IL-6 in inflammatory diseases. Initially constructs that bound directly to IL-6 were tested and showed great target engagement, but very limited clinical efficacy. When constructs targeting the IL-6 receptor were tested they had similar target engagement and great clinical efficacy. This is thought to be reflective of the very large so-called sink of all the IL-6 protein in the body to be bound compared to the much smaller number of IL-6 receptors that needed to be blocked to achieve clinical efficacy.
   (ii) Biomarkers predicting response are an even bigger challenge, for example the use of C-reactive protein(CRP) for targeted therapies in rheumatoid arthritis. CRP has been demonstrated to be a great surrogate predicting response with TNF-targeted constructs, and subsequently also demonstrated to be

very useful for traditional synthetic disease-modifying antirheumatic drugs (DMARDS) such as methotrexate. However, when the IL-6 targeted constructs were developed, CRP was directly reduced, and hence CRP lost its use as a surrogate for clinical response.

(iii) The highest hurdle are biomarkers predicting outcomes, for example the oestrogen receptor status in patients with breast carcinoma. This is a reflection of the intrinsic heterogeneity of the biology underlying the disease and the hence the 'noise' created by the other factors involved in the disease state. Next to that, but reflective of the same principle, biomarkers of outcome can perform on the population level/large groups but underperform in the case of an individual patient.

## 23.5 Platform of Evidence and Probability of Success

During the total duration of a clinical development programme, that can take over a decade, there is no simple equation or single factor that is predictive of success. It is a complex composite that will be different for each molecule and encompasses all the information on the target and molecule from the various disciplines involved, which is termed the platform of evidence. It starts with taking the biology of the target in the patient with the disease and dissecting that into a programme that addresses the challenges facing the teams involved in a structured fashion. Not all challenges will have a similar weight in the likelihood that the programme will succeed, and they will also vary by phase of development. It is good practice to calculate in a structured fashion the hurdles to reach both the next phase and the commercial phase. The goal for success should be changing the patient's life, their ability to thrive and survive, and not whether the next phase of development is achieved, a metric that is frequently used in the industry for resource planning and external communication and unfortunately often confuses teams.

## 23.6 Basic Considerations/Principles Including Statistics

1. Randomization has been discussed before and is used to make sure bias introduced by unequal distribution of patient characteristics does not interfere with the assignment of active *versus* comparators.
2. The size of a trial is very important; if it is too small it will not be able to demonstrate the value of the intervention and if too big it will consume more resources and will take longer. To predict the size of a trial, the sponsor uses power calculations based on the smallest effect that is scientifically or clinically meaningful, and is based on three pillars:

   (i) the alpha level (the significance level) or the acceptable probability of a Type I error (concluding that results are statistically significant when they came about purely by chance or because of unrelated factors) usually set at 0.05 or 5%,

(ii) the effect size (anchored in either comparable trials or assumed),
(iii) the amount of variation in the data, reflected in assumed standard deviation,
(iv) whether you expect the results will only go in a single direction (only improvement) or could go in two directions (both improvement and deterioration are assumed),
(v) the confidence level, or the probability that a parameter will fall between a pair of values around the mean, usually defined between 90 and 99%.

An easy to use calculator can be found on the internet.[5] For example, when you expect a strong signal or an expected difference of 15% between active and control, a very good standard deviation of 10%, and an alpha of 0.05, the data may vary in two directions, and with a confidence level of 90%, you will require a sample size of only 10 subjects per arm. In contrast, with the other assumptions remaining the same, when the delta is half, or 7.5 points and the variation double (20) points it will require 150 subjects per arm.

3. Adaptive design is the technique where there is flexibility built into the design that allows the investigation to proceed depending on a pre-determined outcome.
4. Superiority/inferiority are terms used to describe the pre-set tolerability for difference between two comparators. With a superiority design the expected outcome is that one treatment will demonstrate a benefit over the comparator arm; in an inferiority domain the base assumption is the there is no real difference between the two treatments.
5. Stratification is used when it is known before the start of the clinical investigation that there is significant heterogeneity within the indication studied and allows the analysis plan to be defined up front, recognizing this variability; examples are age in studies in cardiovascular disease or the presence or absence of metastasis in cancer.

## 23.7 Target Product Profile

Very early in the development of an investigational product the development team captures the profile of the aspirational drug in a target product profile or TPP. This TPP describes the targeted disease and if applicable the subsegment of this disease with regard to the disease phenotype, currently available treatment options/unmet medical needs, and the various specifications the future drug is thought to meet.

## 23.8 Study Protocol

Every clinical investigation requires a study protocol. This captures the primary, secondary, and exploratory hypothesis/endpoints the study is aimed to test. Good protocols test only one primary hypothesis. The disease is specified and there are inclusion and exclusion criteria to make sure the patients/subjects are protected against the associated risks.

1. Patient informed consent, language on a level of an 8 year-old child is essential to protect the interests and safety of the study subjects.

2. Validated endpoints and surrogate endpoints.
3. An example of a clinical study protocol is in ref. 6.

## 23.9 Clinical Trial Database

Over the past decades there has been a lot of attention on the transparency around clinical drug research and the results generated. This has resulted in databases that are open source, that each sponsor is obliged to populate and maintain on clinical trials that are actively recruiting, with key items such as disease area, size, intervention, and major inclusion and exclusion criteria. It also keeps this same documentation after the trial has been completed and sponsors are encouraged to include key results, such as the endpoints and safety data. Examples are clinicaltrials.gov for trials that are submitted to the US FDA (https://clinicaltrials.gov) and the EUDRACT database for trials that are submitted to the EMA (https://eudract.ema.europa.eu).

## 23.10 Study Result Reporting

After a study is completed, the data generated in a clinical study report (CSR) is a formally required document by the health authorities; the size and detail depends on whether the study has been completed or not. Frequently the study data are published in peer-reviewed journals. This depends on the initiative taken by the investigators and/or sponsor, there is no legal requirement to publish. When there are multiple publications in the public domain on a comparable topic it can be very informative to compare these data using a structured approach such as a meta-analysis or Cochrane analysis (https://www.cochranelibrary.com, accessed 14 March 2022).

When reviewing a paper on clinical studies, the Cochrane methodology is a good standard to judge confidence in the data provided, based upon levels of evidence (sometimes called the hierarchy of evidence) that are assigned to studies, based on the methodological quality of their design, validity, and applicability to patient care. These decisions give the "grade (or strength) of recommendation":

1. Level I evidence from a systematic review or meta-analysis of all relevant RCTs (randomized controlled trial) or evidence-based clinical practice guidelines based on systematic reviews of RCTs or three or more RCTs of good quality that have similar results.
2. Level II evidence obtained from at least one well-designed RCT (*e.g.* large multisite RCT).
3. Level III evidence obtained from well-designed controlled trials without randomization (*i.e.* quasi-experimental).
4. Level IV evidence from well-designed case-controlled or cohort studies.
5. Level V evidence from systematic reviews of descriptive and qualitative studies (meta-synthesis).

6. Level VI evidence from a single descriptive or qualitative study.
7. Level VII evidence from the opinion of authorities and/or reports of expert committees.

## 23.11 Independent Review Board (IRB)

IRBs are essential for a review of the protocol against the Good Clinical Practice (GCP) guidelines and local practices. Independent Data Review – these boards are generally put into place to independently monitor the safety and efficacy of the investigational product. On the design of clinical programmes, margins are set for the efficacy needed and the tolerability that does not support continuation of the protocol at hand.

## 23.12 Health Authorities and Ethical Considerations

Clinical trials are closely supervised by appropriate regulatory authorities against a well-documented framework of mandatory documents and submissions. The first submission is commonly the request to start dosing in humans and examples are the opening of an investigational dossier (IND) with the Federal Drug Agency (FDA) in the USA, or the Investigation of Medicinal Product Dossier (IMPD) with the European Medicines Agency (EMA) in Europe. Over the past decades the Japanese and Chinese regulatory authorities have become more visible and their input is increasingly solicited from the start of the clinical phase of development. At the end of Phase III, when all relevant data are collected, the sponsor submits a final dossier to these agencies for review, to obtain a label to commercialize on. During the development programme there are a variety of communications possible with the agencies, further details can be found on their respective websites. In addition, many regulatory bodies have established guidelines for many diseases, in which they describe the type of information they are seeking around request for approval and the right to commercialize. Examples are recognized endpoints, acceptable surrogate markers for efficacy and/or safety, and numbers of patients required to justify the claims the sponsor wants to make based upon the clinical data generated. Supportive documentation can be found on the FDA website guidance documents[7] and on the EMA website for guidance documents.[8]

There are some other important items to consider when it comes to the structure in which a clinical investigation is conducted:

1. In addition to the dossier for regulatory bodies, all interventional or observational studies on patients must be approved by a supervising ethics committee before permission is granted to run a clinical investigation. Generally, this body is called the Institutional Review Board (IRB). IRBs can be located at the local investigator's hospital or institution; the alternative is a central (independent/for profit) IRB.
2. To warrant a generally agreed ethical conduct the International Committee for Harmonization (ICH) has developed guidelines for Good Clinical Practice (GCP) that are widely adopted as a framework to conduct clinical investigations. The guidelines aim to ensure the "rights, safety and well-being of trial subjects are protected".[9,10]

3. Investigators must obtain the full and informed consent of participating human subjects. One of the IRB's main functions is to ensure potential patients are adequately informed about the benefits and risks of the clinical investigation they are asked to participate in. If the patient is unable to consent for him/herself, researchers can seek consent from the patient's legally authorized representative. An additional general rule is that when material is collected for genetic testing or that could be used for such purpose, a separate informed consent is obtained.
4. Given that most investigations will collect and document information that is considered private, there are rules and regulations to warrant the privacy of study subjects; for example, in the USA researchers must understand and follow the federal patient privacy (HIPAA) law and good clinical practice. The European community has over recent years been very active as well with the implementation of the General Data Protection Regulation (GDPR).

## 23.13 Investigational Brochure

This is a pivotal document generated by the sponsor of the study on the investigational product that functions as a fact base of all the core data generated, irrespective of the source of the data. It is generally first used at the time of the submission of the IND/IMPD or equivalent, and matures with the drug product throughout the entire life of the molecule. It is a core document in many of the packages that are used to get IRB approval and to inform study staff, investigators, and the like.

## 23.14 Study Teams

The composition of study teams varies between the different phases of development, but also are strongly influenced by the type of trial planned/executed, the disease area, and the various companies. Early development programmes tend to be in a single country at a single site with a relatively small number of subjects (<100), requiring smaller teams, whereas Phase II clinical programmes tend to be at least on a regional scale, and Phase III programmes generally are multinational/on a global scale with very sizable patient populations of up to multiple thousands. Teams consist of supportive scientists (biologists, chemists, pharmacologists, *etc.*) physicians, clinical research associates, statisticians, data managers, and commercial, legal, and operational support. Hence, in early phase trials these teams are usually small, but with the increase in size and complexity they can become very sizable for Phase III pivotal/registrational trials. In Phase IV they tend to become smaller again and usually are not in R&D, but in medical affairs.

## 23.15 Examples of Development Programmes

An example of a traditional development programme is the development of baricitinib for rheumatoid arthritis. Baracitinib is a JAK inhibitor developed by Eli Lilly with the tradename Olumiant.

https://clinicaltrials.gov/ct2/results?term=baricitinib&Search=Clear&age_v=&gndr=&rslt=
(accessed 14 March 2022).

The clinicaltrials.gov website currently lists 114 clinical studies. As reported in the FDA label for baricitinib[11] the clinical development programme included two dose-ranging Phase II trials and four confirmatory Phase III trials. Although other doses have been studied, the recommended dose of baricitinib is 2 mg once daily. The dose-ranging studies (NCT01185353 and NCT01469013) included a 12 week randomized comparison of baricitinib 1, 2, 4, and 8 mg *versus* placebo in 301 and 145 patients, respectively.

The efficacy and safety of baricitinib 2 mg once daily was assessed in two confirmatory Phase III trials. These trials were randomized, double-blind, multicenter studies in patients with active rheumatoid arthritis. The two studies evaluated baricitinib 2 mg and 4 mg. Study NCT01721057 was a 24 week trial in 684 patients with moderately to severely active rheumatoid arthritis who had an inadequate response or intolerance to conventional disease-modifying antirheumatic drugs (DMARDs). Patients received baricitinib 2 mg or 4 mg once daily or placebo added to existing background cDMARD treatment. From Week 16, non-responding patients could be rescued to receive baricitinib 4 mg once daily. The primary endpoint was the proportion of patients who achieved an ACR20 response at Week 12.

Study NCT01721044 was a 24 week trial in 527 patients with moderately to severely active rheumatoid arthritis who had an inadequate response or intolerance to one or more TNF inhibitor therapies with or without other biologic DMARDs. Patients received baricitinib 2 mg or 4 mg once daily or placebo added to background.

cDMARD treatment. From Week 16, non-responding patients could be rescued to receive baricitinib 4 mg once daily. The primary endpoint was the proportion of patients who achieved an ACR20 response at Week 12.

This example includes, besides the core of clinical studies, also the various studies to be done to fully understand the pharmacology (including food effects, drug–drug interaction studies, and effect in race) as well as the efficacy in other indications.

While the best possible clinical experiment is a prospective, randomized, placebo controlled double blind, double dummy, clinical trial, in an oncology setting open-label studies are common This is anchored in the benefit/risk ratio. For targeted therapies, the safety and tolerability profile in healthy volunteers is not relevant, since they do not have the relevant biology, whilst having the off-target effects. Typical Phase I studies are often undertaken in healthy volunteers, allowing rapid recruitment and avoiding the ethical concern of enrolling patients in short-term studies at subtherapeutic doses, when Phase II/III studies would be more appropriate for the patient. But for oncology drugs, patients are often chosen for Phase I studies where the side effect profile may disfavour exposure of healthy volunteers and where the use of patients may provide early indications of efficacy. The following case study illustrates both these points.

Encorafenib (trade name Braftovi) is a second-generation BRAF kinase inhibitor that targets key enzymes in the MAPK signalling pathway, for the treatment of melanomas. Currently 65 clinical studies have been reported for encorafenib.

(https://clinicaltrials.gov/ct2/results/details?term=braftovi). (accessed 14 March 2022).

The clinical development of encorafenib has been described.[12] In 2011 a first time in human Phase I study, NCT01436656, was initiated to establish the maximum tolerated dose (MTD) and/or recommended Phase II dose (RP2D) of daily administered encorafenib (daily, twice daily, and/or every-other-day). The study involved 66 participants who were patients. It was a Phase I, multicenter, open-label, dose escalation study of oral encorafenib in adult patients with locally advanced or metastatic BRAF mutant melanoma patients with locally advanced or metastatic melanoma harbouring the BRAF V600 mutation (during the dose escalation and expansion phases) and patients with metastatic colorectal cancer harbouring the BRAF V600 mutation (during the expansion phase) being enrolled. The study consisted of a dose escalation part, where cohorts of patients received escalating oral doses of encorafenib, followed by a safety dose expansion part where patients were treated with an oral dose of encorafenib given at the MTD or RP2D. Encorafenib 450 mg once daily was defined as the maximum tolerated dose (MTD). Due to frequent occurrence of dose limiting toxicities in patients receiving the MTD in the dose expansion, 300 mg once daily evolved as the recommended Phase II dose for encorafenib monotherapy.

Based on data showing an additional effect on treatment response duration by combining encorafenib with a MEK inhibitor, binimetinib in a BRAF V600E mutant melanoma mouse model, this combination regimen was investigated in a Phase Ib/II open-label clinical study including 23 melanoma patients, NCT01543698. As seen with other BRAF/MEK inhibitor combinations, addition of a MEK inhibitor reduced the occurrence of on-target BRAF inhibitor-related cutaneous adverse events, subsequently allowing for higher dosing of the BRAF inhibitor. Hence, the recommended Phase II doses of encorafenib and binimetinib were defined at 450/600 mg once daily and 45 mg BID, respectively. Preliminary efficacy data were promising, with eight of nine patients with BRAF inhibitor-naive melanoma showing an objective response to combination therapy.

These results led to the initiation of the Phase III open-label COLUMBUS trial, NCT01909453. Comparing a combination of encorafenib plus binimetinib *versus* the BRAF inhibitor, vemurafenib, and LGX818 monotherapy in BRAF mutant melanoma. The major efficacy measure was progression-free survival (PFS) using RECIST 1.1 response criteria and was assessed by blinded independent central review. The median PFS was 14.9 months for patients receiving binimetinib plus encorafenib, and 7.3 months for the vemurafenib monotherapy arm (hazard ratio 0.54, 95% CI: 0.41, 0.71, $p < 0.0001$). In June 2018, based on these results, encorafenib was approved by the FDA in combination with binimetinib for the treatment of patients with unresectable or metastatic BRAF V600E or V600K mutation-positive melanoma.

While Clinicaltrials.gov lists over 60 studies for encorfenib, the pivotal core studies are few in number. Many additional studies are done to support expansions into other disease classes or subclasses, combinations, dosing regimens, and formulations. The interested reader is encouraged to delve deeper into clinicaltrials.gov for further details.

## 23.16 Hints and Tips

The best possible clinical experiment is a prospective, randomized, placebo controlled, double blind, double dummy clinical trial.

Double blind is when neither the patient nor the investigator know whether the active or control (placebo) treatment is being used.

Double dummy means that the active and placebo are identical in colour, type, shape, taste, and appearance.

Patients can be randomized, *i.e.* assigned randomly to treatment options. Within the randomization they can be stratified, *i.e.* assigned to groups based on underlying characteristics that will be relevant to treatment response.

Phase 0 is a study where no unregistered investigational product is used.

Phase I trials are to demonstrate safety and tolerability and this is consequently the phase when humans are first exposed to the investigational product.

Phase IIa studies are for the demonstration of a meaningful effect on the targeted disease. Evidence is sought that the compound hits the projected target (proof of mechanism), that the compound changes the relevant disease biology after engaging the target (proof of principle) and that the disease responds to the compound in a meaningful way (proof of concept). The Phase IIb primary aim is to establish a dose for the Phase III studies.

Phase IV studies are to make sure the potential of the now-approved drug are realized, to understand the benefit/risk profile when the drug is exposed to a wider population, and to explore the impact of any changes to the formulation or manufacturing process.

It is important to ensure studies are appropriately powered to be able to determine the effect, *i.e.* statistically designed with appropriate patient numbers to demonstrate differences between treatment arms or groups.

## Key References

For general guidance you can refer to the regulatory authorities websites:

US FDA, general, http://www.fda.gov/default.htm
US FDA, drugs, http://www.fda.gov/Drugs/default.htm
US FDA, guidance documents, http://www.fda.gov/Drugs/GuidanceComplianceRegulatoryInformation/Guidances/default.htm
EMA, general http://www.ema.europa.eu
Pharmaceuticals and Medical Devices Agency, Japan http://www.pmda.go.jp/english
Pharmaceuticals and Medical Devices Agency, Japan, guidance site http://www.pmda.go.jp/english/service/regulation.html

Clinical trials databases

Submitted to FDA, https://clinicaltrials.gov
Submitted to the EMA, https://eudract.ema.europa.eu
Cochrane analysis, https://www.cochranelibrary.com

## References


1. https://www.drugs.com/monograph/thalidomide.html, accessed 14 March 2022.
2. https://www.fda.gov/regulatory-information/search-fda-guidance-documents/estimating-maximum-safe-starting-dose-initial-clinical-trials-therapeutics-adult-healthy-volunteers, accessed 14 March 2022.
3. H. Attarwala, *J. Young Pharm.*, 2010, **2**(3), 332.
4. O. H. Drummer, D. Gerostamoulos and N. W. Woodford, *Forensic Sci. Int.*, 2019, **298**, 298.
5. https://www.stat.ubc.ca/~rollin/stats/ssize/n2.html, accessed 14 March 2022.
6. https://clinicaltrials.gov/ProvidedDocs/62/NCT03503162/Prot_000.pdf, accessed 14 March 2022.
7. https://www.fda.gov/regulatory-information/search-fda-guidance-documents/clinical-trials-guidance-documents, accessed 14 March 2022.
8. https://www.ema.europa.eu/en/glossary/guideline, accessed 14 March 2022.
9. https://www.ich.org, accessed 14 March 2022.
10. https://www.ema.europa.eu/en/ich-e6-r2-good-clinical-practice, accessed 14 March 2022.
11. https://www.accessdata.fda.gov/drugsatfda_docs/label/2020/207924s002lbl.pdf, accessed 14 March 2022.
12. O. Koelblinger, R. Thuerigen and R. Dummer, *Curr. Opin. Oncol.*, 2018, **30**(2), 125.

# 24 SMN2 Splicing Modification by Small Molecules – A Blueprint to Tackle the Underlying Genetic Cause of Many Underserved Diseases

Hasane Ratni*[a], Martin Ebeling[a], Renata S. Scalco[a], Lutz Mueller[a] and Alexander Stephan[a]

[a]F. Hoffmann-La Roche Ltd, pRED, Pharma Research & Early Development, Roche Innovation Center Basel, Grenzacherstrasse 124, 4070 Basel, Switzerland
*E-mail: ratnih@yahoo.fr

## 24.1 Introduction

Modulation of the natural process of pre-mRNA splicing[1,2] to control the identity of the corresponding protein products is a highly promising approach to treat a number of diseases. A successful example is its application to spinal muscular atrophy, where this is achieved with both an antisense oligonucleotide (ASO) and, potentially more advantageously, with orally bioavailable small molecules. Building on this example and achieving a specific modulation of pre-mRNA splicing with small molecules in a systematic manner would drastically expand the druggable target space in general, and help to develop treatments for a plethora of diseases which remain without therapeutic options as of today.[3,4] Achieving a high selectivity, as outlined for the *SMN2* splicing modifiers below, is a key requirement to deliver an efficacious yet safe treatment.

## 24.2 Spinal Muscular Atrophy and Its Treatment Options

The autosomal recessive disease "proximal spinal muscular atrophy" (SMA) is caused by mutations in or ablation of the survival of motor neuron 1 (*SMN1*) gene.[5,6] It is the most common genetic cause of infant death, with an incidence of about 1 in 6000 to

The Handbook of Medicinal Chemistry: Principles and Practice, 2nd Edition
Edited by Simon E. Ward and Andrew M. Davis

Published by the Royal Society of Chemistry, www.rsc.org

1 in 11 000 live births.[7,8] The disease is characterized by selective loss of spinal motor neurons and skeletal muscle atrophy that causes weakness and paralysis.[9,10]

The product of the *SMN1* gene, SMN protein, is essential for survival. However, gene duplication of *SMN1* creates a highly homologous gene in humans, termed *SMN2*. The *SMN2* gene is nearly identical to *SMN1* in its coding region, with a single translationally synonymous point mutation being responsible for the exclusion of exon 7 from the majority of mature *SMN2* transcripts. This point mutation at position 6 of *SMN2* exon 7 affects a known exonic splicing enhancer (ESE) regulatory site and causes, in the majority of *SMN2* transcripts, skipping of exon 7 during *SMN2* pre-mRNA splicing. Only a small subset of *SMN2* pre-mRNAs is spliced correctly to retain exon 7 in the mature transcript. Thus, the resulting majority of truncated *SMN2* transcripts code for a truncated, unstable SMN protein variant (Figure 24.1). While this has no impact in an unaffected individual with functional output of the *SMN1* gene, the remaining low levels of *SMN2*-derived stable and functional SMN protein are insufficient to fully prevent the SMA disease phenotypes in *SMN1* gene inactivation mutation carriers.[11–13]

Several clinical subgroups have been defined for SMA. In most cases, distinct *SMN2* gene copy numbers segregate with a clinical subgroup and define disease severity. For example, patients with Type 1 SMA, a severe variant of the disease that leads to infant death within the first two years after birth, when left untreated, usually carry two *SMN2* copies. In contrast, patients with the less aggressive forms of Type 2 and Type 3 SMA usually carry three to four *SMN2* copies.[6] The observation that *SMN2* copy number and, thus, SMN protein dosage determine the severity of the disease has: (a) confirmed SMN

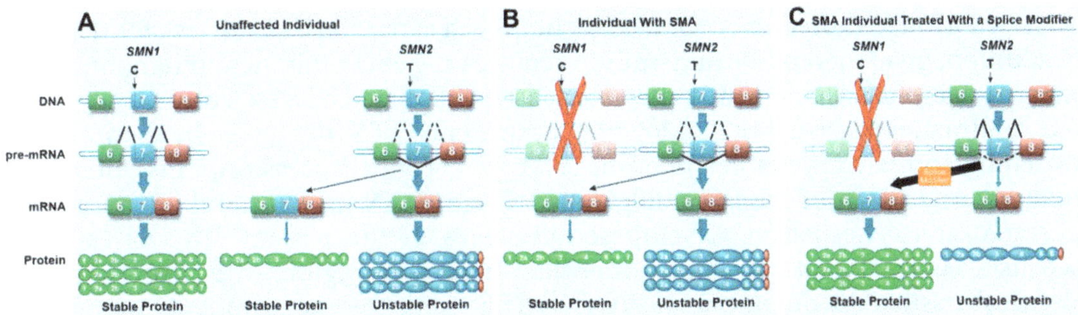


**Figure 24.1** The molecular genetics of SMA and the therapeutic approach of *SMN2* splice modification. (A) In an unaffected individual, the *SMN1* gene produces stable survival motor neuron (SMN) protein. The *SMN2* gene, which is nearly identical to *SMN1*, carries a synonymous point mutation (C>T) in the coding sequence of exon 7 that predominantly leads to exon 7 exclusion during pre-mRNA splicing. In turn, this results in the production of an unstable truncated protein which is rapidly degraded. Only a small portion of *SMN2* mRNA transcripts contain exon 7 and produce stable SMN protein. (B) In individuals with SMA, inactivating mutations in *SMN1* gene or loss of the *SMN1* gene leads to a loss of SMN protein being generated from *SMN1*. The *SMN2* gene produces very limited amounts of stable SMN protein, which leads to manifestation of the disease. (C) *SMN2* splicing modifiers prevent exon 7 exclusion during *SMN2* pre-mRNA processing and force the production of stable SMN protein with the potential to generate near normal SMN protein levels.

protein lowering as cause of SMA and (b) established *SMN2* as a disease-modifying gene.[9]

This SMA-underlying genetic trait has enabled the development of elegant approaches to develop disease-modifying therapeutics. These can be classified into two main categories – gene therapy-dependent ectopic re-expression of stable SMN protein and *SMN2* splicing modification to force exon 7 inclusion and stable SMN protein production.

Virus-mediated ectopic expression of *SMN1* transcripts, utilizing a self-complementary adeno-associated virus serotype 9 (scAAV9) vector, enabled high levels of SMN protein production in motor neurons and peripheral tissues of SMA model mice. This in turn translated into significant rescue of disease-related phenotypes.[14–16]

Subsequently, a study of gene-replacement therapy involving infants with Type 1 SMA, who received a one-time intravenous administration delivering a copy of the scAAV9-SMN1 vector (scAAV9.CB.hSMN, AVXS-101, onasemnogene abeparvovec) confirmed significant benefit for patients in clinical trials.[17] These data enabled the recent FDA and EMA approval for Type 1 SMA patients.

However, AAV-vector immunogenicity, as well as uncontrolled expression with regards to: (a) disease-relevant cell type specificity, (b) SMN expression levels and (c) potential limited duration of expression may bear treatment eligibility limitations or potential risks for SMA patients. In humans with normal output of the *SMN1* gene, the level of the SMN protein decreases with age,[18] but with the current state vector-based gene therapy, the product output of the transgene is uncontrolled and remains highly independent of the host's developmental state. The recently reported[19] toxic gain of function in motor neurons and in sensory pathways several months after transduction of wildtype or SMA model mice with intravenously delivered AAV-*SMN1* cDNA suggest that continued uncontrolled expression of *SMN1* might indeed carry a significant risk for the host. In addition, gene therapy administration requires the concomitant and temporary use of corticosteroids, which could cause corticosteroid-related adverse events.

In contrast, harnessing the endogenous expression of *SMN2* genes by exon 7 splice switching approaches enables relevant cell-type specific expression. This potentially ensures production of the physiologically relevant SMN protein levels required and tolerated at the respective developmental stages of the patient. This is expected because *SMN2* shares an almost identical promoter region with *SMN1*, driving identical tissue-dependent expression.[20,21] That said, the magnitude of such *SMN2* splice-switching treatment benefits will be dependant on the therapeutic modality use (a small molecule or a large molecule), its safety aspect and the level of *SMN2* splicing correction.

A total of three *SMN2* splice modifier molecules are currently in clinical development or have already been approved by health authorities for treatment of SMA patients. These molecules use one of two different molecular mechanisms to achieve SMN2 exon 7 splice switching and exon 7 inclusion to achieve therapeutically relevant increases of SMN protein levels:

(1) Nusinersen, a ribose-*O*-(2-methoxyethyl) (MOE)-modified antisense oligonucleotide (ASO), was approved by the FDA in 2017 as the first disease-modifying SMA treatment and is marketed under the tradename Spinraza by Biogen. It has

shown life-changing benefits for SMA patients, in particular significantly increasing Type 1 SMA patient motor functions, extending patient lives to reach developmental milestones never before seen in untreated SMA Type 1 patients.[22]

Nusinersen targets a splicing silencer element in SMN2 intron 7 to facilitate SMN2 exon 7 inclusion during SMN2 pre-mRNA splicing. *Via* base-paired binding of the ASO nusinersen to the hnRNP-A1/A2-dependent ISS-N1 region in the intron 7 sequence, it blocks access to the sites of negative splicing regulators. Splicing silencer inhibition results in exon 7 inclusion in the SMN2 transcript, thereby resulting in generation of more functional SMN protein.[23] Regular intrathecal (IT) administration of nusinersen is required to enable relevant exposure to the primarily disease-affected motor neurons in the patient's spinal cord. IT administration of nusinersen has been shown to interfere with disease pathology in SMA mouse models and in patients.[22,24]

Lumbar puncture (LP) is an invasive procedure required for IT administration of nusinersen, is associated with risks to patients, requires visits to specialist facilities with trained medical staff and, therefore, may be burdensome for patients, their families and healthcare systems. Patients may require sedation to undergo LP procedures or suffer from LP-related adverse reactions such as headache, backache and post lumbar puncture syndrome. Furthermore, it is not a feasible route of administration for all SMA patients throughout the course of this chronic disease.

(2) Potent small molecule splice modifiers have been developed to utilize an alternative approach to drive *SMN2* exon 7 inclusion and to achieve therapeutically relevant increases of SMN protein levels. Here, two similar but unrelated chemical series have been described that resulted in the creation of Novartis' branaplam (compound **1**, Figure 24.2) and Roche/PTC's risdiplam (compound **2**, Figure 24.2) SMN2 exon 7 splice modifiers.

Both molecules were shown to stabilize the 5′ splice site at the exon 7–intron 7 junction to facilitate exon 7 inclusion during SMN2 pre-mRNA splicing, which led to significant rescue of disease pathology in Type1 SMA-like model mice.[25,26] In particular, risdiplam, which was reported to achieve high target-specific activity through facilitating *SMN2* exon 7 highly selective splicing inclusion by stabilizing an additional ESE element (ESE2) within *SMN2* exon 7, has demonstrated remarkable efficacy in late stage clinical trials.[27]

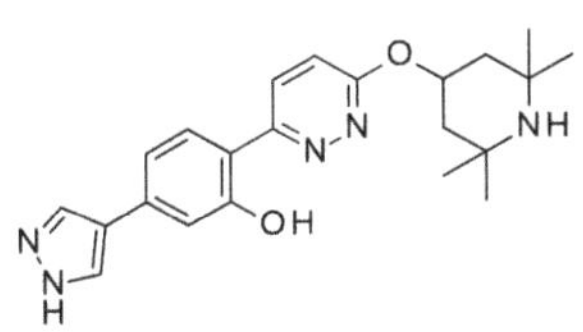

**1, (LMI070)**
**branaplam**

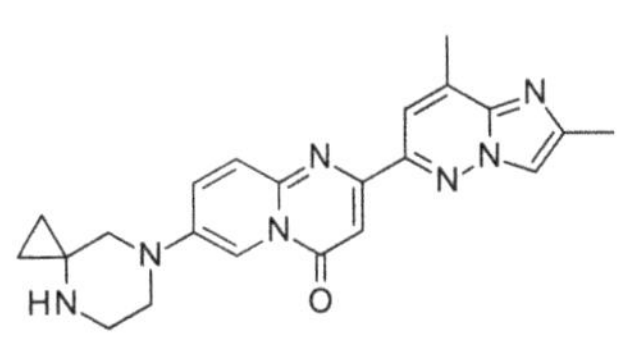

**2, (RG7916)**
**risdiplam**

**Figure 24.2** Branaplam and risdiplam chemical structures.

## 24.3 Systemic Requirement of SMN Rescue for the Treatment of SMA

SMN protein function has been linked to small nuclear ribonuclear protein (snRNP) assembly, pre-mRNA metabolism and RNA trafficking.[28–30] A prominent role for SMN in spinal motor neurons and connected neuronal and neuromuscular circuits is directly linked to the characteristic SMA pathogenesis.[29,31–33]

However, the *SMN1* gene is expressed in many cell types throughout the body, with particular relevance during embryogenesis and early postnatal development. Its ablation without partial rescue through *SMN2* is embryonically lethal in mice and humans.[34] SMN1-deletion studies in distinct tissues have confirmed essential roles for SMN1, and, thus, SMN protein; for example, in the mouse liver and in the muscle of model mice.[35,36]

The first experimental evidence that both rescuing central nervous system (CNS) and peripheral tissue SMN protein levels may translate into the most substantial SMA patient benefit stems from preclinical animal studies with the *SMN2* exon 7 splice modifier ASO nusinersen. Systemic exposure of nusinersen, a route which is not utilized in and approved for SMA patients, has been shown to produce an even more substantial rescue of disease pathology in a Type 1 SMA-like mouse model when compared to IT/CNS exposure alone.[37] In addition, systemic exposure of nusinersen while abolishing its CNS action by utilizing an IT-administered nusinersen-decoy ASO further confirmed the requirement of SMN protein restoration in peripheral organs for a substantial treatment benefit of mild and Type 1 SMA-like severe model mice.[38]

Given the requirement for *SMN2* expression in various tissues to at least survive prenatal development, SMN dosage effects are likely responsible for tissue-dependent phenotypes in SMA patients. This notion is supported by recently published work that confirmed SMN to be required for muscle function and that *SMN2* gene dosage specifically within the *SMN1* ablated mouse muscle defines severity of muscle pathology.[39]

While spinal motor-neuron degeneration is a key feature of SMA pathology, leading to disease-characteristic phenotypes, peripheral organ-related components of the disease are being described in patients, and a growing body of literature is supporting the hypothesis that SMA is likely a systemic disease.[40–42] Thus, restoration of stable SMN protein levels throughout the patient's body may carry the most substantial benefit for disease-modifying treatment of SMA patients. Hence, orally bioavailable and equally systemic distributing *SMN2* splice modifier small molecules like risdiplam are poised to carry the most substantial treatment benefit for SMA patients.

## 24.4 Small Molecule *SMN2* Splicing Modifiers

### 24.4.1 Discovery of Branaplam

The discovery of branaplam started with a high-throughput phenotypic screening (HTS) hit, the pyridazine compound **3** (Figure 24.3).[25,43] The HTS was performed with a library of 1.4 million compounds in a NSC34 motor neuron cell line expressing a SMN2 minigene reporter. Splicing activity assessment through an exon 7 inclusion or

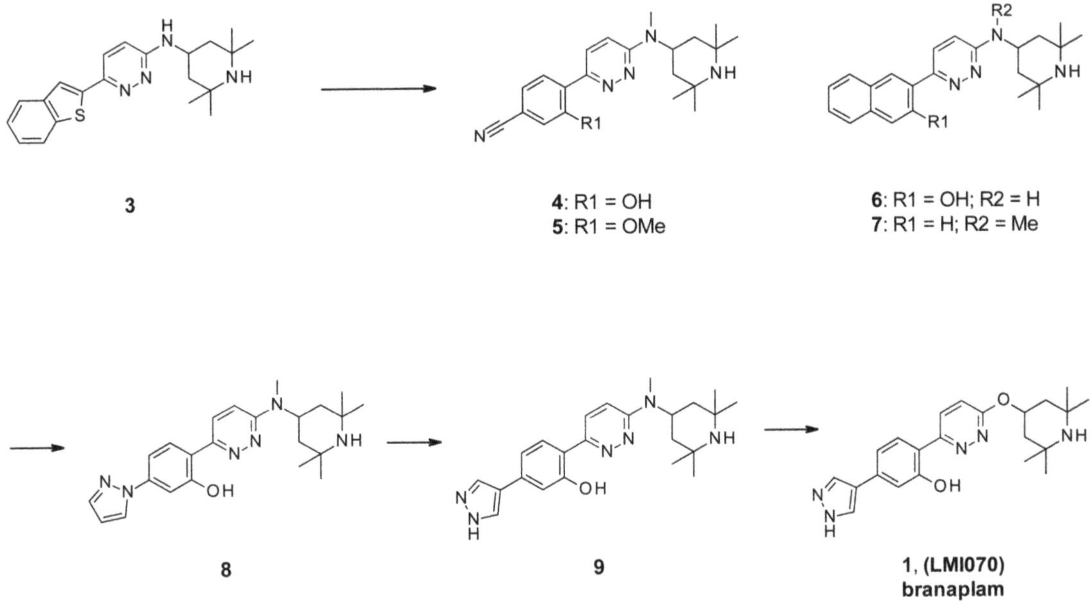


**Figure 24.3** Lead optimization activities from the screening hit **3** to the discovery of branaplam **1**.

exclusion read-out was based on in-frame luciferase expression and dose-dependent activity was confirmed by qPCR. The effect on the endogenous *SMN2* gene in SMNΔ7 mouse myoblasts was confirmed by assessing the SMN protein levels with ELISA. Compound **3** showed promising *in vitro* potency, activating the SMN2 reporter 1700% over DMSO control with an $EC_{50}$ of 3.5 μM and in the ELISA an $EC_{50}$ of 0.6 μM with a 2.5-fold increase. While the compound displayed a favourable physicochemical profile, it also displayed a potent hERG inhibitory activity ($IC_{50}$: 0.6 μM).

The optimization campaign was done in a modular fashion with the structure of the hit being split into three parts:[44] the central core (pyridazine), the left-hand-side moiety with the benzothiophene and finally the nitrogen linked piperidine moiety. Starting with the pyridazine core, it was observed that deletions or shifting of the nitrogen atoms within a six-membered ring resulted in a loss of potency. However, the use of the bioisosteric five-membered ring, 1,3,4 thiadiazole, was equipotent. The pyridazine core was therefore conserved during subsequent modifications of the molecule's left- and right-hand sides. It was also found that methylation of the nitrogen linker was tolerated as both compound **3** and its *N*-methyl analogue had similar potency.

Benzothiophene replacement was tolerant to a wide range of aromatic and heteroaromatic modifications with either bioisosteric naphthalene or substituted phenyl analogues (cpds **4–7**). Of note, the introduction of an *ortho*-hydroxy group on these new left-hand-side moieties resulted in a strongly increased potency potentially due to an intramolecular hydrogen bond with the pyridazine core increasing the planarity of the molecule. (Pair match compounds comparison **4** *versus* **5** and **6** *versus* **7**). But not surprisingly, those derivatives were still potent on hERG. As compound **5** displayed a good

PK profile in mice upon oral administration with good brain penetration and reasonable clearance, it was selected as a tool compound to evaluate its *in vivo* efficacy in the Type I SMA-like SMNΔ7 mouse model to validate the disease-modifying approach. While death typically occurs before postnatal day 15 in these mice, the compound increased SMN protein levels in the brain in a dose-dependent manner which translated into an extension of overall mouse survival.[45]

In order to address the hERG issue associated with compound **5** (hERG $IC_{50}$: 0.3 μM) modifications around the tetra-methyl piperidine moiety were performed as it is a motive shared by potent hERG binders. However, as this group contributed significantly to the SMN potency, any modification led to a substantial drop of potency. On the left-hand-side the replacement of the cyano moiety from compound **4** by a pyrazole (compound **8**, Figure 24.3) did not reduce the hERG affinity, but improved the selectivity *versus* off-targets (*e.g.* PDE3/4). Further exploration of this region using a more polar hetero-aromatic ring system led to a reduced hERG affinity while maintaining the SMN2 potency. A particularly interesting derivative was the regioisomeric carbon-linked pyrazole (compound **9**, Figure 24.3), which exhibited an excellent potency ($EC_{50}$: 0.004 μM, 3.1-fold) and reduced hERG binding ($IC_{50}$: 6.0 μM) while maintaining oral bioavailability.

A final re-evaluation of the amine linker and the tetramethylpiperidine moiety was performed. Among the changes performed was the replacement of the methylamine linker by the oxygen atom linker (compound **1**, branaplam), which showed a significant increase in fold induction to 3.6. Both compounds **9** and **1** had very promising profiles. However, **9** had a greater efflux propensity, as assessed by MDCK-MDR1, which led to a lower brain concentration compared to **1**. This also resulted in a lower effect in the PD model (brain protein increase in mice), therefore compound **1** was taken forward for development.[44]

A Phase 2 study in infants with Type 1 spinal muscular atrophy was initiated with branaplam, using an oral administration protocol.[46] The aim of that study was to assess the safety, PK-PD and efficacy of this compound. The enrolment was subsequently paused and the dose for the enrolled patients reduced as a precautionary measure because the chronic animal toxicity analysis demonstrated a number of unexpected findings, which included signs of peripheral neuropathy.[47] However, the enrolment was later restarted[48] and the Phase 2 study is ongoing as of early 2020.

## 24.5 Discovery of Risdiplam

The discovery of risdiplam (compound **2**, Figure 24.4) also started with a high-throughput screening assay set up to identify small molecules promoting the inclusion of exon 7 during *SMN2* pre-mRNA splicing.[49] This led to the identification of only few hits and among them a promising coumarin derivative **10** with moderate potency (*SMN2* splicing $EC_{1.5x}$: 0.22 μM; SMN protein $EC_{1.5}$: >10 μM). Further optimization of the potency was achieved upon introduction of a basic amine moiety on the left side and of a hydrogen bond acceptor moiety on the right side, concomitantly with an exploration of alternative central cores in place of the coumarin moiety, leading to the derivatives **11–13**.[49,50]

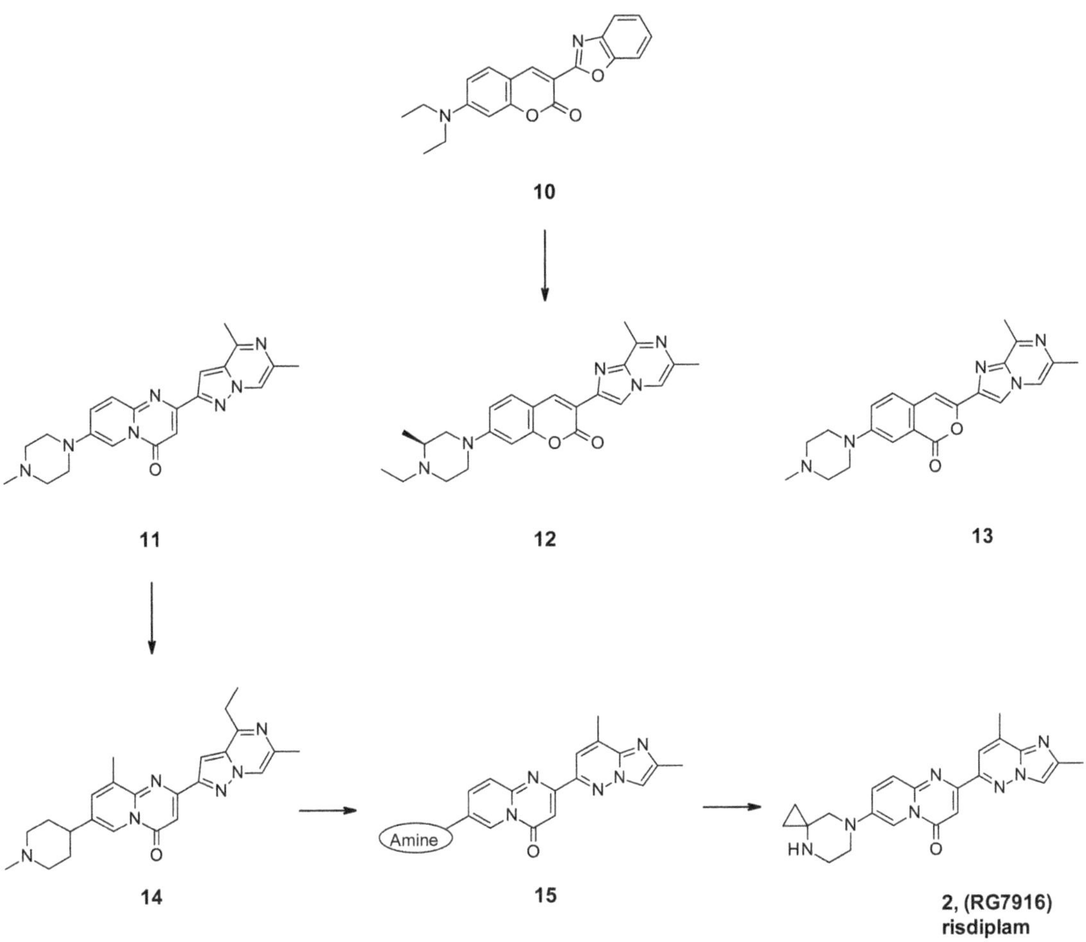


**Figure 24.4** Lead optimization activities from the screening hit **10** to the discovery of risdiplam **2**.

Any potential clinical development of the coumarin or iso-coumarin derivatives **12** and **13** was hampered by data suggestive of mutagenic potential (positive result in an *in vitro* Ames assay) in addition to phototoxicity, as well as poor stability in various *in vitro* assays (chemical stability, in human plasma and metabolic stability).[51] Multiple approaches were undertaken to address those issues in the coumarin and iso-coumarin series, but met with no successes. While the stability could be improved, addressing the potential mutagenic character of those compounds was not feasible, as we either lost the potency on target or maintained the mutagenic Ames profile. In contrast, the pyridopyrimidinone series yielded a different outcome. Multiple analogues of compound **11** were prepared and found to be Ames-negative, while maintaining or further increasing the *in vitro* potency.[51] A key feature was that the combination of the central pyridopyrimidinone moiety together with a suitable right hand-side biaryl moiety led to the absence of an Ames flag *in vitro*. An empirical observation was that the more sterically hindered the right-hand-side moiety was, the better to prevent such a flag.

To achieve the highest clinical efficacy possible, we wanted to design a drug able to increase the SMN protein level in the central nervous system as well as in peripheral tissues (muscles, *etc.*). Therefore, a key parameter was to achieve good brain penetration, hence the molecule should not be a P-gp substrate. To expedite the discovery of such molecules, we looked for simple surrogates to use in the design of our molecules. A good *in vitro* correlation between lipophilicity ($\log D$, coefficient of partition between octanol and aqueous buffer) and P-gp efflux ratio was observed. The great advantage of using lipophilicity as a surrogate for P-gp is that $\log D$ can nowadays be easily predicted using machine learning tools. Compounds with a $\log D$ above 1.5 were generally not P-gp substrates. We also applied a higher limit of 3 to prevent unspecific binding and high clearance issues. Novel molecules were then designed to achieve a $\log D$ between 1.5 and 3. This approach rapidly led to the discovery of compound **14** (RG7800), displaying an excellent tissue distribution and *in vivo* efficacy in mouse models of SMA (C/C allele and Δ7).

Compound **14** was the first small molecule *SMN2* splicing modifier tested in humans, with a Phase 1 study in healthy volunteers demonstrating a dose-dependent effect on *SMN2* alternative splicing. In the subsequent Phase 2 clinical trial in SMA patients (Moonfish),[52,53] proof of mechanism was demonstrated by assessing SMN protein levels in whole blood. Compared to baseline, patients receiving RG7800 had a significant increase of SMN protein to levels which could provide meaningful clinical benefit to SMA patients.[54] However, the clinical development of that molecule was suspended as a precautionary measure because retinal toxicity was observed in cynomolgus monkeys after chronic daily oral dosing (39 weeks) at exposures in excess of those investigated in patients. These eye findings consisted of multifocal peripheral retina degeneration in the photoreceptor layer with hypertrophic retinal pigment epithelium (RPE) and microcystoid spaces in the inner retinal layers in monkeys. This led to the decision to identify a new clinical candidate.

While the aetiology of the retinal finding was unclear, a number of improvements *versus* **14** were targeted, which in turn also impacted positively on the therapeutic window for the retinal finding. Those included a better selectivity *versus* off-target genes for which splicing was affected (particularly *FoxM1*), the reduction of the volume of distribution (Vss) and an on-target potency increase to reduce the efficacious doses/exposures. The optimization started with the replacement of the pyrazolo-pyrazine moiety from compound **14** by a novel right-hand-side group, an imidazo-pyridazine, which led to derivatives of general formula **15** with a much higher potency on *SMN2*.[55] At the same time, this fragment led to a strong improvement of the phototoxicity and the overall good profile was maintained (clearance, fraction unbound). Optimization and selection of the optimal amine moiety was the next key step to strike a balance between maintaining a high potency while having the lowest basicity possible (to reduce drastically the volume of distribution and suppress hERG inhibition), but also preventing the formation of a peripherally restricted active metabolite in order to improve on the therapeutic window between *SMN2* and *FoxM1* modulation *in vivo*. Here as well, we made use of a surrogate for the volume of distribution (Vss) optimization. While the determination of a Vss requires an *in vivo* single dose PK study, we observed that there was a good correlation between the $pK_a$ of the molecule and its Vss value: the lower the basicity, the lower the Vss. Additionally, it is well established that reducing basicity is an efficient way to reduce hERG channel affinity. Using the general formula **15**, we prepared a virtual library based on all commercially available amines, providing us with several thousand compounds. We then reduced this number drastically by using simple machine learning prediction criteria, based on a $\log D$ range of 1.5–3, as previously described, a $pK_a$ range of 6.5–8.5 (minimal $pK_a$ of 6.5 to maintain the on-target potency) and a MW <500 g $mol^{-1}$ for the resulting final products. This led to roughly 100 molecules to consider, and after a visual inspection to remove unwanted amines, we ended up with the preparation of around 40 molecules. Those considerations led to compound **2**, also known as risdiplam.[26] This compound was fully characterized by assessing its distribution, *in vivo* drug levels, effect on SMN protein and expression in tissues in animal models.[56] Safety studies showed that similar retinal findings were also seen with risdiplam (but with a larger window as compared to compound **14**). These lesions were readily detected in-life by spectral domain-optical coherence tomography (sdOCT) and appeared to reach steady-state after a few months of dosing. Further, a clear NOEL (no observed event level) for retinal changes was established for risdiplam in monkeys at high systemic concentrations. The dose/exposure resulting in NOEL was associated with high increase in the SMN2 full length mRNA transcript. This was supported by the data up to this point in the clinical development of risdiplam, as no eye findings representative of the ones observed in monkeys have been identified in patients treated for up to 1 year with this molecule. Based on its full profile, efficacy in preclinical models and favourable safety profile, risdiplam entered clinical development.

## 24.6 Clinical Development of Risdiplam

Risdiplam is currently being evaluated in four multicentre trials in individuals with SMA: FIREFISH (NCT0291348; infants with Type 1 SMA, aged 1–7 months at enrolment),[57] SUNFISH (NCT02908685; children and young adults with Type 2/3 SMA, aged 2–25 years at enrolment),[58] JEWELFISH (NCT03032172; non-naïve patients with SMA, aged 6 months–60 years at enrolment)[59] and RAINBOWFISH (NCT03779334; presymptomatic infants with genetic diagnosis of SMA, from birth to 6 weeks of age at first dose).[60] This comprehensive clinical trial programme was designed to represent the broad, real-world spectrum of people living with SMA with the aim of ensuring access to risdiplam for all appropriate patients.

Initial results of the dose-finding Part 1 of the FIREFISH (Type 1 SMA) and SUNFISH studies (Type 2/3 SMA) demonstrated that risdiplam treatment led to a median 2-fold increase in blood SMN protein levels. In addition, exploratory efficacy analyses provided early evidence of efficacy, illustrating the potential of risdiplam as a therapy for SMA. More recently, these results were confirmed by Part 2 of the FIREFISH and SUNFISH studies. In FIREFISH Part 2, risdiplam treatment was associated with a statistically significant and clinically meaningful improvement in event-free survival, motor milestone achievement and motor function. In SUNFISH Part 2, risdiplam treatment was associated with a statistically significant and clinically meaningful improvement in motor function in a broad and heterogeneous patient population, including older patients with poor motor function, severe scoliosis and contractures. To date, there have been no treatment-related safety findings leading to treatment withdrawal in any risdiplam trial and no preclinical safety findings have been observed in any patient. These positive efficacy findings in combination with the favourable safety profile support risdiplam as a new oral SMA therapy. On 7 August 2020, risdiplam (EVRYSDI™) was approved in the US by the FDA for the treatment of adults and children with SMA, aged 2 months and older.[61]

## 24.7 Assessing Effects of Small Molecule Splicing Modifiers

Modern RNA sequencing technology allows, for the first time, monitoring of all splicing events in any given cell type in one experiment. While this still necessitates studying various different cell types or tissues so as to cover the biological space as comprehensively as possible, it allows for unprecedented analyses of compound specificity.

Here, we describe the analysis of a series of such experiments in the context of developing risdiplam. Human SMA patient fibroblast cells were treated with various compounds known to target the inclusion of SMN2 exon 7, which is not properly spliced in those cells due to the point mutation discussed above.

The compounds, SMN-C3, SMN-C5, RG7800, branaplam and risdiplam, were used in concentrations that demonstrate comparable efficacy towards the targeted splicing event. The aim of the experiment was to identify off-target splicing events that could be responsible for potential side effects.

As a measure of effect size, we used ΔPSI, the change in PSI, between treated samples and untreated controls, where PSI refers to "percent spliced in" and ranges from 0 to 1. The two extreme values 0 and 1 represent splicing events where one of the two possible splice variants is used exclusively; a PSI value of 0.5 indicates equal usage of both options (such as "short form" or "long form" of an exon, "skipping" or "inclusion" of an exon *etc.*). We note that PSI explicitly ignores changes in overall expression: for a gene that is strongly induced by a treatment but keeps the same relative amounts of two splicing isoforms, PSI remains the same.

RNA sequencing reads were generated for all the conditions and mapped to the human transcriptome. For every annotated human alternative splicing event, we identified and quantified reads that uniquely characterize one of the two alternative transcript versions. Relevant reads were found for about 27 000 alternative splicing events in a total of 8277 genes. These were used to calculate PSI and ΔPSI values. Based on the read coverage, we filtered out very low expressed genes and arrived at a total of about 18 000 alternative splicing events in 5666 genes.

Each of these splicing events was then characterized by the value of its largest absolute ΔPSI found in any of the individual experiments. We further simplified the analysis by representing each gene by the one splicing event that has the largest absolute ΔPSI value.

To obtain an overview of the expected effects, we plotted the distribution of these maximum ΔPSI values per gene on a logarithmic scale (Figure 24.5).

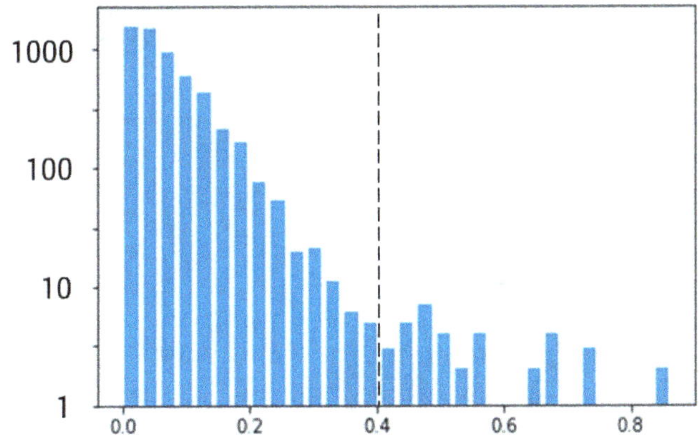


**Figure 24.5** Histogram of the distribution of maximal ΔPSI values across 5666 genes analyzed as described in the text. There is an exponential decline (logarithmic scale) up to a value of around 0.4, above which only 35 genes remain – these are the potential off-target genes (and splicing events).

We obtained a distribution that decreased exponentially with ΔPSI (linear slope in the logarithmic diagram). Based on the shape of this distribution, we selected a cut-off of abs (ΔPSI) = 0.4 (dashed line) to select the most strongly affected splicing events and, hence, genes.

We note that all of these analyses were meant to quantify splicing event changes. They did not allow any conclusions about the biological effects or roles of the events or genes involved. A small ΔPSI value for a critically important exon in a master regulator gene may turn out to be more important than a large ΔPSI value in a structural gene. Any meaningful biological interpretation will have to be based on additional, relevant biological read-outs. Quantitative analysis of splicing events only provides a means to support such interpretations.

For the 35 genes with effects larger than the cut-off defined above, we generated a heat map with all the calculated ΔPSI values for all the compounds tested (Figure 24.6). We have highlighted effects that are larger than our cut-off in yellow and bold font.

Figure 24.6 illustrates impressively how a comprehensive monitoring of splicing effects can be used to gradually improve specificity of a small molecule splicing modifier, *e.g.* from SMN-C5 to risdiplam, a result that was not necessarily expected when the campaign started. Among the secondary splice targets identified, FOXM1 was particularly interesting as to its involvement in cell cycle control. Changes in the balance of splice variants promoting the cell cycle *versus* splice variants resulting in cell cycle arrest could be correlated well with findings such as micronucleus induction in bone marrow and apoptosis in the GI tract and skin in animal toxicity studies.[26] As such changes could have long-term consequences of cell transformation, the tumorigenic potential or risdiplam was assessed subsequently in a suitable transgenic animal model (the rasH2 mouse model) with daily treatment of maximum tolerated doses for a duration of six months. This study did not yield any evidence of a tumorigenic risk for risdiplam.

We note again that, while it is possible to define, measure and calculate objective, quantitative measures for the effects of a treatment on the PSI value of any given splicing

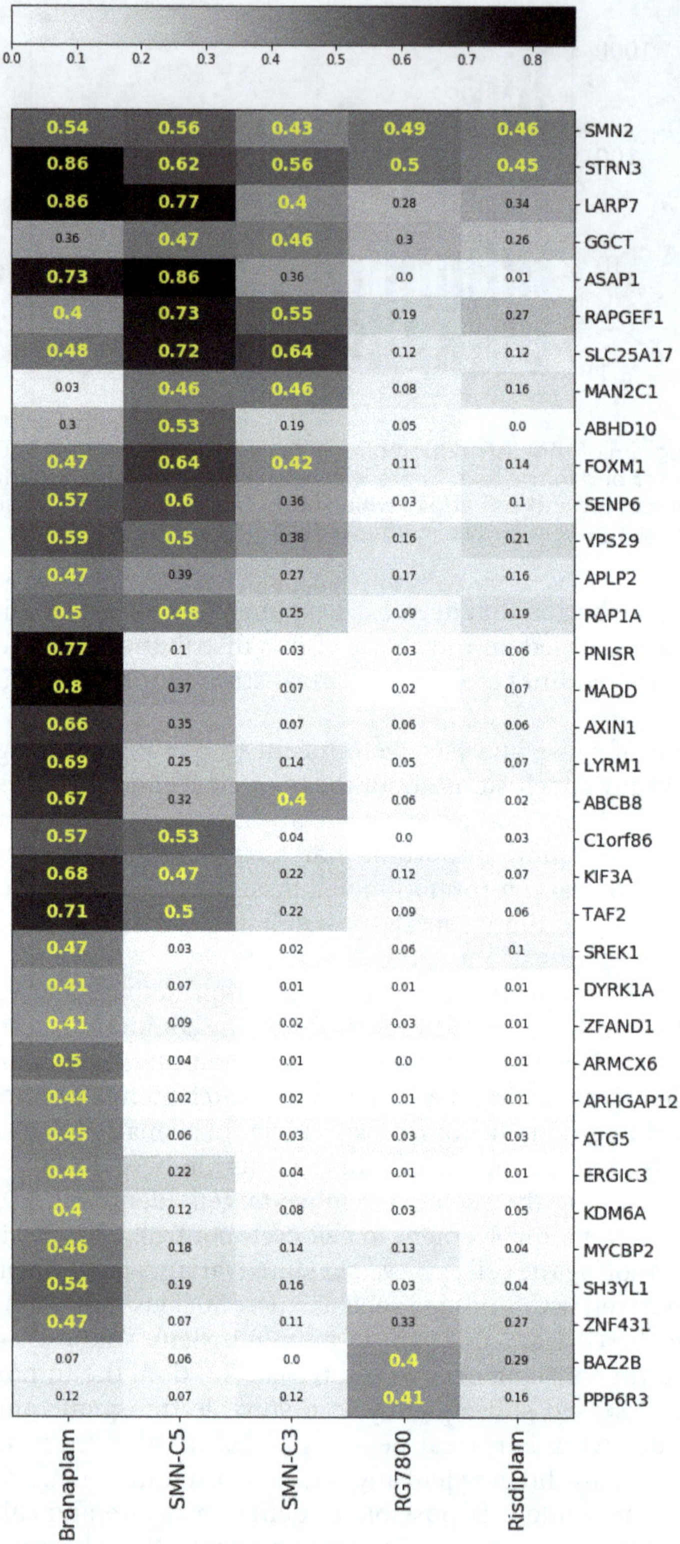


**Figure 24.6** Clustered heat map of the effects of 5 compounds on the 35 genes identified as described in Figure 24.5 above.

event, this does not imply any biological understanding of the biological consequences of such effects, which still have to be assessed in dedicated experiments on cellular systems and relevant animal models.

## 24.8 Conclusions and Future Outlook

Targeting RNA offers a unique opportunity to therapeutically modulate numerous cellular processes implicated in many human diseases. One approach to achieve that is the use of RNA splicing modifiers as a new class of therapeutics, particularly with small molecules. In terms of specificity and safety they represent profound challenges for medicinal chemistry. However, its feasibility has been demonstrated with a first successful application in SMA. Since the discovery of risdiplam, further work on the elucidation of its mode of action has been performed,[62] revealing a dual binding on two sites within SMN2 exon 7, namely ESE2 and 5′ss, potentially explaining its remarkable specificity for the SMN2 target. While the understanding of a binding mode can certainly help to accelerate the optimization of a molecule, its absence by no means precludes the discovery of a medicine. Phenotypic-based projects having already proven to be successful in drug discovery. Finally, this work may pave the way for research and development of future RNA-targeting therapies.

## References


1. Y. Lee and D. C. Rio, Mechanisms and Regulation of Alternative Pre-mRNA Splicing, *Annu. Rev. Biochem.*, 2015, **84**, 291–323.
2. H. Shenasa and K. J. Hertel, Combinatorial regulation of alternative splicing, *Biochim. Biophys. Acta, Gene Regul. Mech.*, 2019, **1862**(11–12), 194392.
3. M. Montes, B. L. Sanford, D. F. Comiskey and D. S. Chandler, RNA Splicing and Disease: Animal Models to Therapies, *Trends Genet.*, 2019, **35**(1), 68–87.
4. A. J. Angelbello, J. L. Chen and M. D. Disney, Small molecule targeting of RNA structures in neurological disorders, *Ann. N. Y. Acad. Sci.*, 2020, **1471**(1), 57–71.
5. S. Lefebvre, L. Burglen, S. Reboullet, O. Clermont, P. Burlet, L. Viollet, B. Benichou, C. Cruaud and P. Millasseau, *et al.*, Identification and characterization of a spinal muscular atrophy-determining gene, *Cell*, 1995, **80**(1), 155–165.
6. S. J. Kolb and J. T. Kissel, Spinal muscular atrophy: a timely review, *Arch. Neurol.*, 2011, **68**(8), 979–984.
7. T. O. Crawford and C. A. Pardo, The neurobiology of childhood spinal muscular atrophy, *Neurobiol. Dis.*, 1996, **3**(2), 97–110.
8. E. A. Sugarman, N. Nagan, H. Zhu, V. R. Akmaev, Z. Zhou, E. M. Rohlfs, K. Flynn, B. C. Hendrickson, T. Scholl, D. A. Sirko-Osadsa and B. A. Allitto, Pan-ethnic carrier screening and prenatal diagnosis for spinal muscular atrophy: clinical laboratory analysis of >72 400 specimens, *Eur. J. Hum. Genet.*, 2012, **20**(1), 27–32.
9. S. Nicole, C. C. Diaz, T. Frugier and J. Melki, Spinal muscular atrophy: Recent advances and future prospects, *Muscle Nerve*, 2002, **26**(1), 4–13.
10. G.-H. Park, S. Kariya and U. R. Monani, Spinal muscular atrophy: new and emerging insights from model mice, *Curr. Neurol. Neurosci. Rep.*, 2010, **10**(2), 108–117.
11. L. Cartegni and A. R. Krainer, Disruption of an SF2/ASF-dependent exonic splicing enhancer in SMN2 causes spinal muscular atrophy in the absence of SMN1, *Nat. Genet.*, 2002, **30**(4), 377–384.
12. S. Cho and G. Dreyfuss, A degron created by SMN2 exon 7 skipping is a principal contributor to spinal muscular atrophy severity, *Genes Dev.*, 2010, **24**(5), 438–442.
13. N. N. Singh and R. N. Singh, Alternative splicing in spinal muscular atrophy underscores the role of an intron definition model, *RNA Biol.*, 2011, **8**(4), 600–606.

14. K. D. Foust, X. Wang, V. L. McGovern, L. Braun, A. K. Bevan, A. M. Haidet, T. T. Le, P. R. Morales, M. M. Rich, A. H. M. Burghes and B. K. Kaspar, Rescue of the spinal muscular atrophy phenotype in a mouse model by early postnatal delivery of SMN, *Nat. Biotechnol.*, 2010, **28**(3), 271–274.
15. C. F. Valori, K. Ning, M. Wyles, R. J. Mead, A. J. Grierson, P. J. Shaw and M. Azzouz, Systemic delivery of scAAV9 expressing SMN prolongs survival in a model of spinal muscular atrophy, *Sci. Transl. Med.*, 2010, **2**(35), 35ra42.
16. N. Armbruster, A. Lattanzi, M. Jeavons, L. Van Wittenberghe, B. Gjata, T. Marais, S. Martin, A. Vignaud, T. Voit, F. Mavilio, M. Barkats and A. Buj-Bello, Efficacy and biodistribution analysis of intracerebroventricular administration of an optimized scAAV9-SMN1 vector in a mouse model of spinal muscular atrophy, *Mol. Ther.--Methods Clin. Dev.*, 2016, 3, 16060/1–16060/8.
17. J. R. Mendell, S. Al-Zaidy, R. Shell, W. D. Arnold, L. R. Rodino-Klapac, T. W. Prior, L. Lowes, L. Alfano, K. Berry, K. Church, J. T. Kissel, S. Nagendran, J. L'Italien, D. M. Sproule, C. Wells, J. A. Cardenas, M. D. Heitzer, A. Kaspar, S. Corcoran, L. Braun, S. Likhite, C. Miranda, K. Meyer, K. D. Foust, A. H. M. Burghes and B. K. Kaspar, Single-dose gene-replacement therapy for spinal muscular atrophy, *N. Engl. J. Med.*, 2017, **377**(18), 1713–1722.
18. D. M. Ramos, C. J. Sumner, C. d'Ydewalle, D. Valdivia, C. L. Hatem, T. O. Crawford, C. J. Sumner, V. Gabbeta, A. Dakka, N. Naryshkin, S. K. Klein, D. A. Norris, J. Matson, F. Rigo, C. F. Bennett, S. J. Taylor, P. G. Zaworski, T. W. Prior, P. J. Snyder, I. Waters, N. Gupte, K. J. Swoboda, S. Paushkin and T. O. Crawford, Age-dependent SMN expression in disease-relevant tissue and implications for SMA treatment, *J. Clin. Invest.*, 2019, **129**(11), 4817–4831.
19. M. Van Alstyne, *et al.*, Gain of toxic function by long-term SMN overexpression in the mouse sensory-motor circuit. *Presented at Cure SMA Virtual Meeting*, 2020.
20. A. Echaniz-Laguna, P. Miniou, D. Bartholdi and J. Melki, The promoters of the survival motor neuron gene (SMN) and its copy (SMNc) share common regulatory elements, *Am. J. Hum. Genet.*, 1999, **64**(5), 1365–1370.
21. U. R. Monani, C. L. Lorson, D. W. Parsons, T. W. Prior, E. J. Androphy, A. H. M. Burghes and J. D. McPherson, A single nucleotide difference that alters splicing patterns distinguishes the SMA gene SMN1 from the copy gene SMN2, *Hum. Mol. Genet.*, 1999, **8**(7), 1177–1183.
22. C. A. Chiriboga, Nusinersen for the treatment of spinal muscular atrophy, *Expert Rev. Neurother.*, 2017, **17**(10), 955–962.
23. N. N. Singh, M. D. Howell, E. J. Androphy and R. N. Singh, How the discovery of ISS-N1 led to the first medical therapy for spinal muscular atrophy, *Gene Ther.*, 2017, **24**(9), 520–526.
24. M. A. Passini, J. Bu, A. M. Richards, C. Kinnecom, S. P. Sardi, L. M. Stanek, Y. Hua, F. Rigo, J. Matson, G. Hung, E. M. Kaye, L. S. Shihabuddin, A. R. Krainer, C. F. Bennett and S. H. Cheng, Antisense oligonucleotides delivered to the mouse CNS ameliorate symptoms of severe spinal muscular atrophy, *Sci. Transl. Med.*, 2011, 3(72), 72ra18/1–72ra18/11.
25. J. Palacino, S. E. Swalley, C. Song, A. K. Cheung, L. Shu, X. Zhang, M. Van Hoosear, Y. Shin, D. N. Chin, C. G. Keller, M. Beibel, N. A. Renaud, T. M. Smith, M. Salcius, X. Shi, M. Hild, R. Servais, M. Jain, L. Deng, C. Bullock, M. McLellan, S. Schuierer, L. Murphy, M. J. J. Blommers, C. Blaustein, F. Berenshteyn, A. Lacoste, J. R. Thomas, G. Roma, G. A. Michaud, B. S. Tseng, J. A. Porter, V. E. Myer, J. A. Tallarico, L. G. Hamann, D. Curtis, M. C. Fishman, W. F. Dietrich, N. A. Dales and R. Sivasankaran, SMN2 splice modulators enhance U1-pre-mRNA association and rescue SMA mice, *Nat. Chem. Biol.*, 2015, **11**(7), 511–517.
26. H. Ratni, M. Ebeling, J. Baird, S. Bendels, J. Bylund, K. S. Chen, N. Denk, Z. Feng, L. Green, M. Guerard, P. Jablonski, B. Jacobsen, O. Khwaja, H. Kletzl, C.-P. Ko, S. Kustermann, A. Marquet, F. Metzger, B. Mueller, N. A. Naryshkin, S. V. Paushkin, E. Pinard, A. Poirier, M. Reutlinger, M. Weetall, A. Zeller, X. Zhao and L. Mueller, Discovery of Risdiplam, a Selective Survival of Motor Neuron-2 (SMN2) Gene Splicing Modifier for the Treatment of Spinal Muscular Atrophy (SMA), *J. Med. Chem.*, 2018, **61**(15), 6501–6517.
27. Roche press release, 7 May, 2019.
28. L. Pellizzoni, J. Yong and G. Dreyfuss, Essential Role for the SMN Complex in the Specificity of snRNP Assembly, *Science (Washington, DC, U. S.)*, 2002, **298**(5599), 1775–1779.
29. A. H. M. Burghes and C. E. Beattie, Spinal muscular atrophy: Why do low levels of survival motor neuron protein make motor neurons sick?, *Nat. Rev. Neurosci.*, 2009, **10**(8), 597–609.
30. R. N. Singh, M. D. Howell, E. W. Ottesen and N. N. Singh, Diverse role of survival motor neuron protein, *Biochim. Biophys. Acta, Gene Regul. Mech.*, 2017, **1860**(3), 299–315.
31. V. L. McGovern, C. C. Iyer, A. W. David, S. E. Gombash, P. G. Zaworski, A. J. Blatnik III, K. D. Foust and A. H. M. Burghes, SMN expression is required in motor neurons to rescue electrophysiological deficits in the SMNΔ7 mouse model of SMA, *Hum. Mol. Genet.*, 2015, **24**(19), 5524–5541.

32. G. Z. Mentis, D. Blivis, W. Liu, E. Drobac, M. E. Crowder, L. Kong, F. J. Alvarez, C. J. Sumner and M. J. O'Donovan, Early Functional Impairment of Sensory-Motor Connectivity in a Mouse Model of Spinal Muscular Atrophy, *Neuron*, 2011, **69**(3), 453–467.
33. S. Kariya, G.-H. Park, Y. Maeno-Hikichi, O. Leykekhman, C. Lutz, M. S. Arkovitz, L. T. Landmesser and U. R. Monani, Reduced SMN protein impairs maturation of the neuromuscular junctions in mouse models of spinal muscular atrophy, *Hum. Mol. Genet.*, 2008, **17**(16), 2552–2569.
34. U. R. Monani, M. Sendtner, D. D. Coovert, D. W. Parsons, C. Andreassi, T. T. Le, S. Jablonka, B. Schrank, W. Rossol, T. W. Prior, G. E. Morris and A. H. M. Burghes, The human centromeric survival motor neuron gene (SMN2) rescues embryonic lethality in Smn-/- mice and results in a mouse with spinal muscular atrophy, *Hum. Mol. Genet.*, 2000, **9**(3), 333–339.
35. C. Cifuentes-Diaz, T. Frugier, F. D. Tiziano, E. Lacene, N. Roblot, V. Joshi, M. H. Moreau and J. Melki, Deletion of murine SMN exon 7 directed to skeletal muscle leads to severe muscular dystrophy, *J. Cell Biol.*, 2001, **152**(5), 1107–1114.
36. J. M. Vitte, B. Davoult, N. Roblot, M. Mayer, V. Joshi, S. Courageot, F. Tronche, J. Vadrot, M. H. Moreau, F. Kemeny and J. Melki, Deletion of murine Smn exon 7 directed to liver leads to severe defect of liver development associated with iron overload, *Am. J. Pathol.*, 2004, **165**(5), 1731–1741.
37. Y. Hua, K. Sahashi, F. Rigo, G. Hung, G. Horev, C. F. Bennett and A. R. Krainer, Peripheral SMN restoration is essential for long-term rescue of a severe spinal muscular atrophy mouse model, *Nature*, 2011, **478**(7367), 123–126.
38. Y. Hua, L. Y. Hsiu, S. Kentaro, R. Frank, B. C. Frank and A. R. Krainer, Motor neuron cell-nonautonomous rescue of spinal muscular atrophy phenotypes in mild and severe transgenic mouse models, *Genes Dev.*, 2015, **29**(3), 288–297.
39. J.-K. Kim, N. N. Jha, Z. Feng, M. R. Faleiro, C. A. Chiriboga, L. Wei-Lapierre, R. T. Dirksen, C.-P. Ko and U. R. Monani, Muscle-specific SMN reduction reveals motor neuron-independent disease in spinal muscular atrophy models, *J. Clin. Invest.*, 2020, **130**(3), 1271–1287.
40. S. L. Lipnick, D. M. Agniel, R. Aggarwal, N. R. Makhortova, S. G. Finlayson, A. Brocato, N. Palmer, B. T. Darras, I. Kohane and L. L. Rubin, Systemic nature of spinal muscular atrophy revealed by studying insurance claims, *PLoS One*, 2019, **14**(3), e0213680.
41. S. E. Matesanz, B. Gross, S. W. Yum, E. A. Kichula, C. Curry, A. I. Rubin, R. Linn, A. I. Rubin, R. Linn, S. W. Yum and E. A. Kichula, Clinical Course in a Patient With Spinal Muscular Atrophy Type 0 Treated With Nusinersen and Onasemnogene Abeparvovec, *J. Child Neurol.*, 2020, 883073820928784.
42. A. Besse, S. Astord, T. Marais, M. Roda, B. Giroux, P. Smeriglio, M. Barkats, F.-X. Lejeune, F. Relaix and M. G. Biferi, AAV9-Mediated Expression of SMN Restricted to Neurons Does Not Rescue the Spinal Muscular Atrophy Phenotype in Mice, *Mol. Ther.*, 2020.
43. A. Cheung, D. N. Chin, N. Dales, A. Fazal, T. B. Hurley, J. Kerrigan, G. O'Brien, L. Shu, R. Sun and M. Sung, Preparation of 1,4-disubstituted pyridazine analogs and methods for treating SMN deficiency related conditions, *WO Pat.*, 2014028459A1, 2014.
44. A. K. Cheung, B. Hurley, R. Kerrigan, L. Shu, D. N. Chin, Y. Shen, G. O'Brien, M. J. Sung, Y. Hou, J. Axford, E. Cody, R. Sun, A. Fazal, R. C. Tomlinson, M. Jain, L. Deng, K. Hoffmaster, C. Song, M. Van Hoosear, Y. Shin, R. Servais, C. Towler, M. Hild, D. Curtis, W. F. Dietrich, L. G. Hamann, K. Briner, K. S. Chen, D. Kobayashi, R. Sivasankaran and N. A. Dales, Discovery of Small Molecule Splicing Modulators of Survival Motor Neuron-2 (SMN2) for the Treatment of Spinal Muscular Atrophy (SMA), *J. Med. Chem.*, 2018, **61**(24), 11021–11036.
45. B. F. El-Khodor, N. Edgar, A. Chen, M. L. Winberg, C. Joyce, D. Brunner, M. Suarez-Farinas and M. P. Heyes, Identification of a battery of tests for drug candidate evaluation in the SMNΔ7 neonate model of spinal muscular atrophy, *Exp. Neurol.*, 2008, **212**(1), 29–43.
46. NCT02268552: An open label study of LMI070 (branaplam) in type 1 spinal muscular atrophy (SMA), 2014, www.clinicaltrials.gov.
47. Novartis press release: Community update on the study of LMI070, 2016.
48. Novartis press release: Update on LMI070(branaplam) clinical trial, 2017.
49. N. A. Naryshkin, M. Weetall, A. Dakka, J. Narasimhan, X. Zhao, Z. Feng, K. K. Y. Ling, G. M. Karp, H. Qi, M. G. Woll, G. Chen, N. Zhang, V. Gabbeta, P. Vazirani, A. Bhattacharyya, B. Furia, N. Risher, J. Sheedy, R. Kong, J. Ma, A. Turpoff, C.-S. Lee, X. Zhang, Y.-C. Moon, P. Trifillis, E. M. Welch, J. M. Colacino, J. Babiak, N. G. Almstead, S. W. Peltz, L. A. Eng, K. S. Chen, J. L. Mull, M. S. Lynes, L. L. Rubin, P. Fontoura, L. Santarelli, D. Haehnke, K. D. McCarthy, R. Schmucki, M. Ebeling, M. Sivaramakrishnan, C.-P. Ko, S. V. Paushkin, H. Ratni, I. Gerlach, A. Ghosh and F. Metzger, SMN2 splicing modifiers improve motor function and longevity in mice with spinal muscular atrophy, *Science*, 2014, **345**(6197), 688–693.

50. M. G. Woll, H. Qi, A. Turpoff, N. Zhang, X. Zhang, G. Chen, C. Li, S. Huang, T. Yang, Y.-C. Moon, C.-S. Lee, S. Choi, N. G. Almstead, N. A. Naryshkin, A. Dakka, J. Narasimhan, V. Gabbeta, E. Welch, X. Zhao, N. Risher, J. Sheedy, M. Weetall and G. M. Karp, Discovery and Optimization of Small Molecule Splicing Modifiers of Survival Motor Neuron 2 as a Treatment for Spinal Muscular Atrophy, *J. Med. Chem.*, 2016, **59**(13), 6070–6085.
51. H. Ratni, G. M. Karp, M. Weetall, N. A. Naryshkin, S. V. Paushkin, K. S. Chen, K. D. McCarthy, H. Qi, A. Turpoff, M. G. Woll, X. Zhang, N. Zhang, T. Yang, A. Dakka, P. Vazirani, X. Zhao, E. Pinard, L. Green, P. David-Pierson, D. Tuerck, A. Poirier, W. Muster, S. Kirchner, L. Mueller, I. Gerlach and F. Metzger, Specific Correction of Alternative Survival Motor Neuron 2 Splicing by Small Molecules: Discovery of a Potential Novel Medicine To Treat Spinal Muscular Atrophy, *J. Med. Chem.*, 2016, **59**(13), 6086–6100.
52. NCT02240355: A study of RO6885247 in adult and pediatric patients with spinal muscular atrophy (Moonfish), 2015, www.clinicaltrials.gov.
53. H. Kletzl, A. Marquet, A. Gunther, I. Gerlach, K. Heinig, S. Dziadek, C. Czech, O. Khwaja, W. Tang, T. Bugawan, J. Heuberger, G. J. Groeneveld, W. Birkhoff, E. Mercuri, H. Lochmuller, C. Wood, D. Fischer and R. Kinch, The oral splicing modifier RG7800 increases full length survival of motor neuron 2 mRNA and survival of motor neuron protein: Results from trials in healthy adults and patients with spinal muscular atrophy, *Neuromuscular Disord.*, 2019, **29**(1), 21–29.
54. C. Czech, W. Tang, T. Bugawan, C. Mano, C. Horn, V. A. Iglesias, S. Frohner, P. G. Zaworski, S. Paushkin, K. Chen and T. Kremer, Biomarker for spinal muscular atrophy: expression of SMN in peripheral blood of SMA patients and healthy controls, *PLoS One*, 2015, **10**(10), e0139950/1–e0139950/11.
55. H. Ratni, L. Green, N. A. Naryshkin and M. L. Weetall, 2-(Imidazo[1,2-*b*]pyridazin-6-yl)pyrido[1,2*a*] pyrimidin-4-one derivatives as SMN modulators and their preparation and use for the treatment of spinal muscular atrophy, *WO Pat.*, 2015173181A1, 2015.
56. A. Poirier, M. Weetall, K. Heinig, F. Bucheli, K. Schoenlein, J. Alsenz, S. Bassett, M. Ullah, C. Senn, H. Ratni, N. Naryshkin, S. Paushkin and L. Mueller, Risdiplam distributes and increases SMN protein in both the central nervous system and peripheral organs, *Pharmacol. Res. Perspect.*, 2018, **6**(6), e00447/1–e00447/12.
57. ClinicalTrials.gov NCT02913482: A study to investigate the safety, tolerability, pharmacokinetics, pharmacodynamics and efficacy of ro7034067 in infants with Type 1 spinal muscular atrophy (FIREFISH). https://clinicaltrials.gov/ct2/show/NCT02913482, accessed September 2020.
58. ClinicalTrials.gov NCT02908685: A study to investigate the safety, tolerability, pharmacokinetics, pharmacodynamics and efficacy of RO7034067 in Type 2 and 3 spinal muscular atrophy participants (SUNFISH), https://clinicaltrials.gov/ct2/show/NCT02908685, accessed September 2020.
59. ClinicalTrials.gov NCT03032172: A study of RO7034067 in adult and pediatric participants with spinal muscular atrophy (JEWELFISH), https://clinicaltrials.gov/ct2/show/NCT03032172, accessed September 2020.
60. ClinicalTrials.gov NCT03779334: A study of risdiplam in infants with genetically diagnosed and presymptomatic spinal muscular atrophy (RAINBOWFISH), https://clinicaltrials.gov/ct2/show/NCT03779334?term=RAINBOWFISH&rank=1, accessed September 2020.
61. Genentech Evrysdi (risdiplam) US Prescribing Information, https://www.gene.com/download/pdf/evrysdi_prescribing.pdf, accessed September 2020.
62. S. Campagne, S. Boigner, S. Rudisser, A. Moursy, L. Gillioz, A. Knorlein, J. Hall, H. Ratni, A. Clery and F. H. T. Allain, Structural basis of a small molecule targeting RNA for a specific splicing correction, *Nat. Chem. Biol.*, 2019, **15**(12), 1191–1198.

# 25 The Discovery of Checkpoint Kinase 1 Inhibitors: From Fragments to Clinical Candidate

Ian Collins*[a]

[a]Cancer Research UK Cancer Therapeutics Unit, The Institute of Cancer Research, London, SM2 5NG, UK
*E-mail: ian.collins02@icr.ac.uk

## 25.1 Introduction

This case history describes the discovery of selective inhibitors of the DNA damage response Checkpoint Kinase 1 (CHK1) for the treatment of cancer, up to the identification and progression into early phase clinical development of the candidate molecule SRA737 (previously CCT245737). Our project started with fragment-based inhibitor discovery, and used extensive structure-based optimisation to generate well-characterised chemical tools to understand the cancer cell and tumour biology of CHK1 inhibition. The tools allowed us to better understand and differentiate the role of functionally related kinases, to validate potential clinical contexts, and in turn to refine the target therapeutic profile and intended trial settings for a candidate CHK1 drug. A salient feature of the project is that we set out to discover inhibitors to use in combination with existing chemotherapies at the outset, driven by the dominant mechanistic understanding of the role of CHK1 in DNA damage repair at the time of initiating the project. The emergence of new biology during the discovery phase highlighted the possibility of additional single agent contexts for CHK1 therapy, which we were able to explore in preclinical models and adapt our early clinical development strategy to exploit.

This case history also exemplifies a project that originated and progressed as a close partnership between an academic, not-for-profit drug discovery laboratory and a biotechnology company. Building effective collaborations between research teams in the partner organisations was critical to the successful identification of a clinical candidate

The Handbook of Medicinal Chemistry: Principles and Practice, 2nd Edition
Edited by Simon E. Ward and Andrew M. Davis

Published by the Royal Society of Chemistry, www.rsc.org

and its subsequent clinical development. The collaboration and its funding structure evolved as the project moved through different stages, bringing in additional partners and new collaborative networks.

## 25.2 CHK1 and Cancer

Despite major advances in targeted drug therapy, genotoxic chemotherapies that damage cellular DNA remain important and widely used in the treatment of cancer. This is particularly so for late stage cancers and metastatic disease, where the continued evolution and migration of cancer cells as the disease progresses leads to tumours consisting of multiple cancer cell populations, in multiple sites within the body, each with potentially different genetics and vulnerabilities. The broad activity of genotoxic chemotherapy, although often leading to severe effects on normal tissues, can still be effective in treating such tumours.

In response to DNA damage, proliferating cells activate a coordinated network of signalling pathways to enable repair of the DNA macromolecule, or to commit the cell to programmed death if repair cannot be achieved[1,2] (see Figure 25.1). The DNA damage response detects the type of damage, for example, single strand or double strand breaks in DNA, and arrests the cell growth and division cycle at defined cell cycle checkpoints to provide time for DNA repair to occur. The checkpoints are active until repair is completed, and the cell cycle can resume. Cancer cells often lose specific cell cycle checkpoint

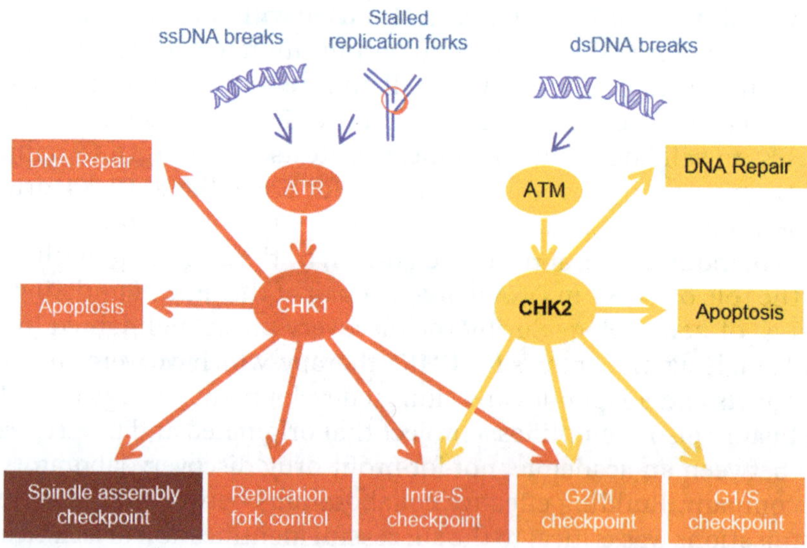


**Figure 25.1** CHK1 and CHK2 signalling in DNA damage response. Single or double strand breaks in DNA arising from radiation, nucleotide mismatches, chemical adducts or stalled replication forks, lead to distinct but overlapping responses mediated by the cell cycle checkpoint kinases CHK1 and CHK2, including cell cycle arrest, activation of DNA repair, senescence or apoptosis. Reproduced from ref. 2 with permission from Springer Nature, Copyright 2018.

functions during oncogenesis, becoming reliant on the remaining processes for successful DNA replication, repair and survival. This differentiates many cancers from untransformed tissue, where cells retain the full complement of cell cycle checkpoint and DNA repair functions, and provides a basis for selective drug targeting of cancer cells.

Loss of function of the tumour suppressor P53 is common in cancer cells and especially compromises the early G1 phase checkpoint, increasing the importance of the later cell cycle checkpoints. The CHK1-dependent S/G2 checkpoint is critical in dealing with single strand breaks in DNA that arise from exogenous DNA-damaging agents and from endogenous errors during DNA replication, a phenomenon known as replication stress.[3] CHK1 and other components of the DNA damage response network can therefore present an intrinsic resistance mechanism to the cytotoxic effects of DNA-damaging chemotherapy, and rescue the deleterious effects of sustained replication stress in tumours.

CHK1 inhibitor discovery projects, including ours, initially sought to test the hypothesis that CHK1 inhibition would potentiate the anti-cancer efficacy of established DNA-damaging chemotherapies, and thus extend the depth or breadth of response to existing clinical treatments. The aim of a combination therapy setting heavily influenced our targeted drug profile and the assay cascade we set up to drive inhibitor discovery. First, we sought to maximise the selectivity of the inhibitors for CHK1 over other kinase and non-kinase off-targets. It is important for drugs acting in target-driven, mechanistic combinations to reduce the accumulation of toxicities arising from off-target pharmacologies of the component therapies. This is a different priority from some single agent, kinase inhibitor anti-cancer therapies, where poly-pharmacology may contribute positively to overall efficacy. Second, we focussed on oral CHK1 inhibitors from the outset to maximise the flexibility for combining with a range of drugs with different dosing routes, dosing durations and schedules. Third, we sought to select cellular assay systems representative of realistic clinical contexts for combination therapy. Thus, our core assay cascade characterised the effects of CHK1 inhibition on cell cycle progression and cell viability in combination with clinically used DNA- damaging agents, initially with topoisomerase inhibitors in colorectal cancer cell lines.

Even with a clear path to the clinic defined from the outset, it is important to acknowledge that basic science did not stand still while our inhibitor discovery progressed. Continued research on the role of CHK1 in the DNA damage response, enabled by the discovery of selective inhibitors, uncovered the potential for single agent efficacy in tumours with high replication stress. Furthermore, combination of CHK1 inhibitors with emerging inhibitors of other DNA damage response mediators also showed preclinical promise.[4] These new findings in turn modified our compound optimisation criteria and informed the strategies for early clinical trials to encompass these additional settings.

## 25.3 Starting Points

### 25.3.1 CHK1 Inhibitor Scaffolds and Target Profile

At the time of starting our project, CHK1 inhibitor scaffolds included the staurosporine analogue UCN-01, and series disclosed by Pfizer, AstraZeneca and Schering-Plough that led to the clinical candidates PF-00477736, AZD7762 and MK-8776 (SCH-900776), respectively (see Figure 25.2). Other CHK1 inhibitors from chemically diverse series subsequently progressed to clinical candidates, including prexasertib, LY2603618, GDC-0425, GDC-0575 and the subject of this case study, SRA737 (CCT245737).[5,6]

The first clinical candidates tended to inhibit both CHK1 and Checkpoint Kinase 2 (CHK2), and some had significant off-target activity against other kinases. Early research had focussed on intravenous drugs suitable for short-term coadministration with intravenous cytotoxic agents. While suitable for some proposed clinical contexts as chemo-sensitisers, intravenous dosing could potentially limit the use of CHK1 inhibitors in combinations, and more especially for chronic inhibition of the target. Emerging

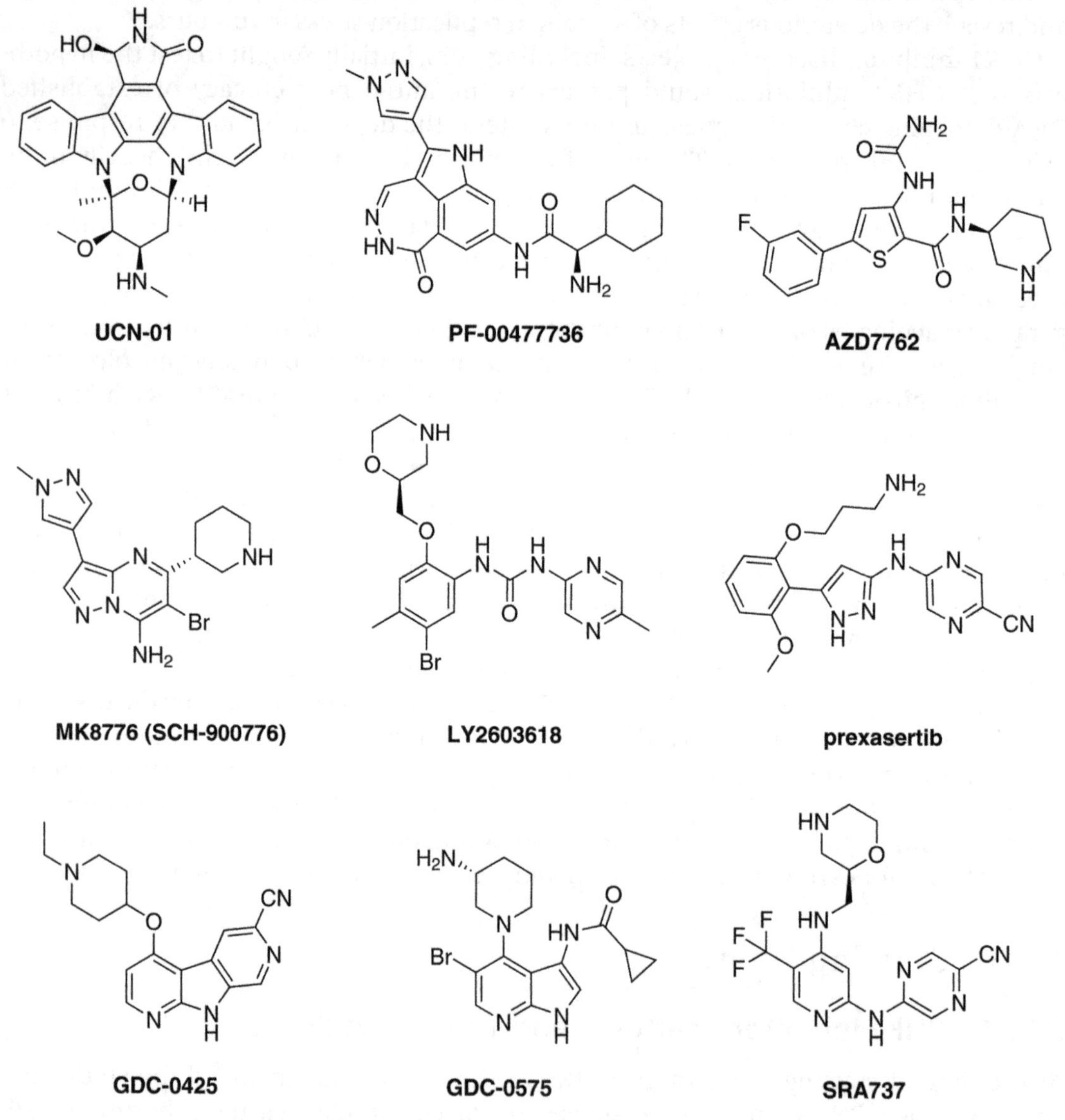


**Figure 25.2** Structures of clinical candidate CHK1 inhibitors from diverse chemical scaffolds.

biology data also suggested that CHK1 and CHK2 had divergent roles in the DNA damage response.[7] Our targeted candidate profile was therefore to develop a selective, orally bioavailable CHK1 inhibitor. As an academic drug discovery group, we also sought to develop highly selective inhibitors for both CHK1 and CHK2 in parallel as chemical tools to enable better understanding the biology of the kinases.[8]

### 25.3.2 Collaborating to Progress CHK1 Fragment Screening

Our academic drug discovery group and colleagues within the structural biology teams at The Institute of Cancer Research (ICR) were already involved in productive collaborations with UK biotechnology companies to apply structure- and fragment-based approaches to inhibitor discovery. These included projects concerning the molecular chaperone heat shock protein 90 (HSP90) and protein kinase B (PKB/AKT) that led to multiple clinical candidates.[9,10] Critical to the success of these collaborations were the complementary expertise and capabilities of the commercial and academic partners, along with mutual alignment on the translational goals of the project, and the drive to deliver clinical benefit. Through actively seeking commercial partners for the CHK1 project, we met scientists at Sareum Ltd, and discovered that both teams were enthused by the prospects for CHK1 as an anti-cancer target and were keen to apply structure-based approaches to inhibitor discovery.

An important ingredient in the success of the collaborative project was the clear complementarity of the scientific partners: The academic group had developed biochemical and mechanistic cellular assays to support the design of CHK1 inhibitors and to understand their impact on cell cycle biology. There were substantial capabilities in medicinal chemistry, drug metabolism and pharmacokinetic (DMPK) studies, and *in vivo* pharmacology in the academic drug discovery group, which included clinicians specialising in early phase clinical trials. Scientists at the commercial partner had established a platform to select screening libraries and apply fragment-based methods and high-throughput protein crystallography to a variety of targets, including CHK1, bringing to bear expertise in *in silico* chemistry, parallel synthesis, medicinal chemistry and kinase pharmacology. An important feature of our collaboration was to enable the academic and company scientists to work closely as a single team, with joint research leadership, sharing of data across the two organisations and day-to-day contact between scientists. The partners each provided financial and infrastructure resources for the joint discovery project, with the academic team funded by substantial grants from Cancer Research UK (CR-UK) to the CR-UK Cancer Therapeutics Unit, and from the ICR.

Multiple CHK1 inhibitor discovery projects have used structure-based approaches to identify adenosine triphosphate (ATP)-competitive ligands, following on from the early determination of the crystal structure of the kinase domain.[11,12] The ATP-binding site of CHK1 contains specific features exploited for the design of selective ligands[13] (see Figure 25.3). Chief among these is the presence of an asparagine residue in the pocket adjacent to the gatekeeper residue. This back pocket, which is not contacted by the endogenous cofactor ATP, is hydrophobic in most kinases and is often involved in lipophilic contacts with inhibitors. In contrast, the polar residue in CHK1 stabilises a network of water molecules within the pocket, creating a hydrophilic environment that

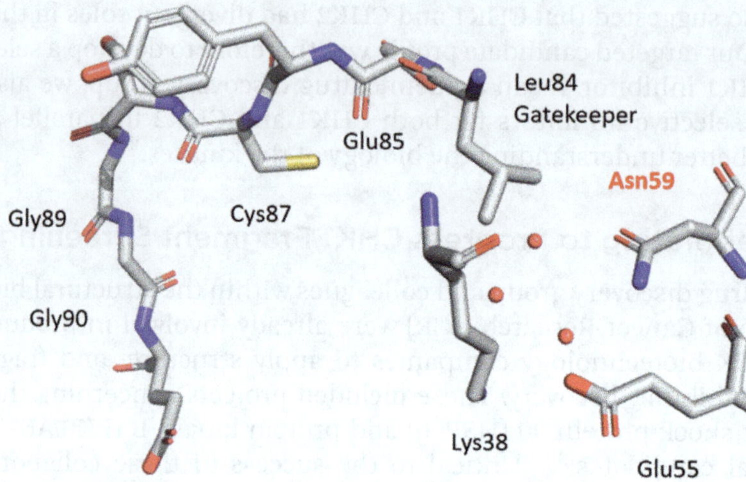


**Figure 25.3** Key features of the ATP-binding pocket of CHK1. Based on the structure of debromohymenialdesine bound to CHK1 (PDB 2C3, ref. 13) with the ligand removed for clarity. Important CHK1 residues shown as grey sticks, including Asn59 and the network of water molecules (red spheres) that can be targeted for CHK1 selective binding.

strongly differentiates CHK1 from most other kinases. The solvent exposed surface at the other side of the CHK1 ATP-binding site contains a glycine–glycine motif that is present in approximately 10% of human kinases, and so presents an additional opportunity for the selective binding of inhibitors.

Our hit finding strategy was to seek ATP-competitive CHK1 fragments binding to the kinase hinge region with the potential to extend into the two regions conferring selectivity, guided by ligand-bound CHK1 crystal structures. We used a biochemical assay adapted for the high concentrations needed to detect the weak binding of low-to-medium molecular weight compounds consisting of 8–24 heavy atoms.[14] A virtual screen of *ca.* 15 000 such commercial compounds using an ATP-site pharmacophore derived from multiple CHK1 structures selected the physical screening set of 361 compounds. Single concentration screening at 250 μM in a CHK1 AlphaScreen format generated 22 primary hits (>25% inhibition with no direct assay interference) which were triaged in a second assay format and counter-screened for interference due to compound aggregation, a significant risk at the high screening concentration. We validated the hits crystallographically by soaking into the apo-CHK1 kinase domain and detected 15 diverse chemical structures in the CHK1 ATP-binding site. Importantly, the rate of crystallographic confirmation was higher for the compounds with lower propensity for aggregation.

## 25.4 From Fragments to *In Vivo* Chemical Tools

### 25.4.1 Evaluating and Growing the Hit Fragments

All of the hit fragments confirmed by crystallography bound to the hinge region of CHK1, as expected from the virtual screening selection. We conducted hit expansion around several of the scaffolds, as it is often the case that not all fragment hits will be suitable for rapid progression. Small sets of compounds were prepared, making use of parallel synthesis where possible, with substitution introduced to target key regions of the ATP-binding site based on the binding poses of the hits in the crystal structures (see Figure 25.4). Iterative crystallography allowed us to follow the effects of new substituents or changes to the core scaffold on binding. Our most detailed studies were on three distinct scaffolds represented by thiazoles, azabicycles and purines.[15–18]

Incorporation of a basic amide substituent to the thiazole scaffold rapidly improved the weak binding to give a micromolar potent hit. However, vectors to contact the bound water molecules in the CHK1 active site were not readily attainable, and the

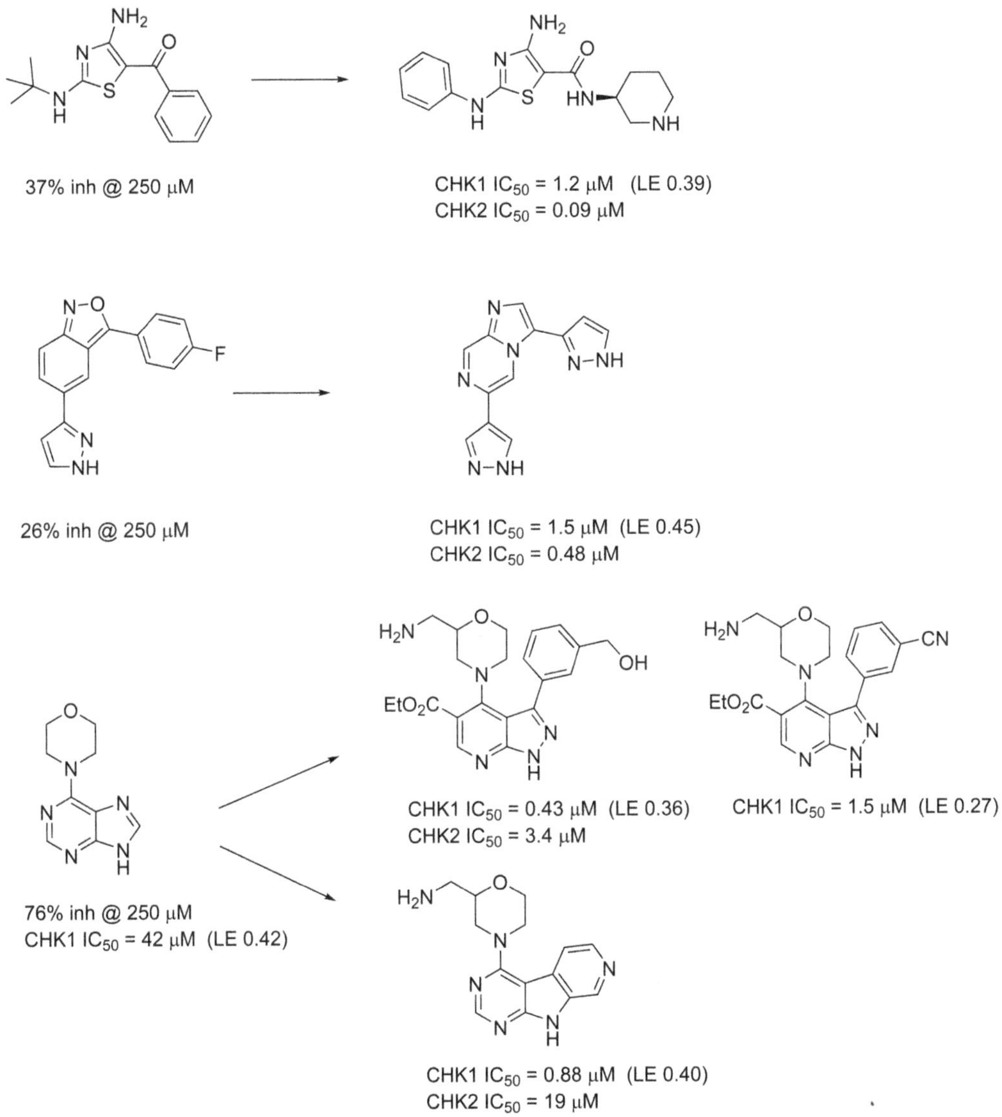


**Figure 25.4** Exploration of thiazole, azabicyclic and purine hit fragments to increase CHK1 potency and explore the potential for CHK1 selectivity.

inhibitors were not selective for inhibition of CHK1 over CHK2. A scaffold hop from a weakly binding benzisoxazole fragment to a series of imidazopyrazines also identified micromolar potent CHK1 inhibitors, but these proved to be generally promiscuous for kinase binding. Better progress was made from 4-(morpholin-4-yl)purine, one of the most ligand efficient fragments identified in the screen. Placement of a basic side chain on the morpholine to interact with acidic residues in the ribose-binding region of the ATP site enhanced affinity for CHK1. A scaffold hop from purine to pyrazolopyridine allowed the addition of a pendant aryl substituent to target the water network, confirmed for a 3-cyanophenyl analogue by crystallography. Despite the promising start, steric congestion of the highly substituted core hindered efficient optimisation of this scaffold. As an alternative, we pursued fusion of the aryl substituent to give a tricyclic core, and found that an optimally placed nitrogen interacted with the bound water network to give a potent and selective CHK1 hit.

### 25.4.2 Scaffold Morphing to Cell Active Leads

The primary assay cascade involved biochemical assays for inhibition of CHK1- and CHK2-mediated peptide substrate phosphorylation. Early in the project, we introduced an off-target screen for cyclin-dependent kinase 1 (CDK1) inhibition, since inhibition of this kinase leads to a general cell cycle arrest that confounds the ability to demonstrate abrogation of the late phase cell cycle checkpoints in cellular assays. We wanted high CHK1 selectivity to ensure a clean, effective mechanism of action and to reduce the potential for unanticipated additive toxicities when used in drug combinations.

To increase potency for CHK1, and selectivity over the other DNA damage response effector CHK2, we made extensive use of structure-based design to target CHK1 specific residues (Section 25.3.2). This indeed led to high CHK1 affinity and selectivity over CHK2. In parallel to the CHK1 inhibitor project, our academic programme to identify selective CHK2 inhibitors also gave insight into the structural attributes of the CHK2 ATP-binding site. Both the preferred core scaffolds and the key interactions with the protein differ between CHK1- and CHK2-selective ligands.[12] Interestingly, reported CHK2 inhibitors include a distinctive sub-set that interact indirectly with the hinge region of the kinase through a bound water molecule, or that replicate this water molecule with a phenolic substituent.

We developed a set of mechanistic cell assays as an integrated approach to measure on-target potency and selectivity, as an efficient alternative to large-scale kinome biochemical screening. We routinely assessed CHK1 inhibition through the ability of the inhibitors to abrogate an etoposide-induced, DNA damage-dependent G2/M cell cycle arrest in HT29 human colon cancer cells. Comparison to the cytotoxicity of the inhibitors in the same cell line indicated the overall selectivity with respect to off-targets causing cell death, since this cell line is not highly sensitive to CHK1 inhibition or depletion alone. Later, we extended this approach to similar paired assays using combinations of the CHK1 inhibitors and other DNA-damaging drugs in cancer cells from different tissues of origin. For compounds with CHK1-dependent activity and phenotypic selectivity in cells, we measured the potentiation of DNA-damaging agents by the CHK1 inhibitors by comparing the cytotoxicity of the single agents to the combination.

The tricyclic scaffold gave a good biochemical and cellular starting profile but had poor physicochemical properties, and developing efficient syntheses proved challenging. We therefore tried a scaffold morphing approach, breaking the five-membered ring to enhance solubility, while simultaneously introducing a second nitrogen atom into the pendant heteroaryl group to permit an overall planar conformation of the bound ligand seen to be favourable from the CHK1 crystal structures (see Figure 25.5). The potency of the resulting *N*-(pyrazin-2-yl)pyrimidin-4-amines was increased through adding a nitrile group to the pyrazine, forming an interaction with the conserved lysine in the ATP-binding site of the kinase, and through varying the position of the basic nitrogen in the side chain.

Guided by crystallographic information, we investigated translocating the basic side chain onto the pyrazine ring while maintaining its interactions in the ribose-binding pocket. This also gave the opportunity to optimise the part of the ligand that extended over the glycine–glycine motif at the entrance to the binding site, through substitution and ring fusion, leading to isoquinoline CHK1 inhibitors with nanomolar potency, exemplified by SAR-020106.

We extensively profiled SAR-020106, and found good CHK1 selectivity against CHK2, CDK1 and a panel of kinases, as expected from the structure-based design and cellular selectivity assays. In fact, when we studied a selection of compounds from the fragment-to-lead sequence in broad kinome biochemical screening, we confirmed that installing the pyrazine nitrile had conferred robust high selectivity for CHK1 in the series.[19]

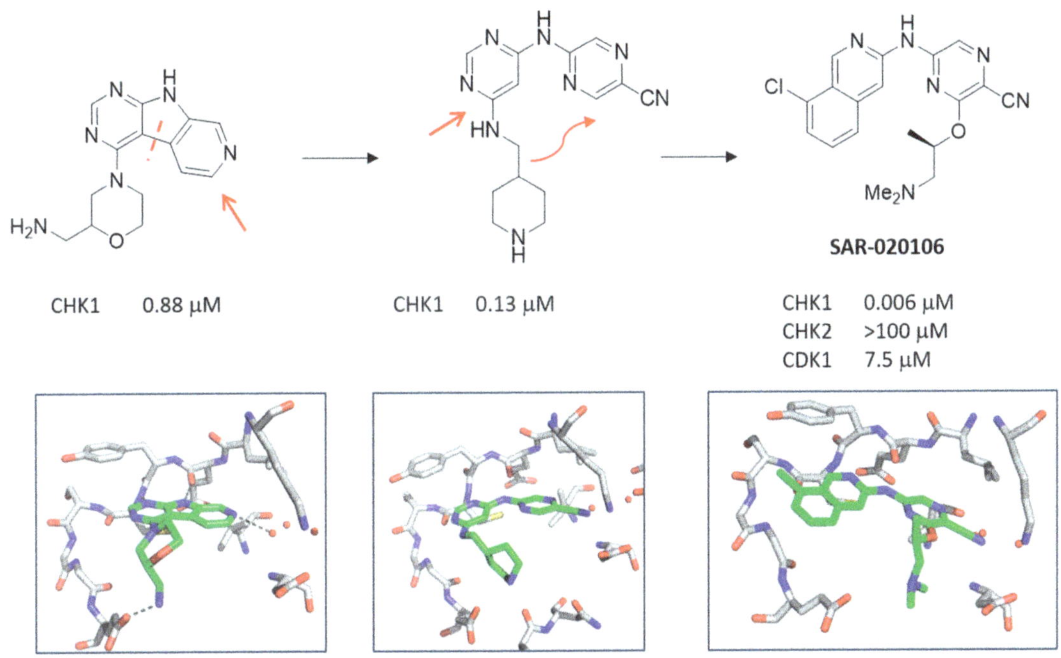


**Figure 25.5** Evolution of the lead CHK1 inhibitor SAR-020106 by a scaffold morphing strategy showing key compounds and their binding modes determined by CHK1 crystallography.

SAR-020106 showed potent abrogation of a DNA-damage-induced S/G2 checkpoint and potentiated the cytotoxicity of various genotoxic chemotherapies in different cancer cells, with induction of apoptosis. While bioavailability and tissue concentrations were limited by high clearance, SAR-020106 had sufficient exposure on intraperitoneal dosing to demonstrate target engagement and potentiation of genotoxic drug efficacy in human tumour xenograft models.[20]

### 25.4.3 From Cell Active Chemical Tools to *In Vivo* Proof of Concept with Oral Agents

To develop orally active agents, we followed a strategy of hybridising the substituted pyrazine driving CHK1 affinity and selectivity with potentially more metabolically stable pyridine scaffolds identified during the scaffold morphing approaches (see Figure 25.6). This generated a series of high affinity, selective *N*-(pyrazin-2-yl)pyridin-4-amines with potent cell activity and reduced *in vitro* microsomal clearance.[21] From this compound set, we used a limited sampling mouse pharmacokinetic (PK) method, involving taking plasma at 1 and 6 hours following intravenous and oral doses, to select efficiently those analogues that had indications of both increased plasma half-life and improved oral bioavailability. Full PK analysis confirmed CCT244747 as having high oral bioavailability, while the compound maintained high CHK1 potency, cellular activity and kinase selectivity.[22]

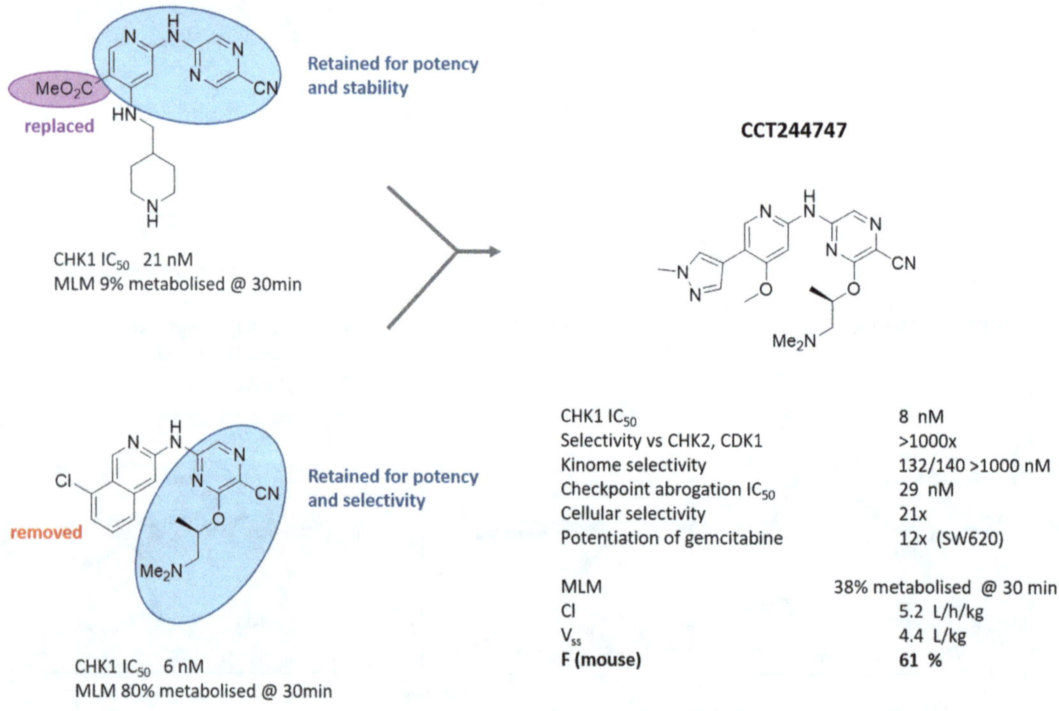


**Figure 25.6** Hybridisation of the potent isoquinoline scaffold with the more metabolically stable *N*-(pyrazin-2-yl)pyridin-4-amines to give orally bioavailable inhibitors.

### 25.4.3.1 Defining the Pharmacodynamic Biomarker Signature of CHK1 Inhibition

The CHK1-selective tool compounds SAR-020106 and CCT244747 allowed us to define the pharmacodynamic biomarker signature of CHK1 inhibition in combination with DNA-damaging agents, and to develop assays to monitor these signals of target engagement and effects on the CHK1 signalling pathway in cells and *in vivo*.[20,22] Importantly, CHK1 auto-phosphorylates on serine 296 when activated by the upstream kinase, ataxia telangiectasia and rad3 related (ATR), which provided direct insight into target inhibition in cells (see Figure 25.7). ATR-dependent phosphorylation of CHK1 reported on the activation of the signalling pathway by the genotoxic agent, and downstream signalling to control cell cycle arrest resulted in increased phospho-CDK1 levels. The biological consequences of unresolved DNA damage and increased DNA strand breaks were shown by increases in chromatin phosphorylation (phosphorylated H2A histone family member X; γH2AX), and cell death through apoptosis (cleaved poly(ADPribose) polymerase; PARP).

### 25.4.3.2 Understanding the Optimum Chemotherapy Combinations

We realised that the precise choice of DNA-damaging chemotherapies for combination with a CHK1 inhibitor could strongly determine the clinical development pathways,

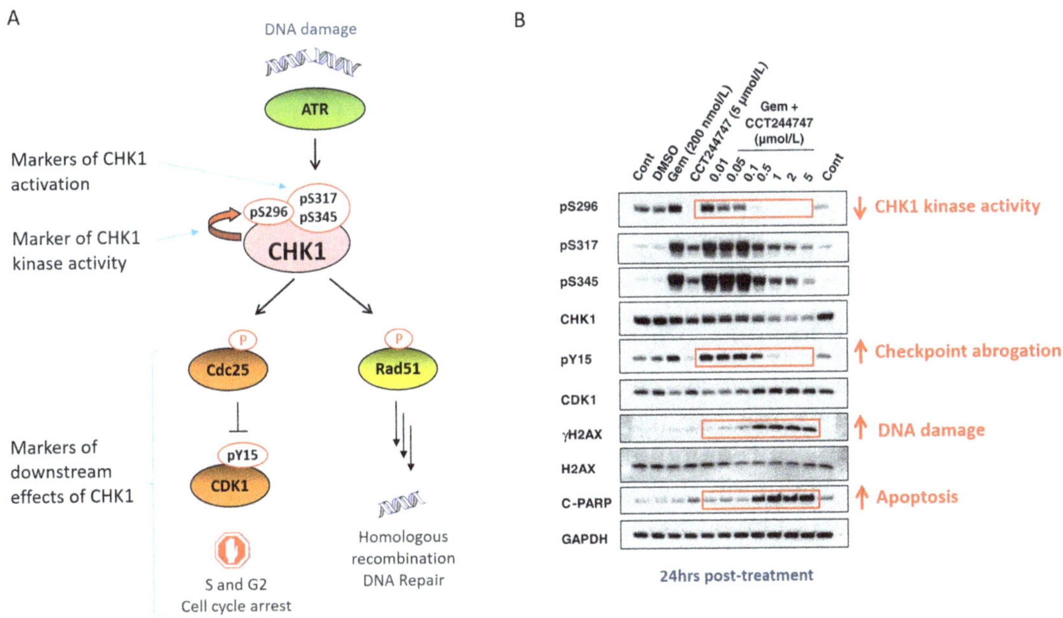


**Figure 25.7** (A) Schematic of the ATR-CHK1 signalling pathway and the components used as pharmacodynamic biomarkers of CHK1 activation, inhibition and downstream effects. (B) The effects of gemcitabine and CCT244747 on the DNA damage response in SW620 human colon cancer cells. Reproduced from ref. 22 with permission from American Association for Cancer Research, Copyright 2012.

as existing genotoxic drugs have well-established clinical populations and dosing regimens, often already combined with other drugs. Early development of inhibitors destined for combinations, benefits from optimisation towards use with chemotherapies recognised as standards of care in defined clinical contexts. This strategy provides a focus for the preclinical pharmacology data needed to support entry of a candidate drug into the clinic. On starting the project, we had concentrated on combinations with topoisomerase inhibitors in colorectal cancer cell lines, as one therapeutic context supported by existing literature, and tractable for development of the cellular and preclinical *in vivo* assays. With the discovery of the advanced, selective tool compounds, we were able to address the choice of target clinical combination more systematically.

We used CCT244747 to screen for the potentiation of a range of DNA-damaging agents including topoisomerase inhibitors, DNA-crosslinking agents, anti-metabolites and ionising radiation.[22] All showed substantial effects, with greatest synergy seen for combinations of our CHK1 inhibitor with the anti-metabolites gemcitabine and 5-fluorodeoxyuridine. This was consistent with the known importance of CHK1 signalling in resolving stalled DNA replication; a stress phenotype exacerbated by anti-metabolites through depletion of the nucleotide intermediate pool and/or incorporation into growing DNA chains. Other CHK1-selective inhibitors were reported to behave similarly.[23] We chose to focus on combinations with the clinical agent gemcitabine, approved for the treatment of pancreatic, non-small cell lung, breast and ovarian cancers.

SAR-020106 and CCT244747 provided evidence of the desired pharmacology from CHK1-selective inhibition. In parallel with our CHK1 research, we had pursued a separate academic project to identify selective inhibitors of CHK2 leading to the cell active tool compound CCT241533.[24] Unlike the CHK1 inhibitors, the CHK2 inhibitor CCT241533 showed no potentiation of the efficacy of a range of DNA-damaging agents.[25] This was consistent with literature reports using RNA interference or other small molecule inhibitors that suggested no benefit from dual CHK1/CHK2 inhibition when combined with most genotoxic agents, and reinforced the desirability of CHK1 selectivity in our target candidate profile.

### 25.4.3.3 Understanding Optimum Drug Combination Schedules

Having selected gemcitabine as the focus of preclinical combination studies, we used the tool compound CCT244747 to study the effects of changing the dosing schedule and duration of CHK1 inhibition on the efficacy of gemcitabine cancer cell models[22] (see Figure 25.8A). We found that starting CHK1 inhibition up to 36 hours after the DNA-damaging agent could be equivalent to simultaneous treatment. Importantly, this predicted flexibility for clinical scheduling that might reduce the potential for additive toxicities due to simultaneous drug dosing. We also found that the duration of inhibition of CHK1 after the initial DNA-damaging therapy was critical, with sustained CHK1 inhibition for 24–48 hours required to achieve maximum potentiation of the cytotoxicity of gemcitabine. This requirement for sustained suppression of the DNA damage response after DNA-damaging treatment reflects the non-synchronised dynamics of the cancer cell population as it passes through the cell cycle to encounter the critical S/

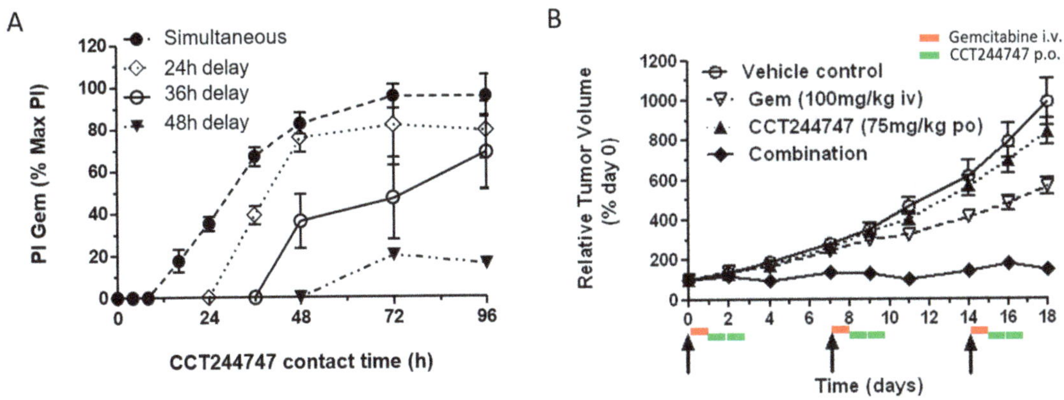


**Figure 25.8** (A) The tool compound CCT244747 elicits maximum potentiation of gemcitabine cytotoxicity in SW620 human colon cancer cells when administered sequentially within 48 h and with sustained exposure. (B) The tool compound potentiates the anti-tumour efficacy of gemcitabine in HT29 human colon cancer xenografts, when dosed orally in a repeating, sequential combination schedule informed by the *in vitro* study. Reproduced from ref. 22 with permission from American Association for Cancer Research, Copyright 2012.

G2-phase checkpoints where the suppression of CHK1 activity manifests, and has been observed with other selective CHK1 inhibitors.[26]

Translation of the sequential, oral dosing schedule of CCT244747 to a repeating cycle in a human tumour xenograft model showed inhibition of tumour growth by the combination therapy while the single agents gave minimal effects (see Figure 25.8B). In parallel, we confirmed inhibition of CHK1 signalling in the xenograft tumours using the target engagement biomarkers, discussed above. These studies validated the desirability of an oral agent to provide the flexibility for two or more days of post-chemotherapy treatment with the CHK1 inhibitor. The intermediate tool molecules SAR-020106 and CCT244747 were therefore very valuable pathfinding tools that helped us refine the target candidate profile, focus the initial choice of clinical context and combination therapy, and develop the later stage *in vivo* assays to guide compound optimisation.

## 25.5 Clinical Candidate Discovery

### 25.5.1 Multi-parameter *In Vitro* and *In Vivo* Optimisation

The tool compounds had clarified that oral activity and sustained pharmacodynamic response were essential in our candidate CHK1 inhibitor. The compound CCT244747, although meeting many of the target criteria, possessed sub-optimal clearance *in vitro* and *in vivo*, leading to predictions of a high and frequent human dose. To address this, we stepped back to the metabolically stable *N*-(pyrazin-2-yl)pyridin-4-amine scaffold with the potency-conferring basic side chain appended to the pyridine ring and sought to re-optimise this series without translocation of the basic group (**1**, Table 25.1). With the 5-aminopyrazine-2-carbonitrile moiety fixed to retain potency, selectivity and

**Table 25.1** Key properties of selected compounds in the 5-(pyridin-2-ylamino)pyrazine-2-carbonitrile lead series, showing evolution of the clinical candidate SRA737 (**7**; CCT245737).

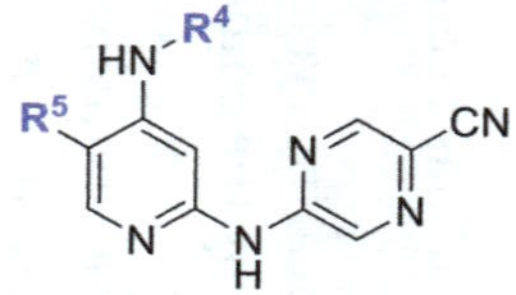


| | $R^4$ | $R^5$ | CHK1 $IC_{50}$ (nM)[a] | Checkpoint abrogation $IC_{50}$ (nM)[b] | Cell selectivity (fold)[c] | HERG (% inh @ 10 μM)[d] | Mouse $C_L$[e] ($L\ h^{-1}\ kg^{-1}$) | Mouse F[f] (%) |
|---|---|---|---|---|---|---|---|---|
| 1 | 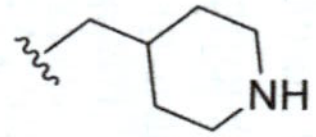 | $MeO_2C$ | 21 | 825 | 3.8 | 39 | — | — |
| 2 | 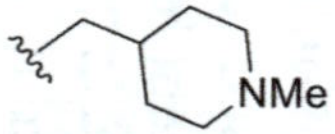 | $MeO_2C$ | 19 | 850 | 4.3 | 82 | — | — |
| 3 | 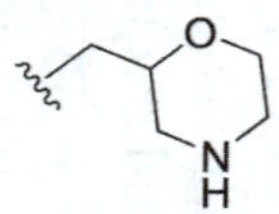 | $MeO_2C$ | 2.2 | 310 | 3.5 | 24 | — | — |
| 4 | 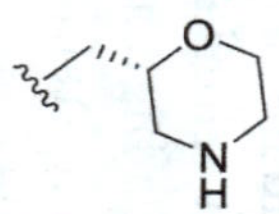 | 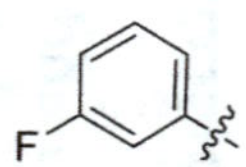 | 6.4 | 120 | 5.8 | 71 $IC_{50}$ 8.8 μM | 6.75 | 53 |
| 5 | 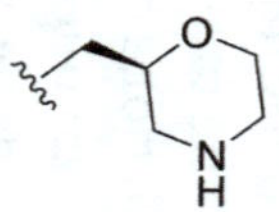 | 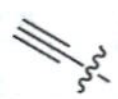 | 5.2 | 100 | 29 | 68 $IC_{50}$ 8.8 μM | 6.35 | 68 |
| 6 | 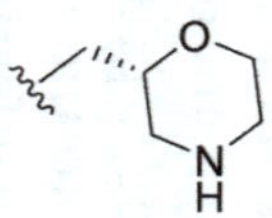 | Cl | 1.9 | 157 | 14 | 83 $IC_{50}$ 6.1 μM | 2.75 | 84 |
| 7 | 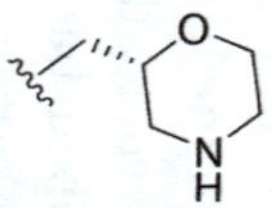 | $F_3C$ | 1.3 | 30 | 23 | 76 $IC_{50}$ 6.2 μM | 2.65 | 105 |

[a]CHK1 biochemical inhibition measured in Caliper microfluidic format.
[b]Abrogation of etoposide-induced G2 checkpoint arrest in HT29 human colon cancer cells.
[c]Ratio of anti-proliferative $GI_{50}$ to $IC_{50}$ for CHK1-mediated abrogation of etoposide-induced G2 checkpoint arrest in HT29 human cancer cells.
[d]Inhibition of hERG ion current in HEK cells overexpressing hERG ion channel.
[e]*In vivo* clearance, calculated based on a 20 g mouse body weight.
[f]Oral bioavailability.

stability, the strategy focussed on variation of the pyridine C4 and C5 substituents. We developed efficient chemical routes for the rapid synthesis of analogues using alkylation, aromatic nucleophilic substitution and palladium-catalysed coupling reactions, with considerable effort applied to find robust conditions for installing the preferred cyanopyrazine group[27] (see Figure 25.9). We later realised the value of this investment in the synthetic chemistry when the general lead optimisation route proved suitable for scale up to prepare multi-gram amounts of potential candidates for preclinical evaluation. The route was also adapted for the manufacture of early batches of the eventual clinical candidate for Phase I trials.

We encountered *in vitro* human ether-a-go-go related gene (HERG) cardiac ion channel inhibition in this series (*e.g.* **2**, Table 25.1) and hypothesised this was due to basicity and overall lipophilicity. Variation of the C4 substitution confirmed this classical HERG structure–activity relationship, and identified that secondary amines with reduced basicity, such as morpholine **3**, minimised the HERG activity, while conferring high affinity for the kinase. At this point, we obtained the final CHK1 crystal structure of the lead optimisation project, which demonstrated a preference for binding of the *R*-enantiomer of the chiral morpholine **3**. Other enantiomer pair comparisons mostly, but not exclusively, showed a similar 2–3 fold preference in CHK1 inhibition for the morpholine *R*-stereochemistry.[27]

With a set of favoured amines identified at the pyridine C4 position, and a larger range of aryl, heteroaryl, alkyl or alkynyl groups possible at the C5 position, we applied a multi-objective *in silico* classification to select substituent combinations for synthesis, using a model trained on the datasets generated so far on the project.[27] We focussed on predicting and optimising three key potency parameters: CHK1 biochemical potency, minimising the ratio of cellular activity to biochemical activity and minimising HERG inhibition. The *in silico* triage of candidates for synthesis helped us to maximise the outputs of the medicinal chemistry team, which was small by contemporary industry standards. While excellent biochemical CHK1 inhibition was achieved with many

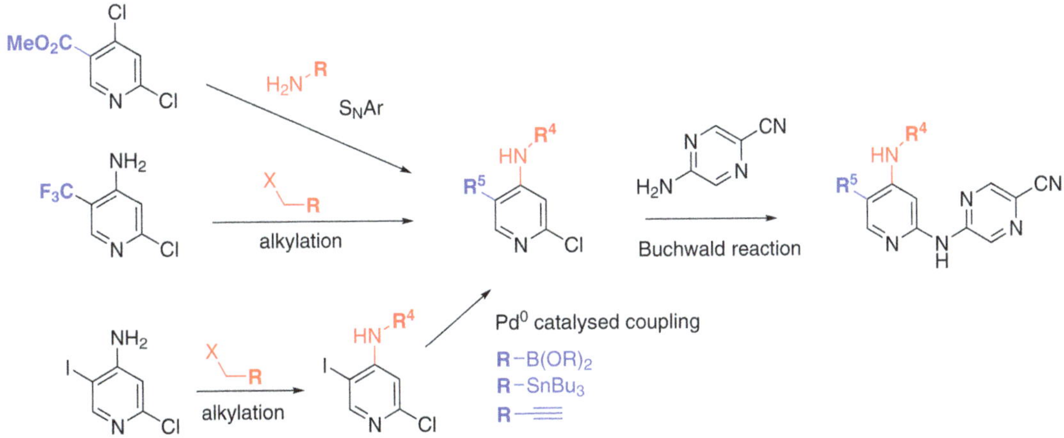


**Figure 25.9** Summary of the synthetic routes developed to support lead optimisation and preclinical candidate evaluation of *N*-(pyrazin-2-yl)pyridin-4-amine CHK1 inhibitors.

substituent combinations, we observed an unexpected profound effect of C5 substituent size on cellular activities, despite equipotent CHK1 inhibition, with larger substituents (*e.g.* **4**) reducing cellular selectivity and potentiation of genotoxic efficacy (see Figure 25.10). We speculated that this cellular behaviour could reflect an off-target activity associated with the larger groups. The larger C5 substituents extended beyond the glycine–glycine surface of CHK1, towards solvent; therefore, restricting the size of the C5 substituent did not compromise the CHK1 kinase affinity or biochemical selectivity.

Compounds with smaller C5 substituents were also favoured for higher oral bioavailability, particularly alkynyl **5**, chloro **6** and trifluoromethyl **7** groups (Table 25.1). We profiled these inhibitors with promising PK profiles for the depth and duration of pharmacodynamic response following a single, high oral dose of the CHK1 inhibitor in combination with gemcitabine in human tumour xenografts, by measuring the inhibition of the gemcitabine-induced CHK1 auto-phosphorylation in tumour samples. Based on the *in vitro* and *in vivo* scheduling studies with the tool compound CCT244747 and the expected clinical contexts, we sought a 24 h duration of action. Both **6** and **7** demonstrated this desired profile, which translated into anti-tumour efficacy including tumour regressions, when dosed with gemcitabine in the HT29 xenograft model using the optimal sequential dosing schedule. While both compounds were effective in the preclinical model, the trifluoromethyl analogue **7** (CCT245737) had better predictions of human PK.

Extensive profiling of CCT245737 (**7**) *in vitro* and *in vivo* showed it to be a potent, selective and metabolically stable CHK1 inhibitor which potentiated the efficacy of a

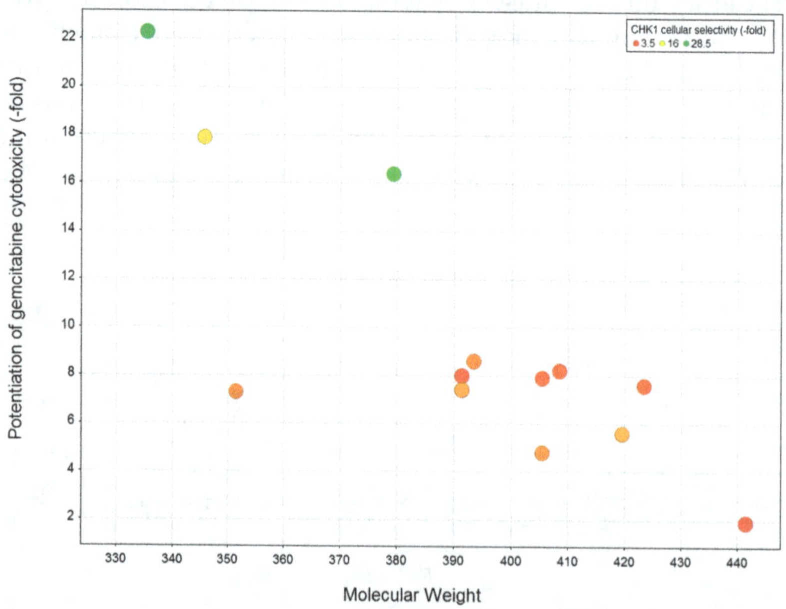


**Figure 25.10** Relationship of efficacy and selectivity in SW620 colon cancer cells to molecular weight for 5-((4-((morpholin-2-ylmethyl)amino)pyridin-2-yl)amino)pyrazine-2-carbonitriles with C5 substituents of various sizes. Reproduced from ref. 27, https://doi.org/10.1021/acs.jmedchem.5b01938, under the terms of the CC BY 4.0 license, https://creativecommons.org/licenses/by/4.0/.

range of genotoxic agents in human cancer cells.[28] The compound had high passive permeability and no efflux in the CaCo2 model of human intestinal absorption.[27] CCT245737 did not inhibit CYP450 enzymes and no susceptibility for metabolic activation was observed. While strongly electron-deficient heterocyclic nitriles can be prone to chemical reaction under physiological conditions, we did not observe this for the 2-amino-5-cyanopyrazine series, likely due to the compensating electron-donating effect of the aniline substituent.[29] The moderately basic morpholine substituent ($pK_a$ 7.87 measured for the whole molecule) conferred aqueous solubility (1.5 mg $mL^{-1}$ at pH 6.5), with good prospects for formulation as a salt. This prediction was borne out during development, where the identification of a stable and soluble organic salt allowed rapid progress in early formulation and toxicology studies.

### 25.5.2 *In Vivo* Pharmacology and Predictions to Human

An important step in the decision to progress a compound as a clinical candidate is to predict the human PK properties and likely clinical efficacious dose, and to relate the required exposure for target engagement to the potential for off-target effects. To enable this for CCT245737, the dose responses for inhibition of CHK1 auto-phosphorylation and anti-tumour efficacy were determined, in combination with gemcitabine given at its maximum tolerated dose in the HT29 tumour xenograft mouse model[28] (see Figure 25.11). These studies established both a preclinical minimum effective dose of CCT245737 in combination (12.5 mg $kg^{-1}$ in mouse xenograft models), and the associated minimum unbound drug concentration in plasma associated with this efficacy and complete inhibition of gemcitabine-induced CHK1 signalling for 24 hours.

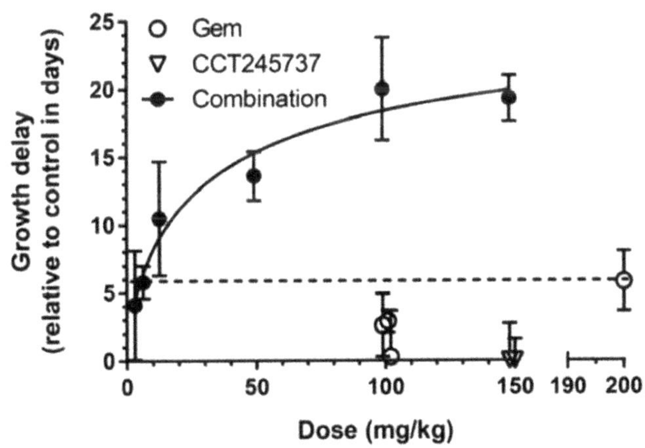


**Figure 25.11** Anti-tumour effects of different oral doses of CCT245737 combined with a fixed dose of gemcitabine (100 mg $kg^{-1}$ i.v.) in HT29 human colon cancer xenografts. The activity of the MTD for single dose gemcitabine (200 mg $kg^{-1}$ i.v.) and CCT245737 (150 mg $kg^{-1}$ p.o.) are also shown (dashed line). Growth delays (days) were determined in several independent experiments and are shown as mean ± SE for $n$ = 6–10 mice per point. Reproduced from ref. 28, https://doi.org/10.18632/oncotarget.4919, under the terms of the CC BY 3.0 license, https://creativecommons.org/licenses/by/3.0/.

Looking at the *in vitro* ADME properties, we found CCT245737 to be approximately ten- to twenty-fold more stable in human than mouse, rat or dog hepatocytes. While mouse microsomal clearance was predictive of mouse *in vivo* pharmacokinetics, due to the difference in hepatocyte stability between preclinical species and humans, we relied on physiological-based PK simulations from the human *in vitro* ADME and physicochemical data, as well as single species scaling from mouse *in vivo* data, to predict human PK properties, rather than multi-species *in vivo* allometric scaling. The various approaches predicted an acceptable low human dose would achieve the unbound drug concentration associated with preclinical target engagement and efficacy.[27] Based on the observed pharmacodynamics of CCT245737 in the human tumour xenograft models, dosing intervals of between 12 and 24 hours were predicted to be capable of achieving sustained CHK1 inhibition in humans.

Broad pharmacological profiling showed minimal interactions across a variety of targets, including cardiovascular ion channels, with only *in vitro* HERG inhibition detected in the micromolar range.[27] We paid particular attention to assessment of the cardiovascular profile, given clinical reports with early CHK1/CHK2 inhibitors that had indicated unwanted effects on heart function. Clinical studies with other CHK1-selective inhibitors have not shown these effects, indicating the cardiac toxicity of early compounds may reflect idiosyncratic off-target activity rather than resulting from CHK1-mediated pharmacology.[30–33] From the predicted minimum effective clinical dose and calculations of the unbound drug concentrations at the peak and trough of the predicted human PK profile, we predicted a suitable therapeutic window over the weak *in vitro* HERG inhibition, according to typical guidelines.[34] This was confirmed in cardiovascular preclinical pharmacology studies. The preclinical pharmacology, PK and physicochemical profile of CCT245737, as well as the predicted effective dose, PK and therapeutic index in humans, met our targets for selection as a clinical candidate for treating solid tumours in combination with the DNA-damaging cytotoxic, gemcitabine.

### 25.5.3 Expanding and Defining Potential Clinical Contexts

To help define potential patient populations for early clinical trials, we investigated the efficacy of the compound in additional human tumour xenograft models. Gemcitabine is used clinically to treat pancreatic ductal adenocarcinoma (PDAC), and in combination with platinum drugs in non-small cell lung cancer (NSCLC). We showed potentiation of the anti-tumour efficacy of gemcitabine by CCT245737 in a genetically engineered mouse model of PDAC, and the potentiation of gemcitabine and cisplatin combined therapy in NSCLC human tumour xenografts.[27,28] These results further supported the proposed early clinical development of CCT245737 in combination with gemcitabine.

During the discovery project, data emerged in the literature suggesting a role for CHK1 inhibitors as single agents, specifically in cancers with high endogenous replication stress. The published results were especially striking in tumours characterised by deregulated MYC oncoproteins, such as MYCN-driven neuroblastoma and MYC-driven lymphoma.[3] We had profiled the early tool compound SAR-020106 for cytotoxicity following three days treatment in the large panel of cancer cell lines set up by the Wellcome Sanger Institute[35] and observed a strong sensitivity of neuroblastoma cell lines to CHK1 inhibition.

A benefit of the situation of our academic drug discovery laboratories within a comprehensive cancer research institute, and part of a wider academic cancer research network, is the ready access to collaborative work with teams of researchers studying specific cancer types and using advanced imaging techniques. In collaboration with paediatric oncology researchers at The Institute of Cancer Research, we quickly tested and confirmed the efficacy of our CHK1 inhibitors as single agents in a genetically engineered mouse model of paediatric MYCN-driven neuroblastoma, where we observed tumour regression upon continuous once-daily oral dosing[27] (see Figure 25.12).

We were also able to collaborate with CRUK-funded colleagues at Newcastle University, to test our inhibitor in a murine allograft model of MYC-driven lymphoma. Single agent efficacy on disease disseminated to multiple lymph nodes was observed following once-daily oral dosing.[28]

The confirmation of preclinical single agent efficacy significantly influenced our early clinical development strategy. With the benefit of an orally bioavailable compound suitable for continuous daily dosing, we decided to plan two parallel tracks for Investigational New Drug enabling studies and Phase I clinical trials. The first would study CCT245737 as a single agent for continuous, daily dosing, reflecting the administration schedules effective in the neuroblastoma and lymphoma preclinical models. This trial would give information on the PK and tolerability of the CHK1 inhibitor alone. The second, informed by our combination preclinical *in vivo* pharmacology studies, would establish the regimen for CCT245737 plus gemcitabine, using an intermittent dose of the CHK1 inhibitor matched to the standard-of-care schedule for the cytotoxic drug, such that CCT2457237 would be dosed for two days after each cycle of chemotherapy.

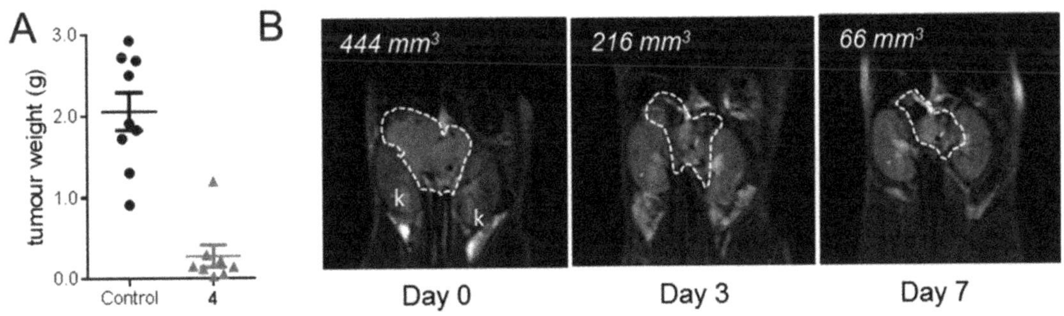


**Figure 25.12** CCT245737 as a single agent (150 mg kg$^{-1}$ po QD7) inhibits the growth of TH-MYCN neuroblastoma. (A) Comparison of tumour weights for vehicle- and compound-treated cohorts (mean ± SEM, $n$ = 8). (B) Pre- and post-treatment T2-weighted MRI assessment of an abdominal tumour in a single mouse treated with CCT245737. k = kidney. Reproduced from ref. 27, https://doi.org/10.1021/acs.jmedchem.5b01938, under the terms of the CC BY 4.0 license, https://creativecommons.org/licenses/by/4.0/.

## 25.6 Preclinical Development, Early Clinical Trials and New Clinical Contexts

Clinical development is considerably more expensive than the preclinical discovery of a new small molecule. Progression of new drug candidates discovered in academic and other not-for-profit laboratories will typically require a larger pharmaceutical company partner to support development, which can also provide access to refined clinical development infrastructures and expertise available in the commercial organisations. The finite number of clinical development compounds that even well-resourced pharmaceutical companies can handle at any time, and the need for in-licensed programmes to fit with existing corporate portfolios and business strategies, can place barriers on this route. Estimated attrition rates for compounds in early phase trials remain high, particularly in oncology,[36] and there is potentially an advantage to progressing through Phase 1 or Phase 1/2 trials independently to substantially de-risk a development candidate. For projects originating in academic laboratories, negotiating the distance between candidate discovery and advanced clinical development is a formidable challenge, sometimes described as a translational medicine "valley of death".[37]

While direct licensing to companies remains an attractive option, the past decade has seen growth in alternative opportunities for academic drug discovery groups to resource early clinical development. These can involve application for major grants from dedicated public or charitable translational funding streams, or the use of venture capital either to form spin-out vehicles for compound development, or to fund individual projects. The development of our CHK1 inhibitor was supported following successful application to a venture capital fund established by Cancer Research Technology, the commercialisation arm of Cancer Research UK, and the European Investment Fund. The Cancer Research Technology Pioneer Fund (CPF), managed by Sixth Element Capital LLP, was formed to accelerate the translation of new anti-cancer agents from late preclinical discovery into early phase trials, and thus to support onward licensing and clinical development.[38] In tandem with the application to the venture capital fund, the project also became part of the Cancer Research UK Centre for Drug Development[39] (CDD) portfolio. The project to develop CCT245737 used a virtual organisation model. This drew on scientific, clinical and project management expertise from within Sixth Element Capital LLP, the CR-UK Centre for Drug Development and CR-UK's clinical science network. Contract research organisations and academic partner laboratories were engaged to deliver specific work packages in synthesis and manufacture, PK and PD analysis development,[40] formulation and toxicology.

Regulatory toxicology was conducted to support the two distinct dosing regimens proposed for Phase 1 trials, and two separate clinical trial applications were made by the development team in partnership with clinical investigators at The Institute of Cancer Research and the Royal Marsden NHS Foundation Trust.[41,42] The trial proposals included multiple dedicated cancer clinical sites that are part of the UK cancer research network. Starting in 2016, the two trials separately investigated a dose escalation for daily monotherapy with CCT245737, and a dose escalation in combination with chemotherapy on an intermittent schedule. The combination trial design involved assessing the doublet therapy of CHK1 inhibitor and gemcitabine, and a triple combination of the CHK1 inhibitor with gemcitabine and cisplatin, representing a common therapy for some lung cancers.

Onward licensing of CCT245737 to Sierra Oncology was achieved shortly after the clinical trials began, accompanied by a change in the compound identifier to SRA737.[38] The commercial partner was rapidly able to assume full responsibility for the two active trials, and to bring additional investment and expertise to adapt and augment the Phase 1/2 clinical plans. Notably, the monotherapy trial was enhanced to include more patients in the expansion phase, and incorporate extensive tumour genetic profiling. Excitingly, additional preclinical studies by colleagues at Sierra Oncology showed that SRA737 potentiated the anti-tumour effect of sub-therapeutic doses of gemcitabine.[42] In this situation, the DNA-damaging anti-metabolite enhances endogenous replication stress in the tumour cells to critical levels, setting up a potential for synthetic lethality with CHK1 inhibition. Dose reduction of the chemotherapy component could have advantages for tolerability, and the combination trial was enhanced to explore combinations of the CHK1 inhibitor with low dose gemcitabine, representing between 10 and 25% of the standard-of-care dose. Once dose escalation was completed, the cohort expansion phase included patients with soft tissue sarcomas, high-grade serous ovarian, small cell lung, and anogenital or cervical cancers.

Preliminary data from the first-in-human monotherapy trial showed PK close to that predicted from the approaches applied during candidate selection.[41] The results demonstrated the safety and tolerability of SRA737, with no evidence of emergent or cumulative toxicity observed with up to nine 28-day cycles of SRA737 administered. A recommended monotherapy dose of 800 mg day$^{-1}$ was determined, where the $C_{min}$ threshold extrapolated from the preclinical efficacy studies was exceed by all doses above 300 mg day$^{-1}$. In the combination trial with low dose gemcitabine (250 mg m$^{-2}$) the recommended Phase 2 dose of SRA737 was determined to be 500 mg day$^{-1}$, administered for two days after each chemotherapy dose.[42] Multiple partial responses were seen in the expansion phase, particularly in a sub-set of patients with advanced anogenital cancer where anti-tumour activity (overall response rate = 30%) including tumour decreases was observed, suggesting a future focus for clinical development.

The properties of our tool compounds SAR-020106 and CCT244747, and the clinical candidate, were disclosed in publications during the discovery project and early development, and the compounds were available to academic and commercial partners to research into new therapeutic indications. This included studying the potential for combining CHK1 inhibition with radiotherapy and oncolytic viral therapy,[43–46] the identification of a new monotherapy context due to synthetic lethality of CHK1 inhibition with tumour cell defects in DNA polymerase activity[47] and the demonstration of efficacy in combination with molecular targeted PARP inhibitors.[48] This last study represents a growing body of data showing anti-tumour efficacy through combining molecular targeted inhibitors of DNA damage response and repair pathways, without the application of explicit DNA-damaging chemotherapies[2] (see Figure 25.13).

The success of cancer immunotherapy and its rapid adoption as a new treatment modality was a major change occurring during the discovery and early development of

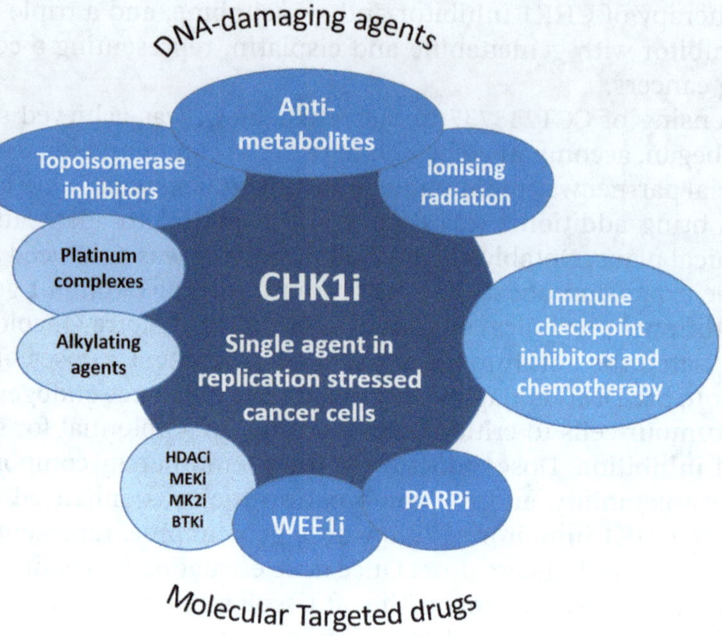


**Figure 25.13** Summary of the potential therapeutic contexts for CHK1 inhibition. Adapted from ref. 2 with permission from Springer Nature, Copyright 2018.

SRA737. Certain tumours remain only modestly tractable to immunotherapy, and there is significant interest in combinations with orthogonal therapies that could enhance efficacy in these cases. In this regard, the combination of low dose gemcitabine and SRA737 identified in the early development phase enhanced the effect of an immune checkpoint inhibitory PD-L1 antibody therapy in multiple preclinical models, especially small cell lung cancer, through modulating the immune microenvironment in the tumours.[49] This illustrates very clearly how the potential clinical contexts for CHK1 inhibition, and the understanding of how to apply the available selective inhibitors, have widened considerably since the outset of our discovery project.

## 25.7 Conclusions

The discovery of the clinical candidate SRA737 was the culmination of a team effort bringing together academic and commercial research organisations in close partnership, leading to the successful transition of the candidate into early phase clinical trials. A fragment-based approach was pursued to generate and optimise chemical hits, where an understanding of the unique structural features of the CHK1 kinase active site allowed highly selective inhibitors to be engineered. Intended from the outset to be used in combination with classical cancer chemotherapy, chemical tool CHK1 inhibitors identified in the project allowed new therapeutic contexts to be explored and validated. This in turn refined the direction taken in lead optimisation and enabled a more diverse early clinical development pathway.

## 25.8 Hints and Tips

Fragment screens often provide many hits and it may be necessary to follow up several series in hit expansion to find the most progressible. Ligand efficiency metrics can help prioritise starting points and monitor how successfully the potency/property optimisation proceeds. Not all fragments retain a consistent binding pose on elaboration and it is important to work this out – usually through iterative structure determination of early compounds in the series.

To explore design hypotheses that introduce interactions with specific residues starting from a ligand-bound protein structure, it is helpful to design a small set of compounds to interrogate each idea, with varying positions of the new functional groups to allow for movements in the amino acid side chains, small flexible regions of the binding site, or the exact ligand pose.

Knowing and quantifying the selectivity of a compound can be a challenge, even if the primary target is part of a protein superfamily with family-wide binding or functional screens available. It can help to pick key off-targets to follow routinely to make efficient use of resources – especially if modulation of those off-targets would confound the interpretation of cellular or tissue assays designed to follow the effect on the primary target. Alternatively, picking a close structural homologue of the primary target can be helpful as selectivity seen here may be more likely (but not guaranteed) to translate to more distantly related proteins.

A set of mechanistic cellular assays can be useful to quantify selectivity and detect unwanted off-target activity that is not expected (an "unknown unknown"). This might involve comparing the effects of the compound in systems engineered to be sensitive to modulation of the target, to matched systems where target modulation should not have an effect. A drawback is that a selectivity issue can be found without knowing how it has arisen, emphasising the desirability of pursuing multiple series early in a project to provide options with different profiles.

Assays to assess target engagement in cells and tissues are extremely valuable. They confirm the target is accessible to the compound in the cell or tissue, and calibrate the biochemical affinity or potency to the biological effect in living systems, informing the target profile. Correlation of target engagement and efficacy in preclinical animal models with the unbound drug concentration profile underpins predictions of the target clinical dose and therapeutic index in humans.

Above, between, below – for drug targets in signal transduction pathways it is helpful to have pharmacodynamic biomarkers that report on the activation of the pathway (above), direct modulation of the target (between) and downstream outputs of the pathway (below).

For many therapeutic areas, and especially for newly discovered targets, developments in basic biological science and therapeutic context will occur during the time taken to discover and develop a candidate drug. A clear idea of the clinical context and intended use is essential at the outset of a drug discovery project, and may need to be adapted as new data emerges. Chemical tools generated during discovery can act as pathfinder molecules to help refine the clinical context during candidate discovery.

## Conflict of Interest Statement

The author is a former employee of The Institute of Cancer Research, which has a commercial interest in the discovery and development of CHK1 inhibitors, including SRA737 and operates a rewards-to-inventors scheme. The author is or has been a consultant for Sierra Oncology, Adorx Ltd, Epidarex LLP, Dunad Therapeutics, and Enterprise Therapeutics Ltd and holds equity in Monte Rosa Therapeutics Inc.

## Acknowledgements

Drug discovery is a team science, and the large number of colleagues involved in this project are authors of the publications cited here from ICR, Sareum Ltd and Sierra Oncology. The author especially acknowledges Professor Michelle Garrett and Professor Udai Banerji, as the ICR biology and clinical project leads, respectively, and Dr John Reader, Dr Tim Mitchell and colleagues at Sareum Ltd. The project team is grateful to CR-UK and the CRT Pioneer Fund, particularly Dr Rob James, for the financial, scientific and logistical support of the project; to colleagues at the CR-UK Centre for Drug Development; and to colleagues at Sierra Oncology. The preclinical discovery project was supported by CR-UK grants C309/A2187, C309/A8274, C309/A11566, by Sareum Ltd, and by the Institute of Cancer Research.

## References

1. M. Garrett and I. Collins, *Trends Pharmacol. Sci.*, 2011, **32**, 308.
2. I. Collins and M. D. Garrett, in *Targeting the DNA Damage Response for Anti-cancer Therapy. Cancer Drug Discovery and Development*, Humana Press, Cham, 1st edn, 2018, pp. 241–276.
3. E. Lecona and O. Fernández-Capetillo, *Exp. Cell Res.*, 2014, **329**, 26.
4. M. Maugeri-Saccà, M. Bartucci and R. De Maria, *Cancer Treat. Rev.*, 2013, **39**, 525.
5. S. Rundle, A. Bradbury, Y. Drew and N. J. Curtin, *Cancers*, 2017, **9**, 41.
6. P. Dent, *Expert Opin. Invest. Drugs*, 2019, **28**, 1095.
7. L. Antoni, N. Sodha, I. Collins and M. D. Garrett, *Nat. Rev. Cancer*, 2007, **7**, 925.
8. P. Workman and I. Collins, *Chem. Biol.*, 2010, **17**, 561.
9. P. A. Brough, W. Aherne, X. Barril, J. Borgognoni, K. Boxall, J. E. Cansfield, K.-M. Cheung, I. Collins, N. G. M. Davies, M. J. Drysdale, B. Dymock, S. A. Eccles, H. Finch, A. Fink, A. Hayes, R. Howes, R. E. Hubbard, K. James, A. M. Jordan, A. Lockie, V. Martins, A. Massey, T. Matthews, E. McDonald, C. J. Northfield, L. H. Pearl, C. Prodromou, S. Ray, F. I. Raynaud, S. D. Roughley, S. Y. Sharp, A. Surgenor, D. L. Walmsley, P. Webb, M. Wood, P. Workman and L. Wright, *J. Med. Chem.*, 2008, **51**, 196218.
10. T. McHardy, J. J. Caldwell, K.-M. Cheung, L. J. Hunter, K. Taylor, M. Rowlands, R. Ruddle, A. Henley, A. de Haven Brandon, M. Valenti, T. G. Davies, L. Fazal, L. Seavers, F. I. Raynaud, S. A. Eccles, G. W. Aherne, M. D. Garrett and I. Collins, *J. Med. Chem.*, 2010, **53**, 2239.
11. P. Chen, C. Luo, Y. Deng, K. Ryan, J. Register, S. Margosiak, A. Tempczyk-Russell, B. Nguyen, P. Myers, K. Lundgren, C.-C. Kan and P. M. O'Connor, *Cell*, 2000, **100**, 681.
12. T. P. Matthews, A. M. Jones and I. Collins, *Expert Opin. Drug Discovery*, 2013, **8**, 621.
13. N. Foloppe, L. M. Fisher, R. Howes, A. Potter, A. G. S. Robertson and A. E. Surgenor, *Bioorg. Med. Chem.*, 2006, **14**, 4792.
14. T. P. Matthews, S. Klair, S. Burns, K. Boxall, G. W. Aherne, M. Cherry, M. Fisher, I. M. Westwood, M. Walton, T. McHardy, D. Williams, R. van Montfort, M. D. Garrett, J. Reader and I. Collins, *J. Med. Chem.*, 2009, **52**, 4810.
15. G. J. Addison, M. Cherry, I. Collins, S. S. Klair and J. C. Reader, *Int. Pat. Appl.*, WO2010007389, 2010.

16. T. P. Matthews, T. McHardy, S. Klair, J. Reader, K. Boxall, M. Fisher, M. Cherry, M. Garrett, C. E. Allen, G. W. Aherne, I. M. Westwood, R. van Montfort and I. Collins, *Bioorg. Med. Chem. Lett.*, 2010, **20**, 4045.
17. T. P. Matthews, S. Klair, S. Burns, K. Boxall, G. W. Aherne, M. Cherry, M. Fisher, I. M. Westwood, M. Walton, T. McHardy, D. Williams, R. van Montfort, M. D. Garrett, J. Reader and I. Collins, *J. Med. Chem.*, 2009, **52**, 4810.
18. J. C. Reader, T. P. Matthews, S. Klair, K.-M. J. Cheung, J. Scanlon, N. Proisy, G. Addison, J. Ellard, N. Piton, S. Taylor, M. Cherry, M. Fischer, K. Boxall, S. Burns, M. I. Walton, I. M. Westwood, A. Hayes, P. Eve, M. Valenti, A. De Haven Brandon, G. Box, R. van Montfort, D. H. Williams, G. W. Aherne, F. I. Raynaud, S. Eccles, M. D. Garrett and I. Collins, *J. Med. Chem.*, 2011, **54**, 8328.
19. C. E. Allen, A. J. Welford, T. P. Matthews, J. J. Caldwell and I. Collins, *Med. Chem. Commun.*, 2014, **5**, 180.
20. M. I. Walton, P. D. Eve, A. Hayes, M. Valenti, A. De Haven Brandon, K. J. Boxall, G. W. Aherne, S. A. Eccles, F. I. Raynaud, D. Williams, J. Reader, I. Collins and M. D. Garrett, *Mol. Cancer Ther.*, 2010, **9**, 89.
21. M. Lainchbury, T. P. Matthews, J. Osborne, T. F. McHardy, K. Boxall, M. I. Walton, A. Hayes, P. Eve, M. Valenti, A. De Haven Brandon, G. Box, G. W. Aherne, J. C. Reader, F. I. Raynaud, S. Eccles, M. D. Garrett and I. Collins, *J. Med. Chem.*, 2012, **55**, 10229.
22. M. I. Walton, P. D. Eve, A. Hayes, M. R. Valenti, A. K. De Haven Brandon, G. Box, A. Hallsworth, E. L Smith, K. J. Boxall, M. Lainchbury, T. P. Matthews, Y. Jamin, S. P. Robinson, G. W. Aherne, J. C. Reader, L. Chesler, F. I. Raynaud, S. A. Eccles, I. Collins and M. D. Garrett, *Clin. Cancer Res.*, 2012, **18**, 5650.
23. Y. Xiao, J. Ramiscal, K. Kowanetz, C. Del Nagro, S. Malek, M. Evangelista, E. Blackwood, P. K. Jackson and T. O'Brien, *Mol. Cancer Ther.*, 2013, **12**, 2285.
24. J. J. Caldwell, E. Welsh, B. Matijssen, V. E. Anderson, L. Antoni, P. Eve, K. Boxall, S. Burns, F. Urban, A. Hayes, F. I. Raynaud, G. W. Aherne, L. H. Pearl, A. W. Oliver, M. D. Garrett and I. Collins, *J. Med. Chem.*, 2011, **54**, 580.
25. V. E. Anderson, M. I. Walton, P. D. Eve, J. J. Caldwell, L. H. Pearl, A. W. Oliver, I. Collins and M. D. Garrett, *Cancer Res.*, 2011, **71**, 463.
26. E. Blackwood, J. Epler, I. Yen, M. Flagella, T. O'Brien, M. Evangelista, S. Schmidt, Y. Xiao, J. Choi, K. Kowanetz, J. Ramiscal, K. Wong, D. Jakubiak, S. Yee, G. Cain, L. Gazzard, K. Williams, J. Halladay, P. K. Jackson and S. Malek, *Mol. Cancer Ther.*, 2013, **12**, 1968.
27. J. D. Osborne, T. P. Matthews, T. McHardy, N. Proisy, K. J. Cheung, M. Lainchbury, N. Brown, M. I. Walton, P. D. Eve, K. J. Boxall, A. Hayes, A. T. Henley, M. R. Valenti, A. K. De Haven Brandon, G. Box, Y. Jamin, S. P. Robinson, I. M. Westwood, R. van Montfort, P. M. Leonard, M. B. A. C. Lamers, J. C. Reader, G. W. Aherne, F. I. Raynaud, S. A. Eccles, M. D. Garrett and I. Collins, *J. Med. Chem.*, 2016, **59**, 5221.
28. M. I. Walton, P. D. Eve, A. Hayes, A. T. Henley, M. R. Valenti, A. K. De Haven Brandon, G. Box, K. J. Boxall, M. Tall, K. Swales, T. P. Matthews, T. McHardy, M. Lainchbury, J. Osborne, J. E. Hunter, N. D. Perkins, G. W. Aherne, J. C. Reader, F. I. Raynaud, S. A. Eccles, I. Collins and M. D. Garrett, *OncoTarget*, 2016, 7, 2329.
29. S. Sinha, D. Ahire, S. Wagh, D. Mullick, R. Sistla, K. Selvakumar, J. C. Cortes, S. P. Putlur, S. Mandlekar and B. M. Johnson, *Chem. Res. Toxicol.*, 2014, **27**, 2052.
30. E. Sausville, P. LoRusso, M. Carducci, J. Carter, M. F. Quinn, L. Malburg, N. Azad, D. Cosgrove, R. Knight, P. Barker, S. Zabludoff, F. Agbo, P. Oakes and A. Senderowicz, *Cancer Chemother. Pharmacol.*, 2014, **73**, 539.
31. T. Seto, T. Esaki, F. Hirai, S. Arita, K. Nosaki, A. Makiyama, T. Kometani, C. Fujimoto, M. Hamatake, H. Takeoka, F. Agbo and X. Shi, *Cancer Chemother. Pharmacol.*, 2013, **72**, 619.
32. A. I. Daud, M. T. Ashworth, J. Strosberg, J. W. Goldman, D. Mendelson, G. Springett, A. P. Venook, S. Loechner, L. S. Rosen, F. Shanahan, D. Parry, S. Shumway, J. A. Grabowsky, T. Freshwater, C. Sorge, S. P. Kang, R. Isaacs and P. N. Munster, *J. Clin. Oncol.*, 2015, **33**, 1060.
33. D. Hong, J. Infante, F. Janku, S. Jones, L. M. Nguyen, H. Burris, A. Naing, T. M. Bauer, S. Piha-Paul, F. M Johnson, R. Kurzrock, L. Golden, S. Hynes, J. Lin, A. Bence Lin and J. Bendell, *J. Clin. Oncol.*, 2016, **34**, 1764.
34. D. J. Leishman, M. M. Abernathy and E. B. Wang, *J. Pharmacol. Toxicol. Methods*, 2020, **105**, 106900.
35. W. Yang, J. Soares, P. Greninger, E. J. Edelman, H. Lightfoot, S. Forbes, N. Bindal, D. Beare, J. A. Smith, I. R. Thompson, S. Ramaswamy, P. A. Futreal, D. A. Haber, M. R. Stratton, C. Benes, U. McDermott and M. J. Garnett, *Nucleic Acids Res.*, 2013, **41**, D955.
36. C. H. Wong, K. W. Siah and A. W. Lo, *Biostatistics*, 2019, **20**, 273.
37. S. W. Hoelder, P. A. Clarke and P. Workman, *Mol. Oncol.*, 2012, **6**, 155.
38. https://www.sixthelementcapital.com/index.php/chk1, accessed 03 January 2020.
39. https://www.cancerresearchuk.org/funding-for-researchers/our-research-infrastructure/our-centre-for-drug-development, accesses 03 January 2020.

40. M. Zangarini, P. Berry, J. Sludden, F. I. Raynaud, U. Banerji, P. Jones, D. Edwards and G. J. Veal, *Bioanalysis*, 2017, **9**, 1001.
41. E. R. Plummer, R. S. Kristeleit, E. Cojocaru, N. M. Haris, L. Carter, R. H. Jones, S. P. Blagden, T. R. J. Evans, H. Arkenau, D. Sarker, S. Danson, S. N. Symeonides, H. Walter, J. Ocen, M. Randhawa, M. M. Kowalski, I. Verdon, A. Dye and U. Banerji, *J. Clin. Oncol.*, 2019, **37**(Suppl. 15), 3094. Abstract of poster presented at the 2019 ASCO annual Meeting I.
42. U. Banerji, E. R. Plummer, V. Moreno, J. E. Ang, A. Quinton, Y. Drew, T. Hernández, D. Roda, L. Carter, A. Navarro, R. S. Kristeleit, H. Arkenau, D. Sarker, D. E. Castellano, H. Walter, P. Roxburgh, S. P. Blagden, A. Anthoney, I. Verdon and R. H. Jones, *J. Clin. Oncol.*, 2019, **37**(Suppl. 15), 3095. Abstract of poster presented at the 2019 ASCO annual Meeting I.
43. R. G. Borst, M. McLaughlin, J. N. Kyula, S. Neijenhuis, A. Khan, J. Good, S. Zaidi, N. G. Powell, P. Meier, I. Collins, M. D. Garrett, M. Verheij and K. J. Harrington, *Int. J. Radiat. Oncol., Biol., Phys.*, 2013, **85**, 1110.
44. H. E. Barker, R. Patel, M. McLaughlin, U. Schick, S. Zaidi, C. M. Nutting, K. L. Newbold, S. Bhide and K. J. Harrington, *Mol. Cancer Ther.*, 2016, **15**, 2042.
45. Y. Touchefeu, A. A. Khan, G. Borst, S. H. Zaidi, M. McLaughlin, V. Roulstone, D. Mansfield, J. Kyula, T. Pencavel, E. M. Karapanagiotou, J. Clayton, M. J. Federspiel, S. J. Russell, M. Garrett, I. Collins and K. J. Harrington, *Radiother. Oncol.*, 2013, **108**, 24.
46. R. Patel, H. E. Barker, J. Kyula, M. McLaughlin, M. T. Dillon, U. Schick, H. Hafsi, A. Thompson, V. Khoo, K. Harrington and S. Zaidi, *Radiother. Oncol.*, 2017, **122**, 470.
47. R. F. Rogers, M. I. Walton, D. L. Cherry, I. Collins, P. A. Clarke, M. D. Garrett and P. Workman, *Cancer Res.*, 2020, **80**, 1735.
48. L. Booth, J. Roberts, A. Poklepovic and P. Dent, *Cancer Biol. Ther.*, 2018, **19**, 786.
49. T. Sen, C. M. Della Corte, S. Milutinovic, R. J. Cardnell, L. Diao, K. Ramkumar, C. M. Gay, C. A. Stewart, Y. Fan, L. Shen, R. J. Hansen, B. Strouse, M. P. Hedrick, C. A. Hassig, J. V. Heymach, J. Wang and L. A. Byers, *J. Thorac. Oncol.*, 2019, **14**, 2152.

# 26 Medicinal Chemistry for Neglected Diseases – Malaria, Tuberculosis, Sleeping Sickness, Leishmaniasis and River Blindness

Jeremy N. Burrows*[a], Christopher B. Cooper[b], Charles Mowbray[c] and Peter Sjö[c]

[a]Medicines for Malaria Venture, Geneva, Switzerland; [b]TB Alliance, New York, NY, USA; [c]Drugs for Neglected Diseases Initiative, Geneva, Switzerland
*E-mail: burrowsj@mmv.org

## 26.1 Introduction: Neglected Tropical Diseases and Diseases of Poverty

Neglected tropical diseases (NTDs) are a defined set of tropical infections affecting predominantly low-income populations in developing regions of the world.[1] They comprise diseases caused by viruses, bacteria, protozoa and parasitic worms (and, recently, snake envenoming was included). Malaria, although a tropical disease, and tuberculosis, affecting large proportions of the world's poor are contrasted with NTDs by virtue of the relative investments in procurement of treatments and research and development (R&D) funding. However, all these diseases share common challenges. First, due to a lack of commercial markets, given the low-income populations commonly afflicted, there is an unacceptably low level of discovery and development innovation and, consequently a dearth of affordable, effective and tolerated medicines for diseases affecting around a quarter of the world's population.[2] Second, given the inability to recoup R&D costs through sales, there is a reluctance from Pharma to engage from the start in discovery and translational activities in what will ultimately be loss-making markets, unless there are risk- and cost-sharing mechanisms. However, there are notable cases of drug donations from Pharma having major impact in the field, for example Merck & Co, Merck

The Handbook of Medicinal Chemistry: Principles and Practice, 2nd Edition
Edited by Simon E. Ward and Andrew M. Davis

Published by the Royal Society of Chemistry, www.rsc.org

KGaA, GSK and Eisai with activities in the development and distribution of ivermectin, praziquantel, albendazole and diethylcarbamazine, to name just a few. Third, on top of a dearth of products and a historical lack of incentives to engage Pharma, there is an inevitable risk of pathogen resistance in areas of infectious disease – providing a scientific challenge in the spectrum of new agents. Fourth, the requirement to deliver low-cost medicines that are simple to administer and often require paediatric formulations places constraints on the complexity of the chemistry, pharmacokinetics, safety, process chemistry and formulation beyond those typically considered in First World disease drug discovery. On the other hand – to some extent adding injury to insult – there is the observation that late-stage, expensive drug discovery failures in infectious diseases are significantly less frequent than in other therapeutic areas.[3] The reasons for this are probably that medicines against pathogens are not designed against human targets (with unpredictable side effects), that there are excellent animal and sometimes human experimental models and that clinical trials have non-ambiguous endpoints, typically measuring pathogen clearance.

Product Development Partnerships (PDPs) such as the Medicines for Malaria Venture (MMV), the Global Alliance for TB Drug Development (GATB) and the Drugs for Neglected Diseases *initiative* (DND*i*) have been founded over the last 20 years to address this market failure. These PDPs are donor-funded organisations seeking to deliver the medicines of their respective disease foci, through global collaboration. The science of drug discovery, however, despite the resource constraints, remains unchanged from that applied to other commercial therapeutic areas. Consequently, MMV, GATB and DND*i* work with partners globally, applying state of the art medicinal chemistry and industrial processes to diseases that affect over 250 million symptomatic and life-threatening cases each year.

This chapter focuses specifically on two of the most prevalent infectious diseases – malaria and tuberculosis – as well as three NTDs which, although impacting fewer patients, cause significant mortality and morbidity, and are incompletely served by existing therapies: sleeping sickness (trypanosomiasis), leishmaniasis and river blindness (onchocerciasis).

Following a description of the disease, the pathogen, the landscape of medicines and the strategies adopted with new discovery research, insights on the drug discovery and medicinal chemistry will be shared, along with at least one case study.

## 26.2 Malaria

### 26.2.1 Disease Overview

Malaria is a parasitic infectious disease caused by the unicellular eukaryotic apicomplexan parasite *Plasmodium*.[4] Whilst there are legion *Plasmodia* infecting numerous vertebrate and insect species, there are six species that are known to infect humans: *P. falciparum*, *P. vivax*, *P. ovale* (actually two sub-species, *P. ovale curtisi* and *P. ovale wallikeri*), *P. malariae*, *P. knowlesi* and *P. cynomolgi*, though infections with the latter are extremely rare. *P. falciparum* is the most lethal among these and is responsible for the vast majority of cases and deaths in Africa, while *P. vivax* is responsible for over 65% of the malaria cases in South America and Asia. In 2019 there were an estimated 229 million cases of malaria and 409 000 deaths, of which approximately 67% were children under the age of 5 years;[5] furthermore, isolated studies suggest the number of asymptomatic but infected individuals is an iceberg compared to these visible "tip" statistics.[6,7] The burden of malaria can be further characterised using the concept of disability-adjusted life years (DALYs), a composite measure that captures premature mortality, prevalence and severity. In 2017 the age-adjusted DALYs for malaria were estimated at a staggering 45 million, but, encouragingly, this had reduced by 34% relative to 2007.[8] The Sustainable Development Goals of the United Nations has called for efforts to end global epidemics, such as malaria.[9] As such the WHO Global Technical Strategy for Malaria has called for a 90% reduction in cases and mortality by 2030 and for ambitious targets for eradication of the key malaria parasites.[10] The good news is that globally, more countries are moving towards zero indigenous cases, and that and the number of countries with fewer than 100 indigenous cases – a strong indicator that elimination is within reach – increased from 17 countries in 2010, to 27 countries in 2019.[5] However, with five countries accounting for over 50% of all worldwide malaria cases (Nigeria 27%, DRC 12%, Uganda 5%, Mozambique 4% and Niger 3%) the challenge of eradication remains evident.

### 26.2.2 *Plasmodium* Lifecycle

Malaria is caused through the transmission of *Plasmodium* parasites from an infected female *Anopheles* mosquito to a human during a blood meal. As shown in Figure 26.1, in the process of feeding, the infected mosquito injects approximately 100 *Plasmodium* sporozoites into the skin, which then burrow in a circular motion to a blood vessel and are carried to the liver, where they invade hepatocytes. Asymptomatic asexual replication is then initiated, which results in a phenomenal clonal expansion: in under six days (in the case of *P. falciparum*) a single sporozoite that has made a successful invasion into a hepatocyte can have multiplied asexually to up to 40 000 new parasites (called merozoites). The merozoites then egress from the hepatocyte, which is lysed, and enter the bloodstream (mmv.org).

In the case of vivax malaria, a small population of liver parasites differentiate into dormant forms called hypnozoites which remain dormant and do not partake in the first round of infection. These hypnozoites can relapse to form liver schizonts and progress to blood-stage infection, even in the absence of a new mosquito bite. This strategy allows *P. vivax* parasites to "wait out" dry or cold winter seasons for many weeks or months, when few biting mosquitoes are around to spread the disease. While *P. falciparum* does not form hypnozoites, recent evidence suggests these parasites can also cause persistent, asymptomatic infections that allow them to "wait" for the end of the dry season in Sahel countries.[11]

Within 30 seconds, a fraction of the merozoites that have just egressed the liver successfully infect erythrocytes, initiating a new asexual process. Whilst the liver-stage infection is asymptomatic and linear (*i.e.* merozoites do not invade new hepatocytes), the blood-stage infection is cyclic and causes disease. In the case of *P. falciparum,* after approximately 48 h, a single merozoite that infects an erythrocyte produces approximately 20–32 new merozoites, at which point the erythrocyte lyses and the new merozoites are able to invade new red cells. During this process, an invading merozoite is

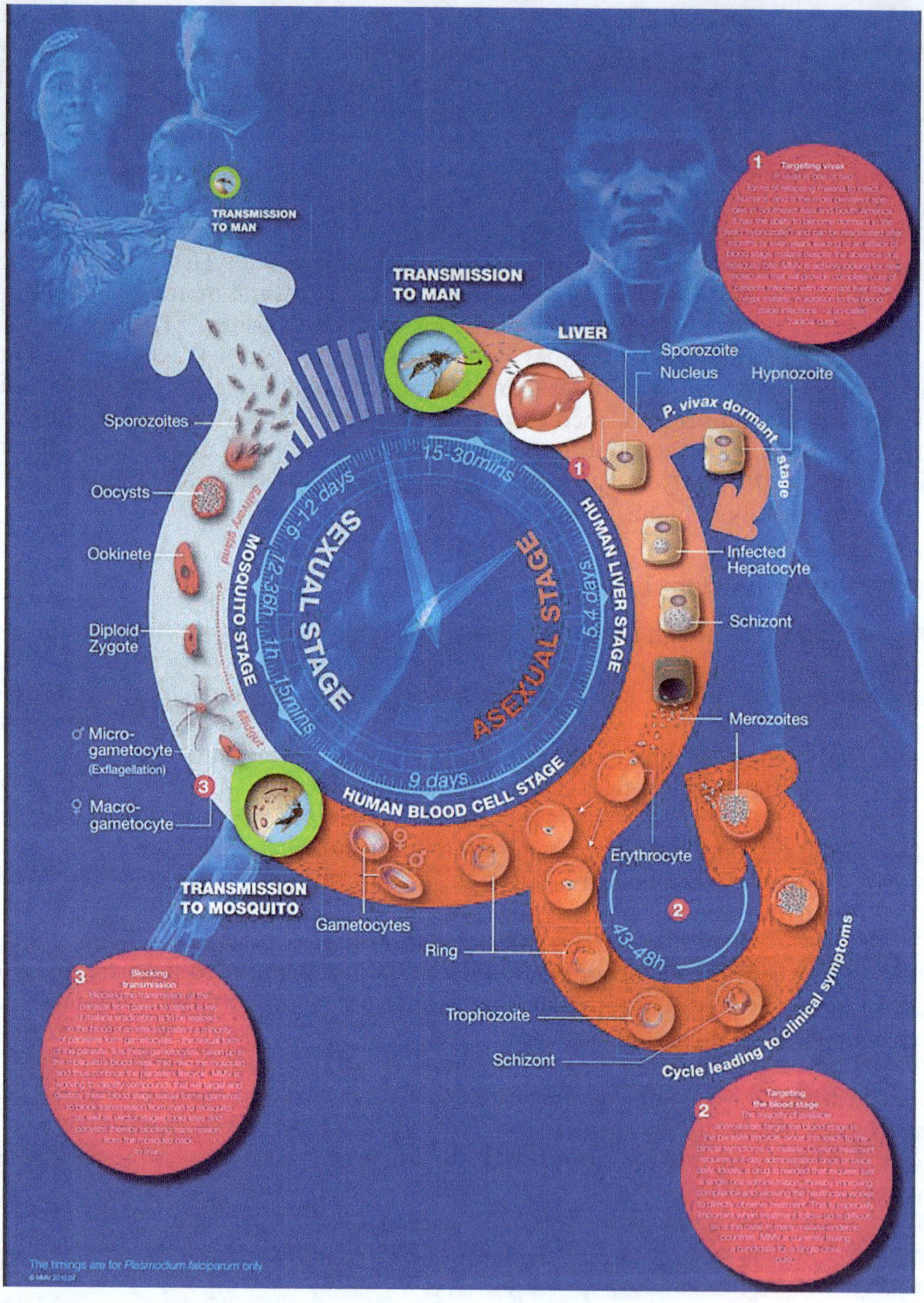


**Figure 26.1** The lifecycle of *Plasmodium*. Image Credit: © mmv.org.

transformed through several intra-erythrocytic stages (called rings at 0–24 h, trophozoites at 24–36 h and schizonts at 36–48 h, approximately) with the schizonts essentially being a biological casing for the multiple new merozoites. Not every blood cell invasion is successful, but every two days, blood parasitaemia increases approximately 10-fold, with a synchronous relentlessness. Spikes of fever in patients coincide with merozoite egress and the body's cytokine response to the transiently vulnerable parasite population. A major cause of fever is the release of "hemozoin",[12] a crystallised, toxic remnant of haemoglobin that the parasite is unable to digest. A seriously ill patient could have as many as $10^{12}$ parasites in their blood (10% parasitaemia *vs.* blood cells) and malaria is recognised as being either *severe* (such that parasitaemia is so high that there is organ failure, where the child is in a coma and cannot swallow oral chemotherapy – thus necessitating parenteral treatment), *uncomplicated* (symptomatic malaria with the patient conscious and able to take oral therapy) or *asymptomatic* (when parasites are only evident by virtue of a specific measurement despite absence of symptoms). Since the asexual blood-stage parasitaemia leads to symptoms, malaria treatments focus on rapid killing and clearance of these parasites in the blood to cure patients. A small proportion, approximately 1% of newly invading merozoites, transition towards a further parasitic form: gametocytes, which are the male and female sexual stages of the parasite able to transmit to the *Anopheles* mosquito. Thus, ring stages that are committed to gametocyte development differentiate over a period of 10–12 days through five stages in which the final and most relevant are the stage V gametocytes. Gametocytes are approximately 20–25% male; early stages sequester to the bone marrow, whereas stage V gametocytes, that are, unlike infected red blood cells able to evade splenic clearance, return to the circulation in the blood, ready to be taken up in a blood meal. Gametocytaemia is asymptomatic, and mature stage V gametocytes can circulate for prolonged periods of time before being cleared (certainly at least 20 days, with examples of microscopic circulation much longer than this[13]). Whilst not metabolically inert, they have very different biology to proliferating forms and subsequently have fewer of the vulnerabilities targeted by existing anti-malarials, making them harder to kill than asexual stages. Thus, an uninfected mosquito taking a blood meal sucks up male and female stage V gametocytes into its midgut. These parasites detect a lower temperature and a pH change, and the presence of xanthurenic acid. They promptly form mature gametes through exflagellation (males) and rounding up (females) leading to sexual reproduction. The diploid zygote differentiates into an ookinete and then an oocyst (similar to a schizont above), which is full of sporozoites, which then migrate to the insect's salivary gland; the duration for the whole mosquito parasite stage takes up to 14 days in the tropics, close to the insect's average life span, but this can be shortened with multiple blood meals.[14] At this point, the transmission cycle can begin again.

The massive mortality caused by *P. falciparum* in very young patients runs counter to the biological dogma that says that, over evolutionary time, parasitic diseases become milder (non-deadly). Malaria parasites employ a series of incompletely understood immune evasion mechanisms, including the serial use of dozens of genes that encode for membrane proteins.[15] Through repeated disease episodes in malaria-endemic countries, many Africans in disease-endemic countries build up a degree of immunity against malaria that reduces the disease to a debilitating, but usually non-deadly condition.[16,17] Pregnant women transmit protective antibodies to their unborn child, and continue to do so during lactation. However, over time this antibody reserve wanes off, putting the very young at extreme risk of death from their first episodes of malaria, until, after a few years, and if they survive, they have built up sufficient immunity to avert death. In this scenario, the parasite dogma only holds for the *adult* generation.

### 26.2.3 Current Landscape and Strategic Focus

The mainstay treatments for uncomplicated falciparum malaria are the artemisinin combination therapies (ACTs); the medicinal chemistry origins of the individual components of ACTs are in two natural products: artemisinin and quinine. Semi-synthetic approaches have delivered more potent and soluble artemisinin derivatives such as dihydroartemisinin and artesunate. Quinine was the inspiration for early 20th C anti-malarial drug discovery ultimately leading, through the century, to chloroquine, piperaquine, amodiaquine, mefloquine, lumefantrine and pyronaridine.[18] ACTs are formulated as fixed-dose combinations that are given to patients over three days. Having a fixed dose in a single formulation promotes compliance (there is no option to take only one drug over the other) and combinations, as stipulated by the WHO, are necessary to reduce the risk of parasite resistance. Indeed, the ACTs artemether-lumefantrine and artesunate-pyronaridine remain efficacious in all regions, even given the emergence and spread in SE Asia and, now, Africa, of partial resistance to the artemisinins and partner drug resistance, in different regions, for chloroquine, piperaquine, amodiaquine and mefloquine. The therapies for severe malaria, as mentioned above, consist of injections of artesunate, artemether or, historically, quinine.[19,20] Rectal suppositories of artesunate have also been delivered as products for children unable to receive i.v. treatment quickly and, thus, are pre-referral life savers prior to receiving formal treatment.[21] Treatment for vivax malaria consists of chloroquine in regions of chloroquine sensitivity, and ACTs in case of chloroquine resistance. To additionally kill hypnozoites and prevent relapses, either primaquine or tafenoquine are given, the latter being preferred due to its single-dose characteristics.[22,23] However, these last two drugs may cause haemolytic anaemia in patients with low G6PD (glucose-6-phosphate dehydrogenase) enzyme activity; administration requires a point-of-care test to ensure safety.[24] There are fewer drugs for malaria prophylaxis. Atovaquone-proguanil remains an effective daily option, with doxycycline and mefloquine as other options; however, the latter has a black-box safety warning on its label due to potential psychiatric side effects. Atovaquone-progaunil is a causal prophylactic (killing liver stage parasites) though is daily, whereas mefloquine is a chemoprohylactic (killing only blood stages) though is weekly.

New anti-malarials must address the existing and future epidemiological landscape as well as the shortcomings and experience with existing interventions. Target Product Profiles (TPP) for combination products, and Target Candidate Profiles (TCP) for individual compounds have been defined to provide criteria and a discovery-development path for such new medicines.[25,26] Their focus is first and foremost on overcoming present and future parasite resistance to drugs, their second is on simpler, cheaper and better tolerated presentations to ensure compliance and third, on delivering a battery of anti-parasitic activities able to not only eliminate symptoms but break the transmission cycle and ultimately contribute to the elimination of the parasite.

Figure 26.2 shows TPP1 – the treatment profile – having relevance in a range of use cases depending on its exact composition, from treatment of uncomplicated or severe malaria to chemoprevention and anti-relapse. TPP2 – the prophylaxis profile – is focused on protecting the vulnerable in areas of endemicity or after potential outbreaks and thus securing the gains in control, leading towards elimination–eradication. The criteria for these TPPs are documented and need to be met based on clinical studies to deliver an effective and community-relevant product. The TCPs that can contribute to these TPPs are also listed and, pragmatically, are linked to a life-cycle stage of the parasite. Thus, TCP1 compounds that kill asexual blood stages are an intrinsic and necessary component of a treatment regimen (TPP1). The criteria for TCP1 both as monotherapy in an early clinical study, and as a candidate drug or even early lead are also defined to aid the Drug Discovery process.

Figure 26.3 shows the portfolio of MMV as of mid-2020. Two decades of investment in discovery, development and delivery of anti-malarials in partnership with Pharma and Academia has resulted in 11 products, and a robust portfolio of medicines in all phases. The symbols indicate the TCP potential of each compound in the portfolio,

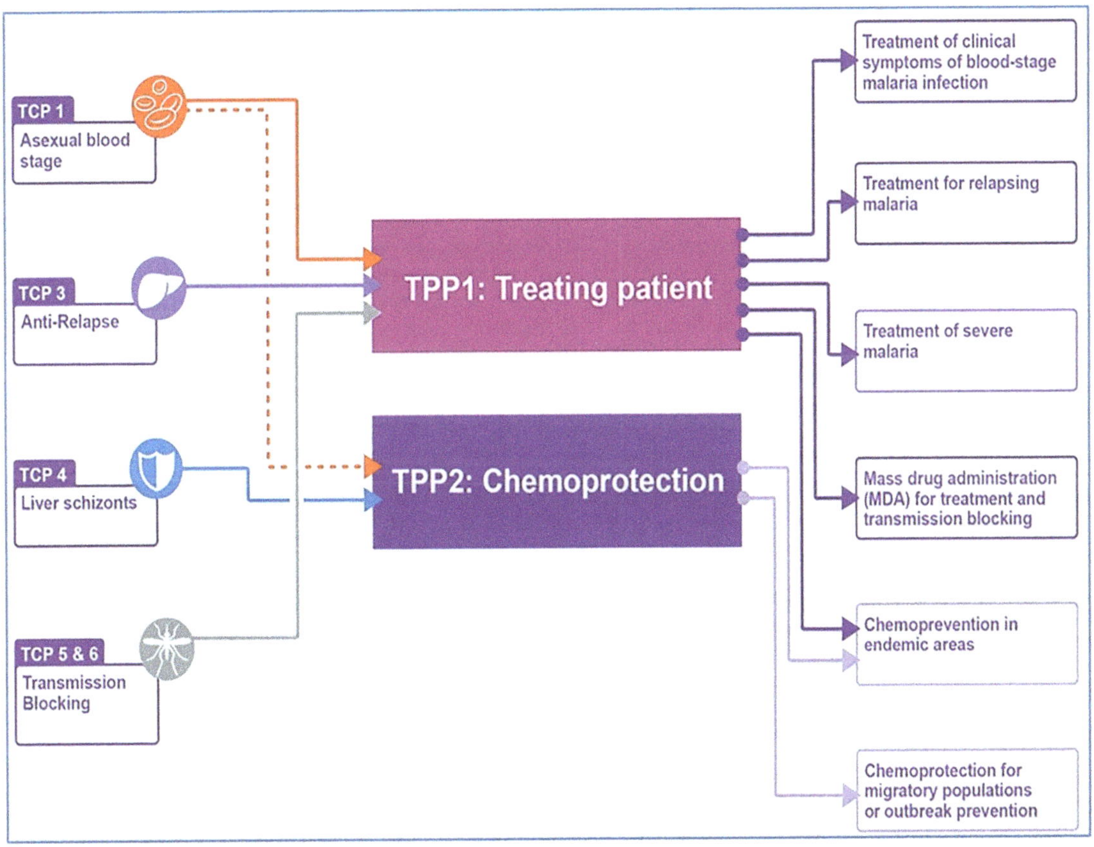


**Figure 26.2** Inter-relationships between the two high-level target product profiles (centre) with the individual target candidate profiles (left) for molecules. Reproduced from ref. 25, https://doi.org/10.1186/s12936-016-1675-x, under the terms of the CC BY 4.0 license, https://creativecommons.org/licenses/by/4.0/.

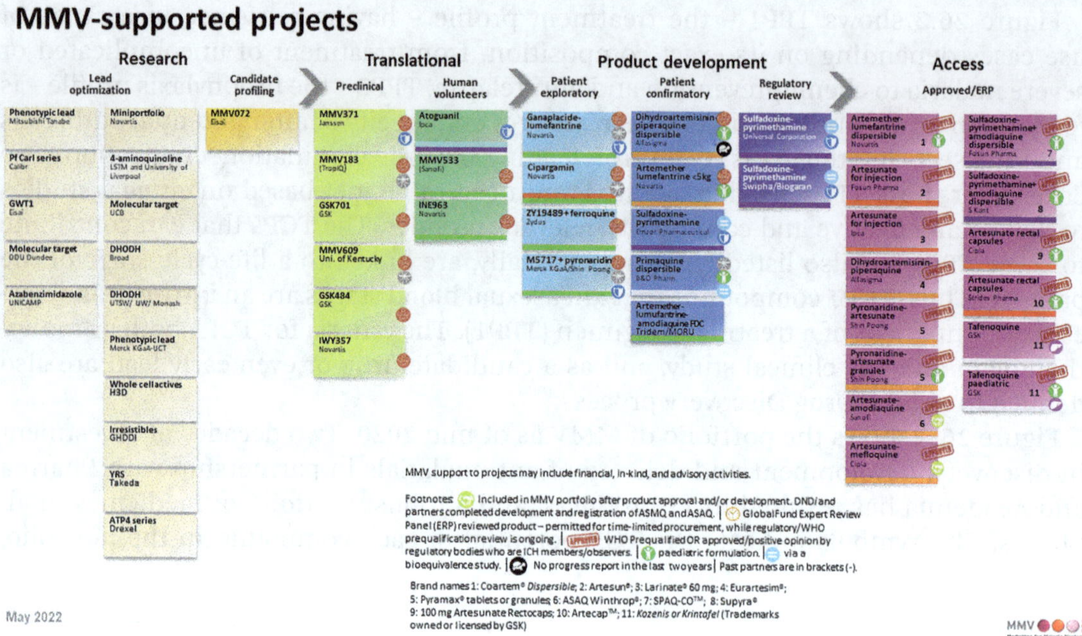


**Figure 26.3** Medicines for Malaria Venture-supported projects as of May 2022. MMV support to projects may include financial, in-kind and advisory activities. MMV has defined Target Product Profiles and Target Candidate Profiles for medicines to support the eradication campaign.[25,26] Colour coding of Target Product Profiles: yellow is 3-day cure, artemisinin-based combination therapies (TPP-1), green is uncomplicated malaria treatments for single exposure radical cure (SERC) and/or resistance management (TPP-1), red is severe malaria treatment/pre-referral intervention (TPP-1), pink is intermittent preventive treatment (TPP-1), white is products targeting prevention of relapse for *P. vivax* (TPP-1), and blue is prophylaxis (TPP-2). Brand names 1: Coartem® Dispersible; 2: Artesun®; 3: Larinate® 60 mg; 4: Eurartesim®; 5: Pyramax® tablets or granules; 6: ASAQ Winthrop®; 7: SPAQ-COTM; 8: Supyra® 9: 100 mg Artesunate Rectocaps; 10: Artecap™; 11: Kozenis or Krintafel (Trademarks owned or licensed by GSK). Image Credit: © mmv.org.

and it is clear that there remain significant gaps and challenges, despite the significant progress. Today's priorities include delivering new medicines against several TCPs:

- TCP3 – new anti-relapse medicines (beyond the 8-aminoquinolines with a G6PD risk)
- TCP1 – low single-dose treatments with a low propensity to select resistance
- TCP5 – drugs with effective gametocytocidal action able to block transmission
- TCP4 – drugs for chemoprophylaxis, particularly with long pharmacological durations of cover.

Over the last 15 years, 31 new candidate drugs have been delivered by the global community, with 25 of those coming from MMV discovery activities. As of mid-2020, 15 candidates remain in active development, with one product (Synriam™, or arterolane–piperaquine), and several in Phase IIa and IIb (with KAF156-lumefantrine as the furthest-progressed combination[27]). Attrition is inevitable, particularly given the constraints of the TPPs on safety, cost, dose size, efficacy and resistance. As such, a healthy and robust discovery portfolio is required to continually fuel the pipeline for the future.

### 26.2.4 Antimalarial Medicinal Chemistry – Key Learnings

In order to progress molecules for anti-malarial drug discovery it is, first, critical to have an appropriate testing cascade; the following is focused mainly on treatment for falciparum malaria. Key features for malaria include a growth inhibition assay able to cope with high test compound numbers and giving good sensitivity and reproducibility.[28] $^3$H-hypoxanthine assays are the gold standard, with LDH (lactate dehydrogenase) activity as a cheaper, second-best assay option with a 72 h endpoint selected, to capture all essential biology. Testing needs to be performed on both sensitive and drug-resistant *P. falciparum* strains, and should include cellular cytotoxicity (on mammalian cells). If the biological target is known, which is increasingly becoming the case, then initial primary biochemical parasite and mammalian orthologue selectivity assays are also relevant in advance of such phenotypic data. Understanding the potential of a compound series from a TCP perspective is then key. To this end, testing in a parasite reduction rate (PRR) assay gives information on the rate of parasite killing and, in a selection experiment, gives information regarding the ease with which resistance develops (important for TCP1); testing on asexual and hypnozoite liver stages gives an indication of a medicine's potential for causal prophylaxis (TCP4) and anti-relapse (TCP3); testing on early and, particularly, mature-stage V gametocytes gives an indication of the potential to block transmission (TCP5). For TCP1, *in vivo* testing involves the engraftment of human erythrocytes, subsequently infected with falciparum malaria, into NSG (immunodeficient NOD SCID Gamma) mice prior to dosing of a compound; this is because *P. falciparum* does not infect mice (although there is a murine species, *P. berghei*). Naturally, the test cascade is tuned to the project goals. In the case of treatment focus, such lifecycle fingerprinting data is routinely performed on improved frontrunners, but is not used for the purpose of optimisation.

If a compound has a specific mode of action, then its rate of kill, lifecycle fingerprint, cross-resistance and frequency of resistance are likely to remain constant across a chemical series. From a medicinal chemistry perspective, it is important to note the presence of Albumax or other protein in assays and thus the potential need to correct for plasma protein binding, to understand the free potency for SAR (structure–activity relationship) purposes. This is important, since all translational work currently suggests that it is the free drug concentrations that drive efficacy, both *in vitro* and *in vivo* – whether in a mouse model or human infection. The major medicinal chemistry drivers are phenotypic potency and predicted human (plasma) half-life, given that a single dose is required to deliver effective exposure for, typically, at least six days in humans. Given the half-life constraints, there is a typical need to drive down drug clearance and to increase its volume of distribution. Consequently, chemical modifications that intrinsically lead to low distribution volumes (such as carboxylic acids) are avoided, and medicinal chemistry teams focus on lowering intrinsic clearances ($Cl_{int}$), an emphasis on low-clearance neutrals and bases, and reasonable lipophilicity to avoid transporters.

All this contributes to an increased volume of distribution (whilst avoiding the usual off-target suspects) using early predictions of human PK (pharmacokinetics) and dose. To that end, MMV has delivered a free online tool to support early quantitative pharmacological predictions that separate into human PK simulations and then the application of translational pharmacodynamic learnings to predict the dose in humans (mmv.org). This tool was designed to help a team focus on the necessary key parameters during Lead Optimisation; however, a detailed work-up of all predicted parameters is independently performed once a potential candidate is identified. Interestingly, whilst permeability is critical for oral absorption, it appears to not be an issue regarding blood-stage potency; in certain cases, an anti-malarial needs to cross as many as four membranes to reach its site of action, yet compounds with low passive permeability (including those with permanent positive charges) appear as hits in screening sets. This permeability is likely due to new permeability pathways in the parasite and other transporters, given the parasites' voracious appetite for certain host nutrients.

Finally, given the targeted patient population for anti-malarials, their safety, low cost and ease of administration are critical. Thus, the complexity of the compound and its chemistry, the solubility and CMC (Chemistry, Manufacturing and Controls) properties that influence the formulation, the dose size, and the safety pharmacology and toxicology (to begin with), and then its reproductive toxicology, become critical. Physical properties, off-target pharmacology, chemical complexity and dose size can all be tackled through responsible medicinal chemistry; however, clinical safety is not always predictable.

## 26.2.5 Portfolio – Case Studies

To illustrate the challenges and, importantly, to communicate lessons from the past, one case study is presented, out of the 25 candidates that MMV has delivered. This example, DSM265, a *Pf* DHODH (dihydroorotate dehydrogenase) inhibitor reached Phase IIa before being terminated.[29–32] Given the extent to which the data on this compound have been reported in the literature,[29–35] a condensed summary of the discovery and development alongside the ten key learnings is the focus of this section.

### 26.2.5.1 DSM265 – Pf DHODH Inhibitor

The malaria parasite is dependent on the *de novo* synthesis of pyrimidines for nucleotide biosynthesis. *Plasmodium falciparum* dihydroorotate dehydrogenase, *Pf* DHODH, is a critical enzyme on this pathway, powered by the electron transport chain within the mitochondria. Phillips *et al.* conducted a high-throughput screen against *Pf* DHODH and identified a triazolopyrimidine hit series with high potency (DSM1;[36]). In time the protein X-ray crystal structure of *Pf* DHODH was solved with members of this series, giving insights on chemical design. The medicinal chemistry challenges focused on: (i) altering the chemistry to remove the mutagenic β-naphthylamine, (ii) optimising potency on the parasite and selectivity to the human and species orthologs used for the GLP (Good Laboratory Practice) safety studies, (iii) optimising the DMPK (drug metabolism and pharmacokinetics), in particular balancing the solubility *vs.* other properties, demonstration of *in vivo* efficacy, and increasing the human plasma half-life prediction through reducing the clearance (given that basic groups to increase volume were not tolerated) and (iv) practically demonstrating sufficient safety for progression into humans.

As such DSM1 was optimised first to DSM191 through exploring aromatic amine replacements;[37] Figure 26.4. DSM191 was the first compound having sufficient mouse PK and potency for an *in vivo* experiment and was the first *in vivo* active *Pf* DHODH inhibitor. With the advent of structural biology (highlighting the feasibility to build off the triazole carbon) and application of QSAR (quantitative SAR; suggesting the logical substituent for the pendant aromatic was $-SF_5$) delivered DSM265 as the preclinical candidate, and the molecule was ultimately tested in Phase I,[38] in a volunteer infection study and in Phase IIa study in Peru,[39]

Key learnings include, first, that target-based drug discovery for malaria is effective once validation of the target from a biological and chemical perspective is without doubt, and significantly aided by multiple species biochemical assays and structural biology. Furthermore, knowing the mechanism of action early, and having phenotypic assays to confirm the killing mechanism, has greatly given confidence in the series and the target. Second, the increased lipophilicity of the candidate and its very high plasma protein binding, along with increased potency means that its intrinsic free potency is significantly improved as compared to earlier compounds and likely to be subnanomolar; in addition, the *in vivo* $EC_{50}$ and MPC (minimal parasiticidal concentration) are in the micromolar range, simply as a result of binding. Third, although selectivity of DSM265 over the human DHODH orthologue was exceptional, the lesser selectivity against rodent DHODH, in particular, led to a need to navigate to non-typical toxicology species for the GLP toxicological studies. Fourth, the reduced potency of DSM265 on vivax field isolates (5-fold) was sufficient to see reduced efficacy on vivax patients compared to falciparum. Fifth, the low intrinsic clearance in all species, in conjunction with *in vivo* clearance in rodents, dogs and monkeys (factoring in binding and partitioning data) was used to estimate a human clearance, volume and plasma half-life. The latter

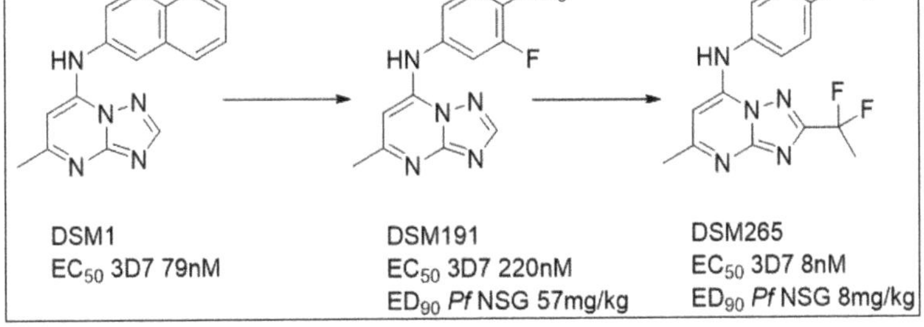


**Figure 26.4** Structures and activities of Hit (DSM1) to Lead (DSM191) to Candidate (DSM265) development. 3D7 is a lab-adapted strain of *P. falciparum* (*Pf*) that is sensitive to most drugs. $EC_{50}$ is the concentration giving 50% inhibition of parasite growth *in vitro*; $ED_{90}$ is the dose giving 90% suppression of parasite growth *in vivo*. NSG is the Nod-SCID-$\gamma$ mouse model.

was approximately 130 h, and the observed human half-life was around 100 h. Sixth, the low solubility and risks associated with variability in systemic exposure translated to a need for significant formulation enhancements – ultimately being "solved" by spray-dried dispersion technology. However, the drug's loading, dose size and cost ultimately contributed to the compound's down-prioritisation. Seventh, the estimation of an efficacious dose from preclinical studies was reinforced with results from the Phase Ib volunteer infection study (predicting a single dose between 200 and 400 mg). In Phase IIa, DSM265 cured 9/10 patients at day 14 with a single dose of 400 mg – demonstrating single-dose potential. Eighth, patients in the aforementioned study had recrudescent resistant parasites in several instances, providing translational validation that *in vitro* selections (which showed a high propensity to select resistance for DSM265) are relevant to the clinic. This is helping to inform new Discovery Criteria. Ninth, the 24 h delay in the onset of efficacy in patients, followed by rapid parasite clearance, ties in well with the *in vitro* PRR data. Indeed, translational modelling has shown that the best preclinical predictor of kill rate is from the PRR experiment. Tenth, the *in vitro* potency on liver stages was recapitulated in the efficacy observed in a clinical sporozoite challenge model, in which DSM265 showed prophylaxis based on a once-weekly dose of 400 mg.[40]

Thus, although DSM265 was ultimately halted for a range of risk factors, including certain toxicities, and high dose and cost (including formulation), as a community there have been substantial learnings from the discovery process.

## 26.3 Tuberculosis

### 26.3.1 Disease Overview

Tuberculosis (TB) is an infectious disease caused by the bacterium *Mycobacterium tuberculosis* (*Mtb*) and is arguably the single most significant bacterial pathogen in the world. It infects one-third of the world's population, and results in 10 million new cases of active tuberculosis (TB) and 1.4 million deaths every year. According to the most recent World Health Organization (WHO) Global Tuberculosis Report, TB is considered the ninth-highest cause of death worldwide, and the leading cause of mortality by a single infectious agent, with the highest rate of infections and death toll rate primarily concentrated in developing and low-income countries.[41]

### 26.3.2 *Mycobacterium tuberculosis* Lifecycle

The cycle of TB infections starts with a pulmonary TB patient coughing and consequently aerosolising *Mtb* bacilli (see Figure 26.5). These infectious droplets are then inhaled by close contacts, and subsequently penetrate the well-ventilated lower part of the lungs. The host immune response attempts to contain the infection, which results in granuloma formation.[42] In approximately 90% of exposed patients, *Mtb* is satisfactorily controlled by such caseated granulomas, and active disease never develops.[43] In a small proportion of such latent TB patients, however, active TB will arise at some point following infection. This may be within months, often as miliary TB, or up to decades later, typically as apical pulmonary TB. The exact perturbation of the immune system

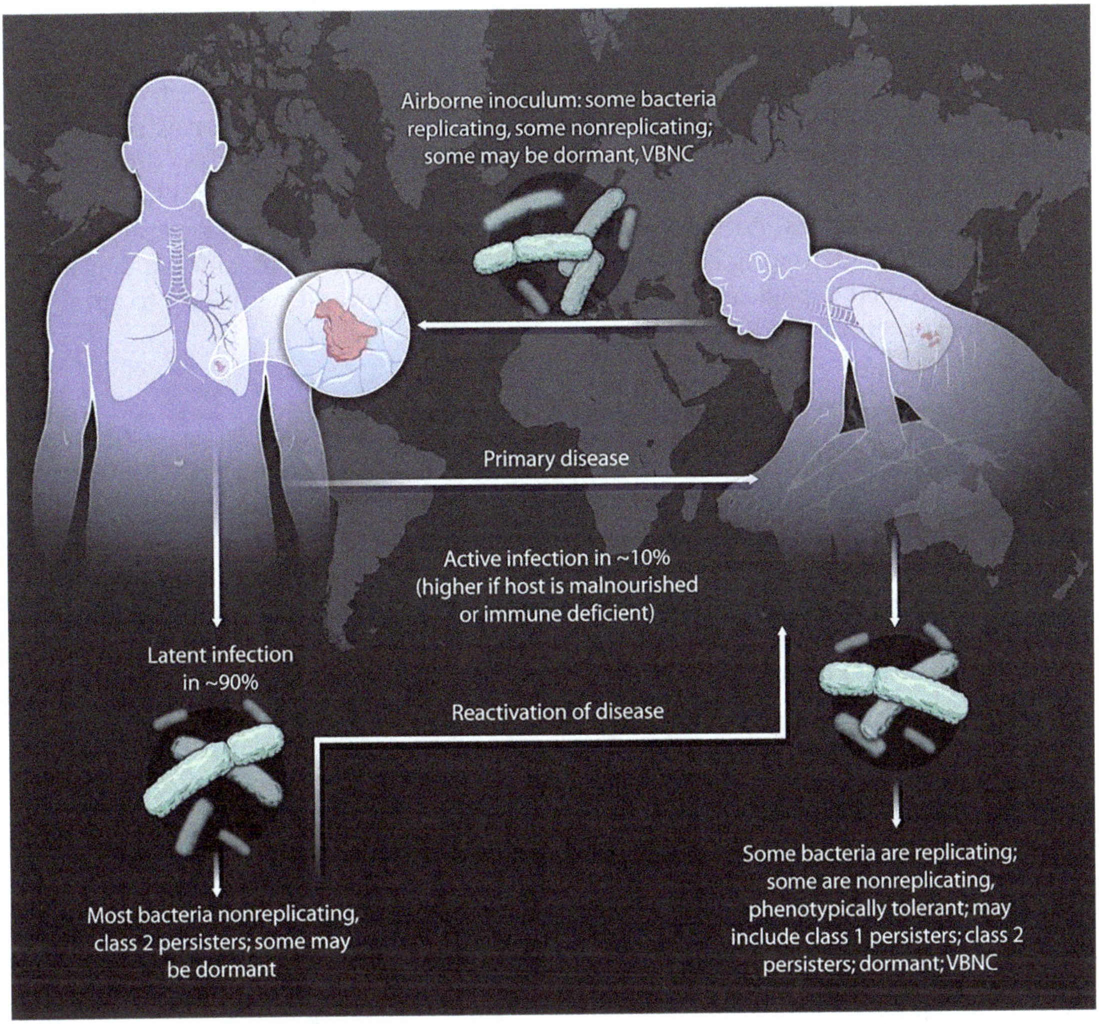


**Figure 26.5** Life cycle of *Mycobacterium tuberculosis*. Of 100 people infected, only 5–10 become ill with tuberculosis. Each of these will infect 10–20 others, and 3–5 will die.[44]

which leads to TB reactivation is uncertain. In some instances, the immune deficiency is apparent, such as HIV co-infection, alcoholism or treatment with anti-TNF antibodies,[43] but in the majority, it remains unclear.

Only patients with pulmonary disease can transmit TB to new hosts, with the very rare exception of laryngeal disease. Other clinical manifestations, such as lymph node TB, TB meningitis, spinal TB or TB of any other organ, are an epidemiological dead end for the bacilli, as they may cause death to the host without onward transmission. Pulmonary TB develops in the apex of the lungs,[45] and therefore bacilli must spread from their initial seeding point in the lung bases to the apex. The precise translocation mechanism is uncertain, but a zebrafish model of *M. marinum* suggests mycobacteria disseminate within infected monocytes.[46]

Once lodged in the lung apex, *Mtb* must subvert the host immune response to drive lung matrix destruction and cavitation, as such cavitation leads to enhanced infectivity.[47] The specific mechanisms which lead to lung cavitation are not well understood, but appear to be driven by host immunity factors, as cavitation is suppressed in advanced HIV infections.[48] Within the walls of pulmonary cavities, the immune response essentially fails,[49] and cavities can contain up to one hundred million bacilli.[50] In the pre-antibiotic era, patients were sometimes symptomatic for several decades, and experienced "fluctuating consumption". This symbiosis was ideal for *Mtb* as it permitted a prolonged period of infectivity, and thereby allowed the disease to spread to many more susceptible individuals.

### 26.3.3 Current Treatments, Portfolio and Gaps

Combination chemotherapy has been the standard of care since the early 1950s, when it was discovered that combining drugs such as streptomycin and isoniazid reduced the incidence of drug resistance, and thus enabled reliable cures with ~18–24 months of treatment. By the 1980s, TB combination therapies were improved with the addition of rifampin and pyrazinamide, which accelerated the eradication of bacterial "persisters", and further shortened the duration of treatment necessary to prevent relapse, resulting in the current WHO recommended 6 month "short course" therapy for drug-sensitive (DS) TB patients.

Current first-line treatment regimens (composed of rifampin [RIF], ethambutol, pyrazinamide, and isoniazid) only provide an ~80% cure rate globally for newly diagnosed individuals with drug-sensitive TB. The prolonged treatment duration plus adverse side effects observed with the four-agent regimen contributes directly to poor overall patient compliance. Inadequate treatment adherence, along with population PK variability, ineffective infection control and geopolitical/logistical distribution issues have led to increased TB drug resistance globally, and fears of a TB epidemic with virtually untreatable *Mtb* strains in growing numbers. According to the 2018 WHO TB Report[51] there were 600 000 new TB cases with resistance to rifampin (RRTB), the most effective first-line drug, of which 490 000 had multidrug-resistant TB (MDR-TB; data for 2016).[51] MDR-TB is a disease caused by *Mtb* which is resistant to both RIF and isoniazid (INH).

Treatment options for drug-resistant TB infections are complex. These often include considerably less effective and more poorly tolerated agents (delivered orally and parenterally), and usually require even longer treatment times with far worse outcomes compared to treatments for drug-sensitive disease. Current regimens for the treatment of MDR-TB and extremely drug-resistant TB (XDR-TB) are not well tolerated, and have significant associated toxicities, such as deafness, severe gastrointestinal or central nervous side effects, and peripheral neuropathies. Furthermore, treatment durations for MDR-TB range from 9 to 20 months with only a ~54% cure rate globally. Even more desperate is the need for regimens to treat XDR-TB, as current treatments are effective only about 20% of the time.[51] Despite these urgent needs, there are sparingly few significantly effective new regimens currently available.[52]

The long, complex treatment regimens employed to cure TB infections are thought to be necessary in part due to the existence of so-called "persister" *Mtb* bacteria that are present during TB infection and are tolerant to many TB drugs due to slower replication rates and altered physiological states.[53] Certain TB drugs (*e.g.* the RNA polymerase [RNAP] inhibitor rifampin) have potent bactericidal activity against these slowly replicating *Mtb* bacteria *in vitro*, and sterilising efficacy *in vivo*, in the clinic, leading to shorter treatment durations. The inability to use rifampin against MDR-TB and XDR-TB (which are, by definition, RIF-resistant) requires the extension of TB treatment schedules to 9–20 months. New TB drugs and regimens that consist of multiple drugs with additive or synergistic activity against persister *Mtb* (as well as replicating *Mtb*), and that are effective against MDR/XDR-TB should result in tissue sterilisation, significantly shorter treatment times and overall improved cure rates for TB patients (Figure 26.6).

With limited commercial potential to be realised with new TB drugs, TB has not been an area of intense drug discovery activity or interest in recent years. In addition, the exodus of much of the pharmaceutical industry from anti-bacterial drug discovery has proven to be a tremendous loss for TB drug research and development efforts, as the TB field no longer benefits from drug candidates developed against other bacteria. Fortunately, some government and non-governmental organisations have taken the initiative to fill this gap, with a turning point occurring with the creation of several not-for-profit PDPs, such as the Global Alliance for TB Drug Development (TB Alliance) founded in 2000. Since then, additional global TB consortia have formed, including the TB Drug Accelerator, the Eli Lilly TB Drug Discovery Initiative, More Medicines for TB (MM4TB) and Orchid. Academic and government laboratories are also involved in translational research to enable TB drug discovery and are in part funded by the National Institutes of Health (NIH) and the Bill & Melinda Gates Foundation. Most recently, the Gates Foundation provided a multiyear grant to underwrite the creation of a new, non-profit biotech organisation, the Gates Medical Research Institute (MRI) to address translational drug development challenges for neglected diseases, including malaria, tuberculosis and diarrheal diseases (gatesmri.org).

The approvals of bedaquiline (TMC-207, Sirturo from Janssen), by the US Food and Drug Administration (FDA) at the end of 2012 (and by the EMA, the European Medicines Agency in March, 2014), delamanid (OPC-67683, Deltyba from Otsuka) by the EMA in December of 2013 and pretomanid (PA-824 from the TB Alliance) by the FDA (August, 2019) and EMA (March, 2020) represent important contributions to MDR- and XDR-TB therapies. However, the current global TB drug discovery pipeline provides too few substrates for the development of treatment-shortening drug regimens to radically change the global TB treatment paradigm. Efforts in recent years (by the TB Alliance [Figure 26.7], and members of the TB Drug Accelerator consortium) have focused on identifying novel biochemical mechanisms – or networks of mechanisms – which may translate into a swifter elimination of TB bacilli under a variety of biological conditions. The challenge remains to identify novel chemical matter to target such systems as well as the integration of appropriate *in vitro*, *in vivo* and *ex vivo* preclinical models to promulgate attractive anti-TB regimens, and similarly dismiss those which do not offer significant improvements over current therapies.

| Regimen | Drug[a] | Intensive Phase: Interval and Dose[b] (Minimum Duration) | Continuation Phase: Drugs | Continuation Phase: Interval and Dose[b,c] (Minimum Duration) | Range of Total Doses | Comments[c,d] | Regimen Effectiveness |
|---|---|---|---|---|---|---|---|
| 1 | INH RIF PZA EMB | 7 d/wk for 56 doses (8 wk), or 5 d/wk for 40 doses (8 wk) | INH RIF | 7 d/wk for 126 doses (18 wk), or 5 d/wk for 90 doses (18 wk) | 182–130 | This is the preferred regimen for patients with newly diagnosed pulmonary tuberculosis. | Greater |
| 2 | INH RIF PZA EMB | 7 d/wk for 56 doses (8 wk), or 5 d/wk for 40 doses (8 wk) | INH RIF | 3 times weekly for 54 doses (18 wk) | 110–94 | Preferred alternative regimen in situations in which more frequent DOT during continuation phase is difficult to achieve. | |
| 3 | INH RIF PZA EMB | 3 times weekly for 24 doses (8 wk) | INH RIF | 3 times weekly for 54 doses (18 wk) | 78 | Use regimen with caution in patients with HIV and/or cavitary disease. Missed doses can lead to treatment failure, relapse, and acquired drug resistance. | |
| 4 | INH RIF PZA EMB | 7 d/wk for 14 doses then twice weekly for 12 doses[e] | INH RIF | Twice weekly for 36 doses (18 wk) | 62 | Do not use twice-weekly regimens in HIV-infected patients or patients with smear-positive and/or cavitary disease. If doses are missed, then therapy is equivalent to once weekly, which is inferior. | Lesser |

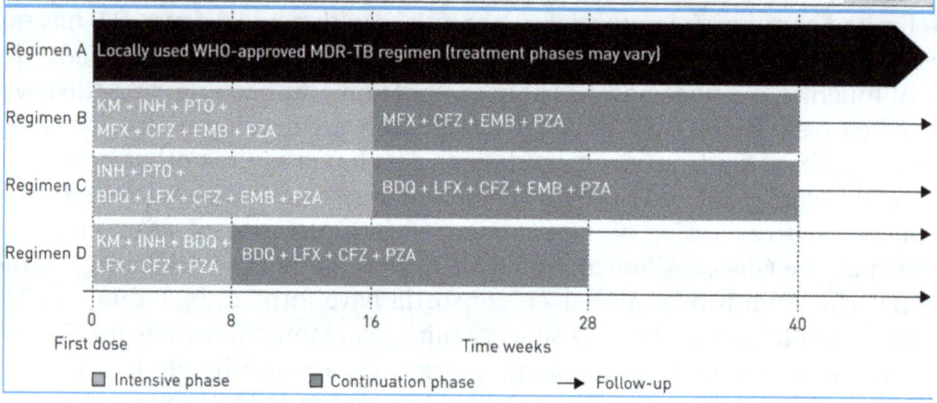


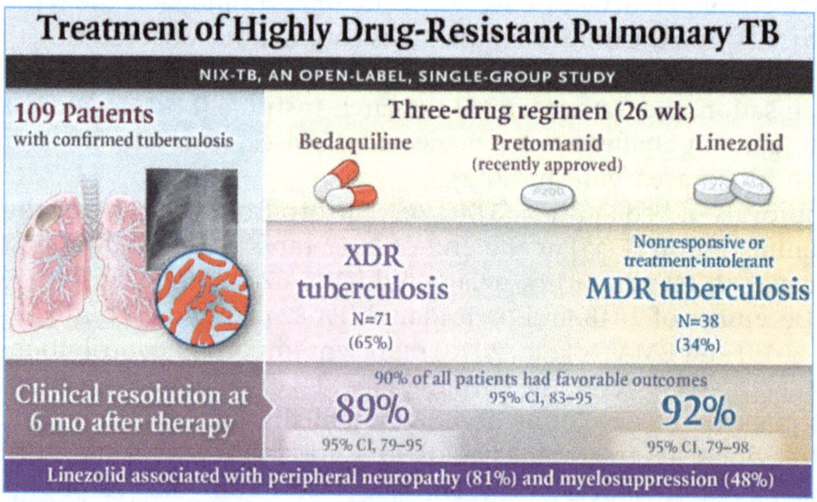


**Figure 26.6** TB treatment regimens. (A) DS-TB.[54] Abbreviations: DOT, directly observed therapy; EMB, ethambutol; HIV, human immunodeficiency virus; INH, isoniazid; PZA, pyrazinamide; RIF, rifampin. [a]Other combinations may be appropriate in certain circumstances. [b]When DOT is used, drugs may be given 5 days per week and the necessary number of doses adjusted accordingly. Although there are no studies that compare 5 with 7 daily doses, extensive experience indicates this would

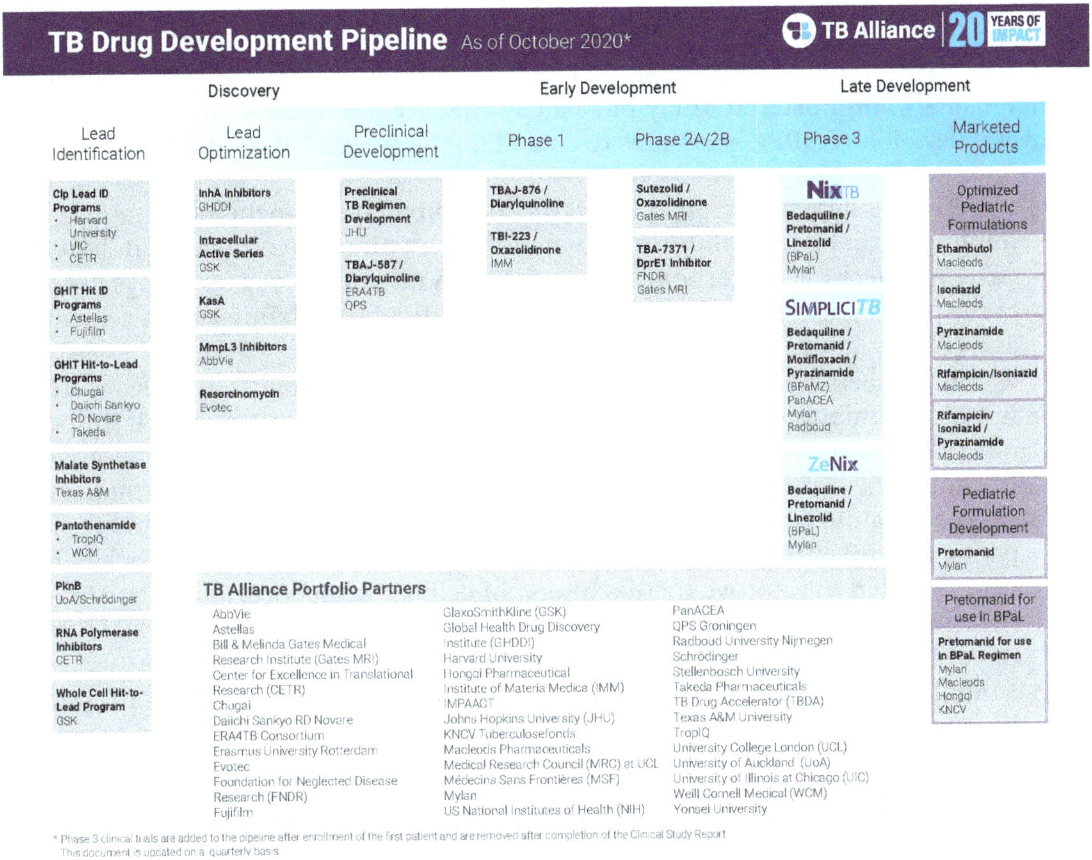


**Figure 26.7** TB Alliance discovery/development portfolio (www.tballiance.org/portfolio).[80] Image Credit: TB Alliance.

be an effective practice. DOT should be used when drugs are administered <7 days per week. $^c$Based on expert opinion, patients with cavitation on initial chest radiograph and positive cultures at completion of 2 months of therapy should receive a 7-month (31-week) continuation phase. $^d$Pyridoxine (vitamin B6), 25–50 mg day$^{-1}$, is given with INH to all persons at risk of neuropathy (*e.g.* pregnant women, breastfeeding infants, persons with HIV, patients with diabetes, alcoholism, malnutrition or chronic renal failure, or patients with advanced age). For patients with peripheral neuropathy, experts recommend increasing pyridoxine dose to 100 mg day$^{-1}$ $^e$Alternatively, some US tuberculosis control programmes have administered intensive-phase regimens 5 days per week for 15 doses (3 weeks), then twice weekly for 12 doses. (B) MDR-TB.[55] STREAM (Evaluation of a Standardised Treatment Regimen of Anti-tuberculosis Drugs for Patients with Multidrug-resistant Tuberculosis) treatment regimens. WHO: World Health Organization; MDR-TB: multidrug-resistant tuberculosis; KM: kanamycin; INH: isoniazid; PTO: prothionamide; MFX: moxifloxacin; CFZ: clofazimine; EMB: ethambutol; PZA: pyrazinamide; BDQ: bedaquiline; LFX: levofloxacin (C) XDR-TB.[51]

### 26.3.4 Antitubercular Medicinal Chemistry – Key Learnings

As noted above, modern TB therapies require multiple (typically three or four) TB agents, usually administered orally once a day. Such requirements immediately point to several key biological/PK attributes to consider for any new TB programme:

(1) Selectivity – depending on the specific anti-tubercular biochemical target, it is imperative that any inhibitor/modulator of such a target does not equally (or comparably) affect the corresponding mammalian target(s). Counter-assays are generally put in place early in any TB testing paradigm to maximise such selectivity, and consequently reduce off-target activities and toxicities.

(2) Whole cell activity – *Mycobacterium tuberculosis* (as is true for all mycobacteria) is unique among Gram-positive bacteria in possessing a reasonably impervious cell envelope, as shown in Figure 26.8. This envelope (which is notable for its abundance of long-chain mycolic acids [MA]) serves as an extremely effective permeability barrier to limit the passive diffusion of various chemotherapeutics of different origins. Modern computational chemistry approaches have been adopted to improve the likelihood of cellular transport/uptake by *Mtb*, but this physical barrier remains a critical challenge in the development of novel target-based anti-tubercular agents.

(3) Solubility/formulation challenges – Perhaps not surprisingly (given the highly lipophilic nature of the *Mtb* outer membrane), many potent TB agents exhibit inordinately high lipophilicities. Indeed, across the entire global TB drug pipeline (see Figure 26.9), over 70% of the agents in discovery and development exhibit clog*P* values of ≥5, and 25% have clog*P* values ≥6.5. The advancement of attractive TB agents through a series of preclinical infection and safety models (including mouse, rat, rabbit, guinea pig, dog and/or monkey) requires adequate dosing formulations, to provide appropriate drug concentrations upon oral administration. The inclusion of various solubilising excipients (*i.e.* Cremophor, Tween 80, PEG 400, Solutol 15 HS, *etc.*) can be considered for improving the oral PK of test

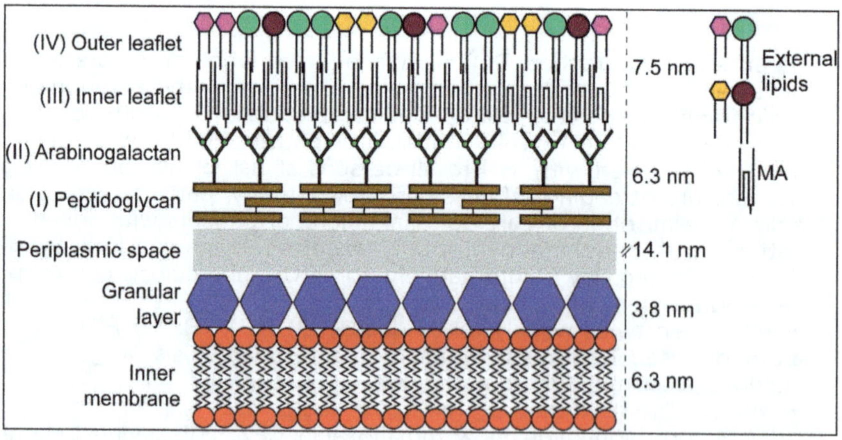


**Figure 26.8** Schematic representation of *Mycobacterium tuberculosis* cell envelope.[56]

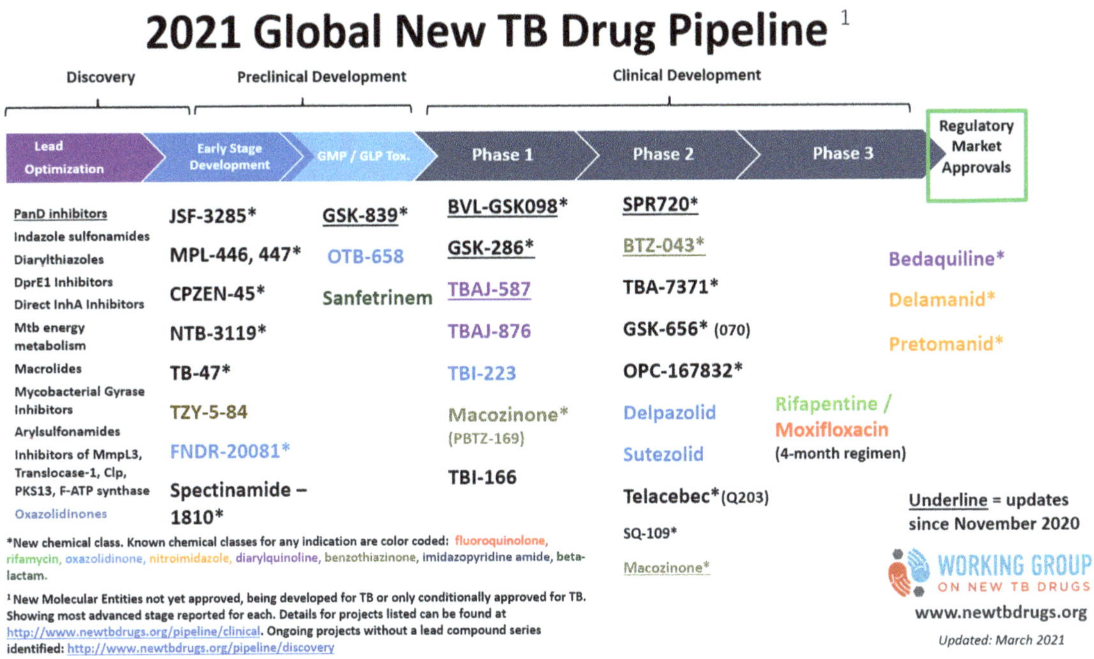


**Figure 26.9** Current global TB programme portfolio (courtesy of Working Group on New TB Drugs, newtbdrugs.com). Image Credit: TB Alliance.

compounds early in lead optimisation, but difficulties may arise in translating original preclinical oral exposures to human exposure when more stable, crystalline polymorphs are identified in later development. Prodrugs may also be considered, but may too drastically affect the overall cost of goods (COG) for any given TB active pharmaceutical ingredient (API).

(4) API cost of goods – Not unlike the previous discussion regarding anti-malarials, the overwhelming majority of TB patients are located in poverty-stricken portions of the world. In fact, the WHO has published estimates that just 22 countries account for over 80% of the TB cases worldwide,[57] and that the vast majority of these high-burden nations represent those with higher poverty levels as well (Figure 26.10). To put the challenge in perspective, the current medication costs for the entire 6 month, four-drug treatment typically prescribed for drug-sensitive TB (*i.e.* rifampicin, isoniazid, ethambutol and pyrazinamide) averages between ~\$40 and \$80 per patient.[58] Against this backdrop, all new TB agents must be evaluated, on their therapeutic potential as well as their COG, and additional process chemistry and CMC considerations must be addressed early in drug development to ensure suitable affordability post-approval.

## 26.3.5 Portfolio – Case Study

As with malaria (*vide supra*), one recent case study is provided here which is exemplary of the challenges faced in the identification and development of novel anti-tubercular agents. The specific example provided below (the identification of TBA-7371, a novel,

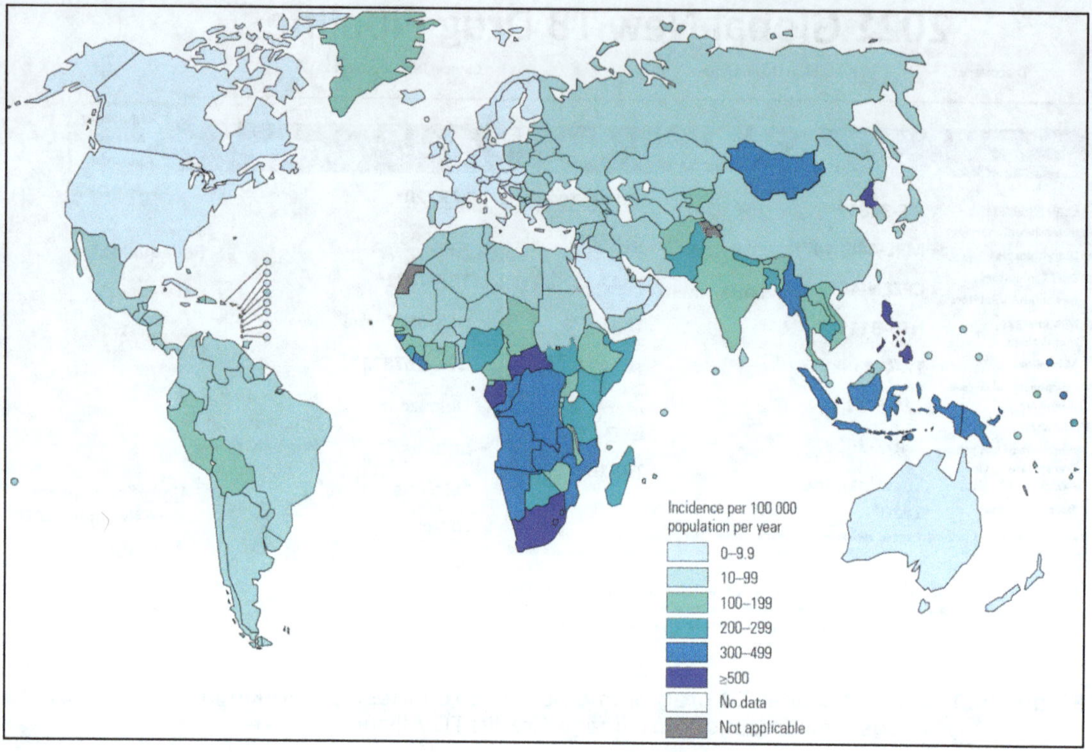


Figure 26.10 Estimated TB incidence rates in 2019 (World Health Organization Report).[41]

non-covalent DprE1 inhibitor) provides a valuable context for the iterative physicochemical and biological property improvements required to advance novel agents to preclinical and clinical trial consideration.

### *26.3.5.1 TBA-7371 – Mtb DprE1 Inhibitor*

As part of a multiyear collaboration between AstraZeneca (AZ) India (Bangalore) and the TB Alliance, several exploratory TB projects were pursued in efforts to identify new chemical matter targeting novel *Mtb* biochemical targets of interest. One such hit identification project grew out of an interest in probing alternative heterocyclic systems based on the previously published University of Notre Dame/Institute Pasteur Korea (IPK) imidazopyridine amides, or IPAs (see Figure 26.11). While the exact biochemical target was poorly understood at the start of the investigation, the AZ team considered whether alternative bicyclic amides might offer comparable or possibly improved anti-TB activities (particularly introducing bactericidal activity which was not observed with the original IPAs). Several "scaffold hopping" exercises were attempted, with one such variant (the 1,4-azaindole system) appearing the most promising. Whole genome sequencing of several azaindole-resistant mutant *Mtb* clones led to the identification of the biochemical target for this series as DprE1 (*i.e.* decaprenylphosphoryl-β-D-ribose-2′-epimerase[59,60]).

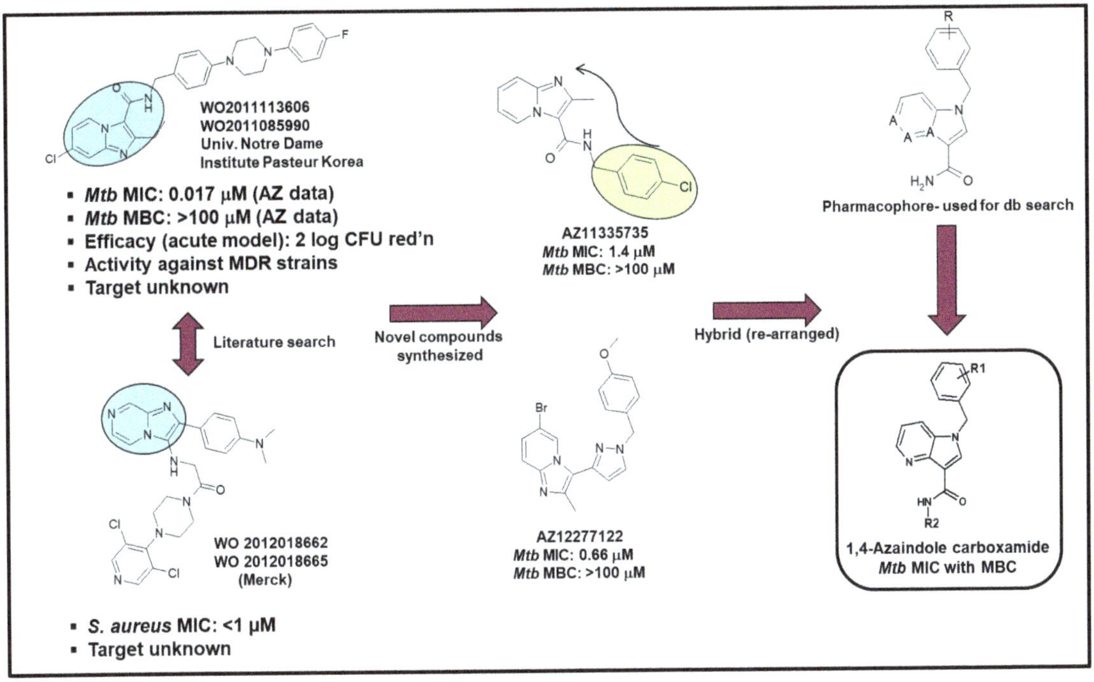


**Figure 26.11** Identification of 1,4-azaindole non-covalent DprE1 inhibitors.

In the absence of crystal structure information, *Mtb* potency of the azaindoles was driven by the development of MIC-based SAR with three points of diversification (*i.e.* amide side chain, hydrophobic pocket group and core ring substitutions – see Figure 26.12). The secondary amide, referred to as the amide side chain, proved to be an essential moiety for maintaining potent MICs, through forming hydrogen bonding with the target DprE1 enzyme.[61] Small hydrophobic or hydrophilic amides such as methyl cyclopropyl, fluoroethyl and hydroxyethyl amides were preferred for cellular potency. The hydrophobic pocket group was found to tolerate a variety of substituted benzyl and heteroarylmethyl groups; however, monosubstituted benzyl groups were less favoured than disubstituted benzyl or heteroarylmethyl groups. Substitution of a methyl or methoxy group at the C-6 position of the 1,4-azaindole also vastly improved their cellular potency.

Although 1,4-azaindoles showed excellent *Mtb* activity *in vitro* and *in vivo*, these compounds in general exhibited poor aqueous solubility, underwent high mouse-specific metabolism, and showed modest inhibition of PDE6. As a result, the major focus of the lead optimisation phase was to retain potency while improving solubility, mouse exposures (PO, orally), mitigating PDE6 inhibition and bringing all the favourable physicochemical and biological properties together in one molecule. The introduction of the hydroxyethyl amide side chain proved crucial to both improving aqueous solubility and modulating the overall physicochemical properties of the 1,4-azaindoles. In addition, the hydroxyethyl amide side chain led to significant improvements in mouse liver microsome (MLM) stability relative to alternative hydrophobic amide side chains. The improved MLM

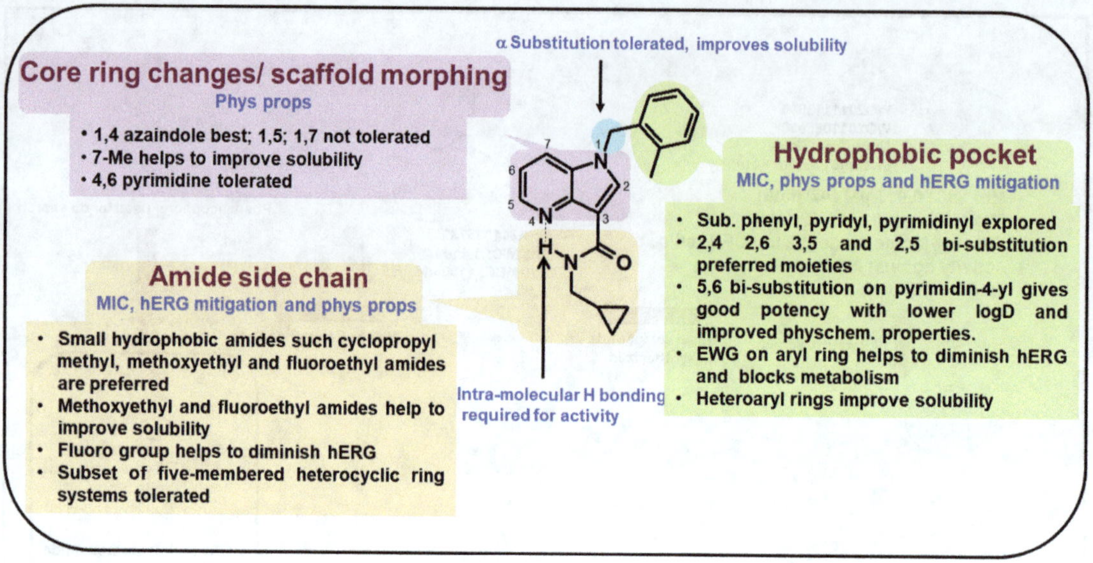


**Figure 26.12** Structure–activity relationship (SAR) for 1,4-azaindole DprE1 inhibitor series.

stability was attributed to compounds with lower lipophilicity, as indicated by measured log$D$ of 2 or less. An additional concern was the observed hERG inhibition[62] observed for many early analogues. The introduction of a range of heterocycles (pyridine, pyrimidine) within the hydrophobic pocket improved the overall aqueous solubility, as well as diminished hERG inhibition liabilities for such analogues (Figure 26.13).

Overall, from an initial *de novo* whole cell active compound, the 1,4-azaindole series was systematically optimised to identify new molecules with low molecular weight, low log$D$, nanomolar DprE1 $IC_{50}$, sub-micromolar MIC, excellent cellular permeability, no CYP inhibition, good oral exposure, low clearance in mice, rats, dogs and humans, and no major safety liabilities.[63] The total synthesis of the 1,4-azaindoles was relatively straightforward, and, with no chiral centre, cGMP API should offer reasonable-to-low cost of goods. The furthest advanced analogue from this programme (TBA-7371; Figure 26.13) has now successfully passed Phase I clinical trials in healthy volunteers. A Phase IIa (Early Bactericidal Activity, EBA) clinical trial for TBA-7371 is currently recruiting patients in Cape Town, South Africa, with an anticipated study completion date of February, 2022. Current TBA-7371 Phase II clinical trials are conducted under the sponsorship and auspices of the Gates MRI (registered as NCT04176250).

## 26.4 Human African Trypanosomiasis and Leishmaniasis

### 26.4.1 Disease Overview

*Sleeping Sickness*

Human African trypanosomiasis (HAT), or sleeping sickness, is caused by eukaryotic unicellular *Trypanosoma brucei* parasites that are transmitted by tsetse flies. HAT is

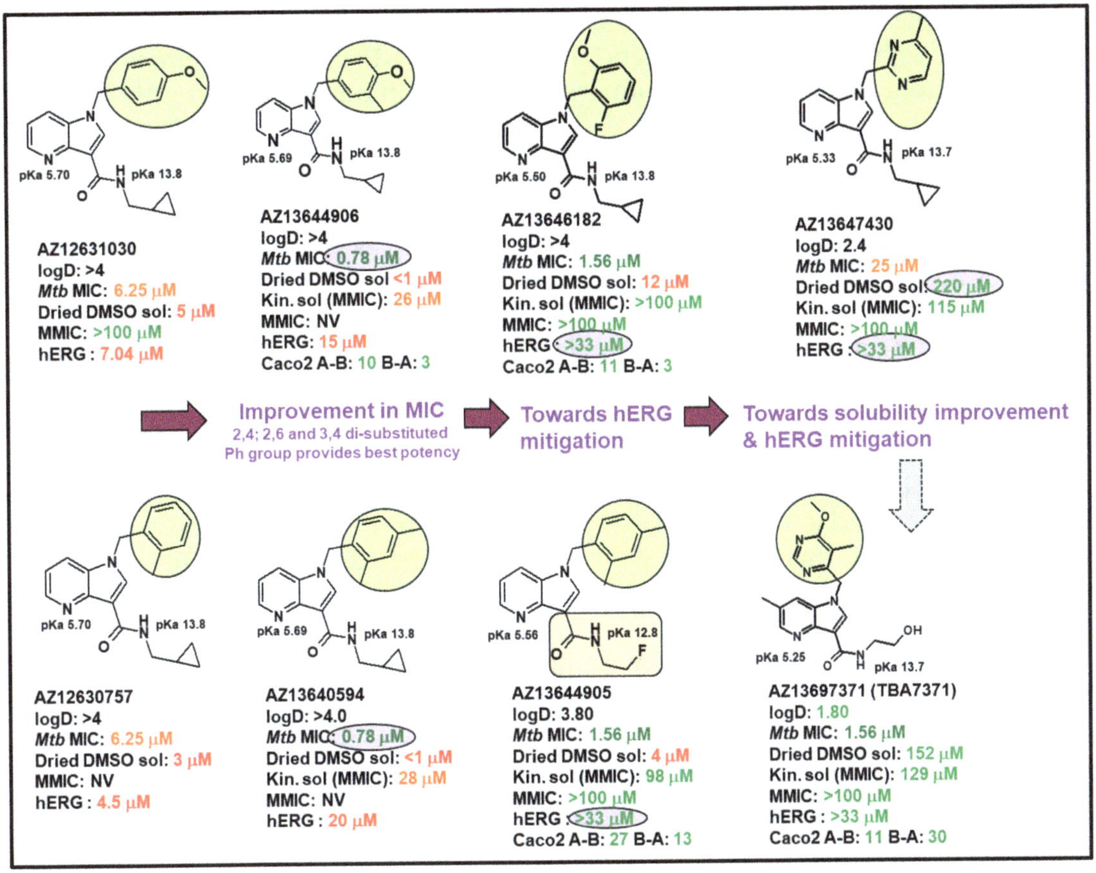


**Figure 26.13** Variations in 1,4-azaindole series leading to clinical candidate TBA-7371.[63]

found only in sub-Saharan Africa. Two sub-species of *Trypanosoma brucei* cause disease: *T. b. gambiense* in West and Central Africa, and *T. b. rhodesiense* in East Africa.

Following infection, trypanosomes multiply in the blood and lymph resulting in stage 1, haemolymphatic, disease. This results in unspecific symptoms such as headache, fever, weakness, joint pain and lymphadenopathy which start to appear after a variable incubation period.

Over time, the parasites cross the blood–brain barrier, invading the central nervous system leading to stage 2, meningo-encephalitic disease, resulting in various neurological disturbances, including sleep disruptions and deep sensory disturbances, abnormal movements, speech difficulties and psychiatric disorders, ultimately resulting in coma and death. Left untreated, HAT caused by *T. b. rhodesiense* is typically acute, progressing to the second stage within a few weeks, and to death within six months. HAT caused by *T. b. gambiense* usually progresses slowly, over around three years.

Since 1995 there has been a significant decrease in the number of cases reported, from more than 25 000 in 1995 to less than 1000 in 2019, thanks to programmes aimed at reducing transmission in sub-Saharan Africa. Transmission can be interrupted by depleting the parasite reservoirs, which is achieved by the detection and treatment of infected people and domestic animals, and by reducing the tsetse fly population and also preventing human-tsetse contacts by other means. However, HAT remains a significant threat to human health, with an estimated 57 million people currently at risk in 36 countries.

*Leishmaniasis*

Leishmaniasis is a disease that threatens an estimated one billion people worldwide, and is endemic in 98 countries. Leishmaniasis is a complex vector-borne disease, transmitted by more than 20 species of the protozoan genus *Leishmania*, and associated with clinical manifestations ranging from relatively benign localised skin ulcers to systemic disease causing severe damage to visceral organs that is fatal if left untreated. The different forms of the disease are categorised as visceral, cutaneous, mucocutaneous and post-kala-azar dermal leishmaniases (PKDL). Leishmaniasis breaks out as "foci", concentrated in geographic areas, and is transmitted by the bite of a sand fly, a vector that is sensitive to environmental changes such as deforestation, building of dams, irrigation schemes and urbanisation. An estimated 700 000 to 1 million new cases of the disease in its various forms occur annually, with an estimated 20 000 to 30 000 associated deaths. The fatality rate of visceral leishmaniasis (VL), also called kala-azar, is over 95% if left untreated.

Visceral leishmaniasis is caused by the protozoan parasites *Leishmania donovani* and *Leishmania infantum*, with a distribution in Asia, East Africa, Latin America and the Mediterranean region. In patients who develop symptoms, presentation is insidious, with development of splenomegaly, irregular fevers, anaemia, pancytopenia, weight loss and weakness occurring progressively over a period of weeks or even months.

Cutaneous leishmaniasis (CL) is endemic to all tropical and subtropical areas of the world. The distribution of this disease is very tightly linked to geography, with a high degree of local variation. Several *Leishmania* species, including *L. amazonensis*, *L. braziliensis*, *L. guyanensis*, *L. mexicana*, *L. panamensis*, *L. aethiopica*, *L. infantum*, *L. major* and *L. tropica*, are known to infect humans and cause CL. The clinical manifestations of CL include skin lesions, which can persist for months, sometimes years. The skin lesions usually develop several weeks or months after the exposure but occasionally first appear years later. The lesions typically evolve from papules to nodular plaques to ulcerative lesions. The healing process typically results in atrophic scarring, which may lead to social stigmatisation.

### 26.4.2 Pathogen Lifecycles of *T. brucei* and *Leishmania* spp.

*Trypanosoma brucei Life Cycle*

*Trypanosoma brucei* parasites are transmitted by tsetse flies (*Glossina* spp.). During a blood meal on the mammalian host the tsetse fly injects metacyclic trypomastigotes into skin tissue. The parasites enter the lymphatic system and pass into the bloodstream. Inside the host, they transform into bloodstream trypomastigotes, which are carried to other sites throughout the body. The trypomastigotes multiply by binary fission in various body fluids, *e.g.* blood, lymph and spinal fluid. The entire life cycle of African trypanosomes in mammals is represented by extracellular stages. The tsetse fly becomes infected with bloodstream trypomastigotes when taking a blood meal on an infected mammalian host. In the fly's midgut, the parasites transform into procyclic trypomastigotes, multiply by binary fission, leave the midgut and transform into epimastigotes. The epimastigotes reach the fly's salivary glands and continue multiplication by binary fission. The cycle in the fly takes approximately three weeks.

Humans are considered to be the main reservoir for *T. b. gambiense*, but other species, *e.g.* other primates and ungulates may also serve as reservoirs. Domestic cattle are considered to be the most epidemiologically relevant animal reservoir of *T. b. rhodesiense*. The only known vector for each form is the tsetse fly.

*Leishmania* Life Cycle

The *Leishmania* spp. parasite, the causal agent of leishmaniasis, is transmitted by the bite of female phlebotomine sandflies. The sandflies inject the infective-stage parasite, promastigotes, during blood meals. Promastigotes that reach the puncture wound are phagocytised by macrophages and transformed into amastigotes. The amastigotes multiply inside infected cells and will affect different tissues, depending in part on the *Leishmania* species, leading to the different clinical manifestations. The parasite lifecycle is completed when the sandflies become infected during blood meals ingesting amastigote-infected macrophages from an infected host. In the sandfly's midgut, the parasites differentiate into promastigotes, which multiply and migrate to the proboscis.

## 26.4.3 Current Treatments for HAT and Leishmaniasis

The treatment opportunities for HAT have significantly improved over recent years through the introduction of novel, optimised intravenous and oral drugs that replaced earlier treatments based on intramuscular pentamidine, intravenous suramin and melarsoprol, an arsenic-based triazine derivative, all associated with significant adverse effects and mortality. A first step towards optimised treatments was the introduction of nifurtimox-eflornithine (NECT; Figure 26.14), an injected treatment with an improved efficacy–safety profile as compared to previous treatments. However, the NECT combination therapy needs to be administered in a hospital setting by trained personnel, which limits its use in remote areas. In 2018, fexinidazole, an optimised short course, oral treatment of HAT caused by *T. b. gambiense* infections was approved by the EMA (Figure 26.14). The introduction of fexinidazole has significantly facilitated the opportunity to also treat patients at primary health facilities. Studies are now ongoing to assess the efficacy of fexinidazole in the treatment of HAT caused by *T. b. rhodesiense.*[64]

Current treatments of VL rely on the use of a small group of drugs, including: meglumine antimoniate, sodium stibogluconate (SSG), liposomal amphotericin B, paromomycin sulfate and miltefosine. Although efficacious against multiple *Leishmania* strains

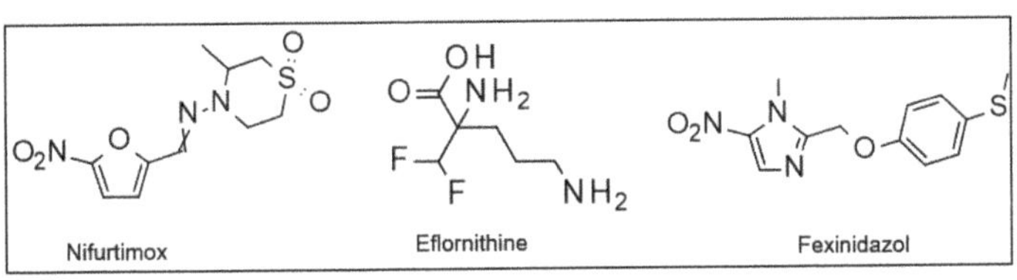


**Figure 26.14** Structures of nifurtimox, eflornithine (the components of NECT) and fexinidazol.

in different populations their use is associated with significant dose-limiting adverse effects and emerging cases of drug resistance observed in specific regions. In addition, limitations related to access and the need for supervised intravenous or intramuscular drug administration restricts their overall use (Table 26.1 and Figure 26.15). Miltefosine, currently the only oral drug available, cannot be administered to female patients of child-bearing age, due to its teratogenicity, unless contraception can be guaranteed. Interestingly, there are significant differences in the clinical response to the same treatment between Asia and Africa, and variations in the clinical response within Africa have also been observed, leading to the development of different regional treatment recommendations.

**Table 26.1** Drugs approved for treatment of visceral leishmaniasis (VL).

| | Meglumine antimoniate (MA) | Sodium stibogluconate (SSG) | Liposomal amphotericin B (AmBisome) | Paromomycin sulfate (PM) | Miltefosine (MF) |
|---|---|---|---|---|---|
| Route of administration | Slow IV or IM infusion | Slow IV or IM infusion | 2 h IV infusion | IM | PO |
| Dose and duration | 20 mg kg$^{-1}$ day$^{-1}$<br>30 days | 20 mg kg$^{-1}$ day$^{-1}$<br>30 days | 10–30 mg kg$^{-1}$ total dose<br>Over 1–10 days | 15–20 mg kg$^{-1}$ day$^{-1}$<br>21 days | 1.5–2.0 mg kg$^{-1}$ day$^{-1}$<br>28 days |
| Treatment efficiency | 35–95% depending on area, resistance in India | 35–95% depending on area, resistance in India | >95% efficacy in India, variable response in Africa | 93–95% India<br>64–85% Africa | 94–97% |
| Side effects | Painful injections<br>Nephro- and cardiotoxicity<br>Pancreatitis | Painful injections<br>Cardiotoxicity<br>Pancreatitis | Rigors and chills<br>Nephrotoxicity<br>Hypokalaemia<br>Anaphylaxis | Painful injections<br>Reversible nephro-, hepato- and ototoxicity | Teratogenic<br>Gastrointestinal, nephro- and hepatotoxicity |

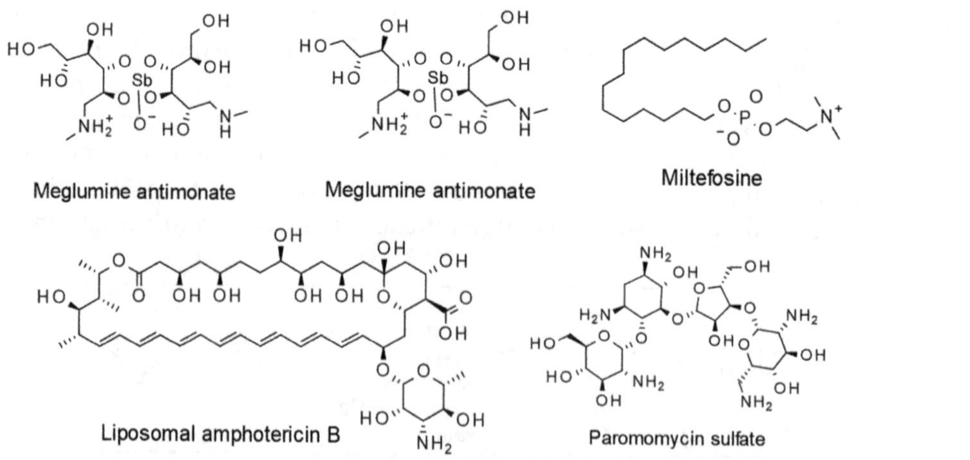


**Figure 26.15** Structures of drugs approved for treatment of visceral leishmaniasis (VL).

### 26.4.4 Challenges in the Discovery of Novel Treatments of HAT and Leishmaniasis

The small number of new drugs targeting kinetoplastid diseases (HAT, leishmaniasis and Chagas disease) that have reached patients over the last decades illustrates the complexity involved in NTD drug discovery both in terms of disease biology and establishing disease-relevant *in vitro* and *in vivo* models that allow the optimisation and evaluation of novel drug candidates. In most cases, kinetoplastid drug discovery relies on phenotypic assays, due to the lack of well-validated biochemical targets allowing for target-based screening. This also limits the possibility to integrate biophysical and structural chemistry methods to support drug design.[81]

Access to well-validated and stable assays able to accurately evaluate SARs is key to progress the optimisation of novel anti-microbials. Fortunately, significant progress has been made over recent years, with the introduction of improved *in vivo* and *in vitro* assays that use, for example, bioluminescence-labelled parasite strains allowing in-life detection of remaining parasites. *In vivo* models exist that reflect both acute and chronic stages of disease, allowing for a well-balanced *in vivo* assessment of compounds and target mechanisms, as well as differentiation *vs.* current standard treatments.

Specific challenges to overcome in kinetoplastid drug discovery includes the need to balance an acceptable physiochemical profile with the need for compounds to reach the parasite target protein residing inside the infected cell, requiring permeation through multiple host cell and parasite membranes. A second challenge is to achieve the selective killing of the parasite, which must be achieved by targeting key parasite housekeeping mechanisms with a high degree of selectivity towards the corresponding mammalian systems, to avoid excessive toxicity.

### 26.4.5 Portfolio Progress and Needs for Novel Treatments of HAT and Leishmaniasis

Significant progress has been made over recent years to replace the existing drug treatments for HAT and leishmaniasis. Based on these efforts, there are now new candidates emerging that can be tested in the clinical trial pipelines, consisting of novel, oral drug treatments with improved safety and efficacy. However, there is a need for novel compounds that expand the mechanistic and chemical diversity to mitigate the risk for late-stage clinical attrition, emerging resistance development, addressing genetic variations both in parasite and host populations (*i.e.* genetic variability in the latter that affects PK). In addition, there is the need to discover and develop new treatments for patient populations not served by the current clinical trial pipeline, *e.g.* HAT caused by *T. b. rhodesiense* and cutaneous leishmaniasis.

#### 26.4.5.1 *Case Study 1: Discovery of DNDI-0690 – a Novel Nitroimidazole for the Treatment of Leishmaniasis*

Nitroimidazoles is a class of compounds with known anti-microbial activity against various parasites, including kinetoplastids. By screening a library of 72 optimised nitroimidazole derivatives for their anti-leishmanial activity, DNDI-VL-2098 was identified and later nominated as a preclinical candidate for the oral treatment of VL. DNDI-VL-2098 showed excellent *in vivo* activity in both mouse and hamster models of VL. Unfortunately, the continued toxicological evaluation identified signs of testicular toxicity in experimental species following prolonged treatment, which led to the decision to stop the progression based on reduced safety margins.[65]

To identify a nitroimidazole back-up series to improve the physicochemical, pharmacological and safety profiles, different nitroimidazole scaffolds were investigated. In particular the 5,6-oxazine-based nitroimidazole scaffold, exemplified by PA-824, appeared attractive, although having poor *in vitro* metabolic stability linked to oxidation of the linker benzylic position. Early attempts to modify the linker attached to the 6-position proved unsuccessful, but finally the stability was improved through a scaffold hop moving the linker from the oxazine 6-position to the 7-position. The resulting compound, X451a, provided good *in vitro* potency (with a *L. don.* $IC_{50}$ of 0.03 μM) and an acceptable metabolic stability *in vitro* (Figure 26.16). Furthermore, modifications identified the two compounds, X451b and X451c, as candidates for an evaluation in the VL mouse and hamster models. Both compounds showed good efficacy in the mouse model when dosed at 25 mg $kg^{-1}$, once a day for 5 days, with 100% and >99% clearance of parasitaemia in mouse and hamster, respectively. However, the overall potency–stability profile was considered better for X451c, thus further work focused on optimising the physiochemical properties of this compound. Replacing the biphenyl for a phenylpyridine improved the aqueous solubility up to 13-fold. This compound, later nominated as DNDI-0690,[67–69] Figure 26.17, displayed an overall profile similar to or slightly improved over DNDI-VL-0298 related to key physicochemical and *in*

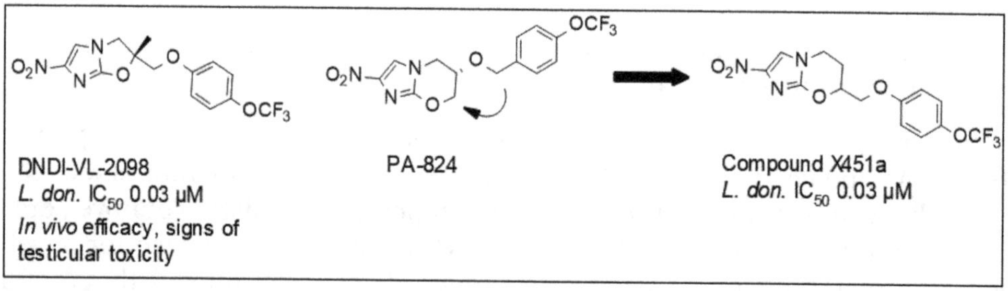


**Figure 26.16** Optimisation of compound X451a.[66]

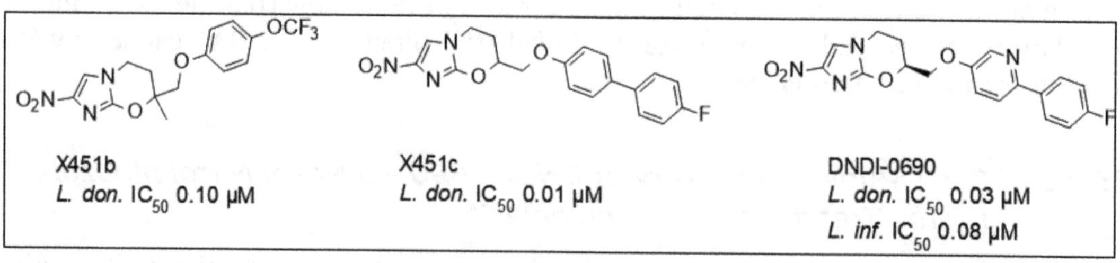


**Figure 26.17** Optimisation of DNDI-0690.

*vitro* selectivity data. DNDI-0690 also showed excellent efficacy in mouse and hamster models of VL. In hamsters infected with *L. infantum* 99.5%, 99.4% and 96.8% parasite clearance was observed in liver, spleen and bone marrow, respectively, when dosing at 12.5 mg $kg^{-1}$ orally twice a day for 5 days. When tested against seven different strains of *L. infantum*, $IC_{50}$ ranging between 0.01 and 0.33 μM was recorded.[70]

Given its excellent safety profile, potent *in vitro* activity and excellent *in vivo* efficacy, the decision was to progress DNDI-0690 into clinical trials for VL with a Phase I single ascending dose study in healthy volunteers initiated in 2019, followed by a multiple ascending dose study in 2020 [ref. https://dndi.org/research-development/portfolio/dndi-0690/, accessed 24 January 2021].

#### 26.4.5.2 Case Study 2: Discovery of Acoziborole for the Treatment of HAT

In the search for novel inhibitors of *T. brucei*, scientists at Anacor Pharmaceuticals screened a focused library of anti-infective benzoxaboroles, which identified a novel inhibitor of *T. brucei* activity ($IC_{50}$ 0.41 μM) that was suitable for further optimisation. Interestingly, X452a was also found to be active in a mouse model of first-stage disease, where clearance parasitaemia and 100% survival were observed 40 days after infection when dosing 50 mg $kg^{-1}$ b.i.d., intraperitoneally (i.p.) for 5 days.[71] Further optimisation of the benzoxaborole led to improved potency and PK properties by varying the linker groups and optimising the phenyl ring substitution. These studies identified the carboxamide-bridged compound SCYX-6759 ($IC_{50}$ 0.21 μM) as a promising candidate for in-depth evaluation in disease models[72] (Figure 26.18).

SCYX-6759 was the first compound with sufficient potency, PK properties and blood–brain barrier permeability to effect a complete cure in a mouse model of stage 2 disease following twice-daily i.p. administration at a dose of 50 mg $kg^{-1}$ for 14 days. Disappointingly however, SCYX-6759 failed to reach similar efficacy when dosed twice-daily orally at 50 mg $kg^{-1}$ for 7 days. Although this compound is well absorbed in the mouse and provides plasma drug levels well in excess of the MIC it fails to reach sufficient brain

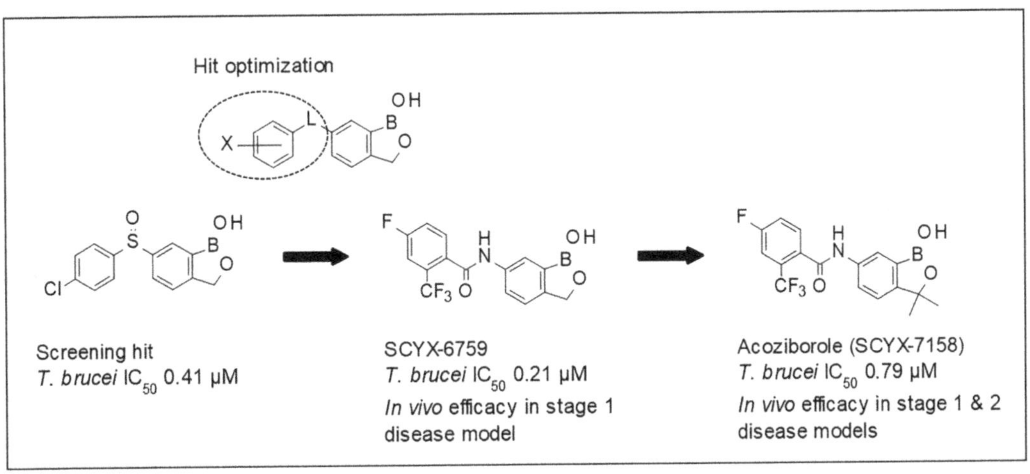


**Figure 26.18** Optimisation of SCYX-7158.[72]

exposure to maintain the MIC between oral dosing, preventing full clearance of parasites residing in the brain.

Consequently, further optimisation of the lead series focused on improving the PK profile, with a particular emphasis on increasing CNS (central nerve system) exposure. The introduction of a C(3) *gem*-methyl group on the oxaborole ring provided the best balance of potency and PK properties. This compound, SCYX-7158 (acoziborole[73–75]), is a potent inhibitor of *T. brucei* activity ($IC_{50}$ 0.79 μM) *in vitro*, and this compound also has similar levels of activity against a panel of different *T. b. rhodesiense* and *T. b. gambiense* strains, with no detectable signs of host cell toxicity. In an *in vitro* washout-out study of the trypanocidal effect, the parasite viability was not restored after 72 h, thus indicating irreversible binding of SCYX-7158 to the target protein (Figure 26.18).

SCYX-7158 is a well-absorbed low-clearance compound that exhibits excellent plasma exposure *in vivo* following oral administration across different species. Importantly, following oral administration, SCYX-7158 produces therapeutically relevant exposure in mouse brains and cerebrospinal fluid.

The *in vivo* efficacy of SCYX-7158 was assessed in a mouse model of stage 2 CNS HAT. In this model, mice are infected with parasites of the *T. b. brucei* TREU 667 strain that produces a persistent haemolymphatic infection within 21 days. When administered as a once-daily oral dose of 12.5 mg $kg^{-1}$ over 7 days starting on day 21 after infection, SCYX-7158 produced an 80% cure rate for *T. b. brucei* infection, with a 100% cure rate observed following 7 daily oral doses of 25 mg $kg^{-1}$.[76]

The mechanism of action of acoziborole is believed to be linked to selective binding to the parasite Cleavage and Polyadenylation Specificity Factor 3 (CPSF3), thereby blocking mRNA processing that is essential for parasite survival.[75]

Acoziborole is currently undergoing clinical Phase IIb/III studies in the Democratic Republic of Congo and Guinea that are expected to finish by the end of 2020. In parallel, non-clinical studies required to meet EMA and US FDA requirements are being progressed.[77]

## 26.5 Onchocerciasis

### 26.5.1 Disease Overview, Filarial Diseases

The filarial worm diseases onchocerciasis (river blindness), *Loa loa* filariasis and lymphatic filariasis (elephantiasis) are causes of substantial morbidity, social stigma and loss of economic growth in tropical and subtropical regions in sub-Saharan Africa. Nearly 150 million people are currently infected with these parasites, of which more than 40 million suffer from symptomatic disease.

Onchocerciasis is an eye and skin disease where symptoms are caused by the early larval forms (microfilariae) residing in the subcutaneous tissue where they evoke intense inflammatory responses when they die. Infected people may show symptoms such as severe itching and various skin changes, and they may also develop eye lesions which can lead to visual impairment and permanent blindness.

### 26.5.2 Pathogen Lifecycle *Onchocerca volvulus*

*Onchocerca volvulus* parasite larvae are transmitted by the female *Simulium* blackfly during blood meals. Following injection, the larvae migrate freely in the subcutaneous tissue where they take residence in subcutaneous nodules. In the nodules, the larvae mature into adult parasites of both sexes. The females dwell in the nodules permanently, while the smaller male worms migrate between nodules to mate. Within 10–12 months of the initial infection the adult worms produce microfilariae that migrate to the skin, eyes and other organs. When a female blackfly bites an infected person during a blood meal it also ingests microfilariae, which develop further in the blackfly and are then transmitted to the next human host during subsequent bites. The reproductive life of the adult worms in humans are about 9–11 years.

### 26.5.3 Current Treatments of Filarial Diseases

There are currently no treatments effective against the *adult* worms, or vaccines preventing *Onchocerca volvulus* infection. However, the *microfilariae* may successfully be targeted by dosing ivermectin every 6 months for up to 15 years, covering the duration of the reproductive lifetime of the adult worms. Ivermectin kills the microfilariae and reduces microfilaridermia by 98–99% after 1–2 months. In areas where *Onchocerca volvulus* co-exists with *Loa loa*, treatment strategies need to be adjusted due to the risk for developing encephalopathy in subjects with high *Loa loa* microfilarial density in blood.

Over the last decades successful prevention programmes have been launched focused on controlling the vector, by spraying insecticides against blackfly larvae and by mass drug administration (MDA) of ivermectin, and more recently, moxidectin (Figure 26.19). These programmes are estimated to have prevented blindness in more than 600 000 people [ref. who.int/news-room/fact-sheets/detail/onchocerciasis, accessed 24 January 2021].

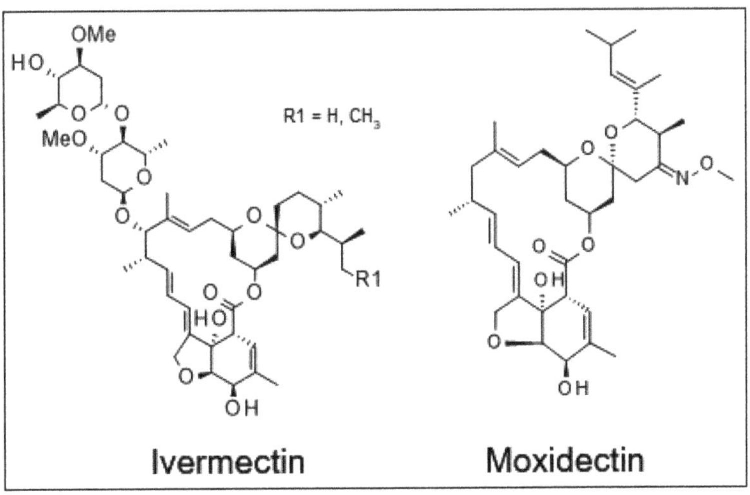


**Figure 26.19** Structures of microfilaricidal compounds.

### 26.5.4 Challenges in the Discovery of Novel Treatments of Onchocerciasis

Current efforts in the discovery of novel agents for treatment of onchocerciasis is limited by access to well-validated assay cascades able to efficiently evaluate the effects against *O. volvulus* microfilariae and adult worms *in vitro* and *in vivo*. The use of insect systems facilitates early-stage identification of agents targeting obligate intracellular bacteria, *Wolbachia* (see below), but for final hit evaluation, filarial *Wolbachia* is required and this continues to represent a bottleneck in drug discovery.

### 26.5.5 Portfolio Progress and Need for Treatments of Filarial Diseases

There is a significant need for improved treatments for onchocerciasis and lymphatic filariasis. In particular, agents able to selectively kill *adult* worms (macrofilaricide) would be highly desirable and is expected to substantially augment the benefits of MDA with current microfilaricides. In addition, access to improved drug treatments could also provide a solution to the treatment of onchocerciasis in the case of *Loa loa* co-infection, where the MDA of ivermectin is restricted.

#### *26.5.5.1 Case Study: Discovery and Development of TylAMac (ABBV-4083) – a Novel Approach to the Treatment of Onchocerciasis*

Filarial worms causing onchocerciasis and lymphatic filariasis carry a symbiotic bacterium, *Wolbachia*, that is essential for worm fertility and ultimate survival. It has been demonstrated that treatment with doxycycline, a broad-spectrum antibiotic, provides an effective treatment of filarial disease through depletion of *Wolbachia*, leading to sterilisation and slow death of the adult worm. In addition, microfilaria depleted of *Wolbachia* are less able to develop in the intermediate blackfly vector. However, doxycycline and other tetracycline-based antibiotics are not well suited for field use as they are contraindicated in children, and in women of child-bearing age. Selective targeting of *Wolbachia* with a safe and efficacious antibiotic would provide an attractive approach to a novel anti-filarial agent.

In an effort to identify novel antibiotics targeting *Wolbachia*, a small collection of 129 antibiotics were tested for antibiotic activity. From the screen, the macrolide Tylosin A (TylA), an antibiotic used in veterinary medicine, was identified as a highly potent anti-*Wolbachia* agent ($EC_{50}$ 28 nM). Other commercially available 16-macrolides were found inactive against *Wolbachia*, similarly 58 synthetic analogues lacking the mycinose sugar residue (Figure 26.20) were also found to be inactive. Notably, tylosin B, containing the mycinose sugar but lacking the mycarose sugar, retained significant anti-*Wolbachia* activity, highlighting the importance of activity linked to the mycinose sugar residue.[78]

Dosed (i.p.) at 200 mg $kg^{-1}$ in a mouse model of filarial disease for 7 days, TylA was found to significantly reduce the length of recovered worms, indicating the suppression of their development. Similar results were obtained when dosing doxycycline for 14 days. However, following oral dosing TylA showed minimal effects on growth, indicating low systemic exposure that could be ascribed to its poor permeability.

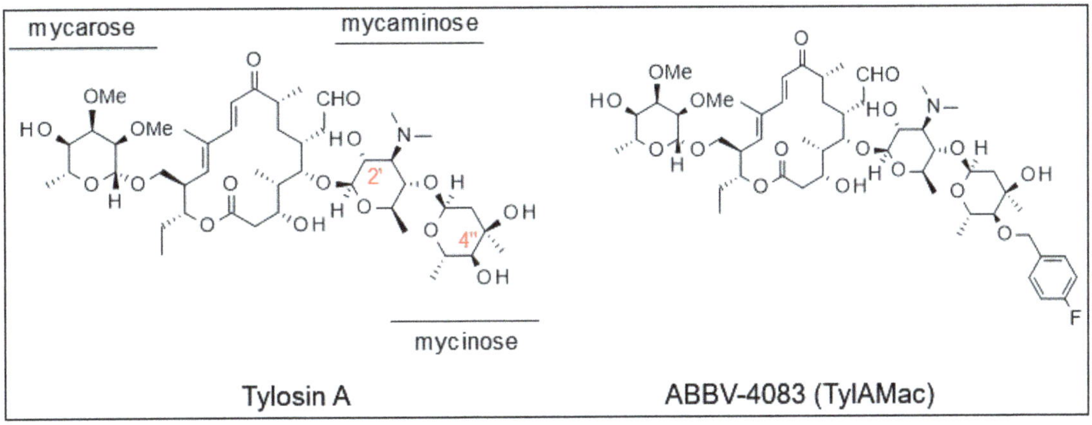


**Figure 26.20** Anti-*Wolbachia* agents.[78]

To address the low permeability of TylA, hypothesised to be linked to the presence of multiple hydroxy groups, the optimisation focused on reducing the number of H-bond donors of TylA by selectively blocking one or more of the hydroxy groups. The initial efforts were focused on acylation of the 2′-hydroxy group, activated by the nearby amino group in the mycaminose sugar fragment, and this led to a 2–3-fold reduction in the anti-*Wolbachia* potency compared to TylA. Importantly, the PK profile significantly improved, compensating for the reduced potency; for example, the 2′-valerate ester provided a ~2.6-fold improvement of the AUC (Area Under the Curve)/$EC_{50}$ compared to TylA, (0.89 *vs.* 0.34). This supported the initial hypothesis and prompted further investigations to modify substitutions on the other chemically accessible hydroxy groups. Modifications to the 4″-hydroxy group on the mycinose sugar residue, similarly to the 2′-hydroxy acylation, led to improved exposure in mice after oral dosing. Interestingly, substitution on the 4″-hydroxy group also led to a significant improvement in the anti-*Wolbachia* potency. This improvement of activity was observed for a range of substitutions: hindered esters, carbamates and benzyl ethers. In particular, the 4-fluorobenzyl substituent provided a significant improvement in both potency and the potency-weighted AUC, with an $EC_{50}$ of 0.019 nM and AUC/$EC_{50}$ of 842. This compound, ABBV-4083, was selected for further studies.

The *in vivo* activity of ABBV-4083 was confirmed in different animal models. When jirds infected with *Litomosoides sigmodontis,* a filarial parasite, were treated with ABBV-4083 at an oral dose of 150 mg $kg^{-1}$, once daily for 14 days, *Wolbachia* levels (measured 16 weeks post-treatment-initiation, pti) were reduced by >99.9% in the recovered female adult worms. As expected, these reductions in *Wolbachia* levels had consequences for worm fertility. At approximately 7 weeks post-treatment-initiation, levels of circulating microfilariae stared to decline and were completely cleared from 12 weeks post-treatment-initiation until the end of this study at 16 weeks post-treatment-initiation. Control animals maintained circulating levels of microfilariae throughout the study. It should be noted that ABBV-4083 is not directly microfilaricidal.

As a preclinical candidate, ABBV-4083 has not produced safety signals in a variety of *in vitro* assays to assess preclinical safety, *e.g.* hERG, *in vitro* genotoxicity and receptor panel screening. ABBV-4083 has been extensively evaluated and found to be safe in 28-day GLP general and reproductive toxicity studies.

Phase I studies have shown that ABBV-4083, now named TylAMac, is safe and well-tolerated and is now prepared for a Phase II proof-of-concept study in the Democratic Republic of Congo.[79]

## 26.6 Conclusion

The drug development portfolios for the diseases covered in this book chapter have been transformed over the last two decades through the work of PDPs and multiple global partnerships focused on delivering against patient-focused target product profiles. At the heart of these innovations is the application of medicinal chemistry and high-quality drug discovery and development thinking. Anti-pathogen medicinal chemistry presents myriad challenges in terms of working with complicated, low-throughput assays, demanding criteria in relation to pharmacokinetics and safety. Furthermore, given the target patient populations, the need to consider dose size, formulations for vulnerable populations, such as children, and cost of goods and cost per dose become critical. Many of these challenges are not considered in the cases of diseases of the First World, and thus there are unique translational learnings for the broader community from the medicinal chemistry and drug discovery work on neglected and tropical diseases.

## 26.7 Hints and Tips

- If you or your organisation wants to join in the fight against diseases of the poor, then contact the authors at the product development partnerships MMV (www.mmv.org), GATB (www.tballiance.org/) and DNDi (www.dndi.org).
- For all neglected and tropical diseases, the key is to focus discovery efforts on chemical series which are not cross-resistant with any clinical or marketed anti-infective (if known). This maximises the potential for efficacy even in resistant populations.
- Drug discovery for malaria, tuberculosis and diseases caused by kinetoplastids or helminths has had a renaissance in the last decade due to increased investment and a focus on following up on hits identified from phenotypic screens that inhibit growth and kill the pathogen.
- Offer your compounds! A huge amount of screening has been done, and finding new, interesting compound sets to interrogate is becoming increasingly difficult. If you have compound libraries with unique qualities or novelty, then these could be particularly interesting to have screened in the anti-parasitic and anti-bacterial assays mentioned in this chapter.
- Medicinal chemistry optimisation focuses on optimising phenotypic potency, minimising known safety risks and optimising pharmacokinetics.
- We still know so little! Knowledge of molecular targets and pathways for all of these diseases is improving dramatically, but is still far removed from the state of biology for human diseases with commercial focus.
- Invite your biology colleagues to join the fight! The corollary is that there is a huge opportunity to advance the basic science and biology, and to apply new technologies; the PDPs mentioned above can help in this regard.
- The quality of a candidate drug for a neglected or tropical disease depends on the nature of the disease and the quality of the standard of care. It is critical that any

new candidate drug improves upon what already exists and shows clear differentiation in key properties such as efficacy, safety and total dose to cure.
- The lower the dose and the fewer the doses the better! Given the targeted patient populations, the affordability of the drug (based on the cost to produce a given dose) and the overall pill burden is critical.
- As with any drug discovery project, the target product profile (TPP) should be defined in advance, along with a testing cascade defining the necessary *in vitro* and *in vivo* assays and milestone criteria necessary for success at every stage. This is particularly important in a disease where research is paid through donor funding, because resource constraints are inevitable.
- When working in large, global collaborations, having centralised testing centres with assays that have been well validated to test critical compounds is extremely important in being able to compare series.
- Get involved! Working on diseases without commercial incentives provides a unique opportunity for sharing of information. In several cases, open-source projects exist that welcome input from external scientists (www.mmv.org/mmv-open/malaria-libre, www.opensourcemalaria.org/, https://dndi.org/partnerships/partnering-with-us/, https://dndi.org/research-development/drug-discovery/)

## Key References

1. M. Phillips, J. Burrows, and C. Manyando, *et al.*, Malaria, *Nat. Rev. Dis. Primers*, 2017, **3**, 17050, DOI: 10.1038/nrdp.2017.50.
2. S. P. S. Rao, M. P. Barrett, and G. Dranoff, *et al.*, Drug Discovery for Kinetoplastid Diseases: Future Directions, *ACS Infect. Dis.*, 2019, **5**, 152, DOI: 10.1021/acsinfecdis.8b00298.
3. B. B. Aldridge, D. Barros-Aguirre, and C. E. Barry, *et al.*, The Tuberculosis Drug Accelerator at year 10: what have we learned?, *Nat. Med.*, 2021, **27**, 1333, DOI: 10.1038/s41591-021-01442-2.
4. F. A. Partridge, R. Forman, and C. J. R. Bataille, *et al.*, Anthelmintic drug discovery: target identification, screening methods and the role of open science, *Beilstein J. Org. Chem.*, 2020, **16**, 1203, DOI: 10.3762/bjoc.16.105.

## Acknowledgements

We wish to thank Rob Hooft for his help with formatting and editing the article.

## References

1. World Health Organization, https://www.who.int/neglected_diseases/diseases/en/, 2020.
2. C. Fitzpatrick, U. Nwankwo, E. Lenk, S. J. de Vlas and D. A. P. Bundy, in *Major Infectious Diseases*, ed. K. K. Holmes, S. Bertozzi, B. R. Bloom and P. Jha, The International Bank for Reconstruction and Development/ The World Bank © 2017 International Bank for Reconstruction and Development/ The World Bank, Washington (DC), 2017.
3. R. K. Harrison, *Nat. Rev. Drug Discovery*, 2016, **15**, 817–818.

4. M. A. Phillips, J. N. Burrows, C. Manyando, R. Hooft van Huijsduijnen, W. C. Van Voorhis and T. N. C. Wells, *Nat. Rev. Dis. Primers*, 2017, **3**, 17050.
5. World Health Organization, https://www.who.int/publications/i/item/9789240015791, 2020.
6. A. M. van Eijk, P. L. Sutton, L. Ramanathapuram, S. A. Sullivan, D. Kanagaraj, G. S. L. Priya, S. Ravishankaran, A. Asokan, V. Sangeetha, P. N. Rao, S. C. Wassmer, N. Tandel, A. Patel, N. Desai, S. Choubey, S. Z. Ali, P. Barla, R. R. Oraon, S. Mohanty, S. Mishra, S. Kale, N. Bandyopadhyay, P. K. Mallick, J. Huck, N. Valecha, O. P. Singh, K. Pradhan, R. Singh, S. K. Sharma, H. C. Srivastava, J. M. Carlton and A. Eapen, *Sci. Rep.*, 2019, **9**, 17095.
7. D. N. R. Roman, N. N. A. Rosalie, A. Kumar, K. M. M. Luther, V. Singh and M. S. Albert, *Parasitol. Int.*, 2018, **67**, 29–33.
8. Hale Collaborators, *Lancet*, 2018, **392**, 1859–1922.
9. World Health Organization, https://www.who.int/neglected_diseases/Revised-Draft-NTD-Roadmap-23Apr2020.pdf, 2020.
10. World Health Organization, http://who.int/malaria/areas/global_technical_strategy/en/, 2016.
11. C. M. Andrade, H. Fleckenstein, R. Thomson-Luque, S. Doumbo, N. F. Lima, C. Anderson, J. Hibbert, C. S. Hopp, T. M. Tran, S. Li, M. Niangaly, H. Cisse, D. Doumtabe, J. Skinner, D. Sturdevant, S. Ricklefs, K. Virtaneva, M. Asghar, M. V. Homann, L. Turner, J. Martins, E. L. Allman, M. E. N'Dri, V. Winkler, M. Llinas, C. Lavazec, C. Martens, A. Farnert, K. Kayentao, A. Ongoiba, T. Lavstsen, N. S. Osorio, T. D. Otto, M. Recker, B. Traore, P. D. Crompton and S. Portugal, *Nat. Med.*, 2020, **26**, 1929–1940.
12. R. R. Schumann, *Proc. Natl. Acad. Sci. U. S. A.*, 2007, **104**, 1743–1744.
13. T. Gebru, A. Lalremruata, P. G. Kremsner, B. Mordmuller and J. Held, *Malar. J.*, 2017, **16**, 330.
14. W. R. Shaw, I. E. Holmdahl, M. A. Itoe, K. Werling, M. Marquette, D. G. Paton, N. Singh, C. O. Buckee, L. M. Childs and F. Catteruccia, *PLoS Pathog.*, 2020, **16**, e1009131.
15. A. Molina-Cruz, G. E. Canepa, N. Kamath, N. V. Pavlovic, J. Mu, U. N. Ramphul, J. L. Ramirez and C. Barillas-Mury, *Proc. Natl. Acad. Sci. U. S. A.*, 2015, **112**, 15178–15183.
16. L. T. Keegan and J. Dushoff, *BMC Infect. Dis.*, 2013, **13**, 428.
17. D. L. Doolan, C. Dobano and J. K. Baird, *Clin. Microbiol. Rev.*, 2009, **22**, 13–36, Table of Contents.
18. N. Harrison, *Lancet Infect. Dis.*, 2015, **15**, 1143.
19. C. J. Woodrow, T. Planche and S. Krishna, *Lancet*, 2006, **367**, 110–111; Author reply 111–112.
20. K. L. Jones, S. Donegan and D. G. Lalloo, *Cochrane Database Syst. Rev.*, 2007, CD005967.
21. L. von Seidlein and J. L. Deen, *Lancet*, 2009, **373**, 522–523.
22. A. Llanos-Cuentas, M. V. G. Lacerda, T. T. Hien, I. D. Vélez, C. Namaik-Larp, C. S. Chu, M. F. Villegas, F. Val, W. M. Monteiro, M. A. M. Brito, M. R. F. Costa, R. Chuquiyauri, M. Casapía, C. H. Nguyen, S. Aruachan, R. Papwijitsil, F. H. Nosten, G. Bancone, B. Angus, S. Duparc, G. Craig, V. M. Rousell, S. W. Jones, E. Hardaker, D. D. Clover, L. Kendall, K. Mohamed, G. C. K. W. Koh, V. M. Wilches, J. J. Breton and J. A. Green, *N. Engl. J. Med.*, 2019, **380**, 229–241.
23. J. D. Berman, *Am. J. Trop. Med. Hyg.*, 2019, **100**(6), 1301–1304.
24. C. S. Chu, D. O. Freedman and W. C. Gorgas, *J. Travel Med.*, 2019, **26**, 1–11.
25. J. N. Burrows, S. Duparc, W. E. Gutteridge, R. Hooft van Huijsduijnen, W. Kaszubska, F. Macintyre, S. Mazzuri, J. J. Mohrle and T. N. C. Wells, *Malar. J.*, 2017, **16**, 26.
26. F. Macintyre, H. Ramachandruni, J. N. Burrows, R. Holm, A. Thomas, J. J. Mohrle, S. Duparc, R. Hooft van Huijsduijnen, B. Greenwood, W. E. Gutteridge, T. N. C. Wells and W. Kaszubska, *Malar. J.*, 2018, **17**, 402.
27. J. G. Kublin, S. C. Murphy, J. Maenza, A. M. Seilie, J. P. Jain, D. Berger, D. Spera, R. Zhao, R. L. Soon, J. L. Czartoski, M. A. Potochnic, E. Duke, M. Chang, A. Vaughan, S. H. I. Kappe, F. J. Leong, P. Pertel and W. T. Prince, *Clin. Infect. Dis.*, 2020, e2407–e2414.
28. K. Katsuno, J. N. Burrows, K. Duncan, R. Hooft van Huijsduijnen, T. Kaneko, K. Kita, C. E. Mowbray, D. Schmatz, P. Warner and B. T. Slingsby, *Nat. Rev. Drug Discovery*, 2015, **14**, 751–758.
29. J. S. McCarthy, T. Ruckle, S. L. Elliott, E. Ballard, K. A. Collins, L. Marquart, P. Griffin, S. Chalon and J. J. Mohrle, *Antimicrob. Agents Chemother.*, 2020, **64**, e01371.
30. S. C. Murphy, E. R. Duke, K. J. Shipman, R. L. Jensen, Y. Fong, S. Ferguson, H. E. Janes, K. Gillespie, A. M. Seilie, A. E. Hanron, L. Rinn, M. Fishbaugher, T. VonGoedert, E. Fritzen, S. H. Kappe, M. Chang, J. C. Sousa, S. R. Marcsisin, S. Chalon, S. Duparc, N. Kerr, J. J. Möhrle, N. Andenmatten, T. Rueckle and J. G. Kublin, *J. Infect. Dis.*, 2018, **217**, 693–702.
31. S. C. Murphy, E. R. Duke, K. J. Shipman, R. L. Jensen, Y. Fong, S. Ferguson, H. E. Janes, K. Gillespie, A. M. Seilie, A. E. Hanron, L. Rinn, M. Fishbaugher, T. VonGoedert, E. Fritzen, S. H. Kappe, M. Chang, J. C. Sousa, S. R. Marcsisin, S. Chalon, S. Duparc, N. Kerr, J. J. Mohrle, N. Andenmatten, T. Rueckle and J. G. Kublin, *J. Infect. Dis.*, 2018, **217**, 693–702.

32. A. Llanos-Cuentas, M. Casapia, R. Chuquiyauri, J.-C. Hinojosa, N. Kerr, M. Rosario, S. Toovey, R. H. Arch, M. A. Phillips, F. D. Rozenberg, J. Bath, C. L. Ng, A. N. Cowell, E. A. Winzeler, D. A. Fidock, M. Baker, J. J. Möhrle, R. Hooft van Huijsduijnen, N. Gobeau, N. Araeipour, N. Andenmatten, T. Rückle and S. Duparc, *Lancet Infect. Dis.*, 2018, **18**, 874–883.
33. K. A. Collins, T. Ruckle, S. Elliott, L. Marquart, E. Ballard, S. Chalon, P. Griffin, J. J. Mohrle and J. S. McCarthy, *Antimicrob. Agents Chemother.*, 2019, **63**, e01837.
34. J. White, S. Dhingra, X. Deng, F. El Mazouni, M. Lee, G. Afanador, A. Lawong, D. R. Tomchick, C. L. Ng, J. Bath, P. K. Rathod, D. A. Fidock and M. A. Phillips, *ACS Infect. Dis.*, 2019, **5**, 90–101.
35. S. Belard and M. Ramharter, *Lancet Infect. Dis.*, 2018, **18**, 819–820.
36. R. Gujjar, A. Marwaha, F. El Mazouni, J. White, K. L. White, S. Creason, D. M. Shackleford, J. Baldwin, W. N. Charman, F. S. Buckner, S. Charman, P. K. Rathod and M. A. Phillips, *J. Med. Chem.*, 2009, **52**, 1864–1872.
37. E. S. H. El Ashry, L. F. Awad, M. Teleb, N. A. Ibrahim, M. M. Abu-Serie and M. N. Abd Al Moaty, *Bioorg. Chem.*, 2020, **96**, 103616.
38. J. S. McCarthy, J. Lotharius, A. Dayan, M. Phillips, K. Marsh, D. Walker, M. Baker, S. Elliott, P. Griffin, C. Ng, D. Fidock, L. Bebrevska, S. Duparc, J. Möhrle and T. Rückle, *ASTMH Annual Meeting*, 2014, **Abstract 675**, 204–205.
39. T. Rückle, S. Duparc, N. Kerr, M. Rosario, P. Qiu, M. A. Phillips, M. Baker, S. Chalon, J. J. Möhrle, M. Casapia, J.-C. Hinojosa and A. Llanos-Cuentas, in *American Society of Tropical Medicine and Hygiene 64th Annual Meeting*, Philadelphia, USA, 2015, vol. 857.
40. M. Sulyok, T. Ruckle, A. Roth, R. E. Murbeth, S. Chalon, N. Kerr, S. S. Samec, N. Gobeau, C. L. Calle, J. Ibanez, Z. Sulyok, J. Held, T. Gebru, P. Granados, S. Bruckner, C. Nguetse, J. Mengue, A. Lalremruata, B. K. L. Sim, S. L. Hoffman, J. J. Mohrle, P. G. Kremsner and B. Mordmuller, *Lancet Infect. Dis.*, 2017, **17**, 636–644.
41. World Health Organization, https://www.who.int/teams/global-tuberculosis-programme/data, 2020.
42. A. M. Cooper, *Annu. Rev. Immunol.*, 2009, **27**, 393–422.
43. T. R. Frieden, T. R. Sterling, S. S. Munsiff, C. J. Watt and C. Dye, *Lancet*, 2003, **362**, 887–899.
44. C. Nathan, *Sci. Transl. Med.*, 2012, **4**, 140sr142.
45. J. F. Murray, *Am. J. Respir. Crit. Care Med.*, 2003, **168**, 1029–1033.
46. J. M. Davis and L. Ramakrishnan, *Cell*, 2009, **136**, 37–49.
47. M. Palaci, R. Dietze, D. J. Hadad, F. K. Ribeiro, R. L. Peres, S. A. Vinhas, E. L. Maciel, V. do Valle Dettoni, L. Horter, W. H. Boom, J. L. Johnson and K. D. Eisenach, *J. Clin. Microbiol.*, 2007, **45**, 4064–4066.
48. C. K. Kwan and J. D. Ernst, *Clin. Microbiol. Rev.*, 2011, **24**, 351–376.
49. G. Kaplan, F. A. Post, A. L. Moreira, H. Wainwright, B. N. Kreiswirth, M. Tanverdi, B. Mathema, S. V. Ramaswamy, G. Walther, L. M. Steyn, C. E. Barry 3rd and L. G. Bekker, *Infect. Immun.*, 2003, **71**, 7099–7108.
50. A. S. Dharmadhikari and E. A. Nardell, *Am. J. Respir. Cell Mol. Biol.*, 2008, **39**, 503–508.
51. F. Conradie, A. H. Diacon, N. Ngubane, P. Howell, D. Everitt, A. M. Crook, C. M. Mendel, E. Egizi, J. Moreira, J. Timm, T. D. McHugh, G. H. Wills, A. Bateson, R. Hunt, C. Van Niekerk, M. Li, M. Olugbosi, M. Spigelman and T. B. T. T. Nix, *N. Engl. J. Med.*, 2020, **382**, 893–902.
52. A. S. Fauci and R. W. Eisinger, *Am. J. Trop. Med. Hyg.*, 2018, **98**, 650–652.
53. Y. Zhang, W. W. Yew and M. R. Barer, *Antimicrob. Agents Chemother.*, 2012, **56**, 2223–2230.
54. P. Nahid, S. E. Dorman, N. Alipanah, P. M. Barry, J. L. Brozek, A. Cattamanchi, L. H. Chaisson, R. E. Chaisson, C. L. Daley, M. Grzemska, J. M. Higashi, C. S. Ho, P. C. Hopewell, S. A. Keshavjee, C. Lienhardt, R. Menzies, C. Merrifield, M. Narita, R. O'Brien, C. A. Peloquin, A. Raftery, J. Saukkonen, H. S. Schaaf, G. Sotgiu, J. R. Starke, G. B. Migliori and A. Vernon, *Clin. Infect. Dis.*, 2016, **63**, e147–e195.
55. R. Moodley, T. R. Godec and S. T. Team, *Eur. Respir. Rev.*, 2016, **25**, 29–35.
56. A. T. Vincent, S. Nyongesa, I. Morneau, M. B. Reed, E. I. Tocheva and F. J. Veyrier, *Front. Microbiol.*, 2018, **9**, 2341.
57. J. Wise, *BMJ*, 1998, **316**, 957.
58. A. Pooran, E. Pieterson, M. Davids, G. Theron and K. Dheda, *PLoS One*, 2013, **8**, e54587.
59. P. S. Shirude, R. Shandil, C. Sadler, M. Naik, V. Hosagrahara, S. Hameed, V. Shinde, C. Bathula, V. Humnabadkar, N. Kumar, J. Reddy, V. Panduga, S. Sharma, A. Ambady, N. Hegde, J. Whiteaker, R. E. McLaughlin, H. Gardner, P. Madhavapeddi, V. Ramachandran, P. Kaur, A. Narayan, S. Guptha, D. Awasthy, C. Narayan, J. Mahadevaswamy, K. G. Vishwas, V. Ahuja, A. Srivastava, K. R. Prabhakar, S. Bharath, R. Kale, M. Ramaiah, N. R. Choudhury, V. K. Sambandamurthy, S. Solapure, P. S. Iyer, S. Narayanan and M. Chatterji, *J. Med. Chem.*, 2013, **56**, 9701–9708.

60. P. S. Shirude, R. K. Shandil, M. R. Manjunatha, C. Sadler, M. Panda, V. Panduga, J. Reddy, R. Saralaya, R. Nanduri, A. Ambady, S. Ravishankar, V. K. Sambandamurthy, V. Humnabadkar, L. K. Jena, R. S. Suresh, A. Srivastava, K. R. Prabhakar, J. Whiteaker, R. E. McLaughlin, S. Sharma, C. B. Cooper, K. Mdluli, S. Butler, P. S. Iyer, S. Narayanan and M. Chatterji, *J. Med. Chem.*, 2014, **57**, 5728–5737.
61. V. Makarov, B. Lechartier, M. Zhang, J. Neres, A. M. van der Sar, S. A. Raadsen, R. C. Hartkoorn, O. B. Ryabova, A. Vocat, L. A. Decosterd, N. Widmer, T. Buclin, W. Bitter, K. Andries, F. Pojer, P. J. Dyson and S. T. Cole, *EMBO Mol. Med.*, 2014, **6**, 372–383.
62. B. T. Priest, I. M. Bell and M. L. Garcia, *Channels*, 2008, **2**, 87–93.
63. M. Chatterji, R. Shandil, M. R. Manjunatha, S. Solapure, V. Ramachandran, N. Kumar, R. Saralaya, V. Panduga, J. Reddy, K. R. Prabhakar, S. Sharma, C. Sadler, C. B. Cooper, K. Mdluli, P. S. Iyer, S. Narayanan and P. S. Shirude, *Antimicrob. Agents Chemother.*, 2014, **58**, 5325–5331.
64. Drugs for Neglected Diseases *initiative*, https://dndi.org/research-development/portfolio/fexinidazole-tb-rhodesiense/, 2020, accessed 15 January 2021.
65. Drugs for Neglected Diseases initiative, https://dndi.org/research-development/portfolio/vl-2098/, 2021, accessed 15 January 2021.
66. S. Gupta, V. Yardley, P. Vishwakarma, R. Shivahare, B. Sharma, D. Launay, D. Martin and S. K. Puri, *J. Antimicrob. Chemother.*, 2015, **70**, 518–527.
67. A. M. Thompson, P. D. O'Connor, A. J. Marshall, V. Yardley, L. Maes, S. Gupta, D. Launay, S. Braillard, E. Chatelain, B. Wan, S. G. Franzblau, Z. Ma, C. B. Cooper and W. A. Denny, *Eur. J. Med. Chem.*, 2021, **209**, 112914.
68. G. J. Wijnant, S. L. Croft, R. de la Flor, M. Alavijeh, V. Yardley, S. Braillard, C. Mowbray and K. Van Bocxlaer, *Antimicrob. Agents Chemother.*, 2019, **63**.
69. K. Van Bocxlaer, D. Caridha, C. Black, B. Vesely, S. Leed, R. J. Sciotti, G. J. Wijnant, V. Yardley, S. Braillard, C. E. Mowbray, J. R. Ioset and S. L. Croft, *Int. J. Parasitol.: Drugs Drug Resist.*, 2019, **11**, 129–138.
70. M. Van den Kerkhof, D. Mabille, E. Chatelain, C. E. Mowbray, S. Braillard, S. Hendrickx, L. Maes and G. Caljon, *Int. J. Parasitol.: Drugs Drug Resist.*, 2018, **8**, 81–86.
71. D. Ding, Y. Zhao, Q. Meng, D. Xie, B. Nare, D. Chen, C. J. Bacchi, N. Yarlett, Y. K. Zhang, V. Hernandez, Y. Xia, Y. Freund, M. Abdulla, K. H. Ang, J. Ratnam, J. H. McKerrow, R. T. Jacobs, H. Zhou and J. J. Plattner, *ACS Med. Chem. Lett.*, 2010, **1**, 165–169.
72. B. Nare, S. Wring, C. Bacchi, B. Beaudet, T. Bowling, R. Brun, D. Chen, C. Ding, Y. Freund, E. Gaukel, A. Hussain, K. Jarnagin, M. Jenks, M. Kaiser, L. Mercer, E. Mejia, A. Noe, M. Orr, R. Parham, J. Plattner, R. Randolph, D. Rattendi, C. Rewerts, J. Sligar, N. Yarlett, R. Don and R. Jacobs, *Antimicrob. Agents Chemother.*, 2010, **54**, 4379–4388.
73. E. A. Dickie, F. Giordani, M. K. Gould, P. Maser, C. Burri, J. C. Mottram, S. P. S. Rao and M. P. Barrett, *Trop. Med. Infect. Dis.*, 2020, **5**.
74. K. J. Meyer, D. J. Meyers and T. A. Shapiro, *J. Antimicrob. Chemother.*, 2019, **74**, 2303–2310.
75. R. J. Wall, E. Rico, I. Lukac, F. Zuccotto, S. Elg, I. H. Gilbert, Y. Freund, M. R. K. Alley, M. C. Field, S. Wyllie and D. Horn, *Proc. Natl. Acad. Sci. U. S. A.*, 2018, **115**, 9616–9621.
76. R. T. Jacobs, B. Nare, S. A. Wring, M. D. Orr, D. Chen, J. M. Sligar, M. X. Jenks, R. A. Noe, T. S. Bowling, L. T. Mercer, C. Rewerts, E. Gaukel, J. Owens, R. Parham, R. Randolph, B. Beaudet, C. J. Bacchi, N. Yarlett, J. J. Plattner, Y. Freund, C. Ding, T. Akama, Y. K. Zhang, R. Brun, M. Kaiser, I. Scandale and R. Don, *PLoS Neglected Trop. Dis.*, 2011, **5**, e1151.
77. Drugs for Neglected Diseases *initiative* https://dndi.org/research-development/portfolio/acoziborole/, 2021, accessed 15 January 2021.
78. T. W. von Geldern, H. E. Morton, R. F. Clark, B. S. Brown, K. L. Johnston, L. Ford, S. Specht, R. A. Carr, D. F. Stolarik, J. Ma, M. J. Rieser, D. Struever, S. J. Frohberger, M. Koschel, A. Ehrens, J. D. Turner, M. P. Hübner, A. Hoerauf, M. J. Taylor, S. A. Ward, K. Marsh and D. J. Kempf, *PLoS Neglected Trop. Dis.*, 2019, **13**, e0007159.
79. Drugs for Neglected Diseases *initiative* https://dndi.org/research-development/portfolio/abbv-4083/, 2021, accessed 15 January 2021.
80. www.tballiance.org/portfolio, accessed February 2022.
81. S. P. S. Rao, M. P. Barrett and G. Dranoff, *et al.*, Drug Discovery for Kinetoplastid Diseases: Future Directions, *ACS Infect. Dis.*, 2019, **5**, 152.
82. B. B. Aldridge, D. Barros-Aguirre and C. E. Barry, *et al.*, The Tuberculosis Drug Accelerator at year 10: what have we learned?, *Nat. Med.*, 2021, **27**, 1333.
83. F. A. Partridge, R. Forman and C. J. R. Bataille, *et al.*, Anthelmintic drug discovery: target identification, screening methods and the role of open science, *Beilstein J. Org. Chem.*, 2020, **16**, 1203.

# 27 New Therapeutic Chemical Modalities: Compositions, Modes-of-action, and Drug Discovery

Eric Valeur*[a]

[a]Roivant Sciences Inc., 451D Street, Boston MA 02210, USA
*E-mail: eric.valeur@roivant.com

## 27.1 Introduction

The opportunity to treat diseases and help patients live a better life is one of the key inspirations for many medicinal chemists. While many successes have been met, from drugs such as Glivec,[1] treating a previously uncurable cancer, to anti-HIV drugs,[2] or rare disease treatment such as for cystic fibrosis,[3] many conditions remain either unaddressed or are merely mitigated by symptom treatment rather than correcting the underlying cause of the disease. The need to address this unmet medical need has pushed scientific investigations into uncharted biology territory, unveiling regulation and signalling pathways and mechanisms of increasing complexity. Unfortunately, while many drug targets are addressable by well-established modalities, namely small molecules and proteins/antibodies, several protein targets are less well suited for these modalities. Indeed, novel biology, augmented by a range of target hypotheses generated through multiple genomic efforts from patient samples, is revealing potential drug targets that require alternative modalities for modulation.[4] Many medicinal chemists have experienced frustration with trying to identify and optimise small molecules against 'undruggable' targets such as transcription factors, phosphatases, and protein–protein interactions.

In the pursuit of learning from nature,[5] a wealth of creative molecules have emerged to address such targets, not only by aiming at modulating a protein function directly, *via* agonism and antagonism, but also intervening prior to protein synthesis. For example, many molecules have been engineered to bind and modulate RNA. Using an oligonucleotide,

The Handbook of Medicinal Chemistry: Principles and Practice, 2nd Edition
Edited by Simon E. Ward and Andrew M. Davis

Published by the Royal Society of Chemistry, www.rsc.org

mRNA levels can be altered for any protein target, in theory. These new classes of molecules, called New Modalities (NMs), have moved from scepticism to marketed drugs (see Table 27.4 in Section 27.7), and in some cases are redefining the therapeutic landscape by fundamentally changing the targetable space. Thus, the so-called 'undruggable' proteins have progressively evolved into 'challenging' or 'hard-to-drug' targets.

The concept of NMs expands beyond synthetically accessible molecules. In this respect, genome-editing approaches are promising to correct any genetic defect, thereby addressing a need difficult to meet with other modalities. Higher-order structures, such as cell therapy,[6–8] and microbes,[9–11] also represent novel modalities. In addition to the development of NMs, additional uses of classical modalities such as some of those described in this book, are contributing to reshaping how diseases can be treated. For example, modulating splicing or blocking translation with small molecules contribute to expanding the range of modes-of-action (MOAs) that medicinal chemists can exploit.

Many NM approaches represent useful strategies to identify and develop chemical probes for hard-to-drug targets. While some of these are described in this chapter, the interested reader is directed to previous reviews from the author.[12–16] This chapter places more emphasis on new chemical modalities that have progressed to late drug discovery, clinical development, or even market. Nevertheless, the first section describes what NMs are made of from a chemical composition standpoint. In particular, beyond individual classes of molecules, fusions or conjugates can also be created to leverage enhanced binding affinities, modulate properties, and even create novel MOAs. Having mapped out the chemical space of NM, the potential MOAs of these modalities are then discussed in Section 27.3. Sections 27.4 and 27.5 then cover drug discovery aspects for these NMs, namely hit finding strategies, and the parameters/limitations to consider during optimisation. Finally, having illustrated all the components, opportunities, and limitations of NMs, Section 27.6 takes a holistic view of drug discovery for project inception and provides a framework for selecting preferred modalities, both classical and new, for a given biological target, with a focus, there again, on more validated modalities.

## 27.2 Chemical Compositions and Architectures

Beyond small molecules/natural products and proteins, nature has created a wealth of other molecules from other areas of the chemical space, including nucleic acids, lipids, and carbohydrates. All of these have been targeted in some form with the potential of forming different therapeutic modalities. In this section, the chemical composition of the most advanced modalities from a drug discovery and development standpoint are described. Other examples, less validated, are also presented to demonstrate the breadth of the types of molecules that can be constructed.

### 27.2.1 Main Chemical Categories of New Modalities as Single Entities

#### *27.2.1.1 Oligonucleotides*

With the blueprint for life on Earth being based on DNA and RNA, nucleic acids are at the centre of biological processes. In fact, protein-coding genes only represent about 2% of the genome,[17] and even proteins themselves originate from DNA and mRNA.

Mimicking the chemical composition and the canonical interaction topology, *i.e.* duplex formation *via* Watson–Crick base pairing, the interest in so-called oligonucleotides (ONs) has surged over the past two decades.[18] These polymers leverage individual building blocks composed of three elements: a core carbohydrate onto which a nucleobase and a phosphate are attached. Elongation into ONs of variable but controlled length occurs *via* linkage of the phosphate group to a hydroxy group from another carbohydrate monomer. Beyond the principle of oligomerisation, nucleic-acid based modalities can be constituted of a single linear strand (antisense oligonucleotides or ASOs, and modified mRNA), double strand (small interfering RNA or siRNA), or folded single strand (aptamers) (Figure 27.1). Depending on the targeted MOA, ONs can vastly vary in length (from ~16 to thousands of nucleotides), and in the composition of the carbohydrate, nucleobase, and phosphate backbone (Figure 27.2). In particular, with the aim of modulating properties such as binding affinity and stability,[19–22] a wealth of modifications have been designed and synthesised.[23]

The phosphate backbone is the central weakness of ONs in terms of stability. Indeed, endo- and exo-nucleases easily hydrolyse these bonds, resulting in short half-lives *in vivo*. Thus, exchanging the natural phosphodiester moiety with a phosphorothioate (PS) linkage can dramatically enhance stability, and this alternate backbone is broadly used.[24] Further backbone modifications, such as phosphoroboran have also been explored, but are to date not present in clinical-stage ONs.[25]

The nucleobase element can also be altered, although Watson–Crick base pairing still needs to be retained,[26–28] and modified nucleobases are primarily pyrimidines, due to the instability of many purine modifications.[29,30] In particular, increased nuclease resistance and enhanced duplex stability can be achieved with methyl, propyne, phenyl, or thiazole moieties installed at position 5 of pyrimidines.[28] One important modification is the substitution of cytidine at the 5 position with a methyl group. This change addresses the common activation of immune responses when CG motifs are present in the ON sequence, and the methyl group has been shown to reduce this issue.[31] In the context of modified mRNA, other important modifications include *N*1-methylpseudouridine and 5-methoxyuridine, in particular to reduce immune activation and enhance translation.[32–34]

Perhaps the most extensively and systematically studied element has been the carbohydrate composition. Indeed, modifications of this component have enabled not only

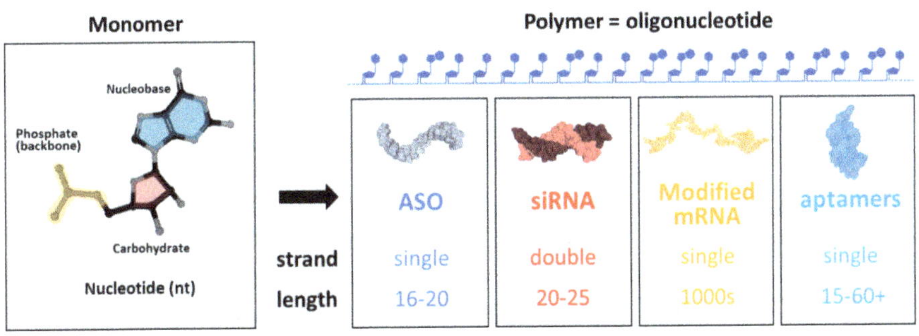


**Figure 27.1** Characteristics of different oligonucleotides.

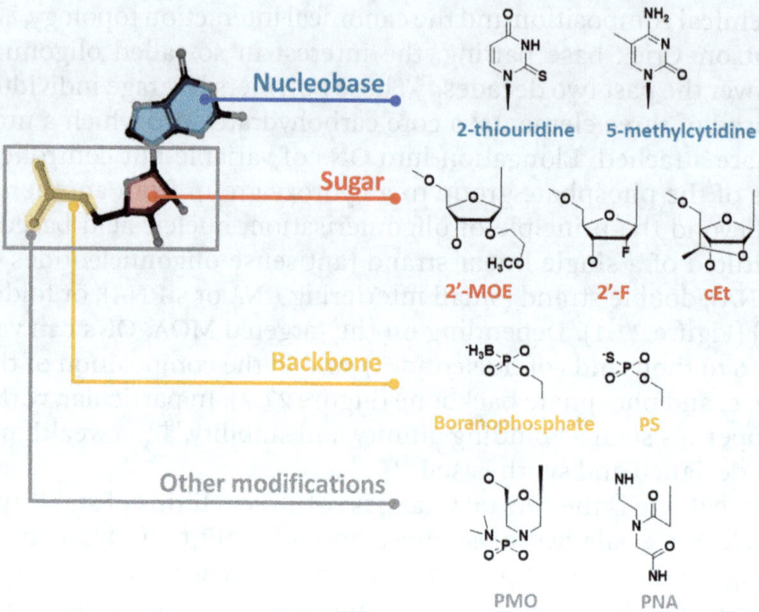


**Figure 27.2** Overview of nucleotide modification.

stronger affinity to the target RNA, but also increased stability by affecting access for nucleases. The 2′-hydroxyposition has been broadly substituted in that respect, with groups of increasing size or with electron-withdrawing groups. Thus, 2′-*O*-methyl, 2′-methoxyethoxy, and 2′-fluoro are regularly used in ONs (Figure 27.2).[35–37] Carbohydrate modifications have generally been aimed at stabilising the 3′-endo conformation of the ribose, which facilitates the preferred A-form of the ON. The conformation can be further rigidified by bridging the 2′ position to the 4′ position and has resulted in the now well-established LNA (locked nucleic acids) and other variations.[38–41] The principle can be further extended by establishing two bridges in the 3′ and 5′ positions, and the 5′ and 6′ positions to form the so-called tricyclic DNA (tcDNA).[42,43]

Finally, the elements that form a nucleotide can be concomitantly modified. For example, phosphorodiamidite morpholino oligomers (PMO) are nucleic acids in which the carbohydrate is replaced by a morpholine while the backbone is made from phosphorodiamidite linkages.[44,45] Another example is replacing the backbone and carbohydrate with peptides to form peptide nucleic acids (PNA).[46]

### *27.2.1.2 Peptide-based New Modalities*

While peptides have been designed and leveraged as therapeutics for several decades, their chemical composition has progressively evolved from polymers of canonical amino acids to modifications providing novel advanced three-dimensional architectures and scaffolds. Thus, the classical linear chain of the monomers that constitute peptides and proteins, while still pursued, has evolved to hypermodified peptides which can address many of the limitations encountered, including plasma stability, further enhanced affinity and specificity, and in some cases cellular uptake.[47] Peptide cyclisation strategies offer many advantages in this respect, and the most prominent approaches will be described in this section.[48–52]

Many monocylic peptide architectures are aimed at mimicking and stabilising existing motifs occurring in particular at protein–protein or protein–ligand interfaces (Figure 27.3). For example, introduction of an unnatural amino acid carrying an alkene group can enable cyclisation *via* ring-closing metathesis, providing so-called 'stapled' peptides when positioned judiciously, and resulting in α-helix mimetics.[53] β-strands are another secondary motif that can be stabilised by cyclisation. In this case, while sidechain to sidechain cyclisation can be implemented, an alternative is to use a turn scaffold such as D-proline-L-proline or a small molecule such as a biaryl or diketopiperazine,[54] and, more recently, 4-mercaptoproline.[55] Cyclic peptides can also be created without any prior structural knowledge. Introducing cysteine on both ends of a peptidic sequence is a trivial way to enable cyclic structures *via* a disulfide bond.[56,57] However, more stable covalent bonds are better suited from a drug discovery standpoint, and, similar to stapled peptides, a cross-link can be generated *via* click chemistry or an increasing number of other methods.[58,59]

Polycyclic peptide architectures have been developed to enhance the stability of peptides (Figure 27.3). One original approach is to mimic scaffolds present in peptide-based natural products.[60–62] Indeed, cysteine-rich peptides such as conotoxins, cyclotides, and sunflower trypsin inhibitor have demonstrated high stability, both against proteases but also chemically.[63–66] Polycyclic scaffolds can also be engineered through unnatural cross-links. For example, in the context of stapled peptides, a second bridge can be generated *via* the incorporation of additional unnatural amino acids and successive, orthogonal cyclisation reactions.[67] Recently, triazole linkages were also incorporated into cyclic peptides, to replace multiple cysteine bridges.[68]

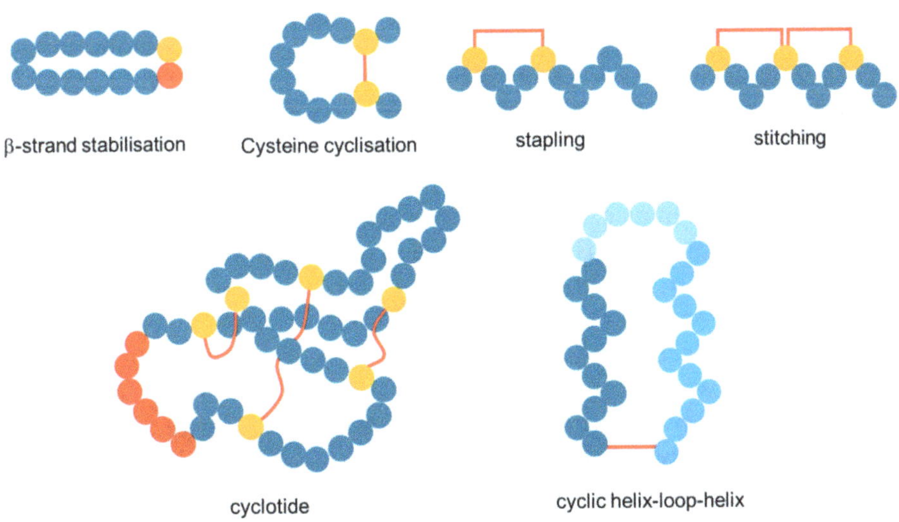


**Figure 27.3** Cyclic peptide architectures.

Even more complex architectures are starting to emerge. In particular, cyclic helix–loop–helix motifs result in mini-protein scaffolds and have been developed to incorporate a cell-penetrating peptide,[69] or, more interestingly, to mimic a regulator of the TEAD transcription factor.[70]

## 27.2.2 Mixed Compositions

Section 27.2.1 has mapped parts of the chemical space for therapeutics that are drastically different from classical modalities. These provide additional opportunities to address a range of MOAs that will be described in Section 27.3. Over the past five years, additional areas of the chemical space have started to be accessed, by combining different modalities.[13] In this section, these original and new compositions are discussed. These chemical entities can generally be designed by either linking the same or different modalities together, or by generating hybrids structures through fusion. The principle of connecting or fusing modalities can also be applied to other drug development challenges such as delivery, but will not be discussed herein, and the interested reader is directed to selected reviews and representative examples.[14,71–73]

Typically, merging or linking modalities can be applied to binding affinity enhancement and to create novel MOAs, especially *via* chemically induced proximity,[74] and these applications will be covered in Section 27.3. The principle can also be used to achieve polypharmacology and will be briefly discussed in this section.

### *27.2.2.1 Merging Chemical Modalities: Homo- and Heterofusions*

The premise of generating novel entities by hybridising or fusing existing molecules is best exemplified with polypharmacology approaches at first. Fusing several molecules of the same modality class, *i.e.* homofusions, to achieve multiple functions has been applied to several chemical entities and biomolecules (Figure 27.4). For example, bi-specific antibodies are aimed at binding different proteins by displaying different epitopes.[75] In the small molecule field, different compounds known to modulate different targets have been fused into a single entity to form the so-called designed multiple ligands (DMLs).[76,77] Similarly, peptide sequences developed for different drug targets have been fused into a single sequence to achieve synergistic effects.[78–81] In addition to fusing modalities in a linear fashion, cyclisation of two molecules is also an approach, as exemplified by macrocyclic peptides discovered against the BIR-2 and BIR-3 domain of the XIAP protein. With the goal of increasing affinity, two macrocyclic peptides targeting adjacent domains were fused, creating an original peptide architecture.[82,83]

While homofusions certainly provide novel scaffolds to modulate biology in innovative ways, merging two different modalities, *i.e.* heterofusions, represents a unique opportunity to access novel areas of the chemical space (Figure 27.5). For example, fusing small molecules with peptides can generate entities displaying the typical strengths of peptides (high affinity and specificity) while modulating conformations. Thus, hybrid macrocycles have been created by leveraging an aromatic oxime

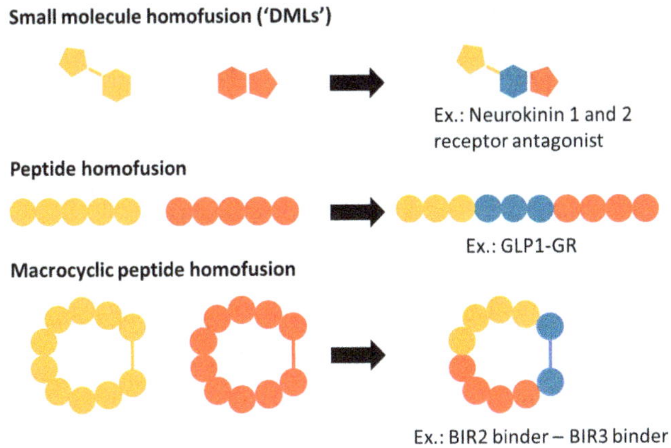


**Figure 27.4** Principles of linear and macrocyclic homofusion.

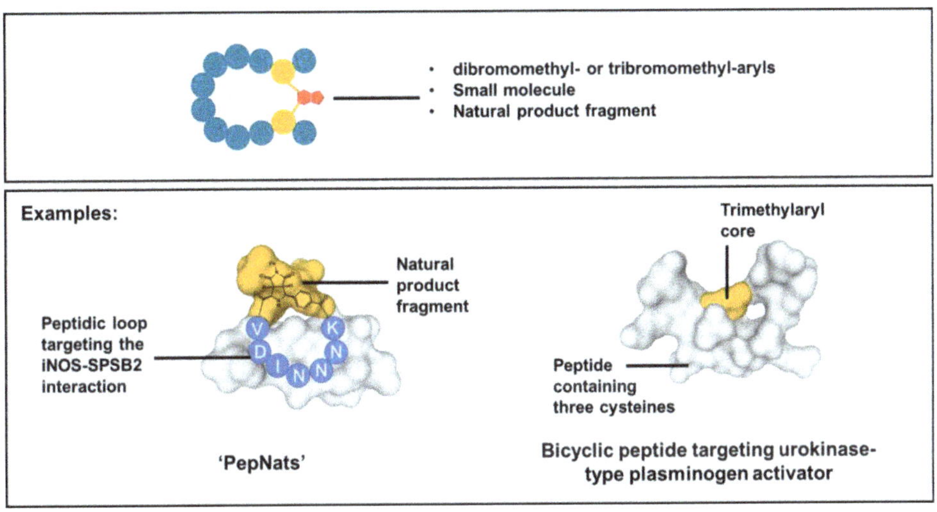


**Figure 27.5** Hybrid architecture examples of heterofusions.

cross-link,[84] and small molecule scaffolds,[85] including dibromomethyl and tribromomethyl aromatic moieties.[86–88] Kritzer and co-workers demonstrated that these small molecule scaffolds produce multiple discrete conformations of the peptide loops that are generated through this strategy. Recently, the small molecules used in these hybrid structures have even been extended to natural product scaffolds. Using on-resin synthesis and cyclisation strategies, libraries of so-called PepNats were generated and applied to protein–protein interactions (PPIs) and receptor selectivity modulation.[89]

### 27.2.2.2 Linking Chemical Modalities: Molecular Conjugates

Novel areas of the chemical space can also be accessed by linking several of the same or different modalities, forming homo- and heteromolecular conjugates, also often referred to as chimera or chimeric molecules (Figure 27.6). A major advantage of connecting modalities is the possibility to enhance binding affinity, a feature particularly useful for challenging targets such as PPIs. For example, linking a small molecule to a peptide has enabled a range of novel inhibitors of the glycoprotein 41 that forms the HIV virus envelope.[90] Another example is the linkage of a small molecule to an ON to inhibit a class of non-coding RNA called microRNA (miRNA) within the so-called RISC complex.[91] In this conjugate, the ON binds the target miRNA while the small molecule exploits a pocket within the argonaute 2 protein from the complex. Achieving synergistic binding by linking several modalities is also illustrated with non-peptidic macrocycles[92] and peptide-ON conjugates.[93]

These examples help to demonstrate the potential of accessing novel parts of the chemical space for classical MOAs. Perhaps the most exciting purpose of fusing and connecting modalities is to enable radically novel MOAs, as will be discussed in Section 27.3. Indeed, linking modalities fosters the concept of chemically-induced proximity.[74] This principle already occurs naturally in single molecules, as exemplified by FK506, which serves as a molecular glue,[15,94] but the engineered connection allows the bringing together of different biomolecules that do not normally interact together, essentially hijacking or rewiring biological processes. The best example in this field is probably the heterobifunctional degraders, also called proteolysis targeted chimeras and known as PROTACs, whose MOA will be detailed in Section 27.3, and which consists of connecting a small molecule binding a first protein, a protein of interest (POI), and another ligand binding to a second protein, an E3 ubiquitin ligase. The resulting small molecule–small molecule conjugate brings the two proteins into proximity, resulting in the ubiquitination of the POI by the E3 ligase and therefore tagging of the POI for proteasomal degradation. This principle is being increasingly explored.[95] Along the same

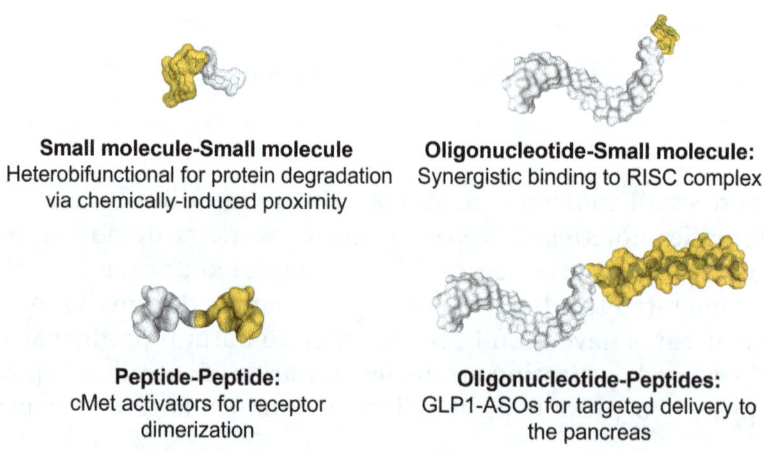


**Figure 27.6** Examples of conjugates and their application.

principle, small molecules can be conjugated to carbohydrates to direct a protein to a specific cellular compartment.[96]

The principle can also be applied to multimeric ligands in order to induce proximity of several copies of a given protein target. For example, conjugation of two macrocyclic peptides binding to the Met protein enables dimerisation of the receptor, resulting in activation of the signalling pathway.[97,98] Other examples include displaying three binders to a cyclic peptidic core to mimic a natural trimeric ligand,[99] and the generation of so-called synthetic antibody mimics, in which conjugation of two copies of a peptidic ligand for immune cells on one hand, and two copies of a small-molecule-like binding motif for cancer cells, brings the two cell types in proximity, resulting in apoptosis.[100] Even in the field of heterobifunctional degraders, multivalency is being extended to trivalent degraders.[101]

In summary, NMs are typically composed of peptidic and ON motifs as single entities, or bring together different parts of the chemical space, either through connection or fusion, forming novel hybrid or chimeric modalities. NMs are also based on linking the same modality, including small molecules, forming a compelling case for chemically induced proximity, which enables radically novel MOAs. Having described the different chemical compositions of NMs, the next section describes their MOAs.

## 27.3 Modes-of-action of New Modalities

Beyond classical small molecules and biologics, NMs are enabling a broader range of MOAs. Historically, drug modalities have been predominantly used as direct agonists or antagonists of protein function. With NMs being able to interact with additional target types, such as RNA, or complexity, such as PPIs,[12,13] more options are available to medicinal chemists to modulate biology and treat diseases, including gene splicing, gene silencing, gene activation, gene correction, chaperones, and protein degradation.[15] Overall, access to novel MOAs has created the opportunity to interfere at multiple levels of biological processes. Thus, in this section, MOAs are organised based on these stages, *i.e.* the DNA, RNA, and protein stages, placing more emphasis on those that are in late-stage drug discovery or in the clinic/marketed.

### 27.3.1 MOAs at the DNA Level

Since all biomolecules originate from DNA, modulating the genome both from a sequence and transcription standpoint represents the most central and most broadly applicable paradigm for drug modalities (Figure 27.7). However, very few modalities have, to date, the potential to achieve an effect in a precise and safe manner. Genome editing approaches to correct loss-of-function genes and other defects constitute the most direct modalities. Since these strategies typically require the use of concomitant biologics, such as proteins, a detailed description falls outside the scope of this chapter. Nevertheless, the CRISPR-CAS9 system is a representative example of how ONs also play a role in biologics.[102–104] In this paradigm, the so-called guide RNA is a key component to direct the CAS9 enzyme to a precise location in the genome for editing *via* sequence

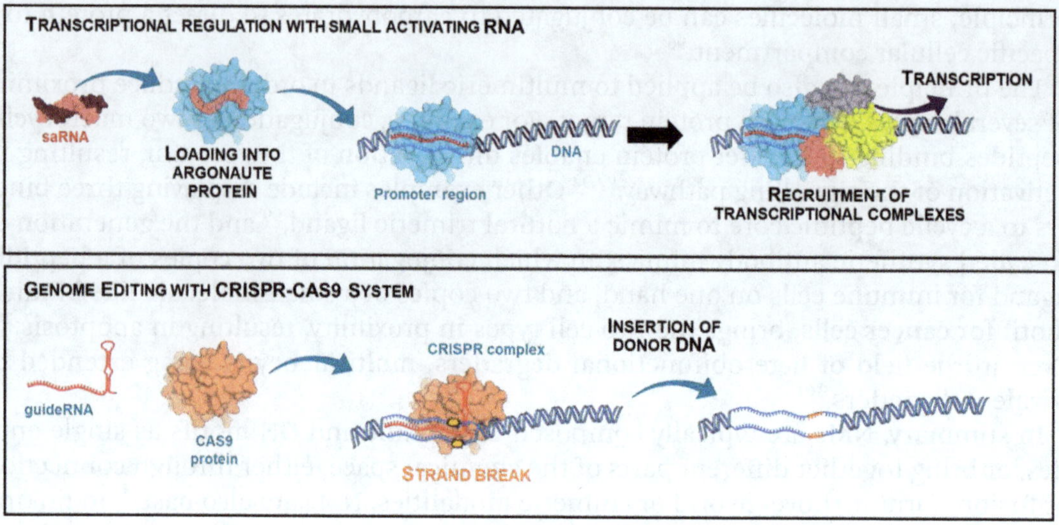


**Figure 27.7** MOA at the DNA level – genome editing and saRNA.

complementarity.[105] Since its inception, the system has evolved to enable insertion of the correct version of a gene, a potential game changer for many rare diseases.[106–108]

An emerging approach at the DNA level does not rely on biologics but exclusively on ONs. The so-called small activating RNA (saRNA) activate the promoter region of genes resulting in upregulation of pre-mRNA levels.[15,109] saRNAs are double-stranded ONs that share some similarity to siRNA. They are indeed processed and loaded into the argonaute protein (see Section 27.3.2) before activating the promoter region as a complex. The most advanced saRNA has entered clinical trials and targets the CEBPA gene, for which lower expression levels have been associated with hepatocellular carcinoma.[110] By systematically targeting and optimising sequences of the saRNAs using 2′-OMe modifications, a 2.5-fold increase in CEBPA mRNA levels was achieved. Other applications are appearing, such as the development of a saRNA targeting HNF4a in the liver, which showed positive impact on dyslipidaemia and metabolic profiles in rats.[111]

## 27.3.2 MOAs at the RNA Level

Due to their direct RNA mimicking nature, ONs are well suited to modulate RNA through a range of MOAs, and dominate RNA-targeted therapeutics, although emerging approaches for RNA editing and small molecule RNA binders have the potential to challenge this supremacy (Figure 27.8).[112–114] MOAs at the RNA level can broadly be classified into direct and indirect modulation of mRNA levels, for either up- or downregulation of protein levels and function.

### *27.3.2.1 Direct Downregulation of mRNA Levels*

With mRNA being the key intermediate to protein levels, many mRNA regulation mechanisms are used by cells. mRNA direct downregulation mechanisms are primarily

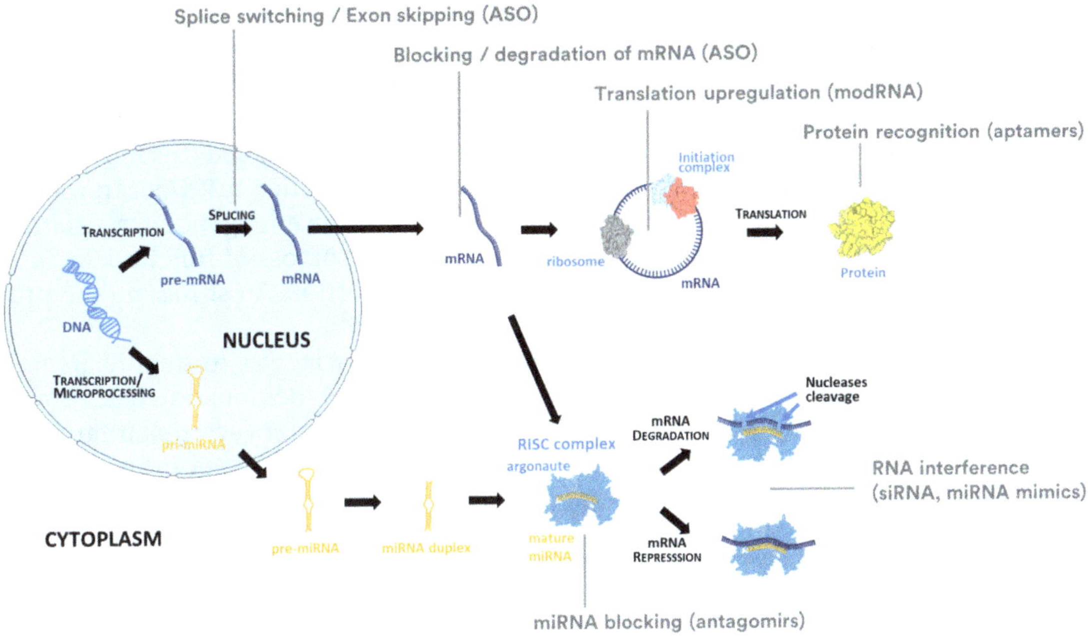


**Figure 27.8** MOAs at the RNA level.

governed *via* non-coding RNAs and protein complexes that degrade or edit mRNA. In particular, the so-called RISC complex plays a central role by enabling repression and degradation of mRNA. In this setting, the argonaute protein is bound by miRNAs, which serve as a guide to recognise an mRNA sequence, usually located at the 3′-untranslated region. Upon binding, the mRNA is either inhibited, when sequence complementarity is incomplete, or degraded by nucleases, when sequence complementarity is complete. Thus, ONs capable of hijacking the RISC complex represent the so-called RNA interference MOA. As discussed in Section 27.2.1, siRNAs are double stranded, 20–25 nucleotide-long ONs, which upon processing by the dicer enzyme load into the argonaute protein and promote degradation of mRNA upon binding. Similarly, an ON that can mimic a miRNA may achieve a similar outcome to the naturally occurring RISC complex.[115–118]

A different MOA consists in degrading mRNA by recruiting RNaseH *via* an ON. An ASO, consisting of a single strand of 16–20 nucleotides and incorporating the so-called gapmer design (see Section 27.4.1), induces formation of a DNA–RNA duplex which is then recognised by RNase-H and results in mRNA degradation.

#### *27.3.2.2 Direct Upregulation of mRNA Levels*

Like many other mechanisms in the discovery of therapeutics, inhibiting function, and, in the case of ASOs and siRNA, degrading mRNA levels, is typically achieved by several means. Upregulation, on the other hand, is much more challenging to enable. By using advanced chemical modifications of nucleotides, particularly on the nucleobases, and combining it with *in vitro* transcription to generate ONs made of 1000s of nucleotides, mimicking mRNA has become a reality and came to fame during the COVID-19 pandemic as potential vaccines.[119,120] Chemical modifications, such as pseudouridine-5′-triphosphate and 5-methylcytidine to replace respectively uridine-5′-triphosphate and cytidine, have also resulted in reduced immune activation and enabled this modality as a viable therapeutic option.[15,32,121,146] These synthetically-modified mRNAs can indeed be delivered into cells and then translated into proteins by the endogenous translation machinery.[122,123] This MOA therefore enables the correction of loss-of-function, or as in the case of coronavirus, the production of viral protein portions to stimulate the production of antibodies.

The first example of a modified mRNA entering clinical trial was to treat heart failure. Preclinical data of an mRNA encoding the VEGF-A protein demonstrated improved heart function upon local administration in a minipig model of myocardial infarction. Subsequently, human testing demonstrated expression of new VEGF-A protein in the forearm of diabetic patient upon intradermal injection, enabling progress to Phase II.[124] Since this landmark, many other modified RNA drug candidates have entered clinical trials, including in the field of cancer vaccines,[125] and with the prominent COVID-19 examples.[120]

#### *27.3.2.3 Correcting Pre-mRNA Splicing*

Another category of MOA at the RNA level consists in rectifying incorrect splicing with ASOs.[126,127] Beyond the gapmer design that results in downregulation of mRNA levels, other designs, that do not induce RNaseH recruitment, can be used to generate stoichiometric binders. Transcription of a given gene results in the generation of pre-mRNAs which then need to be processed by the splicing machinery to separate exonic from intronic regions, combining exons to form a mature mRNA.[128] This process is altered in several diseases, resulting in the generation of mis-spliced mRNA leading to proteins that are truncated or inactive, representing loss-of-function.[129–131] In some cases, mis-splicing can also result in proteins that aggregate creating a gain-of-function phenotype.[132] In either case, stoichiometric binding to pre-mRNA with an ON can result in alternative splicing to the correctly spliced mRNA, by providing steric hindrance at a given portion of the pre-mRNA. This MOA therefore represents an upregulation of mRNA levels, and is best exemplified by nusinersen, approved in 2016 for the treatment of spinal muscular atrophy.[133,134]

#### *27.3.2.4 Indirect Modulation of mRNA Levels via Interaction with Other RNA Species*

Targeting the non-coding RNA species called miRNA, described in Section 27.3.2.1, is a means to indirectly regulate mRNA levels. Indeed, miRNA are a key component of the mRNA downregulation mechanism, driven by the RISC complex. Using an ASO that can either degrade or stoichiometrically repress a miRNA can therefore be a different MOA resulting in upregulation of mRNA by preventing its degradation.[135,135–137] With this prospect in mind, ASOs as antagomirs have been investigated in the clinic, including against miRNA21 for the treatment of Alport syndrome,[138] and miRNA103-107 in diabetic patients.[139] However, the miRNA biology being still poorly understood, limited progress has been seen in this field.

## 27.3.3 MOAs at the Protein Level

Historically, and still today, targeting proteins remains the main point of intervention for therapeutics. However, over the last five years, novel approaches aimed at directly modulating protein levels rather than directly affecting their functions have seen a surge in research. In this subsection, NMs aimed at directly agonising or antagonising protein functions will be discussed, before describing MOAs leveraged for altering protein levels.

### *27.3.3.1 Direct Modulation of Function: Agonism/Antagonism for Challenging Protein Targets*

NMs, especially advanced peptide architectures, are well suited for challenging targets such as PPIs. However, despite many efforts to address poor uptake, which will be discussed in Section 27.5, including in the field of highly structured peptides,[140] accessing intracellular targets often remains difficult. Nevertheless, much progress has been made to address a broader range of protein targets, in particular extracellular or cell-surface-bound. Protein agonism and antagonism being the most established MOA, little explanation is required for how this is generally achieved. Instead, the paragraphs below summarise how NMs can achieve this MOA, and focus on the cases where using these modalities is the most relevant.

#### 27.3.3.1.1 Extracellular Targets

Due to their larger interaction surface than small molecules, peptides are well suited for targets presenting shallow pockets or distant hydrophobic pockets. Considering the natural ligands of certain cell surface receptors, including many GPCRs, peptides are also better suited to achieve not only antagonism but especially agonism for such targets.[141–143] Achieving selectivity can represent a very hard challenge for some target classes.[144] For example, while small molecules have been developed for proteases, immense efforts are required to tune-out activity on closely related family members.[145,146] In this respect, modalities with larger footprints can exploit differences located at the protein surface in proximity to the binding site.[147] Thus, a bicyclic peptide targeted at the human plasma kallikrein inhibitor achieved high selectivity against other proteases, including over 10 000-fold over the closely related factorXIa protein,[87] and this strategy also led to the discovery of the clinical candidate THR-149 from Bicycle Therapeutics.[148] Larger interaction surfaces are also exemplified with the β-strand mimetics described in Section 27.2.1.2. Mimicking the antibacterial peptide protegrin, the antibiotic murepavadin targets the LptD protein and inhibits LPS transport in *Pseudomonas aeruginosa*.[149]

Binding with high specificity to proteins can also be achieved with ONs, in the form of aptamers. Indeed, this modality can form folded structures, much like proteins, leading to secondary and tertiary architectures.[150,151] These three-dimensional arrangements therefore function similarly to antibodies. Their high specificity has been applied to proteins such as Factor IXa and thrombin within the coagulation cascade, or to the VEGF protein, for the treatment of age-related macular degeneration.[152] Interestingly, like antibodies, aptamers are also being directed at agonising proteins, most significantly in immunology (OX40, CD28, CD40).[150]

#### 27.3.3.1.2 Intracellular Targets

With many challenging targets residing inside cells, many NM approaches have been directed at this target space, retaining the classical agonism/antagonism paradigm. Arguably, very few strategies have made significant progress along the drug discovery and development process, although tremendous efforts are being deployed to increase cellular uptake (see Section 27.5.5.2). The only exception is ALRN-6924, a stapled-peptide targeted at the HDM2-p53 interaction.[153] However, progress in the clinic of this drug candidate has been slow.

### *27.3.3.2 Direct Downregulation of Protein Levels*

Targeted protein degradation represents one of the most significant advances of the last decade for NMs.[154–157] Leveraging the principle of chemically-induced proximity,[74] a radically novel MOA has been enabled and has changed the mindset on how protein functions can be modulated. Many proteins, including receptors and enzymes, possess scaffolding functions and regulate PPIs. Therefore, targeting an active site for an enzyme provides a precise means to alter a specific function but does not address any other features of that protein. Thus, protein degradation approaches can provide a broader modulation of target pharmacology.[158] Several approaches have been developed, each representing a new modality and different MOA within the broader spectrum of protein degradation MOAs (Figure 27.9). These will be briefly described, and more emphasis will be placed on E3-ligase-based heterobifunctional degraders, a modality which has now progressed to the clinic.

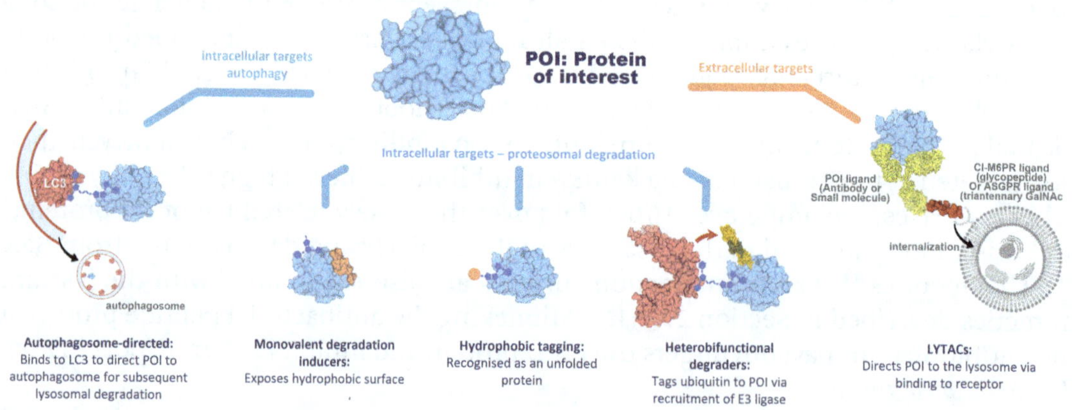


**Figure 27.9** Approaches to protein degradation.

Hydrophobic tagging consists in directly appending a moiety that directs a protein of interest to the proteasome. Thus, adding an adamantyl group or an arginine, protected at the guanidino group with tertiary-butyl carbamate groups ($Boc_3Arg$), to a small molecule protein ligand, mimics protein destabilisation by mirroring a misfolded state, leading to protein degradation.[159,160] The approach has been applied to the degradation of HER3 and the androgen receptor,[161,162] and, beyond leveraging small molecule binders, peptidic ligands such a TAR DNA binding protein 43 (TDP-43) recognition peptide or a TAU targeting peptide have also been used for hydrophobic tagging.[163,164]

The predominant protein degradation strategy is based on conjugates that link a protein of interest (POI) ligand to an E3 ligase ligand.[156,165] This modality therefore chemically induces proximity between the POI and the E3 ligase, resulting in a transfer of ubiquitin to the POI. This tagging then directs the POI to the 26S proteasome for degradation. Several E3 ligase ligands have been exploited, including ligands for MDM2,[166] IAP,[167,168] VHL,[169–171] and CRBN.[172–175] More recently, ligands for KEAP1,[176] and RNF114[177] have also been applied. The next wave of E3 ligase ligands has been discovered by developing novel screening approaches, including *via* covalent handles[178,179] and engineered protein fusion.[180] For example, a electrophilic moiety screen coupled to proteomic analysis led to the identification of DCAF16 as an additional ligase.[181] Another example is the application of affinity-based protein profiling to the discovery of RNF4-based heterobifunctional degraders.[182] Interestingly, differential tissue expression of E3 ligases may be a means to engineer selectivity, creating an additional opportunity for this MOA.[183]

With the premise of the MOA and the associated surge of research in this field, the range of targetable protein classes has rapidly expanded, starting originally with kinases,[184–189] and nuclear receptors,[190–193] to ligases,[194,195] phosphodiesterases,[196] phosphatases,[197] growth factors,[198] transcriptional and epigenetics modulators,[199–209] or even the TAU protein and other challenging protein targets, such as KRAS.[176,198,210]

In addition to approaching degradation by binding to target proteins with small molecules and peptides, additional approaches are being developed to enable the degradation of DNA and RNA binding proteins, which are notoriously difficult to drug. Thus, conjugating an oligonucleotide to an E3 ligase warhead led to the degradation of stem cell factor LIN28 and splicing factor RBFOX1 as proof-of-concept.[211] Following the same principle, double-stranded oligonucleotides were leveraged to bind to transcription factors, and degradation of lymphoid enhancer-binding factor 1 (LEF1) and ETS-related gene (ERG).[212] In a separate effort, these hybrid degraders were applied to the degradation of NF-κB subunit p65 and E2F1,[213] and a chemical genetic approach based on hybrid molecules binding to a Halotag-fused dCAS9 and to transcription factors led to similar outcome.[214]

While heterobifunctional degraders have been applied to the degradation of transmembrane proteins, such as receptor tyrosine kinases EGFR, HER2, and c-MET,[215] and GPCR,[216] the approach remains, to date, limited to intracellular proteins, and other strategies are needed for enabling protein degradation of secreted proteins and expanding the range of targetable cell-surface receptors. To address this gap another approach consists in directing a protein to the lysosome for degradation.[217] This recent strategy is achieved by conjugating a protein ligand such as a small molecule or antibody to glycopeptides that bind to the cation-independent mannose-6-phosphate receptor (CI-M6PR), and these molecules have been called LYTACs.[96] Remarkably, proteins such as apolipoprotein E4, epidermal growth factor receptor, the asialoglycoprotein receptor, CD71, and PDL1 were successfully degraded and the LYTAC approach therefore represents a complementary strategy to heterobifunctional degraders, by enabling the degradation of cell-membrane receptors and circulating proteins. Expanding on the initial proof-of-concept, a triantennary GalNAc ligand to the asialoglycoprotein receptor was conjugated to ligands for EGFR and for integrins to promote lysosomal degradation of the POI.[218]

Finally, targeting a protein to the autophagy system for degradation has also been reported with AUTACs, consisting of a POI ligand conjugated to a guanine derivatives.[219,220] Furthermore, autophagosome-tethering compounds (ATTECs) consisting of ligands binding to the POI and to the autophagosome LC3 protein were developed to degrade the mutant HTT protein for Huntington disease.[221,222]

## 27.4 Hit Finding Strategies and Drug Design of New Modalities

Having described the composition of NMs and the different MOAs that they can enable, the next question is to consider how these are pursued from a drug discovery standpoint. Thus, this section focuses on how starting points can be identified, and on design considerations. Hit finding strategies for NMs have been previously reviewed,[12] and the main aspects will therefore be discussed herein, focusing on the more validated modalities.

### 27.4.1 Oligonucleotides

ONs strategies that leverage the DNA and RNA hybridisation-based MOAs have the major advantage of offering the possibility to programme the sequence for interaction for their nucleic acid target. Indeed, an ON's sequence is always complementary to the target sequence in an antisense direction, when using the conventional 5′-3′ directionality.

Target sequences, for example of an mRNA, can be constituted of thousands of nucleotides and therefore still represent a large search space. Since RNA forms secondary and tertiary structures, regions that are folded tend to represent less well-suited sequences for ONs due to reduced accessibility and the need for an ON to disrupt any duplex already formed in the target RNA.[223] RNA structure prediction still remains broadly elusive, but some algorithms can nevertheless be used to assess the probability of a region to be unstructured and therefore better suited for the design of an ON. From this point, hundreds of sequences can be enumerated and filters such as nucleotide compositions and similarity to other transcript sequences can be used to narrow down the list. Then tens or sometimes hundreds of ONs can be synthesised and screened against their target.

One additional component of the design before synthesis is the targeted MOA and the type of nucleotide modifications used. Within ASOs, most modifications are tolerated, while steric clashes within the RISC complex require siRNA to typically have smaller modifications, such as 2′-F or 2′-OMe. Furthermore, a PS backbone is usually applied in the majority of ASOs and siRNAs. In the case of ASOs, the stoichiometric binder and degrader MOAs require a different design (Figure 27.10). Stoichiometric binders have the advantage to tolerate any arrangement of modifications and are often referred to as mixmers. Degrading ASOs, on the other hand, follow a specific arrangement in which two to five modified nucleotides flank a typically 10-mer DNA sequence. This 'gapmer' design enables formation of a DNA–RNA duplex, leading to RNaseH recruitment and degradation. Using earlier modifications such as 2′-OMe or 2′-MOE, the flanking region consists of 3 to 5 modified nucleotides, while more advanced modifications such as LNA and cEt only require 2–3 modified nucleotides.

In the case of modified RNA used to increase protein levels, the sequence is directly derived from the protein sequence it encodes for. Modifications of the nucleobases are incorporated to tune down immune response and increase half-life. Implementation of these modifications has to take into account the target cells, as protein translation is affected by nucleobase modifications to a different extent in different cell types, and different codons also have more tolerated modifications than others.[34]

Aptamers[150] are the only class of ONs that falls outside sequence programmability, since they fold into highly structured ONs which are still hard to predict *de novo*. The discovery of aptamers therefore relies on an affinity maturation technique called systematic evolution of ligands by exponential enrichment (SELEX).[224] Aptamers do suffer from some of the weaknesses of other ONs, notably stability. Incorporating modified nucleotides is therefore again a classical design approach, and some modifications can even be directly incorporated during screening, by using a modified SELEX protocol.[150]

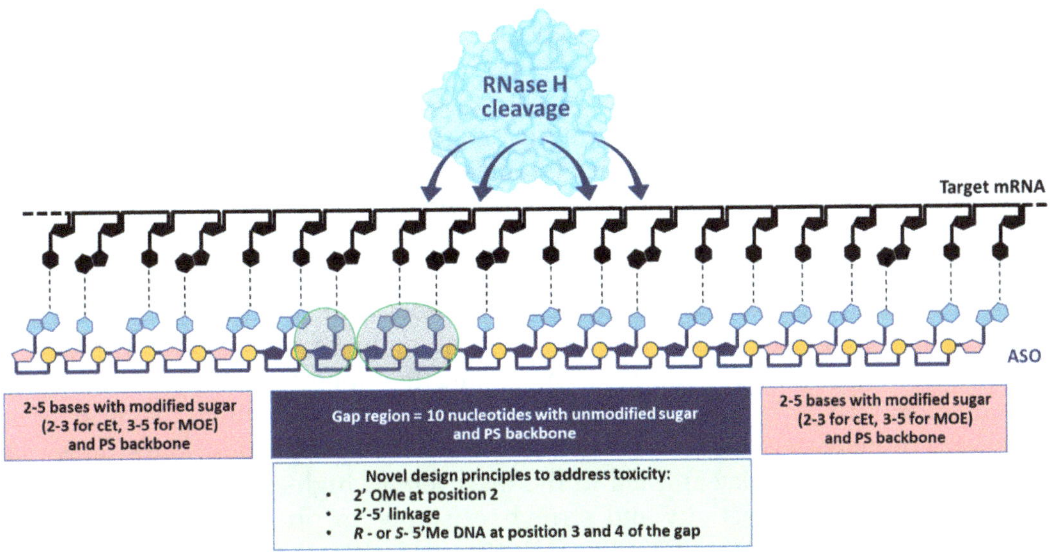


**Figure 27.10** Principles of ASO design for gapmers.

## 27.4.2 Peptides

Similar to small molecules, hit finding for peptides falls broadly into two categories: structure-based drug design and random screening. As described briefly in Section 27.2.1.2, protein structures can form a starting point to derive novel peptide architectures and represent the broad category of protein structure mimetics.[125] In particular, α-helices are displayed in over 60% of protein–protein interfaces.[225] Starting from the amino-acid sequence of the helix, a stabilised peptide can be generated with the 'stapling' strategy described in Section 27.2. In terms of design, the unnatural amino acids used for ring closure are usually positioned at the $(i, i + 3)$, $(i, i + 4)$ and $(i, i + 7)$ positions.[53] In addition, the cross-link can sometimes be utilised to form additional contacts with the protein surface to increase affinity.[13] This approach has been applied to many PPIs, in particular the NOTCH complex,[226] β-catenin,[227] HDM2-p53 inhibitors,[228] and PCKS9.[229] The other secondary structure motif starting from β-sheets can also rapidly lead to a starting point.[54] With a D-Pro-L-Pro motif for cyclisation, followed by optimisation, murepavadin, mentioned in Section 27.3.3.1, was discovered.[149] Other protein structure mimetic approaches are being developed, but remain, to date, in the early stage of drug discovery.[56,86,89]

To leverage highly stable cysteine-rich peptidic scaffolds, existing peptide epitopes for a protein of interest can be inserted within one loop of the scaffold by replacing part of that loop sequence. Thus, the so-called grafting approach can lead to another starting point with enhanced properties compared to the linear peptide.[230] In addition to providing improved stability, the rest of the scaffold can also enhance selectivity against closely related proteins. For example, displaying a pentapeptide within a cyclotide scaffold led to over 100-fold selectivity for the melanocortin receptor type 4 over the 1, 2, and 5 isoforms.[231,232]

Since structural information, either on the protein or on the ligand side, is required for the previous hit finding strategies, other approaches are required for cases lacking such information. In this respect, the well-established technique of phage display has been adapted to the generation of novel peptide architectures. Applying the principle of ring formation from cysteines reacting with halomethyl moieties, extensive libraries can be generated by cyclising directly on the phage, leading to libraries of bicyclic peptides.[27,87] By varying the position of the cysteines and also changing the small molecule core, a wide variety of loop conformations carrying typically 3 to 6 amino acids can be obtained, resulting in high affinity and high specificity, while exhibiting increased proteolytic stability.[28,29,88,233] For example, screening of a billion bicyclic peptide library led to the identification of plasmakalikrein inhibitors with selectivity over the mouse orthologue.[234] This approach can be directed at multiple target classes, including the hard-to-drug NOTCH1[32] and β-catenin,[33] and therapeutic bicyclic peptides have entered clinical trials.[148] A new generation is also emerging, in which two bridges are established to increase scaffold diversity. In the seminal publication, the strategy was transferred to phage display and led to the discovery of high-affinity plasmakalikrein inhibitors, with high selectivity and strong resistance to proteolytic degradation.[235] Moreover, additional adaptions of phage display are leading to even larger libraries of over $10^{10}$ modified peptides.[236,237]

Another high-throughput approach to the discovery of cyclic peptides consists in incorporating unnatural amino acids into an *in vitro* translation system.[238,239] This mRNA display strategy reprograms codons to load amino acids containing a chloroacetyl group which can be cyclised with cysteine residues. Libraries of hundreds of billions of cyclic peptides can be generated with broad size diversity, typically 4 to 25 residues. While very few details are publicly disclosed, the company Peptidream lists some of these peptides as having entered Phase I clinical trials.

Finally, approaches based on high-density microarrays, which can incorporate any non-canonical amino acid,[240] and natural product libraries, in particular venoms,[56] are also viable strategies for identifying constrained peptidic starting points. In addition, genetic encoding of cyclic peptides illustrated by the SICLOPPS (split-intein synthesis of proteins and peptides) approach can be particularly advantageous for challenging targets, despite the requirements of intense molecular biology engineering.[241]

### 27.4.3 Heterobifunctional Degraders

Chemically induced proximity heterobifunctional degrader molecules offer the advantage of directly leveraging all classical hit finding approaches known for small molecules. In theory, any small molecule ligand of a POI can be conjugated to an E3 ligase warhead *via* a linker chain. Thus, existing small molecule inhibitors are the most extensive class of ligands that have been reported. Assuming a ligand to the POI exists or has been identified, two design elements then need to be implemented: the linker and the warhead. With a few warheads currently been established, in particular thalidomide binding CRBN and the VHL ligand binding the VHL E3 ligase,[175,242] libraries of readily conjugatable linker-warhead molecules can be either assembled or purchased. To accelerate library generation for heterobifunctional degraders directed at a given target, one approach consists of systematically producing a library of POI ligand(s) with a reactive handle, and combining this library with a library of pre-made linker-E3 ligase ligands.[243,244] Structural information for the ligand interacting with the POI is particularly useful to identify exit vectors onto which conjugation handles can be appended. In particular, emerging computational approaches based on machine learning are being applied to the construction of degraders by designing the linker connecting the two ligands.[245] While POIs have been shown to be degradable by multiple E3 ligases, degradation is sometimes only observed with a sub-set, which implies that connecting a POI ligand for degrader hit finding may require deployment against multiple E3 ligases in parallel. Interestingly, a cell-based target engagement assay has been developed to screen for permeable E3 ligase ligands before conjugation to a POI ligand, representing a different way to approach heterobifunctional degrader hit finding.[246]

Since the small molecule ligand to the POI does not need to carry out any function *per se*, only a binder is, in theory, required. In this respect, DNA-encoded libraries are an attractive strategy for hit finding in the context of heterobifunctional degraders. Indeed, the binder does not need to be tested for any function, and the DNA tag also already encodes for a conjugation site on the ligand. Thus, the DNA tag can merely be replaced with a linker-warhead to generate a putative degrader molecule. The principle of using ligands deprived of functional activity has been demonstrated by repurposing such existing ligands. As an example, the GSK4027 bromodomain inhibitor of PCAF and GCN5, which lacked functional activity, was transformed into a protein degrader by conjugating it to thalidomide, leading not only to degradation of the two proteins but also functional activity, as demonstrated by cytokine release.[199]

While the principle of designing a putative heterobifunctional degrader is straightforward, achieving activity is not immediate. Indeed formation of a ternary complex between the POI, the degrader molecule and the E3-ligase is a key step to achieve transfer of ubiquitin.[247,248] The linker needs to bring into proximity the two proteins and formation of the ternary complex is a result of a balance between positive cooperativity and negative cooperativity, resulting from the *de novo* protein–protein interactions. While largely determined experimentally, progress in the *in silico* understanding of ternary complexes is being made,[362] in particular by incorporating structural information gained with techniques such as hydrogen–deuterium exchange.[249] Testing a designed degrader molecule also requires one to carefully consider the testing concentration. Indeed, at low concentration, the degrader concentration is too low to bind to both proteins at the same time, with the individual protein concentrations representing an individual titration of the degrader. At high concentrations, binary complexes are formed instead of a ternary complex.[250] This so-called hook effect, with a bell shape curve of activity is therefore typical of heterobifunctional degraders, and, in principle, of any chemically induced proximity approach.

## 27.5 Optimisation of New Modalities

Like any classical small molecules, NMs must be optimised beyond affinity to create drugs. In fact, due to their unique MOAs or architectures, NMs are sometimes easier to optimise for affinity. Other properties such as cellular uptake, stability, or distribution are, on the other hand, often harder to optimise. In many respects, NM optimisation mirrors small molecules, with multiple iterative cycles of Design–Make–Test–Analyse.[251] In this section, the key strengths and limitations of ONs, hyper-modified peptides and heterobifunctional degraders are discussed as a basis for highlighting which parameters need to be monitored, identified, and modulated during the optimisation phase of the drug discovery process. This section is therefore organised along Pharmacokinetics, Safety, and Delivery. Stability is also a key parameter for optimisation but has already been discussed in Section 27.2.1.

### 27.5.1 Pharmacokinetics

#### *27.5.1.1 Tissue Distribution*

Peptides, including hyper-modified, are typically excreted *via* renal filtration. This process is usually rapid and approaches aimed at reducing this route of elimination either by increasing molecular weight, for example with PEG chains, or by increasing plasma protein binding through conjugation to fatty acids have been employed.[252,253] Despite the challenge of rapid extraction, and when compared to larger entities such as proteins and antibodies, peptides have the advantage of being smaller, which helps in penetrating tissues. Nevertheless, some tissues are usually not reachable by classical routes of administration, with synthetic peptides typically not crossing the blood–brain barrier, although examples exist.[254]

ONs have a narrower tissue distribution profile, typically driven by nucleotide modifications. ASOs and siRNA distribute rapidly, predominantly to the liver and kidney. Exposure is also noticeable in spleen and bone marrow, but other tissues usually display significantly lower exposure.[255] Some modifications, such as PMOs have been claimed to allow higher muscle exposure; however, efficacy data has been controversial.[256,257] Separately, the PS backbone has been linked to increased liver concentrations by increasing plasma protein binding and decreasing renal clearance.[255] Overall, ONs distribute to a restricted set of tissues, which limits the number of diseases that can be treated. Nevertheless, higher doses can enable efficacy in peripheral tissues, but is associated with safety concerns due to the resulting even higher exposure in liver and kidney. To circumvent the limited range of reachable tissues, approaches based on targeted delivery are being developed, and need to be considered in any new ON project for optimisation. Conjugating a ligand to a tissue-specific receptor can, in principle, redirect the distribution of the ON to the tissue of interest, and many strategies based on small molecules, carbohydrates, lipids, and NMs have been tested.[13,14,258–266] However, very little actual targeting has typically been observed with the notable exception of GLP1-ASO conjugates.[71,267,268] By linking a peptide agonist for the GLP1 receptor, which displays high levels of expression in pancreatic β-cells, delivery was successfully shifted away from the liver, and resulted in significant uptake of ASO in that cell type. Some targeted delivery approaches, in addition to being of limited efficacy, also suffer from translation gaps between targeting mechanisms in animal models compared to monkeys or humans.[269]

Tissue distribution for modified RNA is different from other ONs since it is driven by formulation. Delivery vehicles such as lipid nanoparticles (LNPs) (see Section 27.5.5) are typically used and these are taken up by the liver and spleen through the phagocytic system.[270]

Finally, biodistribution data for heterobifunctional degraders have not been broadly reported. However, an increasing number of analyses indicate that degraders follow to a large extent a typical small molecule profile, with the potential to achieve broad tissue distribution, although high plasma protein binding (PPB) and therefore low unbound fraction are common.[271–273] Accessing the CNS is being explored, and blood–brain barrier penetration has in particular been demonstrated by Arvinas.[274]

#### *27.5.1.2 Cellular Uptake*

Due to their larger typical size than small molecules, a major challenge for NM optimisation is to overcome poor cellular uptake. Smaller ONs such as ASOs and siRNA can be taken up by certain cell types *via* several mechanisms, believed to be dependent on ON binding to extracellular or membrane-bound proteins.[275–278] However, the majority is trapped in the endosome and less than 2% is believed to escape the endosome and carry its function inside the cell. Despite this low intracellular exposure, high efficacy can be achieved and the efficacious intracellular concentration has be shown to be as low as 200 nM.[279,280] While some nucleotide modifications worsen uptake in many cell lines, as exemplified by PNAs or PMOs,[281] it is unclear whether modifying the carbohydrate component with larger, predominantly hydrophobic groups can improve uptake. However, the PS backbone, which leads to higher protein binding, is believed to increase uptake by binding to endogenous proteins taken up by cells.[276,282] Another approach has been to modify PMOs with basic moieties, forming the so-called 'PMO Plus', carrying charged amines in place of the morpholine.[283] While this approach is being pursued commercially, little has been published on whether this modification is helpful.

Therefore, during ON optimisation, approaches relying on conjugates can be applied to improve uptake, although beyond the example from Section 27.5.2.2 with GLP1 conjugates, little has been successful outside the liver. When targeting hepatocytes, conjugation of ONs to a triantennary carbohydrate, GalNAc, an agonist of the ASGR receptor, can increase productive uptake up to ten-fold, and this approach is being broadly pursued in the clinic.[284–286]

Hyper-modified peptides, despite offering potential for property modulation also face a major challenge in terms of cellular uptake. When pursuing such an approach for intracellular targets, much optimisation effort is to be expected without a guarantee for success. In particular, the rules governing cell permeability are still not fully understood, but progress is being made.[287–289] Many studies have been tailored towards oral absorption, which does not always align with cellular uptake for the targeted cells.[289–291] Nevertheless, these strategies are useful to implement during peptide optimisation. In particular, systematic methylation of the nitrogen backbone can improve intestinal permeability of cyclic peptides,[292–296] and thorough optimisation can achieve peptides with reasonable uptake, as exemplified by macrocyclic CXCR7 receptor binders, displaying nanomolar affinity for their target and 18% bioavailability in rats.[297] Taking advantage of the novel features of hyper-modified peptides, such as the hydrophobic cross-link in stapled peptides, is one approach. The determinants enabling cell permeability of such scaffolds has been investigated, although exploiting the cross-link as a handle is often not sufficient. Understanding how different conformations of a peptide scaffold can mask or expose hydrophilic sections can help to design tailored modifications, and molecular dynamics have in particular been applied to that purpose.[298] Overall, systematic modifications,[299] including by varying the ring size,[300] and polarity adjustments through amphipathic design or lipophilicity increase,[301–304] can help for increasing uptake. Moreover, the development of higher throughput and precise uptake assays is assisting in better understanding of the determinants for permeability.[305]

While being closer to small molecules, heterobifunctional degraders still display, logically, lower cell permeability. However, knowledge on how to optimise these larger molecules is progressing rapidly. In particular, linker optimisation, which already plays a key role in ternary complex formation, is critical for improving cell permeability, including intestinal absorption. Most of the knowledge built to achieve enhanced cellular uptake remains to a large extent proprietary to the companies pursuing degrader approaches. Nevertheless, degraders targeting the pirin proteins were recently described and many properties were considered during optimisation. Indeed, starting from a poorly active starting point, monitoring of hydrogen-bond donor count, log*D* and linker length resulted in compounds showing high pirin degradation in cells.[306] In addition, VH032-based degraders have been studied in a PAMPA assay to elucidate the determinants of cellular permeability.[307] Separately, a systematic analysis of androgen receptor-targeted degraders led the authors to favour CACO-2 over PAMPA assays.[308] These studies certainly help to enhance the view on requirements for cellular permeability, including when combined with analyses of chemical descriptors,[309] or investigating the impact of solution conformations.[310] However, they remain highly context-specific. In this respect, two recent analyses from AstraZeneca and Roche perhaps represents the most useful set of learnings that can be applied more generally, since these compiled hundreds of datapoints.[272,311] They also confirm the experience of many medicinal chemists developing degraders across companies. Like many other molecules, cellular uptake of degraders has more been described in the context of oral delivery, which does not necessary reflect cellular uptake for the cell type of interest. These aspects will be described in Section 27.5.5. Interestingly, specific assessments of permeability have been reported *via* measurement of intracellular heterobifunctional degrader concentration. In the case of BCL6 targeting, degrader concentration was shown to be as low as 50 nM in the nucleus, yet did promote degradation.[206] An approach consisting of using covalent reversible binders to increase intracellular accumulation has also been reported, although the rationale for why accumulation would be increased is surprising.[312]

#### 27.5.1.3 Other Physico-chemical and DMPK Parameters: Solubility, Metabolism and Plasma Protein Binding

Solubility is a critical parameter from a dosing standpoint. In addition, it is also a fundamental parameter for the battery of assays used in optimising molecules. Aggregation, in particular, is a known challenge for peptides that can be assessed routinely.[313] The recent advancement of heterobifunctional degraders has revealed a large challenge in terms of assays. Indeed, these molecules typically possess much lower solubility than classical small molecules, and kinetic solubility is problematic. In this respect, thermodynamic solubility is preferred, but faces the challenge of lower throughput.[311] Interestingly, measuring solubility in buffer such as FASSIF, provides a clearer link to optimisation for oral uptake with better solubility observed in such a regimen.[272]

Another parameter often considered for DMPK optimisation is Plasma Protein Binding (PPB). To some extent, this can be easily triaged for some modalities. Peptides usually display moderate binding, although this can be enhanced to increase half-life, *via* specific conjugation to fatty acids. In particular, this strategy was applied in the development of semaglutide.[314] When considering ONs, and as alluded to previously, several modifications result in very high protein binding, such as phosphorothioates. To that extent, PPB is often not a particularly useful parameter. For NMs such as heterobifunctional degraders, PPB remains, however, very important, perhaps unsurprisingly considering their small molecule nature. However, there again, adapting existing assays is required to address the challenges stemming from the higher lipophilicity range. In particular, scientists at Roche recommend using alternative strategies such as ultracentrifugation methods coupled with high-sensitivity analytical methods.[311]

NMs such as ONs and peptides have well-established metabolism routes. Peptides tend to be rapidly excreted *via* renal filtration and are often metabolised through proteolytic cleavage. ONs have short plasma half-lives following rapid tissue distribution and typically metabolised by intracellular degradation involving enzymes.

Other modalities such as heterobifunctional degraders, on the other hand, display more of a small molecule-like metabolism, but this aspect still remains poorly characterised. In particular, metabolism appears to be specific to the whole entity rather than its fragments.[272,315] Overall, classical liver metabolism rather than biliary or renal clearance is the main route of disposition. Interestingly, in their study on hundreds of degraders, AstraZeneca concluded that there is no significant CYP induction, but recommended to closely monitor CYP inhibition considering the typical high lipophilicity of this type of molecule. Finally, the composition of the linker can have a major impact on metabolism, with PEG chains often being unstable. In addition to these observations, degraders and other bifunctionals require one to carefully consider the implications of metabolites. Indeed, compared to a classical inhibition MOA, a metabolite may completely abolish the targeted MOA by preventing ternary complex formation in a low concentration regimen.

### 27.5.2 Safety

During the identification and development of NMs, safety often represents a major unknown. In particular, ONs are carrying multiple chemical modifications in a systematic way, which runs the risk of class effects, compared to the classical molecule-specific risks of small molecules. With many ASOs and siRNAs in clinical trials, learnings are been captured.[316] For example, PS backbones drive higher unspecific protein binding than phosphodiesters, but also increase the risk of binding specific paraspeckle proteins and thus induction of transcription dysregulation and RNA processing, when used in combination with modifications such as MOE, LNA, and cEt.[317] These binding events can result in the mislocalisation of these proteins, shifting them to the nucleoli compartment and inducing cellular stress and then p53-mediated apoptosis. Recently, a novel design rule was discovered, consisting of modifying the second DNA nucleotide within the gap region of the gapmer, to reduce protein binding and overall hepatotoxicity.[317] Modifying specific backbone linkages has also been shown to modulate these side-effects.[318] Recent learnings are also being applied to further tailor design. These include the introduction of 5′-methyl DNA and 2′-modifications and neutral linkages at judicious positions in the gapmer region.[319–321] These studies are particularly useful for driving optimisation with modifications that can address safety concerns in a systematic way. Immune activation and drug-induced glomerulonephritis have also been on the safety concerns list, but can now be de-risked, both through modifications such as 5-methyl cytosine, but also preclinical testing.[322] Off-target effects through degradation of other transcripts by gapmers has been demonstrated and typically depends on the number of mismatches in the ON sequence.[323,324] Another condition associated with ONs is thrombocytopenia, which was identified in several trials. However, there is no evidence so far supporting a class effect, and efforts are been directed at identifying a possible relationship and mechanism.[325,326] Finally, in the case of modified mRNA, with this modality being less mature, little is still known in terms of overall safety. Immunogenicity risks are usually controlled with bespoke nucleobase modifications and projects have progressed in clinical trials, including the now-approved Covid-19 vaccines, demonstrating that the drug can be tolerated. Importantly, some safety questions may originate more from the formulation used, such as LNPs, than the modality itself.

The safety profile of degraders as a modality is limited, to date. Arguably, since degraders are very close to small molecules, the same safety considerations can and are being applied preclinically, including leveraging the robust palette of *in vitro* and *in vivo* assays. However, MOA-specific safety knowledge remains in its infancy. In particular, knowledge is lacking on the impact of competing with the natural substrates of the E3 ligase. In theory, degraders may indeed induce an accumulation of some proteins, including through saturation of the proteasome, triggering imbalances in many biological pathways.[327] Little is also known about the implication of degrading the POI, or off-target proteins. In theory, even a weak binding event can result in protein degradation, and extensive proteomic assays and analyses are required to define a degradation profile.[328–330] In addition, other protein complexes with the POI may also be ubiquitinated, a process sometimes referred to as the 'bystander effect'. Another theoretical concern in terms of degradation is the risk of enzymes such as CYP being ubiquitinated during degrader metabolism, resulting in similar toxicity to classical time-dependant CYP inhibitors.[272] Another concern is the potential induction of protein degradation with some of the routinely used E3 ligase ligands. For example, thalidomide and analogues can themselves lead to ubiquitination of a range of transcription factors.[172]

Depending on the protein synthesis rate, reversing the effect in case of adverse events may also take longer. In the case of on-target toxicity, the prolonged duration of action of the MOA may render dosing regimen optimisation to mitigate toxicity challenging.[327] Undoubtedly, more knowledge will soon be derived from the degraders that have or are about to enter clinical trials. Separately, opportunities exist for degraders in terms of specificity and therefore safety. Indeed, the additional contacts made by the linker at the POI surface, but also in the POI-E3 ligase cooperativity contacts can increase selectivity against proteins of the same family. In particular, in the case of kinases, selectivity can be dramatically improved.[328,331] Furthermore, due to the requirement for recruiting an E3 ligase in this MOA, the expression levels of different E3 ligases in different tissues are an opportunity for encoding tissue specificity and thus increasing the therapeutic window.

### 27.5.3 Delivery/Route of Administration

The route of administration is a central question and still, often, a limitation of NMs. While the larger size of heterobifunctional degraders was believed to likely limit the opportunity for oral delivery, many efforts have been directed at optimising the linker, as discussed in Section 27.5.2.2. In fact, the first degrader that entered clinical trials is being dosed orally. While optimisation is certainly a larger effort than for classical small molecules, Arvinas' drug candidate demonstrates that oral delivery is a viable option and a reasonable goal to set for a heterobifunctional degrader project. In particular, the learnings shared by AstraZeneca and Roche provide additional guidelines for optimising oral uptake.[272,311] With the challenges faced from high lipophilicity and low solubility, the usual assays have to be adapted, including in terms of incubation conditions. Interestingly, PAMPA assays were found to be of little use. An important aspect is that most heterobifunctional degraders are in the low to medium range in terms of permeability, which increases the role of efflux transporters. When profiling hundreds of degraders, VHL ligands were found to be unsuitable for routinely achieving oral exposure. On the other hand, many other degraders could regularly achieve good oral bioavailability (>30%). Notably, linking bioavailability to physicochemical parameters, such as $\log P$ or $\log D$ required alternative methods, such as chromLog$D$7.4, to circumvent the challenges faced with the classical shake flask method, including compound sticking extensively to assay materials.[272]

For other NMs, with the same problem that their larger size impedes cellular uptake, oral uptake is logically at stake, including when taking into account stability in the gastro-intestinal milieu. Nevertheless, progress has been made, in particular in the peptide field. In addition to a broadening of the range of parenteral routes of administration, such as sub-lingual, inhalation, or transdermal delivery, oral delivery has now been achieved with the first orally administered peptide semaglutide. Taking advantage of the high potency of this peptide to modulate the GLP1-receptor, extensive approaches based on fatty acid conjugation to increase half-life and stability successfully led to the discovery of that once-daily 3 to 14 mg pill.

Systemic and sometimes local delivery, including to the CNS *via* intrathecal injection, are routinely used for ONs,[333] and distribution with this route of administration is being better understood.[334] Sub-cutaneous delivery is also now used, and despite advances for delivery to the lung, muscles and tumours,[335,336] more breakthroughs are needed.[337] Despite the dogma that ONs may not be suitable for oral delivery, progress is been made and the principle has been demonstrated.[338] Excitingly, the first ASO administered orally also progressed to humans, representing a landmark for this modality that few had thought would be possible.[332] While peptides and ASO/siRNAs typically remain below 10 kDa, modified mRNAs are in different category when it comes to size, and delivery is therefore an even bigger challenge. Formulation therefore plays a key role, and LNPs are often used, with the disadvantage of limiting delivery to the liver or to local tissue *via* local injections. Other formulations are therefore being developed, not only to extend the targetable tissues, but also to enable chronic dosing through better-tolerated compositions.[270,339,340]

## 27.6 Selection of Chemical Modalities

In Sections 27.2, 27.3, 27.4, and 27.5, the chemical composition of NMs, which MOAs they can enable, and how to identify starting points and optimising them has been discussed, essentially compiling the targetable space, and the strengths and limitations of all these approaches. Overall, all these NMs expand the range of opportunities to treat diseases by leveraging an extensive repertoire of MOAs, which may be deployed to different disease sub-types for which one modality may be better suited over another. An increased range of opportunities does, however, make the selection of chemical modalities a central question for contemporary drug discovery. Many factors can be taken into account and directly originate from the multi-faceted nature of drug discovery and development. In addition to the scientific aspects, other constrains such as cycle time, differentiation, or even cost of choosing a particular approach also play a role. This last point is unfortunately even more prevalent in the field of NMs, with some modalities being proprietary to some companies, or implicitly having a high barrier to entry, as a result of the required infrastructure and knowledge build. Nevertheless, over the last decade, partnerships have become more common.[12] In this respect, this section describes the more scientific considerations for modality selection, leaving aside any economics. Small molecules and biologics still offer many advantages and are therefore, logically, included in this discussion. Importantly, the framework in this section is based on advanced modalities. Other, less mature, modalities may represent novel opportunities and should be considered as well, but are harder to include into a generic framework due to their limited characterisation.

## 27.6.1 Framework for Modality Selection

### *27.6.1.1 Criteria and MOA Mapping*

Drug discovery's primary goal is to modulate and treat disease, and, leaving aside phenotypic screening for the context of this chapter, selecting a drug target is central to early-stage drug discovery. As discussed earlier, targets are still usually considered to be proteins, or more specifically their function. While non-coding RNAs are increasingly believed to also have a function in themselves,[341,342] the current target-based drug discovery paradigm is still very much aligned along the transcription–translation–function sequence. For this reason, the framework described herein is based on this paradigm.

With an extended set of modalities able to achieve the same outcome *via* different means, *i.e.* modulating function *via* different MOAs, the selection of the MOA represents a critical factor. In addition, classical and NMs display different strengths and weaknesses which can inform the selection of a particular approach. These characteristics, summarised in Table 27.1, are useful for drawing some criteria for modality selection at the inception of a new project. The most central common feature of many NMs is the challenge of achieving cellular uptake, and their common opportunity is to be well suited for hard-to-drug targets.

Based on this, and for each novel drug target, two key questions can be used to define four main scenarios. The target localisation (intra *vs.* extracellular) and the type of effect (up- or downregulation of function/levels) drive the type of MOAs that can be leveraged (Figure 27.11). Localisation helps to separate approaches that can provide high specificity, such as antibodies, but that are to date intractable for intracellular applications. Similarly, some modalities are only applicable to either up- or downregulation. For example, degraders exclusively downregulate protein function/levels.

### *27.6.1.2 Scenario Analysis for Modality Mapping and Selection*

Within each of the scenarios mapped in Figure 27.11, one possible next level assessment is to consider whether this target is classical (*e.g.* kinases and some other enzymes, class A GPCRs *etc.*) or hard-to-drug (PPIs, transcription factors,

**Table 27.1** Summary of strengths and limitations of classical and new modalities.

| Modality | Strengths | Limitations |
|---|---|---|
| Small molecules | • Broad tissue distribution<br>• Oral delivery | • Lower specificity<br>• Requires targetable site |
| Proteins/ antibodies | • High affinity<br>• Long half-life<br>• High specificity | • Tissue penetration<br>• Immunogenicity risk<br>• Extracellular targets only |
| Novel peptide architectures | • High affinity<br>• High specificity<br>• Potential for oral delivery | • Predominantly extracellular targets<br>• Immunogenicity risk |
| ASOs/siRNA | • Programmable<br>• Can be deployed against any target type<br>• Can exhibit long duration of action | • Few tissues reachable<br>• Non-oral<br>• Safety profile not complete yet |
| Modified mRNA | • Unique MOA | • Limited to liver and local administration<br>• Not suitable yet for chronic treatment<br>• Limited overall safety knowledge to date |
| Heterobi-functional degraders | • Unique MOA<br>• May address some 'hard-to-drug' targets<br>• Exploits SM knowledge<br>• Oral delivery possible<br>• Broader pharmacological profile | • Safety profile not complete yet<br>• Extensive optimization required |

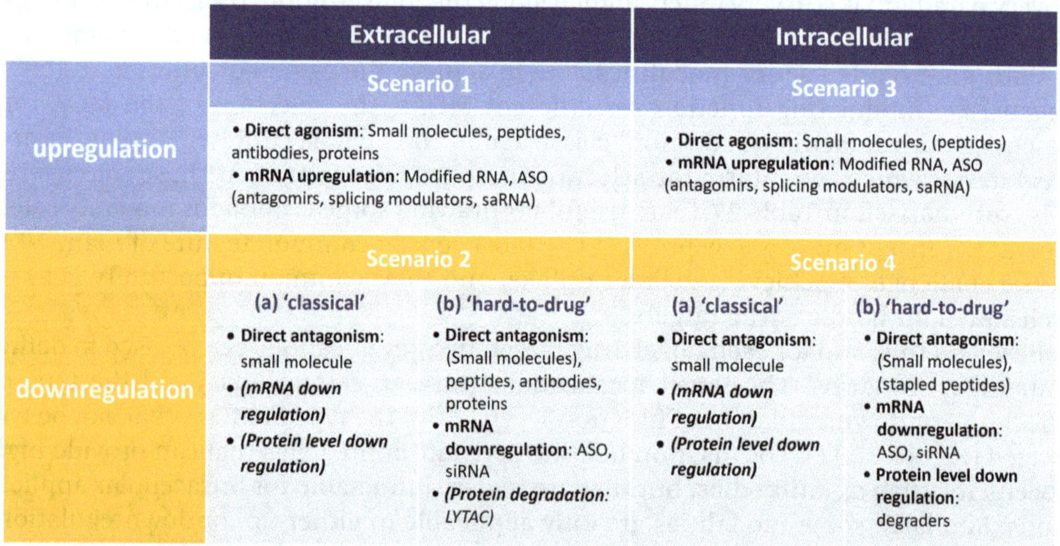


**Figure 27.11** Scenario mapping of targetable MOAs and their associated modalities. Note that some MOAs are listed in parentheses and italic: these are possible, but it is not clear at first glance why the approach would be of advantage if a small molecule can be used. This is also valid for heterobifunctional degraders: the majority of reported degraders to date are in fact targeting proteins with known small molecules. While there may be pharmacological advantages, it is not obvious that degraders are advantageous for many of these targets.

phosphatases *etc.*), which then results in two sub-scenarios. Indeed, this criterion exploits the situation that hard-to-drug targets are often less suitable for classical small molecules and that alternative MOAs may therefore be preferable. However, for upregulation (Scenarios 1 and 3), this type of effect is generally one of the hardest types in drug discovery, apart perhaps for some GPCRs, and the distinction between target types is therefore not as useful. The potential MOAs that can be applied to the six (sub)-scenarios, and their associated modalities that can be considered are also summarised in Figure 27.11.

As summarised in Table 27.1, each modality possesses a different profile of strengths and limitations. Some MOAs also possess specific profiles. The nuances between MOAs and modalities therefore make it challenging to define generic selections with each target requiring bespoke considerations. For example, protein expression from modified mRNA treatment can incorporate endogenous post-translational modifications and therefore be in some cases advantageous over a recombinant protein treatment. Nevertheless, a set of MOA- and/or modality-specific key questions can assist in achieving a shortlist of preferred modalities that can be further analysed based on disease-, target-, and business-specific considerations. These key questions are captured in Table 27.2. Overall, the different steps of the framework of the MOA and modality selection are summarised in Figure 27.12.

## 27.6.2 Examples of Modality Selection

In this section, the framework is placed in the context of real target examples, illustrating the four main categories of scenarios. The mapping step is captured in Table 27.3.

### *27.6.2.1 Example 1: GLP1-receptor (Scenario 1)*

The GLP1 receptor is a glucose-sensitive receptor which, upon binding of the natural GLP1 peptide hormone, triggers insulin secretion. It is therefore an important drug target for glucose level management in diabetic patients.

The MOA and modality selection framework identifies two potential MOAs:

- *Direct agonism*: Small molecules, peptides, and proteins may agonise the GLP1-receptor function.
- *mRNA upregulation*: a modified mRNA may be able to increase the receptor level.

The list of potential modalities and corresponding MOAs is therefore: small molecules, peptides and proteins/antibodies (direct agonism) and modified mRNA (mRNA upregulation).

Next, the MOA/modality-specific key questions are applied:

- *Small molecules/peptide/proteins*:
  - Is there a known mechanism of activation (*e.g.* activators for GPCRs)? What is the chemical composition of the natural ligand? The GLP1 receptor is a class B GPCR, whose ligand is the GLP1 peptide hormone. While possible in theory, a small molecule is less likely to be tractable. Considering the size of the GLP1 peptide (40-mer), proteins and antibodies may be too large.

Table 27.2 Key questions for MOAs and modality to assist selection.

| MOA/modality | Key questions | Reasons/Consequences |
|---|---|---|
| Extracellular direct agonism | • Is there a known mechanism of activation (*e.g.* activators for GPCRs)?<br>• What is the chemical composition of the natural ligand?<br>• Is the target located in a solid tissue? | • Activation is a very hard MOA to enable<br>• Existence of a mechanism may enable mimicking<br>• Knowledge of the endogenous ligand indicates the likely preferred chemical composition or the modality<br>• If the target is predominantly located in a solid tissue, access with antibodies and proteins will likely be more challenging |
| mRNA upregulation | • Are there differentiated splice variants associated with different levels of activity?<br>• Is the mRNA regulation mechanism known and validated? | • Knowledge about splice variants may qualify ASO or SM<br>• Validation of a miRNA regulating the targeted mRNA may enable antagomirs as a modality (ASOs) |
| mRNA downregulation | • Is the mRNA regulation mechanism known and validated (*i.e.* which miRNA is involved)? | • Validation of a miRNA regulating the targeted mRNA may enable miRNA mimics as a modality (ASOs) |
| Protein degradation | • What are the protein levels and half-life?<br>• Where is the POI located? | • Protein having short half-life may be less suitable for protein degradation approaches (rapid turnover)<br>• High levels of the POI, may, depending on the resynthesis rate of the protein, make it less tractable for PROTACs<br>• If the target is extracellular or membrane bound without any intracellular domain, the POI will traffic to the endoplasmic reticulum for folding and packaging, and the proteasome machinery is absent in that compartment. Note that a LYTAC approach may be considered but not well validated yet. |
| Antibodies/ proteins | • Does the route of administration have to be oral? | • If the TPP requires this delivery route, this disables the choice of antibodies or proteins a modality |
| Peptides | • Does the route of administration have to be oral? | • If the TPP requires this delivery route, this would imply the need of intense optimisation without a guarantee for success, and thus decrease the POS of this modality |
| ASOs and siRNA | • Is the target tissue reachable? | • If the target is located outside the liver, kidney, spleen, CNS or eye, this modality would be less preferred. A targeted delivery approach may be required with an overall lower POS. Note that ASO exposure is cell-type dependant in the kidney and other tissues, so a specific cell type may also decrease the POS. |
| Modified RNA | • Is the target tissue reachable or suitable for local delivery?<br>• Is chronic treatment required? | • Modified mRNA delivery is currently restricted.<br>• Chronic treatment has not yet been enabled with tolerated formulations |

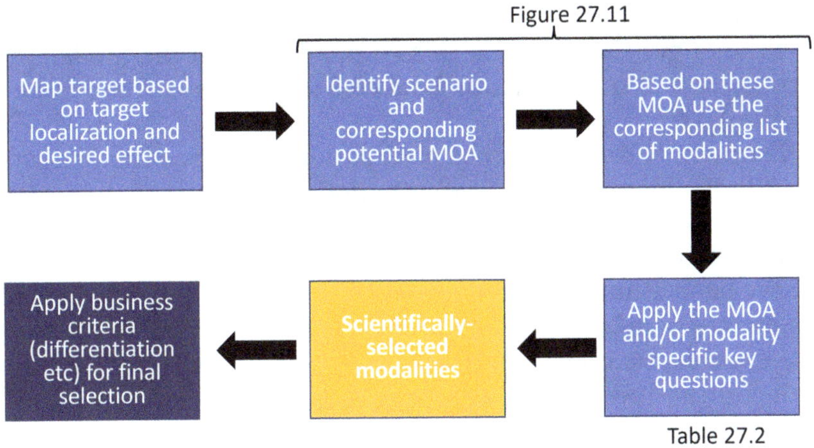


**Figure 27.12** Summary of the MOA and modality selection framework. The tools (figures and tables) are listed for reference.

**Table 27.3** Examples of modality selection for different targets.

| Target | GLP1 receptor | PCSK9 | SMN2 | AR |
|---|---|---|---|---|
| Target localisation | Extracellular (membrane bound) | Extracellular (secreted) | Intracellular | Intracellular (nucleus) |
| Desired effect | Upregulation | Downregulation | Upregulation (correct isoform) | Downregulation |
| Target type | Hard-to-drug (class B GPCR) | Hard-to-drug (PPI) | N/A (Hard-to-drug (MOA)) | Hard-to-drug (Transcription factor/Nuclear receptor) |
| Resulting scenario category | Scenario 1 | Scenario 2b | Scenario 3 | Scenario 4b |
| Potential MOAs | Direct agonism<br>mRNA upregulation | Direct antagonism<br>mRNA down regulation<br>Protein level down regulation | mRNA upregulation | Direct antagonism<br>Protein degradation<br>mRNA downregulation |
| Potential modalities | Peptides<br>Antibodies<br>Modified RNA | Small molecules<br>Peptides<br>ASO/siRNA<br>Antibodies | ASOs (steric blockers)<br>Small molecules (splicing modulators) | Small molecules<br>Heterobifunctional degraders<br>ASO/siRNA |

- Is the target located in a solid tissue? Yes, the GLP1 receptor is located primarily in the pancreas (with some expression in the brain as well). This makes antibodies less favourable.

- *Peptides/antibodies*:
  - Does the route of administration have to be oral? Diabetic patients rely on insulin injections, and an oral profile, while desirable, may not be a must.

- *Modified RNA*:
  - What is the target tissue and is this compatible with the modality? The GLP1-receptor is located on pancreatic beta-cells, which is currently not enabled for modified mRNA.
  - Is the treatment chronic? Glucose modulation requires chronic treatment which is currently challenging to achieve with modified mRNA.

Overall, peptides represent the preferred modality. Interestingly, small molecule approaches have been attempted but the majority failed to deliver clinical candidates, not a surprising outcome considering the less preferred choice of such a modality in this setting. Nevertheless, one small molecule, PF-06882961 recently entered clinical trials.[343] On the other hand, several peptidic agonists have reached the market, including recently semaglutide as the first oral peptide.

#### 27.6.2.2 Example 2: PCSK9 Inhibition (Scenario 2b)

The proprotein convertase subtilisin/kexin type 9 (PCSK9) protein has been a long sought-after drug target due to its high level of target validation and its implications in cardiovascular diseases. PCSK9 is a repressor of the LDL receptor function through induction of its degradation. Following downregulation of the LDL receptor, plasma cholesterol levels increase, with the well-known health consequences.[344] Many approaches have been directed at this target,[345] which has led to approval of alirocumab and evolocumad.

The MOA and modality selection framework identifies three potential MOAs:

- *Direct antagonism*: PCSK9 function modulation implies disrupting the PCK9-LDL receptor interaction. This type of target is typically very hard to drug with small molecules. On the other hand, antibodies and peptides are viable options.
- *mRNA downregulation*: both ASOs gapmers and siRNA can be considered.
- *Protein level downregulation*: PCSK9 being a secreted protein, E3 ligase-based heterobifunctional degrader approaches are to date unsuitable, as the endoplasmic reticulum in which secreted proteins are stored and folded does not possess the machinery for degradation. The LYTAC strategy to degrade extracellular proteins may be considered, but this modality is arguably still in its infancy. Framing protein level downregulation beyond degradation, an additional possibility is to slow down or block translation with modalities that can access the intracellular space, namely small molecules.

The list of potential modalities and corresponding MOA is therefore: peptides and antibodies (direct antagonism), ASOs and siRNAs (mRNA downregulation), small molecules (protein levels downregulation).

Next, the MOA/modality-specific key questions are applied:

- Peptides/antibodies:
  - Does the route of administration have to be oral? Views may vary from one company to the other. Arguably, considering the level of target validation and with part of the patient population already being accustomed to injections (diabetic

patients relying on insulin injections), an oral profile, while desirable, may not be a must. Consequently, peptides and antibodies remain a valid option.

- *ASOs and siRNAs*:
  - Is the target located in a tissue accessible to ONs? PCSK9 is a liver target and is therefore very well suited to ASOs and siRNAs.

The PCSK9 example is particularly useful when considering what eventually happened on this target over the last decade: small molecule antagonists were attempted by several companies without any success for many years, and using this framework, this strategy would have been deprioritised. Peptides and antibodies as antagonists have been targeted at PCSK9, and antibodies eventually reached the market. Additional efforts with peptides are still ongoing.[346] Small molecules to modulate protein levels, an option arguably not considered a decade ago, was successfully implemented by scientists at Pfizer, who designed a cellular assay leading to the identification of such small molecules and deconvolution of the MOA led to translation stalling as the mechanism.[344,347] While this compound series did not progress to the clinic, it nevertheless illustrates how multiple modalities can be aimed at a target, when considering multiple types of MOAs. Moreover, the recent disclosure of direct small molecule modulators of PCSK9 reflects that while the framework enables a rational approach to modality selection, it does not imply that other modalities are impossible.[348]

### 27.6.2.3 Example 3: SMN2 Splicing Correction (Scenario 3)

The survival motor neuron (SMN) protein is a critical determinant of spinal muscular atrophy (SMA), a neuromuscular disease. Indeed, lack of functional SMN, as a result of a genetic mutation, results in loss of motor neurons and muscle atrophy. In order to address the disease, a functional SMN is required, corresponding to the category of function upregulation. To achieve this, leveraging the SMN2 gene and modifying splicing is a way to unable formation of the right mRNA leading to functional SMN protein.

The MOA and modality selection framework identifies three potential MOAs:

- *Direct agonism*: in this very specific case, this is not possible as the functional protein is lacking.
- *mRNA upregulation*: modified RNA would be a direct means to provide the cells with the correct mRNA form. mRNA upregulation could also be achieved by exploiting the SMN2 gene, using putative ASO or small molecules.

The list of potential modalities and corresponding MOA is therefore: modified mRNA (mRNA upregulation), ASOs (mRNA upregulation), small molecules (mRNA upregulation).

Next, the MOA/modality-specific key questions are applied:

- modified RNA:
  - Is the target tissue reachable or suitable for local delivery? SMN2 is a CNS target which is currently not accessible with modified RNA.
  - Is the treatment chronic? The defect being genetic, treatment would need to be repeated, although as neurons are non-dividing cells, longer intervals between doses may be possible if the modality has a long half-life.

- *ASO*:
  - o Is the target located in a tissue accessible to ONs? The answer to this question would have been different at the inception of a SMN2 project a decade ago. Indeed, the currently marketed ASO nusinersen has been developed for SMA and is administered by intrathecal injection.[133,349] It is therefore now established that ASOs can be used for CNS projects.

Overall, small molecules and ASOs represent the preferred modalities. This conclusion is however confounded by the fact that ridisplam and nusinersen are the first examples of small molecules and ASOs modulating splicing and of an ASO being delivered to the CNS.

### 27.6.2.4 Example 4: Androgen Receptor (Scenario 4b)

The androgen receptor (AR) is a transcription factor whose natural ligands are several hormones, including testosterone. Upon binding to one of its ligands, the AR translocates to the nucleus to carry out its transcriptional function. The AR is associated with prostate cancer, and downregulating its function has been a drug target to slow down cancer progression.

The MOA and modality selection framework identifies three potential MOAs:

- *Direct antagonism*: targeting the ligand binding domain with small molecules is a viable approach, despite the sensitivity for this target class to have unpredicted switches between agonism and antagonism when bound to synthetic small molecules.
- *mRNA downregulation*: both ASOs gapmers and siRNA can be considered.
- *Protein level downregulation*: a protein degradation approach such as heterobifunctional degraders can be considered.

The list of potential modalities and corresponding MOA is therefore: small molecules (direct antagonism), ASOs/siRNAs (mRNA downregulation), and heterobifunctional degrader (protein level downregulation).

Next, the MOA/modality-specific key questions are applied:

- *ASO and siRNAs*:
  - o Is the target located in a tissue accessible to ONs? Tumour access still represents a challenge for ON therapies. While possible, this makes ONs less preferred for this target.
- *Protein degradation*:
  - o What are the protein levels and half-life? The AR has a half-life of 3–10 hours in LNCaP cells.[350]
  - o Where is the POI located? The AR is located in the nucleus where the proteasome machinery is present. It is therefore degradable.

Overall, small molecules and degraders represent the preferred modalities, and several small molecules have been approved, such as enzalutamide, while a heterobifunctional degrader targeting the AR is the first example of this modality entering the clinic.

### 27.6.3 Further Considerations

The framework from this section is aimed at providing a guide for medicinal chemists for selecting a set of preferred modalities for a given target. Importantly, no framework can recapitulate and consolidate all the nuances that can tilt a selection towards one over another modality, or even selecting an *a priori* less preferred modality. Many other considerations, such as duration of action and protein half-life, can significantly alter any selection. In addition, new waves of scientific creativity and progress will alter the summaries from this chapter and framework and should be considered when selecting MOAs and modalities for future projects.

## 27.7 Conclusion: Clinical Progress and Perspectives

Over the last decade, NMs have progressively evolved from a state of curiosity, perplexity, or even dismissal, to a position of reshaping the therapeutic landscape. For example, oligonucleotide therapies, such as ASOs and siRNA, long deemed to be intractable, have now resulted in multiple approvals. Modified RNA rapidly raised its status in the context of COVID-19 vaccines, especially from a speed of design-to-clinic standpoint. Peptides, long considered as being not deliverable by oral administration, have demonstrated, *via* semaglutide, that dogma can be broken, a paradigm that is being extended to ASOs. Heterobifunctional degraders are another example, where scepticism (at best) was prevalent for any molecule breaking the Lipinski rules, yet they have highlighted how cell permeability and oral dosing can be enabled through thorough optimisation and a willingness to advance into uncharted territories. Table 27.4 summarises key clinical examples of NMs progress in the clinic and to the market.

While this chapter has aimed to emphasise those NMs that have most significantly progressed towards late-stage drug discovery and through clinical development, the increasing number of innovative approaches also offer many opportunities to develop chemical probes to investigate novel biology.[13] As described in Section 27.2, the different areas of the chemical space can be brought together and combined in the form of fusions and conjugates, not only to exploit the benefits of individual modalities, but also to mimic and hijack biological processes to create unprecedented MOAs. Undoubtedly, creativity in that area will help to further develop these NMs, as well as overcoming some emerging limitations, as seen in the case of degraders with the appearance of novel resistance mechanisms.[351]

Perhaps unsurprisingly, chemically-induced proximity is gaining major attention across multiple range of effect modulations. Thus, heterobifunctional molecules have been developed to induce phosphorylation by recruiting kinases (PHICS),[95] deubiquitinases (DUBTAC),[352] phosphatases (PHORC),[353] and acetylases (ACETAG).[354] The concept is also being deployed at the RNA level, with RIBOTACs, to enable the degradation of RNA species.[355–358] All these exciting developments illustrate how medicinal chemists will significantly shape the future landscape of therapeutic modalities by rewiring biological processes.

In addition to engineering chemical modalities by design, a significant area of opportunities for medicinal and organic chemists is the actual syntheses of such molecules,

**Table 27.4** Overview of representative clinical and marketed drugs, classified by type of new modality.

| Modality | MOA | Name | Target | Disease | Progress | Comment |
|---|---|---|---|---|---|---|
| Peptide (bicyclic conjugate) | Cytotoxic agent (drug-conjugate) | BT1718 | MT1-MMP (receptor) | Cancer | Phase II | |
| Peptide fusion | Agonism | Cotadutide | Dual GLP1/GR | Diabetes | Phase II | |
| Peptide (Stapled) | Antagonism (intracellular) | ARLN-6924 | HDM2-p53 | Cancer | Phase I | |
| Peptide | Direct agonism | Semaglutide | GLP1R | Diabetes | Marketed | First oral peptide active systemically |
| ASO | RNA upregulation (splicing modulation) | Nusinersen | SMN2 | Spinal muscular atrophy | Marketed | |
| ASO | RNA downregulation | Inotersen | Transthyretin | Polyneuropathy of hereditary ATTR amyloidosis | Marketed | |
| siRNA | RNA downregulation | Patisiran | Transthyretin | Hereditary ATTR amyloidosis | Marketed | First siRNA to be approved |
| ASO (antagomir) | RNA upregulation | RG-012 | miR21 | Alport syndrome | Phase II | |
| Modified mRNA | RNA upregulation | AZD8601 | VEGF-A | Heart failure | Phase II | First mRNA therapy that has entered clinical trials |
| Heterobifunctional degraders | Protein degradation | ARV-110 | AR | Cancer | Phase II | |

which typically display increased complexity. There again, the possibility to cross-over the creativity of organic chemists working on small molecules to NMs represents a vast territory for innovation. For example, developing late-stage functionalisation of NMs is particularly valuable considering the efforts sometimes required to synthesise a single molecule.[359] Applying nanoscale chemistry, which is being developed in particular in the context of automation of small molecule synthesis,[360,361] has major implications for NMs, considering the costs associated with some NMs synthesis.

Beyond the direct scientific achievements of NMs, especially over the last 5 years, perhaps an even bigger achievement is how the mindset of many medicinal chemists is evolving, with many young and many experienced scientists embracing the opportunity for creativity and solving therapeutic challenges in innovative ways. As a thought-provoking anecdote, the author was asked a few years ago by another medicinal chemist at a conference, why he had decided to leave medicinal chemistry for NMs… NMs are now an integral part of contemporary medicinal chemistry and drug discovery, and creativity and embracing uncharted territories will undoubtedly benefit many more patients whose conditions require any therapeutics, no matter what their chemical composition or molecular weight.

## 27.8 Hints and Tips

- For a given therapeutic target, consider all modalities, even if those are not enabled in your organisation. This informs the overall opportunity space and whether other groups may be competitors through a different modality, which in some cases may be faster to reach the clinic.
- Carefully consider the target tissue before selecting a modality. If the tissue is not enabled for delivery, then efforts toward solving this specific tissue access should be initiated in parallel with the inception of the project rather than down the line.
- Keep creativity high from a chemical space and engineering standpoint, yet without being fooled by the elusive nature of some modalities when it comes to intracellular access.
- With the development of oral delivery for peptides (semaglutide) and ASOs (PCKS9), remain realistic about the POS for this profile. This is still opportunistic today, so consider first having a viable project with parenteral routes of administration, and if the molecule becomes extremely potent and with long duration of action, then explore oral formulation.
- If target validation is the main goal, consider perhaps a non-classical modality for demonstration, retaining the principle of pharmacological modulation, in particular through measurement of target engagement, keeping in mind though, that different MOAs do not necessarily translate from one another (for example depletion of RNA with an ASO, *versus* inhibition of the protein function with a small molecule).
- While the development of *in silico* models is rapidly progressing across several modalities, there is still a need for substantial empirical data. Notably, modalities such as oligonucleotides and degraders require significantly more *in vivo* studies than classical modalities, due to the challenging translation from *in vitro* to *in vivo* when it comes to DMPK and efficacy.

## Key References


- E. Valeur, S. M. Guéret, H. Adihou, R. Gopalakrishnan, M. Lemurell, H. Waldmann, T. N. Grossmann and A. T. Plowright, *Angew. Chem., Int. Ed.*, 2017, **56**, 10294–10323. *Seminal review of the new modalities field, providing additional examples of new modalities beyond those that are the most advanced preclinically or clinically*
- E. Valeur and P. Jimonet, *J. Med. Chem.*, 2018, **61**, 9004–9029. *Reviews systematically lead generation including for new modalities, and highlights a MOA-centric paradigm for drug discovery, by selecting the point of intervention (DNA, RNA or protein level), modality and the resulting hit finding strategies*
- C. J. Gerry and S. L. Schreiber, *Nat. Chem. Biol.*, 2020, **16**, 369–378. *Describes in detail the premise and principles of chemically induced proximity, hence providing an outlook for how new modalities may further expand in the future*

## List of Abbreviations

| | |
|---|---|
| **ASO** | Antisense oligonucleotide |
| **AUTAC** | Autophagy-targeting chimera |
| **ATTEC** | Autophagosome-tethering compound |
| **DML** | Designed multiple ligand |
| **LNA** | Locked nucleic acid |
| **LNP** | Lipid nanoparticle |
| **miRNA** | Micro RNA |
| **MOA** | Mode of action |
| **NM** | New modality |
| **ON** | Oligonucleotide |
| **PMO** | Phosphorodiamidite morpholino oligomers |
| **PNA** | Peptide nucleic acid |
| **POI** | Protein of interest |
| **POS** | Probability of success |
| **PPI** | Protein–protein interaction |
| **PROTAC** | Proteolysis targeting chimera |
| **PS** | Phosphorothioate |
| **saRNA** | Small activating RNA |
| **siRNA** | Short interference RNA |
| **tcDNA** | Tricyclic DNA |

## References


1. B. J. Druker, F. Guilhot, S. G. O'Brien, I. Gathmann, H. Kantarjian, N. Gattermann, M. W. N. Deininger, R. T. Silver, J. M. Goldman, R. M. Stone, F. Cervantes, A. Hochhaus, B. L. Powell, J. L. Gabrilove, P. Rousselot, J. Reiffers, J. J. Cornelissen, T. Hughes, H. Agis, T. Fischer, G. Verhoef, J. Shepherd, G. Saglio, A. Gratwohl, J. L. Nielsen, J. P. Radich, B. Simonsson, K. Taylor, M. Baccarani, C. So, L. Letvak and R. A. Larson, *N. Engl. J. Med.*, 2006, **355**, 2408–2417.
2. E. De Clercq, *Int. J. Antimicrob. Agents*, 2009, **33**, 307–320.
3. M. Rosenfeld, C. E. Wainwright, M. Higgins, L. T. Wang, C. McKee, D. Campbell, S. Tian, J. Schneider, S. Cunningham, J. C. Davies, M. Rosenfeld, C. E. Wainwright, M. Higgins, L. T. Wang, C. McKee, D. Campbell, S. Tian, J. Schneider, S. Cunningham, J. C. Davies, W. Harris, P. Mogayzel, K. McCoy, C. Milla, R. Rubenstein, S. Walker, P. Black, G. Montgomery, S. McColley, P. Hiatt, G. Sawicki, M. Rock, P. Aurora, F. Ratjen, A. Maitra, A. Ives, E. Gaillard, P. McNalley, H. Selvadurai and P. Robinson, *Lancet Respir. Med.*, 2018, **6**, 545–553.
4. D. M. Hyman, B. S. Taylor and J. Baselga, *Cell*, 2017, **168**, 584–599.
5. A. M. Davis, A. T. Plowright and E. Valeur, *Nat. Rev. Drug Discovery*, 2017, **16**, 681–698.
6. E. Marbán, *Nat. Biomed. Eng.*, 2018, **2**, 353–361.
7. L. Labanieh, R. G. Majzner and C. L. Mackall, *Nat. Biomed. Eng.*, 2018, **2**, 377–391.
8. S. Guedan, M. Ruella and C. H. June, *Annu. Rev. Immunol.*, 2019, **37**, 145–171.
9. P. D. Cani, *Gut*, 2018, **67**, 1716–1725.
10. A. C. Wong and M. Levy, *mSystems*, 2019, **4**, e00122-19.
11. J. L. McQuade, C. R. Daniel, B. A. Helmink and J. A. Wargo, *Lancet Oncol.*, 2019, **20**, e77–e91.
12. E. Valeur and P. Jimonet, *J. Med. Chem.*, 2018, **61**, 9004–9029.
13. E. Valeur, S. M. Guéret, H. Adihou, R. Gopalakrishnan, M. Lemurell, H. Waldmann, T. N. Grossmann and A. T. Plowright, *Angew. Chem., Int. Ed.*, 2017, **56**, 10294–10323.
14. E. Valeur, L. Knerr, M. Ölwegård-Halvarsson and M. Lemurell, *Drug Discovery Today*, 2017, 22, 841–847.
15. E. Valeur, F. Narjes, C. Ottmann and A. T. Plowright, *MedChemComm*, 2019, **10**, 1550–1568.
16. E. Valeur, in *Protein Degradation with New Chemical Modalities*, ed. H. Weinmann and C. Crews, The Royal Society of Chemistry, 2021.

17. I. Dunham, A. Kundaje, S. F. Aldred, P. J. Collins, C. A. Davis, F. Doyle, C. B. Epstein, S. Frietze, J. Harrow, R. Kaul, J. Khatun, B. R. Lajoie, S. G. Landt, B.-K. Lee, F. Pauli, K. R. Rosenbloom, P. Sabo, A. Safi, A. Sanyal, N. Shoresh, J. M. Simon, L. Song, N. D. Trinklein, R. C. Altshuler, E. Birney, J. B. Brown, C. Cheng, S. Djebali, X. Dong, I. Dunham, J. Ernst, T. S. Furey, M. Gerstein, B. Giardine, M. Greven, R. C. Hardison, R. S. Harris, J. Herrero, M. M. Hoffman, S. Iyer, M. Kellis, J. Khatun, P. Kheradpour, A. Kundaje, T. Lassmann, Q. Li, X. Lin, G. K. Marinov, A. Merkel, A. Mortazavi, S. C. J. Parker, T. E. Reddy, J. Rozowsky, F. Schlesinger, R. E. Thurman, J. Wang, L. D. Ward, T. W. Whitfield, S. P. Wilder, W. Wu, H. S. Xi, K. Y. Yip, J. Zhuang, B. E. Bernstein, E. Birney, I. Dunham, E. D. Green, C. Gunter, M. Snyder, M. J. Pazin, R. F. Lowdon, L. A. L. Dillon, L. B. Adams, C. J. Kelly, J. Zhang, J. R. Wexler, E. D. Green, P. J. Good, E. A. Feingold, B. E. Bernstein, E. Birney, G. E. Crawford, J. Dekker, L. Elnitski, P. J. Farnham, M. Gerstein, M. C. Giddings, T. R. Gingeras, E. D. Green, R. Guigó, R. C. Hardison, T. J. Hubbard, M. Kellis, W. J. Kent, J. D. Lieb, E. H. Margulies, R. M. Myers, M. Snyder, J. A. Stamatoyannopoulos, S. A. Tenenbaum, Z. Weng, K. P. White, B. Wold, J. Khatun, Y. Yu, J. Wrobel, B. A. Risk, H. P. Gunawardena, H. C. Kuiper, C. W. Maier, L. Xie, X. Chen, M. C. Giddings, B. E. Bernstein, C. B. Epstein, N. Shoresh, J. Ernst, P. Kheradpour, T. S. Mikkelsen, S. Gillespie, A. Goren, O. Ram, X. Zhang, L. Wang, R. Issner, M. J. Coyne, T. Durham, M. Ku, T. Truong, L. D. Ward, R. C. Altshuler, M. L. Eaton, M. Kellis, S. Djebali, C. A. Davis, A. Merkel, A. Dobin, T. Lassmann, A. Mortazavi, A. Tanzer, J. Lagarde, W. Lin, F. Schlesinger, C. Xue, G. K. Marinov, J. Khatun, B. A. Williams, C. Zaleski, J. Rozowsky, M. Röder, F. Kokocinski, R. F. Abdelhamid, T. Alioto, I. Antoshechkin, M. T. Baer, P. Batut, I. Bell, K. Bell, S. Chakrabortty, X. Chen, J. Chrast, J. Curado, T. Derrien, J. Drenkow, E. Dumais, J. Dumais, R. Duttagupta, M. Fastuca, K. Fejes-Toth, P. Ferreira, S. Foissac, M. J. Fullwood, H. Gao, D. Gonzalez, A. Gordon, H. P. Gunawardena, C. Howald, S. Jha, R. Johnson, P. Kapranov, B. King, C. Kingswood, G. Li, O. J. Luo, E. Park, J. B. Preall, K. Presaud, P. Ribeca, B. A. Risk, D. Robyr, X. Ruan, M. Sammeth, K. S. Sandhu, L. Schaeffer, L.-H. See, A. Shahab, J. Skancke, A. M. Suzuki, H. Takahashi, H. Tilgner, D. Trout, N. Walters, H. Wang, J. Wrobel, Y. Yu, Y. Hayashizaki, J. Harrow, M. Gerstein, T. J. Hubbard, A. Reymond, S. E. Antonarakis, G. J. Hannon, M. C. Giddings, Y. Ruan, B. Wold, P. Carninci, R. Guigó, T. R. Gingeras, K. R. Rosenbloom, C. A. Sloan, K. Learned, V. S. Malladi, M. C. Wong, G. P. Barber, M. S. Cline, T. R. Dreszer, S. G. Heitner, D. Karolchik, W. J. Kent, V. M. Kirkup, L. R. Meyer, J. C. Long, M. Maddren, B. J. Raney, T. S. Furey, L. Song, L. L. Grasfeder, P. G. Giresi, B.-K. Lee, A. Battenhouse, N. C. Sheffield, J. M. Simon, K. A. Showers, A. Safi, D. London, A. A. Bhinge, C. Shestak, M. R. Schaner, S. Ki Kim, Z. Z. Zhang, P. A. Mieczkowski, J. O. Mieczkowska, Z. Liu, R. M. McDaniell, Y. Ni, N. U. Rashid, M. J. Kim, S. Adar, Z. Zhang, T. Wang, D. Winter, D. Keefe, E. Birney, V. R. Iyer, J. D. Lieb, G. E. Crawford, G. Li, K. S. Sandhu, M. Zheng, P. Wang, O. J. Luo, A. Shahab, M. J. Fullwood, X. Ruan, Y. Ruan, R. M. Myers, F. Pauli, B. A. Williams, J. Gertz, G. K. Marinov, T. E. Reddy, J. Vielmetter, E. Partridge, D. Trout, K. E. Varley, C. Gasper, The ENCODE Project Consortium, Overall coordination (data analysis coordination), Data production leads (data production), Lead analysts (data analysis), Writing group, NHGRI project management (scientific management), Principal investigators (steering committee), Boise State University and University of North Carolina at Chapel Hill Proteomics groups (data production and analysis), Broad Institute Group (data production and analysis), U. of G. Cold Spring Harbor Center for Genomic Regulation, Barcelona, RIKEN, Sanger Institute, University of Lausanne, Genome Institute of Singapore group (data production and analysis), Data coordination center at UC Santa Cruz (production data coordination), E. Duke University University of Texas, Austin, University of North Carolina-Chapel Hill group (data production and analysis), Genome Institute of Singapore group (data production and analysis) and C. HudsonAlpha Institute UC Irvine, Stanford group (data production and analysis), *Nature*, 2012, **489**, 57–74.
18. C. F. Bennett and E. E. Swayze, *Annu. Rev. Pharmacol. Toxicol.*, 2010, **50**, 259–293.
19. X. Shen and D. R. Corey, *Nucleic Acids Res.*, 2018, **46**, 1584–1600.
20. V. K. Sharma and J. K. Watts, *Future Med. Chem.*, 2015, **7**, 2221–2242.
21. M. Egli and M. Manoharan, *Acc. Chem. Res.*, 2019, **52**, 1036–1047.
22. A. Khvorova and J. K. Watts, *Nat. Biotechnol.*, 2017, **35**, 238–248.
23. W. B. Wan and P. P. Seth, *J. Med. Chem.*, 2016, **59**, 9645–9667.
24. F. Eckstein, *Antisense Nucleic Acid Drug Dev.*, 2000, **10**, 117–121.
25. A. H. S. Hall, J. Wan, E. E. Shaughnessy, B. Ramsay Shaw and K. A. Alexander, *Nucleic Acids Res.*, 2004, **32**, 5991–6000.
26. W. F. Lima, J. G. Nichols, H. Wu, T. P. Prakash, M. T. Migawa, T. K. Wyrzykiewicz, B. Bhat and S. T. Crooke, *J. Biol. Chem.*, 2004, **279**, 36317–36326.
27. M. E. Østergaard, P. Kumar, J. Nichols, A. Watt, P. K. Sharma, P. Nielsen and P. P. Seth, *Nucleic Acid Ther.*, 2015, **25**, 266–274.

28. P. P. Seth and E. E. Swayze, in *Natural Products in Medicinal Chemistry*, Wiley V.C.H., Weiheim, 2014.
29. C. A. Buhr, R. W. Wagner, D. Grant and B. C. Froehler, *Nucleic Acids Res.*, 1996, **24**, 2974–2980.
30. S. Gryaznov and R. G. Schultz, *Tetrahedron Lett.*, 1994, **35**, 2489–2492.
31. K. Karikó, M. Buckstein, H. Ni and D. Weissman, *Immunity*, 2005, **23**, 165–175.
32. K. Karikó, H. Muramatsu, F. A. Welsh, J. Ludwig, H. Kato, S. Akira and D. Weissman, *Mol. Ther.*, 2008, **16**, 1833–1840.
33. O. Andries, S. Mc Cafferty, S. C. De Smedt, R. Weiss, N. N. Sanders and T. Kitada, *J. Controlled Release*, 2015, **217**, 337–344.
34. B. Li, X. Luo and Y. Dong, *Bioconjugate Chem.*, 2016, **27**, 849–853.
35. T. P. Prakash, *Chem. Biodiversity*, 2011, **8**, 1616–1641.
36. S. Shukla, C. S. Sumaria and P. I. Pradeepkumar, *ChemMedChem*, 2010, **5**, 328–349.
37. S. T. Crooke, *Antisense Drug Technology: Principles, Strategies, and Applications*, 2nd edn, CRC Press, Boca Raton, 2007.
38. A. A. Koshkin, V. K. Rajwanshi and J. Wengel, *Tetrahedron Lett.*, 1998, **39**, 4381–4384.
39. S. Obika, D. Nanbu, Y. Hari, J. Andoh, K. Morio, T. Doi and T. Imanishi, *Tetrahedron Lett.*, 1998, **39**, 5401–5404.
40. D. A. Braasch and D. R. Corey, *Cell Chem. Biol.*, 2001, **8**, 1–7.
41. S. A. Burel, S.-R. Han, H.-S. Lee, D. A. Norris, B.-S. Lee, T. Machemer, S.-Y. Park, T. Zhou, G. He, Y. Kim, A. R. MacLeod, B. P. Monia, S. Lio, T.-W. Kim and S. P. Henry, *Nucleic Acid Ther.*, 2013, **23**, 213–227.
42. K. Relizani, G. Griffith, L. Echevarría, F. Zarrouki, P. Facchinetti, C. Vaillend, C. Leumann, L. Garcia and A. Goyenvalle, *Mol. Ther.--Nucleic Acids*, 2017, **8**, 144–157.
43. A. Goyenvalle, C. Leumann and L. Garcia, *J. Neuromuscul. Dis.*, 2016, **3**, 157–167.
44. A. E. Heald, J. S. Charleston, P. L. Iversen, T. K. Warren, J. B. Saoud, M. Al-Ibrahim, J. Wells, K. L. Warfield, D. L. Swenson, L. S. Welch, P. Sazani, M. Wong, D. Berry, E. M. Kaye and S. Bavari, *N. Engl. J. Med.*, 2015, **373**, 339–348.
45. J. Summerton, *Biochim. Biophys. Acta, Gene Struct. Expression*, 1999, **1489**, 141–158.
46. P. E. Nielsen, M. Egholm, R. H. Berg and O. Buchardt, *Science*, 1991, **254**, 1497–1500.
47. A. A. Vinogradov, Y. Yin and H. Suga, *J. Am. Chem. Soc.*, 2019, **141**, 4167–4181.
48. A. K. Yudin, *Chem. Sci.*, 2014, **6**, 30–49.
49. J. J. Ferrie, J. J. Gruskos, A. L. Goldwaser, M. E. Decker and D. A. Guarracino, *Bioorg. Med. Chem. Lett.*, 2013, **23**, 989–995.
50. A. Rozek, J.-P. S. Powers, C. L. Friedrich and R. E. W. Hancock, *Biochemistry*, 2003, **42**, 14130–14138.
51. R.-Y. Zhang, P. Thapa, M. J. Espiritu, V. Menon and J.-P. Bingham, *Bioorg. Med. Chem.*, 2018, **26**, 1135–1150.
52. S. J. Kaldas and A. K. Yudin, *Chem. - Eur. J.*, 2018, **24**, 7074–7082.
53. P. M. Cromm, J. Spiegel and T. N. Grossmann, *ACS Chem. Biol.*, 2015, **10**, 1362–1375.
54. J. A. Robinson, *Acc. Chem. Res.*, 2008, **41**, 1278–1288.
55. J. R. Pace, B. J. Lampkin, C. Abakah, A. Moyer, J. Miao, K. Deprey, R. A. Cerulli, Y.-S. Lin, J. D. Baleja, D. Baker and J. A. Kritzer, *J. Am. Chem. Soc.*, 2021, **143**, 15039–15044.
56. Z. Zhou, T. Hu, Z. Xu, Z. Lin, Z. Zhang, T. Feng, L. Zhu, Y. Rong, H. Shen, J. M. Luk, X. Zhang and N. Qin, *FASEB J.*, 2014, **29**, 724–732.
57. Z. Zhang, Z. Lin, Z. Zhou, H. C. Shen, S. F. Yan, A. V. Mayweg, Z. Xu, N. Qin, J. C. Wong, Z. Zhang, Y. Rong, D. C. Fry and T. Hu, *ACS Med. Chem. Lett.*, 2014, **5**, 993–998.
58. H. Y. Chow, Y. Zhang, E. Matheson and X. Li, *Chem. Rev.*, 2019, **119**, 9971–10001.
59. L. Reguera and D. G. Rivera, *Chem. Rev.*, 2019, **119**, 9836–9860.
60. L. Cascales, S. T. Henriques, M. C. Kerr, Y.-H. Huang, M. J. Sweet, N. L. Daly and D. J. Craik, *J. Biol. Chem.*, 2011, **286**, 36932–36943.
61. J. Contreras, A. Y. O. Elnagar, S. F. Hamm-Alvarez and J. A. Camarero, *J. Controlled Release*, 2011, **155**, 134–143.
62. B. J. Tombling, C. K. Wang and D. J. Craik, *Angew. Chem., Int. Ed.*, 2020, **59**, 11218–11232.
63. M. Muttenthaler, B. A. Kalyana and P. F. Alewood, *Curr. Pharm. Des.*, 2011, **17**, 4226–4241.
64. M. L. Colgrave, M. J. L. Korsinczky, R. J. Clark, F. Foley and D. J. Craik, *Pept. Sci.*, 2010, **94**, 665–672.
65. D. J. Craik, N. L. Daly, T. Bond and C. Waine, *J. Mol. Biol.*, 1999, **294**, 1327–1336.
66. S. J. de Veer, M.-W. Kan and D. J. Craik, *Chem. Rev.*, 2019, **119**, 12375–12421.
67. G. J. Hilinski, Y.-W. Kim, J. Hong, P. S. Kutchukian, C. M. Crenshaw, S. S. Berkovitch, A. Chang, S. Ham and G. L. Verdine, *J. Am. Chem. Soc.*, 2014, **136**, 12314–12322.
68. A. M. White, S. J. de Veer, G. Wu, P. J. Harvey, K. Yap, G. J. King, J. E. Swedberg, C. K. Wang, R. H. P. Law, T. Durek and D. J. Craik, *Angew. Chem., Int. Ed.*, 2020, **59**, 11273–11277.

69. G. J.-B. Philippe, D. Gaspar, C. Sheng, Y.-H. Huang, A. H. Benfield, N. D. Condon, J. Weidmann, N. Lawrence, A. Löwer, M. A. R. B. Castanho, D. J. Craik and S. Troeira Henriques, *ACS Chem. Biol.*, 2019, **14**, 2071–2087.
70. H. Adihou, R. Gopalakrishnan, T. Förster, S. M. Guéret, R. Gasper, S. Geschwindner, C. Carrillo García, H. Karatas, A. V. Pobbati, M. Vazquez-Chantada, P. Davey, C. M. Wassvik, J. K. S. Pang, B. S. Soh, W. Hong, E. Chiarparin, D. Schade, A. T. Plowright, E. Valeur, M. Lemurell, T. N. Grossmann and H. Waldmann, *Nat. Commun.*, 2020, **11**, 5425.
71. C. Ämmälä, W. J. Drury, L. Knerr, I. Ahlstedt, P. Stillemark-Billton, C. Wennberg-Huldt, E.-M. Andersson, E. Valeur, R. Jansson-Löfmark, D. Janzén, L. Sundström, J. Meuller, J. Claesson, P. Andersson, C. Johansson, R. G. Lee, T. P. Prakash, P. P. Seth, B. P. Monia and S. Andersson, *Sci. Adv.*, 2018, **4**, eaat3386.
72. M. Srinivasarao, C. V. Galliford and P. S. Low, *Nat. Rev. Drug Discovery*, 2015, **14**, 203–219.
73. R. van der Meel, L. J. C. Vehmeijer, R. J. Kok, G. Storm and E. V. B. van Gaal, *Adv. Drug Delivery Rev.*, 2013, **65**, 1284–1298.
74. C. J. Gerry and S. L. Schreiber, *Nat. Chem. Biol.*, 2020, **16**, 369–378.
75. A. F. Labrijn, M. L. Janmaat, J. M. Reichert and P. W. H. I. Parren, *Nat. Rev. Drug Discovery*, 2019, **18**, 585–608.
76. L. L. Kiessling, J. E. Gestwicki and L. E. Strong, *Angew. Chem., Int. Ed.*, 2006, **45**, 2348–2368.
77. R. Morphy and Z. Rankovic, *J. Med. Chem.*, 2005, **48**, 6523–6543.
78. J. Skarbaliene, T. Secher, J. Jelsing, Ansarullah, T. S. R. Neerup, N. Billestrup and K. Fosgerau, *Peptides*, 2015, **69**, 47–55.
79. K. Fosgerau, L. Jessen, J. L. Tolborg, T. Østerlund, K. S. Larsen, K. Rolsted, M. Brorson, J. Jelsing and T. S. R. Neerup, *Diabetes, Obes. Metab.*, 2013, **15**, 62–71.
80. L. N. Axelsen, W. Keung, H. D. Pedersen, E. Meier, D. Riber, A. L. Kjølbye, J. S. Petersen, S. D. Proctor, N.-H. Holstein-Rathlou and G. D. Lopaschuk, *Br. J. Pharmacol.*, 2012, **165**, 2736–2748.
81. B. Finan, B. Yang, N. Ottaway, D. L. Smiley, T. Ma, C. Clemmensen, J. Chabenne, L. Zhang, K. M. Habegger, K. Fischer, J. E. Campbell, D. Sandoval, R. J. Seeley, K. Bleicher, S. Uhles, W. Riboulet, J. Funk, C. Hertel, S. Belli, E. Sebokova, K. Conde-Knape, A. Konkar, D. J. Drucker, V. Gelfanov, P. T. Pfluger, T. D. Müller, D. Perez-Tilve, R. D. DiMarchi and M. H. Tschöp, *Nat. Med.*, 2015, **21**, 27–36.
82. B. A. Seigal, W. H. Connors, A. Fraley, R. M. Borzilleri, P. H. Carter, S. L. Emanuel, J. Fargnoli, K. Kim, M. Lei, J. G. Naglich, M. E. Pokross, S. L. Posy, H. Shen, N. Surti, R. Talbott, Y. Zhang and N. K. Terrett, *J. Med. Chem.*, 2015, **58**, 2855–2861.
83. Y. Zhang, B. A. Seigal, N. K. Terrett, R. L. Talbott, J. Fargnoli, J. G. Naglich, C. Chaudhry, S. L. Posy, R. Vuppugalla, G. Cornelius, M. Lei, C. Wang, Y. Zhang, R. J. Schmidt, D. D. Wei, M. M. Miller, M. P. Allen, L. Li, P. H. Carter, G. D. Vite and R. M. Borzilleri, *ACS Med. Chem. Lett.*, 2015, **6**, 770–775.
84. J. M. Smith, J. R. Frost and R. Fasan, *Chem. Commun.*, 2014, **50**, 5027–5030.
85. J. R. Harjani, B. K. Yap, E. W. W. Leung, A. Lucke, S. E. Nicholson, M. J. Scanlon, D. K. Chalmers, P. E. Thompson, R. S. Norton and J. B. Baell, *J. Med. Chem.*, 2016, **59**, 5799–5809.
86. T. R. Siegert, M. J. Bird, K. M. Makwana and J. A. Kritzer, *J. Am. Chem. Soc.*, 2016, **138**, 12876–12884.
87. C. Heinis, T. Rutherford, S. Freund and G. Winter, *Nat. Chem. Biol.*, 2009, **5**, 502–507.
88. S. Chen, J. Morales-Sanfrutos, A. Angelini, B. Cutting and C. Heinis, *ChemBioChem*, 2012, **13**, 1032–1038.
89. S. M. Guéret, S. Thavam, R. J. Carbajo, M. Potowski, N. Larsson, G. Dahl, A. Dellsén, T. N. Grossmann, A. T. Plowright, E. Valeur, M. Lemurell and H. Waldmann, *J. Am. Chem. Soc.*, 2020, **142**, 4904–4915.
90. C. Wang, W. Shi, L. Cai, L. Lu, Q. Wang, T. Zhang, J. Li, Z. Zhang, K. Wang, L. Xu, X. Jiang, S. Jiang and K. Liu, *J. Med. Chem.*, 2013, **56**, 2527–2539.
91. M. F. Schmidt, O. Korb and C. Abell, *ACS Chem. Biol.*, 2013, **8**, 2122–2126.
92. V. S. Rodrik-Outmezguine, M. Okaniwa, Z. Yao, C. J. Novotny, C. McWhirter, A. Banaji, H. Won, W. Wong, M. Berger, E. de Stanchina, D. G. Barratt, S. Cosulich, T. Klinowska, N. Rosen and K. M. Shokat, *Nature*, 2016, **534**, 272–276.
93. E. Pazos, C. Portela, C. Penas, M. E. Vázquez and J. L. Mascareñas, *Org. Biomol. Chem.*, 2015, **13**, 5385–5390.
94. K. R. Simonetta, J. Taygerly, K. Boyle, S. E. Basham, C. Padovani, Y. Lou, T. J. Cummins, S. L. Yung, S. K. von Soly, F. Kayser, J. Kuriyan, M. Rape, M. Cardozo, M. A. Gallop, N. F. Bence, P. A. Barsanti and A. Saha, *Nat. Commun.*, 2019, **10**, 1402.
95. S. U. Siriwardena, D. N. P. Munkanatta Godage, V. M. Shoba, S. Lai, M. Shi, P. Wu, S. K. Chaudhary, S. L. Schreiber and A. Choudhary, *J. Am. Chem. Soc.*, 2020, **142**, 14052–14057.

96. S. M. Banik, K. Pedram, S. Wisnovsky, G. Ahn, N. M. Riley and C. R. Bertozzi, *Nature*, 2020, **584**, 291–297.
97. K. Ito, K. Sakai, Y. Suzuki, N. Ozawa, T. Hatta, T. Natsume, K. Matsumoto and H. Suga, *Nat. Commun.*, 2015, **6**, 6373.
98. W. Miao, K. Sakai, N. Ozawa, T. Nishiuchi, Y. Suzuki, K. Ito, T. Morioka, M. Umitsu, J. Takagi, H. Suga and K. Matsumoto, *Sci. Rep.*, 2018, **8**, 1–11.
99. N. Trouche, S. Wieckowski, W. Sun, O. Chaloin, J. Hoebeke, S. Fournel and G. Guichard, *J. Am. Chem. Soc.*, 2007, **129**, 13480–13492.
100. P. J. McEnaney, K. J. Fitzgerald, A. X. Zhang, E. F. Douglass, W. Shan, A. Balog, M. D. Kolesnikova and D. A. Spiegel, *J. Am. Chem. Soc.*, 2014, **136**, 18034–18043.
101. S. Imaide, K. M. Riching, N. Makukhin, V. Vetma, C. Whitworth, S. J. Hughes, N. Trainor, S. D. Mahan, N. Murphy, A. D. Cowan, K.-H. Chan, C. Craigon, A. Testa, C. Maniaci, M. Urh, D. L. Daniels and A. Ciulli, *Nat. Chem. Biol.*, 2021, **17**, 1157–1167.
102. C. Fellmann, B. G. Gowen, P.-C. Lin, J. A. Doudna and J. E. Corn, *Nat. Rev. Drug Discovery*, 2017, **16**, 89–100.
103. J. D. Sander and J. K. Joung, *Nat. Biotechnol.*, 2014, **32**, 347–355.
104. D. B. T. Cox, R. J. Platt and F. Zhang, *Nat. Med.*, 2015, **21**, 121–131.
105. M. Adli, *Nat. Commun.*, 2018, **9**, 1–13.
106. S. H. Khan, *Mol. Ther.--Nucleic Acids*, 2019, **16**, 326–334.
107. B. Shui, L. H. Matias, Y. D. Guo and Y. Peng, *Stem Cells Int.*, 2016, **2016**, 8140168.
108. M. H. Porteus, *N. Engl. J. Med.*, 2019, **380**, 947–959.
109. L.-C. Li, S. T. Okino, H. Zhao, D. Pookot, R. F. Place, S. Urakami, H. Enokida and R. Dahiya, *Proc. Natl. Acad. Sci. U. S. A.*, 2006, **103**, 17337–17342.
110. J. Voutila, V. Reebye, T. C. Roberts, P. Protopapa, P. Andrikakou, D. C. Blakey, R. Habib, H. Huber, P. Saetrom, J. J. Rossi and N. A. Habib, *Mol. Ther.*, 2017, **25**, 2705–2714.
111. K.-W. Huang, V. Reebye, K. Czysz, S. Ciriello, S. Dorman, I. Reccia, H.-S. Lai, L. Peng, N. Kostomitsopoulos, J. Nicholls, R. S. Habib, D. A. Tomalia, P. Sætrom, E. Wilkes, P. Cutillas, J. J. Rossi and N. A. Habib, *Mol. Ther.--Nucleic Acids*, 2020, **19**, 361–370.
112. D. B. T. Cox, J. S. Gootenberg, O. O. Abudayyeh, B. Franklin, M. J. Kellner, J. Joung and F. Zhang, *Science*, 2017, **358**, 1019–1027.
113. K. D. Warner, C. E. Hajdin and K. M. Weeks, *Nat. Rev. Drug Discovery*, 2018, **17**, 547–558.
114. J. Palacino, S. E. Swalley, C. Song, A. K. Cheung, L. Shu, X. Zhang, M. Van Hoosear, Y. Shin, D. N. Chin, C. G. Keller, M. Beibel, N. A. Renaud, T. M. Smith, M. Salcius, X. Shi, M. Hild, R. Servais, M. Jain, L. Deng, C. Bullock, M. McLellan, S. Schuierer, L. Murphy, M. J. J. Blommers, C. Blaustein, F. Berenshteyn, A. Lacoste, J. R. Thomas, G. Roma, G. A. Michaud, B. S. Tseng, J. A. Porter, V. E. Myer, J. A. Tallarico, L. G. Hamann, D. Curtis, M. C. Fishman, W. F. Dietrich, N. A. Dales and R. Sivasankaran, *Nat. Chem. Biol.*, 2015, **11**, 511–517.
115. S. M. Elbashir, W. Lendeckel and T. Tuschl, *Genes Dev.*, 2001, **15**, 188–200.
116. N. J. Caplen, S. Parrish, F. Imani, A. Fire and R. A. Morgan, *Proc. Natl. Acad. Sci. U. S. A.*, 2001, **98**, 9742–9747.
117. A. Wittrup and J. Lieberman, *Nat. Rev. Genet.*, 2015, **16**, 543–552.
118. R. L. Setten, J. J. Rossi and S. Han, *Nat. Rev. Drug Discovery*, 2019, **18**, 421–446.
119. U. Sahin, K. Karikó and Ö. Türeci, *Nat. Rev. Drug Discovery*, 2014, **13**, 759–780.
120. L. A. Jackson, E. J. Anderson, N. G. Rouphael, P. C. Roberts, M. Makhene, R. N. Coler, M. P. McCullough, J. D. Chappell, M. R. Denison, L. J. Stevens, A. J. Pruijssers, A. McDermott, B. Flach, N. A. Doria-Rose, K. S. Corbett, K. M. Morabito, S. O'Dell, S. D. Schmidt, P. A. Swanson, M. Padilla, J. R. Mascola, K. M. Neuzil, H. Bennett, W. Sun, E. Peters, M. Makowski, J. Albert, K. Cross, W. Buchanan, R. Pikaart-Tautges, J. E. Ledgerwood, B. S. Graham and J. H. Beigel, *N. Engl. J. Med.*, 2020, **383**, 1920–1931.
121. L. Warren, P. D. Manos, T. Ahfeldt, Y.-H. Loh, H. Li, F. Lau, W. Ebina, P. K. Mandal, Z. D. Smith, A. Meissner, G. Q. Daley, A. S. Brack, J. J. Collins, C. Cowan, T. M. Schlaeger and D. J. Rossi, *Cell Stem Cell*, 2010, 7, 618–630.
122. D. An, J. L. Schneller, A. Frassetto, S. Liang, X. Zhu, J.-S. Park, M. Theisen, S.-J. Hong, J. Zhou, R. Rajendran, B. Levy, R. Howell, G. Besin, V. Presnyak, S. Sabnis, K. E. Murphy-Benenato, E. S. Kumarasinghe, T. Salerno, C. Mihai, C. M. Lukacs, R. J. Chandler, L. T. Guey, C. P. Venditti and P. G. V. Martini, *Cell Rep.*, 2017, **21**, 3548–3558.
123. L. Zangi, K. O. Lui, A. von Gise, Q. Ma, W. Ebina, L. M. Ptaszek, D. Später, H. Xu, M. Tabebordbar, R. Gorbatov, B. Sena, M. Nahrendorf, D. M. Briscoe, R. A. Li, A. J. Wagers, D. J. Rossi, W. T. Pu and K. R. Chien, *Nat. Biotechnol.*, 2013, **31**, 898–907.

124. L.-M. Gan, M. Lagerström-Fermér, L. G. Carlsson, C. Arfvidsson, A.-C. Egnell, A. Rudvik, M. Kjaer, A. Collén, J. D. Thompson, J. Joyal, L. Chialda, T. Koernicke, R. Fuhr, K. R. Chien and R. Fritsche-Danielson, *Nat. Commun.*, 2019, **10**, 871.
125. S. L. Hewitt, A. Bai, D. Bailey, K. Ichikawa, J. Zielinski, R. Karp, A. Apte, K. Arnold, S. J. Zacharek, M. S. Iliou, K. Bhatt, M. Garnaas, F. Musenge, A. Davis, N. Khatwani, S. V. Su, G. MacLean, S. J. Farlow, K. Burke and J. P. Frederick, *Sci. Transl. Med.*, 2019, **11**, eaat9143.
126. M. A. Havens and M. L. Hastings, *Nucleic Acids Res.*, 2016, **44**, 6549–6563.
127. P. Järver, L. O'Donovan and M. J. Gait, *Nucleic Acid Ther.*, 2013, **24**, 37–47.
128. A. G. Matera and Z. Wang, *Nat. Rev. Mol. Cell Biol.*, 2014, **15**, 108–121.
129. R. L. S. Mesman, F. M. G. R. Calléja, M. de la Hoya, P. Devilee, C. J. van Asperen, H. Vrieling and M. P. G. Vreeswijk, *Genet. Med.*, 2020, **22**, 1355–1365.
130. S. Casadei, S. Gulsuner, B. H. Shirts, J. B. Mandell, H. M. Kortbawi, B. S. Norquist, E. M. Swisher, M. K. Lee, Y. Goldberg, R. O'Connor, Z. Tan, C. C. Pritchard, M.-C. King and T. Walsh, *Proc. Natl. Acad. Sci. U. S. A.*, 2019, **116**, 26798–26807.
131. S. J. Bryen, H. Joshi, F. J. Evesson, C. Girard, R. Ghaoui, L. B. Waddell, A. C. Testa, B. Cummings, S. Arbuckle, N. Graf, R. Webster, D. G. MacArthur, N. G. Laing, M. R. Davis, R. Lührmann and S. T. Cooper, *Am. J. Hum. Genet.*, 2019, **105**, 573–587.
132. A. Andreadis, in *Alternative Splicing and Disease*, ed. P. Jeanteur, Springer, Berlin, Heidelberg, 2006, pp. 89–107.
133. R. S. Finkel, E. Mercuri, B. T. Darras, A. M. Connolly, N. L. Kuntz, J. Kirschner, C. A. Chiriboga, K. Saito, L. Servais, E. Tizzano, H. Topaloglu, M. Tulinius, J. Montes, A. M. Glanzman, K. Bishop, Z. J. Zhong, S. Gheuens, C. F. Bennett, E. Schneider, W. Farwell and D. C. De Vivo, *N. Engl. J. Med.*, 2017, **377**, 1723–1732.
134. C. D. Wurster and A. C. Ludolph, *Ther. Adv. Neurol. Disord.*, 2018, **11**, 1–3.
135. J. F. Lima, L. Cerqueira, C. Figueiredo, C. Oliveira and N. F. Azevedo, *RNA Biol.*, 2018, **15**, 338–352.
136. K. A. Lennox and M. A. Behlke, *Pharm. Res.*, 2010, **27**, 1788–1799.
137. M. R. Fabian, N. Sonenberg and W. Filipowicz, *Annu. Rev. Biochem.*, 2010, **79**, 351–379.
138. I. G. Gomez, D. A. MacKenna, B. G. Johnson, V. Kaimal, A. M. Roach, S. Ren, N. Nakagawa, C. Xin, R. Newitt, S. Pandya, T.-H. Xia, X. Liu, D.-B. Borza, M. Grafals, S. J. Shankland, J. Himmelfarb, D. Portilla, S. Liu, B. N. Chau and J. S. Duffield, *J. Clin. Invest.*, 2015, **125**, 141–156.
139. M. Trajkovski, J. Hausser, J. Soutschek, B. Bhat, A. Akin, M. Zavolan, M. H. Heim and M. Stoffel, *Nature*, 2011, **474**, 649–653.
140. H. Yin, Y.-H. Huang, K. Deprey, N. D. Condon, J. A. Kritzer, D. J. Craik and C. K. Wang, *ACS Chem. Biol.*, 2020, **15**, 1650–1661.
141. D. J. Craik, D. P. Fairlie, S. Liras and D. Price, *Chem. Biol. Drug Des.*, 2013, **81**, 136–147.
142. J. J. Nestor Jr, *Curr. Med. Chem.*, 2009, **16**, 4399–4418.
143. Y.-W. Kim, T. N. Grossmann and G. L. Verdine, *Nat. Protoc.*, 2011, **6**, 761–771.
144. K. Namoto, F. Sirockin, H. Sellner, C. Wiesmann, F. Villard, R. J. Moreau, E. Valeur, S. C. Paulding, S. Schleeger, K. Schipp, J. Loup, L. Andrews, R. Swale, M. Robinson and C. J. Farady, *Bioorg. Med. Chem. Lett.*, 2018, **28**, 906–909.
145. A. Schubart, K. Anderson, N. Mainolfi, H. Sellner, T. Ehara, C. M. Adams, A. M. Sweeney, S.-M. Liao, M. Crowley, A. Littlewood-Evans, S. Sarret, G. Wieczorek, L. Perrot, V. Dubost, T. Flandre, Y. Zhang, R. J. H. Smith, A. M. Risitano, R. G. Karki, C. Zhang, E. Valeur, F. Sirockin, B. Gerhartz, P. Erbel, N. Hughes, T. M. Smith, F. Cumin, U. A. Argikar, B. Haraldsson, M. Mogi, R. Sedrani, C. Wiesmann, B. Jaffee, J. Maibaum, S. Flohr, R. Harrison and J. Eder, *Proc. Natl. Acad. Sci. U. S. A.*, 2019, **116**, 7926–7931.
146. N. Mainolfi, T. Ehara, R. G. Karki, K. Anderson, A. Mac Sweeney, S.-M. Liao, U. A. Argikar, K. Jendza, C. Zhang, J. Powers, D. W. Klosowski, M. Crowley, T. Kawanami, J. Ding, M. April, C. Forster, M. Serrano-Wu, M. Capparelli, R. Ramqaj, C. Solovay, F. Cumin, T. M. Smith, L. Ferrara, W. Lee, D. Long, M. Prentiss, A. De Erkenez, L. Yang, F. Liu, H. Sellner, F. Sirockin, E. Valeur, P. Erbel, D. Ostermeier, P. Ramage, B. Gerhartz, A. Schubart, S. Flohr, N. Gradoux, R. Feifel, B. Vogg, C. Wiesmann, J. Maibaum, J. Eder, R. Sedrani, R. A. Harrison, M. Mogi, B. D. Jaffee and C. M. Adams, *J. Med. Chem.*, 2020, **63**, 5697–5722.
147. D. P. Teufel, G. Bennett, H. Harrison, K. van Rietschoten, S. Pavan, C. Stace, F. Le Floch, T. Van Bergen, E. Vermassen, P. Barbeaux, T.-T. Hu, J. H. M. Feyen and M. Vanhove, *J. Med. Chem.*, 2018, **61**, 2823–2836.
148. A Study to Evaluate the Safety of THR-149 in Subjects with Diabetic Macular Edema (DME), https://clinicaltrials.gov/ct2/show/NCT03511898, accessed 20 January 2021.

149. N. Srinivas, P. Jetter, B. J. Ueberbacher, M. Werneburg, K. Zerbe, J. Steinmann, B. V. der Meijden, F. Bernardini, A. Lederer, R. L. A. Dias, P. E. Misson, H. Henze, J. Zumbrunn, F. O. Gombert, D. Obrecht, P. Hunziker, S. Schauer, U. Ziegler, A. Käch, L. Eberl, K. Riedel, S. J. DeMarco and J. A. Robinson, *Science*, 2010, **327**, 1010–1013.
150. J. Zhou and J. Rossi, *Nat. Rev. Drug Discovery*, 2017, **16**, 181–202.
151. H. Sun, X. Zhu, P. Y. Lu, R. R. Rosato, W. Tan and Y. Zu, *Mol. Ther.--Nucleic Acids*, 2014, **3**, e182.
152. S. A. Vinores, *Int. J. Nanomed.*, 2006, **1**, 263–268.
153. A. R. Shustov, S. M. Horwitz, J. Zain, M. R. Patel, S. Goel, L. Sokol, F. Meric-Bernstam, G. Shapiro, S. Dwivedy Nasta, M. Janakiram, D. M. Weinstock, R. Korn, M. Payton, D. A. Annis, D. Pinchasik, M. Aivado and A. Mehta, *Blood*, 2018, **132**, 1623.
154. N. Mainolfi and T. Rasmusson, in *Annual Reports in Medicinal Chemistry*, ed. R. A. Goodnow, Academic Press, 2017, vol. 50, pp. 301–334.
155. Y. Zhang, C. Loh, J. Chen and N. Mainolfi, *Drug Discovery Today: Technol.*, 2019, **31**, 53–60.
156. C. M. Crews, G. Georg and S. Wang, *J. Med. Chem.*, 2016, **59**, 5129–5130.
157. H. Weinmann and C. Crews, *Protein Degradation with New Chemical Modalities*, The Royal Society of Chemistry, 2021.
158. C. M. Olson, B. Jiang, M. A. Erb, Y. Liang, Z. M. Doctor, Z. Zhang, T. Zhang, N. Kwiatkowski, M. Boukhali, J. L. Green, W. Haas, T. Nomanbhoy, E. S. Fischer, R. A. Young, J. E. Bradner, G. E. Winter and N. S. Gray, *Nat. Chem. Biol.*, 2018, **14**, 163–170.
159. T. K. Neklesa and C. M. Crews, *Nature*, 2012, **487**, 308–309.
160. Y. Shi, M. J. C. Long, M. M. Rosenberg, S. Li, A. Kobjack, P. Lessans, R. T. Coffey and L. Hedstrom, *ACS Chem. Biol.*, 2016, **11**, 3328–3337.
161. T. Xie, S. M. Lim, K. D. Westover, M. E. Dodge, D. Ercan, S. B. Ficarro, D. Udayakumar, D. Gurbani, H. S. Tae, S. M. Riddle, T. Sim, J. A. Marto, P. A. Jänne, C. M. Crews and N. S. Gray, *Nat. Chem. Biol.*, 2014, **10**, 1006–1012.
162. J. L. Gustafson, T. K. Neklesa, C. S. Cox, A. G. Roth, D. L. Buckley, H. S. Tae, T. B. Sundberg, D. B. Stagg, J. Hines, D. P. McDonnell, J. D. Norris and C. M. Crews, *Angew. Chem., Int. Ed.*, 2015, **54**, 9659–9662.
163. N. Gao, Y.-P. Huang, T.-T. Chu, Q.-Q. Li, B. Zhou, Y.-X. Chen, Y.-F. Zhao and Y.-M. Li, *Bioorg. Chem.*, 2019, **84**, 254–259.
164. N. Gao, T.-T. Chu, Q.-Q. Li, Y.-J. Lim, T. Qiu, M.-R. Ma, Z.-W. Hu, X.-F. Yang, Y.-X. Chen, Y.-F. Zhao and Y.-M. Li, *RSC Adv.*, 2017, **7**, 40362–40366.
165. D. A. Nalawansha and C. M. Crews, *Cell Chem. Biol.*, 2020, **27**, 998–1014.
166. A. R. Schneekloth, M. Pucheault, H. S. Tae and C. M. Crews, *Bioorg. Med. Chem. Lett.*, 2008, **18**, 5904–5908.
167. K. Sekine, K. Takubo, R. Kikuchi, M. Nishimoto, M. Kitagawa, F. Abe, K. Nishikawa, T. Tsuruo and M. Naito, *J. Biol. Chem.*, 2008, **283**, 8961–8968.
168. Y. Itoh, M. Ishikawa, M. Naito and Y. Hashimoto, *J. Am. Chem. Soc.*, 2010, **132**, 5820–5826.
169. P. Soares, M. S. Gadd, J. Frost, C. Galdeano, L. Ellis, O. Epemolu, S. Rocha, K. D. Read and A. Ciulli, *J. Med. Chem.*, 2018, **61**, 599–618.
170. A. Testa, X. Lucas, G. V. Castro, K.-H. Chan, J. E. Wright, A. C. Runcie, M. S. Gadd, W. T. A. Harrison, E.-J. Ko, D. Fletcher and A. Ciulli, *J. Am. Chem. Soc.*, 2018, **140**, 9299–9313.
171. D. L. Buckley, J. L. Gustafson, I. Van Molle, A. G. Roth, H. S. Tae, P. C. Gareiss, W. L. Jorgensen, A. Ciulli and C. M. Crews, *Angew. Chem., Int. Ed.*, 2012, **51**, 11463–11467.
172. J. Krönke, N. D. Udeshi, A. Narla, P. Grauman, S. N. Hurst, M. McConkey, T. Svinkina, D. Heckl, E. Comer, X. Li, C. Ciarlo, E. Hartman, N. Munshi, M. Schenone, S. L. Schreiber, S. A. Carr and B. L. Ebert, *Science*, 2014, **343**, 301–305.
173. G. Lu, R. E. Middleton, H. Sun, M. Naniong, C. J. Ott, C. S. Mitsiades, K.-K. Wong, J. E. Bradner and W. G. Kaelin, *Science*, 2014, **343**, 305–309.
174. E. S. Fischer, K. Böhm, J. R. Lydeard, H. Yang, M. B. Stadler, S. Cavadini, J. Nagel, F. Serluca, V. Acker, G. M. Lingaraju, R. B. Tichkule, M. Schebesta, W. C. Forrester, M. Schirle, U. Hassiepen, J. Ottl, M. Hild, R. E. J. Beckwith, J. W. Harper, J. L. Jenkins and N. H. Thomä, *Nature*, 2014, **512**, 49–53.
175. G. E. Winter, D. L. Buckley, J. Paulk, J. M. Roberts, A. Souza, S. Dhe-Paganon and J. E. Bradner, *Science*, 2015, **348**, 1376–1381.
176. M. Lu, T. Liu, Q. Jiao, J. Ji, M. Tao, Y. Liu, Q. You and Z. Jiang, *Eur. J. Med. Chem.*, 2018, **146**, 251–259.
177. J. N. Spradlin, X. Hu, C. C. Ward, S. M. Brittain, M. D. Jones, L. Ou, M. To, A. Proudfoot, E. Ornelas, M. Woldegiorgis, J. A. Olzmann, D. E. Bussiere, J. R. Thomas, J. A. Tallarico, J. M. McKenna, M. Schirle, T. J. Maimone and D. K. Nomura, *Nat. Chem. Biol.*, 2019, **15**, 747–755.
178. M. Brand and G. E. Winter, *Nat. Chem. Biol.*, 2019, **15**, 655–656.

179. B. J. Pinch, D. L. Buckley, S. Gleim, S. M. Brittain, L. Tandeske, P. L. D'Alessandro, Z. J. Hauseman, J. Lipps, L. Xu, E. P. Harvey, M. Schirle, E. R. Sprague, W. C. Forrester, D. Dovala, L. M. McGregor and C. R. Thoma, *Cell Chem. Biol.*, 2021, **29**, 57–66.
180. P. Ottis, M. Toure, P. M. Cromm, E. Ko, J. L. Gustafson and C. M. Crews, *ACS Chem. Biol.*, 2017, **12**, 2570–2578.
181. X. Zhang, V. M. Crowley, T. G. Wucherpfennig, M. M. Dix and B. F. Cravatt, *Nat. Chem. Biol.*, 2019, **15**, 737–746.
182. C. C. Ward, J. I. Kleinman, S. M. Brittain, P. S. Lee, C. Y. S. Chung, K. Kim, Y. Petri, J. R. Thomas, J. A. Tallarico, J. M. McKenna, M. Schirle and D. K. Nomura, *ACS Chem. Biol.*, 2019, **14**, 2430–2440.
183. M. Schapira, M. F. Calabrese, A. N. Bullock and C. M. Crews, *Nat. Rev. Drug Discovery*, 2019, **18**, 949–963.
184. J. Popow, H. Arnhof, G. Bader, H. Berger, A. Ciulli, D. Covini, C. Dank, T. Gmaschitz, P. Greb, J. Karolyi-Özguer, M. Koegl, D. B. McConnell, M. Pearson, M. Rieger, J. Rinnenthal, V. Roessler, A. Schrenk, M. Spina, S. Steurer, N. Trainor, E. Traxler, C. Wieshofer, A. Zoephel and P. Ettmayer, *J. Med. Chem.*, 2019, **62**, 2508–2520.
185. C. Zhang, X.-R. Han, X. Yang, B. Jiang, J. Liu, Y. Xiong and J. Jin, *Eur. J. Med. Chem.*, 2018, **151**, 304–314.
186. S. Liu, H. O. Yosief, L. Dai, H. Huang, G. Dhawan, X. Zhang, A. M. Muthengi, J. Roberts, D. L. Buckley, J. A. Perry, L. Wu, J. E. Bradner, J. Qi and W. Zhang, *J. Med. Chem.*, 2018, **61**, 7785–7795.
187. W. Li, C. Gao, L. Zhao, Z. Yuan, Y. Chen and Y. Jiang, *Eur. J. Med. Chem.*, 2018, **151**, 237–247.
188. M. Brand, B. Jiang, S. Bauer, K. A. Donovan, Y. Liang, E. S. Wang, R. P. Nowak, J. C. Yuan, T. Zhang, N. Kwiatkowski, A. C. Müller, E. S. Fischer, N. S. Gray and G. E. Winter, *Cell Chem. Biol.*, 2019, **26**, 300–306.e9.
189. A. H. Miah, I. E. D. Smith, M. Rackham, A. Mares, A. R. Thawani, R. Nagilla, P. A. Haile, B. J. Votta, L. J. Gordon, G. Watt, J. Denyer, D. T. Fisher, P. Dace, P. Giffen, A. Goncalves, I. Churcher, P. Scott-Stevens and J. D. Harling, *J. Med. Chem.*, 2021, **64**, 12978–13003.
190. J. Hu, B. Hu, M. Wang, F. Xu, B. Miao, C.-Y. Yang, M. Wang, Z. Liu, D. F. Hayes, K. Chinnaswamy, J. Delproposto, J. Stuckey and S. Wang, *J. Med. Chem.*, 2019, **62**, 1420–1442.
191. X. Han, C. Wang, C. Qin, W. Xiang, E. Fernandez-Salas, C.-Y. Yang, M. Wang, L. Zhao, T. Xu, K. Chinnaswamy, J. Delproposto, J. Stuckey and S. Wang, *J. Med. Chem.*, 2019, **62**, 941–964.
192. L. Wang, V. S. Guillen, N. Sharma, K. Flessa, J. Min, K. E. Carlson, W. Toy, S. Braqi, B. S. Katzenellenbogen, J. A. Katzenellenbogen, S. Chandarlapaty and A. Sharma, *ACS Med. Chem. Lett.*, 2018, **9**, 803–808.
193. H. Xu, N. Ohoka, H. Yokoo, K. Nemoto, T. Ohtsuki, H. Matsufuji, M. Naito, T. Inoue, G. Tsuji and Y. Demizu, *Front. Chem.*, 2021, **9**, 367.
194. C. Steinebach, H. Kehm, S. Lindner, L. P. Vu, S. Köpff, Á. L. Mármol, C. Weiler, K. G. Wagner, M. Reichenzeller, J. Krönke and M. Gütschow, *Chem. Commun.*, 2019, **55**, 1821–1824.
195. Y. Li, J. Yang, A. Aguilar, D. McEachern, S. Przybranowski, L. Liu, C.-Y. Yang, M. Wang, X. Han and S. Wang, *J. Med. Chem.*, 2019, **62**, 448–466.
196. M. Winzker, A. Friese, U. Koch, P. Janning, S. Ziegler and H. Waldmann, *Angew. Chem., Int. Ed.*, 2020, **59**, 5595–5601.
197. M. Zheng, Y. Liu, C. Wu, K. Yang, Q. Wang, Y. Zhou, L. Chen and H. Li, *Bioorg. Chem.*, 2021, **110**, 104788.
198. Y. Feng, H. Su, Y. Li, C. Luo, H. Xu, Y. Wang, H. Sun, G. Wan, B. Zhou and X. Bu, *Chem. Commun.*, 2020, **56**, 2881–2884.
199. Z. I. Bassi, M. C. Fillmore, A. H. Miah, T. D. Chapman, C. Maller, E. J. Roberts, L. C. Davis, D. E. Lewis, N. W. Galwey, K. E. Waddington, V. Parravicini, A. L. Macmillan-Jones, C. Gongora, P. G. Humphreys, I. Churcher, R. K. Prinjha and D. F. Tough, *ACS Chem. Biol.*, 2018, **13**, 2862–2867.
200. V. Zoppi, S. J. Hughes, C. Maniaci, A. Testa, T. Gmaschitz, C. Wieshofer, M. Koegl, K. M. Riching, D. L. Daniels, A. Spallarossa and A. Ciulli, *J. Med. Chem.*, 2019, **62**, 699–726.
201. B. Zhou, J. Hu, F. Xu, Z. Chen, L. Bai, E. Fernandez-Salas, M. Lin, L. Liu, C.-Y. Yang, Y. Zhao, D. McEachern, S. Przybranowski, B. Wen, D. Sun and S. Wang, *J. Med. Chem.*, 2018, **61**, 462–481.
202. K. Yang, Y. Song, H. Xie, H. Wu, Y.-T. Wu, E. D. Leisten and W. Tang, *Bioorg. Med. Chem. Lett.*, 2018, **28**, 2493–2497.
203. M. Schiedel, D. Herp, S. Hammelmann, S. Swyter, A. Lehotzky, D. Robaa, J. Oláh, J. Ovádi, W. Sippl and M. Jung, *J. Med. Chem.*, 2018, **61**, 482–491.
204. C. Qin, Y. Hu, B. Zhou, E. Fernandez-Salas, C.-Y. Yang, L. Liu, D. McEachern, S. Przybranowski, M. Wang, J. Stuckey, J. Meagher, L. Bai, Z. Chen, M. Lin, J. Yang, D. N. Ziazadeh, F. Xu, J. Hu, W. Xiang, L. Huang, S. Li, B. Wen, D. Sun and S. Wang, *J. Med. Chem.*, 2018, **61**, 6685–6704.

205. L. N. Gechijian, D. L. Buckley, M. A. Lawlor, J. M. Reyes, J. Paulk, C. J. Ott, G. E. Winter, M. A. Erb, T. G. Scott, M. Xu, H.-S. Seo, S. Dhe-Paganon, N. P. Kwiatkowski, J. A. Perry, J. Qi, N. S. Gray and J. E. Bradner, *Nat. Chem. Biol.*, 2018, **14**, 405.
206. W. McCoull, T. Cheung, E. Anderson, P. Barton, J. Burgess, K. Byth, Q. Cao, M. P. Castaldi, H. Chen, E. Chiarparin, R. J. Carbajo, E. Code, S. Cowan, P. R. Davey, A. D. Ferguson, S. Fillery, N. O. Fuller, N. Gao, D. Hargreaves, M. R. Howard, J. Hu, A. Kawatkar, P. D. Kemmitt, E. Leo, D. M. Molina, N. O'Connell, P. Petteruti, T. Rasmusson, P. Raubo, P. B. Rawlins, P. Ricchiuto, G. R. Robb, M. Schenone, M. J. Waring, M. Zinda, S. Fawell and D. M. Wilson, *ACS Chem. Biol.*, 2018, **13**, 3131–3141.
207. J. H.-R. Hsu, T. Rasmusson, J. Robinson, F. Pachl, J. Read, S. Kawatkar, D. H. O'Donovan, S. Bagal, E. Code, P. Rawlins, A. Argyrou, R. Tomlinson, N. Gao, X. Zhu, E. Chiarparin, K. Jacques, M. Shen, H. Woods, E. Bednarski, D. M. Wilson, L. Drew, M. P. Castaldi, S. Fawell and A. Bloecher, *Cell Chem. Biol.*, 2020, **27**, 41–46.e17.
208. A. Dölle, B. Adhikari, A. Krämer, J. Weckesser, N. Berner, L.-M. Berger, M. Diebold, M. M. Szewczyk, D. Barsyte-Lovejoy, C. H. Arrowsmith, J. Gebel, F. Löhr, V. Dötsch, M. Eilers, S. Heinzlmeir, B. Kuster, C. Sotriffer, E. Wolf and S. Knapp, *J. Med. Chem.*, 2021, **64**, 10682–10710.
209. T. Iida, Y. Itoh, Y. Takahashi, Y. Yamashita, T. Kurohara, Y. Miyake, M. Oba and T. Suzuki, *ChemMedChem*, 2021, **16**, 1609–1618.
210. M. J. Bond, L. Chu, D. A. Nalawansha, K. Li and C. M. Crews, *ACS Cent. Sci.*, 2020, **6**, 1367–1375.
211. A. Ghidini, A. Cléry, F. Halloy, F. H. T. Allain and J. Hall, *Angew. Chem., Int. Ed.*, 2021, **60**, 3163–3169.
212. J. Shao, Y. Yan, D. Ding, D. Wang, Y. He, Y. Pan, W. Yan, A. Kharbanda, H. Li and H. Huang, *Adv. Sci.*, 2021, 2102555.
213. J. Liu, H. Chen, H. Ü. Kaniskan, L. Xie, X. Chen, J. Jin and W. Wei, *J. Am. Chem. Soc.*, 2021, **143**, 8902–8910.
214. K. T. G. Samarasinghe, S. Jaime-Figueroa, M. Burgess, D. A. Nalawansha, K. Dai, Z. Hu, A. Bebenek, S. A. Holley and C. M. Crews, *Cell Chem. Biol.*, 2021, **28**, 648–661.e5.
215. G. M. Burslem, B. E. Smith, A. C. Lai, S. Jaime-Figueroa, D. C. McQuaid, D. P. Bondeson, M. Toure, H. Dong, Y. Qian, J. Wang, A. P. Crew, J. Hines and C. M. Crews, *Cell Chem. Biol.*, 2018, **25**, 67–77.e3.
216. Z. Li, Y. Lin, H. Song, X. Qin, Z. Yu, Z. Zhang, G. Dong, X. Li, X. Shi, L. Du, W. Zhao and M. Li, *Acta Pharm. Sin. B*, 2020, **10**, 1669–1679.
217. G. Ahn, S. M. Banik and C. R. Bertozzi, *Cell Chem. Biol.*, 2021, **28**, 1072–1080.
218. G. Ahn, S. M. Banik, C. L. Miller, N. M. Riley, J. R. Cochran and C. R. Bertozzi, *Nat. Chem. Biol.*, 2021, **17**, 937–946.
219. D. Takahashi and H. Arimoto, *Autophagy*, 2020, **16**, 765–766.
220. D. Takahashi, J. Moriyama, T. Nakamura, E. Miki, E. Takahashi, A. Sato, T. Akaike, K. Itto-Nakama and H. Arimoto, *Mol. Cell*, 2019, **76**, 797–810.e10.
221. Z. Li, C. Wang, Z. Wang, C. Zhu, J. Li, T. Sha, L. Ma, C. Gao, Y. Yang, Y. Sun, J. Wang, X. Sun, C. Lu, M. Difiglia, Y. Mei, C. Ding, S. Luo, Y. Dang, Y. Ding, Y. Fei and B. Lu, *Nature*, 2019, **575**, 203–209.
222. Z. Li, C. Zhu, Y. Ding, Y. Fei and B. Lu, *Autophagy*, 2020, **16**, 185–187.
223. W. F. Lima, B. P. Monia, D. J. Ecker and S. M. Freier, *Biochemistry*, 1992, **31**, 12055–12061.
224. M. Darmostuk, S. Rimpelova, H. Gbelcova and T. Ruml, *Biotechnol. Adv.*, 2015, **33**, 1141–1161.
225. A. L. Jochim and P. S. Arora, *Mol. BioSyst.*, 2009, **5**, 924–926.
226. R. E. Moellering, M. Cornejo, T. N. Davis, C. D. Bianco, J. C. Aster, S. C. Blacklow, A. L. Kung, D. G. Gilliland, G. L. Verdine and J. E. Bradner, *Nature*, 2009, **462**, 182–188.
227. T. N. Grossmann, J. T.-H. Yeh, B. R. Bowman, Q. Chu, R. E. Moellering and G. L. Verdine, *Proc. Natl. Acad. Sci. U. S. A.*, 2012, **109**, 17942–17947.
228. Y. S. Chang, B. Graves, V. Guerlavais, C. Tovar, K. Packman, K.-H. To, K. A. Olson, K. Kesavan, P. Gangurde, A. Mukherjee, T. Baker, K. Darlak, C. Elkin, Z. Filipovic, F. Z. Qureshi, H. Cai, P. Berry, E. Feyfant, X. E. Shi, J. Horstick, D. A. Annis, A. M. Manning, N. Fotouhi, H. Nash, L. T. Vassilev and T. K. Sawyer, *Proc. Natl. Acad. Sci. U. S. A.*, 2013, **110**, E3445–E3454.
229. K. Bourbiaux, B. Legrand, P. Verdié, S. Mallart, G. Manette, C. Minoletti, J. D. Stepp, P. Prigent, J.-C. Le Bail, L. Gauzy-Lazo, O. Duclos, J. Martinez and M. Amblard, *J. Med. Chem.*, 2021, **64**, 10834–10848.
230. C. K. Wang and D. J. Craik, *Nat. Chem. Biol.*, 2018, **14**, 417–427.
231. R. Eliasen, N. L. Daly, B. S. Wulff, T. L. Andresen, K. W. Conde-Frieboes and D. J. Craik, *J. Biol. Chem.*, 2012, **287**, 40493–40501.
232. T. Durek, P. M. Cromm, A. M. White, C. I. Schroeder, Q. Kaas, J. Weidmann, A. Ahmad Fuaad, O. Cheneval, P. J. Harvey, N. L. Daly, Y. Zhou, A. Dellsén, T. Österlund, N. Larsson, L. Knerr, U. Bauer, H. Kessler, M. Cai, V. J. Hruby, A. T. Plowright and D. J. Craik, *J. Med. Chem.*, 2018, **61**, 3674–3684.
233. H. van de Langemheen, V. Korotkovs, J. Bijl, C. Wilson, S. S. Kale, C. Heinis and R. M. J. Liskamp, *ChemBioChem*, 2017, **18**, 387–395.

234. V. Baeriswyl, H. Rapley, L. Pollaro, C. Stace, D. Teufel, E. Walker, S. Chen, G. Winter, J. Tite and C. Heinis, *ChemMedChem*, 2012, **7**, 1173–1176.
235. S. S. Kale, C. Villequey, X.-D. Kong, A. Zorzi, K. Deyle and C. Heinis, *Nat. Chem.*, 2018, **10**, 715–723.
236. V. Carle, X.-D. Kong, A. Comberlato, C. Edwards, C. Díaz-Perlas and C. Heinis, *Protein Eng., Des. Sel.*, 2021, gzab018.
237. X.-D. Kong, V. Carle, C. Díaz-Perlas, K. Butler and C. Heinis, *ACS Chem. Biol.*, 2020, **15**, 2907–2915.
238. Y. Huang, M. M. Wiedmann and H. Suga, *Chem. Rev.*, 2019, **119**, 10360–10391.
239. E. S. Iqbal, S. L. Richardson, N. A. Abrigo, K. K. Dods, H. E. O. Franco, H. S. Gerrish, H. K. Kotapati, I. M. Morgan, D. S. Masterson and M. C. T. Hartman, *Chem. Commun.*, 2019, **55**, 8959–8962.
240. V. I. Lyamichev, L. E. Goodrich, E. H. Sullivan, R. M. Bannen, J. Benz, T. J. Albert and J. J. Patel, *Sci. Rep.*, 2017, **7**, 1–10.
241. E. K. Leitch, N. Elumalai, M. Fridén-Saxin, G. Dahl, P. Wan, P. Clarkson, E. Valeur, G. Pairaudeau, H. Boyd and A. Tavassoli, *Chem. Sci.*, 2018, **9**, 5957–5966.
242. D. L. Buckley, I. Van Molle, P. C. Gareiss, H. S. Tae, J. Michel, D. J. Noblin, W. L. Jorgensen, A. Ciulli and C. M. Crews, *J. Am. Chem. Soc.*, 2012, **134**, 4465–4468.
243. B. L. Roberts, Z.-X. Ma, A. Gao, E. D. Leisten, D. Yin, W. Xu and W. Tang, *ACS Chem. Biol.*, 2020, **15**, 1487–1496.
244. C. Steinebach, I. Sosič, S. Lindner, A. Bricelj, F. Kohl, Y. L. D. Ng, M. Monschke, K. G. Wagner, J. Krönke and M. Gütschow, *MedChemComm*, 2019, **10**, 1037–1041.
245. F. Imrie, A. R. Bradley, M. van der Schaar and C. M. Deane, *J. Chem. Inf. Model.*, 2020, **60**, 1983–1995.
246. K. Yang, Y. Zhao, X. Nie, H. Wu, B. Wang, C. M. Almodovar-Rivera, H. Xie and W. Tang, *Cell Chem. Biol.*, 2020, **27**, 866–876.e8.
247. M. S. Gadd, A. Testa, X. Lucas, K.-H. Chan, W. Chen, D. J. Lamont, M. Zengerle and A. Ciulli, *Nat. Chem. Biol.*, 2017, **13**, 514–521.
248. S. L. Fisher and A. J. Phillips, *Curr. Opin. Chem. Biol.*, 2018, **44**, 47–55.
249. S. J. Eron, H. Huang, R. V. Agafonov, M. E. Fitzgerald, J. Patel, R. E. Michael, T. D. Lee, A. A. Hart, J. Shaulsky, C. G. Nasveschuk, A. J. Phillips, S. L. Fisher and A. Good, *ACS Chem. Biol.*, 2021, **16**, 2228–2243.
250. E. F. Douglass, C. J. Miller, G. Sparer, H. Shapiro and D. A. Spiegel, *J. Am. Chem. Soc.*, 2013, **135**, 6092–6099.
251. A. T. Plowright, C. Johnstone, J. Kihlberg, J. Pettersson, G. Robb and R. A. Thompson, *Drug Discovery Today*, 2012, **17**, 56–62.
252. E. M. Bech, S. L. Pedersen and K. J. Jensen, *ACS Med. Chem. Lett.*, 2018, **9**, 577–580.
253. H. Tan, W. Su, W. Zhang, P. Wang, M. Sattler and P. Zou, *Curr. Pharm. Des.*, 2018, **24**, 4932–4946.
254. W. A. Banks, *Peptides*, 2015, **72**, 16–19.
255. R. S. Geary, D. Norris, R. Yu and C. F. Bennett, *Adv. Drug Delivery Rev.*, 2015, **87**, 46–51.
256. V. Sardone, H. Zhou, F. Muntoni, A. Ferlini and M. S. Falzarano, *Molecules*, 2017, **22**, 563.
257. L. Sheng, F. Rigo, C. F. Bennett, A. R. Krainer and Y. Hua, *Nucleic Acids Res.*, 2020, **48**, 2853–2865.
258. M. Manoharan, *Antisense Nucleic Acid Drug Dev.*, 2002, **12**, 103–128.
259. C. Lorenz, P. Hadwiger, M. John, H.-P. Vornlocher and C. Unverzagt, *Bioorg. Med. Chem. Lett.*, 2004, **14**, 4975–4977.
260. B.-S. Herbert, G. C. Gellert, A. Hochreiter, K. Pongracz, W. E. Wright, D. Zielinska, A. C. Chin, C. B. Harley, J. W. Shay and S. M. Gryaznov, *Oncogene*, 2005, **24**, 5262–5268.
261. M. K. Bijsterbosch, E. T. Rump, R. L. A. D. Vrueh, R. Dorland, R. van Veghel, K. L. Tivel, E. A. L. Biessen, T. J. C. van Berkel and M. Manoharan, *Nucleic Acids Res.*, 2000, **28**, 2717–2725.
262. C. Wolfrum, S. Shi, K. N. Jayaprakash, M. Jayaraman, G. Wang, R. K. Pandey, K. G. Rajeev, T. Nakayama, K. Charrise, E. M. Ndungo, T. Zimmermann, V. Koteliansky, M. Manoharan and M. Stoffel, *Nat. Biotechnol.*, 2007, **25**, 1149–1157.
263. A. Aviñó, S. M. Ocampo, R. Lucas, J. J. Reina, J. C. Morales, J. C. Perales and R. Eritja, *Mol. Diversity*, 2011, **15**, 751–757.
264. T. P. Prakash, A. E. Mullick, R. G. Lee, J. Yu, S. T. Yeh, A. Low, A. E. Chappell, M. E. Østergaard, S. Murray, H. J. Gaus, E. E. Swayze and P. P. Seth, *Nucleic Acids Res.*, 2019, **47**, 6029–6044.
265. A. Biscans, A. Coles, R. Haraszti, D. Echeverria, M. Hassler, M. Osborn and A. Khvorova, *Nucleic Acids Res.*, 2019, **47**, 1082–1096.
266. M. F. Osborn, A. H. Coles, A. Biscans, R. A. Haraszti, L. Roux, S. Davis, S. Ly, D. Echeverria, M. R. Hassler, B. M. D. C. Godinho, M. Nikan and A. Khvorova, *Nucleic Acids Res.*, 2019, **47**, 1070–1081.
267. S. F. Dowdy, *Nat. Biotechnol.*, 2017, **35**, 222–229.
268. L. Knerr, T. P. Prakash, R. Lee, W. J. Drury III, M. Nikan, W. Fu, E. Pirie, L. D. Maria, E. Valeur, A. Hayen, M. Ölwegård-Halvarsson, J. Broddefalk, C. Ämmälä, M. E. Østergaard, J. Meuller, L. Sundström, P.

Andersson, D. Janzén, R. Jansson-Löfmark, P. P. Seth and S. Andersson, *J. Am. Chem. Soc.*, 2021, **143**, 3416–3429.

269. M. E. Østergaard, M. Jackson, A. Low, A. E. Chappell, R. G. Lee, R. Q. Peralta, J. Yu, G. A. Kinberger, A. Dan, R. Carty, M. Tanowitz, P. Anderson, T.-W. Kim, L. Fradkin, A. E. Mullick, S. Murray, F. Rigo, T. P. Prakash, C. F. Bennett, E. E. Swayze, H. J. Gaus and P. P. Seth, *Nucleic Acids Res.*, 2019, **47**, 6045–6058.
270. P. S. Kowalski, A. Rudra, L. Miao and D. G. Anderson, *Mol. Ther.*, 2019, **27**, 710–728.
271. D. P. Bondeson, A. Mares, I. E. D. Smith, E. Ko, S. Campos, A. H. Miah, K. E. Mulholland, N. Routly, D. L. Buckley, J. L. Gustafson, N. Zinn, P. Grandi, S. Shimamura, G. Bergamini, M. Faelth-Savitski, M. Bantscheff, C. Cox, D. A. Gordon, R. R. Willard, J. J. Flanagan, L. N. Casillas, B. J. Votta, W. den Besten, K. Famm, L. Kruidenier, P. S. Carter, J. D. Harling, I. Churcher and C. M. Crews, *Nat. Chem. Biol.*, 2015, **11**, 611–617.
272. A. Pike, B. Williamson, S. Harlfinger, S. Martin and D. F. McGinnity, *Drug Discovery Today*, 2020, **25**, 1793–1800.
273. A. Mares, A. H. Miah, I. E. D. Smith, M. Rackham, A. R. Thawani, J. Cryan, P. A. Haile, B. J. Votta, A. M. Beal, C. Capriotti, M. A. Reilly, D. T. Fisher, N. Zinn, M. Bantscheff, T. T. MacDonald, A. Vossenkamper, P. Dace, I. Churcher, A. B. Benowitz, G. Watt, J. Denyer, P. Scott-Stevens and J. D. Harling, *Commun. Biol.*, 2020, **3**, 1–13.
274. A. Cacace, *presented in part at the Targeted Protein Degradation Summit*, October, 2019.
275. E. Linnane, P. Davey, P. Zhang, S. Puri, M. Edbrooke, E. Chiarparin, A. S. Revenko, A. R. Macleod, J. C. Norman and S. J. Ross, *Nucleic Acids Res.*, 2019, **47**, 4375–4392.
276. E. Koller, T. M. Vincent, A. Chappell, S. De, M. Manoharan and C. F. Bennett, *Nucleic Acids Res.*, 2011, **39**, 4795–4807.
277. C. M. Miller, W. B. Wan, P. P. Seth and E. N. Harris, *Nucleic Acid Ther.*, 2018, **28**, 86–96.
278. S. Wang, N. Allen, T. A. Vickers, A. S. Revenko, H. Sun, X. Liang and S. T. Crooke, *Nucleic Acids Res.*, 2018, **46**, 3579–3594.
279. H. Pendergraff, S. Schmidt, J. Vikeså, C. Weile, C. Øverup, M. W. Lindholm and T. Koch, *Nucleic Acid Ther.*, 2019, **30**, 4–13.
280. A. Buntz, T. Killian, D. Schmid, H. Seul, U. Brinkmann, J. Ravn, M. Lindholm, H. Knoetgen, V. Haucke and O. Mundigl, *Nucleic Acids Res.*, 2019, **47**, 953–969.
281. P. L. Iversen, K. M. Aird, R. Wu, M. M. Morse and G. R. Devi, *Curr. Pharm. Biotechnol.*, 2009, **10**, 579–588.
282. S. T. Crooke, P. P. Seth, T. A. Vickers and X. Liang, *J. Am. Chem. Soc.*, 2020, **142**, 14754–14771.
283. P. L. Iversen, T. K. Warren, J. B. Wells, N. L. Garza, D. V. Mourich, L. S. Welch, R. G. Panchal and S. Bavari, *Viruses*, 2012, **4**, 2806–2830.
284. J. K. Nair, J. L. S. Willoughby, A. Chan, K. Charisse, Md. R. Alam, Q. Wang, M. Hoekstra, P. Kandasamy, A. V. Kel'in, S. Milstein, N. Taneja, J. O'Shea, S. Shaikh, L. Zhang, R. J. van der Sluis, M. E. Jung, A. Akinc, R. Hutabarat, S. Kuchimanchi, K. Fitzgerald, T. Zimmermann, T. J. C. van Berkel, M. A. Maier, K. G. Rajeev and M. Manoharan, *J. Am. Chem. Soc.*, 2014, **136**, 16958–16961.
285. T. P. Prakash, M. J. Graham, J. Yu, R. Carty, A. Low, A. Chappell, K. Schmidt, C. Zhao, M. Aghajan, H. F. Murray, S. Riney, S. L. Booten, S. F. Murray, H. Gaus, J. Crosby, W. F. Lima, S. Guo, B. P. Monia, E. E. Swayze and P. P. Seth, *Nucleic Acids Res.*, 2014, **42**, 8796–8807.
286. T. P. Prakash, J. Yu, G. A. Kinberger, A. Low, M. Jackson, F. Rigo, E. E. Swayze and P. P. Seth, *Bioorg. Med. Chem. Lett.*, 2018, **28**, 3774–3779.
287. L. J. Walport, R. Obexer and H. Suga, *Curr. Opin. Biotechnol.*, 2017, **48**, 242–250.
288. P. G. Dougherty, A. Sahni and D. Pei, *Chem. Rev.*, 2019, **119**, 10241–10287.
289. T. Vorherr, I. Lewis, J. Berghausen, S. Desrayaud and M. Schaefer, *Int. J. Pept. Res. Ther.*, 2018, **24**, 35–48.
290. T. Vorherr, *Future Med. Chem.*, 2015, 7, 1009–1021.
291. I. Lewis, M. Schaefer, T. Wagner, L. Oberer, E. Sager, P. Wipfli and T. Vorherr, *Int. J. Pept. Res. Ther.*, 2015, **21**, 205–221.
292. T. R. White, C. M. Renzelman, A. C. Rand, T. Rezai, C. M. McEwen, V. M. Gelev, R. A. Turner, R. G. Linington, S. S. F. Leung, A. S. Kalgutkar, J. N. Bauman, Y. Zhang, S. Liras, D. A. Price, A. M. Mathiowetz, M. P. Jacobson and R. S. Lokey, *Nat. Chem. Biol.*, 2011, **7**, 810–817.
293. J. G. Beck, J. Chatterjee, B. Laufer, M. U. Kiran, A. O. Frank, S. Neubauer, O. Ovadia, S. Greenberg, C. Gilon, A. Hoffman and H. Kessler, *J. Am. Chem. Soc.*, 2012, **134**, 12125–12133.
294. W. M. Hewitt, S. S. F. Leung, C. R. Pye, A. R. Ponkey, M. Bednarek, M. P. Jacobson and R. S. Lokey, *J. Am. Chem. Soc.*, 2015, **137**, 715–721.

295. A. T. Bockus, K. W. Lexa, C. R. Pye, A. S. Kalgutkar, J. W. Gardner, K. C. R. Hund, W. M. Hewitt, J. A. Schwochert, E. Glassey, D. A. Price, A. M. Mathiowetz, S. Liras, M. P. Jacobson and R. S. Lokey, *J. Med. Chem.*, 2015, **58**, 4581–4589.
296. C. L. Ahlbach, K. W. Lexa, A. T. Bockus, V. Chen, P. Crews, M. P. Jacobson and R. S. Lokey, *Future Med. Chem.*, 2015, **7**, 2121–2130.
297. M. Boehm, K. Beaumont, R. Jones, A. S. Kalgutkar, L. Zhang, K. Atkinson, G. Bai, J. A. Brown, H. Eng, G. H. Goetz, B. R. Holder, B. Khunte, S. Lazzaro, C. Limberakis, S. Ryu, M. J. Shapiro, L. Tylaska, J. Yan, R. Turner, S. S. F. Leung, M. Ramaseshan, D. A. Price, S. Liras, M. P. Jacobson, D. J. Earp, R. S. Lokey, A. M. Mathiowetz and E. Menhaji-Klotz, *J. Med. Chem.*, 2017, **60**, 9653–9663.
298. S. Ono, M. R. Naylor, C. E. Townsend, C. Okumura, O. Okada and R. S. Lokey, *J. Chem. Inf. Model.*, 2019, **59**, 2952–2963.
299. A. T. Bockus, J. A. Schwochert, C. R. Pye, C. E. Townsend, V. Sok, M. A. Bednarek and R. S. Lokey, *J. Med. Chem.*, 2015, **58**, 7409–7418.
300. C. R. Pye, W. M. Hewitt, J. Schwochert, T. D. Haddad, C. E. Townsend, L. Etienne, Y. Lao, C. Limberakis, A. Furukawa, A. M. Mathiowetz, D. A. Price, S. Liras and R. S. Lokey, *J. Med. Chem.*, 2017, **60**, 1665–1672.
301. L. Dietrich, B. Rathmer, K. Ewan, T. Bange, S. Heinrichs, T. C. Dale, D. Schade and T. N. Grossmann, *Cell Chem. Biol.*, 2017, **24**, 958–968.e5.
302. A. W. Partridge, H. Y. K. Kaan, Y.-C. Juang, A. Sadruddin, S. Lim, C. J. Brown, S. Ng, D. Thean, F. Ferrer, C. Johannes, T. Y. Yuen, S. Kannan, P. Aronica, Y. S. Tan, M. R. Pradhan, C. S. Verma, J. Hochman, S. Chen, H. Wan, S. Ha, B. Sherborne, D. P. Lane and T. K. Sawyer, *Molecules*, 2019, **24**, 2292.
303. A. Pal, K. Neo, L. Rajamani, F. J. Ferrer, D. P. Lane, C. S. Verma and A. Mortellaro, *Sci. Rep.*, 2019, **9**, 1–15.
304. Y. Wu, A. Kaur, E. Fowler, M. M. Wiedmann, R. Young, W. R. J. D. Galloway, L. Olsen, H. F. Sore, A. Chattopadhyay, T. T.-L. Kwan, W. Xu, S. J. Walsh, P. de Andrade, M. Janecek, S. Arumugam, L. S. Itzhaki, Y. H. Lau and D. R. Spring, *ACS Chem. Biol.*, 2019, **14**, 526–533.
305. K. M. Mientkiewicz, L. Peraro and J. A. Kritzer, *ACS Chem. Biol.*, 2021, **16**, 1184–1190.
306. N. E. A. Chessum, S. Y. Sharp, J. J. Caldwell, A. E. Pasqua, B. Wilding, G. Colombano, I. Collins, B. Ozer, M. Richards, M. Rowlands, M. Stubbs, R. Burke, P. C. McAndrew, P. A. Clarke, P. Workman, M. D. Cheeseman and K. Jones, *J. Med. Chem.*, 2018, **61**, 918–933.
307. V. G. Klein, C. E. Townsend, A. Testa, M. Zengerle, C. Maniaci, S. J. Hughes, K.-H. Chan, A. Ciulli and R. S. Lokey, *ACS Med. Chem. Lett.*, 2020, **11**, 1732–1738.
308. D. E. Scott, T. P. C. Rooney, E. D. Bayle, T. Mirza, H. M. G. Willems, J. H. Clarke, S. P. Andrews and J. Skidmore, *ACS Med. Chem. Lett.*, 2020, **11**, 1539–1547.
309. S. D. Edmondson, B. Yang and C. Fallan, *Bioorg. Med. Chem. Lett.*, 2019, **29**, 1555–1564.
310. Y. Atilaw, V. Poongavanam, C. Svensson Nilsson, D. Nguyen, A. Giese, D. Meibom, M. Erdelyi and J. Kihlberg, *ACS Med. Chem. Lett.*, 2021, **12**, 107–114.
311. C. Cantrill, P. Chaturvedi, C. Rynn, J. Petrig Schaffland, I. Walter and M. B. Wittwer, *Drug Discovery Today*, 2020, **25**, 969–982.
312. W.-H. Guo, X. Qi, X. Yu, Y. Liu, C.-I. Chung, F. Bai, X. Lin, D. Lu, L. Wang, J. Chen, L. H. Su, K. J. Nomie, F. Li, M. C. Wang, X. Shu, J. N. Onuchic, J. A. Woyach, M. L. Wang and J. Wang, *Nat. Commun.*, 2020, **11**, 4268.
313. A. Evers, S. Pfeiffer-Marek, M. Bossart, C. Heubel, U. Stock, G. Tiwari, B. Gebauer, B. Elshorst, A. Pfenninger, U. Lukasczyk, G. Hessler, W. Kamm and M. Wagner, *J. Pharm. Sci.*, 2019, **108**, 1404–1414.
314. L. B. Knudsen and J. Lau, *Front. Endocrinol.*, 2019, **10**, 155.
315. L. Goracci, J. Desantis, A. Valeri, B. Castellani, M. Eleuteri and G. Cruciani, *J. Med. Chem.*, 2020, **63**, 11615–11638.
316. X. Chi, P. Gatti and T. Papoian, *Drug Discovery Today*, 2017, **22**, 823–833.
317. W. Shen, C. L. D. Hoyos, M. T. Migawa, T. A. Vickers, H. Sun, A. Low, T. A. Bell, M. Rahdar, S. Mukhopadhyay, C. E. Hart, M. Bell, S. Riney, S. F. Murray, S. Greenlee, R. M. Crooke, X. Liang, P. P. Seth and S. T. Crooke, *Nat. Biotechnol.*, 2019, **37**, 640–650.
318. M. T. Migawa, W. Shen, W. B. Wan, G. Vasquez, M. E. Oestergaard, A. Low, C. L. De Hoyos, R. Gupta, S. Murray, M. Tanowitz, M. Bell, J. G. Nichols, H. Gaus, X. Liang, E. E. Swayze, S. T. Crooke and P. P. Seth, *Nucleic Acids Res.*, 2019, **47**, 5465–5479.
319. G. Vasquez, G. C. Freestone, W. B. Wan, A. Low, C. L. De Hoyos, J. Yu, T. P. Prakash, M. E. Østergaard, X. Liang, S. T. Crooke, E. E. Swayze, M. T. Migawa and P. P. Seth, *Nucleic Acids Res.*, 2021, **49**, 1828–1839.
320. T. P. Prakash, J. Yu, W. Shen, C. L. De Hoyos, A. Berdeja, H. Gaus, X. Liang, S. T. Crooke and P. P. Seth, *ACS Med. Chem. Lett.*, 2021, **12**, 922–927.

321. M. E. Østergaard, C. L. De Hoyos, W. B. Wan, W. Shen, A. Low, A. Berdeja, G. Vasquez, S. Murray, M. T. Migawa, X. Liang, E. E. Swayze, S. T. Crooke and P. P. Seth, *Nucleic Acids Res.*, 2020, **48**, 1691–1700.
322. K. S. Frazier and L. A. Obert, *Toxicol. Pathol.*, 2018, **46**, 904–917.
323. T. Yoshida, Y. Naito, H. Yasuhara, K. Sasaki, H. Kawaji, J. Kawai, M. Naito, H. Okuda, S. Obika and T. Inoue, *Genes Cells*, 2019, **24**, 827–835.
324. A. T. Watt, G. Swayze, E. E. Swayze and S. M. Freier, *Nucleic Acid Ther.*, 2020, **30**, 215–228.
325. S. T. Crooke, B. F. Baker, J. L. Witztum, T. J. Kwoh, N. C. Pham, N. Salgado, B. W. McEvoy, W. Cheng, S. G. Hughes, S. Bhanot and R. S. Geary, *Nucleic Acid Ther.*, 2017, **27**, 121–129.
326. P. Narayanan, L. Shen, B. R. Curtis, M. A. Bourdon, J. P. Nolan, S. Gupta, C. Hoffmaster, F. Zhou, B. Christian, J. L. Schaubhut, S. Greenlee, S. A. Burel, J. L. Witztum, J. A. Engelhardt and S. P. Henry, *Toxicol. Sci.*, 2018, **164**, 613–626.
327. K. Moreau, M. Coen, A. X. Zhang, F. Pachl, M. P. Castaldi, G. Dahl, H. Boyd, C. Scott and P. Newham, *Br. J. Pharmacol.*, 2020, **177**, 1709–1718.
328. D. P. Bondeson, B. E. Smith, G. M. Burslem, A. D. Buhimschi, J. Hines, S. Jaime-Figueroa, J. Wang, B. D. Hamman, A. Ishchenko and C. M. Crews, *Cell Chem. Biol.*, 2018, **25**, 78–87.e5.
329. P. Grandi and M. Bantscheff, *Drug Discovery Today: Technol.*, 2019, **31**, 99–108.
330. M. M. Savitski, N. Zinn, M. Faelth-Savitski, D. Poeckel, S. Gade, I. Becher, M. Muelbaier, A. J. Wagner, K. Strohmer, T. Werner, S. Melchert, M. Petretich, A. Rutkowska, J. Vappiani, H. Franken, M. Steidel, G. M. Sweetman, O. Gilan, E. Y. N. Lam, M. A. Dawson, R. K. Prinjha, P. Grandi, G. Bergamini and M. Bantscheff, *Cell*, 2018, **173**, 260–274.e25.
331. B. E. Smith, S. L. Wang, S. Jaime-Figueroa, A. Harbin, J. Wang, B. D. Hamman and C. M. Crews, *Nat. Commun.*, 2019, **10**, 131.
332. P. Gennemark, K. Walter, N. Clemmensen, D. Rekić, C. A. M. Nilsson, J. Knöchel, M. Hölttä, L. Wernevik, B. Rosengren, D. Kakol-Palm, Y. Wang, R. Z. Yu, R. S. Geary, S. J. Riney, B. P. Monia, R. Isaksson, R. Jansson-Löfmark, C. S. J. Rocha, D. Lindén, E. Hurt-Camejo, R. Crooke, L. Tillman, T. Rydén-Bergsten, B. Carlsson, U. Andersson, M. Elebring, A. Tivesten and N. Davies, *Sci. Transl. Med.*, 2021, **13**, eabe9117.
333. C. Godfrey, L. R. Desviat, B. Smedsrød, F. Piétri-Rouxel, M. A. Denti, P. Disterer, S. Lorain, G. Nogales-Gadea, V. Sardone, R. Anwar, S. El Andaloussi, T. Lehto, B. Khoo, C. Brolin, W. M. van Roon-Mom, A. Goyenvalle, A. Aartsma-Rus and V. Arechavala-Gomeza, *EMBO Mol. Med.*, 2017, **9**, 545–557.
334. P. Jafar-nejad, B. Powers, A. Soriano, H. Zhao, D. A. Norris, J. Matson, B. DeBrosse-Serra, J. Watson, P. Narayanan, S. J. Chun, C. Mazur, H. Kordasiewicz, E. E. Swayze and F. Rigo, *Nucleic Acids Res.*, 2020, **49**, 657–673.
335. D. Hong, R. Kurzrock, Y. Kim, R. Woessner, A. Younes, J. Nemunaitis, N. Fowler, T. Zhou, J. Schmidt, M. Jo, S. J. Lee, M. Yamashita, S. G. Hughes, L. Fayad, S. Piha-Paul, M. V. P. Nadella, M. Mohseni, D. Lawson, C. Reimer, D. C. Blakey, X. Xiao, J. Hsu, A. Revenko, B. P. Monia and A. R. MacLeod, *Sci. Transl. Med.*, 2015, **7**, 314ra185.
336. S. J. Ross, A. S. Revenko, L. L. Hanson, R. Ellston, A. Staniszewska, N. Whalley, S. K. Pandey, M. Revill, C. Rooney, L. K. Buckett, S. K. Klein, K. Hudson, B. P. Monia, M. Zinda, D. C. Blakey, P. D. Lyne and A. R. Macleod, *Sci. Transl. Med.*, 2017, **9**, aal5253.
337. T. C. Roberts, R. Langer and M. J. A. Wood, *Nat. Rev. Drug Discovery*, 2020, 1–22.
338. L. G. Tillman, R. S. Geary and G. E. Hardee, *J. Pharm. Sci.*, 2008, **97**, 225–236.
339. A. K. Patel, J. C. Kaczmarek, S. Bose, K. J. Kauffman, F. Mir, M. W. Heartlein, F. DeRosa, R. Langer and D. G. Anderson, *Adv. Mater.*, 2019, **31**, 1805116.
340. K. J. Hassett, K. E. Benenato, E. Jacquinet, A. Lee, A. Woods, O. Yuzhakov, S. Himansu, J. Deterling, B. M. Geilich, T. Ketova, C. Mihai, A. Lynn, I. McFadyen, M. J. Moore, J. J. Senn, M. G. Stanton, Ö. Almarsson, G. Ciaramella and L. A. Brito, *Mol. Ther.--Nucleic Acids*, 2019, **15**, 1–11.
341. P. McDonel and M. Guttman, *Cold Spring Harbor Perspect. Biol.*, 2019, **11**, a032151.
342. R.-W. Yao, Y. Wang and L.-L. Chen, *Nat. Cell Biol.*, 2019, **21**, 542–551.
343. D. A. Griffith, D. J. Edmonds, J.-P. Fortin, A. S. Kalgutkar, J. B. Kuzmiski, P. M. Loria, A. R. Saxena, S. W. Bagley, C. Buckeridge, J. M. Curto, D. R. Derksen, J. M. Dias, M. C. Griffor, S. Han, V. M. Jackson, M. S. Landis, D. J. Lettiere, C. Limberakis, Y. Liu, A. M. Mathiowetz, J. C. Patel, D. W. Piotrowski, D. A. Price, R. B. Ruggeri and D. A. Tess, *J. Med. Chem.*, 2022, **65**, 8208–8226.
344. D. N. Petersen, J. Hawkins, W. Ruangsiriluk, K. A. Stevens, B. A. Maguire, T. N. O'Connell, B. N. Rocke, M. Boehm, R. B. Ruggeri, T. Rolph, D. Hepworth, P. M. Loria and P. A. Carpino, *Cell Chem. Biol.*, 2016, **23**, 1362–1371.
345. T. Nishikido and K. K. Ray, *Front. Cardiovasc. Med.*, 2019, **5**, 199.

346. C. Alleyne, R. P. Amin, B. Bhatt, E. Bianchi, J. C. Blain, N. Boyer, D. Branca, M. W. Embrey, S. N. Ha, K. Jette, D. G. Johns, A. D. Kerekes, K. A. Koeplinger, D. LaPlaca, N. Li, B. Murphy, P. Orth, A. Ricardo, S. Salowe, K. Seyb, A. Shahripour, J. R. Stringer, Y. Sun, R. Tracy, C. Wu, Y. Xiong, H. Youm, H. J. Zokian and T. J. Tucker, *J. Med. Chem.*, 2020, **63**, 13796–13824.
347. N. G. Lintner, K. F. McClure, D. Petersen, A. T. Londregan, D. W. Piotrowski, L. Wei, J. Xiao, M. Bolt, P. M. Loria, B. Maguire, K. F. Geoghegan, A. Huang, T. Rolph, S. Liras, J. A. Doudna, R. G. Dullea and J. H. D. Cate, *PLoS Biol.*, 2017, **15**, e2001882.
348. M. H. Serrano-Wu, B. K. Hubbard, V. Kaushik and D. Daniels, *WO Pat.*, 2020150474A1, 2020.
349. M. Bowerman, C. G. Becker, R. J. Yáñez-Muñoz, K. Ning, M. J. A. Wood, T. H. Gillingwater, K. Talbot and T. U. S. R. Consortium, *Dis. Models Mech.*, 2017, **10**, 943–954.
350. D. K. Lee and C. Chang, *J. Clin. Endocrinol. Metab.*, 2003, **88**, 4043–4054.
351. P. Ottis, C. Palladino, P. Thienger, A. Britschgi, C. Heichinger, M. Berrera, A. Julien-Laferriere, F. Roudnicky, T. Kam-Thong, J. R. Bischoff, B. Martoglio and P. Pettazzoni, *ACS Chem. Biol.*, 2019, **14**, 2215–2223.
352. N. J. Henning, L. Boike, J. N. Spradlin, C. C. Ward, G. Liu, E. Zhang, B. P. Belcher, S. M. Brittain, M. J. Hesse, D. Dovala, L. M. McGregor, R. Valdez Misiolek, L. W. Plasschaert, D. J. Rowlands, F. Wang, A. O. Frank, D. Fuller, A. R. Estes, K. L. Randal, A. Panidapu, J. M. McKenna, J. A. Tallarico, M. Schirle and D. K. Nomura, *Nat. Chem. Biol.*, 2022, **18**, 412–421.
353. S. Yamazoe, J. Tom, Y. Fu, W. Wu, L. Zeng, C. Sun, Q. Liu, J. Lin, K. Lin, W. J. Fairbrother and S. T. Staben, *J. Med. Chem.*, 2020, **63**, 2807–2813.
354. W. W. Wang, L.-Y. Chen, J. M. Wozniak, A. M. Jadhav, H. Anderson, T. E. Malone and C. G. Parker, *J. Am. Chem. Soc.*, 2021, **143**, 16700–16708.
355. M. G. Costales, Y. Matsumoto, S. P. Velagapudi and M. D. Disney, *J. Am. Chem. Soc.*, 2018, **140**, 6741–6744.
356. M. G. Costales, H. Aikawa, Y. Li, J. L. Childs-Disney, D. Abegg, D. G. Hoch, S. P. Velagapudi, Y. Nakai, T. Khan, K. W. Wang, I. Yildirim, A. Adibekian, E. T. Wang and M. D. Disney, *Proc. Natl. Acad. Sci. U. S. A.*, 2020, **117**, 2406–2411.
357. M. G. Costales, B. Suresh, K. Vishnu and M. D. Disney, *Cell Chem. Biol.*, 2019, **26**, 1180–1186.e5.
358. H. S. Haniff, Y. Tong, X. Liu, J. L. Chen, B. M. Suresh, R. J. Andrews, J. M. Peterson, C. A. O'Leary, R. I. Benhamou, W. N. Moss and M. D. Disney, *ACS Cent. Sci.*, 2020, **6**, 1713–1721.
359. A. F. M. Noisier, M. J. Johansson, L. Knerr, M. A. Hayes, W. J. Drury, E. Valeur, L. R. Malins and R. Gopalakrishnan, *Angew. Chem., Int. Ed.*, 2019, **58**, 19096–19102.
360. S. Shaabani, R. Xu, M. Ahmadianmoghaddam, L. Gao, M. Stahorsky, J. Olechno, R. Ellson, M. Kossenjans, V. Helan and A. Dömling, *Green Chem.*, 2019, **21**, 225–232.
361. N. J. Gesmundo, B. Sauvagnat, P. J. Curran, M. P. Richards, C. L. Andrews, P. J. Dandliker and T. Cernak, *Nature*, 2018, **557**, 228–232.
362. N. Bai, K. M. Riching, A. Makaju, H. Wu, T. M. Acker, S.-C. Ou, Y. Zhang, X. Shen, D. N. Bulloch, H. Rui, B. W. Gibson, D. L. Daniels, M. Urh, B. M. Rock and S. C. Humphreys, *J. Biol. Chem.*, 2022, **298**, 101653.

# Subject Index

www.ingramcontent.com/pod-product-compliance
Lightning Source LLC
LaVergne TN
LVHW062210200926
848484LV00006B/1368
*9781788018982*